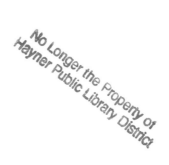
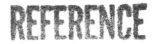

The GALE ENCYCLOPEDIA of MEDICINE

THIRD EDITION

The GALE ENCYCLOPEDIA of MEDICINE

THIRD EDITION

VOLUME

3

G-M

JACQUELINE L. LONGE, PROJECT EDITOR

THOMSON

GALE

Detroit • New York • San Francisco • San Diego • New Haven, Conn. • Waterville, Maine • London • Munich

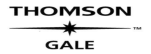

THE GALE ENCYCLOPEDIA OF MEDICINE, THIRD EDITION

Project Editor
Jacqueline L. Longe

Editorial
Shirelle Phelps, Laurie Fundukian, Jeffrey Lehman, Brigham Narins

Editorial Support Services
Luann Brennan, Grant Eldridge, Andrea Lopeman

Rights Acquisition Management
Shalice Caldwell-Shah

Imaging
Randy Bassett, Lezlie Light, Dan Newell, Christine O'Bryan, Robyn V. Young

Product Design
Tracey Rowens

Composition and Electronic Prepress
Evi Seoud, Mary Beth Trimper

Manufacturing
Wendy Blurton, Dorothy Maki

Indexing
Factiva

LIBRARY OF CONGRESS CATALOGING-IN-PUBLICATION DATA

The Gale encyclopedia of medicine / Jacqueline L. Longe, editor.– 3rd ed.
    p. ; cm.
    Includes bibliographical references and index.
    ISBN 1-4144-0368-2 (set hardcover : alk. paper) – ISBN 1-4144-0369-0 (v. 1 : hardcover : alk. paper) – ISBN 1-4144-0370-4 (v. 2 : hardcover : alk. paper) – ISBN 1-4144-0371-2 v. 3 : hardcover : alk. paper) – ISBN 1-4144-0372-0 (v. 4 : hardcover : alk. paper) – ISBN 1-4144-0373-9 (v. 5 : hardcover : alk. paper)
    1. Internal medicine–Encyclopedias.
    [DNLM: 1. Internal Medicine–Encyclopedias–English. 2. Complementary Therapies–Encyclopedias–English. WB 13 G151 2005] I. Title: Encyclopedia of medicine. II. Longe, Jacqueline L. III. Gale Group.
    RC41.G35 2006
    616'.003–dc22
                                                                    2005011418

This title is also available as an e-book
ISBN 1-4144-0485-9 (set)
Contact your Gale sales representative for ordering information.
ISBN 1-4144-0368-2 (set)
    1-4144-0369-0 (Vol. 1)
    1-4144-0370-4 (Vol. 2)
    1-4144-0371-2 (Vol. 3)
    1-4144-0372-0 (Vol. 4)
    1-4144-0373-9 (Vol. 5)

Printed in China
10 9 8 7 6 5 4 3 2 1

CONTENTS

LIST OF ENTRIES

A

Abdominal ultrasound
Abdominal wall defects
Abortion, partial birth
Abortion, selective
Abortion, therapeutic
Abscess incision & drainage
Abscess
Abuse
Acetaminophen
Achalasia
Achondroplasia
Acid phosphatase test
Acne
Acoustic neuroma
Acrocyanosis
Acromegaly and gigantism
Actinomycosis
Acupressure
Acupuncture
Acute kidney failure
Acute lymphangitis
Acute poststreptococcal
  glomerulonephritis
Acute stress disorder
Addiction
Addison's disease
Adenoid hyperplasia
Adenovirus infections
Adhesions
Adjustment disorders
Adrenal gland cancer
Adrenal gland scan
Adrenal virilism
Adrenalectomy
Adrenocorticotropic hormone test
Adrenoleukodystrophy
Adult respiratory distress syndrome
Aging

Agoraphobia
AIDS tests
AIDS
Alanine aminotransferase test
Albinism
Alcoholism
Alcohol-related neurologic disease
Aldolase test
Aldosterone assay
Alemtuzumab
Alexander technique
Alkaline phosphatase test
Allergic bronchopulmonary
  aspergillosis
Allergic purpura
Allergic rhinitis
Allergies
Allergy tests
Alopecia
Alpha$_1$-adrenergic blockers
Alpha-fetoprotein test
Alport syndrome
Altitude sickness
Alzheimer's disease
Amblyopia
Amebiasis
Amenorrhea
Amino acid disorders screening
Aminoglycosides
Amnesia
Amniocentesis
Amputation
Amylase tests
Amyloidosis
Amyotrophic lateral sclerosis
Anabolic steroid use
Anaerobic infections
Anal atresia
Anal cancer
Anal warts
Analgesics, opioid

Analgesics
Anaphylaxis
Anemias
Anesthesia, general
Anesthesia, local
Aneurysmectomy
Angina
Angiography
Angioplasty
Angiotensin-converting enzyme
  inhibitors
Angiotensin-converting enzyme
  test
Animal bite infections
Ankylosing spondylitis
Anorectal disorders
Anorexia nervosa
Anoscopy
Anosmia
Anoxia
Antacids
Antenatal testing
Antepartum testing
Anthrax
Antiacne drugs
Antiandrogen drugs
Antianemia drugs
Antiangina drugs
Antiangiogenic therapy
Antianxiety drugs
Antiarrhythmic drugs
Antiasthmatic drugs
Antibiotic-associated colitis
Antibiotics, ophthalmic
Antibiotics, topical
Antibiotics
Anticancer drugs
Anticoagulant and antiplatelet
  drugs
Anticonvulsant drugs
Antidepressant drugs, SSRI

Epstein-Barr virus test
Erectile dysfunction treatment
Erectile dysfunction
Erysipelas
Erythema multiforme
Erythema nodosum
Erythroblastosis fetalis
Erythrocyte sedimentation rate
Erythromycins
Erythropoietin test
Escherichia coli
Esophageal atresia
Esophageal cancer
Esophageal disorders
Esophageal function tests
Esophageal pouches
Esophagogastroduodenoscopy
Evoked potential studies
Exercise
Exophthalmos
Expectorants
External sphincter electromyography
Extracorporeal membrane
    oxygenation
Eye and orbit ultrasounds
Eye cancer
Eye examination
Eye glasses and contact lenses
Eye muscle surgery
Eyelid disorders

F

Face lift
Factitious disorders
Failure to thrive
Fainting
Familial Mediterranean fever
Familial polyposis
Family therapy
Fanconi's syndrome
Fasciotomy
Fasting
Fatigue
Fatty liver
Fecal incontinence
Fecal occult blood test
Feldenkrais method
Female genital mutilation
Female sexual arousal disorder
Fetal alcohol syndrome
Fetal hemoglobin test
Fever evaluation tests

Fever of unknown origin
Fever
Fibrin split products
Fibrinogen test
Fibroadenoma
Fibrocystic condition of the breast
Fibromyalgia
Fifth disease
Filariasis
Finasteride
Fingertip injuries
Fish and shellfish poisoning
Fistula
Flesh-eating disease
Flower remedies
Fluke infections
Fluoroquinolones
Folic acid deficiency anemia
Folic acid
Follicle-stimulating hormone test
Folliculitis
Food allergies
Food poisoning
Foot care
Foreign objects
Fracture repair
Fractures
Fragile X syndrome
Friedreich's ataxia
Frostbite and frostnip
Fugu poisoning

G

Galactorrhea
Galactosemia
Gallbladder cancer
Gallbladder nuclear medicine scan
Gallbladder x rays
Gallium scan of the body
Gallstone removal
Gallstones
Gammaglobulin
Ganglion
Gangrene
Gas embolism
Gastrectomy
Gastric acid determination
Gastric emptying scan
Gastrinoma
Gastritis
Gastroenteritis
Gastrostomy

Gaucher disease
Gay and lesbian health
Gender identity disorder
Gender reassignment surgery
Gene therapy
General adaptation syndrome
General surgery
Generalized anxiety disorder
Genetic counseling
Genetic testing
Genital herpes
Genital warts
Gestalt therapy
Gestational diabetes
GI bleeding studies
Giardiasis
Ginkgo biloba
Ginseng, Korean
Glaucoma
Glomerulonephritis
Glucose-6-phosphate dehydrogenase
    deficiency
Glycogen storage diseases
Glycosylated hemoglobin test
Goiter
Gonorrhea
Goodpasture's syndrome
Gout drugs
Gout
Graft-vs.-host disease
Granuloma inguinale
Group therapy
Growth hormone tests
Guided imagery
Guillain-Barré syndrome
Guinea worm infection
Gulf War syndrome
Gynecomastia

H

Hair transplantation
Hairy cell leukemia
Hallucinations
Hammertoe
Hand-foot-and-mouth disease
Hantavirus infections
Haptoglobin test
Hartnup disease
Hatha yoga
Head and neck cancer
Head injury
Headache

Proton Pump Inhibitors
Pseudogout
Pseudomonas infections
Pseudoxanthoma elasticum
Psoriasis
Psoriatic arthritis
Psychiatric confinement
Psychoanalysis
Psychological tests
Psychosis
Psychosocial disorders
Psychosurgery
Ptosis
Puberty
Puerperal infection
Pulmonary alveolar proteinosis
Pulmonary artery catheterization
Pulmonary edema
Pulmonary embolism
Pulmonary fibrosis
Pulmonary function test
Pulmonary hypertension
Pulmonary valve insufficiency
Pulmonary valve stenosis
Pyelonephritis
Pyloric stenosis
Pyloroplasty
Pyruvate kinase deficiency

Q

Q fever
Qigong

R

Rabies
Radial keratotomy
Radiation injuries
Radiation therapy
Radical neck dissection
Radioactive implants
Rape and sexual assault
Rashes
Rat-bite fever
Raynaud's disease
Recompression treatment
Rectal cancer
Rectal examination
Rectal polyps
Rectal prolapse

Recurrent miscarriage
Red blood cell indices
Reflex sympathetic dystrophy
Reflex tests
Reflexology
Rehabilitation
Reiki
Reiter's syndrome
Relapsing fever
Relapsing polychondritis
Renal artery occlusion
Renal artery stenosis
Renal tubular acidosis
Renal vein thrombosis
Renovascular hypertension
Respiratory acidosis
Respiratory alkalosis
Respiratory distress syndrome
Respiratory failure
Respiratory syncytial virus
   infection
Restless legs syndrome
Restrictive cardiomyopathy
Reticulocyte count
Retinal artery occlusion
Retinal detachment
Retinal hemorrhage
Retinal vein occlusion
Retinitis pigmentosa
Retinoblastoma
Retinopathies
Retrograde cystography
Retrograde ureteropyelography
Retrograde urethrography
Reye's syndrome
Rheumatic fever
Rheumatoid arthritis
Rhinitis
Rhinoplasty
Riboflavin deficiency
Rickets
Rickettsialpox
Ringworm
Rocky Mountain spotted fever
Rolfing
Root canal treatment
Rosacea
Roseola
Ross River Virus
Rotator cuff injury
Rotavirus infections
Roundworm infections
Rubella test
Rubella

S

Sacroiliac disease
Salivary gland scan
Salivary gland tumors
Salmonella food poisoning
Salpingectomy
Salpingo-oophorectomy
Sarcoidosis
Sarcomas
Saw palmetto
Scabies
Scarlet fever
Scars
Schistosomiasis
Schizoaffective disorder
Schizophrenia
Sciatica
Scleroderma
Sclerotherapy for esophageal varices
Scoliosis
Scrotal nuclear medicine scan
Scrotal ultrasound
Scrub typhus
Scurvy
Seasonal affective disorder
Seborrheic dermatitis
Secondary polycythemia
Sedation
Seizure disorder
Selective serotonin reuptake
   inhibitors
Self-mutilation
Semen analysis
Seniors' health
Sensory integration disorder
Sepsis
Septic shock
Septoplasty
Serum sickness
Severe acute respiratory syndrome
   (SARS)
Severe combined immunodeficiency
Sex hormones tests
Sex therapy
Sexual dysfunction
Sexual perversions
Sexually transmitted diseases
Sexually transmitted diseases cultures
Shaken baby syndrome
Shiatsu
Shigellosis
Shin splints

PLEASE READ—IMPORTANT INFORMATION

The *Gale Encyclopedia of Medicine* is a medical reference product designed to inform and educate readers about a wide variety of disorders, conditions, treatments, and diagnostic tests. Thomson Gale believes the product to be comprehensive, but not necessarily definitive. It is intended to supplement, not replace, consultation with a physician or other healthcare practitioner. While Thomson Gale has made substantial efforts to provide information that is accurate, comprehensive, and up-to-date, Thomson Gale makes no representations or warranties of any kind, including without limitation, warranties of merchantability or fitness for a particular purpose, nor does it guarantee the accuracy, comprehensiveness, or timeliness of the information contained in this product. Readers should be aware that the universe of medical knowledge is constantly growing and changing, and that differences of medical opinion exist among authorities. Readers are also advised to seek professional diagnosis and treatment for any medical condition, and to discuss information obtained from this book with their healthcare provider.

INTRODUCTION

The third edition of the *Gale Encyclopedia of Medicine (GEM3)* is a one-stop source for medical information on over 1,750 common medical disorders, conditions, tests, and treatments, including high-profile diseases such as AIDS, Alzheimer's disease, cancer, and heart attack. This encyclopedia avoids medical jargon and uses language that laypersons can understand, while still providing thorough coverage of each topic. The *Gale Encyclopedia of Medicine 3* fills a gap between basic consumer health resources, such as single-volume family medical guides, and highly technical professional materials.

SCOPE

More than 1,750 full-length articles are included in the *Gale Encyclopedia of Medicine 3*, including disorders/conditions, tests/procedures, and treatments/therapies. Many common drugs are also covered, with generic drug names appearing first and brand names following in parentheses, eg. acetaminophen (Tylenol). Throughout the *Gale Encyclopedia of Medicine 3*, many prominent individuals are highlighted as sidebar biographies that accompany the main topical essays. Articles follow a standardized format that provides information at a glance. Rubrics include:

Disorders/Conditions	Tests/Treatments
Definition	Definition
Description	Purpose
Causes and symptoms	Precautions
Diagnosis	Description
Treatment	Preparation
Alternative treatment	Aftercare
Prognosis	Risks
Prevention	Normal/Abnormal results
Resources	Resources
Key terms	Key terms

In recent years there has been a resurgence of interest in holistic medicine that emphasizes the connection between mind and body. Aimed at achieving and maintaining good health rather than just eliminating disease, this approach has come to be known as alternative medicine. The *Gale Encyclopedia of Medicine 3* includes a number of essays on alternative therapies, ranging from traditional Chinese medicine to homeopathy and from meditation to aromatherapy. In addition to full essays on alternative therapies, the encyclopedia features specific **Alternative treatment** sections for diseases and conditions that may be helped by complementary therapies.

INCLUSION CRITERIA

A preliminary list of diseases, disorders, tests and treatments was compiled from a wide variety of sources, including professional medical guides and textbooks as well as consumer guides and encyclopedias. The general advisory board, made up of public librarians, medical librarians and consumer health experts, evaluated the topics and made suggestions for inclusion. The list was sorted by category and sent to *GEM3* medical advisers, for review. Final selection of topics to include was made by the medical advisors in conjunction with the Thomson Gale editor.

ABOUT THE CONTRIBUTORS

The essays were compiled by experienced medical writers, including physicians, pharmacists, nurses, and other health care professionals. *GEM3* medical advisors reviewed the completed essays to insure that they are appropriate, up-to-date, and medically accurate.

HOW TO USE THIS BOOK

The *Gale Encyclopedia of Medicine 3* has been designed with ready reference in mind.

- Straight **alphabetical arrangement** allows users to locate information quickly.

- Bold faced terms function as **print hyperlinks** that point the reader to related entries in the encyclopedia.

- **Cross-references** placed throughout the encyclopedia direct readers to where information on subjects without entries can be found. Synonyms are also cross-referenced.

- A list of **key terms** are provided where appropriate to define unfamiliar terms or concepts.

- Valuable **contact information** for organizations andsupport groups is included with each entry.

The appendix contains an extensive list of organizations arranged in alphabetical order.

- **Resources section** directs users to additional sources of medical information on a topic.

- A comprehensive **general index** allows users to easily target detailed aspects of any topic, including Latin names.

GRAPHICS

The *Gale Encyclopedia of Medicine 3* is enhanced with over 675 illustrations, including photos, charts, tables, and customized line drawings.

ADVISORS

A number of experts in the library and medical communities provided invaluable assistance in the formulation of this encyclopedia. Our advisory board performed a myriad of duties, from defining the scope of coverage to reviewing individual entries for accuracy and accessibility. The editor would like to express her appreciation to them.

MEDICAL ADVISORS

Rosalyn Carson-DeWitt, M.D.
Durham, NC

Larry I. Lutwick M.D., F.A.C.P.
Director, Infectious Diseases
VA Medical Center
Brooklyn, NY

Samuel Uretsky, Pharm.D.
Pharmacist
Wantagh, NY

CONTRIBUTORS

Margaret Alic, Ph.D.
Science Writer
Eastsound, WA

Janet Byron Anderson
Linguist/Language Consultant
Rocky River, OH

Lisa Andres, M.S., C.G.C.
Certified Genetic Counselor and Medical Writer
San Jose, CA

Greg Annussek
Medical Writer/Editor
New York, NY

Bill Asenjo, Ph.D.
Science Writer
Iowa City, IA

Sharon A. Aufox, M.S., C.G.C.
Genetic Counselor
Rockford Memorial Hospital
Rockford, IL

Sandra Bain Cushman
Massage Therapist, Alexander Technique Practitioner
Charlottesville, VA

Howard Baker
Medical Writer
North York, Ontario

Laurie Barclay, M.D.
Neurological Consulting Services
Tampa, FL

Jeanine Barone
Nutritionist, Exercise Physiologist
New York, NY

Julia R. Barrett
Science Writer
Madison, WI

Donald G. Barstow, R.N.
Clincal Nurse Specialist
Oklahoma City, OK

Carin Lea Beltz, M.S.
Genetic Counselor and Program Director
The Center for Genetic Counseling
Indianapolis, IN

Linda K. Bennington, C.N.S.
Science Writer
Virginia Beach, VA

Issac R. Berniker
Medical Writer
Vallejo, CA

Kathleen Berrisford, M.S.V.
Science Writer

Bethanne Black
Medical Writer
Atlanta, GA

Jennifer Bowjanowski, M.S., C.G.C.
Genetic Counselor
Children's Hospital Oakland
Oakland, CA

Michelle Q. Bosworth, M.S., C.G.C.
Genetic Counselor
Eugene, OR

Barbara Boughton
Health and Medical Writer
El Cerrito, CA

Cheryl Branche, M.D.
Retired General Practitioner
Jackson, MS

Michelle Lee Brandt
Medical Writer
San Francisco, CA

Maury M. Breecher, Ph.D.
Health Communicator/Journalist
Northport, AL

Ruthan Brodsky
Medical Writer
Bloomfield Hills, MI

Tom Brody, Ph.D.
Science Writer
Berkeley, CA

Leonard C. Bruno, Ph.D.
Medical Writer
Chevy Chase, MD

Diane Calbrese
Medical Sciences and Technology Writer
Silver Spring, Maryland

Richard H. Camer
Editor
International Medical News Group
Silver Spring, MD

Rosalyn Carson-DeWitt, M.D.
Medical Writer
Durham, NC

Lata Cherath, Ph.D.
Science Writing Intern
Cancer Research Institute
New York, NY

Linda Chrisman
Massage Therapist and Educator
Oakland, CA

Lisa Christenson, Ph.D.
Science Writer
Hamden, CT

Geoffrey N. Clark, D.V.M.
Editor
Canine Sports Medicine
    Update
Newmarket, NH

Rhonda Cloos, R.N.
Medical Writer
Austin, TX

Gloria Cooksey, C.N.E
Medical Writer
Sacramento, CA

Amy Cooper, M.A., M.S.I.
Medical Writer
Vermillion, SD

David A. Cramer, M.D.
Medical Writer
Chicago, IL

Esther Csapo Rastega, R.N.,
    B.S.N.
Medical Writer
Holbrook, MA

Arnold Cua, M.D.
Physician
Brooklyn, NY

Tish Davidson, A.M.
Medical Writer
Fremont, California

Dominic De Bellis, Ph.D.
Medical Writer/Editor
Mahopac, NY

Lori De Milto
Medical Writer
Sicklerville, NJ

Robert S. Dinsmoor
Medical Writer
South Hamilton, MA

Stephanie Dionne, B.S.
Medical Writer
Ann Arbor, MI

Martin W. Dodge, Ph.D.
Technical Writer/Editor
Centinela Hospital and Medical
    Center
Inglewood, CA

David Doermann
Medical Writer
Salt Lake City, UT

Stefanie B. N. Dugan, M.S.
Genetic Counselor
Milwaukee, WI

Doug Dupler, M.A.
Science Writer
Boulder, CO

Thomas Scott Eagan
Student Researcher
University of Arizona
Tucson, AZ

Altha Roberts Edgren
Medical Writer
Medical Ink
St. Paul, MN

Karen Ericson, R.N.
Medical Writer
Estes Park, CO

L. Fleming Fallon Jr., M.D.,
    Dr.PH
*Associate Professor of Public
    Health*
Bowling Green State University
Bowling Green, OH

Faye Fishman, D.O.
Physician
Randolph, NJ

Janis Flores
Medical Writer
Lexikon Communications
Sebastopol, CA

Risa Flynn
Medical Writer
Culver City, CA

Paula Ford-Martin
Medical Writer
Chaplin, MN

Janie F. Franz
Writer
Grand Forks, ND

Sallie Freeman, Ph.D., B.S.N.
Medical Writer
Atlanta, GA

Rebecca J. Frey, Ph.D.
*Research and Administrative
    Associate*
East Rock Institute
New Haven, CT

Cynthia L. Frozena, R.N.
Nurse, Medical Writer
Manitowoc, WI

Jason Fryer
Medical Writer
San Antonio, TX

Ron Gasbarro, Pharm.D.
Medical Writer
New Milford, PA

Julie A. Gelderloos
Biomedical Writer
Playa del Rey, CA

Gary Gilles, M.A.
Medical Writer
Wauconda, IL

Harry W. Golden
Medical Writer
Shoreline Medical Writers
Old Lyme, CT

Debra Gordon
Medical Writer
Nazareth, PA

Megan Gourley
Writer
Germantown, MD

Jill Granger, M.S.
Senior Research Associate
University of Michigan
Ann Arbor, MI

Alison Grant
Medical Writer
Averill Park, NY

Elliot Greene, M.A.
*former president, American
    Massage Therapy Association*
Massage Therapist
Silver Spring, MD

Peter Gregutt
Writer
Asheville, NC

Laith F. Gulli, M.D.
M.Sc., M.Sc.(MedSci), M.S.A.,
    Msc.Psych, MRSNZ
FRSH, FRIPHH, FAIC, FZS
DAPA, DABFC, DABCI
*Consultant Psychotherapist in
    Private Practice*
Lathrup Village, MI

Kapil Gupta, M.D.
Medical Writer
Winston-Salem, NC

Maureen Haggerty
Medical Writer
Ambler, PA

Clare Hanrahan
Medical Writer
Asheville, NC

Ann M. Haren
Science Writer
Madison, CT

Judy C. Hawkins, M.S.
Genetic Counselor
The University of Texas Medical
 Branch
Galveston, TX

Caroline Helwick
Medical Writer
New Orleans, LA

David Helwig
Medical Writer
London, Ontario

Lisette Hilton
Medical Writer
Boca Raton, FL

Katherine S. Hunt, M.S.
Genetic Counselor
University of New Mexico Health
 Sciences Center
Albuquerque, NM

Kevin Hwang, M.D.
Medical Writer
Morristown, NJ

Holly Ann Ishmael, M.S.,
 C.G.C.
Genetic Counselor
The Children's Mercy Hospital
Kansas City, MO

Dawn A. Jacob, M.S.
Genetic Counselor
Obstetrix Medical Group of
 Texas
Fort Worth, TX

Sally J. Jacobs, Ed.D.
Medical Writer
Los Angeles, CA

Michelle L. Johnson, M.S., J.D.
*Patent Attorney and Medical
 Writer*
Portland, OR

Paul A. Johnson, Ed.M.
Medical Writer
San Diego, CA

Cindy L. A. Jones, Ph.D.
Biomedical Writer
Sagescript Communications
Lakewood, CO

David Kaminstein, M.D.
Medical Writer
West Chester, PA

Beth A. Kapes
Medical Writer
Bay Village, OH

Janet M. Kearney
Freelance writer
Orlando, FL

Christine Kuehn Kelly
Medical Writer
Havertown, PA

Bob Kirsch
Medical Writer
Ossining, NY

Joseph Knight, P.A.
Medical Writer
Winton, CA

Melissa Knopper
Medical Writer
Chicago, IL

Karen Krajewski, M.S., C.G.C.
Genetic Counselor
Assistant Professor of Neurology
Wayne State University
Detroit, MI

Jeanne Krob, M.D., F.A.C.S.
Physician, writer
Pittsburgh, PA

Jennifer Lamb
Medical Writer
Spokane, WA

Richard H. Lampert
Senior Medical Editor
W.B. Saunders Co.
Philadelphia, PA

Jeffrey P. Larson, R.P.T.
Physical Therapist
Sabin, MN

Jill Lasker
Medical Writer
Midlothian, VA

Kristy Layman
Music Therapist
East Lansing, MI

Victor Leipzig, Ph.D.
Biological Consultant
Huntington Beach, CA

Lorraine Lica, Ph.D.
Medical Writer
San Diego, CA

John T. Lohr, Ph.D.
*Assistant Director, Biotechnology
 Center*
Utah State University
Logan, UT

Larry Lutwick, M.D., F.A.C.P.
Director, Infectious Diseases
VA Medical Center
Brooklyn, NY

Suzanne M. Lutwick
Medical Writer
Brooklyn, NY

Nicole Mallory, M.S.
Medical Student
Wayne State University
Detroit, MI

Warren Maltzman, Ph.D.
*Consultant, Molecular
 Pathology*
Demarest, NJ

Adrienne Massel, R.N.
Medical Writer
Beloit, WI

Ruth E. Mawyer, R.N.
Medical Writer
Charlottesville, VA

Richard A. McCartney M.D.
*Fellow, American College of
 Surgeons*
*Diplomat American Board of
 Surgery*
Richland, WA

Bonny McClain, Ph.D.
Medical Writer
Greensboro, NC

Sally C. McFarlane-Parrott
Medical Writer
Ann Arbor, MI

Mercedes McLaughlin
Medical Writer
Phoenixville, CA

Alison McTavish, M.Sc.
Medical Writer and Editor
Montreal, Quebec

Liz Meszaros
Medical Writer
Lakewood, OH

Betty Mishkin
Medical Writer
Skokie, IL

Barbara J. Mitchell
Medical Writer
Hallstead, PA

Mark A. Mitchell, M.D.
Medical Writer
Seattle, WA

Susan J. Montgomery
Medical Writer
Milwaukee, WI

Louann W. Murray, PhD
Medical Writer
Huntington Beach, CA

Bilal Nasser, M.Sc.
Senior Medical Student
Universidad Iberoamericana
Santo Domingo, Domincan
  Republic

Laura Ninger
Medical Writer
Weehawken, NJ

Nancy J. Nordenson
Medical Writer
Minneapolis, MN

Teresa Odle
Medical Writer
Albaquerque, NM

Lisa Papp, R.N.
Medical Writer
Cherry Hill, NJ

Lee Ann Paradise
Medical Writer
San Antonio, TX

Patience Paradox
Medical Writer
Bainbridge Island, WA

Barbara J. Pettersen
Genetic Counselor
Genetic Counseling of Central
  Oregon
Bend, OR

Genevieve Pham-Kanter, M.S.
Medical Writer
Chicago, IL

Collette Placek
Medical Writer
Wheaton, IL

J. Ricker Polsdorfer, M.D.
Medical Writer
Phoenix, AZ

Scott Polzin, M.S., C.G.C.
Medical Writer
Buffalo Grove, IL

Elizabeth J. Pulcini, M.S.
Medical Writer
Phoenix, Arizona

Nada Quercia, M.S., C.C.G.C.
Genetic Counselor
Division of Clinical and
  Metabolic Genetics
The Hospital for Sick Children
Toronto, ON, Canada

Ann Quigley
Medical Writer
New York, NY

Robert Ramirez, B.S.
Medical Student
University of Medicine &
  Dentistry of New Jersey
Stratford, NJ

Kulbir Rangi, D.O.
Medical Doctor and Writer
New York, NY

Esther Csapo Rastegari, Ed.M.,
  R.N./B.S.N.
Registered Nurse, Medical Writer
Holbrook, MA

Toni Rizzo
Medical Writer
Salt Lake City, UT

Martha Robbins
Medical Writer
Evanston, IL

Richard Robinson
Medical Writer
Tucson, AZ

Nancy Ross-Flanigan
Science Writer
Belleville, MI

Anna Rovid Spickler, D.V.M., Ph.D.
Medical Writer
Moorehead, KY

Belinda Rowland, Ph.D.
Medical Writer
Voorheesville, NY

Andrea Ruskin, M.D.
Whittingham Cancer Center
Norwalk, CT

Laura Ruth, Ph.D.
*Medical, Science, & Technology
  Writer*
Los Angeles, CA

Karen Sandrick
Medical Writer
Chicago, IL

Kausalya Santhanam, Ph.D.
Technical Writer
Branford, CT

Jason S. Schliesser, D.C.
Chiropractor
Holland Chiropractic, Inc.
Holland, OH

Joan Schonbeck
Medical Writer
Nursing
Massachusetts Department of
  Mental Health
Marlborough, MA

Laurie Heron Seaver, M.D.
Clinical Geneticist
Greenwood Genetic Center
Greenwood, SC

Catherine Seeley
Medical Writer

Kristen Mahoney Shannon, M.S.,
  C.G.C.
Genetic Counselor
Center for Cancer Risk Analysis
Massachusetts General Hospital
Boston, MA

Kim A. Sharp, M.Ln.
Writer
Richmond, TX

Judith Sims, M.S.
Medical Writer
Logan, UT

Joyce S. Siok, R.N.
Medical Writer
South Windsor, CT

Jennifer Sisk
Medical Writer
Havertown, PA

Patricia Skinner
Medical Writer
Amman, Jordan

Genevieve Slomski, Ph.D.
Medical Writer
New Britain, CT

Stephanie Slon
Medical Writer
Portland, OR

Linda Wasmer Smith
Medical Writer
Albuquerque, NM

Java O. Solis, M.S.
Medical Writer
Decatur, GA

Elaine Souder, PhD
Medical Writer
Little Rock, AR

Jane E. Spehar
Medical Writer
Canton, OH

Lorraine Steefel, R.N.
Medical Writer
Morganville, NJ

Kurt Sternlof
Science Writer
New Rochelle, NY

Roger E. Stevenson, M.D.
Director
Greenwood Genetic Center
Greenwood, SC

Dorothy Stonely
Medical Writer
Los Gatos, CA

Liz Swain
Medical Writer
San Diego, CA

Deanna M. Swartout-Corbeil,
  R.N.
Medical Writer
Thompsons Station, TN

Keith Tatarelli, J.D.
Medical Writer

Mary Jane Tenerelli, M.S.
Medical Writer
East Northport, NY

Catherine L. Tesla, M.S., C.G.C.
Senior Associate, Faculty
Dept. of Pediatrics, Division of
  Medical Genetics
Emory University School of
  Medicine
Atlanta, GA

Bethany Thivierge
Biotechnical Writer/Editor
Technicality Resources
Rockland, ME

Mai Tran, Pharm.D.
Medical Writer
Troy, MI

Carol Turkington
Medical Writer
Lancaster, PA

Judith Turner, B.S.
Medical Writer
Sandy, UT

Amy B. Tuteur, M.D.
Medical Advisor
Sharon, MA

Samuel Uretsky, Pharm.D.
Medical Writer
Wantagh, NY

Amy Vance, M.S., C.G.C.
Genetic Counselor
GeneSage, Inc.
San Francisco, CA

Michael Sherwin Walston
Student Researcher
University of Arizona
Tucson, AZ

Ronald Watson, Ph.D.
Science Writer
Tucson, AZ

Ellen S. Weber, M.S.N.
Medical Writer
Fort Wayne, IN

Ken R. Wells
Freelance Writer
Laguna Hills, CA

Jennifer F. Wilson, M.S.
Science Writer
Haddonfield, NJ

Kathleen D. Wright, R.N.
Medical Writer
Delmar, DE

Jennifer Wurges
Medical Writer
Rochester Hills, MI

Mary Zoll, Ph.D.
Science Writer
Newton Center, MA

Jon Zonderman
Medical Writer
Orange, CA

Michael V. Zuck, Ph.D.
Medical Writer
Boulder, CO

G

Galactorrhea

Definition

Galactorrhea is the secretion of breast milk in men, or in women who are not breastfeeding an infant.

Description

Lactation, or the production of breast milk, is a normal condition occurring in women after delivery of a baby. Many women who have had children may even be able to express a small amount of breast milk from the nipple up to two years after **childbirth**. Galactorrhea, or hyperlactation, however, is a rare condition that can occur in both men and women, where a white or grayish fluid is secreted by the nipples of both breasts. While this condition is not serious in itself, galactorrhea can indicate more serious conditions, including hormone imbalances or the presence of tumors.

Causes and symptoms

Causes

Galactorrhea is associated with a number of conditions. The normal production of breast milk is controlled by a hormone called prolactin, which is secreted by the pituitary gland in the brain. Any condition that upsets the balance of hormones in the blood or the production of hormones by the pituitary gland or sexual organs can stimulate the production of prolactin.

Often, a patient with galactorrhea will have a high level of prolactin in the blood. A tumor in the pituitary gland can cause this overproduction of prolactin. At least 30% of women with galactorrhea, menstrual abnormalities, and high prolactin levels have a pituitary gland tumor. Other types of brain tumors, head injuries, or **encephalitis** (an infection of the brain) can also cause galactorrhea.

Tumors or growths in the ovaries or other reproductive organs in women, or in the testicles or related sexual organs of men, can also stimulate the production of prolactin. Any discharge of fluid from the breast after a woman has passed **menopause** may indicate **breast cancer**. However, most often the discharge associated with breast **cancer** will be from one breast only. In galactorrhea both breasts are usually involved. The presence of blood in the fluid discharged from the breast could indicate a benign growth in the breast tissue itself. In approximately 10–15% of patients with blood in the fluid, carcinoma of the breast tissue is present.

A number of medications and drugs can also cause galactorrhea as a side-effect. Hormonal therapies (like **oral contraceptives**), drugs for treatment of depression or other psychiatric conditions, tranquilizers, morphine, heroin, and some medications for high blood pressure can cause galactorrhea.

Several normal physiologic situations can cause production of breast milk. Nipple stimulation in men or women during sexual intercourse may induce lactation, for women particularly during or just after **pregnancy**.

Even after extensive testing, no specific cause can be determined for some patients with galactorrhea.

Symptoms

The primary symptom of galactorrhea is the discharge of milky fluid from both breasts. In women, galactorrhea may be associated with **infertility**, menstrual cycle irregularities, hot flushes, or amenorrhea–a condition where menstruation stops completely. Men may experience loss of sexual interest and **impotence**. Headaches and visual disturbances have also been associated with some cases of galactorrhea.

Diagnosis

Galactorrhea is generally considered a symptom that may indicate a more serious problem. Collection of a thorough medical history, including pregnancies, surgeries, and consumption of drugs and medications is a first step in diagnosing the cause of galactorrhea. A **physical examination**, along with a breast examination, will usually be conducted. Blood and urine samples may be taken to determine levels of various hormones in the body, including prolactin and compounds related to thyroid function.

A mammogram (an x ray of the breast) or an ultrasound scan (using high frequency sound waves) might be used to determine if there are any tumors or cysts present in the breasts themselves. If a tumor of the pituitary gland is suspected, a series of computer assisted x rays called a computed tomography scan (CT scan) may be done. Another procedure that may be useful is a **magnetic resonance imaging** (MRI) scan to locate tumors or abnormalities in tissues.

Treatment

Treatment for galactorrhea will depend on the cause of the condition and the symptoms. The drug bromocriptine is often prescribed first to reduce the secretion of prolactin and to decrease the size of **pituitary tumors**. This drug will control galactorrhea symptoms and in many cases may be the only therapy necessary. Oral estrogen and progestins (hormone pills, like birth control pills) may control symptoms of galactorrhea for some women. Surgery to remove a tumor may be required for patients who have more serious symptoms of **headache** and vision loss, or if the tumor shows signs of enlargement despite drug treatment. **Radiation therapy** has also been used to reduce tumor size when surgery is not possible or not totally successful. A combination of drug, surgery, and radiation treatment can also be used.

Galactorrhea is more of a nuisance than a real threat to health. While it is important to find the cause of the condition, even if a tumor is discovered in the pituitary gland, it may not require treatment. With very small, slow-growing tumors, some physicians may suggest a "wait and see" approach.

Prognosis

Treatment with bromocriptine is usually effective in stopping milk secretion, however, symptoms may recur if drug therapy is discontinued. Surgical removal or radiation treatment may correct the problem permanently if it is related to a tumor. Frequent monitoring of hormone status and tumor size may be recommended.

Prevention

There is no way to prevent galactorrhea. If the condition is caused by the use of a particular drug, a patient may be able to switch to a different drug that does not have the side-effect of galactorrhea.

Resources

BOOKS

"Galactorrhea." In *Current Medical Diagnosis & Treatment, 1998*. 37th ed. Stamford: Appleton & Lange, 1997.

Altha Roberts Edgren

Galactosemia

Definition

Galactosemia is an inherited disease in which the transformation of galactose to glucose is blocked, allowing galactose to increase to toxic levels in the body. If galactosemia is untreated, high levels of galactose cause **vomiting**, **diarrhea**, lethargy, low blood sugar, brain damage, **jaundice**, liver enlargement, **cataracts**, susceptibility to infection, and **death**.

Description

Galactosemia is a rare but potentially life-threatening disease that results from the inability to metabolize galactose. Serious consequences from galactosemia can be prevented by screening newborns at birth with a simple blood test.

Galactosemia is an inborn error of metabolism. "Metabolism" refers to all chemical reactions that take place in living organisms. A metabolic pathway is a series of reactions where the product of each step in the series is the starting material for the next step. Enzymes are the chemicals that help the reactions occur. Their ability to function depends on their structure, and their structure is determined by the deoxyribonucleic acid (DNA) sequence of the genes that encode them. Inborn errors of metabolism are caused by mutations in these genes which do not allow the enzymes to function properly.

Sugars are sometimes called "the energy molecules," and galactose and glucose are both sugars. For galactose to be utilized for energy, it must be transformed into something that can enter the metabolic pathway that converts glucose into energy (plus water and carbon dioxide). This is important for infants because they typically get most of their nutrient energy from milk, which contains a high level of galactose. Each molecule of lactose, the major sugar constituent of milk, is made up of a molecule of galactose and a molecule of glucose, and so galactose makes up 20% of the energy source of a typical infant's diet.

Three enzymes are required to convert galactose into glucose-1-phosphate (a phosphorylated glucose that can enter the metabolic pathway that turns glucose into energy). Each of these three enzymes is encoded by a separate gene. If any of these enzymes fail to function, galactose build-up and galactosemia result. Thus, there are three types of galactosemia with a different gene responsible for each.

Every cell in a person's body has two copies of each gene. Each of the forms of galactosemia is inherited as a recessive trait, which means that galactosemia is only present in individuals with two mutated copies of one of the three genes. This also means that carriers, with only one copy of a gene mutation, will not be aware that they are carrying a mutation (unless they have had a genetic test), as it is masked by the normal gene they also carry and they have no symptoms of the disease. For each step in the conversion of galactose to glucose, if only one of the two copies of the gene controlling that step is normal (i.e. for carriers), enough functional enzyme is made so that the pathway is not blocked at that step. If a person has galactosemia, both copies of the gene coding for one of the enzymes required to convert glucose to galactose are defective and the pathway becomes blocked. If two carriers of the same defective gene have children, the chance of any of their children getting galactosemia (the chance of a child getting two copies of the defective gene) is 25% (one in four) for each **pregnancy**.

Classic galactosemia occurs in the United States about one in every 50,000–70,000 live births.

Causes and symptoms

Galactosemia I

Galactosemia I (also called classic galactosemia), the first form to be discovered, is caused by defects in both copies of the gene that codes for an enzyme called galactose-1-phosphate uridyl transferase (GALT). There are 30 known different mutations in this gene that cause GALT to malfunction.

Newborns with galactosemia I appear normal at birth, but begin to develop symptoms after they are given milk for the first time. Symptoms include vomiting, diarrhea, lethargy (sluggishness or **fatigue**), low blood glucose, jaundice (a yellowing of the skin and eyes), enlarged liver, protein and amino acids in the urine, and susceptibility to infection, especially from gram negative bacteria. Cataracts (a grayish white film on the eye lens) can appear within a few days after birth. People with galactosemia frequently have symptoms as they grow older even though they have been given a galactose-free diet. These symptoms include **speech disorders**, cataracts, ovarian atrophy, and **infertility** in females, learning disabilities, and behavioral problems.

Galactosemia II

Galactosemia II is caused by defects in both copies of the gene that codes for an enzyme called galactokinase (GALK). The frequency of occurrence of galactosemia II is about one in 100,000–155,000 births.

Galactosemia II is less harmful than galactosemia I. Babies born with galactosemia II will develop cataracts at an early age unless they are given a galactose-free diet. They do not generally suffer from liver damage or neurologic disturbances.

Galactosemia III

Galactosemia III is caused by defects in the gene that codes for an enzyme called uridyl diphosphogalactose-4-epimerase (GALE). This form of galactosemia is very rare.

There are two forms of galactosemia III, a severe form, which is exceedingly rare, and a benign form. The benign form has no symptoms and requires no special diet. However, newborns with galactosemia III, including the benign form, have high levels of galactose-1-phosphate that show up on the initial screenings for elevated galactose and galactose-1-phosphate. This situation illustrates one aspect of the importance of follow-up enzyme function tests. Tests showing normal levels of GALT and GALK allow people affected by the benign form of galactosemia III to enjoy a normal diet.

The severe form has symptoms similar to those of galactosemia I, but with more severe neurological problems, including seizures. Only two cases of this rare form had been reported as of 1997.

Diagnosis

The newborn screening test for classic galactosemia is quick and straightforward; all but three states require testing on all newborns. Blood from a baby who is two to three days old is usually first screened for high levels of galactose and galactose-1-phosphate. If either of these compounds is elevated, further tests are performed to find out which enzymes (GALT, GALK, or GALE) are present or missing. DNA testing may also be performed to confirm the diagnosis.

If there is a strong suspicion that a baby has galactosemia, galactose is removed from the diet right away. In this case, an initial screen for galactose or galactose-1-phosphate will be meaningless. In the absence of galactose in the diet, this test will be negative whether the baby has galactosemia or not. In this case, tests to measure enzyme levels must be given to find out if the suspected baby is indeed galactosemic.

In addition, galactosemic babies who are refusing milk or vomiting will not have elevated levels of galactose or galactose phosphate, and their condition will not be detected by the initial screen. Any baby with symptoms of galactosemia (for example, vomiting) should be given enzyme tests.

Treatment

Galactosemia I and II are treated by removing galactose from the diet. Since galactose is a breakdown product of lactose, the primary sugar constituent of milk, this means all milk and foods containing milk products must be totally eliminated. Other foods like legumes, organ meats, and processed meats also contain considerable galactose and must be avoided. Pills that use lactose as a filler must also be avoided. Soy-based and casein hydrolysate-based formulas are recommended for infants with galactosemia.

Treatment of the severe form of galactosemia III with a galactose-restricted diet has been tried, but this disorder is so rare that the long-term effects of this treatment are unknown.

Prognosis

Early detection in the newborn period is the key to controlling symptoms. Long-term effects in untreated babies include severe **mental retardation**, **cirrhosis** of

---

KEY TERMS

Casein hydrolysate—A preparation made from the milk protein casein, which is hydrolyzed to break it down into its constituent amino acids. Amino acids are the building blocks of proteins.

Catalyst—A substance that changes the rate of a chemical reaction, but is not physically changed by the process.

Enzyme—A protein that catalyzes a biochemical reaction or change without changing its own structure or function.

Galactose—One of the two simple sugars, together with glucose, that makes up the protein, lactose, found in milk. Galactose can be toxic in high levels.

Glucose—One of the two simple sugars, together with galactose, that makes up the protein, lactose, found in milk. Glucose is the form of sugar that is usable by the body to generate energy.

Lactose—A sugar made up of of glucose and galactose. It is the primary sugar in milk.

Metabolic pathway—A sequence of chemical reactions that lead from some precursor to a product, where the product of each step in the series is the starting material for the next step.

Metabolism—The total combination of all of the chemical processes that occur within cells and tissues of a living body.

Recessive trait—An inherited trait or characteristic that is outwardly obvious only when two copies of the gene for that trait are present.

---

the liver, and death. About 75% of the untreated babies die within the first two weeks of life. On the other hand, with treatment, a significant proportion of people with galactosemia I can lead nearly normal lives, although speech defects, learning disabilities, and behavioral problems are common. A 2004 study revealed that children and adolescents with classic galactosemia often have lower quality of life than peers without the disease, exhibiting problems with cognition (thinking and intellectual skills) and social function. In addition, cataracts due to galactosemia II can be completely prevented by a galactose-free diet.

Prevention

Since galactosemia is a recessive genetic disease, the disease is usually detected on a newborn screening test, since most people are unaware that they are carriers of a gene mutation causing the disease. For couples with a previous child with galactosemia, prenatal diagnosis is available to determine whether a pregnancy is similarly affected. Families in which a child has been diagnosed with galactosemia can have DNA testing which can enable other more distant relatives to determine their carrier status. Prospective parents can then use that information to conduct family planning or to prepare for a child with special circumstances. Children born with galactosemia should be put on a special diet right away, to reduce the symptoms and complications of the disease.

Resources

PERIODICALS

Bosch, Annet M., et al. "Living With Classical Galactosmeia: Health-related Quality of Life Consequences." *Pediatrics* May 2004: 1385–1387.

ORGANIZATIONS

Association for Neuro-Metabolic Disorders. 5223 Brookfield Lane, Sylvania, OH 43560. (419) 885-1497.
Metabolic Information Network. PO Box 670847, Dallas, TX 75367-0847. (214) 696-2188 or (800) 945-2188.
Parents of Galactosemic Children, Inc. 2148 Bryton Dr., Powell OH 43065. < http://www.galactosemia.org/index.htm > .

OTHER

"GeneCards: Human Genes, Proteins and Diseases." < http://bioinfo.weizmann.ac.il/cards/ > .
"Vermont Newborn Screening Program: Galactosemia." < http://www.vtmednet.org/~m145037/vhgi_mem/nbsman/galacto.htm > .

Amy Vance, MS, CGC
Teresa G. Odle

Gallbladder cancer

Definition

Cancer of the gallbladder is cancer of the pear-shaped organ that lies on the undersurface of the liver.

Description

Bile from the liver is funneled into the gallbladder by way of the cystic duct. Between meals, the gallbladder stores a large amount of bile. To do this, it must absorb much of the water and electrolytes from the bile. In fact, the inner surface of the gallbladder is the most absorptive surface in the body. After a meal, the gallbladder's muscular walls contract to deliver the bile back through the cystic duct and eventually into the small intestine, where the bile can help digest food.

Demographics

About 5,000 people are diagnosed with gallbladder cancer each year in the United States, making it the fifth most common gastrointestinal cancer. It is more common in females than males and most patients are elderly. Southwest American Indians have a particularly high incidence— six times that of the general population.

Causes and symptoms

Gallstones are the most significant risk factor for the development of gallbladder cancer. Roughly 75 to 90 percent of patients with gallbladder cancer also have gallstones. Larger gallstones are associated with a higher chance of developing gallbladder cancer. Chronic inflammation of the gallbladder from infection also increases the risk for gallbladder cancer.

Unfortunately, sometimes cancer of the gallbladder does not produce symptoms until late in the disease. When symptoms are evident, the most common is **pain** in the upper right portion of the abdomen, underneath the right ribcage. Patients with gallbladder cancer may also report symptoms such as **nausea**, **vomiting**, weakness, **jaundice**, skin **itching**, **fever**, chills, poor appetite, and weight loss.

Diagnosis

Gallbladder cancer is often misdiagnosed because it mimics other more common conditions, such as gallstones, **cholecystitis**, and **pancreatitis**. But the imaging tests that are utilized to evaluate these other conditions can also detect gallbladder cancer. For example, ultrasound is a quick, noninvasive imaging test that reliably diagnoses gallstones and cholecystitis. It can also detect the presence of gallbladder cancer as well as show how far the cancer has spread. If cancer is suspected, a computed tomography scan is useful in confirming the presence of an abnormal mass and further demonstrating the size and extent of the tumor. Cholangiography, usually performed to evaluate a patient with jaundice, can also detect gallbladder cancer.

There are no specific laboratory tests for gallbladder cancer. Tumors can obstruct the normal flow of bile from the liver to the small intestine. Bilirubin, a component of bile, builds up within the liver and is absorbed into the bloodstream in excess amounts. This can be detected in a blood test, but it can also manifest clinically as jaundice. Elevated bilirubin levels and clinical jaundice can also occur with other conditions, such as gallstones.

On occasion, gallbladder cancer is diagnosed incidentally. About one percent of all patients who have their gallbladder removed for symptomatic gallstones are found to have gallbladder cancer. The cancer is found either by the surgeon or by the pathologist who inspects the gallbladder with a microscope.

Treatment

Staging of gallbladder cancer is determined by the how far the cancer has spread. The effectiveness of treatment declines as the stage progresses. Stage I cancer is confined to the wall of the gallbladder. Approximately 25% of cancers are at this stage at the time of diagnosis. Stage II cancer has penetrated the full thickness of the wall, but has not spread to nearby lymph nodes or invaded adjacent organs. Stage III cancer has spread to nearby lymph nodes or has invaded the liver, stomach, colon, small intestine, or large intestine. Stage IV disease has invaded very deeply into two or more adjacent organs or has spread to distant lymph nodes or organs by way of metastasis.

Early Stage I cancers involving only the innermost layer of the gallbladder wall can be cured by simple removal of the gallbladder. Cancers at this stage are sometimes found incidentally when the gallbladder is removed in the treatment of gallstones or cholecystitis. The majority of patients have good survival rates. Late Stage I cancers, which involve the outer muscular layers of the gallbladder wall, are generally treated in the same way as Stage II or III cancers. Removal of the gallbladder is not sufficient for these stages. The surgeon also removes nearby lymph nodes as well as a portion of the adjacent liver (radical surgery). Survival rates for these patients are considerably worse than for those with early Stage I disease. Patients with early Stage IV disease may benefit from radical surgery, but the issue is controversial. Late Stage IV cancer has spread too extensively to allow complete excision. Surgery is not an option for these patients.

Other therapies

When long-term survival is not likely, the focus of therapy shifts to improving quality of life. Jaundice and blockage of the stomach are two problems faced by patients with advanced cancer of the gallbladder.

KEY TERMS

Cholangiography—Radiographic examination of the bile ducts after injection with a special dye

Cholecystitis—Inflammation of the gallbladder, usually due to infection

Computed tomography—A radiology test by which images of cross-sectional planes of the body are obtained

Jaundice—Yellowish staining of the skin and eyes due to excess bilirubin in the bloodstream

Metastasis—The spread of tumor cells from one part of the body to another through blood vessels or lymphatic vessels

Pancreatitis—Inflammation of the pancreas

Stent—Slender hollow catheter or rod placed within a vessel or duct to provide support or maintain patency

Ultrasound—A radiology test utilizing high frequency sound waves

These can be treated with surgery, or alternatively, by special interventional techniques employed by the gastroenterologist or radiologist. A stent can be placed across the bile ducts in order to re-establish the flow of bile and relieve jaundice. A small feeding tube can be placed in the small intestine to allow feeding when the stomach is blocked. Pain may be treated with conventional pain medicines or a celiac **ganglion** nerve block.

Current **chemotherapy** or **radiation therapy** cannot cure gallbladder cancer, but they may offer some benefit in certain patients. For cancer that is too advanced for surgical cure, treatment with chemotherapeutic agents such as 5-fluorouracil may lengthen survival for a few months. The limited benefit of chemotherapy must be weighed carefully against its side effects. Radiation therapy is sometimes used after attempted surgical resection of the cancer to extend survival for a few months or relieve jaundice.

Resources

BOOKS

Abeloff, Martin D. "Gallbladder Carcinoma." In *Clinical Oncology*. 2nd ed. New York: Churchill Livingstone, 2000, pp.1730-1737.

Ahrendt, Steven A., and Henry A. Pitt. "Biliary Tract." In *Sabiston Textbook of Surgery*, edited by Courtney Townsend, Jr., 16th ed. Philadelphia: W.B. Saunders Company, 2001, pp. 1076-1111.

OTHER

National Cancer Institute Cancer Trials web site. < http://
cancertrials.nci.nih.gov/system > . < http://
www.cancertrials.com > .

Kevin O. Hwang, MD

Gallbladder disease *see* **Cholecystitis**

Gallbladder nuclear medicine scan

Definition

A nuclear medicine scan of the gallbladder is used to produce a set of images that look like x rays. The procedure uses a small amount of radioactive dye which is injected into the body. The dye accumulates in the organ, in this case, the gallbladder. A special camera called a scintillation or gamma camera produces images based on how the dye travels through the system and how the radiation is absorbed by the tissues. The procedure is also called cholescintigraphy or a hepatobiliary scan.

Purpose

A nuclear medicine scan can be used to diagnose disease and to find abnormalities in a body organ. A gallbladder scan can detect **gallstones**, tumors, or defects of the gallbladder. It can also be used to diagnose blockages of the bile duct that leads from the gallbladder to the small intestine. Unlike ultrasound, a gallbladder nuclear medicine scan can assess gallbladder function.

Precautions

Women who are pregnant or breastfeeding should tell their doctors before a scan is performed. Some medications or even eating a high fat meal before the procedure can interfere with the results of the scan.

Description

The gallbladder is a small pear-shaped sac located under the liver. The liver produces bile, a yellowish-green mixture of salts, acids, and other chemicals, that are stored in the gallbladder. Bile is secreted into the small intestine to help the body digest fats from foods.

Gallbladder disease, gallstones, **cancer**, or other abnormalities can cause **pain** and other symptoms. A gallbladder condition might be suspected if a patient has chronic or occasional pain in the upper right side of the abdomen. The pain may be stabbing and intense with sudden onset or it may be more of a dull, occasional ache. Loss of appetite, **nausea and vomiting** can also occur. **Fever** may indicate the presence of infection. **Jaundice**, a yellowing of the skin and whites of the eyes, may also indicate that the gallbladder is involved.

A gallbladder nuclear medicine scan may be used to diagnose gallstones, blockage of the bile duct or other abnormalities, and to assess gallbladder functioning and inflammation (**cholecystitis**). The scan is usually performed in a hospital or clinical radiology department. The patient lies on an examination table while a small amount of radioactive dye is injected into a vein in the arm. This dye circulates through the blood and collects in the gallbladder. As the dye moves through the gallbladder, a series of pictures is taken using a special camera called a *scintillation* or *gamma camera*. This procedure produces images that look like x rays. The test usually takes one to two hours to complete, but can last up to four hours.

The results of the scan are read by a radiologist, a doctor specializing in x rays and other types of scanning techniques. A report is sent, usually within 24 hours, to the doctor who will discuss the results with the patient.

Preparation

The patient may be required to withhold food and liquids for up to eight hours before the scan.

Aftercare

No special care is required after the procedure. Once the scan is complete, the patient can return to normal activities.

Risks

Nuclear medicine scans use a very small amount of radioactive material, and the risk of radiation is minimal. Very rarely, a patient may have a reaction to the dye material used.

Normal results

A normal scan shows a gallbladder without gallstones. There will be no evidence of growths or tumors, and no signs of infection or swelling. The normal gallbladder fills with bile and secretes it through the bile duct without blockages.

Abnormal results

An abnormal scan may show abnormal gallbladder emptying (suggesting gallbladder dysfunction or inflammation), or gallstones in the gallbladder or in the bile duct. The presence of tumors, growths or other types of blockages of the duct or the gallbladder itself could also appear on an abnormal scan.

Resources

OTHER

"Gallbladder Scan, Radioisotope." Infonet. < http:// infonet.med.cornell.edu > .

"Nuclear Medicine." Washington Radiology Associates Page. < http://www.wrapc.com > .

Altha Roberts Edgren

Gallbladder surgery *see* **Cholecystectomy**

Gallbladder x rays

Definition

This is an x-ray exam of the gallbladder (GB), a sac-like organ that stores bile that is located under the liver. The study involves taking tablets containing dye (contrast) which outline any abnormalities when x rays are taken the following day. The test was once the standard for diagnosing diseases of the GB such as **gallstones**, but is used less frequently now. This is due to advances in diagnostic ultrasound, which is quick, accurate and doesn't involve exposure to ionizing radiation. When functional parameters of the gallbladder need to be demonstrated, scintigraphy is now the study of choice. OCG, however, can be useful when a gallbladder is contracted down due to

the presence of many, many gallstones. It can also help determine whether the cystic duct is clear, prior to surgical procedures such as **lithotripsy**. OCG may also be used to evaluate gallbladder disease that doesn't involve gallstones, such as adenomyomatosis of the gallbladder or cholesterolosis of the gallbladder.

Purpose

This test, also known as an oral cholecystogram or OCG, is usually ordered to help physicians diagnose disorders of the gallbladder, such as gallstones and tumors, which show up as solid dark structures. It is performed to help in the investigation of patients with upper abdominal **pain**. The test also measures gallbladder function, as the failure of the organ to visualize can signify a non-functioning or diseased gallbladder. The gallbladder may also not visualize if the bilirubin level is over 4 and the study should not be performed under these circumstances.

Precautions

Your physician must be notified if you are pregnant or allergic to iodine. Patients with a history of severe kidney damage, have an increased risk of injury or side effects from the procedure. In those cases, ultrasound is commonly used instead of the x-ray examination. Some people experience side effects from the contrast material (dye tablets), especially **diarrhea**. During preparation for the test, patients should not use any **laxatives**. Diabetics should discuss the need for any adjustment in medication with their physician.

Description

The exam is performed in the radiology department. The night before the test, patients swallow six tablets (one at a time) that contain the contrast (x-ray dye). The following day at the hospital, the radiologist examines the gallbladder with a fluoroscope (a special x ray that projects the image onto a video monitor). Sometimes, patients are then asked to drink a highfat formula that will cause the gallbladder to contract and release bile. X rays will then be taken at various intervals. There is no discomfort from the test. If the gallbladder is not seen, the patient may be asked to return the following day for x rays.

Preparation

The day before the test patients are instructed to eat a high fat lunch (eggs, butter, milk, salad oils, or fatty meats), and a fat-free meal (fruits, vegetables,

KEY TERMS

Bile—A yellow-green liquid produced by the liver, which is released through the bile ducts into the small intestines to help digest fat.

Bilirubin—A reddish-yellow pigment formed from the destruction of red blood cells, and metabolized by the liver. Levels of bilirubin in the blood increase in patients with liver disease or blockage of the bile ducts.

Ultrasound—A non-invasive procedure based on changes in sound waves of a frequency that cannot be heard, but respond to changes in tissue composition. It requires no preparation and no radiation occurs; it has become the "gold standard" for diagnosis of stones in the gallbladder, but is less accurate in diagnosing stones in the bile ducts. Gallstones as small as 2 mm can be identified.

bread, tea or coffee, and only lean meat) in the evening. Two hours after the evening meal, six tablets containing the contrast medium, are taken, one a time. After that, no food or fluid is permitted until after the test.

Aftercare

No special care is required after the study.

Risks

There is a small chance of an allergic reaction to the contrast material. In addition, there is low radiation exposure. X rays are monitored and regulated to provide the minimum amount of radiation exposure needed to produce the image. Most experts feel that the risk is low compared with the benefits. Pregnant women and children are more sensitive to the risks of x rays, and the risk versus benefits should be discussed with the treating physician.

Normal results

The x ray will show normal structures for the age of the patient. The gallbladder should visualize, and be free of any solid structures, such as stones, polyps, etc.

Abnormal results

Abnormal results may show gallstones, tumors, or cholesterol polyps (a tumor growing from the lining that is usually noncancerous). Typically stones will "float" or move around as the patient changes position, whereas tumors will stay in the same place.

Resources

OTHER

"Gall Bladder Exam." Harvard Medical School. < http://www.bih.harvard.edu/radiology/Modalities/Xray/xraysSubdivsf/gallbl.html >.

"Gallstones." National Institutes of Health. < http://www.niddk.nih.gov/health/digest/pubs/gallstns/gallstns.htm >.

"Oral cholecystogram." Healthanswers.com. < http://www.healthanswers.com/database/ami/converted/003821.html >.

Rosalyn Carson-DeWitt, MD

Gallium scan of the body

Definition

A gallium scan of the body is a nuclear medicine test that is conducted using a camera that detects gallium, a form of radionuclide, or radioactive chemical substance.

Purpose

Most gallium scans are ordered to detect cancerous tumors, infections, or areas of inflammation in the body. Gallium is known to accumulate in inflamed, infected, or cancerous tissues. The scans are used to determine whether a patient with an unexplained **fever** has an infection and the site of the infection, if present. Gallium scans also may be used to evaluate **cancer** following **chemotherapy** or **radiation therapy**.

Precautions

Children and women who are pregnant or breastfeeding are only given gallium scans if the potential diagnostic benefits will outweigh the risks.

Description

The patient will usually be asked to come to the testing facility 24–48 hours before the procedure to receive the injection of gallium. Sometimes, the injection will be given only four to six hours before the study or as long as 72 hours before the procedure. The timeframe is based on the area or organs of the body being studied.

For the study itself the patient lies very still for approximately 30–60 minutes. A camera is moved across the patient's body to detect and capture images of concentrations of the gallium. The camera picks up signals from any accumulated areas of the radionuclide. In most cases, the patient is lying down throughout the procedure. Back (posterior) and front (anterior) views will usually be taken, and sometimes a side (lateral) view is used. The camera may occasionally touch the patient's skin, but will not cause any discomfort. A clicking noise may be heard throughout the procedure; this is only the sound of the scanner registering radiation.

Preparation

The intravenous injection of gallium is done in a separate appointment prior to the procedure. Generally, no special dietary requirements are necessary. Sometimes the physician will ask that the patient have light or clear meals within a day or less of the procedure. Many patients will be given **laxatives** or an enema prior to the scan to eliminate any residual gallium from the bowels.

Aftercare

There is generally no aftercare required following a gallium scan. However, women who are breastfeeding who have a scan will be cautioned against breastfeeding for four weeks following the exam.

Risks

There is a minimal risk of exposure to radiation from the gallium injection, but the exposure from one gallium scan is generally less than exposure from x rays.

Normal results

A radiologist trained in nuclear medicine or a nuclear medicine specialist will interpret the exam results and compare them to other diagnostic tests. It is normal for gallium to accumulate in the liver, spleen, bones, breast tissue, and large bowel.

Abnormal results

An abnormal concentration of gallium in areas other than those where it normally concentrates may indicate the presence of disease. Concentrations may be due to inflammation, infection, or the presence of tumor tissue. Often, additional tests are required to determine if the tumors are malignant (cancerous) or benign.

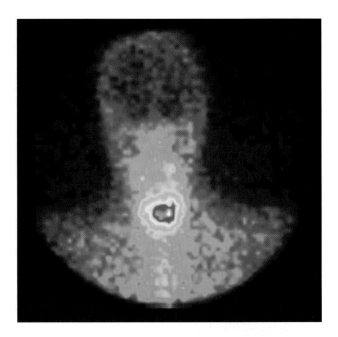

Gallium scan highlighting the thyroid gland. *(Photo Researchers. Reproduced by permission.)*

KEY TERMS

Benign—Not cancerous. Benign tumors are not considered immediate threats, but may still require some form of treatment.

Gallium—A form of radionuclide that is used to help locate tumors and inflammation (specifically referred to as GA67 citrate).

Malignant—This term, usually used to describe a tumor, means cancerous, becoming worse and possibly growing.

Nuclear medicine—A subspecialty of radiology used to show the function and anatomy of body organs. Very small amounts of radioactive substances, or tracers, are detected with a special camera as they accumulate in certain organs and tissues.

Radionuclide—A chemical substance, called an isotope, that exhibits radioactivity. A gamma camera, used in nuclear medicine procedures, will pick up the radioactive signals as the substance gathers in an organ or tissue. They are sometimes referred to as tracers.

Even though gallium normally concentrates in organs such as the liver or spleen, abnormally high concentrations will suggest certain diseases and conditions. For example, Hodgkin's or non-Hodgkin's lymphoma may be diagnosed or staged if there is abnormal gallium activity in the lymph nodes. After a patient receives cancer treatment, such as radiation therapy or chemotherapy, a gallium scan may help to find new or recurring tumors or to record regression of a treated tumor. Physicians can narrow causes of liver problems by noting abnormal gallium activity in the liver. Gallium scans also may be used to diagnose lung diseases or a disease called **sarcoidosis**, in the chest.

Resources

ORGANIZATIONS

American Cancer Society. 1599 Clifton Road NE, Atlanta, GA 30329. (404) 320-3333. < http://www.cancer.org > .

American College of Nuclear Medicine. PO Box 175, Landisville, PA 31906. (717) 898-6006.

American Liver Foundation. 1425 Pompton Avenue, Cedar Grove NJ 07009. (800) GO LIVER (465-4837). < http://www.liverfoundation.org > .

Society of Nuclear Medicine. 1850 Samuel Morse Drive, Reston, VA 10016. (703) 708-9000. < http:// www.snm.org > .

OTHER

"A Patient's Guide to Nuclear Medicine." *University of Iowa Virtual Hospital.* July 2, 2001. < http://www.vh.org/ Patients/IHB/Rad/NucMed/PatGuideNucMed/ PatGuideNucMed.html > .

Teresa Odle

Gallstone removal

Definition

Also known as cholelithotomy, gallstone removal is the medical procedure that rids the gallbladder of calculus buildup.

Purpose

The gallbladder is not a vital organ. Its function is to store bile, concentrate it, and release it during digestion. Bile is supposed to retain all of its chemicals in solution, but commonly one of them crystallizes and forms sand, gravel, and finally stones.

The chemistry of **gallstones** is complex and interesting. Like too much sugar in solution, chemicals in bile will form crystals as the gallbladder draws water out of the bile. The solubility of these chemicals is based on the concentration of three chemicals, not just one–bile acids, phospholipids, and cholesterol. If the chemicals are out of balance, one or the other will not remain in solution. Certain people, in particular the Pima tribe of Native Americans in Arizona, have a genetic predisposition to forming gallstones. Scandinavians also have a higher than average incidence of this disease. Dietary fat and cholesterol are also implicated in their formation. Overweight women in their middle years constitute the vast majority of patients with gallstones in every group.

As the bile crystals aggregate to form stones, they move about, eventually occluding the outlet and preventing the gallbladder from emptying. This creates symptoms. It also results in irritation, inflammation, and sometimes infection of the gallbladder. The pattern is usually one of intermittent obstruction due to stones moving in and out of the way. All the while the gallbladder is becoming more scarred. Sometimes infection fills it with pus–a serious complication.

On occasion a stone will travel down the cystic duct into the common bile duct and get stuck there. This will back bile up into the liver as well as the gallbladder. If the stone sticks at the Ampulla of Vater, the pancreas will also be plugged and will develop **pancreatitis**. These stones can cause a lot of trouble.

Bile is composed of several waste products of metabolism, all of which are supposed to remain in liquid form. The complex chemistry of the liver depends on many chemical processes, which depend in turn upon the chemicals in the diet and the genes that direct those processes. There are greater variations in the output of chemical waste products than there is allowance for their cohabitation in the bile. Incompatible mixes result in the formation of solids.

Gallstones will cause the sudden onset of **pain** in the upper abdomen. Pain will last for 30 minutes to several hours. Pain may move to the right shoulder blade. **Nausea** with or without **vomiting** may accompany the pain.

Precautions

Individuals suffering from sickle cell anemia, children, and patients with large stones may seek other treatments.

Description

Laparoscopic cholecystectomy

Surgery to remove the entire gallbladder with all its stones is usually the best treatment, provided the

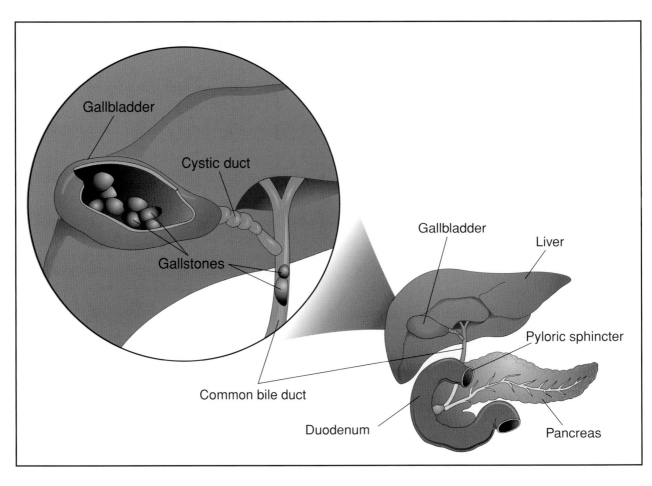

Gallblader

Cystic duct

Gallstones

Common bile duct

Duodenum

Gallbladder

Liver

Pyloric sphincter

Pancreas

Gallstone removal, also known as cholelithotomy, usually involves the surgical removal of the entire gallbladder, but in recent years the procedure done by laparoscopy has resulted in smaller surgical incisions and faster recovery time. *(Illustration by Electronic Illustrators Group.)*

patient is able to tolerate the procedure. Over the past decade, a new technique of removing the gallbladder using a laparoscope has resulted in quicker recovery and much smaller surgical incisions than the six-inch gash under the right ribs that used to be standard. Not everyone is a candidate for this approach.

If a stone is lodged in the bile ducts, additional surgery must be done to remove it. After surgery, the surgeon will ordinarily leave in a drain to collect bile until the system is healed. The drain can also be used to inject contrast material and take x rays during or after surgery.

Endoscopic retrograde cholangiopancreatoscopy (ERCP)

A procedure called endoscopic retrograde cholangiopancreatoscopy (ERCP) allows the removal of some bile duct stones through the mouth, throat, esophagus, stomach, duodenum, and biliary system

without the need for surgical incisions. ERCP can also be used to inject contrast agents into the biliary system, providing superbly detailed pictures.

Cholelithotomy

Rare circumstances require different techniques. Patients too ill for a complete **cholecystectomy** (removal of the gallbladder), sometimes only the stones are removed, a procedure called cholelithotomy. But that does not cure the problem. The liver will go on making faulty bile, and stones will reform, unless the composition of the bile is altered.

Ursodeoxycholic acid

For patients who cannot receive the laparoscopic procedure, there is also a nonsurgical treatment in which ursodeoxycholic acid is used to dissolve the gallstones. Extracorporeal shock-wave **lithotripsy** has also been successfully used to break up gallstones.

KEY TERMS

Cholecystectomy—Surgical removal of the gallbladder.

Cholelithotomy—Surgical incision into the gallbladder to remove stones.

Contrast agent—A substance that causes shadows on x rays (or other images of the body).

Endoscope—One of several instruments designed to enter body cavities. They combine viewing and operating capabilities.

Jaundice—A yellow color of the skin and eyes due to excess bile that is not removed by the liver.

Laparoscopy—Surgery through pencil-sized viewing instruments and tools so that incisions need be less than half an inch long.

During the procedure, high-amplitude sound waves target the stones, slowly breaking them up.

Preparation

There are a number of imaging studies that identify gallbladder disease, but most gallstones will not show up on conventional x rays. That requires contrast agents given by mouth that are excreted into the bile. Ultrasound is very useful and can be enhanced by doing it through an endoscope in the stomach. CT (**computed tomography scans**) and MRI (**magnetic resonance imaging**) scanning are not used routinely but are helpful in detecting common duct stones and complications.

Aftercare

Without a gallbladder, stones rarely reform. Patients who have continued symptoms after their gallbladder is removed may need an ERCP to detect residual stones or damage to the bile ducts caused by the stones before they were removed. Once in a while the Ampulla of Vater is too tight for bile to flow through and causes symptoms until it is opened up.

Resources

BOOKS

Bilhartz, Lyman E., and Jay D. Horton. "Gallstone Disease and Its Complications." In *Sleisenger & Fordtran's Gastrointestinal and Liver Disease*, edited by Mark Feldman, et al. Philadelphia: W. B. Saunders Co., 1998.

J. Ricker Polsdorfer, MD

Gallstones

Definition

A gallstone is a solid crystal deposit that forms in the gallbladder, which is a pear-shaped organ that stores bile salts until they are needed to help digest fatty foods. Gallstones can migrate to other parts of the digestive tract and cause severe **pain** with life-threatening complications.

Description

Gallstones vary in size and chemical structure. A gallstone may be as tiny as a grain of sand or as large as a golf ball. Eighty percent of gallstones are composed of cholesterol. They are formed when the liver produces more cholesterol than digestive juices can liquefy. The remaining 20% of gallstones are composed of calcium and an orange-yellow waste product called bilirubin. Bilirubin gives urine its characteristic color and sometimes causes **jaundice**.

Gallstones are the most common of all gallbladder problems. They are responsible for 90% of gallbladder and bile duct disease, and are the fifth most common reason for hospitalization of adults in the United States. Gallstones usually develop in adults between the ages of 20 and 50; about 20% of patients with gallstones are over 40. The risk of developing gallstones increases with age–at least 20% of people over 60 have a single large stone or as many as several thousand smaller ones. The gender ratio of gallstone patients changes with age. Young women are between two and six times more likely to develop gallstones than men in the same age group. In patients over 50, the condition affects men and women with equal frequency. Native Americans develop gallstones more often than any other segment of the population; Mexican-Americans have the second-highest incidence of this disease.

Definitions

Gallstones can cause several different disorders. Cholelithiasis is defined as the presence of gallstones within the gallbladder itself. Choledocholithiasis is the presence of gallstones within the common bile duct that leads into the first portion of the small intestine (the duodenum). The stones in the duct may have been formed inside it or carried there from the gallbladder. These gallstones prevent bile from flowing into the duodenum. Ten percent of patients with gallstones have choledocholithiasis, which is sometimes called common-duct stones. Patients who don't develop infection usually recover completely from this disorder.

Cholecystitis is a disorder marked by inflammation of the gallbladder. It is usually caused by the passage of a stone from the gallbladder into the cystic duct, which is a tube that connects the gallbladder to the common bile duct. In 5–10% of cases, however, cholecystitis develops in the absence of gallstones. This form of the disorder is called acalculous cholecystitis. Cholecystitis causes painful enlargement of the gallbladder and is responsible for 10–25% of all gallbladder surgery. Chronic cholecystitis is most common in the elderly. The acute form is most likely to occur in middle-aged adults.

Cholesterolosis or cholesterol polyps is characterized by deposits of cholesterol crystals in the lining of the gallbladder. This condition may be caused by high levels of cholesterol or inadequate quantities of bile salts, and is usually treated by surgery.

Gallstone **ileus**, which results from a gallstone's blocking the entrance to the large intestine, is most common in elderly people. Surgery usually cures this condition.

Narrowing (stricture) of the common bile duct develops in as many as 5% of patients whose gallbladders have been surgically removed. This condition is characterized by inability to digest fatty foods and by abdominal pain, which sometimes occurs in spasms. Patients with stricture of the common bile duct are likely to recover after appropriate surgical treatment.

Causes and symptoms

Gallstones are caused by an alteration in the chemical composition of bile. Bile is a digestive fluid that helps the body absorb fat. Gallstones tend to run in families. In addition, high levels of estrogen, insulin, or cholesterol can increase a person's risk of developing them.

Pregnancy or the use of birth control pills can slow down gallbladder activity and increase the risk of gallstones. So can diabetes, **pancreatitis**, and **celiac disease**. Other factors influencing gallstone formation are:

- infection
- obesity
- intestinal disorders

- coronary artery disease or other recent illness
- multiple pregnancies
- a high-fat, low-fiber diet
- smoking
- heavy drinking
- rapid weight loss

Gallbladder attacks usually follow a meal of rich, high-fat foods. The attacks often occur in the middle of the night, sometimes waking the patient with intense pain that ends in a visit to the emergency room. The pain of a gallbladder attack begins in the abdomen and may radiate to the chest, back, or the area between the shoulders. Other symptoms of gallstones include:

- inability to digest fatty foods
- low-grade **fever**
- chills and sweating
- nausea and **vomiting**
- indigestion
- gas
- belching.
- clay-colored bowel movements

Diagnosis

Gallstones may be diagnosed by a family doctor, a specialist in digestive problems (a gastroenterologist), or a specialist in internal medicine. The doctor will first examine the patient's skin for signs of jaundice and feel (palpate) the abdomen for soreness or swelling. After the basic **physical examination**, the doctor will order blood counts or blood chemistry tests to detect evidence of bile duct obstruction and to rule out other illnesses that cause fever and pain, including stomach ulcers, **appendicitis**, and heart attacks.

More sophisticated procedures used to diagnose gallstones include:

- Ultrasound imaging. Ultrasound has an accuracy rate of 96%.
- Cholecystography (cholecystogram, gallbladder series, gallbladder x ray). This type of study shows how the gallbladder contracts after the patient has eaten a high-fat meal.
- Fluoroscopy. This imaging technique allows the doctor to distinguish between jaundice caused by pancreatic **cancer** and jaundice caused by gallbladder or bile duct disorders.

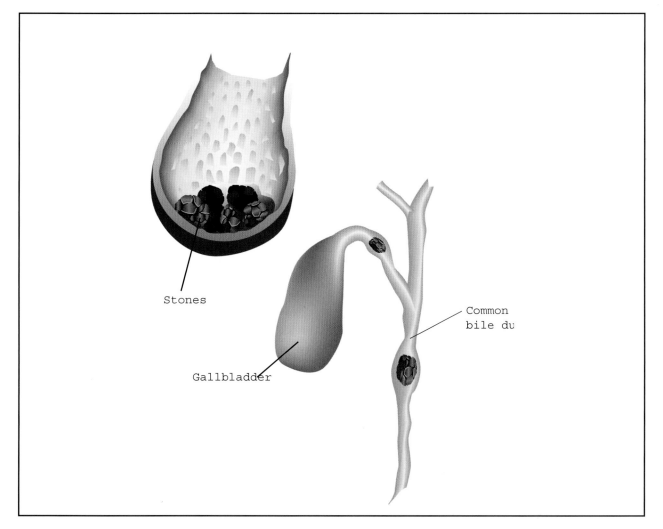

Stones

Common
bile du

Gallbladder

Gallstones form in the gallbladder but can migrate to other parts of the body via the bile duct. *(Illustration by Argosy Inc.)*

- Endoscopy (ERCP). ERCP uses a special dye to outline the pancreatic and common bile ducts and locate the position of the gallstones.

- Radioisotopic scan. This technique reveals blockage of the cystic duct.

Treatment

Watchful waiting

One-third of all patients with gallstones never experience a second attack. For this reason many doctors advise watchful waiting after the first episode. Reducing the amount of fat in the diet or following a sensible plan of gradual weight loss may be the only treatments required for occasional mild attacks. A patient diagnosed with gallstones may be able to manage more troublesome episodes by:

- applying heat to the affected area

- resting and taking occasional sips of water

- using non-prescription forms of **acetaminophen** (Tylenol or Anacin-3)

A doctor should be notified if pain intensifies or lasts for more than three hours; if the patient's fever rises above 101 °F (38.3 °C); or if the skin or whites of the eyes turn yellow.

Surgery

Surgical removal of the gallbladder (**cholecystectomy**) is the most common conventional treatment for recurrent attacks. Laparoscopic surgery, the technique most widely used, is a safe, effective procedure that involves less pain and a shorter recovery period than traditional open surgery. In this technique, the doctor makes a small cut (incision) in the patient's abdomen and removes the gallbladder through a long tube called a laparoscope.

Nonsurgical approaches

LITHOTRIPSY. Shock wave therapy (**lithotripsy**) uses high-frequency sound waves to break up the gallstones. The patient can then take bile salts to dissolve the fragments. Bile salt tablets are sometimes prescribed without lithotripsy to dissolve stones composed of cholesterol by raising the level of bile acids in the gallbladder. This approach requires long-term treatment, since it may take months or years for this method to dissolve a sizeable stone.

CONTACT DISSOLUTION. Contact dissolution can destroy gallstones in a matter of hours. This minimally invasive procedure involves using a tube (catheter) inserted into the abdomen to inject medication directly into the gallbladder.

Alternative treatment

Alternative therapies, like non-surgical treatments, may provide temporary relief of gallstone symptoms. Alternative approaches to the symptoms of gallbladder disorders include homeopathy, Chinese traditional herbal medicine, and **acupuncture**. Dietary changes may also help relieve the symptoms of gallstones. Since gallstones seem to develop more often in people who are obese, eating a balanced diet, exercising, and losing weight may help keep gallstones from forming.

Prognosis

Forty percent of all patients with gallstones have "silent gallstones" that produce no symptoms. Silent stones, discovered only when their presence is indicated by tests performed to diagnose other symptoms, do not require treatment.

Gallstone problems that require treatment can be surgically corrected. Although most patients recover, some develop infections that must be treated with **antibiotics**.

In rare instances, severe inflammation can cause the gallbladder to burst. The resulting infection can be fatal.

Prevention

The best way to prevent gallstones is to minimize risk factors. In addition, a 1998 study suggests that vigorous **exercise** may lower a man's risk of developing gallstones by as much as 28%. The researchers

---

KEY TERMS

Acalculous cholecystitis—Inflammation of the gallbladder that occurs without the presence of gallstones.

Bilirubin—A reddish-yellow waste product produced by the liver that colors urine and is involved in the formation of some gallstones.

Celiac disease—Inability to digest wheat protein (gluten), which causes weight loss, lack of energy, and pale, foul-smelling stools.

Cholecystectomy—Surgical removal of the gallbladder.

Cholecystitis—Inflammation of the gallbladder.

Choledocholithiasis—The presence of gallstones within the common bile duct.

Cholelithiasis—The presence of gallstones within the gallbladder.

Cholesterolosis—Cholesterol crystals or deposits in the lining of the gallbladder.

Common bile duct—The passage through which bile travels from the cystic duct to the small intestine.

Gallstone ileus—Obstruction of the large intestine caused by a gallstone that has blocked the intestinal opening.

Lithotripsy—A nonsurgical technique for removing gallstones by breaking them apart with high-frequency sound waves.

---

have not yet determined whether physical activity benefits women to the same extent.

Resources

ORGANIZATIONS

National Digestive Diseases Clearinghouse (NDDIC). 2 Information Way.

National Institute of Diabetes and Digestive and Kidney Diseases (NIDDK). Building 31, Room 9A04, 31 Center Drive, MSC 2560, Bethesda, MD 208792-2560. (301) 496-3583. < http://www.niddk.nih.gov > .

Maureen Haggerty

Gamete intrafallopian transfer *see* **Infertility therapies**

Gamma-glutamyl transferase test *see* **Liver function tests**

Gammaglobulin

Definition

Gammaglobulin is a type of protein found in the blood. When gammaglobulins are extracted from the blood of many people and combined, they can be used to prevent or treat infections.

Purpose

This medicine is used to treat or prevent diseases that occur when the body's own immune system is not effective against the disease. When disease-causing agents enter the body, they normally trigger the production of antibodies, proteins that circulate in the blood and help fight the disease. Gammaglobulin contains some of these antibodies. When gammaglobulins are taken from the blood of people who have recovered from diseases such as **chickenpox** or hepatitis, they can be given to other people to make them temporarily immune to those diseases. With hepatitis, for example, this is done when someone who has not been vaccinated against hepatitis is exposed to the disease.

Description

Gammaglobulin, also known as immunoglobulin, immune serum globulin or serum therapy, is injected either into a vein or into a muscle. When injected into a vein, it produces results more quickly than when injected into a muscle.

Recommended dosage

Doses are different for different people and depend on the person's body weight and the condition for which he or she is being treated.

Precautions

Anyone who has had unusual reactions to gammaglobulin in the past should let his or her physician know before taking the drugs again. The physician should also be told about any **allergies** to foods, dyes, preservatives, or other substances.

People who have certain medical conditions may have problems if they take gammaglobulins. For example:

- Gammaglobulins may worsen heart problems or deficiencies of immunoglobin A (IgA, a type of antibody)

- Certain patients with low levels of gammaglobulins in the blood (conditions called agammaglobulinemia and hypogammaglobulinemia) may be more likely to have side effects when they take gammaglobulin.

Side effects

Minor side effects such as **headache**, backache, joint or muscle **pain**, and a general feeling of illness usually go away as the body adjusts to this medicine. These problems do not need medical attention unless they continue.

Other side effects, such as breathing problems or a fast or pounding heartbeat, should be brought to a physician's attention as soon as possible.

Anyone who shows the following signs of overdose should check with a physician immediately:

- unusual tiredness or weakness
- dizziness
- nausea
- vomiting
- fever
- chills
- tightness in the chest
- red face
- sweating

Interactions

Anyone who takes gammaglobulin should let the physician know all other medicines he or she is taking and should ask whether interactions with gammaglobulin could interfere with treatment.

Nancy Ross-Flanigan

Ganglion

Definition

A ganglion is a small, usually hard bump above a tendon or in the capsule that encloses a joint. A ganglion is also called a synovial **hernia** or synovial cyst.

Description

A ganglion is a non-cancerous cyst filled with a thick, jelly-like fluid. Ganglions can develop on or beneath the surface of the skin and usually occur between the ages of 20 and 40.

Most ganglions develop on the hand or wrist. This condition is common in people who bowl or who play handball, raquetball, squash, or tennis. Runners and athletes who jump, ski, or play contact sports often develop foot ganglions.

Causes and symptoms

Mild **sprains** or other repeated injuries can irritate and tear the thin membrane covering a tendon, causing fluid to leak into a sac that swells and forms a ganglion.

Ganglions are usually painless, but range of motion may be impaired. Flexing or bending the affected area can cause discomfort, as can continuing to perform the activity that caused the condition.

Cysts on the surface of the skin usually develop slowly but may result from injury or severe strain. An internal ganglion can cause soreness or a dull, aching sensation, but the mass cannot always be felt. Symptoms sometimes become evident only when the cyst causes pressure on a nerve or outgrows the membrane surrounding it.

Diagnosis

Diagnosis is usually made through **physical examination** as well as such imaging studies as x ray, ultrasound, and **magnetic resonance imaging** (MRI). Fluid may be withdrawn from the cyst and evaluated.

Treatment

Some ganglions disappear without treatment, and some reappear despite treatment.

Acetaminophen (Tylenol) or other over-the-counter **analgesics** can be used to control mild **pain**. Steroids or local anesthetics may be injected into cysts that cause severe pain or other troublesome

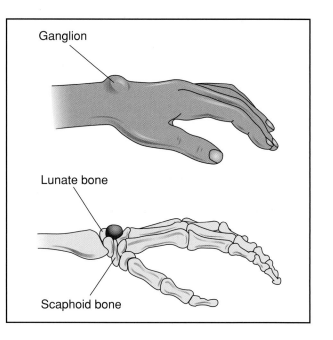

A ganglion is a non-cancerous cyst filled with a thick, jelly-like fluid. Ganglions can develop on or beneath the surface of the skin, most likely on the hand or wrist, although runners and skiers often develop them on the foot. *(Illustration by Electronic Illustrators Group.)*

symptoms. Surgery performed in a hospital operating room or an outpatient facility, is the only treatment guaranteed to remove a ganglion. The condition can recur if the entire cyst is not removed.

A doctor should be notified if the surgical site drains, bleeds, or becomes

- inflamed
- painful
- swollen or if the patient feels ill or develops:
- head or muscle aches
- dizziness
- fever following surgery

The patient may bathe or shower as usual, but should keep the surgical site dry and covered with a bandage for two or three days after the operation. Patients may resume normal activities as soon as they feel comfortable doing so.

Prognosis

Possible complications include excessive postoperative bleeding and infection of the surgical site. Calcification, or hardening, of the ganglion is rare.

Prevention

Exercises that increase muscle strength and flexibility can prevent ganglions. Warming and cooling down before and after workouts may also decrease the rate of developing ganglions.

Resources

OTHER

"Foot Ganglion." ThriveOnline. May 25, 1998. <http://thriveonline.oxygen.com>.

"Hand or Wrist Ganglion." ThriveOnline. May 25, 1998. <http://thriveonline.oxygen.com>.

Maureen Haggerty

Gangrene

Definition

Gangrene is the term used to describe the decay or death of an organ or tissue caused by a lack of blood supply. It is a complication resulting from infectious or inflammatory processes, injury, or degenerative changes associated with chronic diseases, such as **diabetes mellitus**.

Description

Gangrene may be caused by a variety of chronic diseases and post-traumatic, post-surgical, and spontaneous causes. There are three major types of gangrene: dry, moist, and gas (a type of moist gangrene).

Dry gangrene is a condition that results when one or more arteries become obstructed. In this type of gangrene, the tissue slowly dies, due to receiving little or no blood supply, but does not become infected. The affected area becomes cold and black, begins to dry out and wither, and eventually drops off over a period of weeks or months. Dry gangrene is most common in persons with advanced blockages of the arteries (arteriosclerosis) resulting from diabetes.

Moist gangrene may occur in the toes, feet, or legs after a crushing injury or as a result of some other factor that causes blood flow to the area to suddenly stop. When blood flow ceases, bacteria begin to invade the muscle and thrive, multiplying quickly without interference from the body's immune system.

Gas gangrene, also called myonecrosis, is a type of moist gangrene that is commonly caused by bacterial infection with *Clostridium welchii, Cl. perfringes, Cl. septicum, Cl. novyi, Cl. histolyticum, Cl. sporogenes*, or other species that are capable of thriving under conditions where there is little oxygen (anaerobic). Once present in tissue, these bacteria produce gasses and poisonous toxins as they grow. Normally inhabiting the gastrointestinal, respiratory, and female genital tract, they often infect thigh **amputation wounds**, especially in those individuals who have lost control of their bowel functions (incontinence). Gangrene, incontinence, and debility often are combined in patients with diabetes, and it is in the amputation stump of diabetic patients that gas gangrene is often found to occur.

Other causative organisms for moist gangrene include various bacterial strains, including *Streptococcus* and *Staphylococcus*. A serious, but rare form of infection with Group A *Streptococcus* can impede blood flow and, if untreated, can progress to synergistic gangrene, more commonly called necrotizing fasciitis, or infection of the skin and tissues directly beneath the skin.

Chronic diseases, such as diabetes mellitus, arteriosclerosis, or diseases affecting the blood vessels, such as **Buerger's disease** or **Raynaud's disease**, can cause gangrene. Post-traumatic causes of gangrene include compound **fractures**, **burns**, and injections given under the skin or in a muscle. Gangrene may occur following surgery, particularly in individuals with diabetes mellitus or other long-term (chronic) disease. In addition, gas gangrene can be also be a complication of dry gangrene or occur spontaneously in association with an underlying **cancer**.

In the United States, approximately 50% of moist gangrene cases are the result of a severe traumatic injury, and 40% occur following surgery. Car and industrial accidents, crush injuries, and gunshot wounds are the most common traumatic causes. Because of prompt surgical management of wounds with the removal of dead tissue, the incidence of gangrene from trauma has significantly diminished. Surgeries involving the bile ducts or intestine are the most frequent procedures causing gangrene. Approximately two-thirds of cases affect the extremities, and the remaining one-third involve the abdominal wall.

Symptoms

Areas of either dry or moist gangrene are initially characterized by a red line on the skin that marks the border of the affected tissues. As tissues begin to die, dry gangrene may cause some **pain** in the early stages or may go unnoticed, especially in the elderly or in those individuals with diminished sensation to the affected area. Initially, the area becomes cold, numb, and pale before later changing in color to brown, then black. This dead tissue will gradually separate from the healthy tissue and fall off.

Moist gangrene and gas gangrene are distinctly different. Gas gangrene does not involve the skin as much, but usually only the muscle. In moist or gas gangrene, there is a sensation of heaviness in the affected region that is followed by severe pain. The pain is caused by swelling resulting from fluid or gas accumulation in the tissues. This pain peaks, on average, between one to four days following the injury, with a range of eight hours to several weeks. The swollen skin may initially be blistered, red, and warm to the touch before progressing to a bronze, brown, or black color. In approximately 80% of cases, the affected and surrounding tissues may produce crackling sounds (crepitus), as a result of gas bubbles accumulating under the skin. The gas may be felt beneath the skin (palpable). In wet gangrene, the pus is foul-smelling, while in gas gangrene, there is no true pus, just an almost "sweet" smelling watery discharge.

Fever, rapid heart rate, rapid breathing, altered mental state, loss of appetite, **diarrhea**, **vomiting**, and vascular collapse may also occur if the bacterial toxins are allowed to spread in the bloodstream. Gas gangrene can be a life-threatening condition and should receive prompt medical attention

Diagnosis

A diagnosis of gangrene will be based on a combination of the patient history, a **physical examination**, and the results of blood and other laboratory tests. A physician will look for a history of recent trauma, surgery, cancer, or chronic disease. Blood tests will be used to determine whether infection is present and determine the extent to which an infection has spread.

A sample of drainage from a wound, or obtained through surgical exploration, may be cultured with oxygen (aerobic) and without oxygen (anaerobic) to identify the microorganism causing the infection and to aid in determining which antibiotic will be most effective. The sample obtained from a person with gangrene will contain few, if any, white blood cells and, when stained (with Gram stain) and examined under the microscope, will show the presence of purple (Gram positive), rod-shaped bacteria.

X-ray studies and more sophisticated imaging techniques, such as **computed tomography scans** (CT)

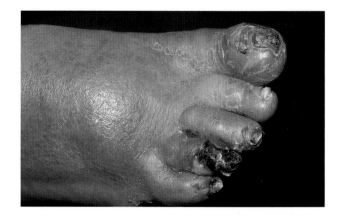

A close-up of gangrene in the toes of a diabetic patient. *(Photo Researchers, Inc. Reproduced by permission.)*

or **magnetic resonance imaging** (MRI), may be helpful in making a diagnosis since gas accumulation and muscle death (myonecrosis) may be visible. These techniques, however, are not sufficient alone to provide an accurate diagnosis of gangrene.

Precise diagnosis of gas gangrene often requires surgical exploration of the wound. During such a procedure, the exposed muscle may appear pale, beefy-red, or in the most advanced stages, black. If infected, the muscle will fail to contract with stimulation, and the cut surface will not bleed.

Treatment

Gas gangrene is a medical emergency because of the threat of the infection rapidly spreading via the bloodstream and infecting vital organs. It requires immediate surgery and administration of **antibiotics**.

Areas of dry gangrene that remain free from infection (aseptic) in the extremities are most often left to wither and fall off. Treatments applied to the wound externally (topically) are generally not effective without adequate blood supply to support wound healing. Assessment by a vascular surgeon, along with x rays to determine blood supply and circulation to the affected area, can help determine whether surgical intervention would be beneficial.

Once the causative organism has been identified, moist gangrene requires the prompt initiation of intravenous, intramuscular, and/or topical broad-spectrum antibiotic therapy. In addition, the infected tissue must be removed surgically (**debridement**), and amputation of the affected extremity may be necessary. Pain medications (**analgesics**) are prescribed to control discomfort. Intravenous fluids and, occasionally, blood transfusions are indicated to counteract

shock and replenish red blood cells and electrolytes. Adequate hydration and **nutrition** are vital to wound healing.

Although still controversial, some cases of gangrene are treated by administering oxygen under pressure greater than that of the atmosphere (hyperbaric) to the patient in a specially designed chamber. The theory behind using hyperbaric oxygen is that more oxygen will become dissolved in the patient's bloodstream, and therefore, more oxygen will be delivered to the gangrenous areas. By providing optimal oxygenation, the body's ability to fight off the bacterial infection are believed to be improved, and there is a direct toxic effect on the bacteria that thrive in an oxygen-free environment. Some studies have shown that the use of hyperbaric oxygen produces marked pain relief, reduces the number of amputations required, and reduces the extent of surgical debridement required. Patients receiving hyperbaric oxygen treatments must be monitored closely for evidence of oxygen toxicity. Symptoms of this toxicity include slow heart rate, profuse sweating, ringing in the ears, **shortness of breath**, **nausea and vomiting**, twitching of the lips/cheeks/eyelids/nose, and convulsions.

The emotional needs of the patient must also be met. The individual with gangrene should be offered moral support, along with an opportunity to share questions and concerns about changes in body image. In addition, particularly in cases where amputation was required, physical, vocational, and **rehabilitation** therapy will also be required.

Prognosis

Except in cases where the infection has been allowed to spread through the blood stream, prognosis is generally favorable. Anaerobic wound infection can progress quickly from initial injury to gas gangrene within one to two days, and the spread of the infection in the blood stream is associated with a 20–25% mortality rate. If recognized and treated early, however, approximately 80% of those with gas gangrene survive, and only 15–20% require any form of amputation. Unfortunately, the individual with dry gangrene most often has multiple other health problems that complicate recovery, and it is usually those other system failures that can prove fatal.

Prevention

Patients with diabetes or severe arteriosclerosis should take particular care of their hands and feet because of the risk of infection associated with even a

KEY TERMS

Aerobic—Organism that grows and thrives only in environments containing oxygen.

Anaerobic—Organism that grows and thrives in an oxygen-free environment.

Arteriosclerosis—Build-up of fatty plaques within the arteries that can lead to the obstruction of blood flow.

Aseptic—Without contamination with bacteria or other microorganisms.

Crepitus—A crackling sound.

Gram stain—A staining procedure used to visualize and classify bacteria. The Gram stain procedure allows the identification of purple (Gram positive) organisms and red (Gram negative) organisms.

Hyperbaric oxygen—Medical treatment in which oxygen is administered in specially designed chambers, under pressures greater than that of the atmosphere, in order to treat specific medical conditions.

Incontinence—A condition characterized by the inability to control urination or bowel functions.

Myonecrosis—The destruction or death of muscle tissue.

Sepsis—The spreading of an infection in the bloodstream.

Thrombosis—The formation of a blood clot in a vein or artery that may obstruct local blood flow or may dislodge, travel downstream, and obstruct blood flow at a remote location.

minor injury. Education about proper **foot care** is vital. Diminished blood flow as a result of narrowed vessels will not lessen the body's defenses against invading bacteria. Measures taken towards the reestablishment of circulation are recommended whenever possible. Any abrasion, break in the skin, or infection tissue should be cared for immediately. Any dying or infected skin must be removed promptly to prevent the spread of bacteria.

Penetrating abdominal wounds should be surgically explored and drained, any tears in the intestinal walls closed, and antibiotic treatment begun early. Patients undergoing elective intestinal surgery should receive preventive antibiotic therapy. Use of antibiotics prior to and directly following surgery has been shown to significantly reduce the rate of infection from 20–30% to 4–8%.

Resources

BOOKS

Berktow, Robert, editor. *The Merck Manual of Diagnosis and Therapy.* 17th ed. Rahway, NJ: Merck Research Laboratories, 1997.

PERIODICALS

Basoglu, M., et al. "Fournier's Gangrene: Review of Fifteen Cases." *American Surgeon* November 1997: 1019-1021.

Kathleen D. Wright, RN

Gas embolism

Definition

Gas **embolism**, also called air embolism, is the presence of gas bubbles in the bloodstream that obstruct circulation.

Description

Gas embolism may occur with decompression from increased pressure; it typically occurs in ascending divers who have been breathing compressed air. If a diver does not fully exhale upon ascent, the air in the lungs expands as the pressure decreases, overinflating the lungs and forcing bubbles of gas (emboli) into the bloodstream. When gas emboli reach the arteries to the brain, the blood blockage causes unconsciousness. Gas embolism is second only to drowning as a cause of **death** among divers.

Gas embolism may also result from trauma or medical procedures such as catheterization and open heart surgery that allow air into the circulatory system.

Causes and symptoms

Gas embolism occurs independent of diving depth; it may occur in as little as 6 ft of water. It is frequently caused by a diver holding his breath during ascent. It may also result from an airway obstruction or other condition that prevents a diver from fully exhaling.

The primary sign of gas embolism is immediate loss of consciousness; it may or may not be accompanied by convulsions.

Diagnosis

Any unconscious diver should be assumed to be the victim of gas embolism, regardless of whether

---

consciousness was lost during or promptly after ascent. A doctor may also find pockets of air in the chest around the lungs and sometimes a collapsed lung from overinflation and rupture. Coughing up blood or a bloody froth around the mouth are visible signs of lung injury.

Treatment

Prompt **recompression treatment** in a hyperbaric (high-pressure) chamber is necessary to deflate the gas bubbles in the bloodstream, dissolve the gases into the blood, and restore adequate oxygenated blood flow to the brain and other organs. Recompression by returning the diver to deeper water will not work, and should not be attempted. The patient should be kept lying down and given oxygen while being transported for recompression treatment.

Before the diver receives recompression treatment, other lifesaving efforts may be necessary. If the diver isn't breathing, artificial respiration (also called mouth-to-mouth resuscitation or rescue breathing) should be administered. In the absence of a pulse, **cardiopulmonary resuscitation (CPR)** must be performed.

Prognosis

The prognosis is dependent upon the promptness of recompression treatment and the extent of the damage caused by oxygen deprivation.

Prevention

All divers should receive adequate training in the use of compressed air and a complete evaluation of fitness for diving. People with a medical history of lung cysts or spontaneous collapsed lung (**pneumothorax**), and those with active **asthma** or other lung disease must not dive, for they would be at extreme risk for gas embolism. Patients with conditions such as **alcoholism** and drug **abuse** are also discouraged from diving. Individuals with certain other medical conditions such as diabetes may be able to dive safely with careful training and supervision.

Resources

ORGANIZATIONS

American College of Hyperbaric Medicine. PO Box 25914-130, Houston, Texas 77265. (713) 528-0657. < http:// www.hyperbaricmedicine.org > .

Divers Alert Network. The Peter B. Bennett Center, 6 West Colony Place, Durham, NC 27705. (800) 446-2671. < http://www.diversalertnetwork.org > .

Undersea and Hyperbaric Medical Society. 10531 Metropolitan Ave., Kensington, MD 20895. (301) 942-2980. < http://www.uhms.org > .

Bethany Thivierge

Gas gangrene *see* **Gangrene**

Gastrectomy

Definition

Gastrectomy is the surgical removal of all or part of the stomach.

Purpose

Gastrectomy is performed for several reasons, most commonly to remove a malignant tumor or to cure a perforated or bleeding stomach ulcer.

Description

Gastrectomy for cancer

Removal of the tumor, often with removal of surrounding lymph nodes, is the only curative treatment for various forms of gastric (stomach) **cancer**. For many patients, this entails removing not just the tumor but part of the stomach as well. The extent to which lymph nodes should also be removed is a subject of some debate, but some studies show additional survival benefit associated with removal of a greater number of lymph nodes.

Gastrectomy, either total or subtotal (also called partial), is the treatment of choice for gastric adenocarcinomas, primary gastric lymphomas (originating in the stomach), and the rare leiomyosarcomas (also called gastric **sarcomas**). Adenocarcinomas are by far the most common form of **stomach cancer** and are less curable than the relatively uncommon lymphomas, for which gastrectomy offers good odds for survival.

After gastrectomy, the surgeon may "reconstruct" the altered portions of the digestive tract so that it continues to function. Several different surgical techniques are used, but, generally speaking, the surgeon attaches any remaining portion of the stomach to the small intestine.

Gastrectomy for gastric cancer is almost always done by the traditional "open" surgery technique, which requires a wide incision to open the abdomen. However, some surgeons use a laparoscopic technique that requires only a small incision. The laparoscope is connected to a tiny video camera that projects a picture of the abdominal contents onto a monitor for the surgeon's viewing. The stomach is operated on through this incision.

The potential benefits of laparoscopic surgery include less postoperative **pain**, decreased hospitalization, and earlier return to normal activities. The use of laparoscopic gastrectomy is limited, however. Only patients with early stage gastric cancers or those whose surgery is only intended for palliation—pain and symptomatic relief rather than cure—should be considered for this minimally invasive technique. It can only be performed by surgeons experienced in this type of surgery.

Gastrectomy for ulcers

Gastrectomy is also occasionally used in the treatment of severe peptic ulcer disease or its complications. While the vast majority of peptic ulcers (gastric ulcers in the stomach or duodenal ulcers in the duodenum) are managed with medication, partial gastrectomy is

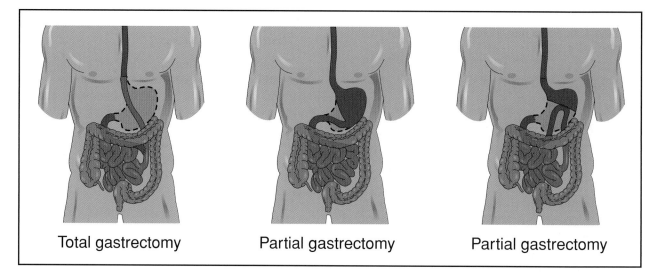

Total gastrectomy   Partial gastrectomy   Partial gastrectomy

Gastrectomy, the surgical removal of all or part of the stomach, is performed primarily to remove a malignant tumor or to cure a bleeding stomach ulcer. Following the gastrectomy, the surgeon may reconstruct the altered portions of the digestive tract so that it continues to function. *(Illustration by Electronic Illustrators Group.)*

sometimes required for peptic ulcer patients who have complications. These include patients who do not respond satisfactorily to medical therapy, those who develop a bleeding or perforated ulcer, and those who develop pyloric obstruction, a blockage to the exit from the stomach.

The surgical procedure for severe ulcer disease is also called an antrectomy, a limited form of gastrectomy in which the antrum, a portion of the stomach, is removed. For duodenal ulcers, antrectomy may be combined with other surgical procedures that are aimed at reducing the secretion of gastric acid, which is associated with ulcer formation. This additional surgery is commonly a **vagotomy**, surgery on the vagus nerve that disables the acid-producing portion of the stomach.

Preparation

Before undergoing gastrectomy, patients may need a variety of tests, such as x rays, **computed tomography scans** (CT scans), ultrasonography, or endoscopic biopsies (microscopic examination of tissue), to assure the diagnosis and localize the tumor or ulcer. **Laparoscopy** may be done to diagnose a malignancy or to determine the extent of a tumor that is already diagnosed. When a tumor is strongly suspected, laparoscopy is often performed immediately before the surgery to remove the tumor; this avoids the need to anesthetize the patient twice and sometimes avoids the need for surgery altogether if the tumor found on laparoscopy is deemed inoperable.

Aftercare

It is important to follow any instructions that have been given for postoperative care. Major surgery usually requires a recuperation time of several weeks.

Risks

Surgery for peptic ulcer is effective, but it may result in a variety of postoperative complications. After gastrectomy, as many as 30% of patients have significant symptoms. An operation called highly selective vagotomy is now preferred for ulcer management, and is safer than gastrectomy.

After a gastrectomy, several abnormalities may develop that produce symptoms related to food intake. This happens largely because the stomach, which serves as a food reservoir, has been reduced in its capacity by the surgery. Other surgical procedures that often accompany gastrectomy for ulcer disease can also contribute to later symptoms: vagotomy, which lessens acid production and slows stomach emptying, and **pyloroplasty**, which enlarges the opening between the stomach and small intestine to facilitate emptying of the stomach.

Some patients experience light-headedness, heart **palpitations** or racing heart, sweating, and **nausea and vomiting** after a meal. These may be symptoms of "dumping syndrome," as food is rapidly "dumped" into the small intestine from the stomach. This is treated by adjusting the diet and pattern of eating, for example, eating smaller, more frequent meals, and limiting liquids.

Patients who have abdominal bloating and pain after eating, frequently followed by **nausea** and **vomiting**, may have what is called the afferent loop syndrome. This is treated by surgical correction. Patients who have early satiety (feeling of fullness after eating), abdominal discomfort, and vomiting may have bile reflux **gastritis** (also called bilious vomiting), which is also surgically correctable. Many patients also experience weight loss.

Reactive **hypoglycemia** is a condition that results when blood sugar becomes too high after a meal, stimulating the release of insulin, about two hours after eating. A high-protein diet and smaller meals are advised.

Ulcers recur in a small percentage of patients after surgery for peptic ulcer, usually in the first few years. Further surgery is usually necessary.

Vitamin and mineral supplementation is necessary after gastrectomy to correct certain deficiencies, especially vitamin B_{12}, iron, and folate. Vitamin D and calcium are also needed to prevent and treat the bone problems that often occur. These include softening and bending of the bones, which can produce pain, and **osteoporosis**, a loss of bone mass. According to one study, the risk for spinal **fractures** may be as high as 50% after gastrectomy.

Depending on the extent of surgery, the risk for post-operative **death** after gastrectomy for gastric cancer has been reported as 1–3% and the risk of non-fatal complications as 9–18%.

Normal results

Overall survival after gastrectomy for gastric cancer varies greatly by the stage of disease at the time of surgery. For early gastric cancer, the five-year survival rate is up to 80–90%; for late-stage disease, the prognosis is bad. For gastric adenocarcinomas that are amenable to gastrectomy, the five-year survival rate is 10–30%, depending on the location of the tumor. The prognosis for patients with gastric lymphoma is better, with five-year survival rates reported at 40–60%.

Most studies have shown that patients can have an acceptable quality of life after gastrectomy for a potentially curable gastric cancer. Many patients will maintain a healthy appetite and eat a normal diet. Others may lose weight and not enjoy meals as much. Some studies show that patients who have total gastrectomies have more disease-related or treatment-related symptoms after surgery and poorer physical function than patients who have subtotal gastrectomies. There does not appear to be much difference, however, in emotional status or social activity level between patients who have undergone total versus subtotal gastrectomies.

Resources

BOOKS

Feldman, Mark., et al., editors. "Stomach and Duodenum: Complications of Surgery for Peptic Ulcer Disease." In *Steisenger & Fordtran's Gastrointestinal and Liver Disease*. Philadelphia: W. B. Saunders Co., 1998.

Caroline A. Helwick

Gastric acid determination

Definition

Gastric acid determination, also known as stomach acid determination, gastric analysis, or basal gastric secretion, is a procedure to evaluate gastric (stomach) function. The test specifically determines the presence of gastric acid, as well as the amount of gastric acid secreted. It is often done in conjunction with the gastric acid stimulation test, a procedure that measures gastric acid output after injection of a drug to stimulate gastric acid secretion.

Purpose

The purpose of the gastric acid determination is to evaluate gastric function by measuring the amount of acid as suctioned directly from the stomach. The complete gastric acid determination includes the basal gastric secretion test, which measures acid secretion while the patient is in a **fasting** state (nothing to eat or drink), followed by the gastric acid stimulation test, which measures the secretion of gastric acid for one hour after injection of pentagastrin or a similar drug that stimulates gastric acid output. The Gastric acid stimulation test is done when the basal secretion test suggests abnormalities in gastric secretion. It is normally performed immediately afterward.

The basal gastric secretion test is indicated for patients with obscure gastric **pain**, loss of appetite, and weight loss. It is also utilized for suspected peptic (related to the stomach) ulcer, severe stomach inflammation (**gastritis**), and Zollinger-Ellison (Z-E) syndrome (a condition in which a pancreatic tumor, called a **gastrinoma**, stimulates the stomach to secrete excessive amounts of acid, resulting in peptic ulcers). Because external factors like the sight or odor of food, as well as psychological **stress**, can stimulate gastric secretion, accurate testing requires that the patient be relaxed and isolated from all sources of sensory stimulation. Abnormal basal secretion can suggest various gastric and duodenal disorders, so further evaluation requires the gastric acid stimulation test.

The gastric acid stimulation test is indicated when abnormalities are found during the basal secretion test. These abnormalities can be caused by a number of disorders, including duodenal ulcer, **pernicious anemia**, and gastric **cancer**. The test will detect abnormalities, but x rays and other studies are necessary for a definitive diagnosis.

Precautions

Because both the basal gastric secretion test and the gastric acid stimulation test require insertion of a gastric tube (intubation) through the mouth or nasal passage, neither test is recommended for patients with esophageal problems, **aortic aneurysm**, severe gastric hemorrhage, or congestive **heart failure**. The gastric acid stimulation test is also not recommended in patients who are sensitive to pentagastrin (the drug used to stimulate gastric acid output).

Description

This test, whether performed for basal gastric acid secretion, gastric acid stimulation, or both, requires the passage of a lubricated rubber tube, either by mouth or through the nasal passage, while the patient is in a sitting or reclining position on the left side. The tube is situated in the stomach, with proper positioning confirmed by fluoroscopy or x ray.

Basal gastric acid secretion

After a wait of approximately 10–15 minutes for the patient to adjust to the presence of the tube, and with the patient in a sitting position, specimens are obtained every 15 minutes for a period of 90 minutes. The first two specimens are discarded to eliminate gastric contents that might be affected by the stress of the intubation process. The patient is allowed no liquids during the test, and saliva must be ejected to avoid diluting the stomach contents.

The four specimens collected during the test constitute the *basal acid output*. If analysis suggests abnormally low gastric secretion, the gastric acid stimulation test is performed immediately afterward.

Gastric acid stimulation test

After the basal samples have been collected, the tube remains in place for the gastric acid stimulation test. Pentagastrin, or a similar drug that stimulates gastric acid output, is injected under the skin (subcutaneously). After 15 minutes, a specimen is collected every 15 minutes for one hour. These specimens are called the *poststimulation specimens*. As is the case with the basal gastric secretion test, the patient can have no liquids during this test, and must eject saliva to avoid diluting the stomach contents.

Preparation

The patient should be fasting (nothing to eat or drink after the evening meal) on the day prior to the test, but may have water up to one hour before the test. **Antacids**, anticholinergics, cholinergics, alcohol, H_2-receptor antagonists (Tagamet, Pepcid, Axid, Zantac), reserpine, adrenergic blockers, and adrenocorticosteroids should be withheld for one to three days before the test, as the physician requests. If pentagastrin is to be administered for the gastric acid secretion test, medical supervision should be maintained, as possible side effects may occur.

Aftercare

Complications such as **nausea**, **vomiting**, and abdominal distention or pain are possible following removal of the gastric tube. If the patient has a **sore throat**, soothing lozenges may be given. The patient may also resume the usual diet and any medications that were withheld for the test(s).

Risks

There is a slight risk that the gastric tube may be inserted improperly, entering the windpipe (trachea) and not the esophagus. If this happens, the patient may have a difficult time breathing or may experience a coughing spell until the tube is removed and reinserted properly. Also, because the tube can be difficult to swallow, if a patient has an overactive gag reflex, there may be a transient rise in blood pressure due to **anxiety**.

KEY TERMS

Achlorhydria—An abnormal condition in which hydrochloric acid is absent from the secretions of the gastric glands in the stomach.

Pernicious anemia—One of the main types of anemia, caused by inadequate absorption of vitamin B_{12}. Symptoms include tingling in the hands, legs, and feet, spastic movements, weight loss, confusion, depression, and decreased intellectual function.

Zollinger-Ellison syndrome—A rare condition characterized by severe and recurrent peptic ulcers in the stomach, duodenum, and upper small intestine, caused by a tumor, or tumors, usually found in the pancreas. The tumor secretes the hormone gastrin, which stimulates the stomach and duodenum to produce large quantities of acid, leading to ulceration. Most often cancerous, the tumor must be removed surgically; otherwise total surgical removal of the stomach is necessary.

Normal results

Reference values for the *basal gastric secretion test* vary by laboratory, but are usually within the following ranges:

- men: 1–5 mEq/h
- women: 0.2–3.8 mEq/h

Reference values for the *gastric acid stimulation test* vary by laboratory, but are usually within the following ranges:

- men: 18–28 mEq/h
- women: 11–21 mEq/h

Abnormal results

Abnormal findings in the *basal gastric secretion test* are considered nonspecific and must be evaluated in conjunction with the results of a gastric acid stimulation test. Elevated secretion may suggest different types of ulcers; when markedly elevated, Zollinger-Ellison syndrome is suspected. Depressed secretion can indicate gastric cancer, while complete absence of secretion (achlorhydria) may suggest pernicious anemia.

Elevated gastric secretion levels in the *gastric acid stimulation test* may be indicative of duodenal ulcer; high levels of secretion again suggest Zollinger-Ellison syndrome.

Resources

BOOKS

Pagana, Kathleen Deska. *Mosby's Manual of Diagnostic and Laboratory Tests*. St. Louis: Mosby, Inc., 1998.

Janis O. Flores

Gastric carcinoma *see* **Stomach cancer**

Gastric emptying scan

Definition

A gastric emptying scan (GES) is an x-ray exam using special radioactive material that allows physicians to identify abnormalities related to emptying of the stomach. Diseases that involve changes in the way the stomach contracts (motility disorders) are best diagnosed by this test.

Purpose

The study is used most frequently to evaluate patients who have symptoms suggestive of decreased, delayed, or rapid gastric emptying, and no visible abnormality to explain their symptoms.

Symptoms pointing to a delay in gastric emptying are non-specific, and may be due to a number of causes, such as ulcers, diabetes, tumors, and others. These symptoms include **nausea**, upper abdominal bloating, and at times **vomiting**. Another significant symptom is called "early satiety," which means feeling full after eating only a small amount of food. In some patients, weight loss is also present. In addition to symptoms, the finding of a large amount of material in the stomach after an overnight fast suggests abnormal emptying, but does not distinguish between an actual blockage or an irregularity in gastric contractions. It is therefore essential to find out what is causing material to remain in the stomach.

Since many diseases can produce the above symptoms, structural lesions (such as tumors or regions of narrowing or scar tissue) need to be ruled out first. This is usually done by upper gastrointestinal series test or by endoscopy (examination of the inside of an organ, in this instance the stomach, with an instrument that has a light at the end of it and an optical system for examination of the organ). Once it is clear that a mechanical or physical lesion is not the cause of symptoms, attempts to document an abnormality in the nervous or muscular function of the stomach is then begun. GES is usually the first step in that evaluation.

Precautions

The exam should not be performed on pregnant women, but is otherwise quite safe. Since eggs are usually used to hold the radioactive material, patients should notify their physician if they are allergic to eggs. However, other materials can be used in place of an egg.

Description

Gastric emptying scans have undergone several changes since the initial studies in the late 1970s. During the study, patients are asked to ingest an egg sandwich containing a radioactive substance (for example, technetium) that can be followed by a special camera. The emptying of the material from the stomach is then followed and displayed both in the form of an image, as well as the percentage emptied over several hours (generally two and four hours). Studies are in progress using substances that are not radioactive, but this procedure is not available to the patient as of yet.

Preparation

The only preparation involved is for the patient to fast overnight before the test.

Risks

The radiation exposure during the study is quite small and safe, unless the patient is pregnant.

Normal results

There are several different measurements considered normal, depending on the radioactive material

and solid meal used. The value is expressed as a percentage of emptying over a period of time. For a technetium-filled egg sandwich, normal emptying is 78 minutes for half the material to leave the stomach, with a variation of 11 minutes either way.

Abnormal results

GES scan studies that show emptying of the stomach in a longer than accepted period is abnormal. Severity of test results and symptoms do not always match; therefore, the physician must carefully interpret these findings. Diabetic injury to the nerves that supply the stomach (called diabetic gastroparesis) is one of the most common causes of abnormal gastric motility. However, up to 30% of patients have no obvious cause to explain the abnormal results and symptoms. These cases are called idiopathic (of unknown cause). GES is often used to follow the effect of medications used for treatment of motility disorders.

Resources

ORGANIZATIONS

American Pseudo-Obstruction and Hirschprung's Disease Society. 158 Pleasant St., North Andover, MA 01845-2797. < http://www.tiac.net/users/aphs > .

David Kaminstein, MD

Gastric lavage *see* **Stomach flushing**

Gastric stapling *see* **Obesity surgery**

Gastric ulcers *see* **Ulcers (digestive)**

Gastrinoma

Definition

Gastrinomas are tumors associated with a rare gastroenterological disorder known as Zollinger-Ellison syndrome (ZES). They occur primarily in the pancreas and duodenum (beginning of the small intestine) and secrete large quantities of the hormone gastrin, triggering gastric acid production that produces ulcers. They may be malignant (cancerous) or benign.

Description

Gastrinomas are an integral part of the Zollinger-Ellison syndrome (ZES). In fact, ZES is also known as gastrinoma. This syndrome consists of ulcer disease in the upper gastrointestinal tract, marked increases in the secretion of gastric acid in the stomach, and tumors of the islet cells in the pancreas. The tumors produce large amounts of gastrin that are responsible for the characteristics of Zollinger-Ellison syndrome, namely severe ulcer disease. Although usually located within the pancreas, they may occur in other organs.

Gastrinomas may occur randomly and sporadically, or they may be inherited as part of a genetic condition called multiple endocrine neoplasia type 1 (MEN-1) syndrome. About half of persons with MEN-1 have gastrinomas, which tend to be more numerous and smaller than tumors in sporadic cases.

About half of ZES patients have multiple gastrinomas, which can vary in size from 1–20 mm. Gastrinomas found in the pancreas are usually much larger than duodenal gastrinomas. About two thirds of gastrinomas are malignant (cancerous). These usually grow slowly, but some may invade surrounding sites rapidly and metastasize (spread) widely. Sometimes, gastrinomas are found only in the lymph nodes, and it is uncertain whether these malignancies have originated in the lymph nodes or have metastasized from a tumor not visible in the pancreas or duodenum.

There is some evidence that the more malignant form of gastrinomas is more frequent in larger pancreatic tumors, especially in females and in persons with a shorter disease symptom duration and higher serum gastrin levels.

Causes and symptoms

Most persons with gastrinomas secrete profound amounts of gastric acid, and almost all develop ulcers, mostly in the duodenum or stomach. Early in the course of the disease, symptoms are typical of peptic ulcers, however once the disease is established, the ulcers become more persistent and symptomatic, and may respond poorly to standard anti-ulcer therapy. Abdominal **pain** is the predominant symptom of ulcer disease. About 40% of patients have **diarrhea** as well. In some patients, diarrhea is the primary symptom of gastrinoma.

Diagnosis

Persons with gastrinomas have many of the same symptoms as persons with ulcers. Their levels of gastric acid, however, are usually far greater than those in common ulcer disease. Gastrinomas are usually diagnosed by a blood test that measures the level of gastrin in the blood. Patients with gastrinomas often have gastrin levels more than 200 pg/mL, which is 4–10

times higher than normal. Serum gastrin levels as high as 450,000 pg/mL have occurred.

When the serum gastrin test does not show these extremely high levels of gastrin, patients may be given certain foods or injections in an attempt to provoke a response that will help diagnose the condition. The most useful of these provocative tests is the secretin injection test (or secretin stimulation or provocative test), which will almost always produce a positive response in persons with gastrinomas but seldom in persons without them.

Surgically, gastrinomas are often difficult to locate, even with careful inspection. They may be missed in at least 10–20% of patients with ZES. Gastrinomas are sometimes found only because they have metastasized and produced symptoms related to the spread of malignancy. Such metastasis may be the most reliable indication of whether the gastrinoma is malignant or benign.

Diagnostic imaging techniques help locate the gastrinomas. The most sophisticated is an x-ray test called radionuclide octreotide scanning (also known as somatostatin receptor scintigraphy or 111In pentetreotide SPECT). A study by the National Institutes of Health (NIH) found this test to be superior to other imaging methods, such as computed tomography scan (CT) or **magnetic resonance imaging** (MRI), in pinpointing the location of tumors and guiding physicians in treatment.

Approximately half of all gastrinomas do not show up on imaging studies. Therefore, exploratory surgery is often recommended to try to locate and remove the tumors.

Treatment

Therapy for gastrinomas should be individualized, since patients tend to have varying degrees of disease and symptoms. Treatment is aimed at eliminating the overproduction of gastric acid and removing the gastrin-producing tumors.

Drugs

Gastrinomas may not be easily treated by the standard anti-ulcer approaches. The medical treatment of choice is with drugs called **proton pump inhibitors**, such as omeprazole or lansoprazole, daily. These drugs are potent inhibitors of gastric acid. High doses of H-2 receptor antagonists may also reduce gastric acid secretion, improve symptoms, and induce ulcer healing. These drugs must be continued indefinitely, since even a brief discontinuation will cause ulcer recurrence. **Antacids** may provide some relief, but it is usually not longlasting or healing.

Surgery

Because of the likelihood that gastrinomas may be malignant, in both sporadic tumors and those associated with the inherited MEN-1 syndrome, surgery to locate and remove gastrinomas is frequently advised. It is now known that complete surgical removal of gastrinomas can cure the overproduction of gastrin, even in patients who have metastases to the lymph nodes. Surgery in patients with MEN-1 and ZES, however, remains controversial since the benefit is less clear.

Freedom from disease after surgery is judged by improved symptoms, reduced gastric acid production, reduced need for drug therapy, normalization of serum gastrin levels, and normalization of results from the secretin stimulation test and imaging studies.

Prognosis

Medical therapy often controls symptoms, and surgery may or may not cure gastrinoma. About 50% of ZES patients in whom gastrinomas are not removed will die from malignant spread of the tumor. In patients with gastrinomas as part of MEN-1 syndrome, the cure rate is extremely low.

A NIH study of patients who had surgical removal of gastrinomas found that 42% were disease-free one year after surgery and 35% were disease-free at five years. Disease recurrences can often be detected with a serum gastrin test or secretin stimulation test.

When gastrinomas are malignant, they often grow slowly. The principal sites of metastasis are the regional lymph nodes and liver, but they may also spread to other structures. About one quarter of patients with gastrinomas have liver metastases at the time of diagnosis. This appears to be more frequent with pancreatic gastrinomas than duodenal gastrinomas.

Metastases of malignant gastrinomas to the liver is very serious. Survival five years after diagnosis is 20–30%, however patients with gastrinomas found only in the lymph nodes have been known to live as long as 25 years after diagnosis, without evidence of further tumor spread. In fact, the life expectancy of patients with gastrinomas that have spread to the lymph nodes is no different from that of patients with gastrinomas that cannot even be found at surgery for about 90%, five years after diagnosis.

KEY TERMS

Gastrin—A hormone secreted in the stomach that is involved in the production of gastric acid. Overproduction of gastric acid contributes to peptic ulcer formation.

Multiple endocrine neoplasia type 1 (MEN-1)—An inherited condition marked by multiple malignancies of the pituitary gland, parathyroid gland, and islet cells of the pancreas. About half of MEN-1 patients with pancreatic islet cell tumors will have gastrinomas, gastrin-producing tumors that lead to ulcer disease.

Peptic ulcer—An eroded area in the stomach lining or in the first part of the duodenum (beginning of the small intestine).

Serum gastrin test—A laboratory test that is performed on a blood sample to determine that level of the hormone gastrin. High levels of gastrin indicate the presence a duodenal ulcer or a gastrinoma.

Sporadic—Occurring at random or by chance, and not as a result of a genetically determined, or inherited, trait.

Resources

ORGANIZATIONS

National Digestive Diseases Information Clearinghouse. 2 Information Way, Bethesda, MD 20892-3570. (800) 891-5389. < http://www.niddk.nih.gov/health/digest/nddic.htm > .

Caroline A. Helwick

▌ Gastritis

Definition

Gastritis commonly refers to inflammation of the lining of the stomach, but the term is often used to cover a variety of symptoms resulting from stomach lining inflammation and symptoms of burning or discomfort. True gastritis comes in several forms and is diagnosed using a combination of tests. In the 1990s, scientists discovered that the main cause of true gastritis is infection from a bacterium called *Helicobacter pylori* (*H. pylori*).

Description

Gastritis should not be confused with common symptoms of upper abdominal discomfort. It has been associated with resulting ulcers, particularly peptic ulcers. And in some cases, chronic gastritis can lead to more serious complications.

Nonerosive H. pylori gastritis

The main cause of true gastritis is *H. pylori* infection. *H. pylori* is indicated in an average of 90% of patients with chronic gastritis. This form of nonerosive gastritis is the result of infection with *Helicobacter pylori* bacterium, a microorganism whose outer layer is resistant to the normal effects of stomach acid in breaking down bacteria.

The resistance of *H. pylori* means that the bacterium may rest in the stomach for long periods of times, even years, and eventually cause symptoms of gastritis or ulcers when other factors are introduced, such as the presence of specific genes or ingestion of **nonsteroidal anti-inflammatory drugs** (NSAIDS). Study of the role of *H. pylori* in development of gastritis and peptic ulcers has disproved the former belief that **stress** lead to most stomach and duodenal ulcers and has resulted in improved treatment and reduction of stomach ulcers. *H. pylori* is most likely transmitted between humans, although the specific routes of transmission were still under study in early 1998. Studies were also underway to determine the role of *H. pylori* and resulting chronic gastritis in development of gastric **cancer**.

Erosive and hemorrhagic gastritis

After *H. pylori*, the second most common cause of chronic gastritis is use of nonsteroidal anti-inflammatory drugs. These commonly used **pain** killers, including **aspirin**, fenoprofen, ibuprofen and naproxen, among others, can lead to gastritis and peptic ulcers. Other forms of erosive gastritis are those due to alcohol and corrosive agents or due to trauma such as ingestion of foreign bodies.

Other forms of gastritis

Clinicians differ on the classification of the less common and specific forms of gastritis, particularly since there is so much overlap with *H. pylori* in development of chronic gastritis and complications of gastritis. Other types of gastritis that may be diagnosed include:

- Acute stress gastritis–the most serious form of gastritis which usually occurs in critically ill patients, such as those in intensive care. Stress erosions may develop suddenly as a result of severe trauma or stress to the stomach lining.

- Atrophic gastritis is the result of chronic gastritis which is leading to atrophy, or decrease in size and wasting away, of the gastric lining. Gastric atrophy is the final stage of chronic gastritis and may be a precursor to gastric cancer.

- Superficial gastritis is a term often used to describe the initial stages of chronic gastritis.

- Uncommon specific forms of gastritis include granulomatous, eosiniphilic and lymphocytic gastritis.

Causes and symptoms

Nonerosive H. pylori gastritis

H. pylori gastritis is caused by infection from the *H. pylori* bacterium. It is believed that most infection occurs in childhood. The route of its transmission was still under study in 1998 and clinicians guessed that there may be more than one route for the bacterium. Its prevalence and distribution differs in nations around the world. The presence of *H. pylori* has been detected in 86–99% of patients with chronic superficial gastritis. However, physicians are still learning about the link of *H. pylori* to chronic gastritis and peptic ulcers, since many patients with *H. pylori* infection do not develop symptoms or peptic ulcers. *H. pylori* is also seen in 90–100% of patients with duodenal ulcers.

Symptoms of *H. pylori* gastritis include abdominal pain and reduced acid secretion in the stomach. However, the majority of patients with *H. pylori* infection suffer no symptoms, even though the infection may lead to ulcers and resulting symptoms. Ulcer symptoms include dull, gnawing pain, often two to three hours after meals and pain in the middle of the night when the stomach is empty.

Erosive and hemorrhagic gastritis

The most common cause of this form of gastritis is use of NSAIDS. Other causes may be **alcoholism** or stress from surgery or critical illness. The role of NSAIDS in development of gastritis and peptic ulcers depends on the dose level. Although even low doses of aspirin or other nonsteroidal anti-inflammatory drugs may cause some gastric upset, low doses generally will not lead to gastritis. However, as many as 10–30% of patients on higher and more frequent doses of NSAIDS, such as those with chronic arthritis, may develop gastric ulcers. In 1998, studies were underway to understand the role of *H. pylori* in gastritis and ulcers among patients using NSAIDS.

Patients with erosive gastritis may also show no symptoms. When symptoms do occur, they may include **anorexia nervosa**, gastric pain, **nausea and vomiting**.

Other Forms of Gastritis

Less common forms of gastritis may result from a number of generalized diseases or from complications of chronic gastritis. Any number of mechanisms may cause various less common forms of gastritis and they may differ slightly in their symptoms and clinical signs. However, they all have in common inflammation of the gastric mucosa.

Diagnosis

Nonerosive H. pylori gastritis

H. pylori gastritis is easily diagnosed through the use of the urea breath test. This test detects active presence of *H. pylori* infection. Other serological tests, which may be readily available in a physician's office, may be used to detect *H. pylori* infection. Newly developed versions offer rapid diagnosis. The choice of test will depend on cost, availability and the physician's experience, since nearly all of the available tests have an accuracy rate of 90% or better. Endoscopy, or the examination of the stomach area using a hollow tube inserted through the mouth, may be ordered to confirm diagnosis. A biopsy of the gastric lining may also be ordered.

Erosive or hemorrhagic gastritis

Clinical history of the patient may be particularly important in the diagnosis of this type of gastritis, since its cause is most often the result of chronic use of NSAIDS, alcoholism, or other substances.

Other forms of gastritis

Gastritis that has developed to the stage of duodenal or gastric ulcers usually requires endoscopy for diagnosis. It allows the physician to perform a biopsy for possible malignancy and for *H. pylori*. Sometimes, an upper gastrointestinal x-ray study with barium is ordered. Some diseases such as Zollinger-Ellison syndrome, an ulcer disease of the upper gastrointestinal tract, may show large mucosal folds in the stomach and duodenum on radiographs or in endoscopy. Other tests check for changes in gastric function.

Treatment

H. pylori gastritis

The discovery of *H. pylori's* role in development of gastritis and ulcers has led to improved treatment of chronic gastritis. In particular, relapse rates for duodenal and gastric ulcers has been reduced with successful treatment of *H. pylori* infection. Since the infection can be treated with **antibiotics**, the bacterium can be completely eliminated up to 90% of the time.

Although *H. pylori* can be successfully treated, the treatment may be uncomfortable for patients and relies heavily on patient compliance. In 1998, studies were underway to identify the best treatment method based on simplicity, patient cooperation and results. No single antibiotic had been found which would eliminate *H. pylori* on its own, so a combination of antibiotics has been prescribed to treat the infection.

DUAL THERAPY. Dual therapy involves the use of an antibiotic and a proton pump inhibitor. **Proton pump inhibitors** help reduce stomach acid by halting the mechanism that pumps acid into the stomach. This also helps promote healing of ulcers or inflammation. Dual therapy has not been proven to be as effective as triple therapy, but may be ordered for some patients who can more comfortably handle the use of less drugs and will therefore more likely follow the two-week course of therapy.

TRIPLE THERAPY. As of early 1998, triple therapy was the preferred treatment for patients with *H. pylori* gastritis. It is estimated that triple therapy successfully eliminates 80–95% of *H. pylori* cases. This treatment regimen usually involves a two-week course of three drugs. An antibiotic such as amoxicillin or tetracycline, and another antibiotic such as clarithomycin or metronidazole are used in combination with bismuth subsalicylate, a substance found in the over-the-counter medication, Pepto-Bismol, which helps protect the lining of the stomach from acid. Physicians were experimenting with various combinations of drugs and time of treatment to balance side effects with effectiveness. Side effects of triple therapy are not serious, but may cause enough discomfort that patients are not inclined to follow the treatment.

OTHER TREATMENT THERAPIES. Scientists have experimented with quadruple therapy, which adds an antisecretory drug, or one which suppresses gastric secretion, to the standard triple therapy. One study showed this therapy to be effective with only a week's course of treatment in more than 90% of patients. Short course therapy was attempted with triple therapy involving antibiotics and a proton pump inhibitor and seemed effective in eliminating *H. pylori* in one week for more than 90% of patients. The goal is to develop the most effective therapy combination that can work in one week of treatment or less.

MEASURING H. PYLORI TREATMENT EFFECTIVENESS. In order to ensure that *H. pylori* has been eradicated, physicians will test patients following treatment. The breath test is the preferred method to check for remaining signs of *H. pylori*.

Treatment of erosive gastritis

Since few patients with this form of gastritis show symptoms, treatment may depend on severity of symptoms. When symptoms do occur, patients may be treated with therapy similar to that for *H. pylori*, especially since some studies have demonstrated a link between *H. pylori* and NSAIDS in causing ulcers. Avoidance of NSAIDS will most likely be prescribed.

Other forms of gastritis

Specific treatment will depend on the cause and type of gastritis. These may include prednisone or antibiotics. Critically ill patients at high risk for bleeding may be treated with preventive drugs to reduce risk of acute stress gastritis. If stress gastritis does occur, the patient is treated with constant infusion of a drug to stop bleeding. Sometimes surgery is recommended, but is weighed with the possibility of surgical complications or **death**. Once torrential bleeding occurs in acute stress gastritis, mortality is as high as greater than 60%.

Alternative treatment

Alternative forms of treatment for gastritis and ulcers should be used cautiously and in conjunction with conventional medical care, particularly now that scientists have confirmed the role of *H. pylori* in gastritis and ulcers. Alternative treatments can help address gastritis symptoms with diet and **nutritional supplements**, herbal medicine and **ayurvedic medicine**. It is believed that zinc, vitamin A and beta-carotene aid in the stomach lining's ability to repair and regenerate itself. Herbs thought to stimulate the immune system and reduce inflammation include **echinacea** (*Echinacea* spp.) and goldenseal (*Hydrastis canadensis*). Ayurvedic medicine involves **meditation**. There are also certain herbs and nutritional supplements aimed at helping to treat ulcers.

Prognosis

The discovery of *H. pylori* has improved the prognosis for patients with gastritis and ulcers. Since

KEY TERMS

Duodenal—Refers to the duodenum, or the first part of the small intestine.

Gastric—Relating to the stomach.

Mucosa—The mucous membrane, or the thin layer which lines body cavities and passages.

Ulcer—A break in the skin or mucous membrane. It can fester and pus like a sore.

treatment exists to eradicate the infection, recurrence is much less common. As of 1998, the only patients requiring treatment for *H. pylori* were those at high risk because of factors such as NSAIDS use or for those with ulcers and other complicating factors or symptoms. Research will continue into the most effective treatment of *H. pylori*, especially in light of the bacterium's resistance to certain antibiotics. Regular treatment of patients with gastric and duodenal ulcers has been recommended, since H. pylori plays such a consistently high role in development of ulcers. It is believed that *H. pylori* also plays a role in the eventual development of serious gastritis complications and cancer. Detection and treatment of *H. pylori* infection may help reduce occurrence of these diseases. The prognosis for patients with acute stress gastritis is much poorer, with a 60 percent or higher mortality rate among those bleeding heavily.

Prevention

The widespread detection and treatment of *H. pylori* as a preventive measure in gastritis has been discussed but not resolved. Until more is known about the routes through which *H. pylori* is spread, specific prevention recommendations are not available. Erosive gastritis from NSAIDS can be prevented with cessation of use of these drugs. An education campaign was launched in 1998 to educate patients, particularly an **aging** population of arthritis sufferers, about risk for ulcers from NSAIDS and alternative drugs.

Resources

PERIODICALS

Podolski, J. L. "Recent Advances in Peptic Ulcer Disease: H. pylori Infection and Its Treatement." *Gastroenterology Nursing* 19, no. 4: 128-136.

ORGANIZATIONS

National Digestive Diseases Information Clearinghouse. 2 Information Way, Bethesda, MD 20892-3570.

Gastroenteritis

(800) 891-5389. <http://www.niddk.nih.gov/health/digest/nddic.htm>.

OTHER

American College of Gastroenterology Page. <http://www.acg.org>.

HealthAnswers.com. <http://www.healthanswers.com>.

Teresa Odle

Gastroduodenostomy (Billroth I) *see* **Ulcer surgery**

Gastroenteritis

Definition

Gastroenteritis is a catchall term for infection or irritation of the digestive tract, particularly the stomach and intestine. It is frequently referred to as the stomach or intestinal flu, although the **influenza** virus is not associated with this illness. Major symptoms include **nausea and vomiting**, **diarrhea**, and abdominal cramps. These symptoms are sometimes also accompanied by **fever** and overall weakness. Gastroenteritis typically lasts about three days. Adults usually recover without problem, but children, the elderly, and anyone with an underlying disease are more vulnerable to complications such as **dehydration**.

Description

Gastroenteritis is an uncomfortable and inconvenient ailment, but it is rarely life-threatening in the United States and other developed nations. However, an estimated 220,000 children younger than age five are hospitalized with gastroenteritis symptoms in the United States annually. Of these children, 300 die as a result of severe diarrhea and dehydration. In developing nations, diarrheal illnesses are a major source of mortality. In 1990, approximately three million deaths occurred worldwide as a result of diarrheal illness.

The most common cause of gastroenteritis is viral infection. Viruses such as rotavirus, adenovirus, astrovirus, and calicivirus and small round-structured viruses (SRSVs) are found all over the world. Exposure typically occurs through the fecal-oral route, such as by consuming foods contaminated by fecal material related to poor sanitation. However, the infective dose can be very low (approximately 100 virus particles), so other routes of transmission are quite probable.

Typically, children are more vulnerable to rotaviruses, the most significant cause of acute watery diarrhea. Annually, worldwide, rotaviruses are estimated to cause 800,000 deaths in children below age five. For this reason, much research has gone into developing a vaccine to protect children from this virus. Adults can be infected with rotaviruses, but these infections typically have minimal or no symptoms.

Children are also susceptible to adenoviruses and astroviruses, which are minor causes of childhood gastroenteritis. Adults experience illness from astroviruses as well, but the major causes of adult viral gastroenteritis are the caliciviruses and SRSVs. These viruses also cause illness in children. The SRSVs are a type of calicivirus and include the Norwalk, Southhampton, and Lonsdale viruses. These viruses are the most likely to produce **vomiting** as a major symptom.

Bacterial gastroenteritis is frequently a result of poor sanitation, the lack of safe drinking water, or contaminated food–conditions common in developing nations. Natural or man-made disasters can make underlying problems in sanitation and food safety worse. In developed nations, the modern food production system potentially exposes millions of people to disease-causing bacteria through its intensive production and distribution methods. Common types of bacterial gastroenteritis can be linked to *Salmonella* and *Campylobacter* bacteria; however, ***Escherichia coli*** 0157 and *Listeria monocytogenes* are creating increased concern in developed nations. **Cholera** and Shigella remain two diseases of great concern in developing countries, and research to develop long-term vaccines against them is underway.

Causes and symptoms

Gastroenteritis arises from ingestion of viruses, certain bacteria, or parasites. Food that has spoiled may also cause illness. Certain medications and excessive alcohol can irritate the digestive tract to the point of inducing gastroenteritis. Regardless of the cause, the symptoms of gastroenteritis include diarrhea, **nausea** and vomiting, and abdominal **pain** and cramps. Sufferers may also experience bloating, low fever, and overall tiredness. Typically, the symptoms last only two to three days, but some viruses may last up to a week.

A usual bout of gastroenteritis shouldn't require a visit to the doctor. However, medical treatment is essential if symptoms worsen or if there are complications. Infants, young children, the elderly, and persons with underlying disease require special attention in this regard.

The greatest danger presented by gastroenteritis is dehydration. The loss of fluids through diarrhea and vomiting can upset the body's electrolyte balance, leading to potentially life-threatening problems such as heart beat abnormalities (arrhythmia). The risk of dehydration increases as symptoms are prolonged. Dehydration should be suspected if a **dry mouth**, increased or excessive thirst, or scanty urination is experienced.

If symptoms do not resolve within a week, an infection or disorder more serious than gastroenteritis may be involved. Symptoms of great concern include a high fever (102 ° F [38.9 °C] or above), blood or mucus in the diarrhea, blood in the vomit, and severe abdominal pain or swelling. These symptoms require prompt medical attention.

Diagnosis

The symptoms of gastroenteritis are usually enough to identify the illness. Unless there is an outbreak affecting several people or complications are encountered in a particular case, identifying the specific cause of the illness is not a priority. However, if identification of the infectious agent is required, a stool sample will be collected and analyzed for the presence of viruses, disease-causing (pathogenic) bacteria, or parasites.

Treatment

Gastroenteritis is a self-limiting illness which will resolve by itself. However, for comfort and convenience, a person may use over-the-counter medications such as Pepto Bismol to relieve the symptoms. These medications work by altering the ability of the intestine to move or secrete spontaneously, absorbing toxins and water, or altering intestinal microflora. Some over-the-counter medicines use more than one element to treat symptoms.

If over-the-counter medications are ineffective and medical treatment is sought, a doctor may prescribe a more powerful anti-diarrheal drug, such as motofen or lomotil. Should pathogenic bacteria or parasites be identified in the patient's stool sample, medications such as **antibiotics** will be prescribed.

It is important to stay hydrated and nourished during a bout of gastroenteritis. If dehydration is absent, the drinking of generous amounts of nonalcoholic fluids, such as water or juice, is adequate. **Caffeine**, since it increases urine output, should be avoided. The traditional BRAT diet–bananas, rice, applesauce, and toast–is tolerated by the tender gastrointestinal system, but it is not particularly nutritious. Many, but not all, medical researchers recommend a diet that includes complex carbohydrates (e.g., rice, wheat, potatoes, bread, and cereal), lean meats, yogurt, fruit, and vegetables. Milk and other dairy products shouldn't create problems if they are part of the normal diet. Fatty foods or foods with a lot of sugar should be avoided. These recommendations are based on clinical experience and controlled trials, but are not universally accepted.

Minimal to moderate dehydration is treated with oral rehydrating solutions that contain glucose and electrolytes. These solutions are commercially available under names such as Naturalyte, Pedialyte, Infalyte, and Rehydralyte. Oral rehydrating solutions are formulated based on physiological properties. Fluids that are not based on these properties–such as cola, apple juice, broth, and sports beverages–are not recommended to treat dehydration. If vomiting interferes with oral rehydration, small frequent fluid intake may be better tolerated. Should oral rehydration fail or severe dehydration occur, medical treatment in the form of intravenous (IV) therapy is required. IV therapy can be followed with oral rehydration as the patient's condition improves. Once normal hydration is achieved, the patient can return to a regular diet.

Alternative treatment

Symptoms of uncomplicated gastroenteritis can be relieved with adjustments in diet, herbal remedies, and homeopathy. An infusion of meadowsweet (*Filipendula ulmaria*) may be effective in reducing nausea and stomach acidity. Once the worst symptoms are relieved, slippery elm (*Ulmus fulva*) can help calm the digestive tract. Of the homeopathic remedies available, *Arsenicum album*, **ipecac**, or *Nux vomica* are three said to relieve the symptoms of gastroenteritis.

Probiotics, bacteria that are beneficial to a person's health, are recommended during the recovery phase of gastroenteritis. Specifically, live cultures of *Lactobacillus acidophilus* are said to be effective in soothing the digestive tract and returning the intestinal flora to normal. *L. acidophilus* is found in live-culture yogurt, as well as in capsule or powder form at health food stores. The use of probiotics is found in folk remedies and has some support in the medical literature. Castor oil packs to the abdomen can reduce inflammation and also reduce spasms or discomfort.

Prognosis

Gastroenteritis is usually resolved within two to three days and there are no long-term effects. If dehydration occurs, recovery is extended by a few days.

KEY TERMS

Dehydration—A condition in which the body lacks the normal level of fluids, potentially impairing normal body functions.

Electrolyte—An ion, or weakly charged element, that conducts reactions and signals in the body. Examples of electrolytes are sodium and potassium ions.

Glucose—A sugar that serves as the body's primary source of fuel.

Influenza—A virus that affects the respiratory system, causing fever, congestion, muscle aches, and headaches.

Intravenous (IV) therapy—Administration of intravenous fluids.

Microflora—The bacterial population in the intestine.

Pathogenic bacteria—Bacteria that produce illness.

Probiotics—Bacteria that are beneficial to a person's health, either through protecting the body against pathogenic bacteria or assisting in recovery from an illness.

Prevention

There are few steps that can be taken to avoid gastroenteritis. Ensuring that food is well-cooked and unspoiled can prevent bacterial gastroenteritis, but may not be effective against viral gastroenteritis.

Resources

PERIODICALS

Hart, C. Anthony, and Nigel A. Cunliffe. "Viral Gastroenteritis." *Current Opinion in Infectious Diseases* 10 (1997): 408.

Moss, Peter J., and Michael W. McKendrick. "Bacterial Gastroenteritis." *Current Opinion in Infectious Diseases* 10 (1997): 402.

Julia Barrett

Gastroesophageal reflux *see* **Heartburn**

Gastrointestinal bleeding studies *see* **GI bleeding studies**

Gastrointestinal study *see* **Liver nuclear medicine scan**

Gastrojejunostomy *see* **Ulcer surgery**

Gastroschisis *see* **Abdominal wall defects**

Gastrostomy

Definition

Gastrostomy is a surgical procedure for inserting a tube through the abdomen wall and into the stomach. The tube is used for feeding or drainage.

Purpose

Gastrostomy is performed because a patient temporarily or permanently needs to be fed directly through a tube in the stomach. Reasons for feeding by gastrostomy include **birth defects** of the mouth, esophagus, or stomach, and problems sucking or swallowing.

Gastrostomy is also performed to provide drainage for the stomach when it is necessary to bypass a long-standing obstruction of the stomach outlet into the small intestine. Obstructions may be caused by peptic ulcer scarring or a tumor.

Precautions

Gastrostomy is a relatively simple procedure. As with any surgery, patients are more likely to experience complications if they are smokers, obese, use alcohol heavily, or use illicit drugs. In addition, some prescription medications may increase risks associated with anesthesia.

Description

Gastrostomy, also called gastrostomy tube insertion, is surgery performed by a general surgeon to give an external opening into the stomach. Surgery is performed either when the patient is under general anesthesia–where the patient feels as if he is in a deep sleep and has no awareness of what is happening–or under **local anesthesia**. With local anesthesia, the patient is awake, but the part of the body cut during the operation is numbed.

A small incision is made on the left side of the abdomen; then, an incision is made through the stomach. A small, flexible, hollow tube, usually made of polyvinylchloride or rubber, is inserted into the stomach. The stomach is stitched closed around the tube, and the incision is closed. The procedure is performed at a hospital or free-standing surgery center.

The length of time the patient needs to remain in the hospital depends on the age of the patient and the patient's general health. In some cases, the hospital stay can be as short as one day, but often is longer.

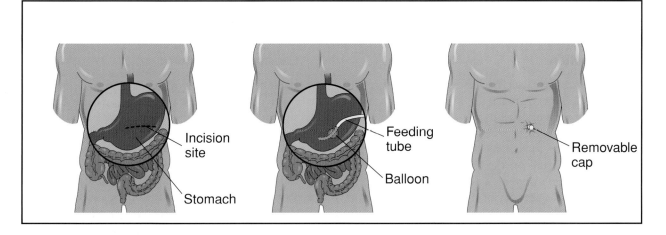

Gastrostomy is a procedure in which the surgeon makes an opening into the stomach and inserts a feeding tube for feeding or for drainage. *(Illustration by Electronic Illustrators Group.)*

Normally, the stomach and abdomen heal in five to seven days.

The cost of the surgery varies, depending on the age and health of the patient. Younger, sicker patients require more intensive, thus more expensive, care.

Preparation

Prior to the operation, the doctor will perform endoscopy and take x rays of the gastrointestinal tract. Blood and urine tests will also be performed, and the patient may meet with the anesthesiologist to evaluate any special conditions that might affect the administration of anesthesia.

Aftercare

Immediately after the operation, the patient is fed intravenously for at least 24 hours. Once bowel sounds are heard, indicating that the gastrointestinal system is working, the patient can begin clear liquid feedings through the tube. Gradually feedings are increased.

Patient education concerning use and care of the gastrostomy tube is very important. Patients and their families are taught how to recognize and prevent infection around the tube, how to feed through the tube, how to handle tube blockage, what to do if the tube pulls out, and what normal activities can be continued.

Risks

There are few risks associated with this surgery. The main complications are infection, bleeding, dislodgment of the tube, stomach bloating, **nausea**, and **diarrhea**.

Normal results

The patient is able to eat through the gastrostomy tube, or the stomach can be drained through the tube.

Resources

OTHER

"Stomach Tube Insertion." HealthAnswers.com. <http://www.healthanswers.com>.

Tish Davidson, A.M.

Gaucher disease

Definition

Gaucher disease is a rare genetic disorder that results in accumulation of fatty molecules called cerebrosides. It can have serious effects on numerous body organs including the liver, spleen, bones and central nervous system. Treatments based on molecular biology are becoming available, but are very expensive.

Description

Gaucher disease was first described by the French physician Philippe Gaucher in 1882. It is the most common of a class of diseases called lysosomal storage diseases, each of which is characterized by the accumulation of a specific chemical substance (a different substance depending on the exact disease). Gaucher disease is characterized by a wide array of different symptoms and the severity of the disease ranges from undetectable to lethal.

Three forms of the disease are recognized: Types I, II and III. Type I is by far the most common and shows the mildest symptoms. It is non-neuronopathic, meaning that the nervous system is not attacked. The onset of Type I can occur at any age in childhood or adult life with the average age of onset at about 21 years. Some affected individuals are have no symptoms throughout adult life. Type II, the infantile form, accounts for less than 1% of patients with Gaucher disease. It is neuronopathic (attacks the nervous system); nervous system effects are severe, and victims often die within the first year of life. Type III most often has its onset during childhood and has some of the features of both the adult and infantile forms. This affects less than 5% of persons with Gaucher disease.

Gaucher disease is caused by the absence, or near absence, of activity of an enzyme called glucocerebrosidase (GC). The normal action of GC is to break down a common molecule called glucocerebroside. If not broken down, glucocerebroside accumulates in certain cells to levels that can cause damage, especially in the spleen, liver, and bone. The common link among these organs is that they house a cell type called a macrophage. A macrophage is a large cell that surrounds and consumes a foreign substance (such as bacteria) in the body. The cellular structures in which glucocerebroside accumulates are called lysosomes.

The three forms of Gaucher disease also differ in their population genetics. Type I is most common in persons of eastern European (Ashkenazi) Jewish descent. Among this population, the disease occurs at a rate of one in 450 live births and about one in 10 to 15 persons are carriers, making it the most common genetic disease affecting Jewish people. The other two types are equally frequent in all ethnic groups. Type II occurs at a rate of one in 100,000 live births,

while Type III is estimated to occur in one in 50,000 live births.

Causes and symptoms

Lack of the GC enzyme is caused by a mutation in the glucocerebrosidase gene. The gene is located on chromosome 1. As of 2000, there have been over 100 mutations described in this gene that causes Gaucher disease. Gaucher disease is inherited in an autosomal recessive pattern. This means that two defective gene copies must be inherited, one from each parent, for the disease to manifest itself. Persons with only one gene mutation are carriers for the disorder. A person who is a carrier for Gaucher disease does not have any symptoms and does not know he or she is a carrier unless he or she has had specific testing. When both parents are carriers for Gaucher disease, there is a one in four chance (25%) in each **pregnancy** for a child to have Gaucher disease. There is a two in three chance that a healthy sibling of an affected child is a carrier.

The results of Gaucher disease are widespread in the body and include excessive growth of the liver and spleen (hepatosplenomegaly), weakening of bones, and, in acute cases, severe nervous system damage. Many patients experience "bone crises," which are episodes of extreme **pain** in their bones.

There is a wide array of other problems that occur with Gaucher disease, such as anemia (fewer than normal red blood cells). Just how these other symptoms are caused is not known. Nor is it known why some patients have very mild disease and others have much more significant problems. Even identical twins with the disease can have differing symptoms.

Diagnosis

Diagnosis of Gaucher disease, based initially on the symptoms described above, can be confirmed by microscopic, enzymatic, and molecular tests. Biopsy (surgical removal of tissue from a problem area) of tissue is helpful for microscopic diagnosis. When biopsy tissue is examined under the microscope, cells will appear swollen and will show characteristic features of the cytoplasm (part of the cell body along with the nucleus) and nucleus. Enzyme tests will show deficiency (<30% of normal levels) of the enzyme GC. Molecular analysis of DNA samples looking at four of the more common mutations will show defects in the gene for GC in 95% of Ashkenazi Jewish individuals and in 75% of non-Jewish people. Diagnosis can be performed prenatally (before birth) if the parents' mutations are known using **amniocentesis** or **chorionic villus sampling**.

Diagnosis as to which of the three types of Gaucher disease an individual has is based on the symptoms, rather than on test results.

Treatment

Until the 1990s, only supportive therapy could be offered. **Analgesics** are used to control pain. Orthopedic treatment is used for bone **fractures**. In some cases, surgical removal of the spleen may be necessary. Several treatments for anemia have been used, including vitamin and iron supplements, blood transfusions, and bone marrow transplants.

The newest form of treatment for Gaucher disease is enzyme replacement therapy, in which GC can be administered intravenously. The enzyme can be prepared either by purification from placentas (alglucerase) or by recombinant DNA manufacturing techniques (imiglucerase). Either way, the cost of treatment ranges from $100,000 to $400,000 per year, which can prevent many from obtaining treatment.

Enzyme replacement is effective at reducing most Gaucher symptoms. The notable exception is neurologic damage in Type II disease, which remains unimproved by this treatment. This treatment is not recommended for individuals who are asymptomatic. As of 2000, the efficacy for the treatment of Type III Gaucher disease is not known. Many questions remain about enzyme replacement therapy in regard to dosage, and method and frequency of administration. The treatment program should be individualized for each patient.

Prognosis

A patient's expected lifespan varies greatly with the type of Gaucher disease. Infants with Type II disease have a life span of one to four years. Patients with Types I and III of the disease have highly variable outcomes with some patients dying in childhood and others living full lives. Little is known about the reasons for this variability.

Prevention

Genetic counseling is advised for individuals with Gaucher disease and for their relatives to accurately assess risk and discuss testing options. For couples who previously had a child with Gaucher or in situations where both parents are carriers for known Gaucher mutations, prenatal diagnosis is available to

---

KEY TERMS

Cerebrosides—Fatty carbohydrates that occur in the brain and nervous system.

Enzymatic replacement therapy—A treatment method used to replace missing enzymes. It is possible to synthesize enzymes and then inject them intravenously into patients.

Glucocerebroside—A cerebroside that contains glucose in the molecule.

---

determine whether a pregnancy is affected. Families in which a person has been diagnosed with Gaucher disease can have DNA testing, which enables other relatives to determine their carrier status. Prospective parents can then use that information to conduct family planning or to prepare for a child who may have special circumstances.

Families in which both parents are known to be a carrier of a mutation for Gaucher disease could consider preimplantation genetic diagnosis. This relatively new procedure can select an embryo without both Gaucher disease mutations prior to implantation of the embryo into the uterus. This technique is only available at selected genetics centers.

As of the early 2000s, population screening for Gaucher disease is not standard of care.

Resources

PERIODICALS

Beutler, E. "Gaucher Disease." *Archives of Internal Medicine* 159 (1999): 881-2.

ORGANIZATIONS

Alliance of Genetic Support Groups. 4301 Connecticut Ave. NW, Suite 404, Washington, DC 20008. (202) 966-5557. Fax: (202) 966-8553. < http:// www.geneticalliance.org > .

Children's Gaucher Research Fund. PO Box 2123, Granite Bay, CA 95746-2123. (916) 797-3700. Fax: (916) 797-3707. < http://www.childrensgaucher.org > .

National Gaucher Foundation. 11140 Rockville Pike, Suite 350, Rockville, MD 20852-3106. (800) 925-8885. < http://www.gaucherdisease.org > .

National Organization for Rare Disorders (NORD). PO Box 8923, New Fairfield, CT 06812-8923. (203) 746-6518 or (800) 999-6673. Fax: (203) 746-6481. < http:// www.rarediseases.org > .

OTHER

"Cerezyme." Genzyme Therapeutics. < http:// www.cerezyme.com > .

"Gaucher Disease: Current Issues in Diagnosis and Treatment." < http://text.nlm.nih.gov/nih/ta/www/16.html > .

"Living with Gaucher Disease: A Guide for Patients, Parents, Relatives, and Friends." < http://neuro-www3.mgh.harvard.edu/gaucher/living.html > .

National Foundation for Jewish Genetic Diseases (NFJGD). < http://www.nfjgd.org/ > .

Amy Vance, MS, CGC

Gay and lesbian health

Definition

Lesbian, gay, bisexual, and transgender (LGBT) individuals are as diverse as the general population in terms of race, ethnicity, age, religion, education, income, and family history. A number of health concerns are unique to or shared by the LGBT community, however, including an increased risk of certain cancers, infectious and **sexually transmitted diseases** (STDs), and mental health disorders; issues relating to **nutrition** and weight, tobacco use, and **substance abuse**; and discrimination by health care and insurance providers.

Description

The definitions of different sexual identities have shifted over the years, as have the perceptions and stereotypes of the general population. Because of the wide range of behaviors and identities that exist in the LGBT community, it is difficult to develop an inclusive definition. It is generally accepted, however, that gay men and lesbians are sexually attracted to or participate in sexual behaviors with individuals of the same gender, while bisexual men and women are sexually attracted to or participate in sexual behaviors with individuals of both genders. Transgender individuals live part- or full-time in a gender role opposite to their genetic sex.

It is estimated that approximately 2.8% of men and 1.4% of women identify as being gay, lesbian, or bisexual while 9.1% of men and 4.3% of women have participated in sexual behavior with someone of the same gender at least once. The true extent of the transgender community has not been well researched in the United States; one study from the Netherlands in 1993 found that one in 11,900 males and one in 30,400 females are transgnder.

There are a number of issues that arise when trying to define sexual orientation. Many gay men and lesbians have participated in or continue to participate in sexual activities with members of the opposite sex but choose not to identify as heterosexuals or bisexuals. Others have never participated in sexual activities at all yet still identify as gay, lesbian, or bisexual. Some men and women identifying as bisexuals are in long-term, monogamous relationships with individuals of the same or opposite sex. Male-to-female (MTF) or female-to-male (FTM) transgender individuals may or may not identify themselves as gay or lesbian.

The implications of these identity issues are far-reaching. Misdiagnoses or improper medical recommendations might come from health care providers who have mistakenly assumed sexual behaviors or risks from the patient's stated identity. For example, a provider might incorrectly assume that a lesbian patient has never had sexual intercourse with a male and therefore would not have contracted STDs not normally transmitted by sexual activities between women. It has been difficult to closely estimate the numbers of LGBT individuals in the United States because of varying definitions. Likewise, the statistics in medical or social studies and surveys on LGBT issues might vary widely depending on what definitions were provided for the respondents. Because of this, many researchers have opted for the more inclusive terms of "men who have sex with men" (MSM) and "women who have sex with women" (WSW) to categorize gay, lesbian, and bisexual respondents.

Important health care issues

Many LGBT individuals have difficulty revealing their sexual identity ("coming out") to their health care providers. They may fear discrimination from providers or believe that their confidentiality might be breached. In some cases health care workers have been poorly trained to address the needs of LGBT individuals or have difficulty communicating with their LGBT patient (one study indicated that 40% of physicians are uncomfortable providing care for gay or lesbian patients). In addition, many questions posed in questionnaires or examinations are heterosexually biased (e.g. asking a lesbian which birth control methods she uses or a gay man if he is married, single, or divorced).

Other reasons why LGBT individuals are often hesitant to share their sexual identity are more logistical. Many insurance companies deny benefits to long-term partners on the basis that they are not married. LGBT patients may have inadequate access to health care, either because they live in a remote rural area or in the crowded inner city. Some same-sex partners encounter discrimination in hospitals and clinics when they are denied the rights usually given to spouses of a patient such as visiting, making medical decisions, and participating in consultations with physicians.

Some of the health concerns and risk factors that are relevant to LBGT individuals may be shared by the general population, while others are more specific to the LGBT community, and still others are specific to different subgroups of LGBT individuals. These health concerns may be grouped into the following areas of concern:

- Sexual behavior issues: STDs such as human **immunodeficiency** virus (HIV) and acquired immune deficiency syndrome (**AIDS**), **hepatitis A** virus (HAV), **hepatitis B** virus (HBV), **bacterial vaginosis**, **gonorrhea**, chlamydia, and **genital warts** (human papillomavirus or HPV); anal, ovarian, and cervical **cancer**.

- Cultural issues: body image, nutrition, weight, and eating disorders; drug and alcohol **abuse**; tobacco use; parenting and family planning.

- Discrimination issues: inadequate medical care; harassment at work, school, or home; difficulty in obtaining housing, insurance coverage, or child custody; violence.

- Sexual identity issues: conflicts with family, friends, and work mates; psychological issues such as **anxiety**, depression, and **suicide**; economic hardship.

CANCER. Cancer is the second leading cause of **death** in the United States. In 2000, it was estimated that 1,220,100 individuals were diagnosed with cancer and 55,200 lost their lives as a result. LBGT individuals are at an increased risk for certain types of cancers. Some researchers believe that those who do not disclose their sexual identity live with an added **stress** that suppresses the immune system, thus leaving them with an increased risk of tumor growth.

Several studies have indicated that lesbians have higher risk for developing **breast cancer**. This is partially related to higher rates of risk factors such as **obesity**, alcohol use, tobacco use, and nulliparity (not bearing children). It has also been shown that lesbians are less likely to be screened for breast cancer than heterosexual women. Lesbians also have additional risk of developing **ovarian cancer**, due to inadequate access to health care, nulliparity, and not using **oral**

contraceptives (use of oral contraceptives has been shown to decrease the risk of getting ovarian cancer).

Gay and bisexual men (or more generally, men who have sex with men [MSM]) are at higher risk of developing non-Hodgkin's lymphoma, **Hodgkin's disease**, and **anal cancer**. **Kaposi's sarcoma**, an AIDS-associated cancer, used to be found in the gay community at rates thousands of times more than the general population before more effective **antiretroviral drugs** became available for people infected with HIV. Anal cancer is associated with transmission of human papillomavirus (HPV); a 1998 study indicated 73% of HIV-positive and 23% of HIV-negative MSM were infected with more than one type of HPV. The risk factors associated with MSM are also associated with increased rates of anal cancer (i.e. **smoking**, having many sexual partners, and receiving anal intercourse).

AIDS. As of 2001, more than 760,000 individuals had been diagnosed with AIDS in the United States. More than 80% are men; about 16% are women, and 1% are children 12 years old or younger. In 2000, more than 30,000 MSM were diagnosed with AIDS. While this number was down from 1999, it remained the highest risk factor for the disease. Other major risk groups associated with AIDS transmission include intravenous drug users (IDUs) who share needles, heterosexuals who engage in high-risk sexual behaviors, inmates at correctional facilities, and neonates (newborns) whose mothers are infected with HIV.

Gender identity disorder is defined as "a strong and persistent cross-gender identification . . . manifested by symptoms such as a stated desire to be the other sex, frequently passing as the other sex, desire to live or be treated as the other sex, or the conviction that he or she as the typical feelings and reactions of the other sex" (DSM-IV, 302.85). Transvestic fetishism is defined as involving "recurrent, intense sexually arousing fantasies, sexual urges, or behaviors involving cross-dressing" (DSM-IV, 302.3). Both disorders lead to a "disturbance that causes clinically significant distress or impairment in social, occupational, or other important areas of functioning." This last point iterates that transgender individuals are not automatically considered under DSM-IV to have a mental disorder.

NUTRITION AND WEIGHT. Diet and nutritional factors are associated with a number of diseases including cancer, **stroke**, diabetes, heart disease, and **osteoporosis**. It has been shown that lesbians are more likely than heterosexual women to be obese, have a higher body mass index (BMI), and have higher rates of smoking, but are also more likely to have a healthier body image

(42% compared to 21% of heterosexual women). Gay men and adolescents, on the other hand, have been shown to have increased rates of eating disorder behaviors than heterosexual men; examples are binge eating (25% compared to 11%), purging behaviors (12% to 4%), and poor body image (28% to 12%).

SUBSTANCE AND TOBACCO USE. Marijuana and **cocaine** use has been shown to be higher among lesbians than heterosexual women. The incidence of the use of some drugs is higher in gay men than heterosexual men; these include marijuana, psychedelic drugs, ecstasy, barbituates, and stimulants such as amyl or butyl nitrate ("poppers"). There is some indication that the use of some illicit drugs speeds up the replication of HIV, although more research needs to be done in this area.

Cigarette smoking is responsible for 430,000 deaths a year in the United States, with an estimated 3,000 nonsmokers dying as a result of exposure to secondhand smoke. In 2004 the rate of smoking among all adults was 28%. In contrast, 50% of gay men, lesbians and bisexuals were noted to be smokers. Lesbians are more than two times as likely to become heavy smokers than heterosexual women. Research shows that lesbians have the toughest time giving up smoking. For many years, efforts to improve health among the LGBT population has focused on AIDS and STDs and smoking cessation has taken a back seat.

Prevention

There are numerous ways that health care providers can improve the access to and experience of health care services for LGBT individuals. These include:

- rewording questionnaires and examinations to be inclusive of LGBT patients

- providing referrals to social service agencies and counseling services that are LGBT-friendly

- taking educational courses that are sensitive to the needs of LGBT patients

- treating the families of LGBT patients as one would the families of heterosexual patients

- maintaining the strictest code of confidentiality

- developing and maintaining health care centers or clinics that address LGBT-specific needs

- asking non-threatening questions to determine if a person is at risk of an STD

- educating patients of risk factors associated with STDs, possible vaccines, and treatments available

- providing services to individuals in the process of disclosing their sexual identity and, if applicable, their families

Resources

PERIODICALS

DuLong, Jessica. "Snuffing Out the Butts: Campaigns to Convince Gay Men and Lesbians to Ditch Cigarettes Tey to Cut Through a Long-held Addiction." *The Advocate* March 16, 2004: 30-32.

ORGANIZATIONS

Gay and Lesbian Medical Association. 459 Fulton Street, Suite 107, San Francisco, CA 94102. (415) 225-4547. < http://www.glma.org > .

Parents, Families, and Friends of Lesbians and Gays. 1726 M Street NW, Suite 400, Washington, DC 20036. (202) 467-8180. < http://www.pflag.org > .

OTHER

Albert, Sarah. "Lesbians and Gays More Likely to Smoke, Survey Says." GayHealth Website. May 16, 2001. < http://www.gayhealth.com/templates/ 99022445042572021484300001/news/ index.html?record = 554 > .

Dean, Laura, Ilan H. Meyer, Kevin Robinson, Randall L. Sell, Robert Sember, Vincent M. B. Silenzio, Deborah J. Bowen, Judith Bradford, Esther Rothblum, Jocelyn White, Patricia Dunn, Ann Lawrence, Daniel Wolfe, and Jessica Xavier. "Lesbian, Gay, Bisexual, and Transgender Health: Findings and Concerns." *Journal of the Gay and Lesbian Medical Association.* October 2000. < http://www.glma.org/pub/jglma/vol4/3/ index.html > .

Garbo, Jon. "FDA Approves Combo Vaccine for Hepatitis A and B." GayHealth Website. May 14, 2001. < http://www.gayhealth.com/templates/ 99022462467343139648300002/news? record = 553 > .

"Healthy People 2010 Companion Document for Lesbian, Gay, Bisexual, and Transgender (LGBT) Health." Gay and Lesbian Medical Association. April 2001. < http://www.glma.org/policy/hp2010/ index.html > .

Stéphanie Dionne
Teresa G. Odle

Gender identity disorder

Definition

The psychological diagnosis gender identity disorder (GID) is used to describe a male or female that feels a strong identification with the opposite sex and experiences considerable distress because of their actual sex.

Description

Gender identity disorder can affect children, adolescents, and adults. Individuals with gender identity disorder have strong cross-gender identification. They believe that they are, or should be, the opposite sex. They are uncomfortable with their sexual role and organs and may express a desire to alter their bodies. While not all persons with GID are labeled as transsexuals, there are those who are determined to undergo sex change procedures or have done so, and, therefore, are classified as transsexual. They often attempt to pass socially as the opposite sex. Transsexuals alter their physical appearance cosmetically and hormonally, and may eventually undergo a sex-change operation.

Children with gender identity disorder refuse to dress and act in sex-stereotypical ways. It is important to remember that many emotionally healthy children experience fantasies about being a member of the opposite sex. The distinction between these children and gender identity disordered children is that the latter experience significant interference in functioning because of their cross-gender identification. They may become severely depressed, anxious, or socially withdrawn.

Causes and symptoms

The cause of gender identity disorder is not known. It has been theorized that a prenatal hormonal imbalance may predispose individuals to the disorder. Problems in the individual's family interactions or family dynamics have also been postulated as having some causal impact.

The *Diagnostic and Statistical Manual of Mental Disorders*, Fourth Edition (*DSM-IV*), the diagnostic reference standard for United States mental health professionals, describes the criteria for gender identity disorder as an individual's strong and lasting cross-gender identification and their persistent discomfort with their biological gender role. This discomfort must cause a significant amount of distress or impairment in the functioning of the individual.

DSM-IV specifies that children must display at least four of the following symptoms of cross-gender identification for a diagnosis of gender identity disorder:

- a repeatedly stated desire to be, or insistence that he or she is, the opposite sex

- a preference for cross-dressing

- a strong and lasting preference to play make-believe and role-playing games as a member of the opposite sex or persistent fantasies that he or she is the opposite sex

- a strong desire to participate in the stereotypical games of the opposite sex

- a strong preference for friends and playmates of the opposite sex

Diagnosis

Gender identity disorder is typically diagnosed by a psychiatrist or psychologist, who conducts an interview with the patient and takes a detailed social history. Family members may also be interviewed during the assessment process. This evaluation usually takes place in an outpatient setting.

Treatment

Treatment for children with gender identity disorder focuses on treating secondary problems such as depression and **anxiety**, and improving self-esteem. Treatment may also work on instilling positive identifications with the child's biological gender. Children typically undergo psychosocial therapy sessions; their parents may also be referred for family or individual therapy.

Transsexual adults often request hormone and surgical treatments to suppress their biological sex characteristics and acquire those of the opposite sex. A team of health professionals, including the treating psychologist or psychiatrist, medical doctors, and several surgical specialists, oversee this transitioning process. Because of the irreversible nature of the surgery, candidates for sex-change surgery are evaluated extensively and are often required to spend a period of time integrating themselves into the cross-gender role before the procedure begins. Counseling and peer support are also invaluable to transsexual individuals.

KEY TERMS

Cross-dressing—Dressing in clothing that is stereo-typical of the opposite sex.

Gender identity disorder (GID)—A strong and lasting cross-gender identification and persistent discomfort with one's biological gender (sex) role. This discomfort must cause a significant amount of distress or impairment in the functioning of the individual.

Transsexual—A person with gender identity disorder who has an overwhelming desire to change anatomic sex; one who seeks hormonal or surgical treatment to change sex.

Prognosis

Long-term follow up studies have shown positive results for many transsexuals who have undergone sex-change surgery. However, significant social, personal, and occupational issues may result from surgical sex changes, and the patient may require psychotherapy or counseling.

Resources

ORGANIZATIONS

American Academy of Child and Adolescent Psychiatry (AACAP). 3615 Wisconsin Ave. NW, Washington, DC 20016. (202) 966-7300. < http://www.aacap.org > .

OTHER

The National Transgender Guide. < http://www.tgguide.com > .

Paula Anne Ford-Martin

Gender reassignment surgery

Definition

Also known as sex change surgery or sex reassignment surgery, gender reassignment surgery is a procedure that changes a person's external genital organs from those of one gender to those of the other.

Purpose

There are two reasons commonly given for altering the genital organs:

- Newborns with intersex deformities must early on be assigned to one sex or the other. These deformities represent intermediate stages between the primordial female genitals and the change into male caused by male hormone stimulation.

- Both men and women occasionally believe they are physically a different sex than they are mentally and emotionally. This dissonance is so profound that they are willing to be surgically altered. This condition is known as **gender identity disorder**; it is thought to be more common in men than in women.

Although technical considerations in the case of babies with ambiguous genitalia would seem to favor surgical conversion to female structures rather than to male, this conclusion has been challenged in the early 2000s. William G. Reiner, a child and adolescent psychiatrist, undertook a study of 29 genetic males who had been born with defective external genitalia and reared as females following surgery. He found that over half of them identified as males by adolescence in spite of the absence of male genitalia. Dr. Reiner has concluded that psychosexual development in genetic and hormonal males is heavily influenced by exposure to androgens prior to birth, and has called for a reevaluation of the practice of routinely assigning male babies with ambiguous genitals to the female sex.

Precautions

Sexual identity is probably the most profound characteristic humans have. Assigning it must take place immediately after birth, both for the child's and the parents' comfort. Changing sexual identity may be the most significant change one can experience. It therefore should be done with every care and caution. By the time most adults come to surgery, they have lived for many years with dissonant identity. The average in one study was 29 years. Nevertheless, even then they may not be fully aware of the implications of becoming a member of the other sex.

Gender identity disorder has been officially defined by the American Psychiatric Associan in the fourth edition of the *Diagnostic and Statistical Manual of Mental Disorders*, or DSM-IV, as a condition in which the affected individual has "a strong and persistent cross-gender identification" combined with "persistent discomfort about one's assigned sex." Because of widespread social disapproval of surgical gender reassignment, researchers do not know the true prevalence of gender identity disorders in the general population. Early estimates were 1:37,000 males and 1:107,000

females. A recent study in the Netherlands, however, maintains that a more accurate estimation is 1:11,900 males and 1:30,400 females. In any case, the number of surgical procedures is lower than the number of patients diagnosed with gender identity disorders.

Description

Converting male to female anatomy requires removal of the penis, reshaping genital tissue to appear more female, and constructing a vagina. A vagina can be successfully formed from a skin graft or an isolated loop of intestine.

Female to male surgery has achieved lesser success, due to the difficulty of building a functioning penis from the much smaller amount of erectile tissue available in the female genitals. Penis construction is not attempted less than a year after the preliminary surgery to remove the female organs. One study in Singapore found that a third of the patients would not undergo the surgery again. Nevertheless, they were all pleased with the change of sex. Besides the genital organs, the breasts need to be surgically altered for a more male appearance. This can be done quite successfully.

Orgasm, or at least a reasonable degree of erogenous sensitivity, can be experienced by patients after surgery.

Preparation

As of the early 2000s, patients requesting gender reassignment surgery must undergo a lengthy process of physical and psychological evaluation before receiving approval for surgery. The Harry Benjamin International Gender Dysphoria Association (HBIGDA), which is presently the largest worldwide professional association dealing with the treatment of gender identity disorders, has published standards of care that are followed by most surgeons who perform genital surgery for gender reassignment. HBIGDA stipulates that a patient must meet the diagnostic criteria for gender identity disorders as defined by either the Diagnostic and Statistical Manual of Mental Disorders, fourth edition (DSM-IV) or the International Classification of Diseases–10 (ICD-10).

Preparation for gender reassignment surgery includes a period of several years of hormonal treatment to change the body contours, vocal pitch, patterns of facial and body hair, etc. to those of the other sex. As the patient's body and voice begin to change, he or she is also asked to practice dressing and acting as a member of that sex.

There is some controversy as of the early 2000s regarding the appropriateness of performing gender reassignment surgery on adolescents, as opposed to either infants or older adults, on the grounds that teenagers are often uncertain about many aspects of their sexuality. The recent case of a thirteen-year-old girl who requested gender reassignment surgery in Australia reflects the intensity of this controversy among surgeons as well as members of the general public.

Aftercare

Social support, particularly from the family, is important for readjustment as a member of the opposite sex. If patients were socially or emotionally unstable before the operation, over 30, or had an unsuitable body build for the new sex, they tend to do poorly. Paul McHugh, the former head of the department of psychiatry at Johns Hopkins University, has reported that people who think that gender reassignment surgery will solve all their emotional and social problems are likely to be disappointed. "[These patients] had much the same problems with relationships, work, and emotions as before. The hope that they would emerge now from their emotional difficulties to flourish psychologically had not been fulfilled."

Risks

All surgery runs the risk of infection, bleeding, and a need to return for repairs. This surgery is irreversible, so the patient must have no doubts about accepting the results.

The most common physical complication of the male to female surgery is narrowing of the new vagina.

There is some risk of patients developing other mental disorders associated with their new sex. Several cases of **anorexia nervosa**, an eating disorder that is far more common in women than in men, have been reported in males who underwent gender reassignment surgery.

Resources

BOOKS

American Psychiatric Association. *Diagnostic and Statistical Manual of Mental Disorders*. 4th ed., revised. Washington, DC: American Psychiatric Association, 2000.

Beers, Mark H., MD, and Robert Berkow, MD., editors. "Psychosexual Disorders." Section 15, Chapter 192 In *The Merck Manual of Diagnosis and Therapy*. Whitehouse Station, NJ: Merck Research Laboratories, 2002.

PERIODICALS

McHugh, Paul, MD. "Surgical Sex." *First Things* 147 (November 2004): 34–38.

Reiner, W. G., and J. P. Gearhart. "Discordant Sexual Identity in Some Genetic Males with Cloacal Exstrophy Assigned to Female Sex at Birth." *New England Journal of Medicine* 350 (January 22, 2004): 333–341.

Reiner, W. G. "Psychosexual Development in Genetic Males Assigned Female: The Cloacal Exstrophy Experience." *Child and Adolescent Psychiatry Clinics of North America* 13 (July 2004): 657–674.

Spriggs, M. P. "Ethics and the Proposed Treatment for a 13-Year-Old with Atypical Gender Identity." *Medical Journal of Australia* 181 (September 20, 2004): 319–321.

Winston, A. P., S. Acharya, S. Chaudhuri, and L. Fellowes. "Anorexia Nervosa and Gender Identity Disorder in Biologic Males: A Report of Two Cases." *International Journal of Eating Disorders* 36 (July 2004): 109–113.

ORGANIZATIONS

American Board of Urology (ABU). 2216 Ivy Road, Suite 210, Charlottesville, VA 22903. (434) 979-0059. < http://www.abu.org > .

American Psychiatric Association (APA). 1400 K Street, NW, Washington, DC 20005. (888) 357-7924. < http://www.psych.org > .

Harry Benjamin International Gender Dysphoria Association, Inc. (HBIGDA). 1300 South Second Street, Suite 180, Minneapolis, MN 55454. (612) 625-1500. < http://www.hbigda.org > .

OTHER

Harry Benjamin International Gender Dysphoria Association (HBIGDA). *Standards of Care for Gender Identity Disorders*, 6th version. February 2001. < http://www.hbigda.org/socv6.html > .

J. Ricker Polsdorfer, MD
Rebecca J. Frey, PhD

Gene therapy

Gene therapy is a rapidly growing field of medicine in which genes are introduced into the body to treat diseases. Genes control heredity and provide the basic biological code for determining a cell's specific functions. Gene therapy seeks to provide genes that correct or supplant the disease-controlling functions of cells that are not, in essence, doing their job. Somatic gene therapy introduces therapeutic genes at the tissue or cellular level to treat a specific individual. Germ-line gene therapy inserts genes into reproductive cells or possibly into embryos to correct genetic defects that could be passed on to future generations. Initially conceived as an approach for treating inherited diseases, like **cystic fibrosis** and Huntington's disease, the scope of potential gene therapies has grown to include treatments for cancers, arthritis, and infectious diseases. Although gene therapy testing in humans has advanced rapidly, many questions surround its use. For example, some scientists are concerned that the therapeutic genes themselves may cause disease. Others fear that germ-line gene therapy may be used to control human development in ways not connected with disease, like intelligence or appearance.

The biological basis of gene therapy

Gene therapy has grown out of the science of genetics or how heredity works. Scientists know that life begins in a cell, the basic building block of all multicellular organisms. Humans, for instance, are made up of trillions of cells, each performing a specific function. Within the cell's nucleus (the center part of a cell that regulates its chemical functions) are pairs of chromosomes. These threadlike structures are made up of a single molecule of DNA (deoxyribonucleic acid), which carries the blueprint of life in the form of codes, or genes, that determine inherited characteristics.

A DNA molecule looks like two ladders with one of the sides taken off both and then twisted around each other. The rungs of these ladders meet (resulting in a spiral staircase-like structure) and are called base pairs. Base pairs are made up of nitrogen molecules and arranged in specific sequences. Millions of these base pairs, or sequences, can make up a single gene, specifically defined as a segment of the chromosome and DNA that contains certain hereditary information. The gene, or combination of genes formed by these base pairs ultimately direct an organism's growth and characteristics through the production of

certain chemicals, primarily proteins, which carry out most of the body's chemical functions and biological reactions.

Scientists have long known that alterations in genes present within cells can cause inherited diseases like cystic fibrosis, sickle-cell anemia, and **hemophilia**. Similarly, errors in the total number of chromosomes can cause conditions such as **Down syndrome** or Turner's syndrome. As the study of genetics advanced, however, scientists learned that an altered genetic sequence also can make people more susceptible to diseases, like **atherosclerosis, cancer,** and even **schizophrenia**. These diseases have a genetic component, but also are influenced by environmental factors (like diet and lifestyle). The objective of gene therapy is to treat diseases by introducing functional genes into the body to alter the cells involved in the disease process by either replacing missing genes or providing copies of functioning genes to replace nonfunctioning ones. The inserted genes can be naturally-occurring genes that produce the desired effect or may be genetically engineered (or altered) genes.

Scientists have known how to manipulate a gene's structure in the laboratory since the early 1970s through a process called gene splicing. The process involves removing a fragment of DNA containing the specific genetic sequence desired, then inserting it into the DNA of another gene. The resultant product is called recombinant DNA and the process is genetic engineering.

There are basically two types of gene therapy. Germ-line gene therapy introduces genes into reproductive cells (sperm and eggs) or someday possibly into embryos in hopes of correcting genetic abnormalities that could be passed on to future generations. Most of the current work in applying gene therapy, however, has been in the realm of somatic gene therapy. In this type of gene therapy, therapeutic genes are inserted into tissue or cells to produce a naturally occurring protein or substance that is lacking or not functioning correctly in an individual patient.

Viral vectors

In both types of therapy, scientists need something to transport either the entire gene or a recombinant DNA to the cell's nucleus, where the chromosomes and DNA reside. In essence, vectors are molecular delivery trucks. One of the first and most popular vectors developed were viruses because they invade cells as part of the natural infection process. Viruses have the potential to be excellent vectors because they have a specific relationship with the host in that they colonize certain cell types and tissues in specific organs. As a result, vectors are chosen according to their attraction to certain cells and areas of the body.

One of the first vectors used was retroviruses. Because these viruses are easily cloned (artificially reproduced) in the laboratory, scientists have studied them extensively and learned a great deal about their biological action. They also have learned how to remove the genetic information that governs viral replication, thus reducing the chances of infection.

Retroviruses work best in actively dividing cells, but cells in the body are relatively stable and do not divide often. As a result, these cells are used primarily for *ex vivo* (outside the body) manipulation. First, the cells are removed from the patient's body, and the virus, or vector, carrying the gene is inserted into them. Next, the cells are placed into a nutrient culture where they grow and replicate. Once enough cells are gathered, they are returned to the body, usually by injection into the blood stream. Theoretically, as long as these cells survive, they will provide the desired therapy.

Another class of viruses, called the adenoviruses, also may prove to be good gene vectors. These viruses can effectively infect nondividing cells in the body, where the desired gene product then is expressed naturally. In addition to being a more efficient approach to gene transportation, these viruses, which cause respiratory infections, are more easily purified and made stable than retroviruses, resulting in less chance of an unwanted viral infection. However, these viruses live for several days in the body, and some concern surrounds the possibility of infecting others with the viruses through sneezing or coughing. Other viral vectors include **influenza** viruses, Sindbis virus, and a herpes virus that infects nerve cells.

Scientists also have delved into nonviral vectors. These vectors rely on the natural biological process in which cells uptake (or gather) macromolecules. One approach is to use liposomes, globules of fat produced by the body and taken up by cells. Scientists also are investigating the introduction of raw recombinant DNA by injecting it into the bloodstream or placing it on microscopic beads of gold shot into the skin with a "gene-gun." Another possible vector under development is based on dendrimer molecules. A class of polymers (naturally occurring or artificial substances that have a high molecular weight and formed by smaller molecules of the same or similar substances), is "constructed" in the laboratory by combining these smaller molecules. They have been used in manufacturing Styrofoam, polyethylene cartons, and Plexiglass. In the laboratory, dendrimers have shown the ability to

transport genetic material into human cells. They also can be designed to form an affinity for particular cell membranes by attaching to certain sugars and protein groups.

The history of gene therapy

In the early 1970s, scientists proposed "gene surgery" for treating inherited diseases caused by faulty genes. The idea was to take out the disease-causing gene and surgically implant a gene that functioned properly. Although sound in theory, scientists, then and now, lack the biological knowledge or technical expertise needed to perform such a precise surgery in the human body.

However, in 1983, a group of scientists from Baylor College of Medicine in Houston, Texas, proposed that gene therapy could one day be a viable approach for treating Lesch-Nyhan disease, a rare neurological disorder. The scientists conducted experiments in which an enzyme-producing gene (a specific type of protein) for correcting the disease was injected into a group of cells for replication. The scientists theorized the cells could then be injected into people with Lesch-Nyhan disease, thus correcting the genetic defect that caused the disease.

As the science of genetics advanced throughout the 1980s, gene therapy gained an established foothold in the minds of medical scientists as a promising approach to treatments for specific diseases. One of the major reasons for the growth of gene therapy was scientists' increasing ability to identify the specific genetic malfunctions that caused inherited diseases. Interest grew as further studies of DNA and chromosomes (where genes reside) showed that specific genetic abnormalities in one or more genes occurred in successive generations of certain family members who suffered from diseases like intestinal cancer, **bipolar disorder**, **Alzheimer's disease**, heart disease, diabetes, and many more. Although the genes may not be the only cause of the disease in all cases, they may make certain individuals more susceptible to developing the disease because of environmental influences, like **smoking**, pollution, and **stress**. In fact, some scientists theorize that all diseases may have a genetic component.

On September 14, 1990, a four-year old girl suffering from a genetic disorder that prevented her body from producing a crucial enzyme became the first person to undergo gene therapy in the United States. Because her body could not produce adenosine deaminase (ADA), she had a weakened immune system, making her extremely susceptible to severe, life-threatening infections. W. French Anderson and colleagues at the National Institutes of Health's Clinical Center in Bethesda, Maryland, took white blood cells (which are crucial to proper immune system functioning) from the girl, inserted ADA producing genes into them, and then transfused the cells back into the patient. Although the young girl continued to show an increased ability to produce ADA, debate arose as to whether the improvement resulted from the gene therapy or from an additional drug treatment she received.

Nevertheless, a new era of gene therapy began as more and more scientists sought to conduct clinical trial (testing in humans) research in this area. In that same year, gene therapy was tested on patients suffering from melanoma (skin cancer). The goal was to help them produce antibodies (disease fighting substances in the immune system) to battle the cancer.

These experiments have spawned an ever growing number of attempts at gene therapies designed to perform a variety of functions in the body. For example, a gene therapy for cystic fibrosis aims to supply a gene that alters cells, enabling them to produce a specific protein to battle the disease. Another approach was used for brain cancer patients, in which the inserted gene was designed to make the cancer cells more likely to respond to drug treatment. Another gene therapy approach for patients suffering from artery blockage, which can lead to strokes, induces the growth of new blood vessels near clogged arteries, thus ensuring normal blood circulation.

Currently, there are a host of new gene therapy agents in clinical trials. In the United States, both nucleic acid based (*in vivo*) treatments and cell-based (*ex vivo*) treatments are being investigated. Nucleic acid based gene therapy uses vectors (like viruses) to deliver modified genes to target cells. Cell-based gene therapy techniques remove cells from the patient in order to genetically alter them then reintroduce them to the patient's body. Presently, gene therapies for the following diseases are being developed: cystic fibrosis (using adenoviral vector), HIV infection (cell-based), **malignant melanoma** (cell-based), Duchenne **muscular dystrophy** (cell-based), hemophilia B (cell-based), **kidney cancer** (cell-based), Gaucher's Disease (retroviral vector), **breast cancer** (retroviral vector), and lung cancer (retroviral vector). When a cell or individual is treated using gene therapy and successful incorporation of engineered genes has occurred, the cell or individual is said to be *transgenic*.

The medical establishment's contribution to transgenic research has been supported by increased government funding. In 1991, the U.S. government

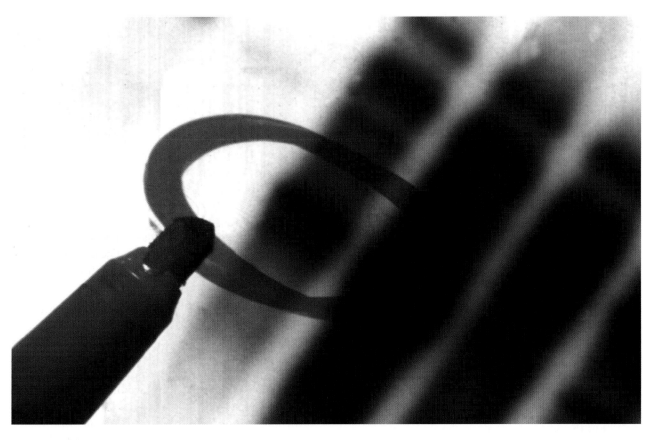

Early detection of cancer. The researcher's pen marks a band on a DNA sequencing autoradiogram confirming a bladder cancer. *(Custom Medical Stock Photo. Reproduced by permission.)*

provided $58 million for gene therapy research, with increases in funding of $15-40 million dollars a year over the following four years. With fierce competition over the promise of societal benefit in addition to huge profits, large pharmaceutical corporations have moved to the forefront of transgenic research. In an effort to be first in developing new therapies, and armed with billions of dollars of research funds, such corporations are making impressive strides toward making gene therapy a viable reality in the treatment of once elusive diseases.

Diseases targeted for treatment by gene therapy

The potential scope of gene therapy is enormous. More than 4,200 diseases have been identified as resulting directly from abnormal genes, and countless others that may be partially influenced by a person's genetic makeup. Initial research has concentrated on developing gene therapies for diseases whose genetic origins have been established and for other diseases that can be cured or improved by substances genes produce.

The following are examples of potential gene therapies. People suffering from cystic fibrosis lack a gene needed to produce a salt-regulating protein. This protein regulates the flow of chloride into epithelial cells, (the cells that line the inner and outer skin layers) that cover the air passages of the nose and lungs. Without this regulation, patients with cystic fibrosis build up a thick mucus that makes them prone to lung infections. A gene therapy technique to correct this abnormality might employ an adenovirus to transfer a normal copy of what scientists call the cystic fibrosis transmembrane conductance regulator, or CTRF, gene. The gene is introduced into the patient by spraying it into the nose or lungs. Researchers announced in 2004 that they had, for the first time, treated a dominant neurogenerative disease called Spinocerebella ataxia type 1, with gene therapy. This could lead to treating similar diseases such as Huntington s disease. They also announced a single intravenous injection could deliver therapy to all muscles, perhaps providing hope to people with muscular dystrophy.

Familial **hypercholesterolemia** (FH) also is an inherited disease, resulting in the inability to process cholesterol properly, which leads to high levels of artery-clogging fat in the blood stream. Patients with FH often suffer heart attacks and strokes because of blocked arteries. A gene therapy approach used to battle FH is much more intricate than most gene therapies because it involves partial surgical removal of patients' livers (*ex vivo* transgene therapy). Corrected copies of a gene that serve to reduce cholesterol build-up are inserted into the liver sections, which then are transplanted back into the patients.

Gene therapy also has been tested on patients with **AIDS**. AIDS is caused by the human **immunodeficiency** virus (HIV), which weakens the body's immune system to the point that sufferers are unable to fight off diseases like pneumonias and cancer. In one approach, genes that produce specific HIV proteins have been altered to stimulate immune system functioning without causing the negative effects that a complete HIV molecule has on the immune system. These genes are then injected in the patient's blood stream. Another approach to treating AIDS is to insert, via white blood cells, genes that have been genetically engineered to produce a receptor that would attract HIV and reduce its chances of replicating. In 2004, researchers reported that had developed a new vaccine concept for HIV, but the details were still in development.

Several cancers also have the potential to be treated with gene therapy. A therapy tested for melanoma, or skin cancer, involves introducing a gene with an anticancer protein called tumor necrosis factor (TNF) into test tube samples of the patient's own cancer cells, which are then reintroduced into the patient. In brain cancer, the approach is to insert a specific gene that increases the cancer cells' susceptibility to a common drug used in fighting the disease. In 2003, researchers reported that they had harnessed the cell killing properties of adenoviruses to treat **prostate cancer**. A 2004 report said that researchers had developed a new DNA vaccine that targeted the proteins expressed in **cervical cancer** cells.

Gaucher disease is an inherited disease caused by a mutant gene that inhibits the production of an enzyme called glucocerebrosidase. Patients with Gaucher disease have enlarged livers and spleens and eventually their bones deteriorate. Clinical gene therapy trials focus on inserting the gene for producing this enzyme.

Gene therapy also is being considered as an approach to solving a problem associated with a surgical procedure known as balloon **angioplasty**. In this procedure, a stent (in this case, a type of tubular scaffolding) is used to open the clogged artery. However, in response to the trauma of the stent insertion, the body initiates a natural healing process that produces too many cells in the artery and results in restenosis, or reclosing of the artery. The gene therapy approach to preventing this unwanted side effect is to cover the outside of the stents with a soluble gel. This gel contains vectors for genes that reduce this overactive healing response.

Regularly throughout the past decade, and no doubt over future years, scientists have and will come up with new possible ways for gene therapy to help treat human disease. Recent advancements include the possibility of reversing **hearing loss** in humans with experimental growing of new sensory cells in adult guinea pigs, and avoiding **amputation** in patients with severe circulatory problems in their legs with angiogenic growth factors.

The Human Genome Project

Although great strides have been made in gene therapy in a relatively short time, its potential usefulness has been limited by lack of scientific data concerning the multitude of functions that genes control in the human body. For instance, it is now known that the vast majority of genetic material does not store information for the creation of proteins, but rather is involved in the control and regulation of gene expression, and is, thus, much more difficult to interpret. Even so, each individual cell in the body carries thousands of genes coding for proteins, with some estimates as high as 150,000 genes. For gene therapy to advance to its full potential, scientists must discover the biological role of each of these individual genes and where the base pairs that make them up are located on DNA.

To address this issue, the National Institutes of Health initiated the Human Genome Project in 1990. Led by James D. Watson (one of the co-discoverers of the chemical makeup of DNA) the project's 15-year goal is to map the entire human genome (a combination of the words gene and chromosomes). A genome map would clearly identify the location of all genes as well as the more than three billion base pairs that make them up. With a precise knowledge of gene locations and functions, scientists may one day be able to conquer or control diseases that have plagued humanity for centuries.

Scientists participating in the Human Genome Project identified an average of one new gene a day, but many expected this rate of discovery to increase. By the year 2005, their goal was to determine the exact location of all the genes on human DNA and the exact sequence of the base pairs that make them up. Some of the genes identified through this project include a gene that predisposes people to **obesity**, one associated with programmed cell death (apoptosis), a gene that guides HIV viral reproduction, and the genes of inherited disorders like Huntington's disease, Lou Gehrig's disease, and some colon and breast cancers. In April 2003, the finished sequence was announced, with 99% of the human genome's gene-containing regions mapped to an accuracy of 99.9%.

The future of gene therapy

Gene therapy seems elegantly simple in its concept: supply the human body with a gene that can correct a biological malfunction that causes a disease. However, there are many obstacles and some distinct questions concerning the viability of gene therapy. For example, viral vectors must be carefully controlled lest they infect the patient with a viral disease. Some vectors, like retroviruses, also can enter cells functioning properly and interfere with the natural biological processes, possibly leading to other diseases. Other viral vectors, like the adenoviruses, often are recognized and destroyed by the immune system so their therapeutic effects are short-lived. Maintaining gene expression so it performs its role properly after vector delivery is difficult. As a result, some therapies need to be repeated often to provide long-lasting benefits.

One of the most pressing issues, however, is gene regulation. Genes work in concert to regulate their functioning. In other words, several genes may play a part in turning other genes on and off. For example, certain genes work together to stimulate cell division and growth, but if these are not regulated, the inserted genes could cause tumor formation and cancer. Another difficulty is learning how to make the gene go into action only when needed. For the best and safest therapeutic effort, a specific gene should turn on, for example, when certain levels of a protein or enzyme are low and must be replaced. But the gene also should remain dormant when not needed to ensure it doesn't oversupply a substance and disturb the body's delicate chemical makeup.

One approach to gene regulation is to attach other genes that detect certain biological activities and then react as a type of automatic off-and-on switch that regulates the activity of the other genes according to biological cues. Although still in the rudimentary stages, researchers are making headway in inhibiting some gene functioning by using a synthetic DNA to block gene transcriptions (the copying of genetic information). This approach may have implications for gene therapy.

The ethics of gene therapy

While gene therapy holds promise as a revolutionary approach to treating disease, ethical concerns over its use and ramifications have been expressed by scientists and lay people alike. For example, since much needs to be learned about how these genes actually work and their long-term effect, is it ethical to test these therapies on humans, where they could have a disastrous result? As with most clinical trials concerning new therapies, including many drugs, the patients participating in these studies usually have not responded to more established therapies and often are so ill the novel therapy is their only hope for long-term survival.

Another questionable outgrowth of gene therapy is that scientists could possibly manipulate genes to genetically control traits in human offspring that are not health related. For example, perhaps a gene could be inserted to ensure that a child would not be bald, a seemingly harmless goal. However, what if genetic manipulation was used to alter skin color, prevent homosexuality, or ensure good looks? If a gene is found that can enhance intelligence of children who are not yet born, will everyone in society, the rich and the poor, have access to the technology or will it be so expensive only the elite can afford it?

The Human Genome Project, which plays such an integral role for the future of gene therapy, also has social repercussions. If individual genetic codes can be determined, will such information be used against people? For example, will someone more susceptible to a disease have to pay higher insurance premiums or be denied health insurance altogether? Will employers discriminate between two potential employees, one with a "healthy" genome and the other with genetic abnormalities?

Some of these concerns can be traced back to the eugenics movement popular in the first half of the twentieth century. This genetic "philosophy" was a societal movement that encouraged people with "positive" traits to reproduce while those with less desirable traits were sanctioned from having children. Eugenics was used to pass strict immigration laws in the United States, barring less suitable people from entering the country lest they reduce the quality of the country's collective gene pool. Probably the most notorious example of eugenics in action was the rise of Nazism in Germany, which resulted in the Eugenic Sterilization Law of 1933. The law required sterilization for those suffering from certain disabilities and even for some who were simply deemed "ugly." To ensure that this novel science is not abused, many governments have

KEY TERMS

Cell—The smallest living unit of the body that groups together to form tissues and help the body perform specific functions.

Chromosome—A microscopic thread-like structure found within each cell of the body, consisting of a complex of proteins and DNA. Humans have 46 chromosomes arranged into 23 pairs. Changes in either the total number of chromosomes or their shape and size (structure) may lead to physical or mental abnormalities.

Clinical trial—The testing of a drug or some other type of therapy in a specific population of patients.

Clone—A cell or organism derived through asexual (without sex) reproduction containing the identical genetic information of the parent cell or organism.

Deoxyribonucleic acid (DNA)—The genetic material in cells that holds the inherited instructions for growth, development, and cellular functioning.

Embryo—The earliest stage of development of a human infant, usually used to refer to the first eight weeks of pregnancy. The term *fetus* is used from roughly the third month of pregnancy until delivery.

Enzyme—A protein that causes a biochemical reaction or change without changing its own structure or function.

Eugenics—A social movement in which the population of a society, country, or the world is to be improved by controlling the passing on of hereditary information through mating.

Gene—A building block of inheritance, which contains the instructions for the production of a particular protein, and is made up of a molecular sequence found on a section of DNA. Each gene is found on a precise location on a chromosome.

Gene transcription—The process by which genetic information is copied from DNA to RNA, resulting in a specific protein formation.

Genetic engineering—The manipulation of genetic material to produce specific results in an organism.

Genetics—The study of hereditary traits passed on through the genes.

Germ-line gene therapy—The introduction of genes into reproductive cells or embryos to correct inherited genetic defects that can cause disease.

Liposome—Fat molecule made up of layers of lipids.

Macromolecules—A large molecule composed of thousands of atoms.

Nitrogen—A gaseous element that makes up the base pairs in DNA.

Nucleus—The central part of a cell that contains most of its genetic material, including chromosomes and DNA.

Protein—Important building blocks of the body, composed of amino acids, involved in the formation of body structures and controlling the basic functions of the human body.

Somatic gene therapy—The introduction of genes into tissue or cells to treat a genetic related disease in an individual.

Vectors—Something used to transport genetic information to a cell.

established organizations specifically for overseeing the development of gene therapy. In the United States, the Food and Drug Administration (FDA) and the National Institutes of Health require scientists to take a precise series of steps and meet stringent requirements before proceeding with clinical trials. As of mid-2004, more than 300 companies were carrying out gene medicine developments and 500 clinical trials were underway. How to deliver the therapy is the key to unlocking many of the researchers discoveries.

In fact, gene therapy has been immersed in more controversy and surrounded by more scrutiny in both the health and ethical arena than most other technologies (except, perhaps, for cloning) that promise to substantially change society. Despite the health and ethical questions surrounding gene therapy, the field will continue to grow and is likely to change medicine faster than any previous medical advancement.

Resources

PERIODICALS

Abella, Harold. "Gene Therapy May Save Limbs." *Diagnostic Imaging* (May 1, 2003): 16.

Christensen R. "Cutaneous Gene Therapy—An Update." *Histochemical Cell Biology* (January 2001): 73-82.

"Gene Therapy Important Part of Cancer Research." *Cancer Gene Therapy Week* (June 30, 2003): 12.

"Initial Sequencing and Analysis of the Human Genome." *Nature* (February 15, 2001): 860-921.

Kingsman, Alan. "Gene Therapy Moves On."
    SCRIP World Pharmaceutical News (July 7, 2004):
    19:ndash;21.

Nevin, Norman. "What Has Happened to Gene Therapy?"
    European Journal of Pediatrics (2000): S240-S242.

"New DNA Vaccine Targets Proteins Expressed in Cervical
    Cancer Cells." *Gene Therapy Weekly* (September 9,
    2004): 14.

"New Research on the Progress of Gene Therapy Presented
    at Meeting." *Obesity, Fitness & Wellness Week* (July 3,
    2004): 405.

Pekkanen, John. "Genetics: Medicine's Amazing Leap."
    Readers Digest (September 1991): 23-32.

Silverman, Jennifer, and Steve Perlstein. "Genome
    Project Completed." *Family Practice News* (May 15,
    2003): 50-51.

"Study Highlights Potential Danger of Gene Therapy."
    Drug Week (June 20, 2003): 495.

"Study May Help Scientists Develop Safer Mthods for Gene
    Therapy." *AIDS Weekly* (June 30, 2003): 32.

Trabis, J. "With Gene Therapy, Ears Grow New Sensory
    Cells." *Science News* (June 7, 2003): 355.

ORGANIZATIONS

National Human Genome Research Institute. The
    National Institutes of Health. 9000 Rockville Pike,
    Bethesda, MD 20892. (301) 496-2433. < http://
    www.nhgri.nih.gov > .

OTHER

Online Mendelian Inheritance in Man. Online genetic testing
    information sponsored by National Center for
    Biotechnology Information. < http://www.ncbi.nlm
    .nih.gov/Omim/ > .

Katherine S. Hunt, MS
Teresa G. Odle

General adaptation syndrome

Definition

General adaptation syndrome, or GAS, is a term used to describe the body's short-term and long-term reactions to **stress**.

Stressors in humans include such physical stressors as **starvation**, being hit by a car, or suffering through severe weather. Additionally, humans can suffer such emotional or mental stressors as the loss of a loved one, the inability to solve a problem, or even having a difficult day at work.

Description

Originally described by Hans Selye (1907–1982), an Austrian-born physician who emigrated to Canada in 1939, the general adaptation syndrome represents a three-stage reaction to stress. Selye explained his choice of terminology as follows: "I call this syndrome *general* because it is produced only by agents which have a general effect upon large portions of the body. I call it *adaptive* because it stimulates defense.... I call it a *syndrome* because its individual manifestations are coordinated and even partly dependent upon each other."

Selye thought that the general adaptation syndrome involved two major systems of the body, the nervous system and the endocrine (or hormonal) system. He then went on to outline what he considered as three distinctive stages in the syndrome's evolution. He called these stages the alarm reaction (AR), the stage of resistance (SR), and the stage of exhaustion (SE).

Stage 1: Alarm reaction (AR)

The first stage of the general adaptation stage, the alarm reaction, is the immediate reaction to a stressor. In the initial phase of stress, humans exhibit a "fight or flight" response, which prepares the body for physical activity. However, this initial response can also decrease the effectiveness of the immune system, making persons more susceptible to illness during this phase.

Stage 2: Stage of resistance (SR)

Stage 2 might also be named the stage of adaptation, instead of the stage of resistance. During this phase, if the stress continues, the body adapts to the stressors it is exposed to. Changes at many levels take place in order to reduce the effect of the stressor. For example, if the stressor is starvation (possibly due to anorexia), the person might experienced a reduced desire for physical activity to conserve energy, and the absorption of nutrients from food might be maximized.

Stage 3: Stage of exhaustion (SE)

At this stage, the stress has continued for some time. The body's resistance to the stress may gradually be reduced, or may collapse quickly. Generally, this means the immune system, and the body's ability to resist disease, may be almost totally eliminated. Patients who experience long-term stress may succumb to heart attacks or severe infection due to their reduced immunity. For example, a person with a stressful job may experience long-term stress that might lead to high blood pressure and an eventual **heart attack**.

Stress, a useful reaction?

The reader should note that Dr. Selye did not regard stress as a purely negative phenomenon; in fact, he frequently pointed out that stress is not only an inevitable part of life but results from intense joy or pleasure as well as fear or **anxiety**. "Stress is not even necessarily bad for you; it is also the spice of life, for any emotion, any activity, causes stress." Some later researchers have coined the term "eustress" or pleasant stress, to reflect the fact that such positive experiences as a job promotion, completing a degree or training program, marriage, travel, and many others are also stressful.

Selye also pointed out that human perception of and response to stress is highly individualized; a job or sport that one person finds anxiety-provoking or exhausting might be quite appealing and enjoyable to someone else. Looking at one's responses to specific stressors can contribute to better understanding of one's particular physical, emotional, and mental resources and limits.

Causes and symptoms

Stress is one cause of general adaptation syndrome. The results of unrelieved stress can manifest as **fatigue**, irritability, difficulty concentrating, and difficulty sleeping. Persons may also experience other symptoms that are signs of stress. Persons experiencing unusual symptoms, such as hair loss, without another medical explanation might consider stress as the cause.

The general adaptation syndrome is also influenced by such universal human variables as overall health and nutritional status, sex, age, ethnic or racial background, level of education, socioeconomic status (SES), genetic makeup, etc. Some of these variables are biologically based and difficult or impossible to change. For example, recent research indicates that men and women respond somewhat differently to stress, with women being more likely to use what is called the "tend and befriend" response rather than the classical "fight or flight" pattern. These researchers note that most of the early studies of the effects of stress on the body were conducted with only male subjects.

Selye's observation that people vary in their perceptions of stressors was reflected in his belief that the stressors themselves are less dangerous to health than people's maladaptive responses to them. He categorized certain diseases, ranging from cardiovascular disorders to inflammatory diseases and mental disorders as "diseases of adaptation," regarding them as "largely due to errors in our adaptaive response to stress" rather than the direct result of such outside factors as germs, toxic substances, etc.

Diagnosis

GAS by itself is not an official diagnostic category but rather a descriptive term. A person who consults a doctor for a stress-related physical illness may be scheduled for blood or urine tests to measure the level of cortisol or other stress-related hormones in their body, or imaging studies to evaluate possible abnormalities in their endocrine glands if the doctor thinks that these tests may help to establish or confirm a diagnosis.

The American Psychiatric Association (APA) recognizes stress as a factor in **anxiety disorders**, particularly **post-traumatic stress disorder** (PTSD) and **acute stress disorder** (ASD). These two disorders are defined as symptomatic reactions to extreme traumatic stressors (war, natural or transportation disasters, criminal assault, **abuse**, hostage situations, etc.) and differ chiefly in the time frame in which the symptoms develop. The APA also has a diagnostic category of **adjustment disorders**, which are characterized either by excessive reactions to stressors within the normal range of experience (e.g. academic examinations, relationship breakups, being fired from a job) or by significant impairment in the person's occupational or social functioning.

Treatment

Treatment of stress-related illnesses typically involves one or more **stress reduction** strategies. Stress reduction strategies generally fall into one of three categories: avoiding stressors; changing one's reaction to the stressor(s); or relieving stress after the reaction to the stressor(s). Many mainstream as well as complementary or alternative (CAM) strategies for stress reduction, such as exercising, listening to music, **aromatherapy**, and massage relieve stress after it occurs.

Many psychotherapeutic approaches attempt to modify the patient's reactions to stressors. These approaches often include an analysis of the patient's individual patterns of response to stress; for example, one commonly used set of categories describes people as "speed freaks," "worry warts," "cliff walkers," "loners," "basket cases," and "drifters." Each pattern has a recommended set of skills that the patient is encouraged to work on; for example, worry **warts** are advised to reframe their anxieties and then identify their core values and goals in order to take concrete action about their worries. In general, persons wishing to improve their management of stress should begin by consulting a medical professional with whom they feel comfortable to discuss which option, or combination of options, they can use.

Selye himself recommended an approach to stress that he described as "living wisely in accordance with natural laws." In his now-classic book *The Stress of Life* (1956), he discussed the following as important dimensions of living wisely:

- Adopting an attitude of gratitude toward life rather than seeking revenge for injuries or slights.

- Acting toward others from altruistic rather than self-centered motives.

- Retaining a capacity for wonder and delight in the genuinely good and beautiful things in life.

- Finding a purpose for one's life and expressing one's individuality in fulfilling that purpose.

- Keeping a healthy sense of modesty about one's goals or achievements.

Resources

BOOKS

American Psychiatric Association. *Diagnostic and Statistical Manual of Mental Disorders*. 4th ed., revised. Washington, D.C.: American Psychiatric Association, 2000.

Beers, Mark H., MD, and Robert Berkow, MD, editors. "Psychiatry in Medicine." Section 15, Chapter 1 85 In *The Merck Manual of Diagnosis and Therapy*. Whitehouse Station, NJ: Merck Research Laboratories, 2004.

PERIODICALS

Benton, Tami D., MD, and Jacqueline Lynch, MSW. "Adjustment Disorders." *eMedicine* September 3, 2004. < http://emedicine.com/med/topic3348.htm > .

Cosen-Binker, L. I., M. G. Binker, G. Negri, and O. Tiscornia. "Influence of Stress in Acute Pancreatitis and Correlation with Stress-Induced Gastric Ulcer." *Pancreatology* 4 (July 2004): 470–484.

Motzer, S. A., and V. Hertig. "Stress, Stress Response, and Health." *Nursing Clinics of North America* 39 (March 2004): 1–17.

Yates, William R., MD. "Anxiety Disorders." *eMedicine* August 15, 2004. < http://emedicine.com/med/topic152.htm > .

ORGANIZATIONS

American Institute of Stress. 124 Park Avenue, Yonkers, NY 10703 (914) 963-1200. Fax: (914) 965-6267. < http://www.stress.org > .

American Psychiatric Association. 1400 K Street NW, Washington DC 20005. (888) 357-7924. < http://www.psych.org > .

Canadian Institute of Stress/Hans Selye Foundation. Medcan Clinic Office, Suite 1500, 150 York Street, Toronto, Ontario, Canada M5H 3S5. (416) 236-4218. < http://www.stresscanada.org > .

National Institute of Mental Health (NIMH). 6001 Executive Boulevard, Room 8184, MSC 9663, Bethesda, MD 20892-9663. (301) 443-4513. < http://www.nimh.nih.gov > .

OTHER

"Stress management, General adaptation syndrome, GAS..." < http://www.holisticonline.com/stress/stress_GAS.htm > .

Michael V. Zuck, PhD
Rebecca J. Frey, PhD

General anesthetic *see* **Anesthesia, general**

General surgery

Definition

General surgery is the treatment of injury, deformity, and disease using operative procedures.

Purpose

General surgery is frequently performed to alleviate suffering when a cure is unlikely through medication alone. It can be used for routine procedures performed in a physician's office, such as **vasectomy**, or for more complicated operations requiring a medical team in a hospital setting, such as laparoscopic **cholecystectomy** (removal of the gallbladder). Areas of the body treated by general surgery include the stomach, liver, intestines, appendix, breasts, thyroid gland, salivary glands, some arteries and veins, and the skin. The brain, heart, eyes, and feet, to name only a few, are areas that require specialized surgical repair.

New methods and techniques are less invasive than previous practices, permitting procedures that were considered impossible in the past. For example, microsurgery has been used in reattaching severed body parts by successfully reconnecting small blood vessels and nerves.

Precautions

Patients who are obese, smoke, have bleeding tendencies, or are over 60, need to follow special precautions, as do patients who have recently experienced an illness such as **pneumonia** or a **heart attack**. Patients on medications such as heart and blood pressure medicine, blood thinners, **muscle relaxants**, tranquilizers, insulin, or sedatives, may require special lab tests prior to surgery and special monitoring during surgery. Special precautions may be necessary for patients using mind-altering drugs such as **narcotics**, psychedelics, hallucinogens, **marijuana**, sedatives, or **cocaine** since these drugs may interact with the anesthetic agents used during surgery.

Description

In earlier times, surgery was a dangerous and dirty practice. Until the middle of the 19th century, as many patients died of surgery as were cured. With the discovery and development of **general anesthesia** in the mid-1800s, surgery became more humane. And as knowledge about infections grew, surgery became more successful as sterile practices were introduced into the operating room. The last 50 years of the 20th century have seen continued advancements.

Types of General Surgery

General surgery experienced major advances with the introduction of the endoscope. This is an instrument for visualizing the interior of a body canal or a hollow organ. Endoscopic surgery relies on this pencil-thin instrument, capable of its own lighting system and small video camera. The endoscope is inserted through tiny incisions called portals. While viewing the procedure on a video screen, the surgeon then operates with various other small, precise instruments inserted through one or more of the portals. The specific area of the body treated determines the type of endoscopic surgery performed. For example, **colonoscopy** uses an endoscope, which can be equipped with a device for obtaining tissue samples for visual examination of the colon. Gastroscopy uses an endoscope inserted through the mouth to examine the interior of the stomach. **Arthroscopy** refers to joint surgery, and abdominal procedures are called laparoscopies.

Endoscopy is used in both treatment and diagnosis especially involving the digestive and female reproductive systems. Endoscopy has advantages over many other surgical procedures, resulting in a quicker recovery and shorter hospital stay. This non-invasive technique is being used for appendectomies, gallbladder surgery, hysterectomies and the repair of shoulder and knee ligaments. However, endoscopy does not come without limitations such as complications and high operating expense. Also, endoscopy doesn't offer advantages over conventional surgery in all procedures. Some literature states that as general surgeons become more experienced in their prospective fields, additional non-invasive surgery will be a more common option to patients.

ONE-DAY SURGERY. One-day surgery is also termed same-day, or outpatient surgery. Surgical procedures usually take two hours or less and involve minimal blood loss and a short recovery time. In the majority of surgical cases, oral medications control postoperative **pain**. Cataract removal, **laparoscopy**, **tonsillectomy**, repair of broken bones, **hernia repair**, and a wide range of cosmetic procedures are common same-day surgical procedures. Many individuals prefer the convenience and atmosphere of one-day surgery centers, as there is less competition for attention with more serious surgical cases. These centers are accredited by the Joint Commission on Accreditation of Healthcare Organizations or the Accreditation Association for Ambulatory Health Care.

Preparation

The preparation of patients has advanced significantly with improved diagnostic techniques and procedures. Before surgery the patient may be asked to undergo a series of tests including blood and urine studies, x rays and specific heart studies if the patient's past medical history and/or physical exam warrants this testing. Before any general surgery the physician will explain the nature of the surgery needed, the reason for the procedure, and the anticipated outcome. The risks involved will be discussed along with the types of anesthesia utilized. The expected length of recovery and limitations imposed during the recovery period are also explained in detail before any general surgical procedure.

Surgical procedures most often require some type of anesthetic. Some procedures require only **local anesthesia**, produced by injecting the anesthetic agent into the skin near the site of the operation. The patient remains awake with this form of medication. Injecting anesthetic agents into a primary nerve located near the surgical site produces block anesthesia (also known as regional anesthesia), which is a more extensive local anesthesia. The patient remains conscious, but is usually sedated. General anesthesia involves injecting anesthetic agents into the blood stream and/or inhaling medicines through a mask placed over the patient's face. During general anesthesia, the patient is asleep and an airway tube is usually placed into the windpipe to help keep the airway open.

As part of the preoperative preparation, the patient will receive printed educational material and may be asked to review audio or videotapes. The patient will be instructed to shower or bathe the evening before or morning of surgery and may be asked to scrub the operative site with a special antibacterial soap. Instructions will also be given to the patient to ingest nothing by mouth for a determined period of time prior to the surgical procedure.

Aftercare

After surgery, blood studies and a laboratory examination of removed fluid or tissue are often performed especially in the case of **cancer** surgery. After the operation, the patient is brought to a recovery room and vital signs, fluid status, dressings and surgical drains are monitored. Pain medications are offered and used as necessary. Breathing exercises are encouraged to maximize respiratory function and leg exercises are encouraged to promote adequate circulation and prevent pooling of blood in the lower extremities. Patients must have a responsible adult accompany them home if leaving the same day as the surgery was performed.

Risks

One of the risks involved with general surgery is the potential for postoperative complications. These complications include—but are not limited to—pneumonia, internal bleeding, and wound infection as well as adverse reactions to anesthesia.

Normal results

Advances in diagnostic and surgical techniques have increased the success rate of general surgery by

---

KEY TERMS

Appendectomy—Removal of the appendix.

Endoscope—Instrument for examining visually the inside of a body canal or a hollow organ such as the stomach, colon, or bladder.

Hysterectomy—Surgical removal of part or all of the uterus.

Laparoscopic cholecystectomy—Removal of the gallbladder using a laparoscope, a fiberoptical instrument inserted through the abdomen.

Microsurgery—Surgery on small body structures or cells performed with the aid of a microscope and other specialized instruments.

Portal—An entrance or a means of entrance.

---

many times compared to the past. Today's less invasive surgical procedures have reduced the length of hospital stays, shortened recovery time, decreased postoperative pain and decreased the size of surgical incision. On the average, a conventional abdominal surgery requires a three to six-day hospital stay and three to six-week recovery time.

Abnormal results

Abnormal results from general surgery include persistent pain, swelling, redness, drainage or bleeding in the surgical area and surgical wound infection resulting in slow healing.

Resources

ORGANIZATIONS

American Medical Association. 515 N. State St., Chicago, IL 60612. (312) 464-5000. < http://www.ama-assn.org > .

Jeffrey P. Larson, RPT

Generalized anxiety disorder

Definition

Generalized **anxiety** disorder is a condition characterized by "free floating" anxiety or apprehension not linked to a specific cause or situation.

Description

Some degree of fear and anxiety is perfectly normal. In the face of real danger, fear makes people more alert and also prepares the body to fight or flee (the so-called "fight or flight" response). When people are afraid, their hearts beat faster and they breathe faster in anticipation of the physical activity that will be required of them. However, sometimes people can become anxious even when there is no identifiable cause, and this anxiety can become overwhelming and very unpleasant, interfering with their daily lives. People with debilitating anxiety are said to be suffering from **anxiety disorders**, such as **phobias**, panic disorders, and generalized anxiety disorder. The person with generalized anxiety disorder generally has chronic (officially, having more days with anxiety than not for at least six months), recurrent episodes of anxiety that can last days, weeks, or even months.

Causes and symptoms

Generalized anxiety disorder afflicts between 2–3% of the general population, and is slightly more common in women than in men. It accounts for almost one-third of cases referred to psychiatrists by general practitioners.

Generalized anxiety disorder may result from a combination of causes. Some people are genetically predisposed to developing it. Psychological traumas that occur during childhood, such as prolonged separation from parents, may make people more vulnerable as well. Stressful life events, such as a move, a major job change, the loss of a loved one, or a divorce, can trigger or contribute to the anxiety.

Psychologically, the person with generalized anxiety disorder may develop a sense of dread for no apparent reason–the irrational feeling that some nameless catastrophe is about to happen. Physical symptoms similar to those found with **panic disorder** may be present, although not as severe. They may include trembling, sweating, heart **palpitations** (the feeling of the heart pounding in the chest), **nausea**, and "butterflies in the stomach."

According to the *Diagnostic and Statistical Manual of Mental Disorders,* 4th edition, a person must have at least three of the following symptoms, with some being present more days than not for at least six months, in order to be diagnosed with generalized anxiety disorder:

- restlessness or feeling on edge
- being easily fatigued
- difficulty concentrating
- irritability
- muscle tension
- sleep disturbance

While generalized anxiety disorder is not completely debilitating, it can compromise a person's effectiveness and quality of life.

Diagnosis

Anyone with chronic anxiety for no apparent reason should see a physician. The physician may diagnose the condition based on the patient's description of the physical and emotional symptoms. The doctor will also try to rule out other medical conditions that may be causing the symptoms, such as excessive **caffeine** use, thyroid disease, **hypoglycemia**, cardiac problems, or drug or alcohol withdrawal. Psychological conditions, such as depressive disorder with anxiety, will also need to be ruled out.

In June 2004, the Anxiety Disorders Association of America released follow-up guidelines to help primary care physicians better diagnose and manage patients with generalized anxiety disorder. They include considering the disorder when medical causes for general, vague physical complaints cannot be ruled out. Since generalized anxiety disorder often co-occurs with **mood disorders** and **substance abuse**, the clinician may have to treat these conditions as well, and therefore must consider them in making the diagnosis.

Treatment

Over the short term, a group of tranquilizers called **benzodiazepines**, such as clonazepam (Klonipin) may help ease the symptoms of generalized anxiety disorder. Sometimes **antidepressant drugs**, such as amitryptiline (Elavil), or **selective serotonin reuptake inhibitors** (SSRIs), such as paroxetine (Paxil), escitalopram (Lexapro), and venlafaxine (Effexor), which also has norepinephrine, may be preferred. Other SSRIs are fluoxetine (Prozac) and sertraline (Zoloft).

Psychotherapy can be effective in treating generalized anxiety disorder. The therapy may take many forms. In some cases, psychodynamically-oriented psychotherapy can help patients work through this anxiety and solve problems in their lives. Cognitive behavioral therapy aims to reshape the way people perceive and react to potential stressors in their lives. Relaxation techniques have also been used in treatment, as well as in prevention efforts.

KEY TERMS

Cognitive behavioral therapy—A psychotherapeutic approach that aims at altering cognitions—including thoughts, beliefs, and images—as a way of altering behavior.

Prognosis

When properly treated, most patients with generalized anxiety disorder experience improvement in their symptoms.

Prevention

While preventive measures have not been established, a number of techniques may help manage anxiety, such as relaxation techniques, breathing exercises, and distraction—putting the anxiety out of one's mind by focusing thoughts on something else.

Resources

PERIODICALS

"Guidelines to.Assist Primary Care Physicians in Diagnosing GAD." *Psychiatric Times* (July 1, 2004): 16.

Sherman, Carl. "GAD Patients Often Require Combined Therapy." *Clinical Psychiatry News* (August 2004): 12–14.

ORGANIZATIONS

American Psychiatric Association. 1400 K Street NW, Washington DC 20005. (888) 357-7924. < http://www.psych.org > .

Anxiety Disorders Association of America. 11900 Park Lawn Drive, Ste. 100, Rockville, MD 20852. (800) 545-7367. < http://www.adaa.org > .

National Institute of Mental Health. Mental Health Public Inquiries, 5600 Fishers Lane, Room 15C-05, Rockville, MD 20857. (888) 826-9438. < http://www.nimh.nih.gov > .

Robert Scott Dinsmoor
Teresa G. Odle

Genetic counseling

Definition

Genetic counseling aims to facilitate the exchange of information regarding a person's genetic legacy. It attempts to:

- accurately diagnose a disorder
- assess the risk of recurrence in the concerned family members and their relatives
- provide alternatives for decision-making
- provide support groups that will help family members cope with the recurrence of a disorder.

Purpose

Genetic counselors work with people concerned about the risk of an inherited disease. The counselor does not prevent the incidence of a disease in a family, but can help family members assess the risk for certain hereditary diseases and offer guidance. Many couples seek genetic counseling because there is a family history of known genetic disorders, **infertility**, **miscarriage**, still births, or early infant mortality. Other reasons for participating in genetic counseling may be the influences of a job or lifestyle that exposes a potential parent to health risks such as radiation, chemicals, or drugs. Any family history of **mental retardation** can be of concern as is a strong family history of heart disease at an early age. Recent statistics show a 3% chance of delivering a baby with **birth defects**. An additional 2% chance of having a baby with **Down syndrome** is present for women in their late thirties and older.

Genetic counseling may take on new emphasis in the near future as genetic research continues to advance. In April 2003, the Human Genome Project announced completion of mapping the entire human genetic makeup. The project identified more than 1,400 disease genes and completed study of the ethical, legal, and social issues raised by this expanded knowledge of human genetics. As knowledge expands and scientists discover more methods to identify and treat various diseases, people will face more difficult decisions about their own genetic information.

Precautions

Amniocentesis, one of the specific tests used to gather information for genetic counseling, is best performed between weeks 15 and 17 of a **pregnancy** and an additional one to four weeks may be required to culture skin cells and analyze them. Thus, these test data are not available to assist prospective parents in decision-making until the second trimester of the pregnancy. Individuals who participate in genetic counseling and associated testing also must be aware that there are no cures or treatments for some of the disorders that may be identified.

Description

With approximately 2,000 genes identified and approximately 5,000 disorders caused by genetic defects, genetic counseling is important in the medical discipline of obstetrics. Genetic counselors, educated in the medical and the psychosocial aspects of genetic diseases, convey complex information to help people make life decisions. There are limitations to the power of genetic counseling, though, since many of the diseases that have been shown to have a genetic basis currently offer no cure (for example, Down syndrome or Huntington's disease). Although a genetic counselor cannot predict the future unequivocally, he or she can discuss the occurrence of a disease in terms of probability.

Genetic counseling also can help people with diseases they may face in their own lifetimes. A 2003 study in Great Britain found that women with a family history of **breast cancer** were less worried about getting the disease if they had genetic counseling.

A genetic counselor, with the aid of the patient or family, creates a detailed family pedigree that includes the incidence of disease in first-degree (parents, siblings, and children) and second-degree (aunts, uncles, and grandparents) relatives. Before or after this pedigree is completed, certain genetic tests are performed using DNA analysis, x ray, ultrasound, urine analysis, **skin biopsy**, and physical evaluation. For a pregnant woman, prenatal diagnosis can be made using amniocentesis or **chorionic villus sampling**.

Family pedigree

An important aspect of the genetic counseling session is the compilation of a family pedigree or medical history. To accurately assess the risk of inherited diseases, information on three generations, including health status and/or cause of **death**, usually is needed. If the family history is complicated, information from more distant relatives may be helpful, and medical records may be requested for any family members who have had a genetic disorder. Through an examination of the family history a counselor may be able to discuss the probability of future occurrence of genetic disorders. In all cases, the counselor provides information in a non-directive way that leaves the decision-making up to the client.

Family history questionnaire

As more detailed genetic information becomes available, physicians and genetic counselors may feel the need to dig more deeply than a family pedigree allows. In 2004, physicians attending an American College of Medical Genetics meeting announced use of a structured questionnaire with 50 items to consistent, thorough gather family history data. Although the questionnaire's format and terminology were confusing to some patients, once a formula was applied to the answers, it still helped reviewers agree on a counseling plan 79% of the time.

Screening tests

Screening blood tests help identify individuals who carry genes for recessive genetic disorders. Screening tests usually are only done if:

- The disease is lethal or causes severe handicaps or disabilities.
- The person is likely to be a carrier due to family pedigree or membership in an at-risk ethnic, geographic or racial group.
- The disorder can be treated or reproductive options exist.
- A reliable test is available.

Genetic disorders such as **Tay-Sachs disease**, sickle-cell anemia, and **thalassemia** meet these criteria, and screening tests are commonly done to identify carriers of these diseases. In addition, screening tests may be done for individuals with family histories of Huntington's disease (a degenerative neurological disease) or **hemophilia** (a bleeding disorder). Such screening tests can eliminate the need for more invasive tests during a pregnancy.

Another screening test commonly used in the United States in the alpha-fetoprotein (AFP) test. This test is done on a sample of maternal blood around week 16 of a pregnancy. An elevation in the serum AFP level indicates that the fetus may have certain birth defects such as neural tube defects (including **spina bifida** and anencephaly). If the test yields an elevated result, it may be run again after seven days. If the level still is elevated after repeat testing, additional diagnostic tests (e.g. ultrasound and/or amniocentesis) are done in an attempt to identify the specific birth defect present.

Ultrasound

Ultrasound is a noninvasive procedure that uses sound waves to produce a reflected image of the fetus upon a screen. It is used to determine the age and position of the fetus, and the location of the placenta. Ultrasound also is useful in detecting visible birth defects such as spina bifida (a defect in the development of the vertebrae of the spinal column and/or the spinal cord). It also is useful for detecting heart defects, and malformations of the head, face, body, and limbs. This procedure, however, cannot detect biochemical or chromosomal alterations in the fetus.

Amniocentesis

Amniocentesis is useful in determining genetic and developmental disorders not detectable by ultrasound. This procedure involves the insertion of a needle through the abdomen and into the uterus of a pregnant woman. A sample of amniotic fluid is withdrawn containing skin cells that have been shed by the fetus. The sample is sent to a laboratory where fetal cells contained in the fluid are isolated and grown in order to provide enough genetic material for testing. This takes about seven to 14 days. The material then is extracted and treated so that visual examination for defects can be made. For some disorders, like Tay-Sachs disease, the simple presence of a telltale chemical compound in the amniotic fluid is enough to confirm a diagnosis.

While it has been routine in recent years to suggest amniocentesis to every pregnant woman age 35 and older to screen for Down syndrome, evidence in 2003 began suggesting that it made more sense and was safer to offer blood test screening. The "triple screen" blood test can identify about three-fourths of Down syndrome cases by measuring certain chemicals in the mother's blood.

Chorionic villus sampling

Chorionic villus sampling involves the removal of a small amount of tissue directly from the chorionic villi (minute vascular projections of the fetal chorion that combine with maternal uterine tissue to form the placenta). In the laboratory, the chromosomes of the fetal cells are analyzed for number and type. Extra chromosomes, such as are present in Down syndrome, can be identified. Additional laboratory tests can be performed to look for specific disorders and the results usually are available within a week after the sample is taken. The primary benefit of this procedure is that it is usually performed between weeks 10 and 12 of a pregnancy, allowing earlier detection of fetal disorders. A 2003 study reported that this test resulted in fewer cases of pregnancy loss, amniotic fluid leakage, or birth defects than early amniocentesis.

Preparation

Genetic diagnosis requires that a couple share information about inherited disorders in their background with the genetic counselor, including details of any genetic diseases in either family. A couple undergoing genetic counseling also reports any past miscarriages and discusses the possibility of exposure to chemicals, radiation (including x rays), or other occupational environmental hazards. The couple also needs to disclose information about personal habits before or during pregnancy such as drug or alcohol **abuse** and the use of prescription or over-the-counter drugs taken by the mother since the beginning of pregnancy. The genetic counselor explains the procedures used in testing that will be done and describes what each test can and cannot reveal.

Aftercare

Genetic counseling provides couples with information that can help them make decisions about future pregnancies. It also gives couples additional time to emotionally prepare if a disorder is detected in the fetus. The counselor discusses the results of testing and informs the couple if a problem is apparent. The doctor or genetic counselor also discusses the treatment options available. Genetic counseling is done in a non-directive way, so that any treatment selected remains the personal choice of the individuals involved. Genetic counseling can provide information essential for family planning and pregnancy management, thus maximizing the chances of a positive outcome.

Risks

Because prenatal testing, such as amniocentesis and chorionic villus sampling, is invasive and carries a 1% risk of miscarriage it should never be considered routine.

Normal results

Screening tests and/or prenatal tests reveal no birth defects or genetic abnormalities.

Abnormal results

A birth defect or genetic disorder is detected. The early diagnosis of birth defects and genetic disorders allows a greater number of treatment options. Some disorders can be treated in utero (before birth while the fetus is still in the uterus), while others may require early delivery, immediate surgery, or **cesarean section** to minimize fetal trauma. Prior warning of fetal difficulties allows parents time to prepare emotionally for the birth of the child. In some instances, termination

KEY TERMS

Sickle-cell anemia—A chronic, inherited blood disorder characterized by crescent-shaped red blood cells. It occurs primarily in people of African descent, and produces symptoms including episodic pain in the joints, fever, leg ulcers, and jaundice.

Tay-Sachs disease—A hereditary disease affecting young children of eastern European Jewish descent. This disease is caused by an enzyme deficiency leading to the accumulation of gangliosides (galactose-containing cerebrosides) found in the surface membranes of nerve cells in the brain and nerve tissue. This deficiency results in mental retardation, convulsions, blindness, and, finally, death.

Thalassemia—An inherited group of anemias occurring primarily among people of Mediterranean descent. It is caused by defective formation of part of the hemoglobin molecule.

of the pregnancy may be chosen. Whatever the test results, this information is essential for family planning and pregnancy management.

Resources

PERIODICALS

"Best Early Test." *Fit Pregnancy* (October-November, 2003): 37.

"Blood Test Screening Reduces Need for Amniocentesis." *Womenós Health Weekly* (December 4, 2003): 51.

Bodenhorn, Nancy, and Gerald Lawson. "Genetic Counseling: Implications for Community Counselors." *Journal of Counseling and Development* (Fall 2003): 497–495.

"Genetic Counseling Questionnaire Helps Assess FamilyÆs Genetic History." *Internal Medicine News* (April 15, 2004): 45.

"Genetic Counseling Reduces WomenÆs Fears." *Womenós Health Weekly* (September 11, 2003): 23.

Wechsler, Jill. "From Genome Exploration to Drug Development." *Pharmaceutical Technology Europe* (June 2003): 18–23.

ORGANIZATIONS

American Medical Association. 515 N. State St., Chicago, IL 60612. (312) 464-5000. <http://www.ama-assn.org>.

American Society of Human Genetics. 9650 Rockville Pike, Bethesda, MD 20814-3998. (301) 571-1825. <http://www.faseb.org/genetics/ashg/ashgmenu.htm>.

March of Dimes Birth Defects Foundation. 1275 Mamaroneck Ave., White Plains, NY 10605. (914) 428-7100. resourcecenter@modimes.org. <http://www.modimes.org>.

Jeffrey P. Larson, RPT
Teresa G. Odle

Genetic studies *see* **Genetic testing**

Genetic testing

Definition

A genetic test examines the genetic information contained inside a person's cells, called DNA, to determine if that person has or will develop a certain disease or could pass a disease to his or her offspring. Genetic tests also determine whether or not couples are at a higher risk than the general population for having a child affected with a genetic disorder.

Purpose

Some families or ethnic groups have a higher incidence of a certain disease than the population as a whole. For example, individuals from Eastern European, Ashkenazi Jewish descent are at higher risk for carrying genes for rare conditions that occur much less frequently in populations from other parts of the world. Before having a child, a couple from such a family or ethnic group may want to know if their child would be at risk of having that disease. Genetic testing for this type of purpose is called genetic screening.

During **pregnancy**, a baby's cells can be studied for certain genetic disorders or chromosomal problems such as **Down syndrome**. Chromosome testing is most commonly offered when the mother is 35 years or older at the time of delivery. When there is a family medical history of a genetic disease or there are individuals in a family affected with developmental and physical delays, genetic testing also may be offered during pregnancy. Genetic testing during pregnancy is called prenatal diagnosis.

Prior to becoming pregnant, couples who are having difficulty conceiving a child or who have suffered multiple miscarriages may be tested to see if a genetic cause can be identified.

A genetic disease may be diagnosed at birth by doing a physical evaluation of the baby and observing characteristics of the disorder. Genetic testing can help to confirm the diagnosis made by the physical evaluation. In addition, genetic testing is used routinely on all newborns to screen for certain genetic diseases that can affect a newborn baby's health shortly after birth.

There are several genetic diseases and conditions in which the symptoms do not occur until adulthood. One such example is Huntington's disease. This is a serious disorder affecting the way in which individuals walk, talk and function on a daily basis. Genetic testing may be able to determine if someone at risk will in fact develop the disease.

Genetic testing may take on new emphasis in the near future as genetic research continues to advance. In April 2003, the Human Genome Project announced completion of mapping the entire human genetic makeup. The project identified more than 1,400 disease genes and completed study of the ethical, legal, and social issues raised by this expanded knowledge of human genetics. As knowledge expands and scientists discover more methods to identify and treat various diseases, people will face more difficult decisions about their own genetic information. In fact, the amount of genetic testing was increasing internationally in 2003, especially for rare diseases.

Some genetic defects may make a person more susceptible to certain types of **cancer**. Testing for these defects can help predict a person's risk. Other types of genetic tests help diagnose and predict and monitor the course of certain kinds of cancer, particularly leukemia and lymphoma.

Precautions

Because genetic testing is not always accurate and because there are many concerns surrounding insurance and employment discrimination for the individual receiving a genetic test, **genetic counseling** should always be performed prior to genetic testing. A genetic counselor is an individual with a master's degree in genetic counseling. A medical geneticist is a physician specializing and board certified in genetics.

A genetic counselor reviews the person's family history and medical records and the reason for the test. The counselor explains the likelihood that the test will detect all possible causes of the disease in question (known as the sensitivity of the test), and the likelihood that the disease will develop if the test is positive (known as the positive predictive value of the test).

Learning about the disease in question, the benefits and risks of both a positive and a negative result, and what treatment choices are available if the result is positive, will help prepare the person undergoing testing. During the genetic counseling session, the individual interested in genetic testing will be asked to consider how the test results will affect his or her life, family, and future decisions.

After this discussion, the person should have the opportunity to indicate in writing that he or she gave informed consent to have the test performed, verifying that the counselor provided complete and understandable information.

Description

Genes and chromosomes

Deoxyribonucleic acid (DNA) is a long molecule made up of two strands of genetic material coiled around each other in a unique double helix structure. This structure was discovered in 1953 by Francis Crick and James Watson.

DNA is found in the nucleus, or center, of most cells (Some cells, such as a red blood cell, don't have a nucleus). Each person's DNA is a unique blueprint, giving instructions for a person's physical traits, such as eye color, hair texture, height, and susceptibility to disease. DNA is organized into structures called chromosomes.

The instructions are contained in DNA's long strands as a code spelled out by pairs of bases, which are four chemicals that make up DNA. The bases occur as pairs because a base on one strand lines up with and is bound to a corresponding base on the other strand. The order of these bases form DNA's code. The order of the bases on a DNA strand is important to ensuring that we are not affected with any genetic diseases. When the bases are out of order, or missing, our cells often do not produce important proteins which can lead to a genetic disorder. While our genes are found in every cell of our body, not every gene is functioning all of the time. Some genes are turned on during critical points in development and then remain silent for the rest of our lives. Other genes remain active all of our lives so that our cells can produce important proteins that help us digest food properly or fight off the **common cold**.

The specific order of the base pairs on a strand of DNA is important in order for the correct protein to be produced. A grouping of three base pairs on the DNA strand is called a codon. Each codon, or three base pairs, comes together to spell a word. A string of many codons together can be thought of as a series of words all coming together to make a sentence. This sentence is what instructs our cells to make a protein that helps our bodies function properly.

Our DNA strands, containing a hundred to several thousand copies of genes, are found on structures called chromosomes. Each cell typically has 46 chromosomes arranged into 23 pairs. Each parent contributes one chromosome to each pair. The first 22 pairs are called autosomal chromosomes, or non-sex chromosomes, and are assigned a number from 1–22. The last pair are the sex chromosomes and include the X and Y chromosomes. If a child receives an X chromosome from each parent, the child is female. If a child receives an X from the mother, and a Y from the father, the child is male.

Just as each parent contributes one chromosome to each pair, so each parent contributes one gene from each chromosome. The pair of genes produces a specific trait in the child. In autosomal dominant conditions, it takes only one copy of a gene to influence a specific trait. The stronger gene is called dominant; the weaker gene, recessive. Two copies of a recessive gene are needed to control a trait while only one copy of a dominant gene is needed. Our sex chromosomes, the X and the Y, also contain important genes. Some genetic diseases are caused by missing or altered genes on one of the sex chromosomes. Males are most often affected by sex chromosome diseases when they inherit an X chromosome with missing or mutated genes from their mother.

TYPES OF GENETIC MUTATIONS. Genetic disease results from a change, or mutation, in a chromosome or in one or several base pairs on a gene. Some of us inherit these mutations from our parents, called hereditary or germline mutations, while other mutations can occur spontaneously, or for the first time in an affected child. For many of the adult on-set diseases, genetic mutations can occur over the lifetime of the individual. This is called acquired or somatic mutations and these occur while the cells are making copies of themselves or dividing in two. There may be some environmental effects, such as radiation or other chemicals, which can contribute to these types of mutations as well.

There are a variety of different types of mutations that can occur in our genetic code to cause a disease. And for each genetic disease, there may be more than one type of mutation to cause the disease. For some genetic diseases, the same mutation occurs in every individual affected with the disease. For example, the most common form of dwarfism, called **achondroplasia**, occurs because of a single base pair substitution. This same mutation occurs in all individuals affected with the disease. Other genetic diseases are caused by different types of genetic mutations that may occur anywhere along the length of a gene. For example, **cystic fibrosis**, the most common genetic disease in

the caucasian population is caused by over hundreds of different mutations along the gene. Individual families may carry the same mutation as each other, but not as the rest of the population affected with the same genetic disease.

Some genetic diseases occur as a result of a larger mutation which can occur when the chromosome itself is either rearranged or altered or when a baby is born with more than the expected number of chromosomes. There are only a few types of chromosome rearrangements which are possibly hereditary, or passed on from the mother or the father. The majority of chromosome alterations where the baby is born with too many chromosomes or missing a chromosome, occur sporadically or for the first time with a new baby.

The type of mutation that causes a genetic disease will determine the type of genetic test to be performed. In some situations, more than one type of genetic test will be performed to arrive at a diagnosis. The cost of genetic tests vary: chromosome studies can cost hundreds of dollars and certain gene studies, thousands. Insurance coverage also varies with the company and the policy. It may take several days or several weeks to complete a test. Research testing where the exact location of a gene has not yet been identified, can take several months to years for results.

Types of Genetic Testing

Direct DNA mutation analysis

Direct DNA sequencing examines the direct base pair sequence of a gene for specific gene mutations. Some genes contain more than 100,000 bases and a mutation of any one base can make the gene nonfunctional and cause disease. The more mutations possible, the less likely it is for a test to detect all of them. This test usually is done on white blood cells from a person's blood but also can be performed on other tissues. There are different ways in which to perform direct DNA mutation analysis. When the specific genetic mutation is known, it is possible to perform a complete analysis of the genetic code, also called direct sequencing. There are several different lab techniques used to test for a direct mutation. One common approach begins by using chemicals to separate DNA from the rest of the cell. Next, the two strands of DNA are separated by heating. Special enzymes (called restriction enzymes) are added to the single strands of DNA and then act like scissors, cutting the strands in specific places. The DNA fragments are then sorted by size through a process called electrophoresis. A special piece of DNA, called a probe, is added to the fragments. The probe is designed to bind to specific mutated portions of the gene. When bound to the probe, the mutated portions appear on x-ray film with a distinct banding pattern.

Indirect DNA Testing

Family linkage studies are done to study a disease when the exact type and location of the genetic alteration is not known, but the general location on the chromosome has been identified. These studies are possible when a chromosome marker has been found associated with a disease. Chromosomes contain certain regions that vary in appearance between individuals. These regions are called polymorphisms and do not cause a genetic disease to occur. If a polymorphism is always present in family members with the same genetic disease, and absent in family members without the disease, it is likely that the gene responsible for the disease is near that polymorphism. The gene mutation can be indirectly detected in family members by looking for the polymorphism.

To look for the polymorphism, DNA is isolated from cells in the same way it is for direct DNA mutation analysis. A probe is added that will detect the large polymorphism on the chromosome. When bound to the probe, this region will appear on x-ray film with a distinct banding pattern. The pattern of banding of a person being tested for the disease is compared to the pattern from a family member affected by the disease.

Linkage studies have disadvantages not found in direct DNA mutation analysis. These studies require multiple family members to participate in the testing. If key family members choose not to participate, the incomplete family history may make testing other members useless. The indirect method of detecting a mutated gene also causes more opportunity for error.

Chromosome analysis

Various genetic syndromes are caused by structural chromosome abnormalities. To analyze a person's chromosomes, his or her cells are allowed to grow and multiply in the laboratory until they reach a certain stage of growth. The length of growing time varies with the type of cells. Cells from blood and bone marrow take one to two days; fetal cells from amniotic fluid take seven to 10 days.

When the cells are ready, they are placed on a microscope slide using a technique to make them burst open, spreading their chromosomes. The slides are stained: the stain creates a banding pattern unique to each chromosome. Under a microscope, the chromosomes are counted, identified, and analyzed based on their size, shape, and stained appearance.

A karyotype is the final step in the chromosome analysis. After the chromosomes are counted, a photograph is taken of the chromosomes from one or more cells as seen through the microscope. Then the chromosomes are cut out and arranged side-by-side with their partner in ascending numerical order, from largest to smallest. The karyotype is done either manually or using a computer attached to the microscope. Chromosome analysis also is called cytogenetics.

Applications for Genetic Testing

Newborn screening

Genetic testing is used most often for newborn screening. Every year, millions of newborn babies have their blood samples tested for potentially serious genetic diseases.

Carrier testing

An individual who has a gene associated with a disease but never exhibits any symptoms of the disease is called a carrier. A carrier is a person who is not affected by the mutated gene he or she possesses, but can pass the gene to an offspring. Genetic tests have been developed that tell prospective parents whether or not they are carriers of certain diseases. If one or both parents are a carrier, the risk of passing the disease to a child can be predicted.

To predict the risk, it is necessary to know if the gene in question is autosomal or sex-linked. If the gene is carried on any one of chromosomes 1–22, the resulting disease is called an autosomal disease. If the gene is carried on the X or Y chromosome, it is called a sex-linked disease.

Sex-linked diseases, such as the bleeding condition **hemophilia**, are usually carried on the X chromosome. A woman who carries a disease-associated mutated gene on one of her X chromosomes, has a 50% chance of passing the gene to her son. A son who inherits that gene will develop the disease because he does not have another normal copy of the gene on a second X chromosome to compensate for the mutated copy. A daughter who inherits the disease associated mutated gene from her mother on one of her X chromosomes will be at risk for having a son affected with the disease.

The risk of passing an autosomal disease to a child depends on whether the gene is dominant or recessive. A prospective parent carrying a dominant gene has a 50% chance of passing the gene to a child. A child needs to receive only one copy of the mutated gene to be affected by the disease.

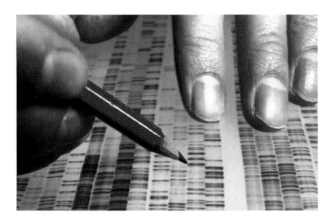

A scientist examines a DNA sequencing autoradiogram on a light box. *(Photo Researchers, Inc. Reproduced by permission.)*

If the gene is recessive, a child needs to receive two copies of the mutated gene, one from each parent, to be affected by the disease. When both prospective parents are carriers, their child has a 25% chance of inheriting two copies of the mutated gene and being affected by the disease; a 50% chance of inheriting one copy of the mutated gene, and being a carrier of the disease but not affected; and a 25% chance of inheriting two normal genes. When only one prospective parent is a carrier, a child has a 50% chance of inheriting one mutated gene and being an unaffected carrier of the disease, and a 50% chance of inheriting two normal genes.

Cystic fibrosis is a disease that affects the lungs and pancreas and is discovered in early childhood. It is the most common autosomal recessive genetic disease found in the caucasian population: one in 25 people of Northern European ancestry are carriers of a mutated cystic fibrosis gene. The gene, located on chromosome 7, was identified in 1989.

The gene mutation for cystic fibrosis is detected by a direct DNA test. More than 600 mutations of the cystic fibrosis gene have been found; each of these mutations causes the same disease. Tests are available for the most common mutations. Tests that check for 86 of the most common mutations in the Caucasian population will detect 90% of carriers for cystic fibrosis. (The percentage of mutations detected varies according to the individual's ethnic background). If a person tests negative, it is likely, but not guaranteed that he or she does not have the gene. Both prospective parents must be carriers of the gene to have a child with cystic fibrosis.

Tay-Sachs disease, also autosomal recessive, affects children primarily of Ashkenazi Jewish descent. Children with this disease die between the ages

of two and five. This disease was previously detected by looking for a missing enzyme. The mutated gene has now been identified and can be detected using direct DNA mutation analysis.

Presymptomatic testing

Not all genetic diseases show their effect immediately at birth or early in childhood. Although the gene mutation is present at birth, some diseases do not appear until adulthood. If a specific mutated gene responsible for a late-onset disease has been identified, a person from an affected family can be tested before symptoms appear.

Huntington's disease is one example of a late-onset autosomal dominant disease. Its symptoms of mental confusion and abnormal body movements do not appear until middle to late adulthood. The chromosome location of the gene responsible for Huntington's chorea was located in 1983 after studying the DNA from a large Venezuelan family affected by the disease. Ten years later the gene was identified. A test now is available to detect the presence of the expanded base pair sequence responsible for causing the disease. The presence of this expanded sequence means the person will develop the disease.

The specific genetic cause of **Alzheimer's disease**, another late onset disease, is not as clear. Although many cases appear to be inherited in an autosomal dominant pattern, many other cases exist as single incidents in a family. Like Huntington's, symptoms of mental deterioration first appear in adulthood. Genetic research has found an association between this disease and genes on four different chromosomes. The validity of looking for these genes in a person without symptoms or without family history of the disease is still being studied.

CANCER SUSCEPTIBILITY TESTING. Cancer can result from an inherited (germline) mutated gene or a gene that mutated sometime during a person's lifetime (acquired mutation). Some genes, called tumor suppressor genes, produce proteins that protect the body from cancer. If one of these genes develops a mutation, it is unable to produce the protective protein. If the second copy of the gene is normal, its action may be sufficient to continue production, but if that gene later also develops a mutation, the person is vulnerable to cancer. Other genes, called oncogenes, are involved in the normal growth of cells. A mutation in an oncogene can cause too much growth, the beginning of cancer.

Direct DNA tests currently are available to look for gene mutations identified and linked to several kinds of cancer. People with a family history of these cancers are those most likely to be tested. If one of these mutated genes is found, the person is more susceptible to developing the cancer. The likelihood that the person will develop the cancer, even with the mutated gene, is not always known because other genetic and environmental factors also are involved in the development of cancer.

Cancer susceptibility tests are most useful when a positive test result can be followed with clear treatment options. In families with **familial polyposis** of the colon, testing a child for a mutated APC gene can reveal whether or not the child needs frequent monitoring for the disease. In 2003, reports showed that genetic testing for high-risk **colon cancer** patients has improved risk assessment. In families with potentially fatal familial medullary **thyroid cancer** or multiple endocrine neoplasia type 2, finding a mutated RET gene in a child provides the opportunity for that child to have preventive removal of the thyroid gland. In the same way, MSH1 and MSH2 mutations can reveal which members in an affected family are vulnerable to familiar colorectal cancer and would benefit from aggressive monitoring.

In 1994, a mutation linked to early-onset familial breast and **ovarian cancer** was identified. BRCA1 is located on chromosome 17. Women with a mutated form of this gene have an increased risk of developing breast and ovarian cancer. A second related gene, BRCA2, was later discovered. Located on chromosome 13, it also carries increased risk of breast and ovarian cancer. Although both genes are rare in the general population, they are slightly more common in women of Ashkenazi Jewish descent.

When a woman is found to have a mutation of one of these genes, the likelihood that she will get breast or ovarian cancer increases, but not to 100%. Other genetic and environmental factors influence the outcome.

Testing for these genes is most valuable in families where a mutation has already been found. BRCA1 and BRCA2 are large genes; BRCA1 includes 100,000 bases. More than 120 mutations to this gene have been discovered, but a mutation could occur in any one of the bases. Studies show tests for these genes may miss 30% of existing mutations. The rate of missed mutations, the unknown disease likelihood in spite of a positive result, and the lack of a clear preventive response to a positive result, make the value of this test for the general population uncertain.

Prenatal and postnatal chromosome analysis

Chromosome analysis can be done on fetal cells primarily when the mother is age 35 or older at the time of delivery, experienced multiple miscarriages, or reports a family history of a genetic abnormality. Prenatal testing is done on the fetal cells from a **chorionic villus sampling** (from the baby's developing placenta) at 9–12 weeks or from the amniotic fluid (the fluid surrounding the baby) at 15–22 weeks of pregnancy. Cells from amniotic fluid grow for seven to 10 days before they are ready to be analyzed. Chorionic villi cells have the potential to grow faster and can be analyzed sooner.

Chromosome analysis using blood cells is done on a child who is born with or later develops signs of **mental retardation** or physical malformation. In the older child, chromosome analysis may be done to investigate developmental delays.

Extra or missing chromosomes cause mental and physical abnormalities. A child born with an extra chromosome 21 (trisomy 21) has Down syndrome. An extra chromosome 13 or 18 also produce well known syndromes. A missing X chromosome causes **Turner syndrome** and an extra X in a male causes **Klinefelter syndrome**. Other abnormalities are caused by extra or missing pieces of chromosomes. **Fragile X syndrome** is a sex-linked disease, causing mental retardation in males.

Chromosome material also may be rearranged, such as the end of chromosome 1 moved to the end of chromosome 3. This is called a chromosomal translocation. If no material is added or deleted in the exchange, the person may not be affected. Such an exchange, however, can cause **infertility** or abnormalities if passed to children.

Evaluation of a man and woman's infertility or repeated miscarriages will include blood studies of both to check for a chromosome translocation. Many chromosome abnormalities are incompatible with life; babies with these abnormalities often miscarry during the first trimester. Cells from a baby that died before birth can be studied to look for chromosome abnormalities that may have caused the **death**.

Cancer diagnosis and prognosis

Certain cancers, particularly leukemia and lymphoma, are associated with changes in chromosomes: extra or missing complete chromosomes, extra or missing portions of chromosomes, or exchanges of material (translocations) between chromosomes. Studies show that the locations of the chromosome breaks are at locations of tumor suppressor genes or oncogenes.

Chromosome analysis on cells from blood, bone marrow, or solid tumor helps diagnose certain kinds of leukemia and lymphoma and often helps predict how well the person will respond to treatment. After treatment has begun, periodic monitoring of these chromosome changes in the blood and bone marrow gives the physician information as to the effectiveness of the treatment.

A well-known chromosome rearrangement is found in chronic myelogenous leukemia. This leukemia is associated with an exchange of material between chromosomes 9 and 22. The resulting smaller chromosome 22 is called the Philadelphia chromosome.

Preparation

Most tests for genetic diseases of children and adults are done on blood. To collect the 5–10 mL of blood needed, a healthcare worker draws blood from a vein in the inner elbow region. Collection of the sample takes only a few minutes.

Prenatal testing is done either on amniotic fluid or a chorionic villus sampling. To collect amniotic fluid, a physician performs a procedure called **amniocentesis**. An ultrasound is done to find the baby's position and an area filled with amniotic fluid. The physician inserts a needle through the woman's skin and the wall of her uterus and withdraws 5–10 mL of amniotic fluid. Placental tissue for a chorionic villus sampling is taken through the cervix. Each procedure takes approximately 30 minutes. A 2003 study comparing the two tests reported that chorionic villus sampling resulted in fewer cases of pregnancy loss, amniotic fluid leakage, and **birth defects**.

Bone marrow is used for chromosome analysis in a person with leukemia or lymphoma. The person is given **local anesthesia**. Then the physician inserts a needle through the skin and into the bone (usually the sternum or hip bone). One-half to 2 mL of bone marrow is withdrawn. This procedure takes approximately 30 minutes.

Aftercare

After blood collection the person can feel discomfort or bruising at the puncture site or may become dizzy or faint. Pressure to the puncture site until the bleeding stops reduces bruising. Warm packs to the puncture site relieve discomfort.

Chorionic villus sampling, amniocentesis and bone marrow procedures are done under a physician's supervision. The person is asked to rest after the procedure and is watched for weakness and signs of bleeding.

Risks

Collection of amniotic fluid and chorionic villus sampling, have the risk of **miscarriage**, infection, and bleeding; the risks are higher for the chorionic villus sampling. Because of the potential risks for miscarriage, 0.5% following the amniocentesis and 1% following the chorionic villus sampling procedure, both of these prenatal tests are offered to couples, but not required. A woman should tell her physician immediately if she has cramping, bleeding, fluid loss, an increased temperature, or a change in the baby's movement following either of these procedures.

After bone marrow collection, the puncture site may become tender and the person's temperature may rise. These are signs of a possible infection.

Genetic testing involves other nonphysical risks. Many people fear the possible loss of privacy about personal health information. Results of genetic tests may be reported to insurance companies and affect a person's insurability. Some people pay out-of-pocket for genetic tests to avoid this possibility. Laws have been proposed to deal with this problem. Other family members may be affected by the results of a person's genetic test. Privacy of the person tested and the family members affected is a consideration when deciding to have a test and to share the results.

A positive result carries a psychological burden, especially if the test indicates the person will develop a disease, such as Huntington's chorea. The news that a person may be susceptible to a specific kind of cancer, while it may encourage positive preventive measures, also may negatively shadow many decisions and activities.

A genetic test result may also be inconclusive, meaning no definitive result can be given to the individual or family. This may cause the individual to feel more anxious and frustrated and experience psychological difficulties.

Prior to undergoing genetic testing, individuals need to learn from the genetic counselor the likelihood that the test could miss a mutation or abnormality.

Normal results

A normal result for chromosome analysis is 46, XX or 46, XY. This means there are 46 chromosomes (including two X chromosomes for a female or one X and one Y for a male) with no structural abnormalities. A normal result for a direct DNA mutation analysis or linkage study is no gene mutation found.

KEY TERMS

Autosomal disease—A disease caused by a gene located on a chromosome other than a sex chromosome (autosomal chromosome).

Carrier—A person who possesses a gene for an abnormal trait without showing signs of the disorder. The person may pass the abnormal gene on to offspring.

Chromosome—A microscopic thread-like structure found within each cell of the body that consists of a complex of proteins and DNA. Humans have 46 chromosomes arranged into 23 pairs. Changes in either the total number of chromosomes or their shape and size (structure) may lead to physical or mental abnormalities.

Deoxyribonucleic acid (DNA)—The genetic material in cells that holds the inherited instructions for growth, development, and cellular functioning.

Dominant gene—A gene, whose presence as a single copy, controls the expression of a trait.

Enzyme—A protein that catalyzes a biochemical reaction or change without changing its own structure or function.

Gene—A building block of inheritance, which contains the instructions for the production of a particular protein, and is made up of a molecular

sequence found on a section of DNA. Each gene is found on a precise location on a chromosome.

Karyotype—A standard arrangement of photographic or computer-generated images of chromosome pairs from a cell in ascending numerical order, from largest to smallest.

Mutation—A permanent change in the genetic material that may alter a trait or characteristic of an individual, or manifest as disease, and can be transmitted to offspring.

Positive predictive value (PPV)—The probability that a person with a positive test result has, or will get, the disease.

Recessive gene—A type of gene that is not expressed as a trait unless inherited by both parents.

Sensitivity—The proportion of people with a disease who are correctly diagnosed (test positive based on diagnostic criteria). The higher the sensitivity of a test or diagnostic criteria, the lower the rate of 'false negatives,' people who have a disease but are not identified through the test.

Sex-linked disorder—A disorder caused by a gene located on a sex chromosome, usually the X chromosome.

There can be some benefits from genetic testing when the individual tested is not found to carry a genetic mutation. Those who learn with certainty they are no longer at risk for a genetic disease may choose not to undergo preventive therapies and may feel less anxious and relieved.

Abnormal results

An abnormal chromosome analysis report will include the total number of chromosomes and will identify the abnormality found. Tests for gene mutations will report the mutations found.

There are many ethical issues to consider with an abnormal prenatal test result. Many of the diseases tested for during a pregnancy cannot be treated or cured. In addition, some diseases tested for during pregnancy may have a late-onset of symptoms or have minimal effects on the affected individual.

Before making decisions based on an abnormal test result, the person should meet again with a genetic

counselor to fully understand the meaning of the results, learn what options are available based on the test result, and the risks and benefits of each of those options.

Resources

PERIODICALS

"Best Early Test." *Fit Pregnancy* (October-November, 2003): 37.

Bodenhorn, Nancy, and Gerald Lawson. "Genetic Counseling: Implications for Community Counselors." *Journal of Counseling and Development* (Fall 2003): 497–495.

"Genetic Testing for High-risk Colon Cancer Patients has Improved Risk Assessment." *Genomics & Genetics Weekly* (August 1, 2003): 18.

"Genetic Testing Increasing Internationally." *Health & Medicine Week* (September 29, 2003): 283.

Wechsler, Jill. "From Genome Exploration to Drug Development." *Pharmaceutical Technology Europe* (June 2003): 18–23.

Yan, Hai. "Genetic Testing-Present and Future." *Science* (September 15, 2000): 1890-1892.

ORGANIZATIONS

Alliance of Genetic Support Groups. 4301 Connecticut Ave. NW, Suite 404, Washington, DC 20008. (202) 966-5557. Fax: (202) 966-8553. < http://www.geneticalliance.org > .

American College of Medical Genetics. 9650 Rockville Pike, Bethesda, MD 20814-3998. (301) 571-1825. < http://www.faseb.org/genetics/acmg/acmgmenu.htm > .

American Society of Human Genetics. 9650 Rockville Pike, Bethesda, MD 20814-3998. (301) 571-1825. < http://www.faseb.org/genetics/ashg/ashgmenu.htm > .

Centers for Disease Control. GDP Office, 4770 Buford Highway NE, Atlanta, GA 30341-3724. (770) 488-3235. < http://www.cdc.gov/genetics > .

March of Dimes Birth Defects Foundation. 1275 Mamaroneck Ave., White Plains, NY 10605. (888) 663-4637. resourcecenter@modimes.org. < http://www.modimes.org > .

National Human Genome Research Institute. The National Institutes of Health, 9000 Rockville Pike, Bethesda, MD 20892. (301) 496-2433. < http://www.nhgri.nih.gov > .

National Society of Genetic Counselors. 233 Canterbury Dr., Wallingford, PA 19086-6617. (610) 872-1192. < http://www.nsgc.org/GeneticCounselingYou.asp > .

OTHER

Blazing a Genetic Trail. Online genetic tutorial. < http://www.hhmi.org/GeneticTrail/ > .

The Gene Letter. Online newsletter. < http://www.geneletter.org > .

Online Mendelian Inheritance in Man. Online genetic testing information sponsored by National Center for Biotechnology Information. < http://www.ncbi.nlm.-nih.gov/Omim/ > .

Understanding Gene Testing. Online brochure produced by the U.S. Department of Health and Human Services. < http://www.gene.com/ae/AE/AEPC/NIH/index.html > .

Katherine S. Hunt, MS
Teresa G. Odle

Genital herpes

Definition

Genital herpes is a sexually transmitted disease caused by a herpes virus. The disease is characterized by the formation of fluid-filled, painful blisters in the genital area.

Description

Genital herpes (herpes genitalis, herpes progenitalis) is characterized by the formation of fluid-filled blisters on the genital organs of men and women. The word "herpes" comes from the Greek adjective *herpestes,* meaning *creeping,* which refers to the serpent-like pattern that the blisters may form. Genital herpes is a sexually transmitted disease which means that it is spread from person-to-person only by sexual contact. Herpes may be spread by vaginal, anal, and oral sexual activity. It is not spread by objects (such as a toilet seat or doorknob), swimming pools, hot tubs, or through the air.

Genital herpes is a disease resulting from an infection by a herpes simplex virus. There are eight different kinds of human herpes viruses. Only two of these, herpes simplex types 1 and 2, can cause genital herpes. It has been commonly believed that herpes simplex virus type 1 infects above the waist (causing cold sores) and herpes simplex virus type 2 infects below the waist (causing genital sores). This is not completely true. Both herpes virus type 1 and type 2 can cause herpes lesions on the lips or genitals, but recurrent cold sores are almost always type 1. The two viruses seem to have evolved to infect better at one site or the other, especially with regard to recurrent disease.

To determine the occurrence of herpes type 2 infection in the United States, the Centers for Disease Control and Prevention (CDC) used information from a survey called the National Health and **Nutrition** Examination Survey III (1988–1994). This survey of 40,000 noninstitutionalized people found that 21.9% of persons age 12 or older had antibodies to herpes type 2. This means that 45 million Americans have been exposed at some point in their lives to herpes simplex virus type 2. More women (25.6%) than men (17.8%) had antibodies. The racial differences for herpes type 2 antibodies were whites, 17.6%; blacks, 45.9%; and Mexican Americans, 22.3%. Interestingly, only 2.6% of adults reported that they have had genital herpes. Over half (50% to 60%) of the white adults in the United States have antibodies to herpes simplex virus type 1. The occurrence of antibodies to herpes type 1 is higher in blacks.

Viruses are different from bacteria. While bacteria are independent and can reproduce on their own, viruses cannot reproduce without the help of a cell. Viruses enter human cells and force them to make more virus. A human cell infected with herpes virus releases thousands of new viruses before it is killed. The cell death and resulting tissue damage causes the actual sores. The highest risk for spreading the virus is the time period beginning with the appearance of blisters and ending with scab formation.

Herpes virus can also infect a cell and instead of making the cell produce new viruses, it hides inside the cell and waits. Herpes virus hides in cells of the nervous system called "neurons." This is called "latency." A latent virus can wait inside neurons for days, months, or even years. At some future time, the virus "awakens" and causes the cell to produce thousands of new viruses which causes an active infection. Sometimes an active infection occurs without visible sores. Therefore, an infected person can spread herpes virus to other people even in the absence of sores.

This process of latency and active infection is best understood by considering the genital sore cycle. An active infection is obvious because sores are present. The first infection is called the "primary" infection. This active infection is then controlled by the body's immune system and the sores heal. In between active infections, the virus is latent. At some point in the future latent viruses become activated and once again cause sores. These are called "recurrent infections" or "outbreaks." Genital sores caused by herpes type 1 recur much less frequently than sores caused by herpes type 2.

Although it is unknown what triggers latent viruses to activate, several conditions seem to bring on infections. These include illness, tiredness, exposure to sunlight, menstruation, skin damage, food allergy and hot or cold temperatures. Although many people believe that **stress** can bring on their genital herpes outbreaks, there is no scientific evidence that there is a link between stress and recurrences. However, at least one clinical study has shown a connection between how well people cope with stress and their belief that stress and recurrent infections are linked.

Newborn babies who are infected with herpes virus experience a very severe, and possibly fatal disease. This is called "neonatal herpes infection." In the United States, one in 3,000–5,000 babies born will be infected with herpes virus. Babies can become infected during passage through the birth canal, but can become infected during the **pregnancy** if the membranes rupture early. Doctors will perform a **Cesarean section** on women who go into labor with active genital herpes.

Causes and symptoms

While anyone can be infected by herpes virus, not everyone will show symptoms. Risk factors for genital herpes include: early age at first sexual activity, multiple sexual partners, and a medical history of other sexually-transmitted diseases.

Most patients with genital herpes experience a prodrome (symptoms of oncoming disease) of **pain**, burning, **itching**, or **tingling** at the site where blisters will form. This prodrome stage may last anywhere from a few hours, to one to two days. The herpes infection prodrome can occur for both the primary infection and recurrent infections. The prodrome for recurrent infections may be severe and cause a severe burning or stabbing pain in the genital area, legs, or buttocks.

Primary genital herpes

The first symptoms of herpes usually occur within two to seven days after contact with an infected person but may take up to two weeks. Symptoms of the primary infection are usually more severe than those of recurrent infections. For up to 70% of the patients, the primary infection causes symptoms which affect the whole body (called "constitutional symptoms") including tiredness, **headache**, **fever**, chills, muscle aches, loss of appetite, as well as painful, swollen lymph nodes in the groin. These symptoms are greatest during the first three to four days of the infection and disappear within one week. The primary infection is more severe in women than in men.

Following the prodrome come the herpes blisters, which are similar on men and women. First, small red bumps appear. These bumps quickly become fluid-filled blisters. In dry areas, the blisters become filled with pus and take on a white to gray appearance, become covered with a scab, and heal within two to three weeks. In moist areas, the fluid-filled blisters burst and form painful ulcers which drain before healing. New blisters may appear over a period of one week or longer and may join together to form very large ulcers. The pain is relieved within two weeks and the blisters and ulcers heal without scarring by three to four weeks.

Women can experience a very severe and painful primary infection. Herpes blisters first appear on the labia majora (outer lips), labia minora (inner lips), and entrance to the vagina. Blisters often appear on the clitoris, at the urinary opening, around the anal opening, and on the buttocks and thighs. In addition, women may get herpes blisters on the lips, breasts, fingers, and eyes. The vagina and cervix are almost always involved which causes a watery discharge. Other symptoms that occur in women are: painful or difficult urination (83%), swelling of the urinary tube (85%), **meningitis** (36%), and throat infection (13%). Most women develop painful, swollen lymph nodes (lymphadenopathy) in the groin and pelvis. About one

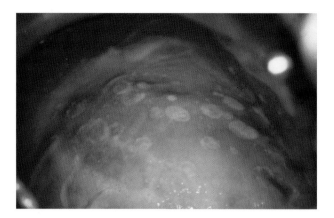

Female cervix covered with herpes lesions *(Photo Researchers. Reproduced by permission.)*

in ten women get a vaginal yeast infection as a complication of the primary herpes infection.

In men, the herpes blisters usually form on the penis but can also appear on the scrotum, thighs, and buttocks. Fewer than half of the men with primary herpes experience the constitutional symptoms. Thirty percent to 40% of men have a discharge from the urinary tube. Some men develop painful swollen lymph nodes (lymphadenopathy) in the groin and pelvis. Although less frequently than women, men too may experience painful or difficult urination (44%), swelling of the urinary tube (27%), meningitis (13%), and throat infection (7%).

Recurrent genital herpes

One or more outbreaks of genital herpes per year occur in 60–90% of those infected with herpes virus. About 40% of the persons infected with herpes simplex virus type 2 will experience six or more outbreaks each year. Genital herpes recurrences are less severe than the primary infection; however, women still experience more severe symptoms and pain than men. Constitutional symptoms are not usually present. Blisters will appear at the same sites during each outbreak. Usually there are fewer blisters, less pain, and the time period from the beginning of symptoms to healing is shorter than the primary infection. One out of every four women experience painful or difficult urination during recurrent infection. Both men and women may develop lymphadenopathy.

Diagnosis

Because genital herpes is so common, it is diagnosed primarily by symptoms. It can be diagnosed and treated by the family doctor, dermatologists (doctors

who specialize in skin diseases), urologists (doctors who specialize in the urinary tract diseases of men and women and the genital organs of men), gynecologists (doctors who specialize in the diseases of women's genital organs) and infectious disease specialists. The diagnosis and treatment of this infectious disease should be covered by most insurance providers.

Laboratory tests may be performed to look for the virus. Because healing sores do not shed much virus, a sample from an open sore would be taken for viral culture. A sterile cotton swab would be wiped over open sores and the sample used to infect human cells in culture. Cells which are killed by herpes virus have a certain appearance under microscopic examination. The results of this test are available within two to ten days. Other areas which may be sampled, depending upon the disease symptoms in a particular patient, include the urinary tract, vagina, cervix, throat, eye tissues, and cerebrospinal fluid.

Direct staining and microscopic examination of the lesion sample may also be used. A blood test may be performed to see if the patient has antibodies to herpes virus. The results of blood testing are available within one day. The disadvantage of this blood test is that it usually does not distinguish between herpes type 1 and 2, and only determines that the patient has had a herpes infection at some point in his or her life. Therefore, the viral culture test must be performed to be absolutely certain that the sores are caused by herpes virus.

Because genital sores can be symptoms of many other diseases, the doctor must determine the exact cause of the sores. The above mentioned tests are performed to determine that herpes virus is causing the genital sores. Other diseases which may cause genital sores are **syphilis**, **chancroid**, **lymphogranuloma venereum**, **granuloma inguinale**, herpes zoster, erythema multiform, Behçet's syndrome, inflammatory bowel disease, **contact dermatitis**, **candidiasis**, and **impetigo**.

Because most newborns who are infected with herpes virus were born to mothers who had no symptoms of infection it is important to check all newborn babies for symptoms. Any skin sore should be sampled to determine if it is caused by herpes simplex. Babies should be checked for sores in their mouth and for signs of herpes infection in their eyes.

Treatment

There is no cure for herpes virus infections. There are **antiviral drugs** available which have some effect in

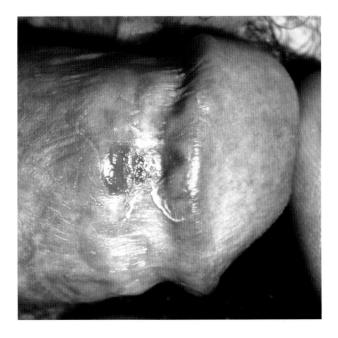

A close-up view of a man's penis with a blister (center of image) caused by the herpes simplex virus. *(Photograph by Dr. P. Marazzi, Custom Medical Stock Photo. Reproduced by permission.)*

lessening the symptoms and decreasing the length of herpes outbreaks. There is evidence that some may also prevent future outbreaks. These antiviral drugs work by interfering with the replication of the viruses and are most effective when taken as early in the infection process as possible. For the best results, drug treatment should begin during the prodrome stage before blisters are visible. Depending on the length of the outbreak, drug treatment could continue for up to 10 days.

Acyclovir (Zovirax) is the drug of choice for herpes infection and can be given intravenously, taken by mouth (orally), or applied directly to sores as an ointment. Acyclovir has been in use for many years and only five out of 100 patients experience side effects. Side effects of acyclovir treatment include **nausea**, **vomiting**, itchy rash, and **hives**. Although acyclovir is the recommended drug for treating herpes infections, other drugs may be used including famciclovir (Famvir), valacyclovir (Valtrex), vidarabine (Vira-A), idoxuridine (Herplex Liquifilm, Stoxil), trifluorothymidine (Viroptic), and penciclovir (Denavir).

Acyclovir is effective in treating both the primary infection and recurrent outbreaks. When taken intravenously or orally, acyclovir reduces the healing time, virus shedding period, and duration of vesicles. The standard oral dose of acyclovir for primary herpes is 200 mg five times daily or 400 mg three times daily for a period of 10 days. Recurrent herpes is treated with the same doses for a period of five days. Intravenous acyclovir is given to patients who require hospitalization because of severe primary infections or herpes complications such as aseptic meningitis or sacral ganglionitis (inflammation of nerve bundles).

Patients with frequent outbreaks (greater than six to eight per year) may benefit from long term use of acyclovir which is called "suppressive therapy." Patients on suppressive therapy have longer periods between herpes outbreaks. The specific dosage used for suppression needs to be determined for each patient and should be reevaluated every few years. Alternatively, patients may use short term suppressive therapy to lessen the chance of developing an active infection during special occasions such as weddings or holidays.

There are several things that a patient may do to lessen the pain of genital sores. Wearing loose fitting clothing and cotton underwear is helpful. Removing clothing or wearing loose pajamas while at home may reduce pain. Soaking in a tub of warm water and using a blow dryer on the "cool" setting to dry the infected area is helpful. Putting an ice pack on the affected area for 10 minutes, followed by five minutes off and then repeating this procedure may relieve pain. A zinc sulfate ointment may help to heal the sores. Application of a baking soda compress to sores may be soothing.

Neonatal herpes

Newborn babies with herpes virus infections are treated with intravenous acyclovir or vidarabine for 10 days. These drugs have greatly reduced deaths and increased the number of babies who appear normal at one year of age. However, because neonatal herpes infection is so serious, even with treatment babies may not survive, or may suffer nervous system damage. Infected babies may be treated with long term suppressive therapy.

Alternative treatment

An imbalance in the amino acids lysine and arginine is thought to be one contributing factor in herpes virus outbreaks. A ratio of lysine to arginine that is in balance (that is more lysine than arginine is present) seems to help the immune system work optimally. Thus, a diet that is rich in lysine may help prevent recurrences of genital herpes. Foods that contain high levels of lysine include most vegetables, legumes, fish, turkey, beef, lamb, cheese, and chicken. Patients may take 500 mg of lysine daily and increase to 1,000 mg three times a day during an outbreak. Intake of the

KEY TERMS

Groin—The region of the body that lies between the abdomen and the thighs.

Latent virus—A nonactive virus which is in a dormant state within a cell. Herpes virus is latent in cells of the nervous system.

Prodrome—Symptoms which warn of the beginning of disease. The herpes prodrome consists of pain, burning, tingling, or itching at a site before blisters are visible.

Recurrence—The return of an active herpes infection following a period of latency.

Ulcer—A painful, pus-draining, depression in the skin caused by an infection.

amino acid arginine should be reduced. Foods rich in arginine that should be avoided are chocolate, peanuts, almonds, and other nuts and seeds.

Clinical experience indicates a connection between high stress and herpes outbreaks. Some patients respond well to **stress reduction** and relaxation techniques. **Acupressure** and massage may relieve tiredness and stress. **Meditation**, **yoga**, **tai chi**, and **hypnotherapy** can also help relieve stress and promote relaxation.

Some herbs, including **echinacea** (*Echinacea* spp.) and garlic (*Allium sativum*), are believed to strengthen the body's defenses against viral infections. Red marine algae (family Dumontiaceae), both taken internally and applied topically, is thought to be effective in treating herpes type I and type II infections. Other topical treatments may be helpful in inhibiting the growth of the herpes virus, in minimizing the damage it causes, or in helping the sores heal. Zinc sulphate ointment seems to help sores heal and to fight recurrence. Lithium succinate ointment may interfere with viral replication. An ointment made with glycyrrhizinic acid, a component of licorice (*Glycyrrhiza glabra*), seems to inactivate the virus. Topical applications of vitamin E or tea tree oil (*Melaleuca* spp.) help dry up herpes sores. Specific combinations of homeopathic remedies may also be helpful treatments for genital herpes.

Prognosis

Although physically and emotionally painful, genital herpes is usually not a serious disease. The primary infection can be severe and may require hospitalization for treatment. Complications of the primary infection may involve the cervix, urinary system, anal opening, and the nervous system. Persons who have a decreased ability to produce an immune response to infection (called "immunocompromised") due to disease or medication are at risk for a very severe, and possibly fatal, herpes infection. Even with antiviral treatment, neonatal herpes infections can be fatal or cause permanent nervous system damage.

Prevention

The only way to prevent genital herpes is to avoid contact with infected persons. This is not an easy solution because many people aren't aware that they are infected and can easily spread the virus to others. Avoid all sexual contact with an infected person during a herpes outbreak. Because herpes virus can be spread at any time, **condom** use is recommended to prevent the spread of virus to uninfected partners. As of early 1998 there were no herpes vaccines available, although new herpes vaccines are being tested in humans.

Resources

BOOKS

Ebel, Charles. *Managing Herpes: How to Live and Love With a Chronic STD*. American Social Health Association, 1998.

Belinda Rowland, PhD

Genital warts

Definition

Genital **warts**, which are also called condylomata acuminata or venereal warts, are growths in the genital area caused by a sexually transmitted papillomavirus. A papillomavirus is a virus that produces papillomas, or benign growths on the skin and mucous membranes.

Description

Genital warts are the most common sexually transmitted disease (STD) in the general population. It is estimated that 1% of sexually active people between the ages of 18 and 45 have genital warts; however, polymerase chain reaction (PCR) testing indicates that as many as 40% of sexually active adults carry the human papillomavirus (HPV) that causes genital warts.

Genital warts vary somewhat in appearance. They may be either flat or resemble raspberries or cauliflower in appearance. The warts begin as small red or pink growths and grow as large as four inches across, interfering with intercourse and **childbirth**. The warts grow in the moist tissues of the genital areas. In women, they occur on the external genitals and on the walls of the vagina and cervix; in men, they develop in the urethra and on the shaft of the penis. The warts then spread to the area behind the genitals surrounding the anus.

Risk factors for genital warts include:

- multiple sexual partners
- infection with another STD
- pregnancy
- anal intercourse
- poor personal hygiene
- heavy perspiration

Causes and symptoms

There are about 80 types of human papillomavirus. Genital warts are caused by HPV types 1, 2, 6, 11, 16, and 18. HPV is transmitted by sexual contact. The incubation period varies from one to six months.

The symptoms include bleeding, **pain**, and odor as well as the visible warts.

Diagnosis

The diagnosis is usually made by examining scrapings from the warts under a darkfield microscope. If the warts are caused by HPV, they will turn white when a 5% solution of white vinegar is added. If the warts reappear, the doctor may order a biopsy to rule out **cancer**.

Treatment

No treatment for genital warts is completely effective because therapy depends on destroying skin infected by the virus. There are no drugs that will kill the virus directly.

Medications

Genital warts were treated until recently with applications of podophyllum resin, a corrosive substance that cannot be given to pregnant patients. A milder form of podophyllum, podofilox (Condylox), has been introduced. Women are also treated with 5-fluorouracil cream, bichloroacetic

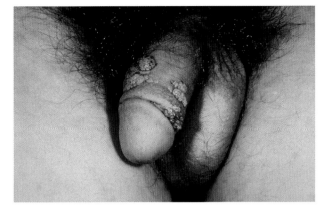

Man with genital warts. (Custom Medical Stock Photo. Reproduced by permission.)

KEY TERMS

Condylomata acuminata—Another name for genital warts.

Papilloma—A benign growth on the skin or mucous membrane. Viruses that cause these growths are called human papillomaviruses (HPVs).

Podophyllum resin—A medication derived from the May apple or mandrake and used to treat genital warts.

---

acid, or trichloroacetic acid. All of these substances irritate the skin and require weeks of treatment.

Genital warts can also be treated with injections of interferon. Interferon works best in combination with podofilox applications.

Surgery

Surgery may be necessary to remove warts blocking the patient's vagina, urethra, or anus. Surgical techniques include the use of liquid nitrogen, electrosurgery, and **laser surgery**.

Prognosis

Genital warts are benign growths and are not cancerous by themselves. Repeated HPV infection in women, however, appears to increase the risk of later **cervical cancer**. Women infected with HPV types 16 and 18 should have yearly cervical smears. Recurrence is common with all present methods of treatment—including surgery—because HPV can remain latent in apparently normal surrounding skin.

Prevention

The only reliable method of prevention is sexual abstinence. The use of condoms minimizes but does not eliminate the risk of HPV transmission. The patient's sexual contacts should be notified and examined.

Resources

BOOKS

Foster, David C. "Vulvar and Vaginal Disease." In *Current Diagnosis*. Vol. 9. edited by Rex B. Conn, et al. Philadelphia: W. B. Saunders Co., 1997.

MacKay, H. Trent. "Gynecology." In *Current Medical Diagnosis and Treatment, 1998,* edited by Stephen McPhee, et al., 37th ed. Stamford: Appleton & Lange, 1997.

Rebecca J. Frey, PhD

Gentamicin *see* **Aminoglycosides**

German measles *see* **Rubella**

Gestalt therapy

Definition

Gestalt therapy is a humanistic therapy technique that focuses on gaining an awareness of emotions and behaviors in the present rather than in the past. The therapist does not interpret experiences for the patient. Instead, the therapist and patient work together to help the patient understand him/herself. This type of therapy focuses on experiencing the present situation rather than talking about what occurred in the past. Patients are encouraged to become aware of immediate needs, meet them, and let them recede into the background. The well-adjusted person is seen as someone who has a constant flow of needs and is able to satisfy those needs.

Purpose

In Gestalt therapy (from the German word meaning *form*), the major goal is self-awareness. Patients work on uncovering and resolving interpersonal issues during therapy. Unresolved issues are unable to fade into the background of consciousness because the needs they represent are never met. In Gestalt therapy, the goal is to discover people connected with a patient's unresolved issues and try to engage those people (or images of those people) in interactions that can lead to a resolution. Gestalt therapy is most useful for patients open to working on self-awareness.

Precautions

The choice of a therapist is crucial. Some people who call themselves "therapists" have limited training in Gestalt therapy. It is important that the therapist be a licensed mental health professional. Additionally, some individuals may not be able to tolerate the intensity of this type of therapy.

Description

Gestalt therapy has developed into a form of therapy that emphasizes medium to large groups, although many Gestalt techniques can be used in one-on-one therapy. Gestalt therapy probably has a greater range of formats than any other therapy technique. It is practiced in individual, couples, and family therapies, as well as in therapy with children.

Ideally, the patient identifies current sensations and emotions, particularly ones that are painful or disruptive. Patients are confronted with their unconscious feelings and needs, and are assisted to accept and assert those repressed parts of themselves.

The most powerful techniques involve role-playing. For example, the patient talks to an empty chair as they imagine that a person associated with an unresolved issue is sitting in the chair. As the patient talks to the "person" in the chair, the patient imagines that the person responds to the expressed feelings. Although this technique may sound artificial and might make some people feel self-conscious, it can be a powerful way to approach buried feelings and gain new insight into them.

Sometimes patients use battacca bats, padded sticks that can be used to hit chairs or sofas. Using a battacca bat can help a patient safely express anger. A patient may also experience a Gestalt therapy marathon, where the participants and one or more facilitators have nonstop **group therapy** over a weekend. The effects of the intense emotion and the lack of sleep can eliminate many psychological defenses and allow significant progress to be made in a short time. This is true only if the patient has adequate psychological strength for a marathon and is carefully monitored by the therapist.

Preparation

Gestalt therapy begins with the first contact. There is no separate diagnostic or assessment period. Instead, assessment and screening are done as part of the ongoing relationship between patient and therapist. This assessment includes determining the patient's willingness and support for work using Gestalt methods, as well as determining the compatibility between the patient and the therapist. Unfortunately, some "encounter groups" led by poorly trained individuals do not provide adequate pre-therapy screening and assessment.

Aftercare

Sessions are usually held once a week. Frequency of sessions held is based on how long the patient can go between sessions without losing the momentum from the previous session. Patients and therapists discuss when to start sessions, when to stop sessions, and what kind of activities to use during a session. However, the patient is encouraged and required to make choices.

Risks

Disturbed people with severe mental illness may not be suitable candidates for Gestalt therapy. Facilities that provide Gestalt therapy and train Gestalt therapists vary. Since there are no national standards for these Gestalt facilities, there are no set national standards for Gestalt therapy or Gestalt therapists.

Normal results

Scientific documentation on the effectiveness of Gestalt therapy is limited. Evidence suggests that this type of therapy may not be reliably effective.

Abnormal results

This approach can be anti-intellectual and can discount thoughts, thought patterns, and beliefs. In the hands of an ineffective therapist, Gestalt procedures can become a series of mechanical exercises, allowing the therapist as a person to stay hidden. Moreover, there is a potential for the therapist to manipulate the patient with powerful techniques, especially in therapy marathons where **fatigue** may make a patient vulnerable.

Resources

ORGANIZATIONS

Association for the Advancement of Gestalt Therapy. 400 East 58th St., New York, NY 10022. (212) 486-1581. < http://www.aagt.org > .

David James Doermann

Gestational diabetes

Definition

Gestational diabetes is a condition that occurs during **pregnancy**. Like other forms of diabetes, gestational diabetes involves a defect in the way the body processes and uses sugars (glucose) in the diet. Gestational diabetes, however, has a number of characteristics that are different from other forms of diabetes.

Description

Glucose is a form of sugar that is present in many foods, including sweets, potatoes, pasta, and breads. The body uses glucose to provide energy. It is stored in the liver, muscles, and fatty tissue. The pancreas produces a hormone (a chemical produced in one part of the body, which travels to another part of the body in order to exert its effect) called insulin. Insulin is required to allow glucose to enter the liver, muscles, and fatty tissues, thus reducing the amount of glucose in the blood. In diabetes, blood levels of glucose remain abnormally high. In many forms of diabetes, this is because the pancreas does not produce enough insulin.

In gestational diabetes, the pancreas is not at fault. Instead, the problem is in the placenta. During pregnancy, the placenta provides the baby with nourishment. It also produces a number of hormones that interfere with the body's usual response to insulin. This condition is referred to as "insulin resistance." Most pregnant women do not suffer from gestational diabetes, because the pancreas works to produce extra quantities of insulin in order to compensate for **insulin resistance**. However, when a woman's pancreas cannot produce enough extra insulin, blood levels of glucose stay abnormally high, and the woman is considered to have gestational diabetes.

About 1–3% of all pregnant women develop gestational diabetes. Women at risk for gestational diabetes include those who:

- are overweight

- have a family history of diabetes

- have previously given birth to a very large, heavy baby

- have previously had a baby who was stillborn, or born with a birth defect

- have an excess amount of amniotic fluid (the cushioning fluid within the uterus that surrounds the developing fetus)

- are over 25 years of age

- belong to an ethnic group known to experience higher rates of gestational diabetes (in the United

States, these groups include Mexican-Americans, American Indians, African-Americans, as well as individuals from Asia, India, or the Pacific Islands)

- have a previous history of gestational diabetes during a pregnancy

Causes and symptoms

Most women with gestational diabetes have no recognizable symptoms. However, leaving gestational diabetes undiagnosed and untreated is risky to the developing fetus. Left untreated, a diabetic mother's blood sugar levels will be consistently high. This sugar will cross the placenta and pour into the baby's system through the umbilical cord. The unborn baby's pancreas will respond to this high level of sugar by constantly putting out large amounts of insulin. The insulin will allow the fetus's cells to take in glucose, where it will be converted to fat and stored. A baby who has been exposed to constantly high levels of sugar throughout pregnancy will be abnormally large. Such a baby will often grow so large that he or she cannot be born through the vagina, but will instead need to be born through a surgical procedure (**cesarean section**).

Furthermore, when the baby is born, the baby will still have an abnormally large amount of insulin circulating. After birth, when the mother and baby are no longer attached to each other via the placenta and umbilical cord, the baby will no longer be receiving the mother's high level of sugar. The baby's high level of insulin, however, will very quickly use up the glucose circulating in the baby's bloodstream. The baby is then at risk for having a dangerously low level of blood glucose (a condition called **hypoglycemia**).

Diagnosis

Since gestational diabetes most often exists with no symptoms detectable by the patient, and since its existence puts the developing baby at considerable risk, screening for the disorder is a routine part of pregnancy care. This screening is usually done between the 24th and 28th week of pregnancy. By this point in the pregnancy, the placental hormones have reached a sufficient level to cause insulin resistance. Screening for gestational diabetes involves the pregnant woman drinking a special solution that contains exactly 50 grams of glucose. An hour later, the woman's blood is drawn and tested for its glucose level. A level less than 140 mg/dl is considered normal.

When the screening glucose level is over 140 mg/dl, a special three-hour glucose tolerance test is performed. This involves following a special diet for three days

prior to the test. This diet is set up to contain at least 150 grams of carbohydrates each day. Just before the test, the patient is instructed to eat and drink nothing (except water) for 10–14 hours. A blood sample is then tested to determine the **fasting** glucose level. The patient then drinks a special solution containing exactly 100 grams of glucose, and her blood is tested every hour for the next three hours. If two or more of these levels are elevated over normal, then the patient is considered to have gestational diabetes.

Treatment

Treatment for gestational diabetes will depend on the severity of the diabetes. Mild forms can be treated with diet (decreasing the intake of sugars and fats, in particular). Many women are put on strict, detailed **diets**, and are asked to stay within a certain range of calorie intake. **Exercise** sometimes is used to keep blood sugar levels lower. Patients often are asked to regularly measure their blood sugar. This is done by poking a finger with a needle called a lancet, putting a drop of blood on a special type of paper, and feeding the paper into a meter that analyzes and reports the blood sugar level. In fact self-monitoring of blood glucose helps manage gestational diabetes and prevent complications. When diet and exercise do not keep blood glucose levels within an acceptable range, a patient may need to take regular shots of insulin.

Many babies born to women with gestational diabetes are large enough to cause more difficult deliveries, and they may require the use of forceps, suction, or cesarean section. Once the baby is born, it is important to carefully monitor its blood glucose levels. These levels may drop sharply and dangerously once the baby is no longer receiving large quantities of sugar from the mother. When this occurs, it is easily resolved by giving the baby glucose.

Prognosis

Prognosis for women with gestational diabetes, and their babies, is generally good. Almost all such women stop being diabetic after the birth of their baby. However, some research has shown that nearly 50% of these women will develop a permanent form of diabetes within 15 years. The child of a mother with gestational diabetes has a greater-than-normal chance of developing diabetes sometime in adulthood, also. A woman who has had gestational diabetes during one pregnancy has about a 66% chance of having it again during any subsequent pregnancies. Women who had gestational diabetes usually are tested for diabetes at the postpartum checkup or after stopping breastfeeding.

KEY TERMS

Glucose—A form of sugar. The final product of the breakdown of carbohydrates (starches).

Insulin—A hormone produced by the pancreas that is central to the processing of sugars and carbohydrates in the diet.

Placenta—An organ that is attached to the inside wall of the mother's uterus and to the fetus via the umbilical cord. The placenta allows oxygen and nutrients from the mother's bloodstream to pass into the unborn baby.

Prevention

There is no known way to actually prevent diabetes, particularly since gestational diabetes is due to the effects of normal hormones of pregnancy. However, the effects of insulin resistance can be best handled through careful attention to diet, avoiding becoming overweight throughout life, and participating in reasonable exercise. A 2003 report also linked **smoking** to increased risk of gestational diabetes.

Resources

PERIODICALS

"Self-monitoring of blood glucose Useful for Managing Gestational Diabetes." *Women's Health Weekly* (August 7, 2003): 42.
"Smoking Tied to Increased Risk of Gestational Diabetes; Dose Response Relationship." *OB GYN News* (September 1, 2003): 5.

ORGANIZATIONS

American Diabetes Association. 1701 North Beauregard Street, Alexandria, VA 22311. (800) 342-2383. < http:// www.diabetes.org > .

Rosalyn Carson-DeWitt, MD
Teresa G. Odle

GI bleeding studies

Definition

GI bleeding studies uses radioactive materials in the investigation of bleeding from the gastrointestinal (GI) tract. These studies go under various names such as "GI bleeding scans" or "Tagged red blood cell scans." They are performed and interpreted by radiologists (physicians who specialize in diagnosis and treatment of diseases by means of x rays or related substances).

Purpose

These studies are designed to find the source of blood loss from the GI tract; that is the stomach, small bowel, or colon. They work best when bleeding is either too slow, intermittent, or too rapid to be identified by other means, such as endoscopy, upper GI series, or **barium enema**.

They are particularly useful when other methods have not been able to determine the site or cause of bleeding.

Precautions

Because of the use of radioactive materials, these studies are best avoided in pregnant patients. Another important relates to the interpretation of these tests, whether normal or abnormal. Since these studies are far from perfect, they can only be used as "guides" as to the cause or site of bleeding. In most instances, further studies must be performed to confirm their findings.

Description

Bleeding scans are based on the accumulation of radioactive material as it exits from the vessels during a bleeding episode. Blood is first withdrawn from the patient. Then, the blood, along with a radioactive substance is injected into a vein and over several hours scans measuring radioactivity are performed. The studies were initially reported to be very sensitive and accurate; however, critical evaluation of these tests have shown them to be less accurate than originally believed.

Preparation

No preparation is needed for these tests. They are often done on an "emergency" basis.

Aftercare

No special care is needed after the exam.

Risks

Bleeding scans are free of any risks or side-effects, aside from the fact that they should best be avoided in **pregnancy**.

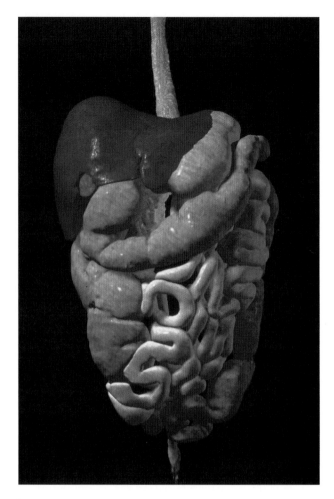

A clay model of the human digestive system. *(Custom Medical Stock Photo. Reproduced by permission.)*

Normal results

A normal exam would fail to show any evidence of accumulation of radioactive material on the scan. However, scans may be normal in as many as 70% of patients who later turn out to have significant causes of bleeding. This is known as a false-negative result. A patient must be bleeding at the same time the scan is performed for it to be seen. Therefore, not finding evidence of a bleeding source during the study, can be misleading.

Abnormal results

The accumulation of radioactive material indicating a "leakage" of blood from the vessels is abnormal. The scan gives a rough, though not exact, guide as to the location of the bleeding. It can tell where the bleeding may be, but usually not the cause. Thus, extreme caution and skill is needed in interpreting these scans, and decisions involving surgery or other treatment should await more definitive tests.

Resources

BOOKS

Lane, Loren. "Radionuclide Scanning." In *Sleisenger & Fordtran's Gastrointestinal and Liver Disease*, edited by Mark Feldman, et al. Philadelphia: W. B. Saunders Co., 1997.

David Kaminstein, MD

Giant-cell arteritis *see* **Temporal arteritis**

Giardia lamblia infection *see* **Giardiasis**

Giardiasis

Definition

Giardiasis is a common intestinal infection spread by eating contaminated food, drinking contaminated water, or through direct contact with the organism that causes the disease, *Giardia lamblia*. Giardiasis is found throughout the world and is a common cause of traveller's **diarrhea**. In the United States it is a growing problem, especially among children in childcare centers.

Description

Giardia is one of the most common intestinal parasites in the world, infecting as much as 20% of the entire population of the earth. It is common in overcrowded developing countries with poor sanitation and a lack of clean water. Recent tests have found *Giardia* in 7% of all stool samples tested nationwide, indicating that this disease is much more widespread than was originally believed. It has been found not only in humans, but also in wild and domestic animals.

Giardiasis is becoming a growing problem in the United States, where it affects three times more children than adults. In recent years, giardiasis outbreaks have been common among people in schools or day-care centers and at catered affairs and large public picnic areas. Children can easily pass on the infection by touching contaminated toys, changing tables, utensils, or their own feces, and then touching other people. For this reason, infection spreads quickly through a daycare center or institution for the developmentally disabled.

Unfiltered streams or lakes that may be contaminated by human or animal wastes are a common source of infection. Outbreaks can occur among campers and hikers who drink untreated water from mountain streams. While 20 million Americans drink unfiltered city water from streams or rivers, giardiasis outbreaks from tainted city water have been rare. Most of these problems have occurred not due to the absence of filters, but because of malfunctions in city water treatment plants, such as a temporary drop in chlorine levels. It is possible to become infected in a public swimming pool, however, since *Giardia* can survive in chlorinated water for about 15 minutes. During that time, it is possible for an individual to swallow contaminated pool water and become infected.

Causes and symptoms

Giardiasis is spread by food or water contaminated by the *Giardia lamblia* protozoan organism found in the human intestinal tract and feces. When the cysts are ingested, the stomach acid degrades the cysts and releases the active parasite into the body. Once within the body, the parasites cling to the lining of the small intestine, reproduce, and are swept into the fecal stream. As the liquid content of the bowel dries up, the parasites form cysts, which are then passed in the feces. Once excreted, the cysts can survive in water for more than three months. The parasite is spread further by direct fecal-oral contamination, such as can occur if food is prepared without adequate hand-washing, or by ingesting the cysts in water or food.

Giardiasis is not fatal, and about two-thirds of infected people exhibit no symptoms. Symptoms will not occur until between one and two weeks after infection. When present, symptoms include explosive, watery diarrhea that can last for a week or more and, in chronic cases, may persist for months. Because the

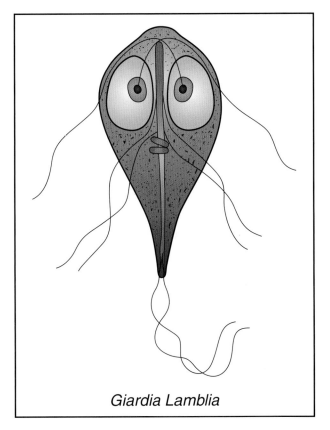
Giardia Lamblia

Infection with the protozoon *Giardia lamblia*, shown above, causes diarrhea in humans. *(Illustration by Electronic Illustrators Group).*

infection interferes with the body's ability to absorb fats from the intestinal tract, the stool is filled with fat. Other symptoms include foul-smelling and greasy feces, stomach pains, gas and bloating, loss of appetite, **nausea and vomiting**. In cases in which the infection becomeschronic, lasting for months or years, symptoms might include poor digestion, problems digesting milk, intermittent diarrhea, **fatigue**, weakness, and significant weight loss.

Diagnosis

Diagnosis can be difficult because it can be easy to overlook the presence of the giardia cysts during a routine inspection of a stool specimen. In the past, the condition has been diagnosed by examining three stool samples for the presence of the parasites. However, because the organism is shed in some stool samples and not others, the infection may not be discovered using this method.

A newer, more accurate method of diagnosing the condition is the enzyme-linked immunosorbent assay

(ELISA) that detects cysts and antigen in stool, and is approximately 90% accurate. While slightly more expensive, it only needs to be done once and is therefore less expensive overall than the earlier test.

Treatment

Acute giardiasis can usually be allowed to run its natural course and tends to clear up on its own. **Antibiotics** are helpful, however, in easing symptoms and preventing the spread of infection. Medications include metronidazole, furazolidone and paromomycin. Healthy carriers with no symptoms do not need antibiotic treatment. If treatment should fail, the patient should wait two weeks and repeat the drug course. Anyone with an impaired immune system (immunocompromised), such as a person with **AIDS**, may need to be treated with a combination of medications.

Prognosis

Giardiasis is rarely fatal, and when treated promptly, antibiotics usually cure the infection. While most people respond quickly to treatment, some have lingering symptoms and suffer with diarrhea and cramps for long periods, losing weight and not growing well. Those most at-risk for a course like this are the elderly, people with a weakened immune system, malnourished children, and anyone with low stomach acid.

Prevention

The best way to avoid giardiasis is to avoid drinking untreated surface water, especially from mountain streams. The condition also can be minimized by practicing the following preventive measures:

- thoroughly washing hands before handling food
- maintaining good personal cleanliness
- boiling any untreated water for at least three minutes
- properly disposing of fecal material

Children with severe diarrhea (and others who are unable to control their bowel habits) should be kept at home until the stool returns to normal. If an outbreak occurs in a daycare center, the director should notify the local health department. Some local health departments require a follow-up stool testing to confirm that the person is no longer contagious. People not in high-risk settings can return to their routine activities after recovery.

Resources

ORGANIZATIONS

Centers for Disease Control and Prevention. 1600 Clifton Rd., NE, Atlanta, GA 30333. (800) 311-3435, (404) 639-3311. < http://www.cdc.gov > .

OTHER

Centers for Disease Control. < http://www.cdc.gov/ncidod/EID/eidtext.htm > .
International Society of Travel Medicine. < http:www.istm.org > .

Carol A. Turkington

Ginkgo biloba

Definition

Ginkgo biloba, known as the maidenhair tree, is one of the oldest trees on Earth, once part of the flora of the Mesozoic period. The ginkgo tree is the only surviving species of the Ginkgoaceae family. This ancient deciduous tree may live for thousands of years. Ginkgo is indigenous to China, Japan, and Korea, but also thrived in North America and Europe prior to the Ice Age. This drastic climate change destroyed the wild ginkgo tree throughout much of the world. In China, ginkgo was cultivated in temple gardens as a sacred tree known as *bai gou*, thus assuring its survival there for over 200 million years. Ginkgo fossils found from the Permian period are identical to the living tree, which is sometimes called a living fossil.

Description

Ginkgo trees may grow to 122 ft (37.2 m) tall and measure 4 ft (1.2 m) in girth. The female trees have a somewhat pointed shape at the top, like a pyramid. The male trees are broader at the crown. The bark of the ornamental ginkgo tree is rough and fissured and may be an ash to dark-brown in color. Distinctive, fan-shaped leaves with long stalks emerge from a sheath on the stem. Leaves are bright green in spring and summer, and turn to golden yellow in the fall. Ginkgo trees may take as long as 30 years to flower. Ginkgo is dioecious, with male and female flowers blooming on separate trees. Blossoms grow singly from the axils of the leaf. The female flowers appear at the end of a leafless branch. The yellow, plum-shaped fruits develop an unpleasant scent as they ripen. They contain an edible inner seed that is available in Asian country marketplaces. Ginkgo's longevity may be due, in part, to its remarkable resistance to disease, pollution, and insect damage. Ginkgo trees are part of the landscape plan in many urban areas throughout the world. Millions of ginkgo trees, grown for harvest of the medicinal leaves, are raised on plantations in the United States, France, South Korea, and Japan, and are exported to Europe for pharmaceutical processing.

Purpose

Ginkgo leaves, fresh or dry, and seeds, separated from the outer layer of the fruit, are used medicinally. Ginkgo has remarkable healing virtues that have been recorded as far back as 2800 B.C. in the oldest Chinese materia medica. Ginkgo seeds were traditionally served to guests along with alcohol drinks in Japan. An enzyme present in the ginkgo seed has been shown in clinical research to speed up alcohol metabolism in the body, underscoring the wisdom of this folk custom. The leaf extract has been used in Asia for thousands of years to treat **allergies**, **asthma**, and **bronchitis**. It is also valued in Chinese medicine as a heart tonic, helpful in the treatment of cardiac arrhythmia. Ginkgo was first introduced to Europe in 1730, and to North America in 1784 where it was planted as an exotic garden ornamental near Philadelphia. Ginkgo medicinal extracts are the primary prescription medicines used in France and Germany.

Ginkgo acts to increase blood flow throughout the body, particularly cerebral blood flow. It acts as a circulatory system tonic, stimulating greater tone in the venous system. The herb is a useful and proven remedy for numerous diseases caused by restricted blood flow. European physicians prescribe the extract for treatment of **Raynaud's disease**, a condition of impaired circulation to the fingers. It is also recommended to treat **intermittent claudication**, a circulatory condition that results in painful cramping of the calf muscles in the leg and impairs the ability to walk. German herbalists recommend ingesting the extract for treatment of leg ulcers, and large doses are used to treat **varicose veins**. Ginkgo is widely recommended in Europe for the treatment of **stroke**. The dried leaf extract may also act to prevent hemmorrhagic stroke by strengthening the blood capillaries throughout the body. In studies of patients with atherosclerotic clogging of the penile artery, long-term therapy with ginkgo extract has provided significant improvement in erectile function. Ginkgo extract also acts to eliminate damaging free-radicals in the body, and has been shown to be effective in treatment of **premenstrual syndrome**, relieving tender or painful breasts.

Ginkgo extract has proven benefits to elderly persons. This ancient herb acts to enhance oxygen utilization and thus improves memory, concentration, and other mental faculties. The herbal extract is used to treat **Alzheimer's disease**. It has been shown to have beneficial effect on the hippocampus, an area of the brain affected by Alzheimer's disease. The herbal extract has also been shown to significantly improve long-distance vision and may reverse damage to the retina of the eye. Studies have also confirmed its value in the treatment of depression in elderly persons. The ginkgo extract may provide relief for persons with **headache**, **sinusitis**, and vertigo. It may also help relieve chronic ringing in the ears known as **tinnitus**.

The active constituents in the ginkgo tree, known as ginkgolides, interfere with a blood protein known as the platelet activating factor, or PAF. Other phytochemicals in ginkgo include flavonoids, biflavonoides, proanthocyanidins, trilactonic diterpenes (including the ginkgolides A, B, C, and M), and bilabolide, a trilactonic sesquiterpene. The therapeutic effects of

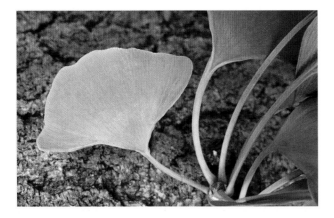

Ginkgo biloba leaves. *(Photograph by Robert J. Huffman. Field Mark Publications. Reproduced by permission.)*

this herb have not been attributed to a single chemical constituent; rather, the medicinal benefits are due to the synergy between the various chemical constituents. The standardized extract of ginkgo must be taken consistently to be effective. A period of at least 12 weeks of use may be required before the beneficial results are evident.

Preparations

Ginkgo's active principles are dilute in the leaves. The herb must be processed to extract the active phytochemicals before it is medicinally useful. It would take an estimated 50 fresh ginkgo leaves to yield one standard dose of the extract. Dry extracts of the leaf, standardized to a potency of 24% flavone glycosides and 6% terpenes, are commercially available. A standard dose is 40 mg, three times daily, though dosages as high as 240 mg daily are sometimes indicated.

Ginkgo extracts are widely used in Europe where they are sold in prescription form or over the counter as an approved drug. This is not the case in the United States, where ginkgo extract is sold as a food supplement in tablet and capsule form.

Precautions

Ginkgo is generally safe and non-toxic in therapeutic dosages. Exceeding a daily dose of 240 mg of the dried extract may result in restlessness, **diarrhea**, and mild gastrointestinal disorders. Those on anticoagulants should have their doctor adjust their dose or should avoid ginkgo in order to avoid over-thinning their blood and hemorrhaging. Ginkgo should be avoided two days before and one to two weeks after surgery to avoid bleeding complications.

Side effects

Severe allergic skin reactions, similar to those caused by poison ivy, have been reported after contact with the fruit pulp of ginkgo. Eating even a small amount of the fruit has caused severe gastrointestinal irritation in some persons. People with persistent headaches should stop taking ginkgo. Some patients on medications for nervous system disease should avoid ginkgo. It can interact with some other medicines, but clinical information is still emerging.

Interactions

The chemically active ginkgolides present in the extract, specifically the ginkgolide B component, act to reduce the clotting time of blood and may interact with antithrombotic medicines, including **aspirin**.

Resources

BOOKS

PDR for Herbal Medicines. Montvale, NJ: Medical Economics Company, 1998.

Clare Hanrahan

Ginseng, Korean

Definition

Korean ginseng is one of the most widely used and acclaimed herbs in the world. Its scientific name is *Panax ginseng*, which is the species from which Chinese, Korean, red, and white ginseng are produced. Chinese and Korean ginseng are the same plant cultivated in different regions, and have slightly different properties according to Chinese medicine. White ginseng is simply the dried or powdered root of Korean ginseng, while red ginseng is the same root that is steamed and dried in heat or sunlight. Red ginseng is said to be slightly stronger and more stimulating in the body than white, according to Chinese herbalism.

Description

Korean ginseng has had a long and illustrious history as an herb for health, and has been used for thousands of years throughout the Orient as a medicine and tonic. Early Chinese medicine texts written in the first century A.D. mention ginseng, and ginseng has long been classified by Chinese medicine as a "superior" herb. This means it is said to promote longevity and vitality. Legends around the world have touted ginseng as an aphrodisiac and sexual tonic. Researchers have found a slight connection between sex drive and consuming ginseng, although a direct link and the mechanism of action are still researched and disputed.

Korean ginseng grows on moist, shaded mountainsides in China, Korea, and Russia. It is a perennial herb that reaches heights of two or more feet, and is distinguished by its dark green leaves and red clusters of berries. The root of the plant is the part valued for its medicinal properties. The root is long and slender and sometimes resembles the shape of the human body. Asian legends claim that this "man-root" has magical powers for those lucky enough to afford or find it, and the roots bearing the closest resemblance to the human body are still the most valuable ones. The word *ren shen* in Chinese means roughly "the essence of the earth in the shape of a man."

Korean ginseng has historically been one of the most expensive of herbs, as it has been highly in demand in China and the Far East for centuries. Wars have been fought in Asia over lands where it grew wild. Wild Korean ginseng is now nearly extinct from many regions. Single roots of wild plants have recently been auctioned in China and New York City for sums approaching $50,000. Most of the world's supply of Korean ginseng is cultivated by farmers in Korea and China.

Because of the number of herbs sold under the name of ginseng, there can be some confusion for the consumer. Korean ginseng is a member of the *Araliaceae* family of plants, which also includes closely related American ginseng (*Panax quinquefolius*) and Siberian ginseng (*Eleutherococcus senticosus*). Both American and Siberian ginseng are considered by Chinese herbalists to be different herbs than Korean ginseng, and are said to have different effects and healing properties in the body. To add more confusion, there are eight herbs in Chinese medicine which are sometimes called ginseng, including black ginseng, purple ginseng, and prince's ginseng, some of which are not at all botanically related to *Panax ginseng*, so consumers should choose ginseng products with awareness.

Purpose

The word *panax* is formed from Greek roots meaning "cure-all," and *Panax ginseng* has long been considered to be one of the great healing and strengthening herbs in natural medicine. Ginseng is classified as an *adaptogen*, which is a substance that helps the body adapt to **stress** and balance itself without causing major side effects. Korean ginseng is used as a tonic for improving overall health and stamina, and Chinese herbalists particularly recommend it for the ill, weak, or elderly. Korean ginseng has long been asserted to have longevity, anti-senility, and memory improvement effects in the aged population. As it helps the body to adapt to stress, athletes may use ginseng as herbal support during rigorous training. Korean ginseng generally increases physical and mental energy. It is a good tonic for the adrenal glands, and is used by those suffering from exhaustion, burnout, or debilitation from chronic illness.

Traditional Chinese medicine also prescribes Korean ginseng to treat diabetes, and research has shown that it enhances the release of insulin from the pancreas and lowers blood sugar levels. Korean ginseng has been demonstrated to lower blood cholesterol levels. It has also been shown to have antioxidant effects and to increase immune system activity, which makes it a good herbal support for those suffering from **cancer** and **AIDS** and other chronic conditions that impair the immune system. Further uses of Korean ginseng in Chinese medicine include treatment of **impotence**, **asthma**, and digestive weakness.

Research

Scientists have isolated what they believe are the primary active ingredients in ginseng, chemicals termed *saponin triterpenoid glycosides*, or commonly called *ginsenocides*. There are nearly 30 ginsenocides in Korean ginseng. Much research on Korean ginseng has been conducted in China, but controlled human experiments with it have not been easily accessible to the English-speaking world. Recent research in China was summarized by Dr. C. Lui in the February 1992 issue of the *Journal of Ethnopharmacology*, where he wrote that *Panax ginseng* was found to contain 28 ginsenocides that "act on the central nervous system, cardiovascular system and endocrine secretion, promote immune function, and have effects on anti-aging and relieving stress."

To summarize other research, Korean ginseng has been shown in studies to have significant effects for the following.

- Physical improvement and performance enhancement for athletes: A study performed over three years in Germany showed athletes given ginseng had favorable improvement in several categories over a control group who took a placebo. Another

1982 study showed that athletes given ginseng had improved oxygen intake and faster recovery time than those given placebos.

- Mental performance improvement and mood enhancement: In general, studies show that ginseng enhances mental performance, learning time, and memory. One study of sixteen volunteers showed improvement on a wide variety of mental tests, including mathematics. Another study showed that those performing intricate and mentally demanding tasks improved performance when given Korean ginseng. Finally, a study has shown improvement of mood in depression sufferers with the use of ginseng.

- Antifatigue and antistress actions: Patients with chronic **fatigue** who were given ginseng showed a statistically significant improvement in physical tests and in mental attention and concentration, when compared with those given placebos.

- Lowering blood sugar: Animal studies have shown that ginseng can facilitate the release of insulin from the pancreas and increase the number of insulin receptors in the body.

- Antioxidant properties: Scientific analysis of ginseng has shown that it has antioxidant effects, similar to the effects of **vitamins** A, C, and E. Thus, ginseng could be beneficial in combating the negative effects of pollution, radiation, and aging.

- Cholesterol reduction: Some studies have shown that Korean ginseng reduces total cholesterol and increases levels of good cholesterol in the body.

- Anticancer effects and immune system stimulation: Several tests have shown that Korean ginseng increases immune cell activity in the body, including the activity of T-cells and lymphocytes, which are instrumental in fighting cancer and other immune system disorders like AIDS. A Korean study indicates that taking ginseng may reduce the chances of getting cancer, as a survey of more than 1,800 patients in a hospital in Seoul showed that those who did not have cancer were more likely to have taken ginseng regularly than those patients who had contracted cancer.

- Physical and mental improvement in the elderly: One study showed significant improvement in an elderly test group in visual and auditory reaction time and cardiopulmonary function when given controlled amounts of Korean ginseng. Korean ginseng has also been shown to alleviate symptoms of menopause.

- Impotence: Studies of human sexual function and Korean ginseng have been generally inconclusive,

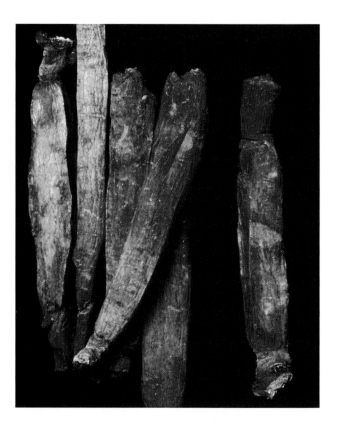

Dried Korean ginseng. *(Custom Medical Stock Photo. Reproduced by permission.)*

despite the wide acclaim of ginseng as a sexual tonic. Tests with lab animals and ginseng have shown some interesting results, indicating that Korean ginseng promotes the growth of male reproductive organs, increases sperm and testoterone levels, and increases sexual activity in laboratory animals. In general, scientists believe the link between ginseng and sex drive is due to ginseng's effect of strengthening overall health and balancing the hormonal system.

Preparations

Korean ginseng can be purchased as whole roots, powder, liquid extracts, and tea. Roots should be sliced and boiled in water for up to 45 minutes to extract all the beneficial nutrients. One to five grams of dry root is the recommended amount for one serving of tea. Herbalists recommend that ginseng not be boiled in metal pots, to protect its antioxidant properties. Ginseng should be taken between meals for best assimilation.

Some high quality Korean ginseng extracts and products are standardized to contain a specified amount of ginsenosides. The recommended dosage for extracts containing four to eight percent of ginsenosides is 100 mg once or twice daily. The recommended dosage for non-standardized root powder or extracts is 1–2 g daily, taken in capsules or as a tea. It is recommended that ginseng be taken in cycles and not continuously; after each week of taking ginseng, a few days without ingesting the herb should be observed. Likewise, Korean ginseng should not be taken longer than two months at a time, after which one month's rest period should be allowed before resuming the cycle again. Chinese herbalists recommend that ginseng be taken primarily in the autumn and winter months.

Precautions

Consumers should be aware of the different kinds of ginseng, and which type is best suited for them. Red Korean ginseng is considered stronger and more stimulating than white, wild ginseng is stronger than cultivated, and Korean ginseng is generally believed to be slightly stronger than Chinese. Furthermore, American and Siberian ginseng have slightly different properties than Korean ginseng, and consumers should make an informed choice as to which herb is best suited for them. Chinese herbalists do not recommend Korean ginseng for those people who have "heat" disorders in their bodies, such as ulcers, high blood pressure, tension headaches, and symptoms associated with high stress levels. Korean ginseng is generally not recommended for those with symptoms of nervousness, mental imbalance, inflammation, or **fever**. Korean ginseng is not recommended for pregnant or lactating women, and women of childbearing age should use ginseng sparingly, as some studies imply that it can influence estrogen levels. Also, Chinese herbalists typically only prescribe ginseng to older people or the weak, as they believe that younger and stronger people do not benefit as much from it and ginseng is "wasted on the young."

Because of the number of and demand for ginseng products on the market, consumers should search for a reputable brand, preferably with a standardized percentage of active ingredients. To illustrate the mislabeling found with some ginseng products, *Consumer*

Reports magazine analyzed ten nationally-distributed ginseng products in 1995. They found that several of them lacked significant amounts of ginsenocides, despite claims on the packaging to the contrary. Ginseng fraud has led the American Botanical Council, publisher of *HerbalGram* magazine, to initiate the Ginseng Evaluation Program, a comprehensive study and standardization of ginseng products on the American market. This study and its labeling standards are still under development, and consumers should watch for it.

Side effects

Korean ginseng acts as a slight stimulant in the body, and in some cases can cause overstimulation, irritability, nervousness and **insomnia**, although strong side effects are generally rare. Taking too high a dosage of ginseng, or taking ginseng for too long without a break, can cause *ginseng intoxication*, for which symptoms might include headaches, insomnia, seeing spots, **dizziness**, shortage of breath and gastrointestinal discomfort. Long term use may cause menstrual abnormalities and breast tenderness in some women.

Interactions

Those taking hormonal drugs should use ginseng with care. Ginseng should not be taken with **caffeine** or other stimulants as these may increase its stimulatory effects and cause uncomfortable side effects.

Resources

BOOKS

Hobbs, Christopher. *Ginseng: The Energy Herb*. Loveland, CO: Botanica Press, 1996.

PERIODICALS

HerbalGram (a quarterly journal of the American Botanical Council and Herb Research Foundation). P.O. Box 144345, Austin, TX 78714-4345. (800) 373-7105.

Douglas Dupler, MA

Glaucoma

Definition

Glaucoma is a group of eye diseases characterized by damage to the optic nerve usually due to excessively high intraocular pressure (IOP).This increased pressure within the eye, if untreated can lead to optic nerve damage resulting in progressive, permanent vision loss, starting with unnoticeable blind spots at the edges of the field of vision, progressing to tunnel vision, and then to blindness.

Description

Between two to three million people in the United States have glaucoma, and 120,000 of those are legally blind as a result. It is the leading cause of preventable blindness in the United States and the most frequent cause of blindness in African-Americans, who are at about a three-fold higher risk of glaucoma than the rest of the population. The risk of glaucoma increases dramatically with age, but it can strike any age group, even newborn infants and fetuses.

Glaucoma can be classified into two categories: open-angle glaucoma and narrow-angle glaucoma. To understand what glaucoma is and what these terms mean, it is useful to understand eye structure.

Eyes are sphere-shaped. A tough, non-leaky protective sheath (the sclera) covers the entire eye, except for the clear cornea at the front and the optic nerve at the back. Light comes into the eye through the cornea, then passes through the lens, which focuses it onto the retina (the innermost surface at the back of the eye). The rods and cones of the retina transform the light energy into electrical messages, which are transmitted to the brain by the bundle of nerves known as the optic nerve.

The iris, the colored part of the eye shaped like a round picture frame, is between the dome-shaped cornea and the lens. It controls the amount of light that enters the eye by opening and closing its central hole (pupil) like the diaphragm in a camera. The iris, cornea, and lens are bathed in a liquid called the aqueous humor, which is somewhat similar to plasma. This liquid is continually produced by nearby ciliary tissues and moved out of the eye into the bloodstream by a system of drainage canals (called the trabecular meshwork). The drainage area is located in front of the iris, in the angle formed between the iris and the point at which the iris appears to meet the inside of the cornea.

Glaucoma occurs if the aqueous humor is not removed rapidly enough or if it is made too rapidly, causing pressure to build-up. The high pressure distorts the shape of the optic nerve and destroys the nerve. Destroyed nerve cells result in blind spots in places where the image from the retina is not being transmitted to the brain.

Open-angle glaucoma accounts for over 90% of all cases. It is called "open-angle" because the angle between the iris and the cornea is open, allowing drainage of the aqueous humor. It is usually chronic and progresses slowly. In narrow-angle glaucoma, the angle where aqueous fluid drainage occurs is narrow, and therefore may drain slowly or may be at risk of becoming closed. A closed-angle glaucoma attack is usually acute, occurring when the drainage area is blocked. This can occur, for example, if the iris and lens suddenly adhere to each other and the iris is pushed forward. In patients with very narrow angles, this can occur when the eyes dilate (e.g., when entering a dark room, or if taking certain medications).

Congenital glaucoma occurs in babies and is the result of incomplete development of the eye's drainage canals during embryonic development. Microsurgery can often correct the defects or they can be treated with a combination of medicine and surgery.

One rare form of open-angle glaucoma, normal tension glaucoma, is different. People with normal-tension glaucoma have optic nerve damage in the presence of normal IOP. As of 1998, the mechanism of this disease is a mystery but is generally detected after an examination of the optic nerve. Those at higher risk for this form of glaucoma are people with a familial history of normal tension glaucoma, people of Japanese ancestry, and people with a history of systemic heart disease such as irregular heart rhythm.

Glaucoma is also a secondary condition of over 60 widely diverse diseases and can also result from injury, inflammation, tumor, or in advanced cases of cataract or diabetes.

Causes and symptoms

Causes

The cause of vision loss in all forms of glaucoma is optic nerve damage. There are many underlying causes and forms of glaucoma. Most causes of glaucoma are not known, but it is clear that a number of different processes are involved, and a malfunction in any one of them could cause glaucoma. For example, trauma to the eye could result in the angle becoming blocked, or, as a person ages, the lens becomes larger and may push the iris forward. The cause of optic nerve damage in normal-tension glaucoma is also unknown, but there is speculation that the optic nerves of these patients are susceptible to damage at lower pressures than what is usually considered to be abnormally high.

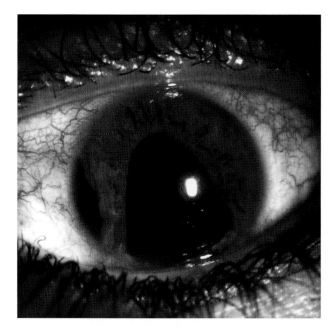

A close-up view of an inflamed eye with acute glaucoma and an irregularly enlarged pupil. *(Custom Medical Stock Photo. Reproduced by permission.)*

It is probable that most glaucoma is inherited. At least ten defective genes that cause glaucoma have been identified.

Symptoms

At first, chronic open-angle glaucoma is without noticeable symptoms. The pressure build-up is gradual and there is no discomfort. Moreover, the vision loss is too gradual to be noticed and each eye fills-in the image where its partner has a blind spot. However, if it is not treated, vision loss becomes evident, and the condition can be very painful.

On the other hand, acute closed-angle glaucoma is obvious from the beginning of an attack. The symptoms are, blurred vision, severe **pain**, sensitivity to light, **nausea**, and halos around lights. The normally clear corneas may be hazy. This is an ocular emergency and needs to be treated immediately.

Similarly, congenital glaucoma is evident at birth. Symptoms are bulging eyes, cloudy corneas, excessive tearing, and sensitivity to light.

Diagnosis

Intraocular pressure, visual field defects, the angle in the eye where the iris meets the cornea, and the appearance of the optic nerve are all considered in the diagnosis of glaucoma. IOP is measured with an instrument known as a tonometer. One type of tonometer involves numbing the eye with an eyedrop that has a yellow coloring in it and touching the cornea with a small probe. This quick test is a routine part of an **eye examination** and is usually included without extra charge in the cost of a visit to an ophthalmologist or optometrist.

Ophthalmoscopes, hand-held instruments with a light source, are used to detect optic nerve damage by looking through the pupil. The optic nerve is examined for changes; the remainder of the back of the eye can be examined as well. Other types of lenses that can be used to examine the back of the eye may also be used. A slit lamp will allow the doctor to examine the front of the eye (i.e., cornea, iris, and lens).

Visual field tests (perimetry) can detect blind spots in a patient's field of vision before the patient is aware of them. Certain defects may indicate glaucoma.

Another test, gonioscopy, can distinguish between narrow-angle and open-angle glaucoma. A gonioscope, which is a hand-held contact lens with a mirror, allows visualization of the angle between the iris and the cornea.

Intraocular pressure can vary throughout the day. For that reason, the doctor may have a patient return for several visits to measure the IOP at different times of the day.

Treatment

Medications

When glaucoma is diagnosed, drugs, typically given as eye drops, are usually tried before surgery. Several classes of medications are effective at lowering IOP and thus preventing optic nerve damage in chronic and neonatal glaucoma. **Beta blockers**, like Timoptic; carbonic anhydrase inhibitors, like acetazolamide; and alpha-2 agonists, such as Alphagan, inhibit the production of aqueous humor. Miotics, like pilocarpine, and prostaglandin analogues, like Xalatan, increase the outflow of aqueous humor. Cosopt is the first eyedrop that is a combined beta blocker (Timoptic) and carbonic anhydrase inhibitor and may be helpful for patients required to take more than one glaucoma medication each day. The Food and drug administration recently approved two new prostaglandin-related drugs, Travatan and Lumigan on March 16, 2001. These drugs work by decreasing intraocular pressure and may be considered for people with glaucoma that are unable to tolerate other IOP lowering drugs. Additionally, Travatan may work best for African-Americans with glaucoma (a population at high risk for glaucoma).

It is important for patients to tell their doctors about any conditions they have or medications they are taking. Certain drugs used to treat glaucoma should not be prescribed for patients with pre-existing conditions. Some of these drugs mentioned have side effects, so patients taking them should be monitored closely, especially for cardiovascular, pulmonary, and behavioral symptoms. Different medications lower IOP by different amounts, and a combination of medications may be necessary. It is important that patients take their medications and that their regimens are monitored regularly, to be sure that the IOP is lowered sufficiently. IOP should be measured three to four times per year.

Normal-tension glaucoma is treated in the same way as chronic high-intraocular-pressure glaucoma. This reduces IOP to less-than-normal levels, on the theory that overly susceptible optic nerves are less likely to be damaged at lower pressures. Research underway may point to better treatments for this form of glaucoma.

Attacks of acute closed-angle glaucoma are medical emergencies. IOP is rapidly lowered by successive deployment of acetazolamide, hyperosmotic agents, a topical beta-blocker, and pilocarpine. Epinephrine should not be used because it exacerbates angle closure.

Surgery

There are several types of **laser surgery** used to treat glaucoma. Laser peripheral iridotomy makes an opening in the iris allowing the fluid to drain, argon laser trabeculoplasty is aimed at the fluid channel opening to help the drainage system function and laser cyclophotocoagulation is used to decrease the amount of fluid made. Microsurgery, also called "filtering surgery" has been used in many different types of glaucoma. A new opening is created in the sclera allowing the intraocular fluid to bypass the blocked drainage canals. The tissue over this opening forms a little blister or bleb on the clear conjuctiva that Doctors monitor ensuring that fluid is draining. These surgeries are usually successful, but the effects often last less than a year. Nevertheless, they are an effective treatment for patients whose IOP is not sufficiently lowered by drugs and for those who can't tolerate the drugs. Because all surgeries have risks, patients should speak to their doctors about the procedure being performed.

Alternative treatment

Vitamin C, vitamin B_1 (thiamine), chromium, zinc,bilberry and rutin may reduce IOP.

There is evidence that medicinal **marijuana** lowers IOP, too. However, marijuana has serious side effects and contains carcinogens, and any IOP-lowering medication must be taken continually to avoid optic nerve damage. Although the Food and Drug Administration (FDA) and National Institutes of Health (NIH) currently recommend against treating glaucoma with marijuana, they are supporting research to learn more about it and to determine the feasibility of separating the components that lower IOP from components that produce side effects and carcinogens.

Any glaucoma patient using alternative methods to attempt to prevent optic nerve damage should also be under the care of a traditionally trained ophthalmologist or optometrist who is licensed to treat glaucoma, so that IOP and optic nerve damage can be monitored.

Prognosis

About half of the people stricken by glaucoma are not aware of it. For them, the prognosis is not good, and many of them will become blind. Sight lost due to glaucoma cannot be restored. On the other hand, the prognosis for treated glaucoma is excellent.

Prevention

Because glaucoma may not initially result in symptoms, the best form of prevention is to have regular eye exams.

Patients with narrow angles should avoid certain medications (even over-the-counter medications, such as some cold or allergy medications).Any person who is glaucoma-susceptible (i.e. narrow angles and borderline IOPs) should read the warning labels on over-the-counter medicines and inform their physicians of products they are considering taking.Steroids may also raise IOP, so patients may need to be monitored more frequently if it is necessary to use steroids for another medical condition.

Not enough is known about the underlying mechanisms of glaucoma to prevent the disease itself. However, prevention of optic nerve damage from glaucoma is essential and can be effectively accomplished when the condition is diagnosed and treated. As more is learned about the genes that cause glaucoma, it will become possible to test DNA and identify

KEY TERMS

Agonist—A drug that mimics one of the body's own molecules.

Alpha-2 agonist (alpha-2 adrenergic receptor agonist)—A class of drugs that bind to and stimulate alpha-2 adrenergic receptors, causing responses similar to those of adrenaline and noradrenaline. They inhibit aqueous humor production and a have a wide variety of effects, including dry mouth, fatigue, and drowsiness.

Aqueous humor—A transparent liquid, contained within the eye, that is composed of water, sugars, vitamins, proteins, and other nutrients.

Betablocker (beta-adrenergic blocker)—A class of drugs that bind beta-adrenergic receptors and thereby decrease the ability of the body's own natural epinephrine to bind to those receptors, leading to inhibition of various processes in the body's sympathetic system. Betablockers can slow the heart rate, constrict airways in the lungs, lower blood pressure, and reduce aqueous secretion by ciliary tissues in the eye.

Carbonic anhydrase inhibitor—A class of diuretic drugs that inhibit the enzyme carbonic anhydrase, an enzyme involved in producing bicarbonate, which is required for aqueous humor production by the ciliary tissues in the eye. Thus, inhibitors of this enzyme inhibit aqueous humor production. Some side effects are urinary frequency, kidney stones, loss of the sense of taste, depression, and anemia.

Cornea—Clear, bowl-shaped structure at the front of the eye. It is located in front of the colored part of the eye (iris). The cornea lets light into the eye and partially focuses it.

Gonioscope—An instrument used to examine the trabecular meshwork; consists of a magnifier and a lens equipped with mirrors, which sits on the patient's cornea.

Hyperosmotic drugs—Refers to a class of drugs for glaucoma that increase the osmotic pressure in the blood, which then pulls water from the eye into the blood.

Iris—The colored part of the eye just behind the cornea and in front of the lens that controls the amount of light sent to the retina.

Lens (the crystalline lens)—A transparent structure in the eye that focuses light onto the retina.

Laser cyclophotocoagulation—A procedure used for severe glaucoma in patients who have not responded well to previous treatments. The laser partially destroys the tissues that make the fluid of the eye.

Laser peripheral iridotomy—This procedure makes a drainage hole in the iris allowing the fluid to drain from the eye

Laser Trabeculoplasty—In this procedure the laser attempts to open the normal drainage channels of the eye so fluid can drain more effectively.

Miotic—A drug that causes pupils to contract.

Ophthalmoscope—An instrument, with special lighting, designed to view structures in the back of the eye.

Optic nerve—The nerve that carries visual messages from the retina to the brain.

Prostaglandin—A group of molecules that exert local effects on a variety of processes including fluid balance, blood flow, and gastrointestinal function.

Prostaglandin analogue—A class of drugs that are similar in structure and function to prostaglandin.

Retina—The inner, light-sensitive layer of the eye containing rods and cones.

Sclera—The tough, fibrous, white outer protective covering that surrounds the eye.

Tonometry—The measurement of pressure.

Trabecular meshwork—A sponge-like tissue located near the cornea and iris that functions to drain the aqueous humor from the eye into the blood.

---

potential glaucoma victims, so they can be treated even before their IOP becomes elevated.

Bonny McClain

Glaucoma surgery *see* **Trabeculectomy**

Glioma *see* **Brain tumor**

Glipizide *see* **Antidiabetic drugs**

Glomerulonephritis

Definition

Acute glomerulonephritis is an inflammatory disease of both kidneys predominantly affecting children from ages two to 12. Chronic glomerulonephritis can develop over a period of 10–20 years and is most often associated with other systemic disease,

including diabetes, **malaria**, hepatitis, or **systemic lupus erythematosus**.

Description

Acute glomerulonephritis is an inflammation of the glomeruli, bundles of tiny vessels inside the kidneys. The damaged glomeruli cannot effectively filter waste products and excess water from the bloodstream to make urine. The kidneys appear enlarged, fatty, and congested.

Causes and symptoms

Acute glomerulonephritis most often follows a streptococcal infection of the throat or skin. In children, it is most often associated with an upper respiratory infection, **tonsillitis**, or **scarlet fever**. Kidney symptoms usually begin two to three weeks after the initial infection. Exposure to certain paints, glue or other organic solvents may also be the causative agent. It is thought that the kidney is damaged with exposure to the toxins that are excreted into the urine.

Mild glomerulonephritis may produce no symptoms, and diagnosis is made with laboratory studies of the urine and blood. Individuals with more severe cases of the disease may exhibit:

- fatigue
- nausea and **vomiting**
- shortness of breath
- disturbed vision
- high blood pressure
- swelling, especially noted in the face, hands, feet, and ankles
- blood and protein in the urine, resulting in a smoky or slightly red appearance

The individual with chronic glomerulonephritis may discover their condition with a routine physical exam revealing high blood pressure, or an eye exam showing vascular or hemorrhagic changes. The kidneys may be reduced to as little as one-fifth their normal size, consisting largely of fibrous tissues.

Diagnosis

Diagnosis of glomerulonephritis is established based on medical history, combined with laboratory studies. A "dipstick" test of urine will reveal increased protein levels. A 24 hour urine collection allows measurement of the excretion of proteins and creatinine. Creatinine clearance from the bloodstream by the

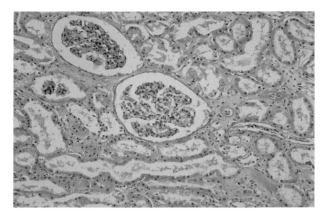

A close-up view of glomerulonephritis affecting the kidney. *(Custom Medical Stock Photo. Reproduced by permission.)*

kidneys is considered an index of the glomerular filtration rate. Blood studies may reveal a low **blood count**, and may also be checked for the presence of a streptococcal antibody titer(a sophisticated blood test indicating presence of streptococcal infection). A **kidney biopsy** may also be performed, using ultrasound to guide the needle for obtaining the specimen.

Treatment

The main objectives in the treatment of acute glomerulonephritis are to:

- decrease the damage to the glomeruli
- decrease the metabolic demands on the kidneys
- improve kidney function

Bedrest helps in maintaining adequate blood flow to the kidney. If residual infection is suspected, antibiotic therapy may be needed. In the presence of fluid overload, **diuretics** may be used to increase output with urination. Iron and vitamin supplements may be ordered if anemia develops, and antihypertensives, if high blood pressure accompanies the illness. In order to rest the kidney during the acute phase, decreased sodium and protein intake may be recommended. The amount of protein allowed is dependent upon the amount lost in the urine, and the requirements of the individual patient. Sodium limitations depend on the amount of **edema** present. Fluid restrictions are adjusted according to the patient's urinary output and body weight.

An accurate daily record of the patient's weight, fluid intake and urinary output assist in estimating kidney function. The patient must be watched for signs of complications and recurrent infection. As edema is reduced and the urine becomes free of protein and red blood cells, the patient is allowed to increase

KEY TERMS

Dialysis—A process of filtering and removing waste products from the bloodstream. Two main types are hemodialysis and peritoneal dialysis. In hemodialysis, the blood flows out of the body into a machine that filters out the waste products and routes the cleansed blood back into the body. In peritoneal dialysis, the cleansing occurs inside the body. Dialysis fluid is injected into the peritoneal cavity and wastes are filtered through the peritoneum, the thin membrane that surrounds the abdominal organs.

Glomeruli—Groups of tiny blood vessels with very thin walls that function as filters in the kidney. Glomeruli become inflamed and are destroyed in the disease process of glomerulonephritis.

Renal—Relating to the kidneys, from the Latin word *renes*.

activity. A woman who has had glomerulonephritis requires special medical attention during **pregnancy**.

Prognosis

In acute glomerulonephritis, symptoms usually subside in two weeks to several months, with 90% of children recovering without complications and adults recovering more slowly. Chronic glomerulonephritis is a disease that tends to progress slowly, so that there are no symptoms until the kidneys can no longer function. The resultant renal failure may require dialysis or kidney transplant.

Prevention

Prevention of glomerulonephritis is best accomplished by avoiding upper respiratory infections, as well as other acute and chronic infections, especially those of a streptococcal origin. Cultures of the infection site, usually the throat, should be obtained and antibiotic sensibility of the offending organism determined. Prompt medical assessment for necessary antibiotic therapy should be sought when infection is suspected. The use of prophylactic immunizations is recommended as appropriate.

Resources

ORGANIZATIONS

American Association of Kidney Patients. 100 S. Ashley Dr., #280, Tampa, FL 33602. (800) 749-2257. < http:// www.aakp.org > .

American Kidney Fund (AKF). Suite 1010, 6110 Executive Boulevard, Rockville, MD 20852. (800) 638-8299. < http://216.248.130.102/Default.htm > .

National Kidney Foundation. 30 East 33rd St., New York, NY 10016. (800) 622-9010. < http://www.kidney.org > .

National Kidney Foundation and Urologic Diseases Information Clearinghouse. 3 Information Way, Bethesda, MD 20892-3580. (800) 891-5390. < http:// www.niddk.nih.gov/health/kidney/nkudic.htm > .

Kathleen D. Wright, RN

Glossopharyngeal neuralgia *see* **Neuralgia**

Glucose-6-phosphate dehydrogenase deficiency

Definition

Glucose-6-phosphate dehydrogenase deficiency is an inherited condition caused by a defect or defects in the gene that codes for the enzyme, glucose-6-phosphate dehydrogenase (G6PD). It can cause **hemolytic anemia**, varying in severity from life-long anemia, to rare bouts of anemia to total unawareness of the condition. The episodes of hemolytic anemia are usually triggered by oxidants, infection, or by eating fava beans.

Description

G6PD deficiency is the most common enzyme deficiency in the world, with about 400 million people living with it. It is most prevalent in people of African, Mediterranean, and Asian ancestry. The incidence in different populations varies from zero in South American Indians to less than 0.1% of Northern Europeans to about 50% of Kurdish males. In the United States, it is most common among African American males; about 11 to 14% are G6PD-deficient.

G6PD deficiency is a recessive sex-linked trait. Thus, males have only one copy of the G6PD gene, but females have two copies. Recessive genes are masked in the presence of a gene that encodes normal G6PD. Accordingly, females with one copy of the gene for G6PD deficiency are usually normal, while males with one copy have the trait.

G6PD is present in all human cells but is particularly important to red blood cells. It is required to make NADPH in red blood cells but not in other cells. It is also required to make glutathione.

Glutathione and NADPH both help protect red blood cells against oxidative damage. Thus, when G6PD is defective, oxidative damage to red blood cells readily occurs, and they break open as a result. This event is called hemolysis, and multiple hemolyses in a short time span constitute an episode of hemolytic anemia.

As of 1998, there are almost 100 different known forms of G6PD enzyme molecules encoded by defective G6PD genes, yet not one of them is completely inactive. This suggests that G6PD is indispensable. Many G6PD defective enzymes are deficient in their stability rather than their initial ability to function. Since red blood cells lack nuclei, they, unlike other cells, cannot synthesize new enzyme molecules to replace defective ones. Hence, we expect young red blood cells to have new, functional G6PD and older cells to have non-functioning G6PD. This explains why episodes of hemolytic anemia are frequently self-limiting; new red blood cells are generated with enzymes able to afford protection from oxidation.

The geographic distribution of G6PD deficiency, allowing for migration, coincides with the geographic distribution of **malaria**. This fact and survival statistics suggest that G6PD deficiency protects against malaria.

Glucose-6-phosphate dehydrogenase deficiency is also known as G6PD deficiency, favism, and primaquine sensitivity.

Causes and symptoms

Causes

G6PD deficiency is caused by one copy of a defective G6PD gene in males or two copies of a defective G6PD gene in females. Hemolytic anemic attacks can be caused by oxidants, infection, and or by eating fava beans.

Symptoms

The most significant consequence of this disorder is hemolytic anemia, which is usually episodic, but the vast majority of people with G6PD deficiency have no symptoms.

The many different forms of G6PD deficiency have been divided into five classes according to severity.

- Class 1–enzyme deficiency with chronic hemolytic anemia
- Class 2–severe enzyme deficiency with less than 10% of normal activity

- Class 3–moderate to mild enzyme deficiency with 10–60% of normal activity
- Class 4–very mild or no enzyme deficiency
- Class 5–increased enzyme activity Fortunately, only a small number of people fall into Class 1.

The major symptoms of hemolytic anemia are **jaundice**, dark urine, abdominal **pain**, back pain, lowered red blood cell count, and elevated bilirubin. People who suffer from severe and chronic forms of G6PD deficiency in addition may have **gallstones**, enlarged spleens, defective white blood cells, and **cataracts**.

Attacks of hemolytic anemia are serious for infants. Brain damage and **death** are possible but preventable outcomes. Newborns with G6PD deficiency are about 1.5 times as likely to get **neonatal jaundice** than newborns without G6PD deficiency.

Diagnosis

Blood tests can detect G6PD deficiency, either by measuring the G6PD enzyme activity between episodes or by measuring bilirubin during an episode. Such tests cost about $50.00. Family histories are helpful, too.

Treatment

In a typical attack of hemolytic anemia, no treatment is needed; the patient will recover in about eight days. However, blood transfusions are necessary in severe cases. Recent success treating elevated bilirubin in newborns by exposing them to bright light has decreased the need for neonatal transfusions.

Alternative treatment

Vitamin E and **folic acid** (both anti-oxidants) may help decrease hemolysis in G6PD-deficient individuals.

Prognosis

The prognosis for almost everyone with G6PD deficiency is excellent. Large studies have shown that G6PD-deficient individuals do not acquire any illnesses more frequently than the rest of the population. In fact the opposite may be true for some diseases like ischemic heart disease and cerebrovascular disease.

KEY TERMS

Bilirubin—A breakdown product derived from hemoglobin; removed from the blood by the liver.

Enzyme—A protein catalyst; one of the two kinds of biological catalysts, which are exceedingly specific; each different enzyme only catalyzes one or two specific reactions.

Enzyme activity—A measure of the ability of an enzyme to catalyze a specific reaction.

Glutathione—A molecule that acts as a co-enzyme in cellular oxidation-reduction reactions.

Hemolysis—Lysis (opening) of red blood cells, with concomitant leakage of cell contents from the cells.

Hemolytic anemia—Anemia due to hemolysis.

Jaundice—Yellowish skin color due to liver disease.

Neonatal—Describes babies just after they are born.

Recessive trait—An inherited trait that is outwardly obvious only when two copies of the gene for that trait are present–as opposed to a dominant trait where one copy of the gene for the dominant trait is sufficient to display the trait. The recessive condition is said to be masked by the presence of the dominant gene when both are present; i.e., the recessive condition is seen only in the absence of the dominant gene.

Sex-linked—Refers to genes or traits carried on one of the sex chromosomes, usually the X.

X chromosome—One of the two types of sex chromosomes, present twice in female cells and once in male cells.

Prevention

Most episodes of hemolytic anemia can be prevented by avoiding fava beans, oxidant drugs, and oxidant chemicals. All of the following oxidants can trigger attacks: acetanilid, dapsone, doxorubicin, furazolidone, methylene blue, nalidixic acid, napthalene, niridazole, nitrofurantoin, phenazopyridine, phenylhydrazine, primaquine, quinidine, quinine, sulfacetamide, sulfamethoxazole, sulfonamide, sulfapyridine, thiazolesulfone, toluidine blue, and trinitrotoluene. Since infections also trigger hemolytic attacks and have other dire consequences, sometimes it is advisable to use one of the listed drugs.

It is especially important to screen newborns who are likely to have G6PD deficiency to ensure that G6PD-deficient babies won't be subjected to any of the triggers of hemolytic anemia. Pregnant women, especially in areas where G6PD deficiency is prevalent, should avoid eating fava beans.

Resources

ORGANIZATIONS

Alliance of Genetic Support Groups. 4301 Connecticut Ave. NW, Suite 404, Washington, D.C. 20008. (202) 966-5557. Fax: (202) 966-8553. < http://www.geneticalliance.org > .

OTHER

Favism Home Page. < http://rialto.com/favism/index.htm > .

Lorraine Lica, PhD

Glucosylcerebroside lipidosis *see* **Gaucher disease**

Gluten enteropathy *see* **Celiac disease**

Glyburide *see* **Antidiabetic drugs**

Glycogen storage diseases

Definition

Glycogen serves as the primary fuel reserve for the body's energy needs. Glycogen storage diseases, also known as glycogenoses, are genetically linked metabolic disorders that involve the enzymes regulating glycogen metabolism. Symptoms vary by the glycogen storage disease (GSD) type and can include **muscle cramps** and wasting, enlarged liver, and low blood sugar. Disruption of glycogen metabolism also affects other biochemical pathways as the body seeks alternative fuel sources. Accumulation of abnormal metabolic by-products can damage the kidneys and other organs. GSD can be fatal, but the risk hinges on the type of GSD.

Description

Most of the body's cells rely on glucose as an energy source. Glucose levels in the blood are very stringently controlled within a range or 70–100 mg/dL, primarily by hormones such as insulin and glucagon. Immediately after a meal, blood glucose levels rise and exceed the body's immediate energy requirements. In a process analogous to putting money in the bank, the body bundles up the extra glucose and stores it as glycogen in the liver and muscles. Later, as the blood glucose levels begin to dip, the body makes a withdrawal from its glycogen savings.

The system for glycogen metabolism relies on a complex system of enzymes. These enzymes are responsible for creating glycogen from glucose, transporting the glycogen to and from storage areas within cells, and extracting glucose from the glycogen as needed. Both creating and tearing down the glycogen macromolecule are multistep processes requiring a different enzyme at each step. If one of these enzymes is defective and fails to complete its step, the process halts. Such enzyme defects are the underlying cause of GSDs.

The enzyme defect arises from an error in its gene. Since the error is in the genetic code, GSDs can be passed down from generation-to-generation. However, all but one GSD are linked to autosomal genes, which means a person inherits one copy of the gene from each parent. Following a Mendelian inheritance pattern, the normal gene is dominant and the defective gene is recessive. As long as a child receives at least one normal gene, there is no risk for a GSD. GSDs appear only if a person inherits a defective gene from both parents.

The most common forms of GSD are Types I, II, III, and IV, which may account for more than 90% of all cases. The most common form is Type I, or von Gierke's disease, which occurs in one out of every 100,000 births. Other forms, such as Types VI and IX, are so rare that reliable statistics are not available. The overall frequency of all forms of glycogen storage disease is approximately one in 20,000–25,000 live births.

Causes and symptoms

GSD symptoms depend on the enzyme affected. Since glycogen storage occurs mainly in muscles and the liver, those sites display the most prominent symptoms.

There are at least 10 different types of GSDs which are classified according to the enzyme affected:

- Type Ia, or von Gierke's disease, is caused by glucose-6-phosphatase deficiency in the liver, kidney, and small intestine. The last step in glycogenolysis, the breaking down of glycogen to glucose, is the transformation of glucose-6-phosphate to glucose. In GSD I, that step does not occur. As a result, the liver is clogged with excess glycogen and becomes enlarged and fatty. Other symptoms include low blood sugar and elevated levels of lactate, lipids,

and uric acid in the blood. Growth is impaired, **puberty** is often delayed, and bones may be weakened by **osteoporosis**. Blood platelets are also affected and frequent nosebleeds and easy bruising are common. Primary symptoms improve with age, but after age 20–30, liver tumors, **liver cancer**, chronic renal disease, and **gout** may appear.

- Type Ib is caused by glucose-6-phosphatase translocase deficiency. In order to carry out the final step of glycogenolysis, glucose-6-phosphate has to be transported into a cell's endoplasmic reticulum. If translocase, the enzyme responsible for that movement, is missing or defective, the same symptoms occur as in Type Ia. Additionally, the immune system is weakened and victims are susceptible to bacterial infections, such as **pneumonia**, mouth and gum infections, and inflammatory bowel disease. Types Ic and Id are also caused by defects in the translocase system.

- Type II, or Pompe's disease or acid maltase deficiency, is caused by lysosomal alpha-D-glucosidase deficiency in skeletal and heart muscles. GSD II is subdivided according to the age of onset. In the infantile form, infants seem normal at birth, but within a few months they develop muscle weakness, trouble breathing, and an enlarged heart. Cardiac failure and **death** usually occur before age 2, despite medical treatment. The juvenile and adult forms of GSD II affect mainly the skeletal muscles in the body's limbs and torso. Unlike the infantile form, treatment can extend life, but there is no cure. **Respiratory failure** is the primary cause of death.

- Type III, or Cori's disease, is caused by glycogen debrancher enzyme deficiency in the liver, muscles, and some blood cells, such as leukocytes and erythrocytes. About 15% of GSD III cases only involve the liver. The glycogen molecule is not a simple straight chain of linked glucose molecules, but rather an intricate network of short chains that branch off from one another. In glycogenolysis, a particular enzyme is required to unlink the branch points. When that enzyme fails, symptoms similar to GSD I occur; in childhood, it may be difficult to distinguish the two GSDs by symptoms alone. In addition to the low blood sugar, retarded growth, and enlarged liver causing a swollen abdomen, GSD III also causes muscles prone to wasting, an enlarged heart, and heightened levels of lipids in the blood. The muscle wasting increases with age, but the other symptoms become less severe.

- Type IV, or Andersen's disease, is caused by glycogen brancher enzyme deficiency in the liver, brain, heart, skeletal muscles, and skin fibroblasts. The glycogen constructed in GSD IV is abnormal and insoluble. As it accumulates in the cells, cell death leads to organ damage. Infants born with GSD IV appear normal at birth, but are diagnosed with enlarged livers and **failure to thrive** within their first year. Infants who survive beyond their first birthday develop **cirrhosis** of the liver by age 3–5 and die as a result of chronic liver failure.

- Type V, or McArdle's disease, is caused by glycogen phosphorylase deficiency in skeletal muscles. Under normal circumstances, muscles cells rely on oxidation of fatty acids during rest or light activity. More demanding activity requires that they draw on their glycogen stockpile. In GSD V, this form of glycogenolysis is disabled and glucose is not available. The main symptoms are muscle weakness and cramping brought on by **exercise**, as well as burgundy-colored urine after exercise due to myoglobin (a breakdown product of muscle) in the urine.

- Type VI, or Hers' disease, is caused by liver phosphorylase deficiency, which blocks the first step of glycogenolysis. In contrast to other GSDs, Type VI seems to be linked to the X chromosome. Low blood sugar is one of the key symptoms, but it is not as severe as in some other forms of GSD. An enlarged liver and mildly retarded growth also occur.

- Type VII, or Tarui's disease, is caused by muscle phosphofructokinase deficiency. Although glucose may be available as a fuel in muscles, the cells cannot metabolize it. Therefore, abnormally high levels of glycogen are stockpiled in the muscle cells. The symptoms are similar to GSD V, but also include anemia and increased levels of uric acid.

- Types VIII and XI are caused by defects of enzymes in the liver phosphorylase activating-deactivating cascade and have symptoms similar to GSD VI.

- Type IX is caused by liver glycogen phosphorylase kinase deficiency and, symptom-wise, is very similar to GSD VI. The main differences are that the symptoms may not be as severe and may also include exercise-related problems in the muscles, such as **pain** and cramps. The symptoms abate after puberty with proper treatment. Most cases of GSD IX are linked to the X chromosome and therefore affect males.

- Type X is caused by a defect in the cyclic adenosine monophosphate-dependent (AMP) kinase enzyme and presents symptoms similar to GSDs VI and IX.

Diagnosis

Diagnosis usually occurs in infancy or childhood, although some milder types of GSD go unnoticed well into adulthood and old age. It is even conceivable that some of the milder GSDs are never diagnosed.

The four major symptoms that typically lead a doctor to suspect GSDs are low blood sugar, enlarged liver, retarded growth, and an abnormal blood biochemistry profile. A definitive diagnosis is obtained by biopsy of the affected organ or organs. The biopsy sample is tested for its glycogen content and assayed for enzyme activity. There are DNA-based techniques for diagnosing some GSDs from more easily available samples, such as blood or skin. These DNA techniques can also be used for prenatal testing.

Treatment

Some GSD types cannot be treated, while others are relatively easy to control through symptom management. In more severe cases, receiving an organ transplant is the only option. In the most severe cases, there are no available treatments and the victim dies within the first few years of life.

Of the treatable types of GSD, many are treated by manipulating the diet. The key to managing GSD I is to maintain consistent levels of blood glucose through a combination of nocturnal intragastric feeding (usually for infants and children), frequent high-carbohydrate meals during the day, and regular oral doses of cornstarch (people over age 2). Juvenile and adult forms of GSD II can be managed somewhat by a high protein diet, which also helps in cases of GSD III, GSD VI, and GSD IX. GSD V and GSD VII can also be managed with a high protein diet and by avoiding strenuous exercise.

For GSD cases in which dietary therapy is ineffective, organ transplantation may be the only viable alternative. Liver transplants have been effective in reversing the symptoms of GSD IV.

Advances in genetic therapy offer hope for effective treatment in the future. This therapy involves using viruses to deliver a correct form of the gene to affected cells. Another potential therapy utilizes transgenic animals to produce correct copies of the defective enzyme in their milk. In late 1997, a Dutch pharmaceutical company, Pharming Health Care Products, began clinical trials to treat GSD II with human alpha-glucosidase derived from the milk of transgenic rabbits. Researchers at Duke University in North Carolina are also focusing on a treatment for Pompe's disease and, aided by Synpac Pharmaceuticals Limited of the United Kingdom, plan to begin clinical trials of a recombinant form of the enzyme in 1998.

KEY TERMS

Amniocentesis—A medical test done during pregnancy in which a small sample of the amniotic fluid is taken from around the fetus. The fluid contains fetal cells that can be examined for genetic abnormalities.

Autosomal gene—A gene found on one of the 22 autosomal chromosome pairs; i.e., not on a sex (X or Y) chromosome.

Chorionic villus sampling—A medical test done during pregnancy in which a sample of the membrane surrounding the fetus is removed for examination. This examination can reveal genetic fetal abnormalities.

Glucose—A form of sugar that serves as the body's main energy source.

Glycogen—A macromolecule composed mainly of glucose that serves as the storage form of glucose that is not immediately needed by the body.

Glycogenolysis—The process of tearing-down a glycogen molecule to free up glucose.

Glycogenosis—An alternate term for glycogen storage disease. The plural form is glycogenoses.

Gout—A painful condition in which uric acid precipitates from the blood and accumulates in joints and connective tissues.

Mendelian inheritance—An inheritance pattern for autosomal gene pairs. The genetic trait displayed results from one parent's gene dominating over the gene inherited from the other parent.

Osteoporosis—A disease in which the bones become weak and brittle.

Renal disease—Kidney disease.

Transgenic animal—Animals that have had genes from other species inserted into their genetic code.

Prognosis

People with well-managed, treatable types of GSD can lead long, relatively normal lives. This goal is accomplished with the milder types of GSD, such as Types VI, IX, and X. As the GSD type becomes more severe, a greater level of vigilance against infections and other complications is required. Given current treatment options, complications such as **liver disease**, **heart failure**, and respiratory failure may not be warded-off indefinitely. Quality of life and life expectancy are substantially decreased.

Prevention

Because GSD is an inherited condition, it is not preventable. If both parents carry the defective gene, there is a one-in-four chance that their offspring will inherit the disorder. Other children may be carriers or they may miss inheriting the gene altogether.

Through chorionic villi sampling and **amniocentesis**, the disorder can be detected prior to birth. Some types of GSD can be detected even before conception occurs, if both parents are tested for the presence of the defective gene. Before undergoing such testing, the prospective parents should meet with a genetic counselor and other professionals in order to make an informed decision.

Resources

ORGANIZATIONS

Acid Maltase Deficiency Association. PO Box 700248, San Antonio, TX 78270-0248. (210) 494-6144. < http://www.amda-pompe.org > .

American Liver Foundation. 1425 Pompton Ave., Cedar Grove, NJ 07009. (800) 223-0179. < http://www.liverfoundation.org > .

Association for Glycogen Storage Disease. PO Box 896, Durant, Iowa 52747-9769. (319) 785-6038.

Julia Barrett

▌Glycosylated hemoglobin test

Definition

Glycosylated hemoglobin is a test that indicates how much sugar has been in a person's blood during the past two to four months. It is used to monitor the effectiveness of diabetes treatment.

Purpose

Diabetes is a disease in which a person cannot effectively use sugar in the blood. Left untreated, blood sugar levels can be very high. High sugar levels increase risk of complications, such as damage to eyes, kidneys, heart, nerves, blood vessels, and other organs.

A routine blood sugar test reveals how close to normal a sugar level is at the time of the test. The glycosylated **hemoglobin test** reveals how close to normal it has been during the past several months.

This information helps a physician evaluate how well a person is responding to diabetes treatment and to determine how long sugar levels have been high in a person newly diagnosed with diabetes.

Description

The Diabetes Control and Complications Trial (DCCT) demonstrated that people with diabetes who maintained blood glucose (sugar) and total **fasting** hemoglobin levels at or close to a normal range decreased their risk of complications by 50–75%. Based on results of this study, the American Diabetes Association (ADA) recommends routine glycosylated hemoglobin testing to measure long-term control of blood sugar.

Glycosylated hemoglobin measures the percentage of hemoglobin bound to glucose. Hemoglobin is a protein found in every red blood cell. As hemoglobin and glucose are together in the red blood cell, the glucose gradually binds to the A1c form of hemoglobin in a process called glycosylation. The amount bound reflects how much glucose has been in the blood during the past average 120-day lifespan of red cells.

Several methods are used to measure the amount of bound hemoglobin and glucose. They are electrophoresis, chromatography, and immunoassay. All are based on the separation of hemoglobin bound to glucose from that without glucose.

The ADA recommends glycosylated hemoglobin be done during a person's first diabetes evaluation, again after treatment is begun and sugar levels are stabilized, then repeated at least semiannually. If the person does not meet treatment goals or sugar levels have not stabilized, the test should be repeated quarterly.

Other names for the test include: Hemoglobin A1c, Diabetic control index, GHb, glycosylated hemoglobin, and glycated hemoglobin. The test is covered by insurance. Results usually are available the following day.

Preparation

A person does not need to fast before this test. A healthcare worker ties a tourniquet on the person's upper arm, locates a vein in the inner elbow region, and inserts a needle into the vein. Vacuum action draws the blood through the needle into an attached tube. Collection of the sample takes only a few minutes. This test requires 5 mL of blood.

KEY TERMS

Diabetes mellitus—A disease in which a person can't effectively use sugar in the blood to meet the needs of the body. It is caused by a lack of the hormone insulin.

Glucose—The main form of sugar used by the body for energy.

Glycosylated hemoglobin—A test that measures the amount of hemoglobin bound to glucose. It is a measure of how much glucose has been in the blood during the past two to four months.

In 2004, more convenient fingerstick methods of the test were being developed. An over-the-counter, at-home test kit was in the beginning stages of approval. People with diabetes could stick their own fingers, draw the blood and send the sample by mail for results within five to seven days.

Aftercare

Discomfort or bruising may occur at the puncture site, or the person may feel dizzy or faint. Pressure to the puncture site until bleeding stops reduces bruising. Warm packs relieve discomfort.

Normal results

Diabetes treatment should achieve glycosylated hemoglobin levels of less than 7.0%. Normal value for a non-diabetic person is 4.0–6.0%.

Because laboratories use different methods, results from different laboratories can not always be compared. The National Glycosylation Standardization Program gives a certification to laboratories using tests standardized to those used in the DCCT study.

Abnormal results

Results require interpretation by a physician with knowledge of the person's clinical condition, as well as the test method used. Some methods give false high or low results if the person has an abnormal hemoglobin, such as hemoglobin S or F.

Conditions that increase the lifespan of red cells, such as a **splenectomy** (removal of the spleen), falsely increase levels. Conditions that decrease the lifespan, such as hemolysis (disruption of the red blood cell membrane), falsely decrease levels.

Resources

PERIODICALS

"Simple Choice A1c." *Diabetes Forecast* January 2004: RG7.

ORGANIZATIONS

American Diabetes Association. 1701 North Beauregard Street, Alexandria, VA 22311. (800) 342-2383. < http://www.diabetes.org >.

Centers for Disease Control and Prevention. 1600 Clifton Rd., NE, Atlanta, GA 30333. (800) 311-3435, (404) 639-3311. < http://www.cdc.gov >.

National Diabetes Information Clearinghouse. 1 Information Way, Bethesda, MD 20892-3560. (800) 860-8747. < http://www.niddk.nih.gov/health/diabetes/ndic.htm >.

Nancy J. Nordenson
Teresa G. Odle

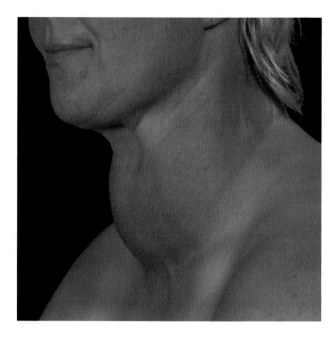

This woman's goiter may have been caused by an insufficient intake of iodine. *(Custom Medical Stock Photo. Reproduced by permission.)*

Goiter

Definition

Goiter refers to any visible enlargement of the thyroid gland.

Description

The thyroid gland sits astride the trachea (windpipe) and is shaped like a butterfly. It makes thyroxin, a hormone that regulates the metabolic activity of the body, rather like the gas pedal on a car. Too much thyroxin increases the metabolism, causing weight loss, temperature elevation, nervousness, and irritability. Too little thyroxin slows the metabolism down, deepens the voice, causes weight gain and water retention, and retards growth and mental development in children. Both conditions also alter hair and skin growth, bowel function, and menstrual flow.

Curiously, the thyroid gland is often enlarged whether it is making too much hormone, too little, or sometimes even when it is functioning normally. The thyroid is controlled by the pituitary gland, which secretes thyroid stimulating hormone (TSH) in response to the amount of thyroxin it finds in the blood. TSH increases the amount of thyroxin secreted by the thyroid and also causes the thyroid gland to grow.

- Hyperthyroid goiter–If the amount of stimulating hormone is excessive, the thyroid will both enlarge and secrete too much thyroxin. The result–hyperthyroidism with a goiter. Graves' disease is the most common form of this disorder.

- Euthyroid goiter–The thyroid is the only organ in the body to use iodine. If dietary iodine is slightly inadequate, too little thyroxin will be secreted, and the pituitary will sense the deficiency and produce more TSH. The thyroid gland will enlarge enough to make sufficient thyroxin.

- Hypothyroid goiter–If dietary iodine is severely reduced, even an enlarged gland will not be able to make enough thyroxin. The gland will keep growing under the influence of TSH, but it may never be able to make enough thyroxin.

Causes and symptoms

Excess TSH (or similar hormones), cysts, and tumors will enlarge the thyroid gland. Of these, TSH enlarges the entire gland while cysts and tumors enlarge only a part of it.

The only symptom from a goiter is the large swelling just above the breast bone. Rarely, it may constrict the trachea (windpipe) or esophagus and cause difficulty breathing or swallowing. The rest of the symptoms come from thyroxin or the lack of it.

KEY TERMS

Cyst—A liquid-filled structure developing abnormally in the body.

Euthyroid—Having the right amount of thyroxin stimulation.

Hyperthyroid—Having too much thyroxin stimulation.

Hypothyroid—Having too little thyroxin stimulation.

Pituitary gland—The master gland, located in the middle of the head, that controls most of the other glandss by secreting stimulating hormones.

Radiotherapy—The use of ionizing radiation, either as x rays or radioactive isotopes, to treat disease.

Thyroxin—The hormone secreted by the thyroid gland.

Diagnosis

The size, shape, and texture of the thyroid gland help the physician determine the cause. A battery of blood tests are required to verify the specific thyroid disease. Functional imaging studies using radioactive iodine determine how active the gland is and what it looks like.

Treatment

Goiters of all types will regress with treatment of the underlying condition. Dietary iodine may be all that is needed. However, if an iodine deficient thyroid that has grown in size to accommodate its deficiency is suddenly supplied an adequate amount of iodine, it could suddenly make large amounts of thyroxin and cause a thyroid storm, the equivalent of racing your car motor at top speed.

Hyperthyroidism can be treated with medications, therapeutic doses of radioactive iodine, or surgical reduction. Surgery is much less common now than it used to be because of progress in drugs and radiotherapy.

Prognosis

Although goiters diminish in size, the thyroid may not return to normal. Sometimes thyroid function does not return after treatment, but thyroxin is easy to take as a pill.

Prevention

Euthyroid goiter and hypothyroid goiter are common around the world because many regions have inadequate dietary iodine, including some places in the United States. International relief groups are providing iodized salt to many of these populations. Because **mental retardation** is a common result of **hypothyroidism** in children, this is an extremely important project.

Resources

ORGANIZATIONS

International Council for the Control of Iodine Deficiency Disorders. 43 Circuit Road, Chester Hill, MA, 02167. (207) 335-2221. < http://www.tulane.edu/~icec/icciddhome.htm > .

Micronutrient Initiative (c/o International Development Research Centre). 250 Albert St., Ottawa, Ontario, Canada K1G 3H9. (613) 236-6163, ext. 2050. < http://www.idrc.ca/mi/index.htm > .

J. Ricker Polsdorfer, MD

Gonadal dysgenesis *see* **Turner syndrome**

Gonorrhea

Definition

Gonorrhea is a highly contagious sexually transmitted disease that is caused by the bacterium *Neisseria gonorrhoeae*. The mucous membranes of the genital region may become inflamed without the development of any other symptoms. When symptoms occur, they are different in men and women. In men, gonorrhea usually begins as an infection of the vessel that carries urine and sperm (urethra). In women, it will most likely infect the narrow part of the uterus (cervix). If untreated, gonorrhea can result in serious medical complications.

Description

Gonorrhea is commonly referred to as "the clap." The incidence of gonorrhea has steadily declined since the 1980s, largely due to increased public awareness campaigns and the risk of contracting other **sexually transmitted diseases**, such as **AIDS**. Still, current estimates range from 400,000 to as many as one million projected cases of gonorrhea in the United States each year. These estimates vary due to the private nature of the disease and the consequent underreporting that

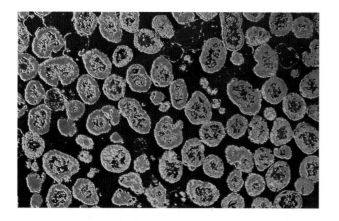

A transmission electron microscopy (TEM) image of *Neisseria gonorrhoeae*. *(Custom Medical Stock Photo. Reproduced by permission.)*

occurs. The majority of reported cases of gonorrhea come from public health clinics.

The disease affects people of all ages, races, and socioeconomic levels, but some individuals are more at-risk than others. Adolescents and young adults are the highest risk group, with more than 80% of the reported cases each year occurring in the 15–29 age group. Those individuals with multiple sexual partners and who use no barrier **contraception**, such as condoms, are most at-risk. Reported rates vary among racial and ethnic groups.

The risk factors for gonorrhea are not unlike those for all sexually transmitted diseases. Both men and women can become infected through a variety of sexual contact behaviors, including oral, anal, or vaginal intercourse. The disease is transmitted very efficiently. In fact, women run a 60–90% chance of contracting the disease after just one sexual encounter with an infected male. The disease can also be transmitted from an infected mother to her infant during delivery.

Causes and symptoms

If treated early, gonorrhea can be cured. Unfortunately, many individuals with gonorrhea, particularly women, will experience no symptoms to alert them to the possibility that they have contracted gonorrhea, and therefore, many do not seek treatment. When present, the symptoms and complications of gonorrhea are primarily limited to the genital, urinary, and gastrointestinal systems and usually begin between one day and two weeks following infection. If left untreated, serious complications can result if the disease spreads to the bloodstream and infects the brain, heart valves, and joints. Untreated gonorrhea

can also result in severe damage to the reproductive system, making an individual unable to conceive a child (sterile).

Symptoms of gonorrhea in women

As many as 80% of women with gonorrhea show no symptoms. If present, symptoms may include the following:

- bleeding between menstrual periods
- chronic abdominal **pain**
- painful urination
- vaginal discharge, often cloudy and yellow
- in the case of oral infection, there may be no symptoms or only a sore throat.
- anal infection may cause rectal **itching** or discharge.

Because women often do not show any symptoms, complications are more likely to occur as the disease progresses. The most common complication is **pelvic inflammatory disease** (PID). PID can occur in up to 40% of women with gonorrhea and may result in damage to the fallopian tubes, a **pregnancy** developing outside the uterus (**ectopic pregnancy**), or sterility. If an infected woman is pregnant, gonorrhea can be passed on to her newborn through the birth canal during delivery. These infants may experience eye infections that could lead to blindness.

Symptoms of gonorrhea in men

Men are more likely to experience the following symptoms:

- thick and cloudy discharge from the penis
- burning or pain during urination
- more frequent urination
- in the case of oral infection, there may be no symptoms or only a sore throat
- anal infection may cause rectal itching or discharge

In men, complications can affect the prostate, testicles, and surrounding glands. Inflammation, tissue death and pus formation (abscesses), and scarring can occur and result in sterility.

Diagnosis

The diagnosis of gonorrhea can be made at a public health clinic or a family physician office. First, the doctor will discuss symptoms and the patient's known contact or at-risk behavior. There are three methods available to test for the presence of

Neisseria gonorrhoeae. These include a culture, a Gram stain, and an ELISA test. Culture of secretions from the infected area is the preferred method for gonorrhea screening in patients with or without symptoms. A cotton swab can be used to collect enough sample for a culture. The sample is incubated for up to two days, providing enough time for the bacteria to multiply and be accurately identified. This test is nearly 100% accurate.

Gram stains are more accurate in the diagnosis of gonorrhea in men than in women. To perform this test, a small amount of discharge from the infected area will be placed on a slide, stained with a special dye, and examined under a microscope for the presence of the gonococcus bacteria. The advantage to this test is that results can be obtained very quickly at the initial visit. Because it requires that the physician or technician be able to recognize and accurately identify the bacteria simply by looking at it under a microscope, however, this test is only about 70% accurate. As a result, one of the other methods may also be used to confirm the diagnosis.

ELISA, or enzyme-linked immunosorbent assay, has emerged as a rapid and sensitive test for gonorrhea. It is much more sensitive than the gram stain and is more convenient than the culture test, which involves the transport and storage of samples. As of late 1997, several other diagnostic tests were being researched with the goal of providing a cost-effective method of screening for a variety of sexually transmitted diseases. One of the most interesting of these is a home test that can be taken by the patient themselves, allowing for a degree of privacy and confidentiality.

When a patient suspects exposure to or experiences symptoms of gonorrhea, he or she may see a public health provider or family practice physician. Physicians trained in obstetrics or gynecology may also be involved, particularly if gynecological complications occur. Men who experience complications may be referred to a urologist. There are also infectious disease physicians who specialize in the treatment and research of all infectious diseases, including those transmitted sexually. All physicians must report this highly contagious disease to public health officials, and patients are asked to provide the names of sex partners during the suspected period of infection so that they can be notified of the risk.

Treatment

Gonorrhea has become more difficult and expensive to treat since the 1970s, due to the increased resistance of gonorrhea to certain **antibiotics**. In fact, according to projections from the Centers for Disease Control and Prevention, 30% of the strains of gonorrhea were resistant to routine antibiotics in 1994, and resistance has been increasing steadily. Furthermore, many patients have both gonorrhea and chlamydial infections. Therefore, two drug treatment regimens are common. Medications used to treat gonorrhea include ceftriaxone, cefixime, spectinomycin, ciprofloxacin, and ofloxacin. Ceftriaxone and doxycycline or azithromycin are often given simultaneously to treat possible co-existing chlamydia (in pregnant women, erythromycin should be substituted for the aforementioned anti-chlamydial agents). In 2004, reports said that oral antibiotics were preferred over intramuscular forms of the drugs. Also, researchers reported that cefixime had not been available and that fluoroquinolone had been used by more physicians to treat gonorrhea. However, fluoroquinolone resistance was rising among patients with gonorrhea, and in June 2004 the Centers for Disease Control recommended that clinicians no longer prescribe the drug as first-line treatment for gonorrhea in men who have sex with men.

An extremely important consideration is to make sure that all of the prescribed medication is taken. If a course of antibiotics is not completed, the medication will only kill those organisms that are susceptible to the antibiotic, allowing those that are resistant to the effects of that particular antibiotic to multiply and possibly cause a new infection that will be more difficult to treat. Patients should refrain from sexual intercourse until treatment is complete and return for follow-up testing. Any sexual partners during the time of infection, even if those partners do not show symptoms, should be notified and treated when any sexually transmitted disease is involved.

Alternative treatment

Although there is no known alternative to antibiotics in the treatment of gonorrhea, there are herbs and **minerals** that may be used to supplement antibiotic treatment:

- *Lactobacillus acidophilus* or live-culture yogurts are helpful, while taking antibiotics, to replenish gastrointestinal flora.

- The following supplements may be used to improve the body's immune function: zinc, multivitamins and mineral complexes, vitamin C, and garlic (*Allium sativum*).

- Several herbs may reduce some symptoms or help speed healing: kelp has balanced **vitamins** and minerals. Calendula (*Calendula officinalis*), myrrh (*Commiphora molmol*), and thuja (*Thuja occidentalis*) may help reduce discharge and inflammation when used as a tea or douche.

- Hot baths may also help reduce pain and inflammation.

- A variety of herbs may help with symptoms of the reproductive and urinary systems.

- If a physician approves, **fasting**, combined with certain juices, may help cleanse the urinary and gastro-intestinal systems.

- There may be **acupressure** and **acupuncture** points that will help with system cleansing. These exact pressure points can be provided and treated by an acupressurist or acupuncturist.

Prognosis

The prognosis for patients with gonorrhea varies based on how early the disease is detected and treated. If treated early and properly, patients can be entirely cured of the disease. Up to 40% of female patients who are not treated early may develop pelvic inflammatory disease (PID) and the possibility of resulting sterility. Although the risk of **infertility** is higher in women than in men, men may also become sterile if the urethra becomes inflamed (**urethritis**) as a result of an untreated gonorrhea infection. Following an episode of PID, a woman is six to 10 times more likely, should a pregnancy occur, to have a pregnancy develop outside the uterus (ectopic pregnancy), which can result in death. Liver infection may also occur in untreated women. In approximately 2% of patients with untreated gonorrhea, the gonococcal infection may spread throughout the body and can cause **fever**, arthritis-like joint pain, and **skin lesions**.

Prevention

Currently, there is no vaccine for gonorrhea, but several are under development. The best prevention is to abstain from having sex or to engage in sex only when in a mutually monogamous relationship in which both partners have been tested for gonorrhea, AIDS, and other sexually transmitted diseases. The next line of defense is the use of condoms, which have been shown to be highly effective in preventing disease (and unwanted pregnancies). To be 100% effective, condoms must be used properly. A female birth-control device that

---

KEY TERMS

Cervix—The narrow part or neck of the uterus.

Chlamydia—The most common bacterial sexually transmitted disease in the United States that often accompanies gonorrhea and is known for its lack of evident symptoms in the majority of women.

Ectopic pregnancy—A pregnancy that occurs outside the uterus, such as in the fallopian tubes. Although the fetus will not survive, in some cases, ectopic pregnancy can also result in the death of the mother.

ELISA—Enzyme-linked immunosorbent assay. This test has been used a screening test for AIDS for many years and has also been used to detect gonorrhea bacteria.

HIV—Human immunodeficiency virus, the virus that causes AIDS. The risk of acquiring AIDS is increased by the presence of gonorrhea or other sexually transmitted diseases.

Neisseria gonorrhoeae—The bacterium that causes gonorrhea. It cannot survive for any length of time outside the human body.

Pelvic inflammatory disease (PID)—An infection of the upper genital tract that is the most serious threat to a woman's ability to reproduce. At least 25% of women who contract the disease, which can be a complication of gonorrhea, will experience long-term consequences such as infertility or ectopic pregnancy.

Sexually transmitted diseases (STDs)—A group of diseases which are transmitted by sexual contact. In addition to gonorrhea, this groups generally includes chlamydia, HIV (AIDS), herpes, syphilis, and genital warts.

Sterile—Unable to conceive a child.

Urethra—The canal leading from the bladder, and in men, also a path for sperm fluid.

Urethritis—Inflammation of the urethra.

---

blocks the entry of sperm into the cervix (**diaphragm**) can also reduce the risk of infection. The risk of contracting gonorrhea increases with the number of sexual partners. Any man or woman who has sexual contact with more than one partner is advised to be tested regularly for gonorrhea and other sexually transmitted diseases.

Resources

BOOKS

Sparling, P. Fredrick. "Gonococcal Infections." In *Cecil Textbook of Medicine*, edited by Russel L. Cecil, et al. Philadelphia: W.B. Saunders Company, 2000.

PERIODICALS

"Fluoroquinolone-resistant Gonorrhea on the Rise: Exposure History is Critical." *Emergency Medicine Alert* July 2004: 11–12.

Georgia, Kristen. "Revised Approach to Gonorrhea Treatment." *Patient Care* July 2004: 11.

ORGANIZATIONS

American Foundation for the Prevention of Venereal Disease, Inc. 799 Broadway, Suite 638, New York, NY 10003. (212) 759-2069.

National Institute of Allergy and Infectious Diseases. National Institutes of Health, Bethesda, MD 20892.

Teresa G. Odle

Goodpasture's syndrome

Definition

An uncommon and life-threatening hypersensitivity disorder believed to be an autoimmune process related to antibody formation in the body. Goodpasture's syndrome is characterized by renal (kidney) disease and lung hemorrhage.

Description

The disorder is characterized by autoimmune reaction which deposits of antibodies in the membranes of both the lung and kidneys, causing both inflammation of kidney (**glomerulonephritis**) and lung bleeding. It is typically a disease of young males.

Causes and symptoms

The exact cause is unknown. It is an autoimmune disorder; that is, the immune system is fighting the body's own normal tissues through creating antibodies that attack the lungs and kidneys. Sometimes the disorder is triggered by a viral infection, or by the inhalation of gasoline or other hydrocarbon solvents. An association also exists between cigarette **smoking** and the syndrome. The target antigen of the Goodpasture's antibodies has been localized to a protein chain (type IV collagen).

Symptoms include foamy, bloody, or dark colored urine, decreased urine output, **cough** with bloody sputum, difficulty breathing after exertion, weakness, **fatigue**, **nausea** or **vomiting**, weight loss, nonspecific chest **pain** and/or pale skin.

Diagnosis

The clinician will perform a battery of tests to confirm a diagnosis. These tests include a complete **blood count** (CBC) to confirm anemia, iron levels to check for blood loss and blood urea nitrogen (BUN) and creatinine levels to test the kidney function. A **urinalysis** will be done to check for damage to the kidneys. A sputum test will be done to look for specific antibodies. A **chest x ray** will be done to assess the amount of fluid in the lung tissues. A lung needle biopsy and a **kidney biopsy** will show immune system deposits. The kidney biopsy can also show the presence of the harmful antibodies that attack the lungs and kidneys.

Treatment

Treatment is focused on slowing the progression of the disease. Treatment is most effective when begun early, before kidney function has deteriorated to a point where the kidney is permanently damaged, and dialysis is necessary. **Corticosteroids**, such as prednisone, or other anti-inflammatory medications may be used to reduce the immune response. Immune suppressants such as cyclophosphamide or azathioprine are used aggressively to reduce immune system effects.

A procedure whereby blood plasma, which contains antibodies, is removed from the body and replaced with fluids or donated plasma (**plasmapheresis**) may be performed daily for two or more weeks to remove circulating antibodies. It is fairly effective in slowing or reversing the disorder. Dialysis to clean the blood of wastes may be required if kidney function is poor. A kidney transplant may be successful, especially if performed after circulating antibodies have been absent for several months.

Prognosis

The probable outcome is variable. Most cases progress to severe renal failure and end-stage renal disease within months. Early diagnosis and treatment makes the probable outcome more favorable.

Prevention

No known prevention of Goodpasture's syndrome exists. People should avoid glue sniffing and the siphoning gasoline. Stopping smoking, if a family history of renal failure exists, may prevent some cases. Early diagnosis and treatment may slow progression of the disorder.

KEY TERMS

Antibody—A protein molecule produced by the immune system in response to a protein that is not recognized as belonging in the body.

Antigen—Any substance that, as a result of coming in contact with appropriate cells,induces a state of sensitivity and/or immune responsiveness after a period of time and that reacts in a demonstrable way with antibodies.

Autoimmune disorder—An abnormality within the body whereby the immune system incorrectly attacks the body's normal tissues, thereby causing disease or organ dysfunction.

Blood urea nitrogen (BUN)—A test used to measure the blood level of urea nitrogen, a waste that is normally filtered from the kidneys.

Creatinine—A test used to measure the blood level of creatinine, a waste product filtered out of the blood by the kidneys. Higher than usual levels of this substance may indicate kidney disease.

Glomerulus (glomeruli)—A small tuft of blood capillaries in the kidney, responsible for filtering out waste products.

Resources

BOOKS

Tierney, Lawrence, et. al. *Current Medical Diagnosis and Treatment*. Los Altos: Lange Medical Publications, 2001.

ORGANIZATIONS

American Kidney Fund. 6110 Executive Boulevard, Suite 1010, Rockville, MD 20852. (800) 638-8299. < http://www.akfinc.org > .

National Kidney Foundation. 30 East 33rd Street, New York, NY 10016. (800) 622-9010. < http://www.kidney.org > .

Kim A. Sharp, M.Ln.

Gout

Definition

Gout is a form of acute arthritis that causes severe **pain** and swelling in the joints. It most commonly affects the big toe, but may also affect the heel, ankle, hand, wrist, or elbow. It affects the spine often enough to be a factor in back pain. Gout usually comes on suddenly, goes away after 5–10 days, and can keep recurring. Gout is different from other forms of arthritis because it occurs when there are high levels of uric acid circulating in the blood, which can cause urate crystals to settle in the tissues of the joints.

Description

Uric acid, which is found naturally in the blood stream, is formed as the body breaks down waste products, mainly those containing purine, a substance that is produced by the body and is also found in high concentrations in some foods, including brains, liver, sardines, anchovies, and dried peas and beans. Normally, the kidneys filter uric acid out of the blood and excrete it in the urine. Sometimes, however, the body produces too much uric acid or the kidneys aren't efficient enough at filtering it from the blood, and it builds up in the blood stream, a condition known as hyperuricemia. A person's susceptibility to gout may increase because of the inheritance of certain genes or from being overweight and eating a rich diet. In some cases, another disease (such as lymphoma, leukemia, or **hemolytic anemia**) may be the underlying cause of the uric acid buildup that results in gout. An additional factor is occupational or environmental; it is now known that chronic exposure to high levels of lead decreases the body's excretion of urates, allowing uric acid to accumulate in the blood.

Hyperuricemia doesn't always cause gout. Over the course of years, however, sharp urate crystals build up in the synovial fluid of the joints. Often, some precipitating event, such as an infection, surgery, the **stress** of hospitalization, a stubbed toe, or even a heavy drinking binge can cause inflammation. White blood cells, mistaking the urate crystals for a foreign invader, flood into the joint and surround the crystals, causing inflammation—in other words, the redness, swelling, and pain that are the hallmarks of a gout attack.

Causes and symptoms

As a result of high levels of uric acid in the blood, needle-like urate crystals gradually accumulate in the joints. Urate crystals may be present in the joint for a long time without causing symptoms. Infection, injury to the joint, surgery, drinking too much, or eating the wrong kinds of foods may suddenly bring on the symptoms, which include pain, tenderness, redness, warmth, and swelling of the joint. In many cases, the gout attack begins in the middle of the night. The pain is often so excruciating that the sufferer cannot bear weight on the joint or tolerate the pressure of bed-covers. The inflamed skin over the joint may be red, shiny, and dry, and the inflammation may be accompanied by a mild **fever**. These symptoms may go away in about a week and disappear for months or years at a time. However, over the course of time, attacks of gout recur more and more frequently, last longer, and affect more joints. Eventually, stone-like deposits known as tophi may build up in the joints, ligaments, and tendons, leading to permanent joint deformity and decreased motion. (In addition to causing the tophi associated with gout, hyperuricemia can also cause **kidney stones**, also called renal calculi or uroliths.)

Gout affects an estimated one million Americans; according to the National Institutes of Health, it accounts for about 5% of all cases of arthritis. It occurs more often in men than in women; the sex ratio is about 4:1. Uric-acid levels tend to increase in men at **puberty**, and, because it takes 20 years of hyperuricemia to cause gout symptoms, men commonly develop gout in their late 30s or early 40s. Women more typically develop gout later in life, starting in their 60s. According to some medical experts, estrogen protects against hyperuricemia, and when estrogen levels fall during **menopause**, urate crystals can begin to build up in the joints. Excess body weight, regular excessive alcohol intake, the use of blood pressure medications called **diuretics**, and high levels of certain fatty substances in the blood (serum triglycerides) associated with an increased risk of heart disease can all increase a person's risk of developing gout.

Gout appears to be on the increase in the American population. According to a study published in November 2002, there was a twofold increase in the incidence of gout over the 20 years between 1977 and 1997. It is not yet known whether this increase is the result of improved diagnosis or whether it is associated with risk factors that have not yet been identified.

Diagnosis

Usually, physicians can diagnose gout based on the **physical examination** and medical history (the patient's description of symptoms and other information). Doctors can also administer a test that measures the level of uric acid in the blood. While normal uric acid levels don't necessarily rule out gout and high levels don't confirm it, the presence of hyperuricemia increases the likelihood of gout. The development of a tophus can confirm the diagnosis of gout. The most definitive way to diagnose gout is

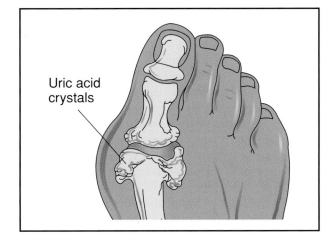

Uric acid crystals

Gout, a form of acute arthritis, most commonly occurs in the big toe. It is caused by high levels of uric acid in the blood, in which urate crystals settle in the tissues of the joints and produce severe pain and swelling. (Illustration by Electronic Illustrators Group.)

to take a sample of fluid from the joint and test it for urate crystals.

Treatment

The goals of treatment for gout consist of alleviating pain, avoiding severe attacks in the future, and preventing long-term joint damage. In addition to taking pain medications as prescribed by their doctors, people having gout attacks are encouraged to rest and to increase the amount of fluids that they drink.

Acute attacks of gout can be treated with nonaspirin, **nonsteroidal anti-inflammatory drugs** (NSAIDs) such as naproxen sodium (Aleve), ibuprofen (Advil), or indomethacin (Indocin). In some cases, these drugs can aggravate a peptic ulcer or existing **kidney disease** and cannot be used. Doctors sometimes also use colchicine (Colbenemid), especially in cases where nonsteroidal anti-inflammatory drugs cannot be used. Colchicine may cause **diarrhea**, which tends to go away once the patient stops taking it. **Corticosteroids** such as prednisone (Deltasone) and adrenocorticotropic hormone (Acthar) may be given orally or may be injected directly into the joint for a more concentrated effect. While all of these drugs have the potential to cause side effects, they are used for only about 48 hours and are not likely to cause major problems. However, **aspirin** and closely related drugs (salicylates) should be avoided because they can ultimately worsen gout.

Once an acute attack has been successfully treated, doctors try to prevent future attacks of gout and long-term joint damage by lowering uric acid levels in the blood. There are two types of drugs for correcting hyperuricemia. Such uricosuric drugs as probenecid (Benemid) and sulfinpyrazone (Anturane) lower the levels of urate in the blood by increasing its removal from the body (excretion) through the urine. These drugs may promote the formation of kidney stones, however, and they may not work for all patients, especially those with kidney disease. Allopurinol (Zyloprim), a type of drug called a xanthine-oxidase inhibitor, blocks the production of urate in the body, and can dissolve kidney stones as well as treating gout. The potential side effects of allopurinol include rash, a skin condition known as **dermatitis**, and liver dysfunction. In 2004, the FDA was seeking trial data on a new drug called oxypurinol (Oxyprim) for treating chronic gout. These medications may have to be taken for life to prevent further gout attacks.

New quality of care indicators were released in 2004 to improve care for patients with gout. The aim of the guidelines was to prevent repeat gout attacks and to reduce medication errors associated with intravenous colchicine in hospitals.

Alternative treatment

Alternative approaches to gout focus on correcting hyperuricemia by encouraging weigt loss and limiting the intake of alcohol and purine-rich foods. In addition, consuming garlic (*Allium sativum*) has been recommended to help prevent gout. Increasing fluid intake, especially by drinking water, is also recommended. During an acute attack, contrast **hydrotherapy** (alternating three-minute hot compresses with 30–second cold compresses) can help dissolve the crystals and resolve the pain faster.

Prognosis

Gout cannot be cured but usually it can be managed successfully. As tophi dissolve, joint mobility generally improves. (In some cases, however, medicines alone do not dissolve the tophi and they must be removed surgically.) Lowering uric acid in the blood also helps to prevent or improve the kidney problems that may accompany gout.

Prevention

For centuries, gout has been known as a "rich man's disease" or a disease caused by overindulgence in food and drink. While this view is perhaps a little overstated and oversimplified, lifestyle factors clearly influence a person's risk of developing gout. Since

obesity and excessive alcohol intake are associated with hyperuricemia and gout, losing weight and limiting alcohol intake can help ward off gout. **Dehydration** may also promote the formation of urate crystals, so people taking diuretics or "water pills" may be better off switching to another type of blood pressure medication. Everyone should be sure to drink at least six to eight glasses of water each day. Since purine is broken down in the body into urate, it may also be helpful to avoid foods high in purine, such as organ meats, sardines, anchovies, red meat, gravies, beans, beer, and wine. A 2004 study revealed that eating more low-fat dairy products could reduce risk of developing gout.

Resources

BOOKS

Parker, James N., M.D., and Philip M. Parker, Ph. D. *The 2002 Official Patient's Sourcebook on Gout.* San Diego, CA: ICON Health Publications, 2002.

PERIODICALS

Arromdee, E., C. J. Michet, C. S. Crowson, et al. "Epidemiology of Gout: Is the Incidence Rising?"

Journal of Rheumatology 29 (November 2002): 2403–2406.

Coghill, Kim. "FDA Panel Discusses Endpoints for Approval of Gout Products." *Bioworld Today* (June 3, 2004).

"Dairy-rich Diet May Help Prevent Gout." *Tufts University Health & Nutrition Letter* (June 2004): 2.

Hsu, C. Y., T. T. Shih, K. M. Huang, et al. "Tophaceous Gout of the Spine: MR Imaging Features." *Clinical Radiology* 57 (October 2002): 919–925.

Lin, J. L., D. T. Tan, H. H. Ho, and C. C. Yu. "Environmental Lead Exposure and Urate Excretion in the General Population." *American Journal of Medicine* 113 (November 2002): 563–568.

MacReady, Norma. "New Gout Quality-of-care Standards Take Aim at Medication-related Errors." *Internal Medicine News* (June 1, 2004): 18.

Perez-Ruiz, F., M. Calabozo, G. G. Erauskin, et al. "Renal Underexcretion of Uric Acid is Present in Patients with Apparent High Urinary Uric Acid Output." *Arthritis and Rheumatism* 47 (December 15, 2002): 610–613.

Raj, J. M., S. Sudhakar, K. Sems, and R. W. Carlson. "Arthritis in the Intensive Care Unit." *Critical Care Clinics* 18 (October 2002): 767–780.

Shekarriz, B., and M. L. Stoller. "Uric Acid Nephrolithiasis: Current Concepts and Controversies." *Journal of Urology* 168, no. 4, Part 1 (October 2002): 1307–1314.

ORGANIZATIONS

Arthritis Foundation. 1300 W. Peachtree St., Atlanta, GA 30309. (800) 283-7800. < http://www.arthritis.org > .

National Institute of Arthritis and Musculoskeletal and Skin Diseases (NIAMS). National Institutes of Health (NIH), 1 AMS Circle, Bethesda, MD 20892-3675. < www.niams.nih/gov > .

OTHER

National Institute of Arthritis and Musculoskeletal and Skin Diseases (NIAMS). *Questions and Answers About Gout.* Bethesda, MD: NIAMS, 2002. NIH Publication No. 02-5027. < www.niams.nih.gov/hi/topics/gout/gout/htm > .

Robert Scott Dinsmoor
Rebecca J. Frey, PhD
Teresa G. Odle

Gout drugs

Definition

Gout drugs are medicines that prevent or relieve the symptoms of gout, a disease that affects the joints and kidneys.

Purpose

Gout is a disease in which uric acid, a waste product that normally passes out of the body in urine, collects and forms crystals in the joints and the kidneys. When uric acid crystals build up in the joints, the tissue around the joint becomes inflamed, and nerve endings in the area become irritated, causing extreme **pain**. Uric acid crystals in the kidneys can lead to **kidney stones** and eventually to kidney failure.

The symptoms of gout–severe pain, usually in the hand or foot (often at the base of the big toe), but sometimes in the elbow or knee–should be reported to a health care professional. If not treated, gout can lead to high blood presssure, deformed joints, and even **death** from kidney failure. Fortunately, the condition is easily treated. For patients who have just had their first attack, physicians may prescribe only medicine to reduce the pain and inflammatin, such as **nonsteroidal anti-inflammatory drugs**, **corticosteroids**, or colchicine. Patients may also be advised to change their eating and drinking habits, avoiding organ meats and other protein-rich foods, cutting out alcoholic beverages, and drinking more water. Some people never have another gout attack after the first. For those who do, physicians may prescribe additional drugs that either help the body get rid of uric acid or reduce the amount of uric acid the body produces. These drugs will not relieve gout attacks that already have started, but will help prevent attacks when taken regularly.

Description

Three main types of drugs are used in treating gout. Colchicine helps relieve the symptoms of gout by reducing inflammation. Allopurinol (Lopurin, Zyloprim) reduces the amount of uric acid produced in the body. Probenecid (Benemid, Probalan) and sulfinpyrazone (Anturane) help the body get rid of excess uric acid. Physicians may recommend that patients take more than one type of gout drug at the same time. Some of these medicines may also be prescribed for other medical conditions that are caused by too much uric acid in the body.

Recommended dosage

The recommended dosage depends on the type of gout drug. Check with the physician who prescribed the drug or the pharmacist who filled the prescription for the correct dosage.

Always take gout drugs exactly as directed. Never take larger or more frequent doses than recommended. Patients who are told to take more than one gout drug should carefully follow the physician's directions for taking all medicines.

Gout drugs such as allopurinol, probenecid, and sulfinpyrazone must be taken regularly to prevent gout attacks. The medicine may take some time to begin working, so gout attacks may continuee for awhile after starting to take the drug. Continuing to take the drug is important, even if it does not seem to be working t first.

Colchicine may be taken regularly in low doses to help prevent gout attacks or in high doses for only a few hours at a time to relieve an attack. The chance of serious side effects is greater when this medicine is taken in high doses for short periods.

Precautions

Seeing a physician regularly while taking gout drugs is important. The physician will check to make sure the medicine is working as it should and will watch for unwanted side effects. Blood tests may be ordered to help the physician monitor how well the drug is working.

Drinking alcohol, including beer and wine, may increase the amount of uric acid in the body and may interfere with the effects of gout medicine. People with gout (or other conditions that result from excess uric acid) may need to limit the amount of alcohol they drink or stop drinking alcohol altogether.

Some people feel drowsy or less alert when taking gout drugs. Anyone who takes this type of medicine should not drive, use machines or do anything else that might be dangerous until they have found out how the drugs affect them.

Some gout drugs may change the results of certain medical tests. Before having medical tests, anyone taking this medicine should alert the health care professional in charge.

Older people may be especially sensitive to the effects of colchicine. The drug may also stay in their bodies longer than it does in younger people. Both the increased sensitivity to the drug and the longer time for the drug to leave the body may increase the chance of side effects.

Special conditions

People who have certain medical conditions or who are taking certain other medicines can have problems if they take gout drugs. Before taking these drugs, be sure to let the physician know about any of these conditions:

ALLERGIES. Anyone who has ever had unusual reactions to gout drugs or to medicines used to relieve pain or inflammation should let his or her physician know before taking gout drugs. The physician should also be told about any **allergies** to foods, dyes, preservatives, or other substances.

DIABETES. Some gout drugs may cause false results on certain urine sugar tests, but not on others. Diabetic patients who take gout drugs should check with their physicians to find out if their medicine will affect the results of their urine sugar tests.

PREGNANCY. The effects of taking gout drugs during **pregnancy** are not fully understood. Women who are pregnant or who may become pregnant should check with their physicians before using gout drugs.

BREASTFEEDING. Gout drugs may pass into breast milk. Women who are taking this medicine and want to breastfeed their babies should check with their physicians.

OTHER MEDICAL CONDITIONS. Gout drugs may cause problems for people with certain medical conditions. For example, the risk of severe allergic reactions or other serious side effects is greater when people with these medical conditions take certain gout drugs:

- congestive heart disease
- high blood pressure
- blood disease
- diabetes
- kidney disease or kidney stones
- cancer being treated with drugs or radiation
- stomach or intestinal problems, including stomach ulcer (now or in the past)

Before using gout drugs, people with any of medical problems listed above should make sure their physicians are aware of their conditions.

USE OF CERTAIN MEDICINES. Taking gout drugs with certain other drugs may affect the way the drugs work or may increase the chance of side effects.

Side effects

A skin rash that develops during treatment with gout drugs may be a sign of a serious and possibly life-threatening reaction. If any of these symptoms occur, stop taking the medicine and check with a physician immediately:

- skin rash, **itching**, or **hives**
- scaly or peeling skin

- chills, **fever, sore throat, nausea and vomiting**, yellow skin or eyes, joint pain, muscle aches or pains–especially if these symptoms occur at the same time or shortly after a skin rash

Patients taking colchicine should stop taking it immediately if they have **diarrhea**, stomach pain, **nausea**, or **vomiting**. If these symptoms continue for 3 hours or more after the medicine is stopped, check with a physician.

Other side effects of may also need medical attention. If any of the following symptoms occur while taking gout drugs, check with the physician who prescribed the medicine as soon as possible:

- pain in the side or lower back
- painful urination
- blood in the urine

Less serious side effects, such as **headache**, loss of appetite, and joint pain and inflammation usually go away as the body adjusts to the drug and do not need medical treatment.

Other side effects may occur. Anyone who has unusual symptoms while taking gout difficult to interpret. Even so, each individual cell in the body carries thousands of genes coding for proteins, with some estimates as high as 150,000 genes. For **gene therapy** to advance to its full potential, scientists must discover the biological role of each of these individual genes and where the base pairs that make them up are located on DNA.

To address this issue, the National Institutes of Health initiated the Human Genome Project in 1990. Led by James D. Watson (one of the co-discoverers of the chemical makeup of DNA) the project's 15-year goal is to map the entire human genome (a combination of the words gene and chromosomes). A genome map would clearly identify the location of all genes as well as the more than three billion base pairs that make them up. With a precise knowledge of gene locations and functions, scientists may one day be able to conquer or control diseases that have plagued humanity for centuries.

Scientists participating in the Human Genome Project have identified an average of one new gene a day, but many expect this rate of discovery to increase. By the year 2005, their goal is to determine the exact location of all the genes on human DNA and the exact sequence of the base pairs that make them up. Some of the genes identified through this project include a gene that predisposes people to **obesity**, one associated with programmed cell death (apoptosis), a gene that guides HIV viral reproduction, and the genes of inherited

disorders like Huntington's disease, Lou Gehrig's disease, and some colon and breast cancers. In February of 2001, scientists published a rought draft of the complete human genome. With fewer than the anticipated number of genes found, between 30,000–40,000, the consequences of this announcement are enormous. Scientists caution however, that the initial publication is only a draft of the human genome and much more work is still ahead for the completion of the project. As the human genome is completed, there will be more information available for gene therapy research and implementation.

The future of gene therapy

Gene therapy seems elegantly simple in its concept: supply the human body with a gene that can correct a biological malfunction that causes a disease. However, there are many obstacles and some distinct questions concerning the viability of gene therapy. For example, viral vectors must be carefully controlled lest they infect the patient with a viral disease. Some vectors, like retroviruses, can also enter cells functioning properly and interfere with the natural biological processes, possibly leading to other diseases. Other viral vectors, like the adenoviruses, are often recognized and destroyed by the immune system so their therapeutic effects are short-lived. Maintaining gene expression so it performs its role properly after vector delivery is difficult. As a result, some therapies need to be repeated often to provide long-lasting benefits.

One of the most pressing issues, however, is gene regulation. Genes work in concert to regulate their functioning. In other words, several genes may play a part in turning other genes on and off. For example, certain genes work together to stimulate cell division and growth, but if these are not

Nancy Ross-Flanigan

Gouty arthritis *see* **Gout**

Graft-vs.-host disease

Definition

Graft-vs.-host disease is an immune attack on the recipient by cells from a donor.

Description

The main problem with transplanting organs and tissues is that the recipient host does not recognize the new tissue as its own. Instead, it attacks it as foreign in the same way it attacks germs, to destroy it.

If immunogenic cells from the donor are transplanted along with the organ or tissue, they will attack the host, causing graft vs. host disease.

The only transplanted tissues that house enough immune cells to cause graft vs. host disease are the blood and the bone marrow. Blood transfusions are used every day in hospitals for many reasons. Bone marrow transplants are used to replace blood forming cells and immune cells. This is necessary for patients whose **cancer** treatment has destroyed their own bone marrow. Because bone marrow cells are among the most sensitive to radiation and **chemotherapy**, it often must be destroyed along with the cancer. This is true primarily of leukemias, but some other cancers have also been treated this way.

Causes and symptoms

Even if the donor and recipient are well matched, graft-vs.-host disease can still occur. There are many different elements involved in generating immune reactions, and each person is different, unless they are identical twins. Testing can often find donors who match all the major elements, but there are many minor ones that will always be different. How good a match is found also depends upon the urgency of the need and some good luck.

Blood **transfusion** graft-vs.-host disease affects mostly the blood. Blood cells perform three functions: carrying oxygen, fighting infections, and clotting. All of these cell types are decreased in a transfusion graft-vs.-host reaction, leading to anemia (lack of red blood cells in the blood), a decrease in resistance to infections, and an increase in bleeding. The reaction occurs between four to 30 days after the transfusion.

The tissues most affected by bone marrow graft-vs.-host disease are the skin, the liver, and the intestines. One form or the other occurs in close to half of the patients who receive bone marrow transplants.

Bone marrow graft-vs.-host disease comes in an acute and a chronic form. The acute form appears within two months of the transplant; the chronic form usually appears within three months. The acute disease produces a skin rash, liver abnormalities, and **diarrhea** that can be bloody. The skin rash is primarily a patchy thickening of the skin. Chronic disease can produce a similar skin rash, a tightening or an

inflammation of the skin, lesions in the mouth, drying of the eyes and mouth, hair loss, liver damage, lung damage, and **indigestion**. The symptoms are similar to an autoimmune disease called **scleroderma**.

Both forms of graft-vs.-host disease bring with them an increased risk of infections, either because of the process itself or its treatment with cortisone-like drugs and immunosuppressives. Patients can die of liver failure, infection, or other severe disturbances of their system.

Treatment

Both the acute and the chronic disease are treated with cortisone-like drugs, immunosuppressive agents like cyclosporine, or with **antibiotics** and immune chemicals from donated blood (gamma globulin). Infection with one particular virus, called cytomegalovirus (CMV) is so likely a complication that some experts recommend treating it ahead of time.

Prognosis

Children with **acute leukemias** have greatly benefited from the treatment made possible by **bone marrow transplantation**. Survival rates have climbed by 15–50%. It is an interesting observation that patients who develop graft-vs.-host disease are less likely to have a recurrence of the leukemia that was being treated. This phenomenon is called graft-vs.-leukemia.

Bone marrow transplant patients who do not have a graft-vs.-host reaction gradually return to normal immune function in a year. A graft-vs.-host reaction may prolong the diminished immune capacity indefinitely, requiring supplemental treatment with immunoglobulins (gamma globulin).

Somehow the grafted cells develop a tolerance to their new home after six to 12 months, and the medications can be gradually withdrawn. Graft-vs.-host disease is not the only complication of blood transfusion or bone marrow transplantation. Host-vs.-graft or rejection is also common and may require a repeat transplant with another donor organ. Infections are a constant threat in bone marrow transplant because of the disease being treated, the prior radiation or chemotherapy and the medications used to treat the transplant.

Prevention

For recipients of blood transfusions who are especially likely to have graft-vs.-host reactions, the

KEY TERMS

Anemia—Too few red blood cells, or too little hemoglobin in them.

Immunoglobulin—Chemicals in the blood that defend against infections.

Immunosuppressive—A chemical which suppresses an immune response.

Inflammation—The body's immune reaction to presumed foreign substances like germs. Inflammation is characterized by increased blood supply and activation of defense mechanisms. It produces redness, swelling, heat, and pain.

Lesion—Localized disease or damage.

Scleroderma—Progressive disease of the connective tissue of the skin and internal organs.

red blood cells can safely be irradiated (using x rays) to kill all the immune cells. The red blood cells are less sensitive to radiation and are not harmed by this treatment.

Much current research is directed towards solving the problem of graft-vs.-host disease. There are efforts to remove the immunogenic cells from the donor tissue, and there are also attempts to extract and purify bone marrow cells from the patient before treating the cancer. These cells are then given back to the patient after treatment has destroyed all that were left behind.

Resources

BOOKS

Armitage, James O. "Bone Marrow Transplantation." In *Harrison's Principles of Internal Medicine*, edited by Anthony S. Fauci, et al. New York: McGraw-Hill, 1997.

J. Ricker Polsdorfer, MD

Grafts and grafting *see* **Bone grafting; Coronary artery bypass graft surgery; Graft-vs.-host disease; Skin grafting**

Granular conjunctivitis *see* **Trachoma**

Granulocytic ehrlichiosis *see* **Ehrlichiosis**

Granulocytopenia *see* **Neutropenia**

Granuloma inguinale

Definition

Granuloma inguinale is a sexually transmitted infection that affects the skin and mucous membranes of the anal and genital areas. Its name is derived from granuloma, a medical term for a mass or growth of granulation tissue, and *inguinale*, a Latin word that means located in the groin. Granulation tissue is tissue formed during wound healing that is rich in blood capillaries and has a rough or lumpy surface.

Description

Granuloma inguinale is a chronic infection with frequent relapses caused by a rod-shaped bacterium. It occurs worldwide but is most common in tropical or subtropical countries, where it is associated with poverty and poor hygiene. As many as 20% of male patients with **sexually transmitted diseases** (STDs) in tropical countries have granuloma inguinale. The disease is less common in the United States, with fewer than 100 reported cases per year. Most patients are between the ages of 20 and 40 years, with a 2:1 male-to-female ratio.

Although granuloma inguinale is relatively uncommon in the United States in comparison with other STDs, it is still a significant public health problem. It can be acquired through casual sexual contacts when traveling abroad. Moreover, patients with granuloma inguinale are vulnerable to superinfection (infection by other disease agents) with other STDs, especially **syphilis**. Patients with granuloma inguinale are also a high-risk group for Acquired Immune Deficiency Syndrome (**AIDS**) transmission, because the disease causes open genital ulcers that can be easily invaded by the AIDS virus.

Granuloma inguinale is spread primarily through heterosexual and male homosexual contact; however, its occurrence in children and sexually inactive adults indicates that it may also be spread by contact with human feces. Granuloma inguinale is not highly contagious; however, persons with weakened immune systems are at greater risk of infection.

Causes and symptoms

Granuloma inguinale, which is sometimes called donovanosis, is caused by *Calymmatobacterium granulomatis*, a rod-shaped bacterium formerly called *Donovania granulomatis*. The bacterium has an incubation period ranging from eight days to 12 weeks, with an average of two to four weeks. The disease has a slow and gradual onset, beginning with an inconspicuous pimple or lumpy eruption on the skin. In 90% of patients, the initial sign of infection is in the genital region, but a minority of patients will develop the sore in their mouth or anal area if their sexual contact involved those parts of the body. Many patients do not notice the sore because it is small and not usually painful. In some women, the first symptom of granuloma inguinale is bleeding from the genitals.

The initial pimple or sore is typically followed by three stages of disease. In the first stage, the patient develops a mass of pink or dull red granulation tissue in the area around the anus. In the second stage, the bacteria erode the skin to form shallow, foul-smelling ulcers which spread from the genital and anal areas to the thighs and lower abdomen. The edges of the ulcers are marked by granulation tissue. In the third stage, the ulcerated areas form deep masses of keloid or scar tissue that may spread slowly for many years.

Patients with long-term infections are at risk for serious complications. The ulcers in second-stage granuloma inguinale often become superinfected with syphilis or other STD organisms. Superinfected ulcers become painful to touch, filled with pus and dead tissue, and are much more difficult to treat. There may be sizable areas of tissue destruction in superinfected patients. In addition, the scar tissue produced by third-stage infection can grow until it closes off parts of the patient's urinary tract. It is also associated with a higher risk of genital **cancer**.

Diagnosis

The most important aspect of diagnosis is distinguishing between granuloma inguinale and other STDs, particularly since many patients will be infected with more than one STD. Public health officials recommend that patients tested for granuloma inguinale be given a blood test for syphilis as well. In addition, the doctor will need to distinguish between granuloma inguinale and certain types of skin cancer, **amebiasis**, fungal infections, and other bacterial ulcers. The most significant distinguishing characteristic of granuloma inguinale is the skin ulcer, which is larger than in most other diseases, painless, irregular in shape, and likely to bleed when touched.

The diagnosis of granuloma inguinale is made by finding Donovan bodies in samples of the patient's skin tissue. Donovan bodies are oval rod-shaped organisms that appear inside infected tissue cells under a microscope. The doctor obtains a tissue sample either by cutting a piece of tissue from the edge of

---

KEY TERMS

Donovan bodies—Rod-shaped oval organisms found in tissue samples from patients with granuloma inguinale. Donovan bodies appear deep purple when stained with Wright's stain.

Granulation tissue—A kind of tissue formed during wound healing, with a rough or irregular surface and a rich supply of blood capillaries.

Granuloma—An inflammatory swelling or growth composed of granulation tissue, as in granuloma inguinale.

Keloid—An unusual or abnormal growth of scar tissue, as in the third stage of granuloma inguinale.

Punch biopsy—A method of obtaining skin samples under local anesthesia using a surgical skin punch.

Superinfection—A condition in which a patient with a contagious disease acquires a second infection, as when a patient with granuloma inguinale is also infected with syphilis.

Wright's stain—A chemical used to stain tissue samples for laboratory analysis.

---

an skin ulcer with a scalpel or by taking a punch biopsy. To make a punch biopsy, the doctor will inject a local anesthetic into an ulcerated area and remove a piece of skin about 1/16 of an inch in size with a surgical skin punch. The tissue sample is then air-dried and stained with Wright's stain, a chemical that will cause the Donovan bodies to show up as dark purple safety pin-shaped objects inside lighter-staining capsules.

Treatment

Granuloma inguinale is treated with oral **antibiotics**. Three weeks of treatment with erythromycin, streptomycin, or tetracycline, or 12 weeks of treatment with ampicillin are standard forms of therapy. Although the skin ulcers will start to show signs of healing in about a week, the patient must take the full course of medication to minimize the possibility of relapse.

Prognosis

Most patients with granuloma inguinale recover completely, although superinfected ulcers may require lengthy courses of medication. Early treatment prevents the complications associated with second- and third-stage infection.

Prevention

Prevention of granuloma inguinale has three important aspects:

• Avoidance of casual sexual contacts, particularly among homosexual males, in countries with high rates of the disease

• Tracing and examination of an infected person's recent sexual contacts

• Monitoring the patient's ulcers or scar tissue for signs of reinfection for a period of six months after antibiotic treatment

Resources

BOOKS

Chambers, Henry F. "Infectious Diseases: Bacterial & Chlamydial." In *Current Medical Diagnosis and Treatment, 1998.* edited by Stephen McPhee, et al., 37th ed. Stamford: Appleton & Lange, 1997.

Rebecca J. Frey, PhD

Granulomatous ileitis *see* **Crohn's disease**

Graves' disease *see* **Hyperthyroidism**

Greenfield filter *see* **Vena cava**

Grippe *see* **Influenza**

Group A streptococcus infection *see* **Streptococcal infections**

Group B streptococcus infection *see* **Streptococcal infections**

Group therapy

Definition

Group therapy is a form of psychosocial treatment where a small group of patients meet regularly to talk, interact, and discuss problems with each other and the group leader (therapist).

Purpose

Group therapy attempts to give individuals a safe and comfortable place where they can work out problems and emotional issues. Patients gain insight into their own thoughts and behavior, and offer suggestions and support to others. In addition, patients who have a difficult time with interpersonal relationships can benefit from the social interactions that are a basic part of the group therapy experience.

Precautions

Patients who are suicidal, homicidal, psychotic, or in the midst of a major acute crisis are typically not referred for group therapy until their behavior and emotional state have stabilized. Depending on their level of functioning, cognitively impaired patients (like patients with organic brain disease or a traumatic brain injury) may also be unsuitable for group therapy intervention. Some patients with sociopathic traits are not suitable for most groups.

Description

A psychologist, psychiatrist, social worker, or other healthcare professional typically arranges and conducts group therapy sessions. In some therapy groups, two co-therapists share the responsibility of group leadership. Patients are selected on the basis of what they might gain from group therapy interaction and what they can contribute to the group as a whole.

Therapy groups may be homogeneous or heterogeneous. Homogeneous groups have members with similar diagnostic backgrounds (for example, they may all suffer from depression). Heterogeneous groups have a mix of individuals with different emotional issues. The number of group members varies widely, but is typically no more than 12. Groups may be time limited (with a predetermined number of sessions) or indefinite (where the group determines when therapy ends). Membership may be closed or open to new members once sessions begin.

The number of sessions in group therapy depends on the makeup, goals, and setting of the group. For example, a therapy group that is part of a **substance abuse** program to rehabilitate inpatients would be called short-term group therapy. This term is used because, as patients, the group members will only be in the hospital for a relatively short period of time. Long-term therapy groups may meet for six months, a year, or longer. The therapeutic approach used in therapy depends on the focus of the group and the psychological training of the therapist. Some common techniques include psychodynamic, cognitive-behavioral, and **Gestalt therapy**.

In a group therapy session, group members are encouraged to openly and honestly discuss the issues that brought them to therapy. They try to help other group members by offering their own suggestions, insights, and empathy regarding their problems.

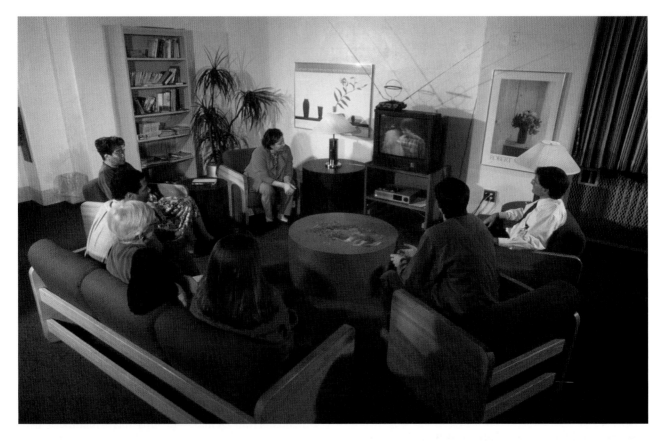

Group therapy is practiced in a variety of settings, including both inpatient and outpatient facilities, and is used to treat anxiety, mood, and personality disorders as well as psychoses. *(Photo Researchers, Inc. Reproduced by permission.)*

There are no definite rules for group therapy, only that members participate to the best of their ability. However, most therapy groups do have some basic ground rules that are usually discussed during the first session. Patients are asked not to share what goes on in therapy sessions with anyone outside of the group. This protects the confidentiality of the other members. They may also be asked not to see other group members socially outside of therapy because of the harmful effect it might have on the dynamics of the group.

The therapist's main task is to guide the group in self-discovery. Depending on the goals of the group and the training and style of the therapist, he or she may lead the group interaction or allow the group to take their own direction. Typically, the group leader does some of both, providing direction when the group gets off track while letting them set their own agenda. The therapist may guide the group by simply reinforcing the positive behaviors they engage in. For example, if a group member shows empathy to another member, or offers a constructive suggestion, the therapist will point this out and explain the value of these actions to the group. In almost all group therapy situations, the therapist will attempt to emphasize the common traits among group members so that members can gain a sense of group identity. Group members realize that others share the same issues they do.

The main benefit group therapy may have over individual psychotherapy is that some patients behave and react more like themselves in a group setting than they would one-on-one with a therapist. The group therapy patient gains a certain sense of identity and social acceptance from their membership in the group. Suddenly, they are not alone. They are surrounded by others who have the same anxieties and emotional issues that they have. Seeing how others deal with these issues may give them new solutions to their problems. Feedback from group members also offers them a unique insight into their own behavior, and the group provides a safe forum in which to practice new behaviors. Lastly, by helping others in the group work through their problems, group therapy members can gain more self-esteem. Group therapy may also simulate family experiences of patients and will allow family dynamic issues to emerge.

KEY TERMS

Cognitive-behavioral—A therapy technique that focuses on changing beliefs, images, and thoughts in order to change maladjusted behaviors.

Gestalt—A humanistic therapy technique that focuses on gaining an awareness of emotions and behaviors in the present rather than in the past.

Psychodynamic—A therapy technique that assumes improper or unwanted behavior is caused by unconscious, internal conflicts and focuses on gaining insight into these motivations.

Self-help groups like Alcoholics Anonymous and Weight Watchers fall outside of the psychotherapy realm. These self-help groups do offer many of the same benefits of social support, identity, and belonging that make group therapy effective for many. Self-help group members meet to discuss a common area of concern (like **alcoholism**, eating disorders, **bereavement**, parenting). Group sessions are not run by a therapist, but by a nonprofessional leader, group member, or the group as a whole. Self-help groups are sometimes used in addition to psychotherapy or regular group therapy.

Preparation

Patients are typically referred for group therapy by a psychologist or psychiatrist. Some patients may need individual therapy first. Before group sessions begin, the therapist leading the session may conduct a short intake interview with the patient to determine if the group is right for the patient. This interview will also allow the therapist to determine if the addition of the patient will benefit the group. The patient may be given some preliminary information on the group before sessions begin. This may include guidelines for success (like being open, listening to others, taking risks), rules of the group (like maintaining confidentiality), and educational information on what group therapy is about.

Aftercare

The end of long-term group therapy may cause feelings of grief, loss, abandonment, anger, or rejection in some members. The group therapist will attempt to foster a sense of closure by encouraging members to explore their feelings and use newly acquired coping techniques to deal with them.

Working through this termination phase of group therapy is an important part of the treatment process.

Risks

Some very fragile patients may not be able to tolerate aggressive or hostile comments from group members. Patients who have trouble communicating in group situations may be at risk for dropping out of group therapy. If no one comments on their silence or makes an attempt to interact with them, they may begin to feel even more isolated and alone instead of identifying with the group. Therefore, the therapist usually attempts to encourage silent members to participate early on in treatment.

Normal results

Studies have shown that both group and individual psychotherapy benefit about 85% of the patients that participate in them. Optimally, patients gain a better understanding of themselves, and perhaps a stronger set of interpersonal and coping skills through the group therapy process. Some patients may continue therapy after group therapy ends, either individually or in another group setting.

Resources

ORGANIZATIONS

American Psychiatric Association. 1400 K Street NW, Washington DC 20005. (888) 357-7924. < http://www.psych.org > .
American Psychological Association (APA). 750 First St. NE, Washington, DC 20002-4242. (202) 336-5700. < ttp://www.apa.org > .

Paula Anne Ford-Martin

Growth hormone suppression test *see* **Growth hormone tests**

Growth hormone tests

Definition

Growth hormone (hGH), or somatotropin, is a hormone responsible for normal body growth and development by stimulating protein production in muscle cells and energy release from the breakdown of fats. Tests for growth hormone include Somatotropin hormone test, Somatomedin C, Growth hormone suppression test (glucose loading test), and Growth hormone stimulation test (Arginine test or Insulin tolerance test).

Purpose

Growth hormone tests are ordered for the following reasons:

- to identify growth deficiencies, including delayed **puberty** and small stature in adolescents that result from pituitary or thyroid malfunction

- to aid in the diagnosis of hyperpituitarism that is evident in gigantism or acromegaly

- to screen for inadequate or reduced pituitary gland function

- to assist in the diagnosis of **pituitary tumors** or tumors related to the hypothalamus, an area of the brain

- to evaluate hGH therapy

Precautions

Taking certain drugs such as amphetamines, dopamine, **corticosteroids**, and phenothiazines may increase and decrease growth hormone secretion, respectively. Other factors influencing hGH secretion include **stress**, **exercise**, diet, and abnormal glucose levels. These tests should not be done within a week of any radioactive scan.

Description

Several hormones play important roles in human growth. The major human growth hormone (hGH), or somatotropin, is a protein made up of 191 amino acids that is secreted by the anterior pituitary gland and coordinates normal growth and development. Human growth is characterized by two spurts, one at birth and the other at puberty. hGH plays an important role at both of these times. Normal individuals have measurable levels of hGH throughout life. Yet levels of hGH fluctuate during the day and are affected by eating and exercise. Receptors that respond to hGH exist on cells and tissues throughout the body. The most obvious effect of hGH is on linear skeletal development. But the metabolic effects of hGH on muscle, the liver, and fat cells are critical to its function. Surprisingly, a 2004 study reported that obese people have lower-than-normal levels of human growth hormone in their bodies. Humans have two forms of hGH, and the functional difference between the two is unclear. They are both formed from the same gene, but one lacks the amino acids in positions 32–46.

hGH is produced in the anterior portion of the pituitary gland by somatotrophs under the control of hormonal signals in the hypothalamus. Two hypothalamic hormones regulate hGH; they are growth hormone-releasing hormone (GHRH) and growth hormone—inhibiting hormone (GHIH). When blood glucose levels fall, GHRH triggers the secretion of stored hGH. As blood glucose levels rise, GHRH release is turned off. Increases in blood protein levels trigger a similar response. As a result of this hypothalamic feedback loop, hGH levels fluctuate throughout the day. Normal plasma hGH levels average 1–3 ng/ML with peaks as high as 60 ng/ML. In addition, plasma glucose and amino acid availability for growth is also regulated by the hormones adrenaline, glucagon, and insulin.

Most hGH is released at night. Peak spikes of hGH release occur around 10 P.M., midnight, and 2 A.M. The logic behind this night-time release is that most of hGH's effects are controlled by other hormones, including the somatomedins, IGH-I and IGH-II. As a result, the effects of hGH are spread out more evenly during the day.

A number of hormonal conditions can lead to excessive or diminished growth. Because of its critical role in producing hGH and other hormones, an abnormal pituitary gland will often yield altered growth. Dwarfism (very small stature) can be due to underproduction of hGH, lack of IGH-I, or a flaw in target tissue response to either of these growth hormones. Overproduction of hGH or IGH-I, or an exaggerated response to these hormones can lead to gigantism or acromegaly, both of which are characterized by a very large stature.

Gigantism is the result of hGH overproduction in early childhood leading to a skeletal height up to 8 feet (2.5m) or more. Acromegaly results when hGH is overproduced after the onset of puberty. In this condition, the epiphyseal plates of the long bone of the body do not close, and they remain responsive to additional stimulated growth by hGH. This disorder is characterized by an enlarged skull, hands and feet, nose, neck, and tongue.

Somatotropin

Somatotropin is used to identify hGH deficiency in adolescents with short stature, delayed sexual maturity, and other growth deficiencies. It also aids in documenting excess hGH production that is responsible for gigantism or acromegaly, and confirms underactivity or overproduction of the pituitary gland (**hypopituitarism** or hyperpituitarism). However, due to the episodic secretion of hGH, as well as hGH production in response to stress, exercise, or other factors, random assays are not an adequate determination of hGH deficiency. To negate these variables and obtain more accurate readings, a blood sample can be drawn one to 1.5 hours after sleep (hGH levels increase during sleep), or strenuous exercise can be performed for 30 minutes before blood is drawn (hGH levels increase after exercise). The hGH levels at the end of an exercise period are expected to be maximal.

Somatomedin C

The somatomedin C test is usually ordered to detect pituitary abnormalities, hGH deficiency, and acromegaly. Also called insulin-like growth factor (IGF-1), somatomedin C is considered a more accurate reflection of the blood concentration of hGH because such variables as time of day, activity levels, or diet do not influence the results. Somatomedin C is part of a group of peptides, called somatomedins, through which hGH exerts its effects. Because it circulates in the bloodstream bound to long-lasting proteins, it is more stable than hGH. Levels of somatomedin C depend on hGH levels, however. As a result, somatomedin C levels are low when hGH levels are deficient. Abnormally low test results of somatomedin C require an abnormally reduced or absent hGH during an hGH stimulation test in order to diagnose hGH deficiency. Nonpituitary causes of reduced somatomedin C include **malnutrition**, severe chronic illness, severe **liver disease**, **hypothyroidism**, and Laron's dwarfism.

Growth hormone stimulation test

The hGH stimulation test, also called hGH Provocation test, Insulin Tolerance, or Arginine test, is performed to test the body's ability to produce human growth hormone, and to identify suspected hGH deficiency. A normal patient can have low hGH levels, but if hGH is still low after stimulation, a diagnosis can be more accurately made.

Insulin-induced **hypoglycemia** (via intravenous injection of insulin) stimulates hGH and corticotropin secretion as well. If such stimulation is unsuccessful, then there is a malfunction of the anterior pituitary gland. Blood samples may be obtained following an energetic exercise session lasting 20 minutes.

A substance called hGH-releasing factor has recently been used for hGH stimulation. This approach promises to be more accurate and specific for hGH deficiency caused by the pituitary. Growth

hormone deficiency is also suspected when x ray determination of bone age indicates retarded growth in comparison to chronologic age. At present, the best method to identify hGH-deficient patients is a positive stimulation test followed by a positive response to a therapeutic trial of hGH.

Growth hormone suppression test

Also called the glucose loading test, this procedure is used to evaluate excessive baseline levels of human growth hormone, and to confirm diagnosis of gigantism in children and acromegaly in adults. The procedure requires two different blood samples, one drawn before the administration of 100 g of glucose (by mouth), and a second sample two hours after glucose ingestion.

Normally, a glucose load suppresses hGH secretion. In a patient with excessive hGH levels, failure of suppression indicates anterior pituitary dysfunction and confirms a diagnosis of **acromegaly and gigantism**.

Preparation

Somatotropin: This test requires a blood sample. The patient should be **fasting** (nothing to eat or drink from midnight the night before the test). Stress and/or exercise increases hGH levels, so the patient should be at complete rest for 30 minutes before the blood sample is drawn. If the physician has requested two samples, they should be drawn on consecutive days at approximately the same time on both days, preferably between 6 A.M. and 8 A.M.

Somatomedin C: This test requires a blood sample. The patient should have nothing to eat or drink from midnight the night before the test.

Growth hormone stimulation: This test requires intravenous administration of medications and the withdrawal of frequent blood samples, which are obtained at 0, 60, and 90 minutes after injection of arginine and/or insulin. The patient should have nothing to eat or drink after midnight the night before the test.

Growth hormone suppression: This test requires two blood samples, one before the test and another two hours after administration of 100 g of glucose solution by mouth. The patient should have nothing to eat or drink after midnight, and physical activity should be limited for 10–12 hours before the test.

Risks

Growth hormone stimulation: Only minor discomfort is associated with this test, and results from the insertion of the IV line and the low blood sugar (hypoglycemia) induced by the insulin injection. Some patients may experience sleepiness, sweating and/or nervousness, all of which can be corrected after the test by ingestion of cookies, juice, or a glucose infusion. Severe cases of hypoglycemia may cause ketosis (excessive amounts of fatty acid byproducts in the body), acidosis (a disturbance of the body's acid-base balance), or **shock**. With the close observation required for the test, these are unlikely.

Growth hormone suppression: Some patients experience **nausea** after the administration of this amount of glucose. Ice chips can alleviate this symptom.

Normal results

Normal results may vary from laboratory to laboratory but are usually within the following ranges:

Somatotropin:

• men: 5 ng/ml

• women: less than 10 ng/ml

• children: 0–10 ng/ml

• newborn: 10–40 ng/ml.

Somatomedin C:

• adult: 42–110 ng/ml

• Child:

• 0–8 years: Girls 7–110 ng/ml; Boys 4–87 ng/ml

• 9–10 years: Girls 39–186 ng/ml; Boys 26–98 ng/ml

• 11–13 years: Girls 66–215 ng/ml; Boys 44–207 ng/ml

• 14–16 years: Girls 96–256 ng/ml; Boys 48 255 ng/ml.

Growth hormone stimulation: greater than 10 ng/ml.

Growth hormone suppression: Normally, glucose suppresses hGH to levels of undetectable to 3 ng/ml in 30 minutes to two hours. In children, rebound stimulation may occur after two to five hours.

Abnormal results

Somatotropin hormone: Excess hGH is responsible for the syndromes of gigantism and acromegaly. Excess secretion is stimulated by **anorexia nervosa**, stress, hypoglycemia, and exercise. Decreased levels

---

are seen in hGH deficiency, dwarfism, hyperglycemia, **failure to thrive**, and delayed sexual maturity.

Somatomedin C: Increased levels contribute to the syndromes of gigantism and acromegaly. Stress, major surgery, hypoglycemia, **starvation**, and exercise stimulate hGH secretion, which in turn stimulates somatomedin C.

Growth hormone stimulation: Decreased levels are seen in pituitary deficiency and hGH deficiency. Diseases of the pituitary can result in failure of the pituitary to secrete hGH and/or all the pituitary hormones. As a result, the hGH stimulation test will fail to stimulate hGH secretion.

Growth hormone suppression: The acromegaly syndrome elevates base hGH levels to 75 ng/ml, which in turn are not suppressed to less than 5 ng/ml during the test. Excess hGH secretion may cause unchanged or rising hGH levels in response to glucose loading, confirming a diagnosis of acromegaly or gigantism. In such cases, verification of results is required by repeating the test after a one-day rest.

Resources

PERIODICALS

"Weight-loss Hormone." *Better Nutrition* (May 2004): 32.

Janis O. Flores
Teresa G. Odle

G6PD deficiency *see* **Glucose-6-phosphate dehydrogenase deficiency**

Guaifenesin *see* **Expectorants**

Guided imagery

Definition

Guided imagery is the use of relaxation and mental visualization to improve mood and/or physical well-being.

Purpose

The connection between the mind and physical health has been well documented and extensively studied. Positive mental imagery can promote relaxation and reduce **stress**, improve mood, control high blood pressure, alleviate **pain**, boost the immune system, and lower cholesterol and blood sugar levels. Through guided imagery techniques, patients can learn to control functions normally controlled by the autonomic nervous system, such as heart rate, blood pressure, respiratory rate, and body temperature.

One of the biggest benefits of using guided imagery as a therapeutic tool is its availability. Imagery can be used virtually anywhere, anytime. It is also an equal opportunity therapy. Although some initial training in the technique may be required, guided imagery is accessible to virtually everyone regardless of economic status, education, or geographical location.

Guided imagery also gives individuals a sense of empowerment, or control. The technique is induced by a therapist who guides the patient. The resulting mental imagery used is solely a product of the individual's imagination. Some individuals have difficulty imagining. They may not get actual clear images but perhaps vague feelings about the guided journey. However these individuals' brains and nervous systems responses seem to be the same as those with more detailed imaginings.

Patients who feel uncomfortable "opening up" in a traditional therapist-patient session may feel more at ease with a self-directed therapy like guided imagery.

Description

Guided imagery is simply the use of one's imagination to promote mental and physical health. It can be self-directed, where the individual puts himself into a relaxed state and creates his own images, or directed by others. When directed by others, an individual listens to a therapist, video, or audiotaped **exercise** that leads him through a relaxation and imagery exercise. Some therapists also use guided imagery in group settings.

Guided imagery is a two-part process. The first component involves reaching a state of deep relaxation through breathing and muscle relaxation techniques. During the relaxation phase, the person closes her eyes and focuses on the slow, in and out sensation of breathing. Or, she might focus on releasing the feelings of tension from her muscles, starting with the toes and working up to the top of the head. Relaxation tapes often feature soft music or tranquil, natural sounds such as rolling waves and chirping birds in order to promote feelings of relaxation.

Once complete relaxation is achieved, the second component of the exercise is the imagery, or visualization, itself. There are a number of different types of guided imagery techniques, limited only by the imagination. Some commonly used types include relaxation imagery, healing imagery, pain control imagery, and mental rehearsal.

Relaxation imagery

Relaxation imagery involves conjuring up pleasant, relaxing images that rest the mind and body. These may be experiences that have already happened, or new situations.

Healing imagery

Patients coping with diseases and injuries can imagine **cancer** cells dying, **wounds** healing, and the body mending itself. Or, patients may picture themselves healthy, happy, and symptom-free. Another healing imagery technique is based on the idea of *qi*, or energy flow, an idea borrowed from **traditional Chinese medicine**. Chinese medicine practitioners believe that illness is the result of a blockage or slowing of energy flow in the body. Individuals may use guided imagery to imagine energy moving freely throughout the body as a metaphor for good health.

Pain control imagery

Individuals can control pain through several imagery techniques. One method is to produce a mental image of the pain and then transform that image into something less frightening and more manageable. Another is to imagine the pain disappearing, and the patient as completely pain-free. Or, one may imagine the pain as something over which he has complete control. For example, patients with back problems may imagine their pain as a high voltage electric current surging through their spine. As they use guided imagery techniques, they can picture themselves reaching for an electrical switch and turning down the power on the current to alleviate the pain.

Mental rehearsal

Mental rehearsal involves imagining a situation or scenario and its ideal outcome. It can be used to reduce **anxiety** about an upcoming situation, such as labor and delivery, surgery, or even a critical life event such as an important competition or a job interview. Individuals picture themselves going through each step of the anxiety-producing event and then successfully completing it.

Preparations

For a successful guided imagery session, individuals should select a quiet, relaxing location where there is a comfortable place to sit or recline. If the guided imagery session is to be prompted with an audiotape or videotape, a stereo, VCR, or portable tape player should be available. Some people find that quiet background music improves their imagery sessions.

The session, which can last anywhere from a few minutes to an hour, should be uninterrupted. Taking the phone off the hook and asking family members for solitude can ensure a more successful and relaxing session.

Imagery combined with other relaxation techniques such as **yoga**, massage, or **aromatherapy** can greatly enhance the effects of these therapies. It can be done virtually anywhere.

Precautions

Because of the state of extreme relaxation involved in guided imagery, individuals should never

KEY TERMS

Aromatherapy—The therapeutic use of plant-derived, aromatic essential oils to promote physical and psychological well-being.

Autonomic nervous system—The part of the nervous system that controls so-called involuntary functions such as heart rate, salivary gland secretion, respiratory function, and pupil dilation.

attempt to use guided imagery while driving or operating heavy machinery.

Side effects

Guided imagery can induce sleepiness, and some individuals may fall asleep during a session. Other than this, there are no known adverse side effects to guided imagery.

Research and general acceptance

Use of guided imagery is a widely accepted practice among mental healthcare providers and is gaining acceptance as a powerful pain control tool across a number of medical disciplines. Results of a study conducted at The Cleveland Clinic Foundation and published in 1999 found that cardiac surgery patients who used a guided imagery tape prior to surgery experienced less pain and anxiety. These patients also left the hospital earlier following surgery than patients who used pain medication only.

Another study conducted by Harvard Medical School researchers found that for more than 200 patients undergoing invasive vascular or renal surgery, guided imagery controlled pain and anxiety more effectively than medication alone.

Resources

BOOKS

Battino, Rubin. *Guided Imagery and Other Approaches to Healing*. Carmarthen, United Kingdom: Crown House Publishing, 2000.

PERIODICALS

Lang, Elvira, et al. "Adjunctive non-pharmacological analgesia for invasive medical procedures: a randomized trial." *The Lancet*. 355, no. 9214, (April 2000): 1486-1490.

ORGANIZATIONS

The Academy for Guided Imagery. P.O. Box 2070, Mill Valley, CA 94942. (800) 726-2070.

OTHER

Brennan, Patricia. "Stress First Aid Kit." (Guided imagery audiotape set.) Available from Inside Out Publishing at (888) 727-3296 or < http://www.facingthedawn.com > .

Paula Anne Ford-Martin

Guillain-Barré syndrome

Definition

Guillain-Barré syndrome (GBS) causes progressive muscle weakness and **paralysis** (the complete inability to use a particular muscle or muscle group), which develops over days or up to four weeks, and lasts several weeks or even months.

Description

The classic scenario in GBS involves a patient who has just recovered from a typical, seemingly uncomplicated viral infection. Symptoms of muscle weakness appear one to four weeks later. The most common preceding infections are cytomegalovirus, herpes, Epstein-Barr virus, and viral hepatitis. A gastrointestinal infection with the bacteria *Campylobacter jejuni* is also common and may cause a severe type of GBS from which it is particularly difficult to recover. About 5% of GBS patients have a surgical procedure as a preceding event. Patients with lymphoma, **systemic lupus erythematosus**, or **AIDS** have a higher than normal risk of GBS. Other GBS patients have recently received an immunization, while still others have no known preceding event. In 1976–77, there was a vastly increased number of GBS cases among people who had been recently vaccinated against the Swine flu. The reason for this phenomenon has never been identified, and no other flu vaccine has caused such an increase in GBS cases.

Causes and symptoms

The cause of the weakness and paralysis of GBS is the loss of myelin, which is the material that coats nerve cells (the loss of myelin is called demyelination). Myelin is an insulating substance which is wrapped around nerves in the body, serving to speed conduction of nerve impulses. Without myelin, nerve conduction slows or stops. GBS has a short, severe course. It causes inflammation and destruction of the myelin sheath, and it disturbs multiple nerves. Therefore, it is considered an acute inflammatory demyelinating polyneuropathy.

The reason for the destruction of myelin in GBS is unknown, although it is thought that the underlying problem is autoimmune in nature. An autoimmune disorder is one in which the body's immune system, trained to fight against such foreign invaders as viruses and bacteria, somehow becomes improperly programmed. The immune system becomes confused, and is not able to distinguish between foreign invaders and the body itself. Elements of the immune system are unleashed against areas of the body, resulting in damage and destruction. For some reason, in the case of GBS, the myelin sheath appears to become a target for the body's own immune system.

The first symptoms of GBS consist of muscle weakness (legs first, then arms, then face), accompanied by prickly, **tingling** sensations (paresthesias). Symptoms affect both sides of the body simultaneously, a characteristic that helps distinguish GBS from other causes of weakness and paresthesias. Normal reflexes are first diminished, then lost. The weakness eventually affects all the voluntary muscles, resulting in paralysis. When those muscles necessary for breathing become paralyzed, the patient must be placed on a mechanical ventilator which takes over the function of breathing. This occurs about 30% of the time. Very severely ill GBS patients may have complications stemming from other nervous system abnormalities which can result in problems with fluid balance in the body, severely fluctuating blood pressure, and heart rhythm irregularities.

Diagnosis

Diagnosis of GBS is made by looking for a particular cluster of symptoms (progressively worse muscle weakness and then paralysis), and by examining the fluid that bathes the brain and spinal canal through **cerebrospinal fluid (CSF) analysis**. This fluid is obtained by inserting a needle into the lower back (lumbar region). When examined in a laboratory, the CSF of a GBS patient will reveal a greater-than-normal quantity of protein, with normal numbers of white blood cells and a normal amount of sugar. Electrodiagnostic studies may show slowing or block of conduction in nerve endings in parts of the body other than the brain. Minor abnormalities will be present in 90% of patients.

KEY TERMS

Autoimmune—The body's immune system directed against the body itself.

Demyelination—Disruption or destruction of the myelin sheath, leaving a bare nerve. Results in a slowing or stopping of impulses traveling along that nerve.

Inflammatory—Having to do with inflammation, the body's response to either invading foreign substances (such as viruses or bacteria) or to direct injury of body tissue.

Myelin—The substance that is wrapped around nerves, and which is responsible for speed and efficiency of impulses traveling through those nerves.

Treatment

There is no direct treatment for GBS. Instead, treatments are used that support the patient with the disabilities caused by the disease. The progress of paralysis must be carefully monitored, in order to provide mechanical assistance for breathing if it becomes necessary. Careful attention must also be paid to the amount of fluid the patient is taking in by drinking and eliminating by urinating. Blood pressure, heart rate, and heart rhythm also must be monitored.

A procedure called **plasmapheresis**, performed early in the course of GBS, has been shown to shorten the course and severity of GBS. Plasmapheresis consists of withdrawing the patient's blood, passing it through an instrument that separates the different types of blood cells, and returning all the cellular components (red and white blood cells and platelets) along with either donor plasma or a manufactured replacement solution. This is thought to rid the blood of the substances that are attacking the patient's myelin.

It has also been shown that the use of high doses of immunoglobulin given intravenously (by drip through a needle in a vein) may be just as helpful as plasmapheresis. Immunoglobulin is a substance naturally manufactured by the body's immune system in response to various threats. It is interesting to note that corticosteroid medications (such as prednisone), often the mainstay of anti-autoimmune disease treatment, are not only unhelpful, but may in fact be harmful to patients with GBS.

Prognosis

About 85% of GBS patients make reasonably good recoveries. However, 30% of adult patients, and a greater percentage of children, never fully regain their previous level of muscle strength. Some of these patients suffer from residual weakness, others from permanent paralysis. About 10% of GBS patients begin to improve, then suffer a relapse. These patients suffer chronic GBS symptoms. About 5% of all GBS patients die, most from cardiac rhythm disturbances.

Patients with certain characteristics tend to have a worse outcome. These include people of older age, those who required breathing support with a mechanical ventilator, and those who had their worst symptoms within the first seven days.

Prevention

Because so little is known about what causes GBS to develop, there are no known methods of prevention.

Resources

ORGANIZATIONS

American Academy of Neurology. 1080 Montreal Ave., St. Paul, MN 55116. (612) 695-1940. < http://www.aan.com > .

Guillain-Barré Syndrome Foundation International. PO Box 262, Wynnewood, PA 19096. (610) 667-0131. (610) 667-0131. < http://www.webmast.com/gbs > .

Rosalyn Carson-DeWitt, MD

Guinea worm infection

Definition

Infection occurs when the parasitic guinea worm resides within the body. Infection is not apparent until a pregnant female worm prepares to expel embryos. The infection is rarely fatal, but the latter stage is painful. The infection is also referred to as dracunculiasis, and less commonly as dracontiasis.

Description

Before the early 1980s, guinea worms infected 10–15 million people annually in central Africa and parts of Asia. By 1996, worldwide incidence of infection fell to fewer than 153,000 cases per year.

Complete eradication of guinea worm infection is a goal of international water safety programs.

To survive, guinea worms require three things: water during the embryo stage, an intermediate host during early maturation, and a human host during adulthood. In bodies of water, such as ponds, guinea worm embryos are eaten by tiny, lobster-like water fleas. Once ingested, the embryos mature into larvae.

Humans become hosts by consuming water containing infected water fleas. Once in the human intestine, larvae burrow into surrounding tissue. After three to four, the worms mate. Males die soon after, but pregnant females continue to grow. As adults, each threadlike worm can be three feet long and harbor three million embryos. More than one guinea worm can infect a person at the same time.

About eight months later, the female prepares to expel mature embryos by migrating toward the skin surface. Until this point, most people are unaware that they are infected. Extreme **pain** occurs as the worm emerges from under the skin, often around the infected person's ankle. The pain is temporarily relieved by immersing the area in water, an act that contaminates the water and starts the cycle again.

Causes and symptoms

Dracunculus medinensis, or guinea worm, causes infection. Symptoms are commonly absent until a pregnant worm prepares to expel embryos. By secreting an irritating chemical, the worm causes a blister to form on the skin surface. This chemical also causes **nausea**, **vomiting**, **dizziness**, and **diarrhea**. The blister is accompanied by a burning, stabbing pain and can form anywhere on the body; but, the usual site is the lower leg or foot. Once the blister breaks, an open sore remains until the worm has expelled all the embryos.

Diagnosis

Guinea worm infection is identified by the symptoms.

Treatment

Most people infected with guinea worm rely on traditional medicine. The worm is extracted by gently and gradually pulling the worm out and winding it around a small strip of wood. Surgical removal is possible, but rarely done in rural areas. Extraction is complemented by herbs and oils to treat the wound site. Such treatment can ease extraction and may help prevent secondary infections.

KEY TERMS

Guinea worm embryo—The guinea worm at its earliest life stage prior to or shortly after being expelled from an adult female worm.

Guinea worm larvae—The guinea worm during its middle life stage as it matures within a water flea. The larvae can only grow to adulthood within a human host.

Host—With regard to guinea worm infection, either the water flea or human from which the worm gets nourishment and shelter as it matures.

Secondary infection—An illness–typically caused by bacteria–that follows from a guinea worm infection.

Modern medicine offers safe surgical removal of the guinea worm, and drug therapy can prevent infection and pain. Using drugs to combat the worms has had mixed results.

Prognosis

If the worm is completely removed, the wound heals in approximately two to four weeks. However, if a worm emerges from a sensitive area, such as the sole of a foot, or if several worms are involved, healing requires more time. Recovery is also complicated if the worm breaks during extraction. Serious secondary infections frequently occur in such situations. There is the risk of permanent disability in some cases, and having one guinea worm infection does not confer immunity against future infections.

Prevention

Guinea worn infection is prevented by disrupting transmission. Wells and other protected water sources are usually safe from being contaminated with worm embryos. In open water sources, poisons may be used to kill water fleas. Otherwise, water must be boiled or filtered.

Resources

OTHER

World Health Organization. June 7, 1998. < http://www.who.int/home-page/index.en.shtml >.

Julia Barrett

Gulf War syndrome

Definition

Gulf War syndrome describes a wide spectrum of illnesses and symptoms ranging from **asthma** to **sexual dysfunction** that have been reported by U.S. and U.S. allied soldiers who served in the Persian Gulf War in 1990–1991.

Description

Between 1994 and 1999, 145 federally funded research studies on Gulf War-related illnesses were undertaken at a cost of over $133 million. Despite this investment and the data collected from over 100,000 veterans who have registered with the Department of Defense (DOD) and/or Veterans Administration (VA) as having Gulf War-related illnesses, there is still much debate over the origin and nature of Gulf War syndrome. As of early 2001, the DOD has failed to establish a definite cause for the disorder. Veterans who have the illness experience a wide range of debilitating symptoms that elude a single diagnosis. Common symptoms include **fatigue**, trouble breathing, headaches, disturbed sleep, memory loss, and lack of concentration. Similar experiences among Gulf War veterans have been reported in the United Kingdom and Canada.

Causes and symptoms

There is much current debate over a possible causative agent for Gulf War syndrome other than the **stress** of warfare. Intensive efforts by the Veterans Administration and other public and private institutions have investigated a wide range of potential factors. These include chemical and biological weapons, the immunizations and preventive treatments used to protect against them, smoke from oil well fires, exposure to depleted uranium, and diseases endemic to the Arabian peninsula. So far investigators have not approached a consensus. In its final report released in December 2000, the Presidential Special Oversight Board for Department of Defense Investigations of Gulf War Chemical and Biological Incidents cited combat stress as a possible causative factor, but called for further research. There is also a likelihood that U.S. and allied forces were exposed to low levels of sarin and/or cyclosarin (nerve gases) released during the destruction of Iraqi munitions at Kharnisiyah, Iraq, and that these chemicals might be linked to the syndrome. In July 1997, the VA informed approximately 100,000 U.S. servicemen of their possible exposure to the nerve agents.

In October 1999, the U.S. Pentagon released a report that hypothesized that an experimental drug known as pyriostigmine bromide (PB) might be linked to the physical symptoms manifested in Gulf War Syndrome. The experimental drug was given to U.S. and Canadian troops during the war to protect soldiers against the effects of the chemical nerve agent soman. It has also been suggested that botulinum toxoid and **anthrax** vaccinations administered to soldiers during the conflict may be responsible for some manifestations of the syndrome.

Some studies have shown that Gulf War veterans have a higher incidence of positive tests for *Mycoplasma fermentans*, a bacteria, in their bloodstream. However, other clinical studies have not found a link between the bacterial infection and Gulf War-related illnesses.

Statistical analysis tells us that the following symptoms are about twice as likely to appear in Gulf War veterans than in their non-combat peers: depression, posttraumatic stress disorder (PTSD), chronic fatigue, cognitive dysfunction (diminished ability to calculate, order thoughts, evaluate, learn, and remember), **bronchitis**, asthma, **fibromyalgia**, alcohol **abuse**, **anxiety**, and sexual discomfort. PTSD is the modern equivalent of shell shock (World War I) and battle fatigue (World War II). It encompasses most of the psychological symptoms of war veterans, including nightmares, panic at sudden loud noises, and inability to adjust to peacetime living. **Chronic fatigue syndrome** has a specific medical definition that attempts to separate common fatigue from a more disabling illness in hope of finding a specific cause. Fibromyalgia is another newly defined syndrome, and as such it has arbitrarily rigid defining characteristics. These include a certain duration of illness, a specified minimum number of joint and muscle **pain** located in designated areas of the body, sleep disturbances, and other associated symptoms and signs.

Researchers have identified three distinct syndromes and several variations in Gulf War veterans. Type one patients suffer primarily from impaired thinking. Type two patients have a greater degree of confusion and ataxia (loss of coordination). Type three patients were the most affected by joint pains, muscle pains, and extremity paresthesias (unnatural sensations like burning or tingling in the arms and legs). In each of the three types, researchers found different but measurable impairments on objective testing of neurological function. The business of the nervous system is much more complex and subtle than other body functions. Measuring it requires equally complex effort. The tests used in this study carefully measured and compared localized nerve performance at several different tasks against the same values in normal subjects. Brain wave response to noise and touch, eye muscle response to spinning, and caloric testing (stimulation of the ear with warm and cold water, which causes vertigo) were clearly different between the normal and the test subjects. The researchers concluded that there was "a generalized injury to the nervous system." Another research group concluded their study by stating that there was "a spectrum of neurologic injury involving the central, peripheral, and autonomic nervous systems."

Diagnosis

Until there is a clear definition of the disease, diagnosis is primarily an **exercise** in identifying those Gulf War veterans who have undefined illness in an effort to learn more about them and their symptoms. Both the Department of Defense and the Veterans Administration currently have programs devoted to this problem. Both the DOD's Comprehensive Clinical Evaluation Program and the VA's Persian Gulf Registry provide free, in-depth medical evaluations to Gulf War veterans and their families. In addition to providing individual veterans with critical medical care, these organizations use the cumulative data from these programs to advance research on Gulf War Syndrome itself.

Treatment

Specific treatment awaits specific diagnosis and identification of a causative agent. Meanwhile, veterans can benefit from the wide variety of supportive and non-specific approaches to this and similar problems. There are many drugs available for symptomatic relief. Psychological counseling by those specializing in this area can be immensely beneficial, even life-saving for those contemplating **suicide**. Veterans' benefits are available for those who are impaired by their symptoms.

Alternative treatment

The symptoms can be worked with using many modalities of alternative health care. The key to working successfully with people living their lives with Gulf War syndrome is long-term, ongoing care, whether it be **hypnotherapy**, **acupuncture**, homeopathy, **nutrition**, vitamin/mineral therapy, or bodywork.

Experimental treatment with **antibiotics** is advocated by some healthcare professionals who believe that Gulf War illness is related to a *Mycoplasma*

KEY TERMS

Ataxia—Lack of coordination.

Caloric testing—Flushing warm and cold water into the ear stimulates the labyrinth and causes vertigo and nystagmus if all the nerve pathways are intact.

Endemic—Always there.

Paresthesia—An altered sensation often described as burning, tingling, or pin pricks.

Syndrome—Common features of a disease or features that appear together often enough to suggest they may represent a single, as yet unknown, disease entity. When a syndrome is first identified, an attempt is made to define it as strictly as possible, even to the exclusion of some cases, in order to separate out a pure enough sample to study. This process is most likely to identify a cause, a positive method of diagnosis, and a treatment. Later on, less typical cases can be considered.

---

fermentans bacterial infection. However, a conclusive link has not been clinically proven.

Prognosis

The outlook for Persian Gulf War veterans is unclear, but will hopefully improve as more information is gathered about the illness. Gradual return to a functioning life may take many years of work and much help. It is important to note that even in the absence of an identifiable and curable cause, recovery is possible.

Resources

BOOKS

Wheelwright, Jeff. *The Irritable Heart.* New York: W.W. Norton & Co., 2001.

ORGANIZATIONS

The American Legion. Gulf War Veteran Issues. < http://www.legion.org/gulftoc.htm >.

Office of the Special Assistant for Gulf War Illnesses. 5113 Leesburg Pike, Suite 901, Falls Church, VA, 22041. (703) 578-8518. < http://www.gulflink.osd.mil >.

U.S. Department of Defense. Comprehensive Clinical Evaluation Program (CCEP). (800) 796-9699.

Veterans Administration. Persian Gulf Medical Information Helpline. 400 South 18th Street, St. Louis, Missouri 63103-2271. (800)749-8387.

Veterans Administration. Persian Gulf Registry. (800)PGW-VETS (800) 749-8387. < http:// www.va.gov > .

OTHER

Office of the Special Assistant for Gulf War Illnesses. *Fourth Annual Report: Office of the Special Assistant for Gulf War Illnesses.* Falls Church, VA: Office of the Special Assistant for Gulf War Illnesses, 2000. < http:// www.gulflink.osd.mil/library/annual/ 4thannual_report_jan01.htm > .

Paula Anne Ford-Martin

Gum disease *see* **Periodontal disease**

Günther's disease *see* **Porphyrias**

Gynecomastia

Definition

Gyne refers to female, and mastia refers to the breast. Gynecomastia is strictly a male disease and is any growth of the adipose (fatty) and glandular tissue in a male breast. Not all breast growth in men is considered abnormal, just excess growth.

Causes and symptoms

Breast growth is directed exclusively by female hormones–estrogens. Although men have some estrogen in their system, it is usually insufficient to cause much breast enlargement because it is counterbalanced by male hormones–androgens. Upsetting the balance, either by more of one or less of the other, results in the male developing female characteristics, breast growth being foremost.

At birth both male and female infants will have little breast buds from their mother's hormones. These recede until adolescence, when girls always, and boys sometimes, have breast growth. At this time, the boy's breast growth is minimal, often one-sided and temporary.

Extra or altered sex chromosomes can produce intersex problems of several kinds. Breast growth along with male genital development is seen in Klinefelter syndrome–the condition of having an extra X (female) chromosome–and a few other chromosomal anomalies. One of the several glands that produce hormones can malfunction for reasons other than chromosomes. Failure of androgen production is as likely to produce gynecomastia as overabundant

KEY TERMS

Androgen—Male sex hormone.

Cirrhosis—Diffuse scarring caused by alcohol or chronic hepatitis often leading to liver failure.

Estrogen—Sex hormone responsible for stimulating female sexual characteristics.

Klinefelter syndrome—A condition in a male characterized by having an extra X (female) chromosome and suffering from infertility and gynecomastia.

Thyroid—A gland in the neck that makes thyroxin. Thyroxin regulates the speed of metabolism.

estrogen production. Testicular failure and castration can also be a cause. Some cancers and some benign tumors can make estrogens. Lung **cancer** is known to increase estrogens.

If the hormone manufacturing organs are functioning properly, problems can still arise elsewhere. The liver is the principle chemical factory in the body. Other organs like the thyroid and kidneys also effect chemical processes. If any of these organs are diseased, a chemical imbalance can result that alters the manufacturing process. Men with **cirrhosis** of the liver will often develop gynecomastia from increased production of estrogens.

Finally, drugs can also cause breast enlargement. Estrogens are given to men to treat **prostate cancer** and a few other diseases. **Marijuana** and heroin, along with some prescription drugs, have estrogen effects in some men. On the list are methyldopa (for blood pressure), cimetidine (for peptic ulcers), diazepam (Valium), antidepressants, and spironolactone (a diuretic).

Diagnosis

Carefully feeling the area beneath the nipple of an adolescent boy with breast enlargement will reveal a discreet and sometimes tender lump the size of a fat nickel or quarter. For more serious gynecomastia, the underlying disease will require evaluation, if it is not already well understood.

Treatment

This condition is usually not treated. If it is the result of endocrine disease, hormone manipulations may reduce the effects of the imbalance. There are a number of medical and surgical interventions possible. Radiation of misbehaving organs and cancers is considered an effective treatment.

Prognosis

The progress of gynecomastia is determined by its cause.

Resources

BOOKS

Wilson, Jean D. "Endocrine Disorders of the Breast." In *Harrison's Principles of Internal Medicine*, edited by Anthony S. Fauci, et al. New York: McGraw-Hill, 1997.

J. Ricker Polsdorfer, MD

H

H-2 blockers

Definition

Histamine H-2 receptor blockers act by stopping the pathway that leads to the secretion of stomach acid. There are two kinds of pathways that react to stimulation by histamine. Histamine is produced in the body and released by mast cells in response to some types of injury or to the presence of an antigen. When histamine reaches the H-1 receptors, the reaction results in dilation of capillaries, leading to redness and swelling, along with **itching**. These reactions can be controlled with traditional **antihistamines**.

Histamine that reaches the H-2 receptors causes increased secretion of stomach acid.

Purpose

H2 receptor blockers are used to treat conditions associated with excess amounts of stomach acid, although in some cases they have been replaced by the **proton pump inhibitors**, which have a greater effect on reducing acid secretions.

H2 receptor blockers are used to treat the following conditions:

- duodenal ulcer, as short term therapy and maintenance
- gastric ulcer, as short term therapy and maintenance
- gastroesophageal reflux disease (GERD), including endoscopically diagnosed erosive esophagitis
- pathological hypersecretory conditions such as Zollinger-Ellison syndrome, systemic **mastocytosis**, and multiple endocrine adenomas
- upper GI bleeding
- **heartburn**, acid **indigestion**, and sour stomach

None of the drugs in this class has been approved for use by children under the age of 12 years. However, standard pediatric texts have reported on use by infants and children.

Description

There are four H2 receptor blockers on the market. Although they all work in the same manner and have similar effects, they are not all approved for the same uses.

Cimetidine (Tagamet) is available in both prescription and over-the-counter forms. The oldest of the group and the most studied, this drug is the least potent of the H2 receptor blockers, which means that higher dosages are required to provide comparable effects. There is no evidence that higher potency improves therapeutic results.

Cimetidine is the only drug in its class which is approved for prevention of upper gastro-intestinal bleeding. It has been reported on for a number of uses, with varying degrees of success. Cimetidine, like ranitidine, has shown some benefit in treatment of colorectal **cancer**. Although some claims have been made that cimetidine is useful in treatment of **acetaminophen** overdose, the evidence for this use is lacking, and cimetidine should not be used. Because cimetidine is a mild antiandrogen, it has been of some use in treatment of **hirsutism** (abnormal growth of hair on a woman's face and body).

The three other H2 receptor blockers, famotidine (Pepcid, Pepcid AC), nizatidine (Axid), and ranitidine (Zantac), are similar in their uses. All are approved for treatment of duodenal ulcer both acute treatment and maintenance therapy, gastro-esophageal reflux disease, including erosive esophagitis and gastric ulcer short term treatment, although in this group ranitidine alone is approved for maintenance treatment.

In their over-the-counter (non-prescription) forms, cimetidine and famotidine are approved for treatment of heartburn, acid indigestion, and sour stomach.

Drugs in this class are similar in other respects as well. Although study results vary, cimetidine will usually show its effects within one hour and last for about five hours after a single dose; famotidine and nizatidine also show effects within one hour but may act for up to 12 hours at maximum dosing. Ranitidine has a comparable onset of action and duration in adults but may be slower in the elderly. Onset and duration of action will vary with the individual, the dose of medication, and the presence or absence of food or **antacids** in the stomach.

When *Facts and Comparisons*, a widely used on-line drug information resource, compared the published reports on cure rates for duodenal ulcers, it found that after eight weeks of treatment, all drugs showed healing rates in the range of 82% to 95%. These results were based on comparing separate studies and did not represent comparative trials of the drugs against each other.

Recommended dosage

Cimetidine doses for patients over the age of 12 years, for oral administration.

- Short-term treatment of active duodenal ulcer: 800 mg at bedtime. Other dose regimens are sometimes used.

- Heartburn, acid indigestion, and sour stomach using the over-the-counter product: 100 to 200 mg with water when symptoms start. The dose may be repeated once in 24 hours.

- Prevention of heartburn, acid indigestion, and sour stomach using the over-the-counter product: 100 to 200 mg with water up to one hour before eating food or drinking beverages expected to cause symptoms. Dose should not exceed 400 mg in 24 hours.

- Treatment of hypersecretory conditions: 300 mg four times a day, with meals and at bedtime.

- Gastroesophageal reflux disease: 800 to 1600 mg a day, divided into smaller doses. Treatment usually lasts 12 weeks.

Famotidine doses for patients over the age of 12 years, for oral administration.

- Treatment of duodenal ulcers: 40 mg once a day at bedtime. If necessary, 20 milligrams two times a day may be used.

- Prevention of duodenal ulcers: 20 mg once a day at bedtime.

- Gastric ulcers: 40 mg once a day at bedtime.

- To treat heartburn, acid indigestion, and sour stomach using the over-the-counter product: 10 mg with water when symptoms start. The dose may be repeated once in 24 hours.

- Hypersecretory conditions: 20 mg every six hours.

- Gastroesophageal reflux disease: 20 mg two times a day, usually for up to six weeks.

Nizatidine doses for patients over the age of 12 years, for oral administration.

- Treatment of duodenal or gastric ulcers: 300 mg once a day at bedtime. Alternately, 150 mg two times a day.

- Prevention of duodenal ulcers: 150 mg once a day at bedtime.

- Prevention of heartburn, acid indigestion, and sour stomach: 75 mg taken thirty to sixty minutes before meals which may cause symptoms. The dose may be repeated once in 24 hours.

- Gastroesophageal reflux disease: 150 mg two times a day.

Ranitidine doses for patients over the age of 12 years, for oral administration.

- Duodenal ulcers, treatment: 150 mg two times a day. Alternately, 300 mg once a day at bedtime.

- Duodenal ulcers, prevention: 150 mg at bedtime.

- Gastric ulcers, treatment: 150 mg two times a day.

- Heartburn, acid indigestion, and sour stomach, treatment: 75 mg with water when symptoms start. The dose may be repeated once in 24 hours.

- Heartburn, acid indigestion, and sour stomach, prevention: 75 mg with water taken thirty to sixty minutes before meals or beverages which may cause symptoms. The dose may be repeated once in 24 hours.

- Hypersecretory conditions: 150 mg two times a day.

- Gastroesophageal reflux disease: 150 mg two times a day. The dose may be increased as needed.

Precautions

Overall, the histamine H2 receptor blockers are a safe class of drugs. However, some patients may be particularly susceptible to adverse effects of these drugs. H2 receptor blockers are metabolized in the liver and excreted through the kidneys. Therefore, patients with kidney or liver problems may require reduced doses in order to maintain safe blood levels of the drugs.

Although the safety and effectiveness of H2 receptor blockers in patients over the age of 65 appears to be similar to that seen in younger patients, age-associated reductions in kidney function may lead to elevated blood levels.

Allergic reactions to these drugs are rare but have been reported.

The histamine H2 receptor blockers are **Pregnancy** category B. There are no adequate and well-controlled studies with these agents in pregnant women. Women should use them only when clearly needed and when the potential benefits outweigh the potential hazards to the fetus. Cimetidine is known to cross the placenta.

All drugs in this class are excreted into breast milk and should not be taken by nursing women. Decide whether to discontinue nursing, or discontinue the drug, taking into account the importance of the drug to the mother.

These drugs may mask the symptoms of **stomach cancer**.

Side effects

Although side effects due to the H2 receptor blockers are relatively rare and usually mild, a large number of adverse effects have been reported, in part because of the high use of these drugs. For example, the most common single adverse effect of cimetidine has been a 4% incidence of breast enlargement among males taking the drug in high doses for hypersecretory conditions. Similarly, the incidence of **headache** among high-dose cimetidine patients was 3.5%. Among patients taking lower doses, the frequency of headache was 2.1% compared to 2.3% in a placebo control group. Decreased white blood cell count was reported in 1 in 1,000,000 patients.

The reported side effects from the H2 receptor blocks are:

- abdominal **pain**
- back, leg, or stomach pain
- bleeding or crusting sores on lips
- blistering, burning, redness, scaling, or tenderness of skin
- blisters on palms of hands and soles of feet
- changes in vision or blurred vision
- coughing or difficulty in swallowing
- dark-colored urine
- dizziness

- fainting
- fast, pounding, or irregular heartbeat
- fever and/or chills
- flu-like symptoms
- general feeling of discomfort or illness
- hives
- inflammation of blood vessels
- joint pain
- light-colored stools
- mood or mental changes, including **anxiety**, agitation, confusion, **hallucinations** (seeing, hearing, or feeling things that are not there), mental depression, nervousness, or severe mental illness
- muscle cramps or aches
- nausea, **vomiting**, or loss of appetite
- pain
- peeling or sloughing of skin
- red or irritated eyes
- shortness of breath
- skin rash or itching
- slow heartbeat
- sore throat
- sores, ulcers, or white spots on lips, in mouth, or on genitals
- sudden difficult breathing
- swelling of face, lips, mouth, tongue, or eyelids
- swelling of hands or feet
- swollen or painful glands
- tightness in chest
- troubled breathing, unusually slow or irregular breathing
- unusual bleeding or bruising
- unusual tiredness or weakness
- wheezing
- yellow eyes or skin

    Less frequently reported are

- constipation
- decreased sexual ability (especially in patients with Zollinger-Ellison disease who have received high doses of cimetidine for at least 1 year)
- decrease in sexual desire

- diarrhea
- difficult urination
- dizziness
- drowsiness
- dryness of mouth or skin
- headache
- increased or decreased urination
- increased sweating
- loss of hair
- ringing or buzzing in ears
- runny nose
- swelling of breasts or breast soreness in females and males
- trouble in sleeping

Not all of these adverse effects have been reported with all of the H2 receptor blockers, and some of the adverse effects may not have been drug related. However, because of the high similarity between drugs in this class, any of the reported adverse effects may be considered a possible result of therapy.

Interactions

Cimetidine and ranitidine are both metabolized in the liver using the cytochrome P450 oxidase enzyme system. Since the same enzymes metabolize many drugs, taking two or more drugs that affect the same group of enzymes may cause one of the drugs to be retained in the body longer than would have been expected. The following is a partial list of drugs which may interact with cimetidine, or to a lesser extent with ranitidine.

- benzodiazepines, including Valium, Librium and Xanax
- caffeine
- calcium channel blockers, including Adalat, Calan, Procadia, and others
- carbamazepine
- chloroquine
- labetolol
- lidocaine
- metoprolol
- metronidazole
- phenytoin
- propranolol

- quinidine
- quinine
- sulfonylureas (includes many of the drugs used to treat diabetes)
- theophyllines (used to treat **asthma**; Dyphylline, a member of this group, does not interact with cimetidine)
- triamterene (a diuretic drug rarely used alone but may be found in fixed combinations, including Dyazide and Maxzide)
- tricyclic antidepressants (a group that includes amitriptyline, imipramine, and others)
- valproic acid
- warfarin

Additional drugs may also interact with the H2 receptor blockers, particularly those which might have a similar mechanism or action or adverse effects.

Resources

BOOKS

Beers, Mark H., ed. *Merck Manual of Medical Information: Home Edition.* Riverside, NJ: Simon & Schuster, 2004.

Physicians' Desk Reference 2005. Montvale, NJ: Thomson Healthcare, 2004.

Robertson, Jason, et al. *The Harriet Lane Handbook: A Manual for Pediatric House Officers.* Orlando, FL: Mosby Inc., 2005.

PERIODICALS

Black, R. A., and D. A. Hill. "Over-the-counter medications in pregnancy." *American Family Physician* 67, no. 12 (June 15, 2003): 2517–24.

Chandramouli, J. "What is the most effective therapy for preventing NSAID-induced gastropathy?" *Journal of Pain and Palliative Care Pharmacotherapy* 16, no. 2 (2002): 23–36.

ORGANIZATION

American College of Gastroenterology. PO Box 342260, Bethesda, MD 20827–2260. (301)263-9000. < www.acg.gi.org >.

American Gastroenterological Association. 4930 Del Ray Avenue, Bethesda, MD 20814. (301)654-2055. < www.gastro.org >.

Samuel D. Uretsky, Pharm.D.

Habitual abortion *see* **Recurrent miscarriage**

Hair transplantation

Definition

Hair transplantation is a surgical procedure used to treat baldness or hair loss. Typically, tiny patches of scalp are removed from the back and sides of the head and implanted in the bald spots in the front and top of the head.

Purpose

Hair transplantation is a cosmetic procedure performed on men (and occasionally on women) who have significant hair loss, thinning hair, or bald spots where hair no longer grows. In men, hair loss and baldness are most commonly due to genetic factors (a tendency passed on in families) and age. Male pattern baldness, in which the hairline gradually recedes to expose more and more of the forehead, is the most common form. Men may also experience a gradual thinning of hair at the crown or very top of the skull. For women, hair loss is more commonly due to hormonal changes and is more likely to be a thinning of hair from the entire head. An estimated 50,000 men get transplants each year. Transplants can also be done to replace hair lost due to **burns**, injury, or diseases of the scalp.

Precautions

Although hair transplantation is a fairly simple procedure, some risks are associated with any surgery. It is important to inform the physician about any medications currently being used and about previous allergic reactions to drugs or anesthetic agents. Patients with blood clotting disorders also need to inform their physician before the procedure is performed.

Description

Hair transplantation surgery is performed by a physician in an office, clinic, or hospital setting. Each surgery lasts two to three hours during which approximately 250 grafts will be transplanted. A moderately balding man may require up to 1,000 grafts to get good coverage of a bald area, so a series of surgeries scheduled three to four months apart is usually required. The patient may be completely awake during the procedure with just a local anesthetic drug applied to numb the areas of the scalp. Some patients may be given a drug to help them relax or may be given an anesthetic drug that puts them to sleep.

The most common transplant procedure uses a thin strip of hair and scalp from the back of the head. This strip is cut into smaller clumps of five or six hairs. Tiny cuts are made in the balding area of the scalp and a clump is implanted into each slit. The doctor performing the surgery will attempt to recreate a natural looking hairline along the forehead. Minigrafts, micrografts, or implants of single hair follicles can be used to fill in between larger implant sites and can provide a more natural-looking hairline. The implants will also be arranged so that thick and thin hairs are interspersed and the hair will grow in the same direction.

Another type of hair replacement surgery is called scalp reduction. This involves removing some of the skin from the hairless area and "stretching" some of the nearby hair-covered scalp over the cutaway area.

Health insurance will not pay for hair transplants that are done for cosmetic reasons. Insurance may pay for hair replacement surgery to correct hair loss due to accident, burn, or disease.

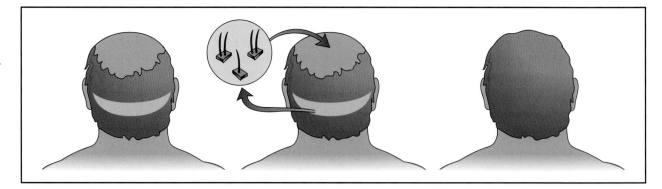

The most common hair transplant procedure involves taking small strips of scalp containing hair follicles from the donor area, usually at the sides or back of the head. These strips are then divided into several hundred smaller grafts. The surgeon relocates these grafts containing skin, follicle, and hair to tiny holes in the balding area by using microsurgical instruments or lasers. *(Illustration by Electronic Illustrators Group.)*

It is important to be realistic about what the final result of a hair transplant will look like. This procedure does not create new hair, it simply redistributes the hair that the patient still has. Some research has been conducted where chest hair has been transplanted to the balding scalp, but this procedure is not widely practiced.

Preparation

It is important to find a respected, well-established, experienced surgeon and discuss the expected results prior to the surgery. The patient may need blood tests to check for bleeding or clotting problems and may be asked not to take **aspirin** products before the surgery. The type of anesthesia used will depend on how extensive the surgery will be and where it will be performed. The patient may be awake during the procedure, but may be given medication to help them relax. A local anesthetic drug which numbs the area will be applied or injected into the skin at the surgery sites.

Aftercare

The area may need to be bandaged overnight. The patient can return to normal activities; however, strenuous activities should be avoided in the first few days after the surgery. On rare occasions, the implants can be "ejected" from the scalp during vigorous **exercise**. There may be some swelling, bruising, **headache**, and discomfort around the graft areas and around the eyes. These symptoms can usually be controlled with a mild **pain** reliever like aspirin. Scabs may form at the graft sites and should not be scraped off. There may be some numbness at the sites, but it will diminish within two to three months.

Risks

Although there are rare cases of infection or scarring, the major risk is probably that the grafted area does not look the way the patient expected it to look.

Normal results

The transplanted hair will fall out within a few weeks, however, new hair will start to grow in the graft sites within about three months. A normal rate of hair growth is about 0.25–0.5 in (6–13 mm) per month.

Abnormal results

Major complications as a result of hair transplantation are extremely rare. Occasionally, a patient may have problems with delayed healing, infection, scarring, or rejection of the graft; but this is uncommon.

Resources

ORGANIZATIONS

American Academy of Cosmetic Surgery. 401 N. Michigan Ave., Chicago, IL 60611-4267. (313) 527-6713. < http://www.cosmeticsurgeryonline.com >.

American Academy of Facial Plastic and Reconstructive Surgery. 1110 Vermont Avenue NW, Suite 220, Washington, DC 20005. (800) 332-3223.

OTHER

"Hair Transplant." Ienhance. < http://www.ienhance.com >.

"Transplants; Flap Surgery; and The Perfect Candidate." Transplant Network. < http://www.hair-transplants.net >.

Altha Roberts Edgren

Hairy cell leukemia

Definition

Hairy cell leukemia is a disease in which a type of white blood cell called the lymphocyte, present in the blood and bone marrow, becomes malignant and proliferates. It is called hairy cell leukemia because the cells have tiny hair-like projections when viewed under the microscope.

Description

Hairy cell leukemia (HCL) is a rare **cancer**. It was first described in 1958 as *leukemic reticuloendotheliosis*, erroneously referring to a red blood cell because researchers were unsure of the cell of origin. It became more easily identifiable in the 1970s. There are approximately 600 new cases diagnosed every year in the United States, making up about 2% of the adult cases of leukemia each year.

HCL is found in cells located in the blood. There are three types of cells found in the blood: the red blood cells that carry oxygen to all the parts of the body; the white blood cells that are responsible for fighting infection and protecting the body from diseases; and the platelets that help in the clotting of blood. Hairy cell leukemia affects a type of white blood cell called the lymphocyte. Lymphocytes are made in the bone marrow, spleen, lymph nodes, and other organs. It specifically affects B-lymphocytes,

which mature in the bone marrow. However, extremely rare variants of HCL have been discovered developing from T-lymphocytes, which mature in the thymus.

When hairy cell leukemia develops, the white blood cells become abnormal both in the way they appear (by acquiring hairy projections) and in the way they act (by proliferating without the normal control mechanisms). Further, the cells tend to accumulate in the spleen, causing it to become enlarged. The cells may also collect in the bone marrow and prevent it from producing normal blood cells. As a result, there may not be enough normal white blood cells in the blood to fight infection.

The median age at which people develop HCL is 52 years. Though it occurs in all ages, HCL more commonly develops in the older population. Men are four times more likely to develop HCL than women. There have been reports of familial aggregation of disease, with higher occurrences in Ashkenazi Jewish men. A potential genetic link is undergoing further investigation.

Causes and symptoms

The cause of hairy cell leukemia is not specifically known. However, exposure to radiation is a known cause of leukemia in general. Familial involvement is another theory, suggesting that there is a genetic component associated with this disease.

HCL is a chronic (slowly progressing) disease, and the patients may not show any symptoms for many years. As the disease advances, the patients may suffer from one or more of the following symptoms:

- weakness
- **fatigue**
- recurrent infections
- **fever**
- anemia
- bruising
- **pain** or discomfort in the abdominal area
- weight loss (uncommon)
- night sweats (uncommon)

Pain and discomfort are caused by an enlarged spleen, which results from the accumulation of the abnormal hairy cells in the spleen. Blood tests may show abnormal counts of all the different types of cells. This happens because the cancerous cells invade the bone marrow as well and prevent it from producing normal blood cells. Because of the low white cell count in the blood, the patient may have frequent infections. Fever often accompanies the infections. The patient is most susceptible to bacterial infections, but infections of any kind are the major cause of **death**. The low red cell count may cause anemia, fatigue, and weakness, and the low **platelet count** may cause the person to bruise and bleed easily.

Diagnosis

When a patient suffers from the above symptoms, the doctor will palpate the abdomen and may order scans to see if the spleen is enlarged (splenomegaly). An enlarged spleen is present in 80% of patients. An enlarged liver is less common, but can occur.

If the spleen is enlarged, the doctor may order several blood tests. In these tests, the total numbers of each of the different types of blood cells (CBC) are reported. Sixty to eighty percent of patients suffer from pancytopenia, which is a dramatic reduction in the number of red blood cells, white blood cells, and platelets circulating in the blood.

If the blood tests are abnormal, the doctor may order a bone marrow aspiration and biopsy. In order to establish a diagnosis, hairy cells must be present in the bone marrow.

Treatment

When physicians perform blood tests, they will determine the level of hemoglobin (the oxygen-transporting molecule of red blood cells). Serum hemoglobin levels and the size of the spleen, which can be measured on exam and by using an x ray, are proposed criteria for determining the stage of HCL. The following are the three proposed stages and their criteria:

- Stage I: Hemoglobin greater than 12 g/dL (1 g = approximately 0.02 pint and 1 dL = approximately 0.33 ounce) and spleen less than or equal to 10 cm (3.9 inches).

- Stage II: Hemoglobin between 8.5 and 12 g/dL and spleen greater than 10 cm (3.9 inches).

- Stage III: Hemoglobin less than 8.5 g/dL and spleen greater than 10 cm (3.9 inches).

Since there is generally no accepted staging system, another method for evaluating the progression of HCL is to group patients into two categories: untreated HCL and progressive HCL, in which hairy cells are present after therapy has been administered.

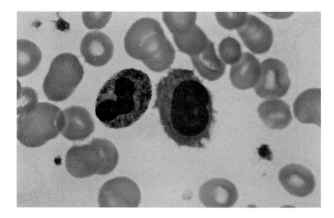

A magnified image of white blood cells with "hairy" projections. *(Photograph by M. Abbey. Photo Researchers, Inc. Reproduced by permission.)*

Some people with hairy cell leukemia have very few or no symptoms at all, and it is reasonable to expect that 10% of patients may not need any treatment. However, if the patient is symptomatic and needs intervention, HCL is especially responsive to treatment.

There are three main courses of treatment: chemotherapy, splenectomy (surgical removal of the spleen), and immunotherapy. Once a patient meets treatment criteria, purine analogues, particularly the drugs, pentostatin and cladribine, are the first-line therapy. Pentostatin is administered at $5mg/m^2$ for two days every other week until total remission is achieved. Patients may experience side effects such as fever, **nausea**, **vomiting**, **photosensitivity**, and kerato-conjuctivitis. However, follow-up studies estimate a relapse-free survival rate at 76%. Cladribine (2-CdA) taken at 0.1mg/kg/day for seven days also has an impressive response. Eighty-six percent of patients experience complete remission after treatment, while 16% experience partial remission. Fever is the principal side effect of 2-CdA.

Biological therapy or immunotherapy, where the body's own immune cells are used to fight cancer, is also being investigated in clinical trials for hairy cell leukemia. A substance called interferon that is produced by the white blood cells of the body was the first systemic treatment that showed consistent results in fighting HCL. The FDA approved inter-feron-alpha (INF-alpha) to fight HCL. The mechanism by which INF-alpha works is not clearly understood. However, it is known that interferon stimulates the body's natural killer cells that are suppressed during HCL. The standard dosage is $2 \ MU/m^2$ three times a week for 12 months. Side

KEY TERMS

Anemia—A condition in which there is low iron in the blood due to a deficiency of red blood cells.

Bone marrow—The spongy tissue inside the large bones in the body that is responsible for making the red blood cells, white blood cells, and platelets.

Bone marrow aspiration and biopsy—A procedure in which a needle is inserted into the large bones of the hip or spine and a small piece of marrow is removed for microscopic examination.

Immunotherapy—A mode of cancer treatment in which the immune system is stimulated to fight the cancer.

Leukemia—A disease in which the cells that constitute the blood become cancerous or abnormal.

Lymph nodes—Oval-shaped organs that are the size of peas, located throughout the body, and contain clusters of cells called lymphocytes. They filter out and destroy the bacteria, foreign particles, and cancerous cells from the blood.

Malignant—Cells that have the ability to invade locally, cause destruction of surrounding tissue, and travel to other sites in the body.

Keratoconjunctivitis—Inflammation of the conjunctiva and cornea of the eye.

Spleen—An organ that lies next to the stomach. Its function is to remove the worn-out blood cells and foreign materials from the blood stream.

Splenectomy—A surgical procedure that involves the surgical removal of the spleen.

effects include fever, myalgia, malaise, **rashes**, and gastrointestinal complaints.

If the spleen is enlarged, it may be removed in a surgical procedure known as splenectomy. This usually causes a remission of the disease. However, 50% of patients that undergo splenectomy require some type of systemic treatment such as **chemotherapy** or immunotherapy. Splenectomy is not the most widely used course of treatment as it was many years ago. Although the spleen is not an indispensable organ, it is responsible for helping the body fight infection. Therefore, other therapies are preferred in order to salvage the spleen and its functions.

Most patients have excellent prognosis and can expect to live 10 years or longer. The disease may remain silent for years with treatment. Continual

follow-up is necessary to monitor the patient for relapse and determine true cure rates.

Alternative treatment

Many individuals choose to supplement traditional therapy with complementary methods. Often, these methods improve the tolerance of side effects and symptoms as well as enrich the quality of life. The American Cancer Society recommends that patients talk to their doctor to ensure that the methods they are using are safely supplementing traditional therapy. Some complementary treatments include the following:

- yoga
- meditation
- religious practices and prayer
- music therapy
- art therapy
- massage therapy
- aromatherapy

Prevention

Since the cause for the disease is unknown and there are no specific risk factors, there is no known prevention.

Resources

BOOKS

Bast, Robert C. *Cancer Medicine.* Lewiston, NY:B.C. Decker Inc., 2000.

Haskell, Charles M. *Cancer Treatment.* 5th ed. Philadephia: W.B. Saunders Company, 2001.

ORGANIZATIONS

American Cancer Society. 1599 Clifton Road, N.E. Atlanta, Georgia 30329. (800) 227-2345. <http://www.cancer.org>.

Cancer Research Institute (National Headquarters). 681 Fifth Avenue, New York, N.Y. 10022. (800) 992-2623. <http://www.cancerresearch.org>.

Hairy Cell Leukemia Research Foundation. 2345 County Farm Lane, Schaumburg, IL 60194. (800) 693-6173.

Leukemia Society of America, Inc. 600 Third Ave, New York, NY 10016. (800) 955-4572.

National Cancer Institute. 9000 Rockville Pike, Building 31, Room 10A16, Bethesda, Maryland, 20892. (800) 422-6237. <http://wwwicic.nci.nih.gov>.

Oncolink. University of Pennsylvania Cancer Center. <http://cancer.med.upenn.edu>.

OTHER

"Coping With Side Effects." National Cancer Institute. July 2, 2001. <http://cancernet.nci.nih.gov/chemotherapy/chemoside.html>.

NCI/PDQ Patient Statement, "Hairy cell leukemia." National Cancer Institute, 2001.

Lata Cherath, PhD
Sally C. McFarlane-Parrott

Halitosis *see* **Bad breath**

Hallucinations

Definition

Hallucinations are false or distorted sensory experiences that appear to be real perceptions. These sensory impressions are generated by the mind rather than by any external stimuli, and may be seen, heard, felt, and even smelled or tasted.

Description

A hallucination occurs when environmental, emotional, or physical factors such as **stress**, medication, extreme **fatigue**, or mental illness cause the mechanism within the brain that helps to distinguish conscious perceptions from internal, memory-based perceptions to misfire. As a result, hallucinations occur during periods of consciousness. They can appear in the form of visions, voices or sounds, tactile feelings (known as haptic hallucinations), smells, or tastes.

Patients suffering from **dementia** and psychotic disorders such as **schizophrenia** frequently experience hallucinations. Hallucinations can also occur in patients who are not mentally ill as a result of stress overload or exhaustion, or may be intentionally induced through the use of drugs, **meditation**, or sensory deprivation. A 1996 report, published in the *British Journal of Psychiatry*, noted that 37% of 4,972 people surveyed experienced hypnagogic hallucinations (hallucinations that occur as a person is falling to sleep). Hypnopomic hallucinations (hallucinations that occur just upon waking) were reported by 12% of the sample.

Causes and symptoms

Common causes of hallucinations include:

- Drugs. Hallucinogenics such as ecstasy (3,4-methylenedioxymethamphetamine, or MDMA), **LSD (lysergic acid diethylamide**, or acid), mescaline

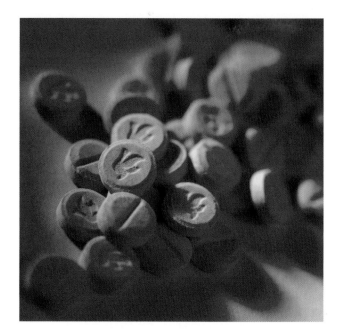

Ecstasy tablets. *(Corbis. Reproduced by permission)*

(3,4,5-trimethoxyphenethylamine, or peyote), and psilocybin (4-phosphoryloxy-N, N-dimethyltryptamine, or mushrooms) trigger hallucinations. Other drugs such as **marijuana** and PCP have hallucinatory effects. Certain prescription medications may also cause hallucinations. In addition, drug withdrawal may induce tactile and visual hallucinations; as in an alcoholic suffering from **delirium** tremens (DTs).

- Stress. Prolonged or extreme stress can impede thought processes and trigger hallucinations.

- Sleep deprivation and/or exhaustion. Physical and emotional exhaustion can induce hallucinations by blurring the line between sleep and wakefulness.

- Meditation and/or sensory deprivation. When the brain lacks external stimulation to form perceptions, it may compensate by referencing the memory and form hallucinatory perceptions. This condition is commonly found in blind and deaf individuals.

- Electrical or neurochemical activity in the brain. A hallucinatory sensation—usually involving touch—called an aura, often appears before, and gives warning of, a migraine. Also, auras involving smell and touch (tactile) are known to warn of the onset of an epileptic attack.

- Mental illness. Up to 75% of schizophrenic patients admitted for treatment report hallucinations.

- Brain damage or disease. Lesions or injuries to the brain may alter brain function and produce hallucinations.

Diagnosis

Aside from hypnogogic and hypnopompic hallucinations, more than one event suggests a person should seek evaluation. A general physician, psychologist, or psychiatrist will try to rule out possible organic, environmental, or psychological causes through a detailed medical examination and social history. If a psychological cause such as schizophrenia is suspected, a psychologist will typically conduct an interview with the patient and his family and administer one of several clinical inventories, or tests, to evaluate the mental status of the patient.

Occasionally, people who are in good mental health will experience a hallucination. If hallucinations are infrequent and transitory, and can be accounted for by short-term environmental factors such as sleep deprivation or meditation, no treatment may be necessary. However, if hallucinations are hampering an individual's ability to function, a general physician, psychologist, or psychiatrist should be consulted to pinpoint their source and recommend a treatment plan.

Treatment

Hallucinations that are symptomatic of a mental illness such as schizophrenia should be treated by a psychologist or psychiatrist. Antipsychotic medication such as thioridazine (Mellaril), haloperidol (Haldol), chlorpromazine (Thorazine), clozapine (Clozaril), or risperidone (Risperdal) may be prescribed.

Prognosis

In many cases, chronic hallucinations caused by schizophrenia or some other mental illness can be controlled by medication. If hallucinations persist, psychosocial therapy can be helpful in teaching the patient the coping skills to deal with them. Hallucinations due to sleep deprivation or extreme stress generally stop after the cause is removed.

Resources

ORGANIZATIONS

American Psychological Association (APA). 750 First St. NE, Washington, DC 20002-4242. (202) 336-5700. < ttp://www.apa.org >.
National Alliance for the Mentally Ill (NAMI). Colonial Place Three, 2107 Wilson Blvd., Ste. 300, Arlington, VA 22201-3042. (800) 950-6264. < http://www.nami.org >.

Paula Anne Ford-Martin

KEY TERMS

Aura—A subjective sensation or motor phenomenon that precedes and indicates the onset of a neurological episode, such as a migraine or an epileptic seizure.

Hypnogogic hallucination—A hallucination, such as the sensation of falling, that occurs at the onset of sleep.

Hypnopompic hallucination—A hallucination that occurs as a person is waking from sleep.

Sensory deprivation—A situation where an individual finds himself in an environment without sensory cues. Also, (used here) the act of shutting one's senses off to outside sensory stimuli to achieve hallucinatory experiences and/or to observe the psychological results.

Hallucinogen *see* **Lysergic acid diethylamide**

Hallux valgus *see* **Bunion**

Haloperidol *see* **Antipsychotic drugs**

Hammertoe

Definition

Hammertoe is a condition in which the toe is bent in a claw-like position. It can be present in more than one toe but is most common in the second toe.

Description

Hammertoe is described as a deformity in which the toes bend downward with the toe joint usually enlarged. Over time, the joint enlarges and stiffens as it rubs against shoes. Other foot structures involved include the overlying skin and blood vessels and nerves connected to the involved toes.

Causes and symptoms

The shortening of tendons responsible for the control and movement of the affected toe or toes cause hammertoe. Top portions of the toes become callused from the friction produced against the inside of shoes. This common foot problem often results from improper fit of footwear. This is especially the case with high-heeled shoes placing pressure on the front part of the foot that compresses the smaller toes tightly together. The condition frequently stems from muscle imbalance, and usually leaves the affected individual with impaired balance.

Diagnosis

A thorough medical history and physical exam by a physician is always necessary for the proper diagnosis of hammertoe and other foot conditions. Because the condition involves bony deformity, x rays can help to confirm the diagnosis.

Treatment

Conservative

Wearing proper footwear and stockings with plenty of room in the toe region can provide treatment for hammertoe. Stretching exercises may be helpful in lengthening the excessively tight tendons.

Surgery

In advanced cases, where conservative treatment is unsuccessful, surgery may be recommended. The tendons that attach to the involved toes are located and an incision is made to free the connective tissue to the foot bones. Additional incisions are made so the toes no longer bend in a downward fashion. The middle joints of the affected toes are connected together permanently with surgical hardware such as pins and wire sutures. The incision is then closed with fine sutures. These sutures are removed approximately seven to ten days after surgery.

Alternative treatment

Various soft tissue and joint treatments offered by **chiropractic** and **massage therapy** may be useful to decrease the tightness of the affected structures.

Prognosis

If detected early, hammertoe can be treated non-surgically. If surgery becomes necessary, surgical risks are minimal with the overall outcome providing good results.

Prevention

Wearing comfortable shoes that fit well can prevent many foot ailments. Foot width may increase with

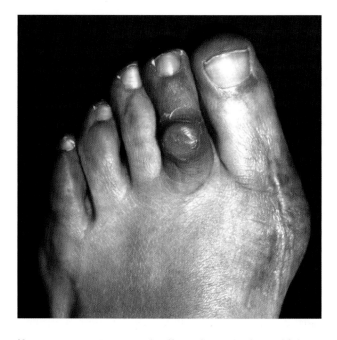

Hammertoe most commonly affects the second toe which, as shown, often develops a corn over the deformity. *(Photograph by Dr. H.C. Robinson, Custom Medical Stock Photo. Reproduced by permission.)*

age. Feet should always be measured before buying shoes. The upper part of the shoes should be made of a soft, flexible material to match the shape of the foot. Shoes made of leather can reduce the possibility of skin irritations. Soles should provide solid footing and not be slippery. Thick soles lessen pressure when walking on hard surfaces. Low-heeled shoes are more comfortable, safer, and less damaging than high-heeled shoes.

Resources

ORGANIZATIONS

American Orthopedic Foot and Ankle Society. 222 South Prospect, Park Ridge, IL 60068.
American Podiatry Medical Association. 9312 Old Georgetown Road, Bethesda, MD 20814.

Jeffrey P. Larson, RPT

Hand-foot-and-mouth disease

Definition

Hand-foot-and-mouth disease is an infection of young children in which characteristic fluid-filled blisters appear on the hands, feet, and inside the mouth.

Description

Coxsackie viruses belong to a family of viruses called enteroviruses. These viruses live in the gastro-intestinal tract, and are therefore present in feces. They can be spread easily from one person to another when poor hygiene allows the virus within the feces to be passed from person to person. After exposure to the virus, development of symptoms takes only four to six days. Hand-foot-and-mouth disease can occur year-round, although the largest number of cases are in summer and fall months.

An outbreak of hand-foot-and-mouth disease occurred in Singapore in 2000, with more than 1,000 diagnosed cases, all in children, resulting in four deaths. A smaller outbreak occurred in Malaysia in 2000. In 1998, a serious outbreak of enterovirus 71 in Taiwan resulted in more than one million cases of hand-foot-and-mouth disease. Of these, there were 405 severe cases and 78 deaths, 71 of which were children younger than five years of age.

Hand-foot-and-mouth should not be confused with foot and mouth disease, which infects cattle but is extremely rare in humans. An outbreak of foot and mouth disease swept through Great Britain and into other parts of Europe and South America in 2001.

Causes and symptoms

Hand-foot-and-mouth disease is very common among young children, and often occurs in clusters of children who are in daycare together. It is spread when poor hand-washing after a diaper change or contact with saliva (drool) allows the virus to be passed from one child to another.

Within about four to six days of acquiring the virus, an infected child may develop a relatively low-grade **fever**, ranging from 99–102 °F (37.2–38.9 °C). Other symptoms include **fatigue**, loss of energy, decreased appetite, and a sore sensation in the mouth that may interfere with feeding. After one to two days, fluid-filled bumps (vesicles) appear on the inside of the mouth, along the surface of the tongue, on the roof of the mouth, and on the insides of the cheeks. These are tiny blisters, about 3–7 mm in diameter. Eventually, they may appear on the palms of the hands and on the soles of the feet. Occasionally, these vesicles may occur in the diaper region.

The vesicles in the mouth cause the majority of discomfort, and the child may refuse to eat or drink due to **pain**. This phase usually lasts for an average of a week. As long as the bumps have clear fluid within them, the disease is at its most contagious. The fluid

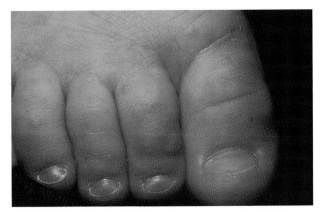

A child's foot with pustules on toes, indicating hand-foot-mouth disease. (Custom Medical Stock Photo. Reproduced by permission.)

within the vesicles contains large quantities of the causative viruses. Extra care should be taken to avoid contact with this fluid.

Diagnosis

Diagnosis is made by most practitioners solely on the basis of the unique appearance of blisters of the mouth, hands, and feet, in a child not appearing very ill.

Treatment

There are no treatments available to cure or decrease the duration of the disease. Medications like **acetaminophen** or ibuprofen may be helpful for decreasing pain, and allowing the child to eat and drink. It is important to try to encourage the child to take in adequate amounts of fluids, in the form of ice chips or popsicles if other foods or liquids are too uncomfortable.

Alternative treatment

There are no effective alternative treatments for hand-foot-and-mouth disease.

Prognosis

The prognosis for a child with hand-foot-and-mouth disease is excellent. The child is usually completely better within about a week of the start of the illness.

Prevention

Prevention involves careful attention to hygiene. Thorough, consistent hand-washing practices, and discouraging the sharing of clothes, towels, and stuffed toys are all helpful. Virus continues to be passed in the feces for several weeks after infection, so good hygiene should be practiced long after all signs of infection have passed.

Resources

BOOKS

Morag, Abraham, and Pearay L. Ogra. "Viral Infections." In *Nelson Textbook of Pediatrics.* edited by Richard Behrman, 16th ed. Philadelphia: W.B. Saunders Co., 2000.

PERIODICALS

"New Tricks for an Old Enterovirus." *Infectious Disease Alert* (December 15, 1999): 45.

Rosalyn Carson-DeWitt, MD
Ken R. Wells

Hand-Schüller-Christian syndrome *see* **Histiocytosis X**

Hansen's disease *see* **Leprosy**

Hantavirus infections

Definition

Hantavirus infection is caused by a group of viruses that can infect humans with two serious illnesses: hemorrhagic **fever** with renal syndrome (HFRS), and Hantavirus pulmonary syndrome (HPS).

Description

Hantaviruses are found without causing symptoms within various species of rodents and are passed to humans by exposure to the urine, feces, or saliva of those infected rodents. Ten different hantaviruses have been identified as important in humans. Each is found in specific geographic regions, and therefore is spread by different rodent carriers. Further, each type

of virus causes a slightly different form of illness in its human hosts:

- Hantaan virus is carried by the striped field mouse, and exists in Korea, China, Eastern Russia, and the Balkans. Hantaan virus causes a severe form of hemorrhagic fever with renal syndrome (HFRS).

- Puumula virus is carried by bank voles, and exists in Scandinavia, western Russia, and Europe. Puumula virus causes a milder form of HFRS, usually termed *nephropathia epidemica*.

- Seoul virus is carried by a type of rat called the Norway rat, and exists worldwide, but causes disease almost exclusively in Asia. Seoul virus causes a form of HFRS that is slightly milder than that caused by Hantaan virus, but results in liver complications.

- Prospect Hill virus is carried by meadow voles and exists in the United States, but has not been found to cause human disease.

- Sin Nombre virus, the most predominant strain in the United States, is carried by the deer mouse. This virus was responsible for severe cases of HPS that occurred in the Southwestern United States in 1993.

- Black Creek Canal virus has been found in Florida. It is predominantly carried by cotton rats.

- New York virus strain has been documented in New York State. The vectors for this virus seem to be deer mice and white-footed mice.

- Bayou virus has been reported in Louisiana and Texas and is carried by the marsh rice rat.

- Blue River virus has been found in Indiana and Oklahoma and seems to be associated with the white-footed mouse.

- Monongahela virus, discovered in 2000, has been found in Pennsylvania and is transmitted by the white-footed mouse.

Causes and symptoms

Hemorrhagic fever with renal syndrome (HFRS)

Hantaviruses that produce forms of hemorrhagic fever with renal syndrome (HFRS) cause a classic group of symptoms, including fever, malfunction of the kidneys, and low **platelet count**. Because platelets are blood cells important in proper clotting, low numbers of circulating platelets can result in spontaneous bleeding, or hemorrhage.

Patients with HFRS have **pain** in the head, abdomen, and lower back, and may report bloodshot eyes and blurry vision. Tiny pinpoint hemorrhages, called petechiae, may appear on the upper body and the soft palate in the mouth. The patient's face, chest, abdomen, and back often appear flushed and red, as if sunburned.

After about five days, the patient may have a sudden drop in blood pressure; often it drops low enough to cause the clinical syndrome called **shock**. Shock is a state in which blood circulation throughout the body is insufficient to deliver proper quantities of oxygen. Lengthy shock can result in permanent damage to the body's organs, particularly the brain, which is very sensitive to oxygen deprivation.

Around day eight of HFRS, kidney involvement results in multiple derangements of the body chemistry. Simultaneously, the hemorrhagic features of the illness begin to cause spontaneous bleeding, as demonstrated by bloody urine, bloody vomit, and in very serious cases, brain hemorrhages with resulting changes in consciousness.

Day eleven often brings further chemical derangements, with associated confusion, **hallucinations**, seizures, and lung complications. Those who survive this final phase usually begin to turn the corner toward recovery at this time, although recovery takes approximately six weeks.

Hantavirus pulmonary syndrome (HPS)

Hantavirus pulmonary syndrome (HPS) develops in four stages. They are:

- The incubation period. This lasts from one to five weeks from exposure. Here, the patient may exhibit no symptoms.

- The prodrome, or warning signs, stage. Symptoms begin with a fever, muscle aches, **headache**, **dizziness**, and abdominal pain and upset. Sometimes there is **vomiting** and diarrhea.

- The cardiopulmonary stage. The patient slips into this stage rapidly, sometimes within a day or two of initial symptoms; sometimes as long as 10 days later. There is a drop in blood pressure, shock, and leaking of the blood vessels of the lungs, which results in fluid accumulation in the lungs, and subsequent **shortness of breath**. The fluid accumulation can be so rapid and so severe as to put the patient in **respiratory failure** within only a few hours. Some patients experience severe abdominal tenderness.

- The convalescent stage. If the patient survives the respiratory complications of the previous stage, there is a rapid recovery, usually within a day or two. However, abnormal liver and lung functioning may persist for six months.

Diagnosis

Serologic techniques help diagnose a hantavirus infection. The patient's blood is drawn, and the ELISA (enzyme-linked immunosorbent assay) is done in a laboratory to identify the presence of specific immune substances (antibodies)—substances which an individual's body would only produce in response to the hantavirus.

It is very difficult to demonstrate the actual virus in human tissue, or to grow cultures of the virus within the laboratory, so the majority of diagnostic tests use indirect means to demonstrate the presence of the virus.

Treatment

Treatment of hantavirus infections is primarily supportive, because there are no agents available to kill the viruses and interrupt the infection. Broad-spectrum **antibiotics** are given until the diagnosis is confirmed. Supportive care consists of providing treatment in response to the patient's symptoms. Because both HFRS and HPS progress so rapidly, patients must be closely monitored, so that treatment may be started at the first sign of a particular problem. Low blood pressure is treated with medications. Blood transfusions are given for both hemorrhage and shock states. Hemodialysis is used in kidney failure. (Hemodialysis involves mechanically cleansing the blood outside of the body, to replace the kidney's normal function of removing various toxins form the blood.) Rapid respiratory assistance is critical, often requiring intubation.

The anti-viral agent ribavirin has been approved for use in early treatment of hantavirus infections.

Prognosis

The diseases caused by hantaviruses are extraordinarily lethal. About 6–15% of people who contract HFRS have died. Almost half of all people who contract HPS will die. This gives HPS one of the highest fatality rates of any acute viral disease. It is essential that people living in areas where the hantaviruses exist seek quick medical treatment should they begin to develop an illness that might be due to a hantavirus.

Prevention

There are no immunizations currently available against any of the hantaviruses. In 2003, developments in genetic science were helping researchers work on a possible **vaccination** and therapy for several versions of hantavirus, including the Sin Nombre virus that causes HPS. With further work, a gene-based vaccine could become available in the future. However, the only known forms of hantavirus prevention involve rodent control within the community and within individual households. The following is a list of preventive measures:

- Avoiding areas known to be infested by rodents is essential.

- Keeping a clean home and keeping food in rodent-proof containers.

- Disposing of garbage and emptying pet food dishes at night.

- Setting rodent traps around baseboards and in tight places. Disposing of dead animals with gloves and disinfecting the area with bleach.

- Using rodenticide as necessary.

- Sealing any entry holes 0.25 inch wide or wider around foundations with screen, cement, or metal flashing.

- Clearing brush and junk from house foundations.

- Putting metal flashing around house foundations.

- Elevating hay, woodpiles, and refuse containers.

- Airing out all sealed outbuildings or cabins 30 minutes before cleaning for the season.

- When camping, avoiding sleeping on the bare ground. It is advised to sleep on a cot or in a tent with a floor.

Resources

BOOKS

Harper, David R., and Andrea S. Meyer. *Of Mice, Men, and Microbes: Hantavirus.* San Diego: Academic Press, 1999.

PERIODICALS

"DNA Vaccine Protects Against Hantavirus Pulmonary Syndrome." *Heart Disease Weekly* November 2, 2003: 31.

Jones, Amy. "Setting a Trap for Hantavirus." *Nursing* September 2000: 20.

Monroe, Martha C., Sergey P. Morzunov, Angela M. Johnson, Michael De. Bowen, et al. "Genetic Diversity and Distribution of Peromyscus-Borne Hantaviruses in North America." *Nursing* January-February 1999: 75–86.

Naughton, Laurie. "Hantavirus Infection in the United States: Are We Prepared?" *Physician Assistant* May 2000: 33.

Rhodes III, Luther V., Cinnia Huang, Angela J. Sanchez, Stuart T. Nichol, et al. "Hantavirus Pulmonary Syndrome Associated with Monongahela Virus, Pennsylvania." *Emerging Infectious Diseases* November 2000: 616.

Van Bevern, Pamela A. "Hantavirus Pulmonary Syndrome." *Clinician Reviews* July 2000: 108.

Janie F. Franz
Teresa G. Odle

▍Haptoglobin test

Definition

This test is done to help evaluate a person for **hemolytic anemia**.

Purpose

Haptoglobin is a blood protein made by the liver. The haptoglobin levels decrease in hemolytic anemia. Hemolytic **anemias** include a variety of conditions that result in hemolyzed, or burst, red blood cells.

Decreased values can also indicate a slower type of red cell destruction unrelated to anemia. For example, destruction can be caused by mechanical heart valves or abnormal hemoglobin, such as **sickle cell disease** or **thalassemia**.

Haptoglobin is known as an acute phase reactant. Its level increases during acute conditions such as infection, injury, tissue destruction, some cancers, **burns**, surgery, or trauma. Its purpose is to remove damaged cells and debris and rescue important material such as iron. Haptoglobin levels can be used to monitor the course of these conditions.

Description

Hemoglobin is the protein in the red blood cell that carries oxygen throughout the body. Iron is an essential part of hemoglobin; without iron, hemoglobin can not function. Haptoglobin's main role is to save iron by attaching itself to any hemoglobin released from a red cell.

When red blood cells are destroyed, the hemoglobin is released. Haptoglobin is always present in the blood waiting to bind to released hemoglobin. White blood cells (called macrophages) bring the haptoglobin-hemoglobin complex to the liver, where the haptoglobin and hemoglobin are separated and the iron is recycled.

In hemolytic anemia, so many red cells are destroyed that most of the available haptoglobin is needed to bind the released hemoglobin. The more severe the hemolysis, the less haptoglobin remains in the blood.

Haptoglobin is measured in several different ways. One way is called rate nephelometry. A person's serum is mixed with a substance that will bind to haptoglobin. The amount of bound haptoglobin is measured using a rate nephelometer, which measures the amount of light scattered by the bound haptoglobin. Another way of measuring haptoglobin is to measure it according to how much hemoglobin it can bind.

Preparation

This test requires 5 mL of blood. The person being tested should avoid taking **oral contraceptives** or androgens before this test. A healthcare worker ties a tourniquet on the person's upper arm, locates a vein in the inner elbow region, and inserts a needle into that vein. Vacuum action draws the blood through the needle into an attached tube. Collection of the sample takes only a few minutes.

Aftercare

Discomfort or bruising may occur at the puncture site or the person may feel dizzy or faint. Pressure to the

---

KEY TERMS

Acute phase reactant—A substance in the blood that increases as a response to an acute condition such as infection, injury, tissue destruction, some cancers, burns, surgery, or trauma.

Haptoglobin—A blood protein made by the liver. Its main role is to save iron by attaching itself to any hemoglobin released from a red cell.

Hemoglobin—The protein in the red blood cell that carries oxygen.

Hemolytic anemia—A variety of conditions that result in hemolyzed, or burst, red blood cells.

---

puncture site until the bleeding stops reduces bruising. Warm packs to the puncture site relieve discomfort.

Normal results

Normal results vary based on the laboratory and test method used. Haptoglobin is not present in newborns at birth, but develop adult levels by 6 months.

Abnormal results

Decreased haptoglobin levels usually indicates hemolytic anemia. Other causes of red cell destruction also decrease haptoglobin: a blood **transfusion** reaction; mechanical heart valve; abnormally shaped red cells; or abnormal hemoglobin, such as thalassemia or sickle cell anemia.

Haptoglobin levels are low in **liver disease**, because the liver can not manufacture normal amounts of haptoglobin. Low levels may also indicate an inherited lack of haptoglobin, a condition found particularly in African Americans.

Haptoglobin increases as a reaction to illness, trauma, or rheumatoid disease. High haptoglobin values should be followed-up with additional tests. Drugs can also effect haptoglobin levels.

Normal results vary widely from person to person. Unless the level is very high or very low, haptoglobin levels are most valuable when the results of several tests done on different days are compared.

Nancy J. Nordenson

Hardening of the arteries *see* **Atherosclerosis**

Harelip *see* **Cleft lip and palate**

Hartnup disease

Definition

Hartnup disease is an inherited nutritional disorder with primary symptoms including a red, scaly rash and sensitivity to sunlight.

Description

Hartnup disease was first identified in the 1950s in the Hartnup family in London. A defect in intestines and kidneys makes it difficult to break down and absorb protein in the diet. This causes a condition very similar to pellegra (niacin deficiency). The condition occurs in about one of every 26,000 live births.

Causes and symptoms

Hartnup disease is an in-born error of metabolism, that is, a condition where certain nutrients cannot be digested and absorbed properly. The condition is passed on genetically in families. It occurs when a person inherits two recessive genes for the disease, one from each parent. People with Hartnup disease are not able to absorb some of the amino acids (the smaller building blocks that make up proteins) in their intestines. One of the amino acids that is not well absorbed is tryptophan, which the body uses to make its own form of niacin.

The majority of people with this disorder do not show any symptoms. About 10–20% of people with Hartnup disease do have symptoms. The most prominent symptom is a red, scaly rash that gets worse when the patient is exposed to sunlight. **Headache**, **fainting**, and **diarrhea** may also occur. Mental retardation, cerebral ataxia (muscle weakness), and **delirium** (a confused, agitated, delusional state) are some of the more serious complications that can occur. Short stature has also been noted in some patients. Although this is an inherited disease, the development of symptoms depends on a variety of factors including diet, environment, and other genetic traits controlling amino acid levels in the body. Symptoms can be brought on by exposure to sunlight, fever, drugs, or other stresses. Poor **nutrition** frequently precedes an attack of symptoms. The frequency of attacks usually decreases as the patient gets older.

Diagnosis

The symptoms of this disease suggest a deficiency of a B vitamin called niacin. A detailed diet history can

KEY TERMS

Amino acids—Proteins are made up of organic compounds called amino acids. The human body uses amino acids to build and repair body tissue. The body can make some of its own amino acids from other nutrients in the diet; these are called non-essential amino acids. Essential amino acids are those that cannot be made by the body but must be consumed in the diet. Animal proteins (like meat, eggs, fish, and milk) provide all of the amino acids.

Aminoaciduria—A condition confirmed by laboratory tests where high levels of amino acids are found in the urine.

Pellegra—A condition caused by a dietary deficiency of one of the B vitamins, called niacin.

Tryptophan—An essential amino acid that has to consumed in the diet because it cannot be manufactured by the body. Tryptophan is converted by the body to niacin, one of the B vitamins.

be used to assess if there is adequate protein and **vitamins** in the diet. The diagnosis of Hartnup disease is confirmed by a laboratory test of the urine which will contain an abnormally high amount of amino acids (aminoaciduria).

Treatment

The vitamin niacin is given as a treatment for Hartnup disease. The typical dosage ranges from 40–200 mg of nicotinamide (a form of niacin) per day to prevent pellagra-like symptoms. Some patients may require dietary supplements of tryptophan.

Eating a healthy, high protein diet can relieve the symptoms and prevent them from recurring.

Prognosis

The prognosis for a healthy life is good once the condition has been identified and treated.

Prevention

Hartnup disease is an inherited condition. Parents may not have the disease themselves, but may pass the genes responsible for it on to their children. Genetic testing can be used to identify carriers of the genes. Symptoms can usually be controlled with a high protein diet, vitamin supplements of niacin, and by avoiding the stresses that contribute to attacks of symptoms.

Resources

ORGANIZATIONS

National Organization for Rare Disorders. PO Box 8923, New Fairfield, CT 06812-8923. (800) 999-6673. < http://www.rarediseases.org >.

NIH/National Institute of Diabetes, Digestive and Kidney Diseases. Building 31, Room 9A04, 31 Center Drive, Bethesda MD 20892-2560. (301) 496-3583.

OTHER

"Hartnup disorder." OMIM Homepage, Online Mendelian Inheritance in Man. < http://www.ncbi.nlm.nih.gov/Omim >.

"Nephrology: Hartnup disease." Medstudents.com. < http://www.medstudents.com >.

Altha Roberts Edgren

Hashimoto's disease *see* **Thyroiditis**

Hatha yoga

Definition

Hatha **yoga** is the most widely practiced form of yoga in America. It is the branch of yoga which concentrates on physical health and mental well-being. Hatha yoga uses bodily postures (*asanas*), breathing techniques (*pranayama*), and **meditation** (*dyana*) with the goal of bringing about a sound, healthy body and a clear, peaceful mind. There are nearly 200 hatha yoga postures, with hundreds of variations, which work to make the spine supple and to promote circulation in all the organs, glands, and tissues. Hatha yoga postures also stretch and align the body, promoting balance and flexibility.

Purpose

In a celebrated 1990 study, *Dr. Dean Ornish's Program for Reversing Heart Disease* (Random House), a cardiologist showed that yoga and meditation combined with a low-fat diet and group support could significantly reduce the blockage of coronary arteries. Other studies have shown yoga's benefit in reducing stress-related problems such as high blood pressure and cholesterol. Meditation has been adopted by medical schools and clinics as an effective **stress** management technique. Hatha yoga is also used

by physical therapists to improve many injuries and disabilities, as the gentleness and adaptability of yoga make it an excellent **rehabilitation** program.

Yoga has been touted for its ability to reduce problems with such varying conditions as **asthma**, backaches, diabetes, **constipation**, **menopause**, **multiple sclerosis**, **varicose veins**, and **carpal tunnel syndrome**. A vegetarian diet is the dietary goal of yoga, and this change of lifestyle has been shown to significantly increase longevity and reduce heart disease.

Yoga as a daily **exercise** program can improve fitness, strength, and flexibility. People who practice yoga correctly every day report that it can promote high levels of overall health and energy. The mental component of yoga can clarify and discipline the mind, and yoga practitioners say its benefits can permeate all facets of a person's life and attitude, raising self-esteem and self-understanding.

Description

Origins

Yoga was developed in ancient India as far back as 5,000 years ago; sculptures detailing yoga positions have been found in India which date back to 3000 B.C. Yoga is derived from a Sanskrit word which means "union." The goal of classical yoga is to bring self-transcendence, or enlightenment, through physical, mental and spiritual health. Many people in the West mistakenly believe yoga to be a religion, but its teachers point out that it is a system of living designed to promote health, peace of mind, and deeper awareness of ourselves. There are several branches of yoga, each of which is a different path and philosophy toward self-improvement. Some of these paths include service to others, pursuit of wisdom, non-violence, devotion to God, and observance of spiritual rituals. Hatha yoga is the path which has physical health and balance as a primary goal, for its practitioners believe that greater mental and spiritual awareness can be brought about with a healthy and pure body.

The origins of hatha yoga have been traced back to the eleventh century A.D. The Sanskrit word *ha* means "sun" and *tha* means "moon," and thus hatha, or literally sun-moon yoga, strives to balance opposing parts of the physical body, the front and back, left and right, top and bottom. Some yoga masters (*yogis*) claim that hatha yoga was originally developed by enlightened teachers to help people survive during the Age of Kali, or the spiritual dark ages, in which Hindus believe we are now living.

The original philosophers of yoga developed it as an eight-fold path to complete health. These eight steps include moral and ethical considerations (such as honesty, non-aggression, peacefulness, non-stealing, generosity, and sexual propriety), self-discipline (including purity, simplicity, devotion to God, and self-knowledge), posture, breath control, control of desires, concentration, meditation, and happiness. According to yogis, if these steps are followed diligently, a person can reach high levels of health and mental awareness.

As it has subsequently developed, hatha yoga has concentrated mainly on two of the eight paths, breathing and posture. Yogis believe breathing to be the most important metabolic function; we breathe roughly 23,000 times per day and use about 4,500 gallons of air, which increases during exercise. Thus, breathing is extremely important to health, and *prana*, or life-force, is found most abundantly in the air and in the breath. If we are breathing incorrectly, we are hampering our potential for optimal health. *Pranayama*, literally the "science of breathing" or "control of life force," is the yogic practice of breathing correctly and deeply.

In addition to breathing, hatha yoga utilizes asanas, or physical postures, to bring about flexibility, balance and strength in the body. Each of these postures has a definite form and precise steps for achieving the desired position and for exiting it. These postures, yogis maintain, have been scientifically developed to increase circulation and health in all parts of the body, from the muscular tissues to the glands and internal organs. Yogis claim that although hatha yoga can make the body as strong and fit as any exercise program, its real benefits come about because it is a system of maintenance and balance for the whole body.

Yoga was brought to America in the late 1800s, when Swami Vivekananda, an Indian yogi, presented a lecture on yoga in Chicago. Hatha yoga captured the imagination of the Western mind, because accomplished yogis could demonstrate incredible levels of fitness, flexibility, and control over their bodies and metabolism. Yoga has flourished in the West. Americans have brought to yoga their energy and zest for innovation, which troubles some Indian yogis and encourages others, as new variations and schools of yoga have developed. For instance, power yoga is a recent Americanized version of yoga which takes hatha yoga principles and speeds them up into an extremely rigorous aerobic workout, and many strict hatha yoga teachers oppose this sort of change to their philosophy. Other variations of hatha yoga

in America now include Iyengar, Ashtanga, Kripalu, Integral, Viniyoga, Hidden Language, and Bikram yoga, to name a few. Sivananda yoga was practiced by Lilias Folen, who was responsible for introducing many Americans to yoga through public television.

Iyengar yoga was developed by B.K.S. Iyengar, who is widely accepted as one of the great living yogis. Iyengar uses classical hatha yoga asanas and breathing techniques, but emphasizes great precision and strict form in the poses, and uses many variations on a few postures. Iyengar allows the use of props such as belts, ropes, chairs, and blocks to enable students to get into postures they otherwise couldn't. In this respect, Iyengar yoga is good for physical therapy because it assists in the manipulation of inflexible or injured areas.

Ashtanga yoga, made popular by yogi K. Patabhi Jois, also uses hatha yoga asanas, but places an emphasis on the sequences in which these postures are performed. Ashtanga routines often unfold like long dances with many positions done quickly one after the other. Ashtanga is thus a rigorous form of hatha yoga, and sometimes can resemble a difficult aerobic workout. Ashtanga teachers claim that this form of yoga uses body heat, sweating, and deep breathing to purify the body.

Kripalu yoga uses hatha yoga positions but emphasizes the mental and emotional components of each asana. Its teachers believe that tension and long-held emotional problems can be released from the body by a deep and meditative approach to the yoga positions. Integral yoga seeks to combine all the paths of yoga, and is generally more meditative than physical, emphasizing spirituality and awareness in everyday life. Viniyoga tries to adapt hatha yoga techniques to each individual body and medical problem. Hidden Language yoga was developed by Swami Sivananda Radha, a Western man influenced by Jungian psychology. It emphasizes the symbolic and psychological parts of yoga postures and techniques. Its students are encouraged to write journals and participate in group discussions as part of their practice. Bikram yoga has become very popular in the late 1990s, as its popular teacher, Bikram Choudury, began teaching in Beverly Hills and has been endorsed by many famous celebrities. Bikram yoga uses the repetition of 26 specific poses and two breathing techniques to stretch and tone the whole body.

A hatha yoga routine consists of a series of physical postures and breathing techniques. Routines can take anywhere from 20 minutes to two hours, depending on the needs and ability of the practitioner. Yoga should always be adapted to one's state of health; that is, a shorter and easier routine should be used when a person is fatigued. Yoga is ideally practiced at the same time every day, to encourage the discipline of the practice. It can be done at any time of day; some prefer it in the morning as a wake-up routine, while others like to wind down and de-stress with yoga at the end of the day.

Yoga asanas consist of three basic movements: backward bends, forward bends, and twisting movements. These postures are always balanced; a back bend should be followed with a forward bend, and a leftward movement should be followed by one to the right. Diaphragm breathing is important during the poses, where the breath begins at the bottom of the lungs. The stomach should move outward with the inhalation and relax inward during exhalation. The breath should be through the nose at all times during hatha asanas. Typically, one inhales during backward bends and exhales during forward bending movements.

The mental component in yoga is as important as the physical movements. Yoga is not a competitive sport, but a means to self-awareness and self-improvement. An attitude of attention, care, and non-criticism is important; limitations should be acknowledged and calmly improved. Patience is important, and yoga stretches should be slow and worked up to gradually. The body should be worked with, and never against, and a person should never overexert. A yoga stretch should be done only so far as proper form and alignment of the whole body can be maintained. Some yoga stretches can be uncomfortable for beginners, and part of yoga is learning to distinguish between sensations that are beneficial and those that can signal potential injury. A good rule is that positions should be stopped when there is sharp **pain** in the joints, muscles, or tendons.

Preparations

All that is needed to perform hatha yoga is a flat floor and adequate space for stretching out. A well-ventilated space is preferable, for facilitating proper breathing technique. Yoga mats are available which provide non-slip surfaces for standing poses. Loose, comfortable clothing should be worn. Yoga should be done on an empty stomach; a general rule is to wait three hours after a meal.

Yoga is an exercise that can be done anywhere and requires no special equipment. Yoga uses only gravity and the body itself as resistance, so it is a low-impact activity excellent for those who don't do well with other types of exercise. The mental component of yoga can appeal to those who get bored easily with

---

KEY TERMS

Asana—Yoga posture or stance.

Diaphragm breathing—Method of deep breathing using the entire lungs.

Dyana—Yoga meditation.

Meditation—Technique of mental relaxation.

Prana—Yoga term for life-enhancing nutrient found in air, food and water.

Pranayama—Yoga method of breathing.

---

exercise. By the same token, yoga can be a good stress management tool for those who prefer movement to sitting meditation.

Precautions

As with any exercise program, people should check with their doctors before starting yoga practice for the first time. Those with medical conditions, injuries or spinal problems should find a yoga teacher familiar with their conditions before beginning yoga. Pregnant women, particularly after the third month of **pregnancy**, should only perform a few yoga positions with the supervision of an experienced teacher. Some yoga asanas can be very difficult, and potentially injurious, for beginners, so teachers should always be consulted as preparation for advanced yoga positions. Certain yoga positions should not be performed by those with fevers, or during menstruation.

Side effects

Those just beginning hatha yoga programs often report **fatigue** and soreness throughout the body, as yoga stretches and exercises muscles and tendons which are often long-neglected. Some yogic breathing and meditation techniques can be difficult for beginners and can cause **dizziness** or disorientation; these are best performed under the guidance of a teacher.

Resources

BOOKS

Feuerstein, Georg. *Yoga for Dummies*. New York: IDG Books, 1999.

PERIODICALS

Yoga International Magazine. R.R. 1 Box 407, Honesdale, PA 18431. < http://www.yimag.com >.

Yoga Journal. P.O. Box 469088, Escondido, CA 92046. < http://www.yogajournal.com >.

ORGANIZATIONS
International Association of Yoga Therapists (IAYT). 4150 Tivoli Ave., Los Angeles, CA 90066.

Douglas Dupler, MA

Haverhill fever *see* **Rat-bite fever**

Hay fever *see* **Allergic rhinitis**

HBF test *see* **Fetal hemoglobin test**

HCG *see* **Infertility drugs**

Head and neck cancer

Definition

The term head and neck cancers refers to a group of cancers found in the head and neck region. This includes tumors found in:

- The oral cavity (mouth). The lips, the tongue, the teeth, the gums, the lining inside the lips and cheeks, the floor of the mouth (under the tongue), the roof of the mouth and the small area behind the wisdom teeth are all included in the oral cavity.

- The oropharynx (which includes the back one-third of the tongue, the back of the throat and the tonsils).

- Nasopharynx (which includes the area behind the nose).

- Hypopharynx (lower part of the throat).

- The larynx (voice box, located in front of the neck, in the region of the Adam's apple). In the larynx, the **cancer** can occur in any of the three regions: the glottis (where the vocal cords are); the supraglottis (the area above the glottis); and the subglottis (the area that connects the glottis to the windpipe).

The most frequently occurring cancers of the head and neck area are oral cancers and laryngeal cancers. Almost half of all the head and neck cancers occur in the oral cavity, and a third of the cancers are found in the larynx. By definition, the term "head and neck cancers" usually excludes tumors that occur in the brain.

Description

Head and neck cancers involve the respiratory tract and the digestive tract; and they interfere with the functions of eating and breathing. Laryngeal cancers affect speech. Loss of any of these functions is significant. Hence, early detection and appropriate treatment of head and neck cancers is of utmost importance.

Roughly 10% of all cancers are related to the head and the neck. It is estimated that more than 55,000 Americans will develop cancer of the head and neck in 1998, and nearly 13,000 will die from the disease. The American Cancer Society estimates that in 1998, approximately, 11,100 new cases of **laryngeal cancer** alone will be diagnosed and 4,300 people will die of this disease. Oral cancer is the sixth most common cancer in the United States. Approximately 40,000 new cases are diagnosed each year and it causes at least 8,000 deaths. Among the major cancers, the survival rate for head and neck cancers is one of the poorest. Less than 50% of the patients survive five years or more after initial diagnosis. This is because the early signs of head and neck cancers are frequently ignored. Hence, when it is first diagnosed, it is often in an advanced stage and not very amenable to treatment.

The risk for both oral cancer and laryngeal cancer seems to increase with age. Most of the cases occur in individuals over 40 years of age, the average age at diagnosis being 60. While oral cancer strikes men twice as often as it does women, laryngeal cancer is four times more common in men than in women. Both diseases are more common in black Americans than among whites.

Causes and symptoms

Although the exact cause for these cancers is unknown, tobacco is regarded as the single greatest risk factor: 75–80% of the oral and laryngeal cancer cases occur among smokers. Heavy alcohol use has also been included as a risk factor. A combination of tobacco and alcohol use increases the risk for oral cancer by 6–15 times more than for users of either substance alone. In rare cases, irritation to the lining of the mouth, due to jagged teeth or ill-fitting dentures, has been known to cause oral cancer. Exposure to asbestos appears to increase the risk of developing laryngeal cancer.

In the case of lip cancer, just like skin cancer, exposure to sun over a prolonged period has been shown to increase the risk. In the Southeast Asian countries (India and Sri Lanka), chewing of betel nut has been associated with cancer of the lining of the cheek. An increased incidence of nasal cavity cancer has been observed among furniture workers, probably due to the inhalation of wood dust. A virus (Epstein-Barr) has been shown to cause nasopharyngeal cancer.

Head and neck cancers are one of the easiest to detect. The early signs can be both seen and felt. The signs and symptoms depend on the location of the cancer:

- Mouth and oral cavity: a sore that does not heal within two weeks, unusual bleeding from the teeth or gums, a white or red patch in the mouth, a lump or thickening in the mouth, throat, or tongue.

- Larynx: persistent hoarseness or **sore throat**, difficulty breathing, or **pain**.

- Hypopharynx and oropharynx: difficulty in swallowing or chewing food, ear pain.

- Nose, sinuses, and nasopharyngeal cavity: pain, bloody discharges from the nose, blocked nose, and frequent sinus infections that do not respond to standard **antibiotics**.

When detected early and treated appropriately, head and neck cancers have an excellent chance of being cured completely.

Diagnosis

Specific diagnostic tests used depend on the location of the cancer. The standard tests are:

Physical examination

The first step in diagnosis is a complete and thorough examination of the oral and nasal cavity, using mirrors and other visual aids. The tongue and the back of the throat are examined as well. Any suspicious looking lumps or lesions are examined with fingers (palpation). In order to look inside the larynx, the doctor may sometimes perform a procedure known as **laryngoscopy**. In indirect laryngoscopy, the doctor looks down the throat with a small, long handled mirror. Sometimes the doctor inserts a lighted tube (laryngoscope or a fiberoptic scope) through the patient's nose or mouth. As the tube goes down the throat, the doctor can observe areas that cannot be seen by a simple mirror. This procedure is called a direct laryngoscopy. Sometimes patients may be given a mild sedative to help them relax, and a local anesthetic to ease any discomfort.

Blood tests

The doctor may order blood or other immunological tests. These tests are aimed at detecting antibodies to the Epstein-Barr virus, which has been known to cause cancer of the nasopharynx.

Imaging tests

X rays of the mouth, the sinuses, the skull, and the chest region may be required. A computed tomography scan (CT scan), a procedure in which a computer takes a series of x-ray pictures of areas inside the body, may be done. Ultrasonograms (images generated using sound waves) or an MRI (**magnetic resonance imaging**, a procedure in which a picture is created using magnets linked to a computer), are alternate procedures which a doctor may have done to get detailed pictures of the areas inside the body.

Biopsy

When a sore does not heal or a suspicious patch or lump is seen in the mouth, larynx, nasopharynx, or throat, a biopsy may be performed to rule out the possibility of cancer. The biopsy is the most definitive diagnostic tool for detecting the cancer. If cancerous cells are detected in the biopsied sample, the doctor may perform more extensive tests in order to find whether, and to where, the cancer may have spread.

Treatment

The cancers can be treated successfully if diagnosed early. The choice of treatment depends on the size of the tumor, its location, and whether it has spread to other parts of the body.

In the case of lip and mouth cancers, sometimes surgery is performed to remove the cancer. Radiation therapy, which destroys the cancerous cells, is also one of the primary modes of treatment, and may be used alone or in combination with surgery. If lip surgery is drastic, **rehabilitation** cosmetic or reconstructive surgery may have to be considered.

Cancers of the nasal cavity are often diagnosed late because they have no specific symptoms in their early stages, or the symptoms may just resemble chronic **sinusitis**. Hence, treatment is often complex, involving a combination of radiotherapy and surgery. Surgery is generally recommended for small tumors. If the cancer cannot be removed by surgery, radiotherapy is used alone.

Treatment of oropharynx cancers (cancers that are either in the back of the tongue, the throat, or the tonsils) generally involves **radiation therapy** and/or surgery. After aggressive surgery and radiation, rehabilitation is often necessary and is an essential part of the treatment. The patient may experience difficulties with swallowing, chewing, and speech and may require a team of health care workers, including speech therapists, prosthodontists, occupational therapists, etc.

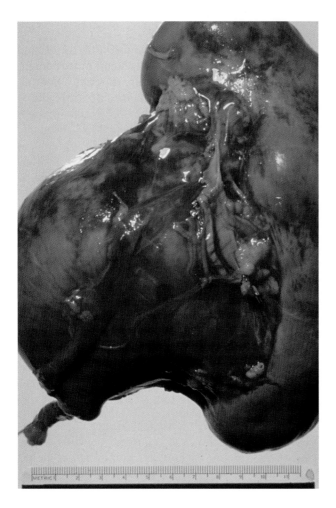

A specimen of a squamous cell carcinoma of the tongue and jaw. *(Custom Medical Stock Photo. Reproduced by permission.)*

Cancers of the nasopharynx are different from the other head and neck cancers in that there does not appear to be any association between alcohol and tobacco use and the development of the cancer. In addition, the incidence is seen primarily in two age groups: young adults and 50–70 year-olds. The Epstein-Barr virus has been implicated as the causative agent in most patients. While 80–90% of small tumors are curable by radiation therapy, advanced tumors that have spread to the bone and cranial nerves are difficult to control. Surgery is not very helpful and, hence, is rarely attempted. Radiation remains the only treatment of choice to treat the cancer that has metastasized (traveled) to the lymph nodes in the neck.

In the case of cancer of the larynx, radiotherapy is the first choice to treat small lesions. This is done in an attempt to preserve the voice. If the cancer recurs later, surgery may be attempted. If the cancer is limited to one of the two vocal cords, laser excision surgery is used. In order to treat advanced cancers, a combination of surgery and radiation therapy is often used. Because the chances of a cure in the case of advanced laryngeal cancers are rather low with current therapies, the patient may be advised to participate in clinical trials so they may get access to new experimental drugs and procedures, such as chemotherapy, that are being evaluated.

When only part of the larynx is removed, a relatively slight change in the voice may occur—the patient may sound slightly hoarse. However, in a total **laryngectomy**, the entire voice box is removed. The patients then have to re-learn to speak using different approaches, such as esophageal speech, tracheo-esophageal (TE) speech, or by means of an artificial larynx.

In esophageal speech, the patients are taught how to create a new type of voice by forcing air through the esophagus (food pipe) into the mouth. This method has a high success rate of approximately 65% and patients are even able to go back to jobs that require a high level of verbal communication, such as telephone operators and salespersons.

In the second approach, TE speech, a small opening, called a **fistula**, is created surgically between the trachea (breathing tube to the lungs) and the esophagus (tube into the stomach) to carry air into the throat. A small tube, known as the "voice prosthesis," is placed in the opening of the fistula to keep it open and to prevent food and liquid from going down into the trachea. In order to talk, the stoma (or the opening made at the base of the neck) must be covered with one's thumb during exhalation. As the air is forced out from the trachea into the esophagus, it vibrates the walls of the esophagus. This produces a sound that is then modified by the lips and tongue to produce normal sounding speech.

In the third approach, an artificial larynx, a battery driven vibrator, is placed on the outside of the throat. Sound is created as air passes through the stoma (opening made at the base of the neck) and the mouth forms words.

Prognosis

Oral Cavity

With early detection and immediate treatment, survival rates can be dramatically improved. For lip and oral cancer, if detected at its early stages, almost 80% of the patients survive five years or more. However, when diagnosed at the advanced stages, the five year survival rate drops to a mere 18%.

Nose and sinuses

Cancers of the nasal cavity often go undetected until they reach an advanced stage. If diagnosed at the early stages, the five-year survival rates are 60–70%. However, if cancers are more advanced, only 10–30% of the patients survive five years or more.

Oropharynx

In cancer of the oropharynx, 60–80% of the patients survive five years or more if the cancer is detected in the early stages. As the cancer advances, the survival rate drops to 15–30%.

Nasopharynx

Patients who are diagnosed with early stage cancers that have originated in the nasopharynx have an excellent chance of a complete cure (almost 95%). Unfortunately, most of the time, the patients are in an advanced stage at the time of initial diagnosis. With the new **chemotherapy** drugs, the five year survival rate has improved and 5–40% of the patients survive five years or longer.

Larynx

Small cancers of the larynx have an excellent five-year survival rate of 75–95%. However, as with most of the head and neck cancers, the survival rates drop dramatically as the cancer advances. Only 15–25% of the patients survive five years or more after being initially diagnosed with advanced laryngeal cancer.

Prevention

Refraining from the use of all tobacco products (cigarettes, cigars, pipe tobacco, chewing tobacco), consuming alcohol in moderation, and practicing good oral hygiene are some of the measures that one can take to prevent head and neck cancers. Since there is an association between excessive exposure to the sun and lip cancer, people who spend a lot of time outdoors in the sun should protect themselves from the sun's harmful rays. Regular physical examinations, or mouth examination by the patient himself, or by the patient's doctor or dentist, can help detect oral cancer in its very early stages.

Since working with asbestos has been shown to increase one's risk of getting cancer of the larynx, asbestos workers should follow safety rules to avoid inhaling asbestos fibers. Also, malnutrition and vitamin deficiencies have been shown to have some association with an increased incidence of head and neck

---

KEY TERMS

Biopsy—The surgical removal and microscopic examination of living tissue for diagnostic purposes.

Chemotherapy—Treatment of cancer with synthetic drugs that destroy the tumor either by inhibiting the growth of the cancerous cells or by killing the cancer cells.

Clinical trials—Highly regulated and carefully controlled patient studies, where either new drugs to treat cancer or novel methods of treatment are investigated.

Computerized tomography scan (CT scan)—A medical procedure where a series of X-rays are taken and put together by a computer in order to form detailed pictures of areas inside the body.

Laryngoscopy—A medical procedure that uses flexible, lighted, narrow tubes inserted through the mouth or nose to examine the larynx and other areas deep inside the neck.

Magnetic resonance imaging (MRI)—A medical procedure used for diagnostic purposes where pictures of areas inside the body can be created using a magnet linked to a computer.

Radiation therapy—Treatment using high energy radiation from x-ray machines, cobalt, radium, or other sources.

Stoma—When the entire larynx must be surgically removed, an opening is surgically created in the neck so that the windpipe can be brought out to the neck. This opening is called the stoma.

Ultrasonogram—A procedure where high-frequency sound waves that cannot be heard by human ears are bounced off internal organs and tissues. These sound waves produce a pattern of echoes which are then used by the computer to create sonograms, or pictures of areas inside the body.

X rays—High energy radiation used in high doses, either to diagnose or treat disease.

---

cancers. The American Cancer Society, therefore, recommends eating a healthy diet, consisting of at least five servings of fruits and vegetables every day, and six servings of food from other plant sources such as cereals, breads, grain products, rice, pasta and beans. Reducing one's intake of high-fat food from animal sources is advised.

Resources

ORGANIZATIONS

American Association of Oral and Maxillofacial Surgeons. 9700 West Bryn Mawr Ave., Rosemont, IL 60018-5701. (847) 678-6200. < http://www.aaoms.org >.

International Association of Laryngectomees (IAL). 7440 North Shadeland Ave., Suite 100, Indianapolis, IN 46250. < http://www.larynxlink.com/ >.

National Cancer Institute. Building 31, Room 10A31, 31 Center Drive, MSC 2580, Bethesda, MD 20892-2580. (800) 422-6237. < http://www.nci.nih.gov >.

National Oral Health Information ClearingHouse; 1 NOHIC Way, Bethesda, MD 20892-3500. (301)-402-7364.

Oral Health Education Foundation, Inc. 5865 Colonist Drive, P.O. Box 396, Fairburn, GA 30213. (770) 969-7400.

Lata Cherath, PhD

Head injury

Definition

Injury to the head may damage the scalp, skull or brain. The most important consequence of head trauma is traumatic brain injury. Head injury may occur either as a closed head injury, such as the head hitting a car's windshield, or as a penetrating head injury, as when a bullet pierces the skull. Both may cause damage that ranges from mild to profound. Very severe injury can be fatal because of profound brain damage.

Description

External trauma to the head is capable of damaging the brain, even if there is no external evidence of damage. More serious injuries can cause skull fracture, **blood clots** between the skull and the brain, or bruising and tearing of the brain tissue itself.

Injuries to the head can be caused by traffic accidents, sports injuries, falls, workplace accidents, assaults, or bullets. Most people have had some type of head injury at least once in their lives, but rarely do they require a hospital visit.

However, each year about two million people suffer from a more serious head injury, and up to 750,000 of them are severe enough to require hospitalization. Brain injury is most likely to occur in males between ages 15 and 24, usually as a result of car and motorcycle accidents. About 70% of all accidental deaths are due to head injuries, as are most of the disabilities that occur after trauma.

A person who has had a head injury and who is experiencing the following symptoms should seek medical care immediately:

- serious bleeding from the head or face
- loss of consciousness, however brief
- confusion and lethargy
- lack of pulse or breathing
- clear fluid drainage from the nose or ear

Causes and symptoms

A head injury may cause damage both from the direct physical injury to the brain and from secondary factors, such as lack of oxygen, brain swelling, and disturbance of blood flow. Both closed and penetrating head injuries can cause swirling movements throughout the brain, tearing nerve fibers and causing widespread bleeding or a blood clot in or around the brain. Swelling may raise pressure within the skull (intracranial pressure) and may block the flow of oxygen to the brain.

Head trauma may cause a **concussion**, in which there is a brief loss of consciousness without visible structural damage to the brain. In addition to loss of consciousness, initial symptoms of brain injury may include:

- memory loss and confusion
- **vomiting**
- **dizziness**
- partial **paralysis** or **numbness**
- shock
- anxiety

After a head injury, there may be a period of impaired consciousness followed by a period of confusion and impaired memory with disorientation and a breakdown in the ability to store and retrieve new information. Others experience temporary amnesia following head injury that begins with memory loss over a period of weeks, months, or years before the injury (retrograde **amnesia**). As the patient recovers, memory slowly returns. Post-traumatic amnesia refers to loss of memory for events during and after the accident.

Epilepsy occurs in 2–5% of those who have had a head injury; it is much more common in people who have had severe or penetrating injuries. Most cases of epilepsy appear right after the accident or within the first year, and become less likely with increased time following the accident.

Closed head injury

Closed head injury refers to brain injury without any penetrating injury to the brain. It may be the result of a direct blow to the head; of the moving head being rapidly stopped, such as when a person's head hits a windshield in a car accident; or by the sudden deceleration of the head without its striking another object. The kind of injury the brain receives in a closed head injury is determined by whether or not the head was unrestrained upon impact and the direction, force, and velocity of the blow. If the head is resting on impact, the maximum damage will be found at the impact site. A moving head will cause a "contrecoup injury" where the brain damage occurs on the side opposite the point of impact, as a result of the brain slamming into that side of the skull. A closed head injury also may occur without the head being struck, such as when a person experiences **whiplash**. This type of injury occurs because the brain is of a different density than the skull, and can be injured when delicate brain tissues hit against the rough, jagged inner surface of the skull.

Penetrating head injury

If the skull is fractured, bone fragments may be driven into the brain. Any object that penetrates the skull may implant foreign material and dirt into the brain, leading to an infection.

Skull fracture

A skull fracture is a medical emergency that must be treated promptly to prevent possible brain damage. Such an injury may be obvious if blood or bone fragments are visible, but it's possible for a fracture to have occurred without any apparent damage. A skull fracture should be suspected if there is:

- blood or clear fluid leaking from the nose or ears
- unequal pupil size
- bruises or discoloration around the eyes or behind the ears
- swelling or depression of part of the head

Intracranial hemorrhage

Bleeding (hemorrhage) inside the skull may accompany a head injury and cause additional damage to the brain. A blood clot (hematoma) may occur if a blood vessel between the skull and the brain ruptures; when the blood leaks out and forms a clot, it

can press against brain tissue, causing symptoms from a few hours to a few weeks after the injury. If the clot is located between the bones of the skull and the covering of the brain (dura), it is called an epidural hematoma. If the clot is between the dura and the brain tissue itself, the condition is called a **subdural hematoma**. In other cases, bleeding may occur deeper inside the brain. This condition is called intracerebral hemorrhage or intracerebral contusion (from the word for bruising).

In any case, if the blood flow is not stopped, it can lead to unconsciousness and **death**. The symptoms of bleeding within the skull include:

- nausea and vomiting
- **headache**
- loss of consciousness
- unequal pupil size
- lethargy

Postconcussion syndrome

If the head injury is mild, there may be no symptoms other than a slight headache. There also may be confusion, dizziness, and blurred vision. While the head injury may seem to have been quite mild, in many cases symptoms persist for days or weeks. Up to 60% of patients who sustain a mild brain injury continue to experience a range of symptoms called "postconcussion syndrome," as long as six months or a year after the injury.

The symptoms of postconcussion syndrome can result in a puzzling interplay of behavioral, cognitive, and emotional complaints that can be difficult to diagnose, including:

- headache
- dizziness
- mental confusion
- behavior changes
- memory loss
- cognitive deficits
- depression
- emotional outbursts

Diagnosis

The extent of damage in a severe head injury can be assessed with computed tomography (CT) scan, **magnetic resonance imaging** (MRI), **positron emission tomography** (PET) scans, electroencephalograms experts warn that there is a good chance that patient complaints after a mild head injury will be downplayed or dismissed. In the case of mild head injury or postconcussion syndrome, CT and MRI scans, electroencephalograms (EEG), and routine neurological evaluations all may be normal because the damage is so subtle. In many cases, these tests can't detect the microscopic damage that occurs when fibers are stretched in a mild, diffuse injury. In this type of injury, the axons lose some of their covering and become less efficient. This mild injury to the white matter reduces the quality of communication between different parts or the brain. A PET scan, which evaluates cerebral blood flow and brain metabolism, may be of help in diagnosing mild head injury.

Patients with continuing symptoms after a mild head injury should call a local chapter of a head-injury foundation that can refer patients to the best nearby expert.

Treatment

If a concussion, bleeding inside the skull, or skull fracture is suspected, the patient should be kept quiet in a darkened room, with head and shoulders raised slightly on pillow or blanket.

After initial emergency treatment, a team of specialists may be needed to evaluate and treat the problems that result. A penetrating wound may require surgery. Those with severe injuries or with a deteriorating level of consciousness may be kept hospitalized for observation. If there is bleeding inside the skull, the blood may need to be surgically drained; if a clot has formed, it may need to be removed. Severe skull **fractures** also require surgery. Supportive care and specific treatments may be required if the patient experiences further complications. People who experience seizures, for example, may be given **anticonvulsant drugs**, and people who develop fluid on the brain (**hydrocephalus**) may have a shunt inserted to drain the fluid.

In the event of long-term disability as a result of head injury, there are a variety of treatment programs available, including long-term **rehabilitation**, coma treatment centers, transitional living programs, behavior management programs, life-long residential or day treatment programs and independent living programs.

Prognosis

Prompt, proper diagnosis and treatment can help alleviate some of the problems after a head injury.

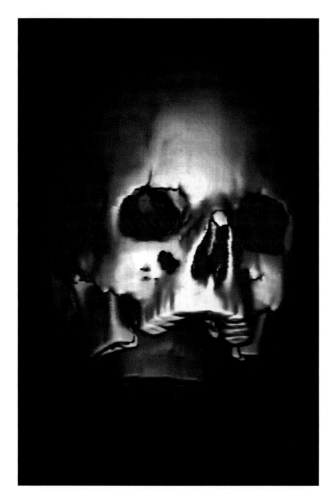

A three-dimensional computed tomography (CT) scan of a human skull showing a depressed skull fracture above the right eye. *(Custom Medical Stock Photo. Reproduced by permission.)*

(EEG), and routine neurological and neuropsychological evaluations.

Doctors use the Glasgow **Coma** Scale to evaluate the extent of brain damage based on observing a patient's ability to open his or her eyes, respond verbally, and respond to stimulation by moving (motor response). Patients can score from three to 15 points on this scale. People who score below eight when they are admitted usually have suffered a severe brain injury and will need rehabilitative therapy as they recover. In general, higher scores on the Glasgow Coma Scale indicate less severe brain injury and a better prognosis for recovery.

Patients with a mild head injury who experience symptoms are advised to seek out the care of a specialist; unless a family physician is thoroughly familiar with medical literature in this newly emerging area,

KEY TERMS

Computed tomography scan (CT)—A diagnostic technique in which the combined use of a computer and x rays produce clear cross-sectional images of tissue. It provides clearer, more detailed information than x rays alone.

Electroencephalogram (EEG)—A record of the tiny electrical impulses produced by the brain's activity. By measuring characteristic wave patterns, the EEG can help diagnose certain conditions of the brain.

Magnetic resonance imaging (MRI)—A diagnostic technique that provides high quality cross-sectional images of organs within the body without x rays or other radiation.

Positron emission tomography (PET) scan—A computerized diagnostic technique that uses radioactive substances to examine structures of the body. When used to assess the brain, it produces a three-dimensional image that reflects the metabolic and chemical activity of the brain.

However, it usually is difficult to predict the outcome of a brain injury in the first few hours or days; a patient's prognosis may not be known for many months or even years.

The outlook for someone with a minor head injury generally is good, although recovery may be delayed and symptoms such as headache, dizziness, and cognitive problems can persist for up to a year or longer after an accident. This can limit a person's ability to work and cause strain in personal relationships.

Serious head injuries can be devastating, producing permanent mental and physical disability. Epileptic seizures may occur after a severe head injury, especially a penetrating brain injury, a severe skull fracture, or a serious brain hemorrhage. Recovery from a severe head injury can be very slow, and it may take five years or longer to heal completely. Risk factors associated with an increased likelihood of memory problems or seizures after head injury include age, length and depth of coma, duration of post-traumatic and retrograde amnesia, presence of focal brain injuries, and initial Glasgow Coma Scale score.

As researchers learn more about the long-term effects of head injuries, they have begun to uncover links to later conditions. A 2003 report found that mild brain injury during childhood could speed up expression of **schizophrenia** in those who were already likely to get the disorder because of genetics. Those with a history of a childhood brain injury, even a minor one, were more likely to get familial schizophrenia than a sibling and to have earlier onset. Another study in 2003 found that people who had a history of a severe head injury were four times more likely to develop Parkinson's disease than the average population. Those requiring hospitalization for their head injuries were 11 times as likely. The risk did not increase for people receiving mild head injuries.

Prevention

Many severe head injuries could be prevented by wearing protective helmets during certain sports, or when riding a bike or motorcycle. Seat belts and airbags can prevent many head injuries that result from car accidents. Appropriate protective headgear always should be worn on the job where head injuries are a possibility.

Resources

PERIODICALS

"Childhood Head Injury Tied to Later Schizophreia." *The Brown University Child and Adolescent Behavior Letter* June 2003: 5.

"Link to Head Injury Found." *Pain & Central Nervous System Week* June 9, 2003: 3.

ORGANIZATIONS

American Epilepsy Society. 342 North Main Street, West Hartford, CT 06117-2507. (860) 586-7505. < http:// www.aesnet.org >.

Brain Injury Association. 1776 Massachusetts Ave. NW, Ste. 100, Washington, DC 20036. (800) 444-6443.

Family Caregiver Alliance. 425 Bush St., Ste. 500, San Francisco, CA 94108. (800) 445-8106. < http:// www.caregiver.org >.

Head Injury Hotline. PO Box 84151, Seattle WA 98124. (206) 621- 8558. < http://www.headinjury.com >.

Head Trauma Support Project, Inc. 2500 Marconi Ave., Ste. 203, Sacramento, CA 95821. (916) 482-5770.

National Head Injury Foundation. 333 Turnpike Rd., Southboro, MA 01722. (617) 485-9950.

Carol A. Turkington
Teresa G. Odle

Head lice *see* **Lice infestation**

Head trauma *see* **Head injury**

Headache

Definition

A headache involves **pain** in the head which can arise from many disorders or may be a disorder in and of itself.

Description

There are three types of primary headaches: tension-type (muscular contraction headache), migraine (vascular headaches), and cluster. Virtually everyone experiences a tension-type headache at some point. An estimated 18% of American women suffer migraines, compared to 6% of men. Cluster headaches affect fewer than 0.5% of the population, and men account for approximately 80% of all cases. Headaches caused by illness are secondary headaches and are not included in these numbers.

Approximately 40–45 million people in the United States suffer chronic headaches. Headaches have an enormous impact on society due to missed workdays and productivity losses.

Causes and symptoms

Traditional theories about headaches link tension-type headaches to muscle contraction, and migraine and cluster headaches to blood vessel dilation (swelling). Pain-sensitive structures in the head include blood vessel walls, membranous coverings of the brain, and scalp and neck muscles. Brain tissue itself has no sensitivity to pain. Therefore, headaches may result from contraction of the muscles of the scalp, face or neck; dilation of the blood vessels in the head; or brain swelling that stretches the brain's coverings. Involvement of specific nerves of the face and head may also cause characteristic headaches. Sinus inflammation is a common cause of headache. Keeping a headache diary may help link headaches to stressful occurrences, menstrual phases, food triggers, or medication.

Tension-type headaches are often brought on by stress, overexertion, loud noise, and other external factors. The typical tension-type headache is described as a tightening around the head and neck, and an accompanying dull ache.

Migraines are intense throbbing headaches occurring on one or both sides of the head, usually on one side. The pain is accompanied by other symptoms such as **nausea**, **vomiting**, blurred vision, and aversion to light, sound, and movement. Migraines often are triggered by food items, such as red wine, chocolate, and aged cheeses. For women, a hormonal connection is likely, since headaches occur at specific points in the menstrual cycle, with use of oral contraceptives, or the use of hormone replacement therapy after **menopause**. Research shows that a complex interaction of nerves and neurotransmitters in the brain act to cause migraine headaches.

Cluster headaches cause excruciating pain. The severe, stabbing pain centers around one eye, and eye tearing and nasal congestion occur on the same side. The headache lasts from 15 minutes to four hours and may recur several times in a day. Heavy smokers are more likely to suffer cluster headaches, which also are associated with alcohol consumption.

Diagnosis

Since headaches arise from many causes, a physical exam assesses general health and a neurologic exam evaluates the possibility of neurologic disease as a cause for the headache. If the headache is the primary illness, the doctor asks for a thorough history of the headache. Questions revolve around its frequency and duration, when it occurs, pain intensity and location, possible triggers, and any prior symptoms. This information aids in classifying the headache.

Warning signs that should point out the need for prompt medical intervention include:

- "Worst headache of my life." This may indicate subarachnoid hemorrhage from a ruptured aneurysm (swollen blood vessel) in the head or other neurological emergency.

- Headache accompanied by one-sided weakness, **numbness**, visual loss, speech difficulty, or other signs. This may indicate a **stroke**. Migraines may include neurological symptoms.

- Headache that becomes worse over a period of 6 months, especially if most prominent in the morning or if accompanied by neurological symptoms. This may indicate a **brain tumor**.

- Sudden onset of headache. If accompanied by **fever** and stiff neck, this can indicate **meningitis**.

Headache diagnosis may include neurological imaging tests such as computed tomography scan (CT scan) or **magnetic resonance imaging** (MRI).

Treatment

Headache treatment is divided into two forms: abortive and prophylactic. Abortive treatment addresses a headache in progress, and prophylactic treatment prevents headache occurrence.

Tension-type headaches can be treated with **aspirin**, **acetaminophen**, ibuprofen, or naproxen. In early 1998, the FDA approved extra-strength Excedrin, which includes **caffeine**, for mild migraines. Physicians continue to investigate and monitor the best treatment for migraines and generally prefer a stepped approach, depending on headache severity, frequency and impact on the patient's quality of life. A group of drugs called triptans are usually preferred for abortive treatment. About seven triptans are available in the United States and the pill forms are considered most effective. They should be taken as early as possible during the typical migraine attack. The most common prophylactic therapies include antidepressants, **beta blockers**, **calcium channel blockers** and antiseizure medications. Antiseizure medications have proven particularly effective at blocking the actions of neurotransmitters that start migraine attacks. Topiramate (Topamax) was shown effective in several combined clinical trials in 2004 at 50 to 200 mg per day.

In 2004, a new, large study added evidence to show the effectiveness of botulinum toxin type A (Botox) treatment to prevent headache pain for those with frequent, untreatable tension and migraine headaches. Patients were treated every three months, with two to five injections each time. They typically received relief within two to three weeks.

Cluster headaches may also be treated with ergotamine and sumatriptan, as well as by inhaling pure oxygen. Prophylactic treatments include prednisone, calcium channel blockers, and methysergide.

Alternative treatment

Alternative headache treatments include:

• acupuncture or **acupressure**

• biofeedback

• chiropractic

• herbal remedies using feverfew (*Chrysanthemum parthenium*), valerian (*Valeriana officinalis*), white willow (*Salix alba*), or skullcap (*Scutellaria lateriflora*), among others

• homeopathic remedies chosen specifically for the individual and his/her type of headache

• hydrotherapy

• massage

• magnesium supplements

KEY TERMS

Abortive—Referring to treatment that relieves symptoms of a disorder.

Analgesics—A class of pain-relieving medicines, including aspirin and Tylenol.

Biofeedback—A technique in which a person is taught to consciously control the body's response to a stimulus.

Chronic—Referring to a condition that occurs frequently or continuously or on a regular basis.

Prophylactic—Referring to treatment that prevents symptoms of a disorder from appearing.

Transcutaneous electrical nerve stimulation—A method that electrically stimulates nerve and blocks the transmission of pain signals, called TENS.

• regular physical **exercise**

• relaxation techniques, such as **meditation** and **yoga**

• transcutaneous **electrical nerve stimulation** (TENS) (A procedure that electrically stimulates nerves and blocks the signals of pain transmission.)

Prognosis

Headaches are typically resolved through the use of **analgesics** and other treatments. Research in 2004 showed that people who have migraine headaches more often than once a month may be at increased risk for stroke.

Prevention

Some headaches may be prevented by avoiding triggering substances and situations, or by employing alternative therapies, such as yoga and regular exercise. Since **food allergies** often are linked with headaches, especially cluster headaches, identification and elimination of the allergy-causing food(s) from the diet can be an important preventive measure.

Resources

PERIODICALS

Kruit, Mark C., et al. "Migraine as a Risk Factor for Subclinical Brain Lesions." *JAMA, Journal of the American Medical Association* January 28, 2004: 427–435.

Norton, Patrice G. W. "Botox Stops Headache Pain in Recalcitrant Cases." *Clinical Psychiatry News* March 2004: 72.

Taylor, Frederick, et al. "Diagnosis and Management of Migraine in Family Practice." *Journal of Family Practice* January 2004: S3–S25.

ORGANIZATIONS

American Council for Headache Education (ACHE). 19 Mantua Road, Mt. Royal, NJ 08061. (800) 255-2243. < http://www.achenet.org >.

National Headache Foundation. 428 W. St. James Place, Chicago, IL 60614. (800) 843-2256. < http://www.headaches.org >.

Julia Barrett
Teresa G. Odle

Hearing aids

Definition

A hearing aid is a device that can amplify sound waves in order to help a deaf or hard-of-hearing person hear sounds more clearly.

Purpose

Recent technology can help most people with hearing loss understand speech better and achieve better communication.

Precautions

It's important that a person being fitted for a hearing aid understand what an aid can and can't do. An aid can help a person hear better, but it won't return hearing to normal levels. Hearing aids boost all sounds, not just those the person wishes to hear. Especially when the source of sound is far away (such as up on a stage), environmental noise can interfere with good speech perception. And while the aid amplifies sound, it doesn't necessarily improve the clarity of the sound. A hearing aid is a machine, and can never duplicate the true sound that people with normal hearing experience, but it will help the person take advantage of the hearing that remains.

Description

More than 1,000 different models are available in the United States. All of them include a microphone (to pick up sound), amplifier (to boost sound strength), a receiver or speaker (to deliver sound to the ear), and are powered by a battery. Depending on the style, it's possible to add features to filter or block out background noise, minimize feedback, lower sound in noisy settings, or boost power when needed.

Hearing aids are either "monaural" (a hearing aid for one ear), or "binaural" (for two ears); more than 65% of all users have binaural aids. Hearing aids are divided into several different types:

- digital
- in-the-ear
- in-the-canal
- behind-the-ear
- on-the-body

Digital aids are sophisticated, very expensive aids that borrow computer technology to allow a person to tailor an aid to a specific **hearing loss** pattern. Using miniature computer chips, the aids can selectively boost certain frequencies while leaving others alone. This means a person could wear such an aid to a loud party, and screen out unwanted background noise, while tuning in on one-on-one conversations. The aid is programmed by the dealer to conform to the patient's specific hearing loss. Some models can be programmed to allow the wearer to choose different settings depending on the noise of the environment.

In-the-ear aids are lightweight devices whose custom-made housings contain all the components; this device fits into the ear canal with no visible wires or tubes. It's possible to control tone but not volume with these aids, so they are helpful only for people with mild hearing loss. Some people find these aids are easier to put on and take off than behind-the-ear aids. However, because they are custom-fit to a person's ear, it is not possible to try on before ordering. Some people find them uncomfortable in hot weather.

In-the-canal aids fit far into the ear canal, with only a small bit extending into the external ear. The smallest is the MicroCanal, which fits out of sight down next to the eardrum and is removed with a small transparent wire. These are extremely expensive, but they are not visible, offer better acoustics, and are easier to maintain. They can more closely mimic natural sound because of the position of the microphone; this position also cuts down on wind noise. But their small size makes them harder to handle, and their battery is especially small and difficult to insert. Adjusting the volume may be hard, since a person must stick a finger down into the ear to adjust volume, and this very tiny aid doesn't have the power of other, larger, aids.

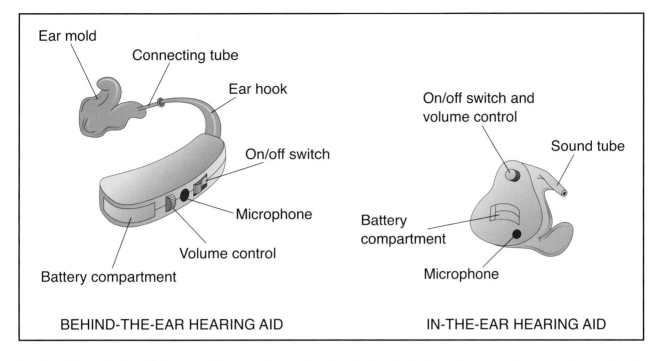

Ear mold
Connecting tube
Ear hook
On/off switch
Microphone
Volume control
Battery compartment

BEHIND-THE-EAR HEARING AID

On/off switch and volume control
Sound tube
Battery compartment
Microphone

IN-THE-EAR HEARING AID

Hearing aids are devices that can amplify sound waves to help a deaf or hard-of-hearing person hear sounds more clearly. *(Illustration by Electronic Illustrators Group.)*

Behind-the-ear aids include a microphone, amplifier and receiver inside a small curved case worn behind the ear; the case is connected to the earmold by a short plastic tube. The earmold extends into the ear canal. Some models have both tone and volume control, plus a telephone pickup device. However, many users think them unattractive and out of date; and people who wear glasses find that the glasses interfere with the aid's fit. Others don't have space behind the ear for the mold to fit comfortably. However, they do offer a few advantages.

Behind-the-ear aids:

• don't require as much maintenance

• are easily interchangeable if they need to be serviced

• are more powerful

• are easier to handle than smaller aids

• can provide better sound quality

• tend to be more reliable

Eyeglass models are the same as behind-the-ear devices, except that the case fits into an eyeglass frame instead of resting behind the ears. Not many people buy this type of aid, but those who do believe it's less obvious, although there is a tube that travels from the temple of the glasses to the earmold. But it can be hard to fit this type of aid, and repairs can be problematic.

Also, if the aid breaks, the person also loses the benefit of the glasses.

CROS or the crossover system type of hearing aid is often used in conjunction with the eyeglass model. The CROS (contralateral routing of signal) system features a microphone behind the ear that feeds the amplified signal to the better ear, eliminating "head shadow," which occurs when the head blocks sound from the better ear. This type may help make speech easier to understand for people with a high-frequency loss in both ears.

A BI-CROS system uses two microphones (one above each ear) that send signals to a single amplifier. Sound then travels to a single receiver, which transfers it to the better ear via a conventional earmold.

On-the-body aids feature a larger microphone, amplifier, and power supply inside a case carried inside the pocket, or attached to clothing. The receiver attaches directly to the earmold; its power comes through a flexible wire from the amplifier. Although larger than other aids, the on-the-body aids are more powerful and easier to adjust than other devices. While not popular for everyone, they are often used by those with a profound hearing loss, or by very young children. Some people who are almost totally deaf find they need the extra power boost available only from a body aid.

The latest aids on the market may eliminate the amplifier and speaker in favor of a tiny magnet mounted on a silicone disk, similar to a contact lens, which rests right on the eardrum. Called the Earlens, it is designed to be held in place by a thin film of oil. Users wear a wireless microphone, either in the ear or on a necklace, that picks up sounds and converts them into magnetic signals, making the magnet vibrate. As the Earlens vibrates, so does the eardrum, transmitting normal-sounding tones to the middle and inner ears.

Other researchers are bypassing the middle ear completely; they surgically implant a tiny magnet in the inner ear. By attaching a magnet to the round window, they open a second pathway to the inner ear. An electromagnetic coil implanted in bone behind the ear vibrates the implanted magnet. Unlike the Earlens, this magnetic implant would not block the normal hearing pathway.

Preparation

The fist step in getting a hearing aid is to have a medical exam and a hearing evaluation. (Most states prohibit anyone selling a hearing aid until the patient has been examined by a physician to rule out medical problems.) After performing a hearing evaluation, an audiologist should be able to determine whether a hearing aid will help, and which one will do the most good. This is especially important because aids can be very expensive (between $500 and $4,000), and are often not covered by health insurance. Hearing aids come in a wide range of styles and types, requiring careful testing to make sure the aid is the best choice for a particular hearing loss.

Some audiologists sell aids; others can make a recommendation, or give one a list of competent dealers in one's area. Patients should shop around and compare prices. In all but three states, hearing aids must be fitted and sold only by licensed specialists called dealers, specialists, dispensers, or dispensing audiologists.

The hearing aid dealer will make an impression of the consumer's ears using a putty-like material, from which a personalized earmold will be created. It's the dealer's job to make sure the aid fits properly. The person may need several visits to find the right hearing aid and learn how to use it. The dealer will help the consumer learn how to put the aid on, adjust the controls, and maintain the device. The dealer should be willing to service the aid and provide information about what to do if sensitivity to the earmold develops. (Some people are allergic to the materials in the mold.)

Aftercare

Within several weeks, the wearer should return to the dealer to have the aid checked, and to discuss the progress in wearing the aid. About 40% of all aids need some modification or adjustment in the beginning.

Within the first month of getting an aid, the patient should make an appointment for a full hearing examination to determine if the aid is functioning properly.

Risks

While there are no medical risks to hearing aids, there is a risk associated with hearing aids: many people end up not wearing their aids because they say everything seems loud when wearing them. This is because they have lived for so long with a hearing problem that they have forgotten how loud "normal" sound can be. Other potential problems with hearing aids include earmold discomfort, and a build up of excess ear wax after getting a hearing aid.

Normal results

A hearing aid will boost the loudness of sound, which can improve a person's ability to understand speech.

Resources

ORGANIZATIONS

American Academy of Otolaryngology-Head and Neck Surgery, Inc. One Prince St., Alexandria VA 22314-3357. (703) 836-4444. <http://www.entnet.org>.
Better Hearing Institute. 515 King Street, Suite 420, Alexandria, VA 22314. (703) 684-3391.

Hearing Industries Association. 1800 M St. NW, Washington, DC 20036. (202) 651-5258.

Hear Now. 9745 E. Hampden Ave., Ste. 300, Denver, CO 80231. (800) 648-HEAR. (202) 651-5258.

National Hearing Aid Society. 20361 Middlebelt, Livonia, MI 48152. (800) 521-5247 or (313) 478-2610.

National Information Center on Deafness. Gallaudet College, 800 Florida Ave. NE, Washington, DC 20002. (202) 651-5051; (202) 651-5052 (TDD).

Carol A. Turkington

Decibel Ratings And Hazardous Levels Of Noise	
Decibel Level	**Example Of Sounds**
30	Soft whisper
35	Noise may prevent the listener from falling asleep
40	Quiet office noise level
50	Quiet conversation
60	Average television volume, sewing machine, lively conversation
70	Busy traffic, noisy restaurant
80	Heavy city traffic, factory noise, alarm clock
90	Cocktail party, lawn mower
100	Pneumatic drill
120	Sandblasting, thunder
140	Jet airplane
180	Rocket launching pad

Above 110 decibels, hearing may become painful
Above 120 decibels is considered deafening
Above 135 decibels, hearing will become extremely painful and hearing loss may result if exposure is prolonged Above 180 decibels, hearing loss is almost certain with any exposure

Hearing loss

Definition

Hearing loss is any degree of impairment of the ability to apprehend sound.

Description

Sound can be measured accurately. The term decibel (dB) refers to an amount of energy moving sound from its source to our ears or to a microphone. A drop of more than 10 dB in the level of sound a person can hear is significant.

Sound travels through a medium like air or water as waves of compression and rarefaction. These waves are collected by the external ear and cause the tympanic membrane (ear drum) to vibrate. The chain of ossicles connected to the ear drum—the incus, malleus, and stapes—carries the vibration to the oval window, increasing its amplitude 20 times on the way. There the energy causes a standing wave in the watery liquid (endolymph) inside the Organ of Corti. (A standing wave is one that does not move. A vibrating cup of coffee will demonstrate standing waves.) The configuration of the standing wave is determined by the frequency of the sound. Many thousands of tiny nerve fibers detect the highs and lows of the standing wave and transmit their findings to the brain, which interprets the signals as sound.

To summarize, sound energy passes through the air of the external ear, the bones of the middle ear and the liquid of the inner ear. It is then translated into nerve impulses, sent to the brain through nerves and understood there as sound. It follows that there are five steps in the hearing process:

- air conduction through the external ear to the ear drum

- bone conduction through the middle ear to the inner ear

- water conduction to the Organ of Corti

- nerve conduction into the brain

- interpretation by the brain.

Hearing can be interrupted in several ways at each of the five steps.

The external ear canal can be blocked with ear wax, foreign objects, infection, and tumors. Overgrowth of the bone, a condition that occurs when the ear canal has been flushed with cold water repeatedly for years, can also narrow the passageway, making blockage and infection more likely. This condition occurs often in Northern Californian surfers and is therefore called "surfer's ear."

The ear drum is so thin a physician can see through it into the middle ear. Sharp objects, pressure from an infection in the middle ear, even a firm cuffing or slapping of the ear, can rupture it. It is also susceptible to pressure changes during scuba diving.

Several conditions can diminish the mobility of the ossicles (small bones) in the middle ear. **Otitis media** (an infection in the middle ear) occurs when fluid cannot escape into the throat because of blockage of the eustachian tube. The fluid that accumulates, whether it be pus or just mucus and dampens the motion of the ossicles. A disease called **otosclerosis** can bind the stapes in the oval window and thereby cause deafness.

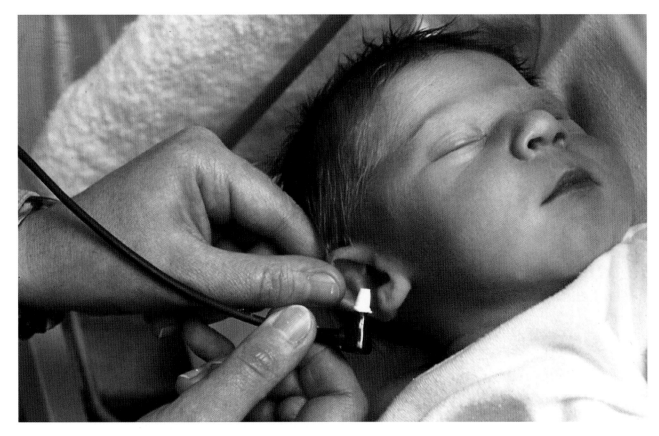

An Oto-Acoustic Emission (OAE) hearing test being perfomred on a newborn baby. The probe emits harmless sound into the baby's ear, and the response of the inner ear is detected and registered on a computer. Early diagnosis of a hearing disorder is important in young children, who may experience difficulties in speech and language development. *(Photograph by James King-Holmes, Photo Researchers, Inc. Reproduced by permission.)*

All the conditions mentioned so far, those that occur in the external and middle ear, are causes of conductive hearing loss. The second category, sensory hearing loss, refers to damage to the Organ of Corti and the acoustic nerve. Prolonged exposure to loud noise is the leading cause of sensory hearing loss. A million people have this condition, many identified during the military draft and rejected as being unfit for duty. The cause is often believed to be prolonged exposure to rock music. Occupational noise exposure is the other leading cause of noise induced hearing loss (NIHL) and is ample reason for wearing ear protection on the job. A third of people over 65 have presbycusis—sensory hearing loss due to **aging**. Both NIHL and presbycusis are primarily high frequency losses. In most languages, it is the high frequency sounds that define speech, so these people hear plenty of noise, they just cannot easily make out what it means. They have particular trouble selecting out speech from background noise. Brain infections like **meningitis**, drugs such as the aminoglycoside **antibiotics** (streptomycin, gentamycin, kanamycin, tobramycin),

and Meniere's disease also cause permanent sensory hearing loss. Meniere's disease combines attacks of hearing loss with attacks of vertigo. The symptoms may occur together or separately. High doses of salicylates like **aspirin** and quinine can cause a temporary high-frequency loss. Prolonged high doses can lead to permanent deafness. There is an hereditary form of sensory deafness and a congenital form most often caused by rubella (German **measles**).

Sudden hearing loss—at least 30dB in less than three days—is most commonly caused by cochleitis, a mysterious viral infection.

The final category of hearing loss is neural. Damage to the acoustic nerve and the parts of the brain that perform hearing are the most likely to produce permanent hearing loss. Strokes, multiple sclerosis, and acoustic neuromas are all possible causes of neural hearing loss.

Hearing can also be diminished by extra sounds generated by the ear, most of them from the same kinds of disorders that cause diminished hearing.

These sounds are referred to as **tinnitus** and can be ringing, blowing, clicking, or anything else that no one but the patient hears.

Diagnosis

An examination of the ears and nose combined with simple hearing tests done in the physician's office can detect many common causes of hearing loss. An audiogram often concludes the evaluation, since these simple means often produce a diagnosis. If the defect is in the brain or the acoustic nerve, further neurological testing and imaging will be required.

The audiogram has many uses in diagnosing hearing deficits. The pattern of hearing loss across the audible frequencies gives clues to the cause. Several alterations in the testing procedure can give additional information. For example, speech is perceived differently than pure tones. Adequate perception of sound combined with inability to recognize words points to a brain problem rather than a sensory or conductive deficit. Loudness perception is distorted by disease in certain areas but not in others. Acoustic neuromas often distort the perception of loudness.

Treatment

Conductive hearing loss can almost always be restored to some degree, if not completely.

- matter in the ear canal can be easily removed with a dramatic improvement in hearing.
- surfer's ear gradually regresses if cold water is avoided or a special ear plug is used. In advanced cases, surgeons can grind away the excess bone.
- middle ear infection with fluid is also simple to treat. If medications do not work, surgical drainage of the ear is accomplished through the ear drum, which heals completely after treatment.
- traumatically damaged ear drums can be repaired with a tiny skin graft.
- surgical repair of otosclerosis through an operating microscope is one of the most intricate of procedures, substituting tiny artificial parts for the original ossicles.

Sensory and neural hearing loss, on the other hand, cannot readily be cured. Fortunately it is not often complete, so that **hearing aids** can fill the deficit.

In-the-ear hearing aids can boost the volume of sound by up to 70 dB. (Normal speech is about 60 dB.) Federal law now requires that they be dispensed only

upon a physician's prescription. For complete conduction hearing loss there are now available bone conduction hearing aids and even devices that can be surgically implanted in the cochlea.

Tinnitus can sometimes be relieved by adding white noise (like the sound of wind or waves crashing on the shore) to the environment.

Decreased hearing is such a common problem that there are legions of organizations to provide assistance. Special language training, both in lip reading and signing, special schools and special camps for children are all available in most regions of the United States.

Alternative treatment

Conductive hearing loss can be treated with alternative therapies that are specific to the particular condition. Sensory hearing loss may be helped by homeopathic therapies. Oral supplementation with essential fatty acids such as flax oil and omega 3 oil can help alleviate the accumulation of wax in the ear.

Prevention

Prompt treatment and attentive follow-up of middle ear infections in children will prevent this cause of conductive hearing loss. Control of infectious childhood diseases such as measles has greatly reduced sensory hearing loss as a complication of epidemic diseases. Laws that require protection from loud noise in the workplace have achieved substantial reduction in noise induced hearing loss. Surfers should use the right kind of ear plugs.

Resources

ORGANIZATIONS

Alexander Graham Bell Association for the Deaf. 3417 Volta Place NW, Washington, DC 20007. (202) 337-5220. <http://www.agbell.org>.

Auditory-Verbal International. 2121 Eisenhower Ave., Suite 402, Alexandria, VA 22314. (703) 739-1049. <avi@auditory-verbal.org> <http://www.auditory-verbal.org/contact.htm>.

Better Hearing Institute. 515 King Street, Suite 420, Alexandria, VA 22314. (703) 684-3391.

Central Institute for the Deaf. Washington University. St. Louis, Missouri. <http://cidmac.wustl.edu>.

League for the Hard of Hearing. 71 West 23rd St., New York, New York 10010-4162. (212) 741-7650. <http://www.lhh.org>.

National Association of the Deaf. 814 Thayer Ave., Silver Spring, MD, 20910. (301) 587-1788. <http://nad.policy.net>.

Self Help for Hard of Hearing People, Inc. 7800 Wisconsin Ave., Bethesda, MD 20814. (301) 657-2248. <http://www.shhh.org>.

The Sight & Hearing Association (SHA). <http://www.sightandhearing.org>.

World Recreation Association of the Deaf (WRAD). <http://www.wrad.org>.

J. Ricker Polsdorfer, MD

Hearing test with an audiometer *see* **Audiometry**

Hearing tests with a tuning fork

Definition

A tuning fork is a metal instrument with a handle and two prongs or tines. Tuning forks, made of steel, aluminum, or magnesium-alloy will vibrate at a set frequency to produce a musical tone when struck. The vibrations produced can be used to assess a person's ability to hear various sound frequencies.

Purpose

A vibrating tuning fork held next to the ear or placed against the skull will stimulate the inner ear to vibrate, and can help determine if there is **hearing loss**.

Precautions

No special precautions are necessary when tuning forks are used to conduct a hearing test.

Description

Two types of hearing tests with tuning forks are typically conducted. In the Rinne test, the vibrating tuning fork is held against the skull, usually on the bone behind the ear (mastoid process) to cause vibrations through the bones of the skull and inner ear. It is also held next to, but not touching, the ear, to cause vibrations in the air next to the ear. The patient is asked to determine which sound is louder, the sound heard through the bone or through the air. A second hearing test using a tuning fork is the Weber test. For this test, the stem or handle of the vibrating tuning fork is placed at various points along the midline of the skull and face. The patient is then asked to identify which ear hears the sound created by the vibrations. Tuning forks of different sizes produce different frequencies of vibrations and can be used to establish the range of hearing for an individual patient.

Preparation

No special preparation is required for a hearing test with tuning forks.

Aftercare

No special aftercare is required. If hearing loss is revealed during testing with tuning forks, the patient may require further testing to determine the extent of the hearing loss.

Risks

There are no risks associated with the use of tuning forks to screen for hearing loss.

Normal results

With the Rinne test, a person will hear the tone of the vibration longer and louder when the tuning fork is held next to the ear, rather than when it is held against the mastoid bone. For the Weber test, the tone produced when the tuning fork is placed along the center of the skull, or face, sounds about the same volume in each ear.

Abnormal results

The Rinne test detects a hearing loss when a patient hears a louder and longer tone when the vibrating tuning fork is held against the mastoid bone than when it is held next to the ear. The volume of sound vibrations conducted through parts of the skull and face in the Weber test can indicate which ear may have a hearing loss.

Resources

ORGANIZATIONS

American Academy of Otolaryngology-Head and Neck Surgery, Inc. One Prince St., Alexandria VA 22314-3357. (703) 836-4444. <http://www.entnet.org>.

Ear Foundation. 1817 Patterson St., Nashville, TN 37203. (800) 545-4327. <http://www.earfoundation.org>.

Altha Roberts Edgren

Heart arrest *see* **Sudden cardiac death**

Heart arrhythmias *see* **Arrhythmias**

Heart attack

Definition

A heart attack is the death of, or damage to, part of the heart muscle because the supply of blood to the heart muscle is severely reduced or stopped.

Description

Heart attack is the leading cause of death in the United States. More than 1.5 million Americans suffer a heart attack every year, and almost half a million die, according to the American Heart Association. Most heart attacks are the end result of years of silent but progressive **coronary artery disease**, which can be prevented in many people. A heart attack often is the first symptom of coronary artery disease. According to the American Heart Association, 63% of women and 48% of men who died suddenly of coronary artery disease had no previous symptoms. Heart attacks also are called myocardial infarctions (MIs).

A heart attack occurs when one or more of the coronary arteries that supply blood to the heart are completely blocked and blood to the heart muscle is cut off. The blockage usually is caused by **atherosclerosis**, the build-up of plaque in the artery walls, and/or by a blood clot in a coronary artery. Sometimes, a healthy or atherosclerotic coronary artery has a spasm and the blood flow to part of the heart decreases or stops. Why this happens is unclear, but it can result in a heart attack.

About half of all heart attack victims wait at least two hours before seeking help. This increases their chance of sudden death or being disabled. The longer the artery remains blocked during a heart attack, the more damage will be done to the heart. If the blood supply is cut off severely or for a long time, muscle cells suffer irreversible injury and die. This can cause the patient to die. That is why it is important to recognize the signs of a heart attack and seek prompt medical attention at the nearest hospital with 24-hour emergency cardiac care.

About one-fifth of all heart attacks are silent, that is, the victim does not know one has occurred. Although the victim feels no **pain**, silent heart attacks still can damage the heart.

The outcome of a heart attack also depends on where the blockage is, whether the heart rhythm is disturbed, and whether another coronary artery supplies blood to that part of the heart. Blockages in the left coronary artery usually are more serious than in the right coronary artery. Blockages that cause an arrhythmia, an irregular heartbeat, can cause sudden death.

Causes and symptoms

Heart attacks generally are caused by severe coronary artery disease. Most heart attacks are caused by **blood clots** that form on atherosclerotic plaque. This blocks a coronary artery from supplying oxygen-rich blood to part of the heart. A number of major and contributing risk factors increase the risk of developing coronary artery disease. Some of these can be changed and some cannot. People with more risk factors are more likely to develop coronary artery disease.

Major risk factors

Major risk factors significantly increase the risk of coronary artery disease. Those which cannot be changed are:

- Heredity. People whose parents have coronary artery disease are more likely to develop it. African Americans also are at increased risk, due to their higher rate of severe **hypertension** than whites.

- Sex. Men under the age of 60 years of age are more likely to have heart attacks than women of the same age.

- Age. Men over the age of 45 and women over the age of 55 are considered at risk. Older people (those over 65) are more likely to die of a heart attack. Older women are twice as likely to die within a few weeks of a heart attack as a man. This may be because of other co-existing medical problems.

Major risk factors that can be changed are:

- **Smoking**. Smoking greatly increases both the chance of developing coronary artery disease and the change of dying from it. Smokers have two to four times the risk of non-smokers of **sudden cardiac death** and are more than twice as likely to have a heart attack. They also are more likely to die within an hour of a heart attack. Second-hand smoke also may increase risk.

- **High cholesterol**. Cholesterol is a soft, waxy substance that is produced by the body, as well as obtained from eating foods such as meat, eggs, and other animal products. Cholesterol level is affected by age, sex, heredity, and diet. Risk of developing coronary artery disease increases as blood cholesterol levels increase. When combined with other factors, the risk is even greater. Total cholesterol of 240 mg/dL and over poses a high risk, and 200–239 mg/dL a borderline high risk. In LDL cholesterol, high risk starts at 130–159 mg/dL, depending on other risk factors. HDL (healthy cholesterol) can lower or raise the coronary risk also.

- High blood pressure. High blood pressure makes the heart work harder, and over time, weakens it. It increases the risk of heart attack, **stroke**, kidney failure, and congestive **heart failure**. A blood pressure of 140 over 90 or above is considered high. As the numbers increase, high blood pressure goes from Stage 1 (mild) to Stage 4 (very severe). When combined with obesity, smoking, high cholesterol, or diabetes, the risk of heart attack or stroke increases several times.

- Lack of physical activity. This increases the risk of coronary artery disease. Even modest physical activity is beneficial if done regularly.

- Use of certain drugs or supplements. Extreme caution is advised in the use of the herbal supplement ephedra. The supplement, which was marketed for weight loss and to improve athletic performance, was found to contribute to heart attack, seizure, stoke and death. In April 2003, the U.S. Food and Drug Administration (FDA) investigating controlling or banning the substance. While it was once believed that **hormone replacement therapy** (HRT) helped prevent heart disease in women, a large clinical trial called the Women's Health Initiative found the opposite to be true. In 2003, the FDA began requiring manufacturers of HRT to place warnings on the box listing adverse effects of estrogen, including increased risk of heart attack, stroke and blood clots. The labels also must mention that HRT should not be used as a preventive medicine for heart disease.

Contributing risk factors

Contributing risk factors have been linked to coronary artery disease, but their significance or prevalence cannot always be demonstrated. Contributing risk factors are:

- Diabetes mellitus. The risk of developing coronary artery disease is seriously increased for diabetics. More than 80% of diabetics die of some type of heart or blood vessel disease.

- **Obesity**. Excess weight increases the strain on the heart and increases the risk of developing coronary artery disease, even if no other risk factors are present. Obesity increases both blood pressure and blood cholesterol, and can lead to diabetes.

- **Stress** and anger. Some scientists believe that stress and anger can contribute to the development of coronary artery disease. Stress, the mental and physical reaction to life's irritations and challenges, increases the heart rate and blood pressure, and can injure the lining of the arteries. Evidence shows that anger increases the risk of dying from heart disease and more than doubles the risk of having a heart attack right after an episode of anger.

- **Rheumatoid arthritis** in women. A report released in 2003 noted that women with rheumatoid arthritis has a higher risk of heart attach than those without the condition. The reason is most likely the inflammation arthritis causes.

More than 60% of heart attack victims experience symptoms before the heart attack occurs. These sometimes occur days or weeks before the heart attack. Sometimes, people do not recognize the symptoms of a heart attack or are in denial that they are having one. Symptoms are:

- Uncomfortable pressure, fullness, squeezing, or pain in the center of the chest. This lasts more than a few minutes, or may go away and return.
- Pain that spreads to the shoulders, neck, or arms.
- Chest discomfort accompanied by lightheadedness, fainting, sweating, **nausea**, or **shortness of breath**.

All of these symptoms do not occur with every heart attack. Sometimes, symptoms disappear and then reappear. A person with any of these symptoms should immediately call an emergency rescue service or be driven to the nearest hospital with a 24-hour cardiac care unit, whichever is quicker.

Diagnosis

Experienced emergency care personnel usually can diagnose a heart attack simply by looking at the patient. To confirm this diagnosis, they talk with the patient, check heart rate and blood pressure, perform an electrocardiogram, and take a blood sample. The electrocardiogram shows which coronary artery is blocked. Electrodes covered with conducting jelly are placed on the patient's chest, arms, and legs. They send impulses of the heart's activity through an oscilloscope (a monitor) to a recorder, which traces them on paper. The blood test shows the leak of enzymes or other biochemical markers from damaged cells in the heart muscle. In 2003, the FDA cleared a new test for ruling out heart attacks in people who come to emergency rooms with severe chest pains. It is the first new blood test for evaluation of heart attacks since 1994 and is used along with an electrocardiogram.

Treatment

Heart attacks are treated with cardiopulmonary resuscitation (CPR) when necessary to start and keep the patient breathing and his heart beating. Additional treatment can include close monitoring, electric shock, drug therapy, re-vascularization procedures, percutaneous transluminal coronary **angioplasty** and coronary artery bypass surgery. Upon arrival at the hospital, the patient is closely monitored. An electrical-shock device, a defibrillator, may be used to restore a normal rhythm if the heartbeat is fluttering uncontrollably. Oxygen often is used to ease the heart's workload or to help victims of severe heart attack breathe easier. If oxygen is used within hours of the heart attack, it may help limit damage to the heart.

Drugs to stabilize the patient and limit damage to the heart include thrombolytics, aspirin, anticoagulants, painkillers and tranquilizers, beta-blockers, ace-inhibitors, nitrates, rhythm-stabilizing drugs, and diuretics. Drugs that limit damage to the heart work only if given within a few hours of the heart attack. Thrombolytic drugs that break up blood clots and enable oxygen-rich blood to flow through the blocked artery increase the patient's chance of survival if given as soon as possible after the heart attack. Thrombolytics given within a few hours after a heart attack are the most effective. Injected intravenously, these include anisoylated plasminogen streptokinase activator complex (APSAC) or anistreplase (Eminase), recombinant tissue-type plasminogen activator (r-tPA, Retevase, or Activase), and streptokinase (Streptase, Kabikinase).

To prevent additional heart attacks, **aspirin** and an anticoagulant drug often follow the thrombolytic drug. These prevent new blood clots from forming and existing blood clots from growing. **Anticoagulant drugs** help prevent the blood from clotting. The most common anticoagulants are heparin and warfarin. Heparin is given intravenously while the patient is in the hospital. Warfarin, taken orally, often is given later. Aspirin helps to prevent the dissolved blood clots from reforming.

To relieve pain, a nitroglycerine tablet taken under the tongue may be given. If the pain continues, morphine sulfate may be prescribed. Tranquilizers such as diazepam (Valium) and alprazolam (Ativan) may be prescribed to lessen the trauma of a heart attack.

To slow down the heart rate and give the heart a chance to heal, beta-blockers often are given intravenously right after the heart attack. These can also help prevent sometimes fatal ventricular fibrillation. Beta-blockers include atenolol (Tenormin), metoprolol (Lopressor), nadolol, pindolol (Visken), propranolol (Inderal), and timolol (Blocadren).

Nitrates, a type of vasodilator, also are given right after a heart attack to help improve the delivery of blood to the heart and ease heart failure symptoms. Nitrates include isosorbide mononitrate (Imdur), isosorbide dinitrate (Isordil, Sorbitrate), and nitroglycerin (Nitrostat).

When a heart attack causes an abnormal heartbeat, arrhythmia drugs may be given to restore the heart's normal rhythm. These include: amiodarone (Cordarone), atropine, bretylium, disopyramide (Norpace), lidocaine (Xylocaine), procainamide (Procan), propafenone (Rythmol), propranolol (Inderal), quinidine, and sotalol (Betapace). Angiotensin-converting enzyme (ACE) inhibitors reduce the resistance against which the heart beats and are used to manage and prevent heart failure.

They are used to treat heart attack patients whose hearts do not pump well or who have symptoms of heart failure. Taken orally, they include Altace, Capoten, Lotensin, Monopril, Prinivil, Vasotec, and Zestril. Angiotensin receptor blockers, such as losartan (Cozaar) may substitute. **Diuretics** can help get rid of excess fluids that sometimes accumulate when the heart is not pumping effectively. Usually taken orally, they cause the body to dispose of fluids through urination. Common diuretics include: bumetanide (Bumex), chlorthalidone (Hygroton), chlorothiazide (Diuril), furosemide (Lasix), hydrochlorothiazide (HydroDIRUIL, Esidrix), spironolactone (Aldactone), and triamterene (Dyrenium).

Percutaneous transluminal coronary angioplasty and coronary artery bypass surgery are invasive revascularization procedures that open blocked coronary arteries and improve blood flow. They usually are performed only on patients for whom clot-dissolving drugs do not work, or who have poor **exercise** stress tests, poor left ventricular function, or **ischemia**. Generally, angioplasty is performed before coronary artery bypass surgery.

Percutaneous transluminal coronary angioplasty, usually called coronary angioplasty, is a non-surgical procedure in which a catheter (a tiny plastic tube) tipped with a balloon is threaded from a blood vessel in the thigh or arm into the blocked artery. The balloon is inflated and compresses the plaque to enlarge the blood vessel and open the blocked artery. The balloon is then deflated and the catheter is removed. Coronary angioplasty is performed in a hospital and generally requires a two-day stay. It is successful about 90% of the time. For one third of patients, the artery narrows again within six months after the procedure. The procedure can be repeated. It is less invasive and less expensive than coronary artery bypass surgery.

In coronary artery bypass surgery, called bypass surgery, a detour is built around the coronary artery blockage with a healthy leg or chest wall artery or vein. The healthy vein then supplies oxygen-rich blood to the heart. Bypass surgery is major surgery appropriate for patients with blockages in two or three major coronary arteries or severely narrowed left main coronary arteries, as well as those who have not responded to other treatments. It is performed in a hospital under **general anesthesia** using a heart-lung machine to support the patient while the healthy vein is attached to the coronary artery. About 70% of patients who have bypass surgery experience full relief from **angina**; about 20% experience partial relief. Long term, symptoms recur in only about three or four percent of patients per year. Five years after bypass surgery, survival expectancy is 90%, at 10 years it is about 80%, at 15 years it is about 55%, and at 20 years it is about 40%.

There are several experimental surgical procedures for unblocking coronary arteries under study including: **atherectomy**, where the surgeon shaves off and removes strips of plaque from the blocked artery; laser angioplasty, where a catheter with a laser tip is inserted to burn or break down the plaque; and insertion of a metal coil called a stent that can be implanted permanently to keep a blocked artery open.

Prognosis

The aftermath of a heart attack is often severe. Two-thirds of heart attack patients never recover fully. Within one year, 27% of men and 44% of women die. Within six years, 23% of men and 31% of women have another heart attack, 13% of men and 6% of women experience sudden death, and about 20% have heart failure. People who survive a heart attack have a chance of sudden death that is four to six times greater than others and a chance of illness and death that is two to nine times greater. Older women are more likely than men to die within a few weeks of a heart attack. In 2003, a new drug showed some promise in helping patients who have had a heart attack and developed heart failure. Called eplerenone, it lowered the death rate and risk of sudden death among patients tested.

Prevention

Many heart attacks can be prevented through a healthy lifestyle, which can reduce the risk of developing coronary artery disease. For patients who have already had a heart attack, a healthy lifestyle and carefully following doctor's orders can prevent another heart attack. A heart healthy lifestyle includes eating right, regular exercise, maintaining a healthy weight, no smoking, moderate drinking, no illegal drugs, controlling hypertension, and managing stress.

A healthy diet includes a variety of foods that are low in fat (especially saturated fat), low in cholesterol, and high in fiber; plenty of fruits and vegetables; and limited sodium. Some foods are low in fat but high in cholesterol, and some are low in cholesterol but high in fat. Saturated fat raises cholesterol, and, in excessive amounts, it increases the amount of the proteins in blood that form blood clots. Polyunsaturated and monounsaturated fats are relatively good for the heart. Fat should comprise no more than 30 percent of total daily calories.

Cholesterol, a waxy, lipid-like substance, comes from eating foods such as meat, eggs, and other animal products. It also is produced in the liver. Soluble fiber can help lower cholesterol. Cholesterol should be limited to about 300 mg per day. Many popular lipid-lowering drugs can reduce LDL-cholesterol by an average of 25–30% when combined with a low-fat, low-cholesterol diet. Fruits and vegetables are rich in fiber, **vitamins**, and **minerals**. They are also low calorie and nearly fat free. Vitamin C and beta-carotene, found in many fruits and vegetables, keep LDL-cholesterol from turning into a form that damages coronary arteries. Excess sodium can increase the risk of high blood pressure. Many processed foods contain large amounts of sodium, which should be limited to a daily intake of 2,400 mg—about the amount in a teaspoon of salt.

The "Food Guide" Pyramid developed by the U.S. Departments of Agriculture and Health and Human Services provides easy to follow guidelines for daily heart-healthy eating: six to 11 servings of bread, cereal, rice, and pasta; three to five servings of vegetables; two to four servings of fruit; two to three servings of milk, yogurt, and cheese; and two to three servings of meat, poultry, fish, dry beans, eggs, and nuts. Fats, oils, and sweets should be used sparingly.

Regular aerobic exercise can lower blood pressure, help control weight, and increase HDL ("good") cholesterol. It may keep the blood vessels more flexible. Moderate intensity aerobic exercise lasting about 30 minutes four or more times per week is recommended for maximum heart health, according to the Centers for Disease Control and Prevention and the American College of Sports Medicine. Three 10-minute exercise periods also are beneficial. Aerobic exercise—activities such as walking, jogging, and cycling—uses the large muscle groups and forces the body to use oxygen more efficiently. It also can include everyday activities such as active gardening, climbing stairs, or brisk housework.

Maintaining a desirable body weight also is important. About one-fourth of all Americans are overweight, and nearly one-tenth are obese, according to the Surgeon General's Report on Nutrition and Health. People who are 20% or more over their ideal body weight have an increased risk of developing coronary artery disease. Losing weight can help reduce total and LDL cholesterol, reduce triglycerides, and boost relative levels of HDL cholesterol. It also may reduce blood pressure.

Smoking has many adverse effects on the heart. It increases the heart rate, constricts major arteries, and can create irregular heartbeats. It also raises blood pressure, contributes to the development of plaque, increases the formation of blood clots, and causes blood platelets to cluster and impede blood flow. Heart damage caused by smoking can be repaired by quitting–even heavy smokers can return to heart health. Several studies have shown that ex-smokers face the same risk of heart disease as non-smokers within five to 10 years of quitting.

Drinking should be done in moderation. Modest consumption of alcohol can actually protect against coronary artery disease. This is believed to be because alcohol raises HDL cholesterol levels. The American Heart Association defines moderate consumption as one ounce of alcohol per day—roughly one cocktail, one 8-ounce glass of wine, or two 12-ounce glasses of beer. A study released in 2003 reported that risk of heart attack in men was reduced 30% to 35 % if they drank moderate amounts of alcoholic beverages three or four times a week. In some people, however, moderate drinking can increase risk factors for heart disease, such as raising blood pressure. Excessive drinking is always bad for the heart. It usually raises blood pressure, and can poison the heart and cause abnormal heart rhythms or even heart failure. Illegal drugs, like **cocaine**, can seriously harm the heart and should never be used.

High blood pressure, one of the most common and serious risk factors for coronary artery disease, can be completely controlled through lifestyle changes and medication. People with moderate hypertension may be able to control it through lifestyle changes such as reducing sodium and fat, exercising regularly, managing stress, quitting smoking, and drinking alcohol in moderation. If these changes do not work, and for people with severe hypertension, there are eight types of drugs that provide effective treatment.

Stress management means controlling mental and physical reactions to life's irritations and challenges. Techniques for controlling stress include: taking life more slowly, spending time with family and friends, thinking positively, getting enough sleep, exercising, and practicing relaxation techniques.

Daily aspirin therapy has been proven to help prevent blood clots associated with atherosclerosis. It also can prevent heart attacks from recurring, prevent heart attacks from being fatal, and lower the risk of strokes.

KEY TERMS

Angina—Chest pain that happens when diseased blood vessels restrict the flow of blood to the heart. Angina often is the first symptom of coronary artery disease.

Atherosclerosis—A process in which the walls of the coronary arteries thicken due to the accumulation of plaque in the blood vessels. Atherosclerosis is the cause of coronary artery disease.

Coronary arteries—The two arteries that provide blood to the heart. The coronary arteries surround the heart like a crown, coming out of the aorta, arching down over the top of the heart, and dividing into two branches. These are the arteries where coronary artery disease occurs.

Myocardial infarction—The technical term for heart attack. Myocardial means heart muscle and infarction means death of tissue from lack of oxygen.

Plaque—A deposit of fatty and other substances that accumulate in the lining of the artery wall.

Resources

PERIODICALS

"First New Blood Test to Evaluate Heart Attacks." *Biomedical Market Newsletter* January-February 2003: 42.

"Heart Attacks Reduced by Alchohol." *The Lancet* January 11, 2003: 149.

Kirn, Timothy F. "FDA Probes Ephedra, Proposes Warning Label (Risk of Heart Attack, Seizure, Stroke)." *Clinical Psychiatry News* April 2003: 49.

Pitt, Bertram, et al. "Eplerenone, a Selective Aldosterone Blocker, in Patients with Left Ventricular Dysfunction after Myocardial Infarction." *The New England Journal of Medicine* April 3, 2003: 1309-1313.

Stephenson, Joan. "FDA Orders Estrogen Safety Warnings: Agency Offers Guidance for HRT Use." *JAMA* February 5, 2003: 537.

ORGANIZATIONS

American Heart Association. 7320 Greenville Ave. Dallas, TX 75231. (214) 373-6300. <http://www.americanheart.org>.

National Heart, Lung and Blood Institute. PO Box 30105, Bethesda, MD 20824-0105. (301) 251-1222. <http://www.nhlbi.nih.gov>.

Texas Heart Institute. Heart Information Service. PO Box 20345, Houston, TX 77225-0345. <http://www.tmc.edu/thi>.

Lori De Milto
Teresa G. Odle

Heart block

Definition

Heart block refers to a delay in the normal flow of electrical impulses that cause the heart to beat. They are further classified as first-, second-, or third-degree block.

Description

The muscles of the heart contract in a rhythmic order for each heart beat, because electrical impulses travel along a specific route called the conduction system. The main junction of this system is called the atrioventricular node (AV node). Just as on a highway, there are occasionally some delays getting the impulse from one point to another. These delays are classified according to their severity.

In first-degree heart block, the signal is just slowed down a little as it travels along the defective part of the conduction system so that it arrives late traveling from the atrium to the ventricle.

In second-degree heart block, not every impulse reaches its destination. The block may affect every other beat, every second or third beat, or be very rare. If the blockage is frequent, it results in an overall slowing of the heart called bradycardia.

Third-degree block, also called complete heart block, is the most serious. When no signals can travel through the AV node, the heart uses its backup impulse generator in the lower portion of the heart. Though this impulse usually keeps the heart from stopping entirely, it is too slow to be an effective pump.

Causes and symptoms

First-degree heart block is fairly common. It is seen in teenagers, young adults and in well-trained athletes. The condition may be caused by rheumatic fever, some types of heart disease and by some drugs. First-degree heart block produces no symptoms.

Some cases of second-degree heart block may benefit from an artificial pace-maker. Second-degree block can occasionally progress to third-degree.

Third-degree heart block is a serious condition that affects the heart's ability to pump blood effectively. Symptoms include **fainting**, **dizziness** and sudden **heart failure**. If the ventricles beat more than 40 times per minute, symptoms are not as severe, but include tiredness, low blood pressure on standing, and **shortness of breath**.

Young children who have received a forceful blunt chest injury, can experience first-, or second-degree heart block.

Diagnosis

Diagnosis of first-, and second-degree heart block is made by observing it on an electrocardiograph (ECG).

Third-degree heart block usually results in symptoms such as fainting, dizziness and sudden heart failure, which require immediate medical care. A physical exam and ECG confirm the presence of heart block.

Treatment

Some second- and almost all third-degree heart blocks require an artificial pacemaker. In an emergency, a temporary pacemaker can be used until an implanted device is advisable. Most people need the pacemaker for the rest of their lives.

Prognosis

Most people with first- and second-degree heart block don't even know they have it. For people with third-degree block, once the heart has been restored to its normal, dependable rhythm, most people live full and comfortable lives.

Resources

ORGANIZATIONS

American Heart Association. 7320 Greenville Ave. Dallas, TX 75231. (214) 373-6300. < http:// www.americanheart.org >.

Dorothy Elinor Stonely

Heart catheterization *see* **Cardiac catheterization**

Heart failure

Definition

Heart failure is a condition in which the heart has lost the ability to pump enough blood to the body's tissues. With too little blood being delivered, the organs and other tissues do not receive enough oxygen and nutrients to function properly.

Description

According to the American Heart Association, about 4.9 million Americans are living with congestive heart failure. Of these, 2.5 million are males and 2.4 million are females. Ten of every 1,000 people over age 65 have this condition. There are about 400,000 new cases each year.

Heart failure happens when a disease affects the heart's ability to deliver enough blood to the body's tissues. Often, a person with heart failure may have a buildup of fluid in the tissues, called **edema**. Heart failure with this kind of fluid buildup is called congestive heart failure. Where edema occurs in the body depends on the part of the heart that is affected by heart failure. Heart failure caused by abnormality of the lower left chamber of the heart (left ventricle) means that the left ventricle cannot pump blood out to the body as fast as it returns from the lungs. Because blood cannot get back to the heart, it begins to back up in the blood vessels of the lungs. Some of the fluid in the blood is forced into the breathing space of the lungs, causing **pulmonary edema**. A person with pulmonary edema has shortness of breath, which may be acute, severe and life threatening. A person with congestive heart failure feels tired because not enough blood circulates to supply the body's tissues with the oxygen and nutrients they need. Abnormalities of the heart structure and rhythm also can be responsible for left ventricular congestive heart failure.

In right-sided heart failure, the lower right chamber of the heart (right ventricle) cannot pump blood to the lungs as fast as it returns from the body through the veins. Blood then engorges the right side of the heart and the veins. Fluid backed up in the veins is forced out into the tissues, causing swelling (edema), usually in the feet and legs. Congestive heart failure of the right ventricle often is caused by abnormalities of the heart valves and lung disorders.

When the heart cannot pump enough blood, it tries to make up for this by becoming larger. By becoming enlarged (hypertrophic) the ventricle can contract more strongly and pump more blood. When this happens, the heart chamber becomes larger and the muscle in the heart wall becomes thicker. The heart also compensates by pumping more often to improve blood output and circulation. The kidneys try to compensate for a failing heart by retaining more salt and water to increase the volume of blood. This extra fluid also can cause edema. Eventually, as the condition worsens over time these measures are not enough to keep the heart pumping enough blood needed by the body. Kidneys often weaken under these circumstances, further aggravating the situation and making therapy more difficult.

For most people, heart failure is a chronic disease with no cure. However, it can be managed and treated with medicines and changes in diet, exercise, and lifestyle habits. **Heart transplantation** is considered in some cases.

Causes and symptoms

The most common causes of heart failure are:

- **coronary artery disease** and heart attack (which may be "silent")

- **cardiomyopathy**

- high blood pressure (**hypertension**)

- heart valve disease

- congenital heart disease

- **alcoholism** and drug **abuse**

The most common cause of heart failure is coronary artery disease. In coronary artery disease, the arteries supplying blood to the heart become narrowed or blocked. When blood flow to an area of the heart is completely blocked, the person has a **heart attack**. Some heart attacks go unrecognized. The heart muscle suffers damage when its blood supply is reduced or blocked. If the damage affects the heart's ability to pump blood, heart failure develops.

Cardiomyopathy is a general term for disease of the heart muscle. Cardiomyopathy may be caused by coronary artery disease and various other heart problems. Sometimes the cause of cardiomyopathy cannot be found. In these cases the heart muscle disease is called idiopathic cardiomyopathy. Whatever the cause, cardiomyopathy can weaken the heart, leading to heart failure.

High blood pressure is another common cause of heart failure. High blood pressure makes the heart work harder to pump blood. After a while, the heart

cannot keep up and the symptoms of heart failure develop.

Defects of the heart valves, congenital heart diseases, alcoholism, and drug abuse cause damage to the heart that can all lead to heart failure.

A person with heart failure may experience the following:

- **shortness of breath**

- frequent coughing, especially when lying down

- swollen feet, ankles, and legs

- abdominal swelling and **pain**

- fatigue

- **dizziness** or **fainting**

- sudden **death**

A person with left-sided heart failure may have shortness of breath and coughing caused by the fluid buildup in the lungs. Pulmonary edema may cause the person to **cough** up bubbly phlegm that contains blood. With right-sided heart failure, fluid build-up in the veins and body tissues causes swelling in the feet, legs, and abdomen. When body tissues, such as organs and muscles, do not receive enough oxygen and nutrients they cannot function as well, leading to tiredness and dizziness.

Diagnosis

Diagnosis of heart failure is based on:

- symptoms

- medical history

- **physical examination**

- **chest x ray**

- electrocardiogram (ECG; also called EKG)

- other imaging tests

- **cardiac catheterization**

A person's symptoms can provide important clues to the presence of heart failure. Shortness of breath while engaging in activities and episodes of shortness of breath that wake a person from sleep are classic symptoms of heart failure. During the physical examination, the physician listens to the heart and lungs with a stethoscope for telltale signs of heart failure. Irregular heart sounds, "gallops," a rapid heart rate, and murmurs of the heart valves may be heard. If there is fluid in the lungs a crackling sound may be heard. Rapid breathing or other changes in breathing may also be present. Patients with heart failure also may have a rapid pulse.

By pressing on the abdomen, the physician can feel if the liver is enlarged. The skin of the fingers and toes may have a bluish tint and feel cool if not enough oxygen is reaching them.

A chest x ray can show if there is fluid in the lungs and if the heart is enlarged. Abnormalities of heart valves and other structures also may be seen on chest x ray.

An electrocardiogram gives information on the heart rhythm and the size of the heart. It can show if the heart chamber is enlarged and if there is damage to the heart muscle from blocked arteries.

Besides chest x ray, other imaging tests may help make a diagnosis. **Echocardiography** uses sound waves to make images of the heart. These images can show if the heart wall or chambers are enlarged and if there are any abnormalities of the heart valves. An echocardiogram also can be used to find out how much blood the heart is pumping. It determines the amount of blood in the ventricle (ventricular volume) and the amount of blood the ventricle pumps each time it beats (called the ejection fraction). A healthy heart pumps at least one-half the amount of blood in the left ventricle with each heartbeat. Radionuclide ventriculography also measures the ejection fraction by imaging with very low doses of an injected radioactive substance as it travels through the heart.

A new test that measures the level of a particular hormone in the blood was introduced in 2003 and researchers said the test may be useful for testing for heart failure in physicians' offices because it could provide results in 15 minutes.

Cardiac catheterization involves using a small tube (catheter) that is inserted through a blood vessel into the heart. It is used to measure pressure in the heart and the amount of blood pumped by the heart. This test can help find abnormalities of the coronary arteries, heart valves, and heart muscle, and other blood vessels. Combined with echocardiography and other tests, cardiac catheterization can help find the cause of heart failure. It is not always necessary, however.

Treatment

Heart failure usually is treated with lifestyle changes and medicines. Sometimes surgery is needed to correct abnormalities of the heart or heart valves. Heart transplantation is a last resort to be considered in certain cases.

Dietary changes to maintain proper weight and reduce salt intake may be needed. Reducing salt intake helps to lessen swelling in the legs, feet, and abdomen. Appropriate **exercise** also may be recommended, but it is important that heart failure patients only begin an exercise program with the advice of their doctors. Walking, bicycling, swimming, or low-impact aerobic exercises may be recommended. There are good heart **rehabilitation** programs at most larger hospitals.

Other lifestyle changes that may reduce the symptoms of heart failure include stopping smoking or other tobacco use, eliminating or reducing alcohol consumption, and not using harmful drugs.

One or more of the following types of medicines may be prescribed for heart failure:

- **diuretics**
- digitalis
- **vasodilators**
- beta blockers
- angiotensin converting enzyme inhibitors (ACE inhibitors)
- angiotensin receptor blockers (ARBs)
- calcium channel blockers

Diuretics help eliminate excess salt and water from the kidneys by making patients urinate more often. This helps reduce the swelling caused by fluid buildup in the tissues. Digitalis helps the heart muscle to have stronger pumping action. Vasodilators, ACE inhibitors, ARBs, and calcium channel blockers lower blood pressure and expand the blood vessels so blood can move more easily through them. This action makes it easier for the heart to pump blood through the vessels. Cholesterol-lowering drugs called statins can help prevent death from heart failure. A 2003 study showed a 62% drop in mortality rate among patients with severe heart failure who took statin therapy.

In 2003, a new noninvasive procedure was being tested for patients with congestive heart failure. Called enhanced external counterpulsation (EECP), it consisted of inflating three sets of pneumatic cuffs attached to the patient's legs. The therapy had positive effects on the blood pressure and reduced frequency of episodes of **angina** (pain) in a clinical trial by as much as 70%.

Surgery is used to correct certain heart conditions that cause heart failure. Congenital heart defects and abnormal heart valves can be repaired with surgery. Blocked coronary arteries usually can be treated with **angioplasty** or coronary artery bypass surgery.

KEY TERMS

Angioplasty—A technique for treating blocked coronary arteries by inserting a catheter with a tiny balloon at the tip into the artery and inflating it.

Angiotensin-converting enzyme (ACE) inhibitor—A drug that relaxes blood vessel walls and lowers blood pressure.

Arrhythmias—Abnormal heartbeat.

Atherosclerosis—Buildup of a fatty substance called a plaque inside blood vessels.

Calcium channel blocker—A drug that relaxes blood vessels and lowers blood pressure.

Cardiac catheterization—A diagnostic test for evaluating heart disease; a catheter is inserted into an artery and passed into the heart.

Cardiomyopathy—Disease of the heart muscle.

Catheter—A thin, hollow tube.

Congenital heart defects—Abnormal formation of structures of the heart or of its major blood vessels present at birth.

Congestive heart failure—A condition in which the heart cannot pump enough blood to supply the body's tissues with sufficient oxygen and nutrients; back up of blood in vessels and the lungs causes buildup of fluid (congestion) in the tissues.

Coronary arteries—Arteries that supply blood to the heart muscle.

Coronary artery bypass—Surgical procedure to reroute blood around a blocked coronary artery.

Coronary artery disease—Narrowing or blockage of coronary arteries by atherosclerosis.

Digitalis—A drug that helps the heart muscle to have stronger pumping action.

Diuretic—A type of drug that helps the kidneys eliminate excess salt and water.

Edema—Swelling caused by fluid buildup in tissues.

Ejection fraction—A measure of the portion of blood that is pumped out of a filled ventricle.

Heart valves—Valves that regulate blood flow into and out of the heart chambers.

Hypertension—High blood pressure.

Hypertrophic—Enlarged.

Idiopathic cardiomyopathy—Cardiomyopathy without a known cause.

Pulmonary edema—Buildup of fluid in the tissue of the lungs.

Vasodilator—Any drug that relaxes blood vessel walls.

Ventricles—The two lower chambers of the heart.

With severe heart failure, the heart muscle may become so damaged that available treatments do not help. Patients with this stage of heart failure are said to have end-stage heart failure. Heart transplant usually is considered for patients with end-stage heart failure when all other treatments have stopped working.

Prognosis

Most patients with mild or moderate heart failure can be successfully treated with dietary and exercise programs and the right medications. In fact, in 2003, the American Heart Association said that even those awaiting heart transplants could benefit from exercise. Many people are able to participate in normal daily activities and lead relatively active lives.

Patients with severe heart failure may eventually have to consider heart transplantation. Approximately 50% of patients diagnosed with congestive heart

failure live for five years with the condition. Women with heart failure usually live longer than men with heart failure.

Prevention

Heart failure usually is caused by the effects of some type of heart disease. The best way to try to prevent heart failure is to eat a healthy diet and get regular exercise, but many causes of heart failure cannot be prevented. People with risk factors for coronary disease (such as high blood pressure and **high cholesterol** levels) should work closely with their physician to reduce likelihood of heart attack and heart failure.

Heart failure sometimes can be avoided by identifying and treating any conditions that might lead to heart disease. These include high blood pressure, alcoholism, and coronary artery disease. Regular blood pressure checks and obtaining immediate medical care for symptoms of coronary artery disease, such as chest pain, will help to get these conditions found and treated early, before they can damage the heart muscle.

A 2003 initiative called OPTIMIZE H-F was aimed at preventing severe heart failure and deaths among patients discharge from hospitals. The project created a registry or database of patients with heart failure that could be shared among hospitals. Finally, diagnosing and treating heart failure before the heart becomes severely damaged can improve the prognosis. With proper treatment, many patients may continue to lead active lives for a number of years.

Resources

PERIODICALS

"Even Heart Failure Patients Should Exercise." *Clinician Reviews* April 2003: 50-52.

Jancin, Bruce. "Noninvasive Procedure Eyed for Heart Failure: Enhanced External Counterpulsation." *Family Practice News* June 1, 2003: 12.

"New Care Initiative to Improve Outcomes for Heart Failure Patients." *Heart Disease Weekly* April 20, 2003: 45.

"Rapid Congestive Heart Failure Test a Useful Tool in Physician Offices." *Heart Disease Weekly* June 15, 2003: 19.

Zoler, Michael N. "Heart Failure Deaths Plunge with Statins." *Internal Medicine News* April 15, 2003: 35-41.

ORGANIZATIONS

American Heart Association. 7320 Greenville Ave. Dallas, TX 75231. (214) 373-6300. <http://www.americanheart.org>.

National Heart, Lung and Blood Institute. PO Box 30105, Bethesda, MD 20824-0105. (301) 251-1222. <http://www.nhlbi.nih.gov>.

Texas Heart Institute. Heart Information Service. PO Box 20345, Houston, TX 77225-0345. <http://www.tmc.edu/thi>.

Toni Rizzo
Teresa G. Odle

▌ Heart murmurs

Definition

A heart murmur is an abnormal, extra sound during the heartbeat cycle made by blood moving through the heart and its valves. It is detected by the physician's examination using a stethoscope.

Description

A heart which is beating normal makes two sounds, "lubb" when the valves between the atria and ventricles close, and "dupp" when the valves between the ventricles and the major arteries close. A heart murmur is a series of vibratory sounds made by turbulent blood flow. The sounds are longer than normal heart sounds and can be heard between the normal sounds of the heart.

Heart murmurs are common in children and can also result from heart or valve defects. Nearly two thirds of heart murmurs in children are produced by a normal heart and are harmless. This type of heart murmur is usually called an "innocent" heart murmur. It can also be called "functional" or "physiologic." Innocent heart murmurs are usually very faint, intermittent, and occur in a small area of the chest. Pathologic heart murmurs may indicate the presence of a serious heart defect. They are louder, continual, and may be accompanied by a click or gallop.

Some heart murmurs are continually present; others happen only when the heart is working harder than usual, including during **exercise** or certain types of illness. Heart murmurs can be diastolic or systolic. Those which occur during relaxation of the heart between beats are called diastolic murmurs. Those which occur during contraction of the heart muscle are called systolic murmurs. The characteristics of the murmur may suggest specific alterations in the heart or its valves.

Causes and symptoms

Innocent heart murmurs are caused by blood flowing through the chambers and valves of the heart or the blood vessels near the heart. Sometimes anxiety, stress, **fever**, anemia, overactive thyroid, and **pregnancy** will cause innocent murmurs that can be heard by a physician using a stethoscope. Pathologic heart murmurs, however, are caused by structural abnormalities of the heart. These include defective heart valves or holes in the walls of the heart. Valve problems are more common. Valves that do not open completely cause blood to flow through a smaller opening than normal, while those that do not close properly may cause blood to go back through the valve. A hole in the wall between the left and right sides of the heart, called a septal defect, can cause heart murmurs. Some septal defects close on their own; others require surgery to prevent progressive damage to the heart.

The symptoms of heart murmurs differ depending on the cause of the heart murmur. Innocent heart murmurs and those which do not impair the function of the heart have no symptoms. Murmurs that are due to severe abnormalities of a heart valve may cause shortness of breath, **dizziness**, chest pains, **palpitations**, and lung congestion.

Diagnosis

Heart murmurs can be heard when a physician listens to the heart through a stethoscope during a regular check-up. Very loud heart murmurs and those with clicks or extra heart sounds should be evaluated further. Infants with heart murmurs who do not thrive, eat, or breath properly and older children who lose consciousness suddenly or are intolerant to exercise should also be evaluated. If the murmur sounds suspicious, the physician may order a chest x ray, an electrocardiogram, and an echocardiogram.

An electrocardiogram (ECG) shows the heart's activity and may reveal muscle thickening, damage, or a lack of oxygen. Electrodes covered with conducting jelly are placed on the patient's chest, arms, and legs. They send impulses of the heart's activity through a monitor (oscilloscope) to a recorder which traces them on paper. The test takes about 10 minutes and is commonly performed in a physician's office. An exercise ECG can reveal additional information.

An echocardiogram (cardiac ultrasound), may be ordered to identify a structural problem that is causing the heart murmur. An echocardiogram uses sound waves to create an image of the heart's chambers and valves. The technician applies gel to a hand-held transducer then presses it against the patient's chest. The sound waves are converted into an image that can be displayed on a monitor. Performed in a cardiology outpatient diagnostic laboratory, the test takes 30 minutes to an hour.

Treatment

Innocent heart murmurs do not affect the patient's health and require no treatment. Heart murmurs due to scptal defects may require surgery. Those due to valvular defects may require antibiotics to prevent infection during certain surgical or dental procedures. Severely damaged or diseased valves can be repaired or replaced through surgery.

Alternative treatment

If a heart murmur requires surgical treatment, there are no alternative treatments, although there are alternative therapies that are helpful for pre- and

---

KEY TERMS

Atria—The upper two chambers of the heart.

Echocardiogram—A non-invasive ultrasound test that shows an image of the inside of the heart. An echocardiogram can be performed to identify any structural problems which cause a heart murmur.

Electrocardiogram—A test that shows the electrical activity of the heart by placing electronic sensors on the patient. This test can be used to confirm the presence of a heart murmur.

Pathologic—Characterized by disease or the structural and functional changes due to disease. Pathologic heart murmurs may indicate a heart defect.

Ventricles—The lower two chambers of the heart.

---

post-surgical support of the patient. If the heart murmur is innocent, heart activity can be supported using the herb hawthorn (*Crataegus laevigata* or *C. oxyacantha*) or coenzyme Q10. These remedies improve heart contractility and the heart's ability to use oxygen. If the murmur is valvular in origin, herbs that act like **antibiotics** as well as options that build resistance to infection in the valve areas may be considered.

Prognosis

Most children with innocent heart murmurs grow out of them by the time they reach adulthood. Severe causes of heart murmurs may progress to severe symptoms and **death**.

Resources

ORGANIZATIONS

American Heart Association. 7320 Greenville Ave. Dallas, TX 75231. (214) 373-6300. <http://www.americanheart.org>.

Texas Heart Institute. Heart Information Service. PO Box 20345, Houston, TX 77225-0345. <http://www.tmc.edu/thi>.

Lori De Milto

Heart muscle infection *see* **Myocarditis**

Heart scan *see* **Echocardiography**

Heart septal defect *see* **Atrial septal defect**

Heart sonogram *see* **Echocardiography**

Heart surgery for congenital defects

Definition

A variety of surgical procedures that are performed to repair the many types of heart defects that may be present at birth.

Purpose

Heart surgery for congenital defects is performed to repair a defect as much as possible and improve the flow of blood and oxygen to the body. While congenital heart defects vary in their severity, most require surgery. Surgery is recommended for congenital heart defects that result in a lack of oxygen, a poor quality of life, or a patient who does not thrive. Some types of congenital heart defects that don't cause symptoms are treated surgically because they can lead to serious complications.

Precautions

There are many types of surgery for congenital heart defects and many considerations in the decision to operate. The patient's cardiologist or surgeon will discuss these issues on an individual basis.

Description

There are many types of congenital heart defects. Most obstruct the flow of blood in the heart, or the vessels near it, or cause an abnormal flow of blood through the heart. Rarer types include newborns born with one ventricle, one side of the heart that is not completely formed, or the pulmonary artery and the aorta coming out of the same ventricle. Most congenital heart defects require surgery during infancy or childhood. Recommended ages for surgery for the most common congenital heart defects are:

- atrial septal defects: during the preschool years

- patent ductus arteriosus: between ages one and two

- coarctation of the aorta: in infancy, if it's symptomatic, at age four otherwise

- tetralogy of Fallot: age varies, depending on the patient's signs and symptoms

- transposition of the great arteries: often in the first weeks after birth, but before the patient is 12 months old

Surgical procedures seek to repair the defect as much as possible and restore circulation to as close to normal as possible. Sometimes, multiple, serial, surgical procedures are necessary. Smaller congenital heart defects can now be repaired in a cardiac catheterization lab instead of an operating room. Catheterization procedures include balloon atrial septostomy and **balloon valvuloplasty**. Surgical procedures include arterial switch, Damus-Kaye-Stansel procedure, Fontan procedure, Ross procedure, shunt procedure, and venous switch or intra-atrial baffle.

Catheterization procedures

Balloon atrial septostomy and balloon valvuloplasty are cardiac catheterization procedures. **Cardiac catheterization** procedures can save the lives of critically ill neonates and in some cases eliminate or delay more invasive surgical procedures. It is expected that catheterization procedures will continue to replace more types of surgery for congenital heart defects in the future. A thin tube called a catheter is inserted into an artery or vein in the leg, groin, or arm and threaded into the area of the heart which needs repair. The patient receives a local anesthetic at the insertion site and is awake but sedated during the procedure.

BALLOON ATRIAL SEPTOSTOMY. Balloon atrial septostomy is the standard procedure for correcting transposition of the great arteries; it is sometimes used in patients with mitral, pulmonary, or tricupsid atresia (atresia is a defect that causes the blood to carry too little oxygen to the body). Balloon atrial septostomy enlarges the atrial opening. A special balloon-tipped catheter is inserted into the right atrium and inflated to create a large opening in the atrial septum.

BALLOON VALVULOPLASTY. Balloon valvuloplasty uses a balloon-tipped catheter to open a narrowed heart valve, improving the flow of blood. It is the procedure of choice in pulmonary stenosis and is sometimes used in aortic stenosis. Balloons made of plastic polymers are placed at the end of the catheter and inflated to relieve the obstruction in the heart valve. Long-terms results are excellent in most cases. The operative **death** rate is 2–4%.

Surgical procedures

These procedures are performed under **general anesthesia**. Some require the use of a heart-lung machine, which cools the body to reduce the need for oxygen and takes over for the heart and lungs during the procedure.

ARTERIAL SWITCH. Arterial switch is performed to correct transposition of the great arteries, where the position of the pulmonary artery and the aorta are reversed. The procedure involves connecting the aorta to the left ventricle and the pulmonary artery to the right ventricle.

DAMUS-KAYE-STANSEL PROCEDURE. Transposition of the great arteries can also be corrected by the Damus-Kaye-Stansel procedure, in which the pulmonary artery is cut in two and connected to the ascending aorta and right ventricle.

FONTAN PROCEDURE. For tricuspid atresia and pulmonary atresia, the Fontan procedure connects the right atrium to the pulmonary artery directly or with a conduit, and the atrial defect is closed. Survival is over 90%.

PULMONARY ARTERY BANDING. Pulmonary artery banding is narrowing the pulmonary artery with a band to reduce blood flow and pressure in the lungs. It is used for ventricular septal defect, atrioventricular canal defect, and tricuspid atresia. Later, the band can be removed and the defect corrected with open heart surgery.

ROSS PROCEDURE. To correct aortic stenosis, the Ross procedure grafts the pulmonary artery to the aorta.

SHUNT PROCEDURE. For Tetralogy of Fallot, tricuspid atresia, or pulmonary atresia, the shunt procedure creates a passage between blood vessels, sending blood into parts of the body that need it.

VENOUS SWITCH. For transposition of the great arteries, venous switch creates a tunnel inside the atria to re-direct oxygen-rich blood to the right ventricle and aorta and venous blood to the left ventricle and pulmonary artery.

OTHER TYPES OF SURGERY. These surgical procedures are also used to treat common congenital heart defects. A medium to large ventricular or **atrial septal defect** can be closed by suturing it or covering it with a Dacron patch. For patent ductus arteriosus, surgery consists of dividing the ductus into two and tying off the ends. If performed within the patient's first few years, there is practically no risk associated with this operation. Surgery for coarctation of the aorta involves opening the chest wall, removing the defect, and reconnecting the ends of the aorta. If the defect is too long to be reconnected, a Dacron graft is used to replace the missing piece. In uncomplicated cases, the risk of the operation is 1–2%.

Preparation

Before surgery for congenital heart defects, the patient will receive a complete evaluation, which includes a physical exam, a detailed family history, a chest x ray, an electrocardiogram, an echocardiogram, and usually cardiac catheterization. For six to eight hours before the surgery, the patient cannot eat or drink anything. An electrocardiogram shows the heart's activity and may reveal a lack of oxygen. Electrodes covered with conducting jelly are placed on the patient's chest, arms, and legs and the heart's impulses are traced on paper. An echocardiogram uses sound waves to create an image of the heart's chambers and valves. Gel is applied to a hand-held transducer and then pressed against the patient's chest. Cardiac catheterization is an invasive diagnostic technique used to evaluate the heart in which a long tube is inserted into a blood vessel and guided into the heart. A contrast solution is injected to make the heart visible on x rays.

Aftercare

After heart surgery for congenital defects, the patient goes to an intensive care ward where he or she is connected to a variety of tubes and monitors, including a ventilator. Patients are monitored every 15 minutes until vital signs are stable. Heart sounds, oxygenation, and the electrocardiogram are monitored. Chest tubes will be checked to ensure that they're draining properly and there is no hemorrhage. **Pain** medications will be administered. Complications such as **stroke**, lung **blood clots**, and reduced blood flow to the kidneys will be watched for. After the ventilator and breathing tube are removed, **chest physical therapy** and exercises to improve circulation will be started.

Risks

Complications from heart surgery for congenital defects can be severe. They include shock, congestive **heart failure**, lack of oxygen or too much carbon dioxide in the blood, irregular heartbeat, stroke, infection, kidney damage, lung blood clot, low blood pressure, hemorrhage, cardiac arrest, and death.

Resources

ORGANIZATIONS

American Heart Association. 7320 Greenville Ave. Dallas, TX 75231. (214) 373-6300. < http:// www.americanheart.org >.

Children's Health Information Network. 1561 Clark Drive, Yardley, PA 19067. (215) 493-3068. < http://www.tchin.org >.

Congenital Heart Anomalies Support, Education & Resources, Inc. 2112 North Wilkins Road, Swanton, OH 43558. (419) 825-5575. < http://www.csun.edu/~hfmth006/chaser >.

Texas Heart Institute. Heart Information Service. PO Box 20345, Houston, TX 77225-0345. < http://www.tmc.edu/thi >.

Lori De Milto

Heart transplantation

Definition

Heart transplantation, also called cardiac transplantation, is the replacement of a patient's diseased or injured heart with a healthy donor heart.

Purpose

Heart transplantation is performed on patients with end-stage heart failure or some other life-threatening heart disease. Before a doctor recommends heart transplantation for a patient, all other possible treatments for his or her disease must have been tried. The purpose of heart transplantation is to extend and improve the life of a person who would otherwise die from **heart failure**. Most patients who receive a new heart were so sick before transplantation that they could not live a normal life. Replacing a patient's diseased heart with a healthy, functioning donor heart often allows the recipient to return to normal daily activities.

Precautions

Because healthy donor hearts are in short supply, strict rules dictate who should or should not get a heart transplant. Patients who have conditions that might cause the new heart to fail should not have a heart transplant. Similarly, patients who may be too sick to survive the surgery or the side effects of the drugs they must take to keep their new heart working would not be good transplant candidates.

Patients who have any of the following conditions may not be eligible for heart transplantation:

- active infection
- pulmonary **hypertension**
- chronic lung disease with loss of more than 40% of lung function
- untreatable liver or **kidney disease**
- diabetes that has caused serious damage to vital organs
- disease of the blood vessels in the brain, such as a stroke
- serious disease of the arteries
- mental illness or any condition that would make a patient unable to take the necessary medicines on schedule
- continuing alcohol or drug abuse

Description

Patients with end-stage heart disease that threatens their life even after medical treatment may be considered for heart transplantation. Potential candidates must have a complete medical examination before they can be put on the transplant waiting list. Many types of tests are done, including blood tests, x rays, and tests of heart, lung, and other organ function. The results of these tests indicate to doctors how serious the heart disease is and whether or not a patient is healthy enough to survive the transplant surgery.

Organ waiting list

A person approved for heart transplantation is placed on the heart transplant waiting list of a heart transplant center. All patients on a waiting list are registered with the United Network for Organ Sharing (UNOS). UNOS has organ transplant specialists who run a national computer network that connects all the transplant centers and organ-donation organizations.

When a donor heart becomes available, information about it is entered into the UNOS computer and compared to information from patients on the waiting list. The computer program produces a list of patients ranked according to blood type, size of the heart, and how urgently they need a heart. Because the heart must be transplanted as quickly as possible, the list of local patients is checked first for a good match. After that, a regional list, and then a national list, are checked. The patient's transplant team of heart and transplant specialists makes the final decision as to whether a donor heart is suitable for the patient.

The transplant procedure

When a heart becomes available and is approved for a patient, it is packed in a sterile cold solution and rushed to the hospital where the recipient is waiting.

Heart transplant surgery involves the following basic steps:

- A specialist in cardiovascular anesthesia gives the patient **general anesthesia**.

- Intravenous **antibiotics** are usually given to prevent bacterial wound infections.

- The patient is put on a heart/lung machine, which performs the functions of the heart and lungs and pumps the blood to the rest of the body during surgery. This procedure is called cardiopulmonary bypass.

National Transplant Waiting List By Organ Type (June 2000)	
Organ Needed	**Number Waiting**
Kidney	48,349
Liver	15,987
Heart	4,139
Lung	3,695
Kidney-Pancreas	2,437
Pancreas	942
Heart-Lung	212
Intestine	137

- After adequate blood circulation is established, the patient's diseased heart is removed.

- The donor heart is attached to the patient's blood vessels.

- After the blood vessels are connected, the new heart is warmed up and begins beating. If the heart does not begin to beat immediately, the surgeon may start it with an electrical shock.

- The patient is taken off the heart/lung machine.

- The new heart is stimulated to maintain a regular beat with medications for two to five days after surgery, until the new heart functions normally on its own.

Heart transplant recipients are given immunosuppressive drugs to prevent the body from rejecting the new heart. These drugs are usually started before or during the heart transplant surgery. Immunosuppressive drugs keep the body's immune system from recognizing and attacking the new heart as foreign tissue. Normally, immune system cells recognize and attack foreign or abnormal cells, such as bacteria, **cancer** cells, and cells from a transplanted organ. The drugs suppress the immune cells and allow the new heart to function properly. However, they can also allow infections and other adverse effects to occur to the patient.

Because the chance of rejection is highest during the first few months after the transplantation, recipients are usually given a combination of three or four immunosuppressive drugs in high doses during this time. Afterwards, they must take maintenance doses of immunosuppressive drugs for the rest of their lives.

Cost and insurance coverage

The total cost for heart transplantation varies, depending on where it is performed, whether transportation and lodging are needed, and on whether there are any complications. The costs for the surgery and

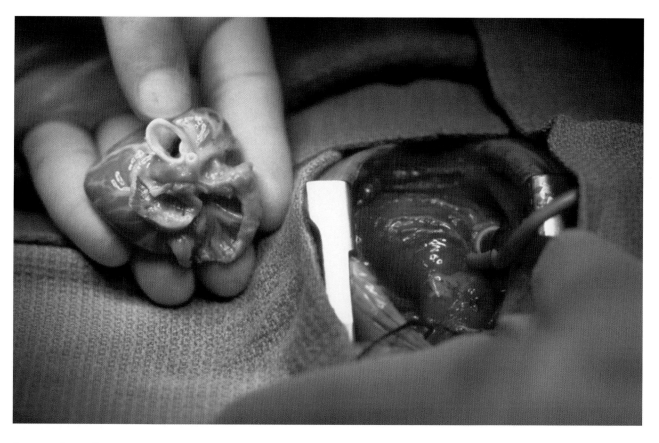

A comparison of the old and new hearts of Dylan Stork, the smallest heart transplant recipient in the world. Dylan was seven weeks old and weighed 5.5 pounds (2.5 kg) at the time of the operation. *(Photograph by Alexander Tsiaras, Photo Researchers, Inc. Reproduced by permission.)*

first year of care are estimated to be about $250,000. The medical tests and medications after the first year cost about $21,000 per year.

Insurance coverage for heart transplantation varies depending on the policy. Most commercial insurance companies pay a certain percentage of heart transplant costs. Medicare pays for heart transplants if the surgery is performed at Medicare-approved centers. Medicaid pays for heart transplants in 33 states and in the District of Colombia.

Preparation

Before patients are put on the transplant waiting list, their blood type is determined so a compatible donor heart can be found. The heart must come from a person with the same blood type as the patient, unless it is blood type O. A blood type O heart can be transplanted into a person with any type of blood.

A panel reactive antibodies (PRA) test is also done before heart transplantation. This test tells doctors whether or not the patient is at high risk for having a hyperacute reaction against a donor heart. A hyperacute reaction is a strong immune response against the new heart that happens within minutes to hours after the new heart is transplanted. If the PRA shows that a patient has a high risk for this kind of reaction, then a crossmatch is done between a patient and a donor heart before transplant surgery. A crossmatch checks how close the match is between the patient's tissue type and the tissue type of the donor heart.

Most people are not high risk and a crossmatch usually is not done before the transplant because the surgery must be done as quickly as possible after a donor heart is found.

While waiting for heart transplantation, patients are given treatment to keep the heart as healthy as possible. They are regularly checked to make sure the heart is pumping enough blood. Intravenous medications may be used to improve cardiac output. If these drugs are not effective, a mechanical pump can help keep the heart functioning until a donor heart becomes available. Inserted through an artery into the aorta, the pump assists the heart in pumping blood.

Aftercare

Immediately following surgery, patients are monitored closely in the intensive care unit (ICU) of the hospital for 24–72 hours. Most patients need to receive oxygen for four to 24 hours following surgery. Blood pressure, heart function, and other organ functions are carefully monitored during this time.

Heart transplant patients start taking immunosuppressive drugs before or during surgery to prevent immune rejection of the heart. High doses of immunosuppressive drugs are given at this time, because rejection is most likely to happen within the first few months after the surgery. A few months after surgery, lower doses of immunosuppressive drugs usually are given and must be taken for the rest of the patient's life.

For six to eight weeks after the transplant surgery, patients usually come back to the transplant center twice a week for physical examinations and medical tests. These tests check for any signs of infection, rejection of the new heart, or other complications.

In addition to **physical examination**, the following tests may be done during these visits:

- laboratory tests to check for infection
- chest x ray to check for early signs of lung infection
- electrocardiogram (ECG) to check heart function
- echocardiogram to check the function of the ventricles in the heart
- blood tests to check liver and kidney function
- complete blood counts (CBC) to check the numbers of blood cells
- taking of a small tissue sample from the donor heart (endomyocardial biopsy) to check for signs of rejection.

During the physical examination, the blood pressure is checked and the heart sounds are listened to with a stethoscope to determine if the heart is beating properly and pumping enough blood. Kidney and liver function are checked because these organs may lose function if the heart is being rejected.

An endomyocardial biopsy is the removal of a small sample of the heart muscle. This is done with a very small instrument that is inserted through an artery or vein and into the heart. The heart muscle tissue is examined under a microscope for signs that the heart is being rejected. Endomyocardial biopsy is usually done weekly for the first four to eight weeks after transplant surgery and then at longer intervals after that.

Risks

The most common and dangerous complications of heart transplant surgery are organ rejection and infection. Immunosuppressive drugs are given to prevent rejection of the heart. Most heart transplant patients have a rejection episode soon after transplantation, but doctors usually diagnose it immediately when it will respond readily to treatment. Rejection is treated with combinations of immunosuppressive drugs given in higher doses than maintenance immunosuppression. Most of these rejection situations are successfully treated.

Infection can result from the surgery, but most infections are a side effect of the immunosuppressive drugs. Immunosuppressive drugs keep the immune system from attacking the foreign cells of the donor heart. However, the suppressed immune cells are also unable to adequately fight bacteria, viruses, and other microorganisms. Microorganisms that normally do not affect persons with healthy immune systems can cause dangerous infections in transplant patients taking immunosuppressive drugs.

Patients are given antibiotics during surgery to prevent bacterial infection. Patients may also be given an antiviral drug to prevent virus infections. Patients who develop infections may need to have their immunosuppressive drugs changed or the dose adjusted. Infections are treated with antibiotics or other drugs, depending on the type of infection.

Other complications that can happen immediately after surgery are:

- bleeding
- pressure on the heart caused by fluid in the space surrounding the heart (pericardial tamponade)
- irregular heart beats
- reduced cardiac output
- increased amount of blood in the circulatory system
- decreased amount of blood in the circulatory system

About half of all heart transplant patients develop coronary artery disease 1–5 years after the transplant. The coronary arteries supply blood to the heart. Patients with this problem develop chest pains called **angina**. Other names for this complication are coronary allograft vascular disease and chronic rejection.

Outcomes

Heart transplantation is an appropriate treatment for many patients with end-stage heart failure.

KEY TERMS

Anesthesia—Loss of the ability to feel pain, caused by administration of an anesthetic drug.

Angina—Characteristic chest pain which occurs during exercise or stress in certain kinds of heart disease.

Cardiopulmonary bypass—Mechanically circulating the blood with a heart/lung machine that bypasses the heart and lungs.

Cardiovascular—Having to do with the heart and blood vessels.

Complete blood count (CBC)—A blood test to check the numbers of red blood cells, white blood cells, and platelets in the blood.

Coronary artery disease—Blockage of the arteries leading to the heart.

Crossmatch—A test to determine if patient and donor tissues are compatible.

Donor—A person who donates an organ for transplantation.

Echocardiogram—A test that visualizes and records the position and motion of the walls of the heart using ultrasound waves.

Electrocardiogram (ECG)—A test that measures electrical conduction of the heart.

End-stage heart failure—Severe heart disease that does not respond adequately to medical or surgical treatment.

Endomyocardial biopsy—Removal of a small sample of heart tissue to check it for signs of damage caused by organ rejection.

Fatigue—Loss of energy; tiredness.

Graft—A transplanted organ or other tissue.

Immunosuppressive drug—Medication used to suppress the immune system.

Inotropic drugs—Medications used to stimulate the heart beat.

Pulmonary hypertension—An increase in the pressure in the blood vessels of the lungs.

Recipient—A person who receives an organ transplant.

The outcomes of heart transplantation depend on the patient's age, health, and other factors. About 73% of heart transplant patients are alive four years after surgery.

After transplant, most patients regain normal heart function, meaning the heart pumps a normal amount of blood. A transplanted heart usually beats slightly faster than normal because the heart nerves are cut during surgery. The new heart also does not increase its rate as quickly during exercise. Even so, most patients feel much better and their capacity for **exercise** is dramatically improved from before they received the new heart. About 85% of patients return to work and other daily activities. Many are able to participate in sports.

Resources

ORGANIZATIONS

American Council on Transplantation. P.O. Box 1709, Alexandria, VA 22313. 1-800-ACT-GIVE.

Health Services and Resources Administration, Division of Organ Transplantation. Room 11A-22, 5600 Fishers Lane, Rockville, MD 20857.

United Network for Organ Sharing (UNOS). 1100 Boulders Parkway, Suite 500, P.O. Box 13770, Richmond, VA 23225-8770. (804) 330-8500. < http://www.unos.org >.

OTHER

"What Every Patient Needs to Know." *United Network forOrgan Sharing (UNOS)*. < http://www.unos.org/ frame_Default.asp?Category = Patients >.

Toni Rizzo

Heart tumors *see* **Myxoma**

Heart valve repair

Definition

Heart valve repair is a surgical procedure used to correct a malfunctioning heart valve. Repair usually involves separating the valve leaflets (the one-way "doors" of the heart valve which open and close to pump blood through the heart) or forcing them open with a balloon catheter, a technique known as *balloon valvuloplasty*.

Purpose

To correct damage to the mitral, aortic, pulmonary, or tricuspid heart valves caused by a systemic infection, **endocarditis**, rheumatic heart disease, a congenital heart defect, or mitral and/or aortic valve disease. Damaged valves may not open properly (stenosis) or they may not close adequately (valve regurgitation, insufficiency, or incompetence).

Precautions

Patients who have a diseased heart valve that is badly scarred or calcified may be better candidates for valve replacement surgery.

Description

Heart valve repair is performed in a hospital setting by a cardiac surgeon. During valve repair surgery, the patient's heart is stopped, and his/her blood is circulated outside of the body through an *extracorporeal bypass circuit*, also called heart-lung machine or just "the pump." The extracorporeal circuit consists of tubing and medical devices that take over the function of the patient's heart and lungs during the procedure. As blood passes through the circuit, carbon dioxide is removed from the bloodstream and replaced with oxygen. The oxygenated blood is then returned to the body. Other components may also be added to the circuit to filter fluids from the blood or concentrate red blood cells.

In cases of valve disease where the leaflets have become fused together, a procedure known as a valvulotomy is performed. In valvulotomy, the leaflets of the valves are surgically separated, or partially resected, with an incision to increase the size of the valve opening. The surgeon may also make adjustments to the chordae, the cord-like tissue that connects the valve leaflets to the ventricle muscles, to improve valve function.

Another valve repair technique, **balloon valvuloplasty**, is used in patients with pulmonary, aortic, and **mitral valve stenosis** to force open the valve. Valvuloplasty is similar to a cardiac **angioplasty** procedure in that it involves the placement of a balloon-tipped catheter into the heart. Once inserted into the valve, the balloon is inflated and the valve dilates, or opens. Valvuloplasty does not require a bypass circuit.

Preparation

A number of diagnostic tests may be administered prior to valve repair surgery. **Magnetic resonance imaging** (MRI), echocardiogram, angiogram, and/or scintigram are used to help the surgeon get an accurate picture of the extent of damage to the heart valve and the status of the coronary arteries.

Aftercare

The patient's blood pressure and vital signs will be carefully monitored following a valve repair procedure, and he or she watched closely for signs of edema or congestive **heart failure**.

Echocardiography or other diagnostic tests are ordered for the patient at some point during or after surgery to evaluate valvular function. A **cardiac rehabilitation** program may also be recommended to assist the patient in improving **exercise** tolerance after the procedure.

Risks

As with any invasive surgical procedure, hemorrhage, infarction, **stroke**, **heart attack**, and infection are all possible complications of heart valve repair. The overall risks involved with the surgery depend largely on the complexity of the procedure and physical condition of the patient.

Normal results

Ideally, a successful heart valve repair procedure will return heart function to age-appropriate levels. If valvuloplasty is performed, a follow-up valve repair or replacement surgery may be necessary at a later date.

Resources

BOOKS

DeBakey, Michael E., and Antonio Gotto, Jr. *The New Living Heart.* Holbrook, MA: Adams Media Corporation, 1997.

Paula Anne Ford-Martin

Heart valve replacement

Definition

Heart valve replacement is a surgical procedure during which surgeons remove a damaged valve from the heart and substitute a healthy one.

Purpose

Four valves direct blood to and from the body through the heart: the aortic valve, the pulmonic valve, the tricuspid valve, and the mitral valve. Any of these valves may malfunction because of a birth defect, infection, disease, or trauma. When the malfunction is so severe that it interferes with blood flow, an individual will have heart **palpitations**, **fainting** spells, and/or difficulty breathing. These symptoms will progressively worsen and cause **death** unless the damaged valve is replaced surgically.

Precautions

Abnormal tricuspid valves usually are not replaced because they do not cause serious symptoms. Mildly or even moderately diseased mitral valves may not need to be replaced because their symptoms are tolerable or they can be treated with such drugs as beta blockers or calcium antagonists, which slow the heart rate. However, a severely diseased mitral valve should be repaired or replaced unless the person is too ill to tolerate the operation because of another condition or illness.

Description

After cutting through and separating the breastbone and ribs, surgeons place the patient on a cardio-pulmonary bypass machine, which will perform the functions of the heart and lungs during the operation. They then open the heart and locate the faulty valve. Slicing around the edges of the valve, they loosen it from the tendons that connect it to the rest of the heart and withdraw it. The new valve is inserted and sutured into place. The patient is then taken off the bypass machine and the chest is closed. The surgery takes three to five hours and is covered by most insurance plans.

There are three types of replacement valves. One class is made from animal tissue, usually a pig's aortic valve. Another is mechanical and is made of metal and plastic. The third, includes human valves that have been removed from an organ donor or that, rarely, are the patient's own pulmonic valve.

There is no single ideal replacement valve. The choice between an animal valve or a mechanical valve depends largely on the age of the patient. Because valves obtained from animals have a life expectancy of 7–15 years, they usually are given to older patients. Mechanical valves are used in younger patients because they are more durable. Because mechanical valves are made of foreign material, however, **blood clots** can form on their surface. Therefore, patients who receive these valves must take anticoagulants the rest of their lives.

Donor or pulmonic valves are given only to those patients who will deteriorate rapidly because of a narrowing of the passageway between the aorta and the left ventrical (aortic stenosis). These valves are limited in their use because of the small supply available from donors and the strain that could be caused by removing and transferring a patient's own pulmonic valve.

Preparation

Before patients undergo heart valve replacement, they must be evaluated carefully for any signs that they may not tolerate the surgery.

Preoperative tests include:

- electrocardiography, which assesses the electrical activity of the heart
- echocardiography, which uses sound waves to show the extent of the obstruction of blood flow through the heart and determine the degree of loss of heart function due to the malfunctioning valve
- chest x ray, which provides an overall view of the anatomy of the heart and the lungs

Cardiac catheterization may also be performed to further asses the valve and to determine if coronary bypass surgery should also be done.

Aftercare

A patient usually spends one to three days in the hospital intensive care unit (ICU) after heart valve replacement so that the working of his or her heart and circulation can be monitored closely. When first brought to the ICU after surgery, the patient undergoes a neurological examination to be sure he or she has not suffered a **stroke**. The patient continues to breathe by means of a tube inserted in the trachea at the time of surgery. This mechanical ventilation is not withdrawn until the patient is fully awake from anesthesia, shows signs that he or she can breathe

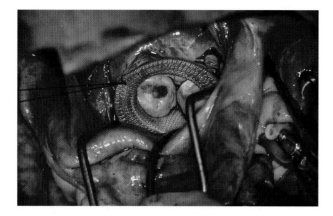

Open heart surgery showing replacement of a valve. *(Photograph by David Leah. Photo Researchers. Reproduced by permission.)*

satisfactorily without mechanical support, and has steadfast circulation.

Once stablilized, the patient is transferred to a standard medical/surgical unit where he or she receives drugs that will prevent excess fluid from building up around the heart. As soon as possible, the patient begins walking and exercising to regain strength. He or she is also placed on a diet that is low in salt and cholesterol.

After being released from the hospital, the patient continues a daily **exercise** program that includes vigorous walking, and he or she may also join a recommended **cardiac rehabilitation** program. He or she usually can return to work or other normal activities within two months of the surgery.

Risks

Complications following heart valve replacement are not common, but can be serious. All valves made from animal tissue will develop calcium deposits over time. If these deposits hamper the function of the valve, it must be replaced. Valves may become dislodged. Blood clots may form on the surface of the substitute valve, break off into the general circulation, and become wedged in an artery supplying blood to the brain, kidneys, or legs. These blood clots may cause fainting spells, stroke, kidney failure, or loss of circulation to the legs. These blood clots can be treated with drugs or surgery.

Infection of heart muscle affects up to 2% of patients who have heart valve replacement. Such an infection is treated with intravenous **antibiotics**. If the infection persists, the new valve may have to be replaced.

Anticoagulants—Drugs that prevent blood clots from forming.

Aortic valve—A fold in the channel leading from the aorta to the left ventricle of the heart. The aortic valve directs blood flow that has received oxygen from the lungs to the aorta which transmits blood to the rest of the body.

Cardiac catheterization—A thin tube called a catheter is inserted into an artery or vein in the leg, groin or arm. The catheter tube is carefully threaded into the area of the heart needing surgical repair. A local anaesthesia is used at the insertion sites.

Cardiopulmonary bypass machine—A mechanical instrument that takes over the circulation of the body while heart surgery is taking place.

Echocardiography—A diagnostic instrument that assesses the structure of the heart using sound waves.

Electrocardiography—A diagnostic instrument that evaluates the function of the heart by measuring the electrical activity generated by the beating of the heart.

Mitral valve—A fold in between the left atrium and the left ventricle of the heart that directs blood that has received oxygen from the lungs to the aortic valve and the aorta.

Pulmonic valve—A fold in the pulmonary artery that directs blood to the lungs. It may be transferred to replace a severely diseased aortic valve during heart valve replacement surgery for aortic stenosis.

Tricuspid valve—A fold in between the right atrium and the right ventricle of the heart that directs blood that needs oxygen to the lungs.

Normal results

Few patients die as a result of the surgery. Approximately 3% of all patients die during or immediately after heart valve replacement, and less than 1% of patients below the age of 65 die because of the operation. The vast majority of patients who have heart valve replacement return to normal activity after the surgery. Depending on the type of valve they receive, these patients will have no symptoms of valve abnormality for at least seven years. Also, their quality of life will improve because they may no longer have difficulty breathing, fainting spells, or palpitations.

Resources

BOOKS

American Heart Association. *American HeartAssociation's Your Heart: An Owner's Manual.* Englewood Cliffs, NJ: Prentice Hall, 1991.

ORGANIZATIONS

The American College of Cardiology. 9111 Old Georgetown Road, Bethesda, MD 20814. (800) 253-4636. <http://www.acc.org>.

American College of Surgeons. 55 E. Erie St., Chicago, IL 60611. (312) 202-5000. <http://www.facs.org>.

American Heart Association. 7320 Greenville Ave. Dallas, TX 75231. (214) 373-6300. <http://www.americanheart.org>.

Karen Marie Sandrick

Heartburn

Definition

Heartburn is a burning sensation in the chest that can extend to the neck, throat, and face; it is worsened by bending or lying down. It is the primary symptom of gastroesophageal reflux, which is the movement of stomach acid into the esophagus. On rare occasions, it is due to gastritis (stomach lining inflammation).

Description

More than one-third of the population is afflicted by heartburn, with about one-tenth afflicted daily. Infrequent heartburn is usually without serious consequences, but chronic or frequent heartburn (recurring more than twice per week) can have severe consequences. Accordingly, early management is important.

Understanding heartburn depends on understanding the structure and action of the esophagus. The esophagus is a tube connecting the throat to the stomach. It is about 10 in (25 cm) long in adults, lined with squamous (plate-like) epithelial cells, coated with mucus, and surrounded by muscles that push food to the stomach by sequential waves of contraction (peristalsis). The lower esophageal sphincter (LES) is a thick band of muscles that encircles the esophagus just above the uppermost part of the stomach. This sphincter is usually tightly closed and normally opens only when food passes from the esophagus into the stomach. Thus, the contents of the stomach are normally kept from moving back into the esophagus.

The stomach has a thick mucous coating that protects it from the strong acid it secretes into its interior when food is present, but the much thinner esophageal coating doesn't provide protection against acid. Thus, if the LES opens inappropriately or fails to close completely, and stomach contents leak into the esophagus, the esophagus can be burned by acid. The resulting burning sensation is called heartburn.

Occasional heartburn has no serious long-lasting effects, but repeated episodes of gastroesophageal reflux can ultimately lead to esophageal inflammation (esophagitis) and other damage. If episodes occur more frequently than twice a week, and the esophagus is repeatedly subjected to acid and digestive enzymes from the stomach, ulcerations, scarring, and thickening of the esophagus walls can result. This thickening of the esophagus wall causes a narrowing of the interior of the esophagus. Such narrowing affects swallowing and peristaltic movements. Repeated irritation can also result in changes in the types of cells that line the esophagus. The condition associated with these changes is termed Barrett's syndrome and can lead to **esophageal cancer**.

Causes and symptoms

Causes

A number of different factors may contribute to LES malfunction with its consequent gastroesophageal acid reflux:

- The eating of large meals that distend the stomach can cause the LES to open inappropriately.

- Lying down within two to three hours of eating can cause the LES to open.

- Obesity, **pregnancy**, and tight clothing can impair the ability of the LES to stay closed by putting pressure on the abdomen.

- Certain drugs, notably nicotine, alcohol, diazepam (Valium), meperidine (Demerol), theophylline, morphine, prostaglandins, calcium channel blockers, nitrate heart medications, anticholinergic and adrenergic drugs (drugs that limit nerve reactions), including dopamine, can relax the LES.

- Progesterone is thought to relax the LES.

- Greasy foods and some other foods such as chocolate, coffee, and peppermint can relax the LES.

- Paralysis and **scleroderma** can cause the LES to malfunction.

- Hiatus **hernia** may also cause heartburn according to some gastroenterologists. (Hiatus hernia is a protrusion of part of the stomach through the diaphragm to a position next to the esophagus.)

Symptoms

Heartburn itself is a symptom. Other symptoms also caused by gastroesophageal reflux can be associated with heartburn. Often heartburn sufferers salivate excessively or regurgitate stomach contents into their mouths, leaving a sour or bitter taste. Frequent gastroesophageal reflux leads to additional complications including difficult or painful swallowing, sore throat, hoarseness, coughing, **laryngitis**, **wheezing**, **asthma**, **pneumonia**, gingivitis, **bad breath**, and earache.

Diagnosis

Gastroenterologists and internists are best equipped to diagnose and treat gastroesophageal reflux. Diagnosis is usually based solely on patient histories that report heartburn and other related symptoms. Additional diagnostic procedures can confirm the diagnosis and assess damage to the esophagus, as well as monitor healing progress. The following diagnostic procedures are appropriate for anyone who has frequent, chronic, or difficult-to-treat heartburn or any of the complicating symptoms noted in the previous paragraph.

X rays taken after a patient swallows a barium suspension can reveal esophageal narrowing, ulcerations or a reflux episode as it occurs. However, this procedure cannot detect the structural changes associated with different degrees of esophagitis. This diagnostic procedure has traditionally been called the "upper GI series" or "barium swallow" and costs about $250.00.

Esophagoscopy is a newer procedure that uses a thin flexible tube to view the inside of the esophagus directly. It should be done by a gastroenterologist or gastrointestinal endoscopist and costs about $700. It gives an accurate picture of any damage present and gives the physician the ability to distinguish between different degrees of esophagitis.

Other tests may also be used. They include pressure measurements of the LES; measurements of esophageal acidity (pH), usually throughout a 24-hour period; and microscopic examination of biopsied tissue from the esophageal wall (to inspect esophageal cell structure for Barrett's syndrome and malignancies).

New technology introduced by 2003 allows for continuous monitoring of pH levels to help determine the cause. A tiny wireless capsule can be delivered to the lining of the esophagus through a catheter and data recorder on a device the size of a pager that is clipped to the patient's belt or purse for 48 hours. The capsule eventually sloughs off and passes harmlessly through the gastrointestinal tract in seven to 10 days.

Note: A burning sensation in the chest is usually heartburn and is not associated with the heart. However, chest **pain** that radiates into the arms and is not accompanied by regurgitation is a warning of a possible serious heart problem. Anyone with these symptoms should contact a doctor immediately.

Treatment

Drugs

Occasional heartburn is probably best treated with over-the-counter **antacids**. These products go straight to the esophagus and immediately begin to decrease acidity. However, they should not be used as the sole treatment for heartburn sufferers who either have two or more episodes per week or who suffer for periods of more than three weeks. There is a risk of kidney damage and other metabolic changes.

H2 blockers (histamine receptor blockers, such as Pepsid AC, Zantac, Tagamet) decrease stomach acid production and are effective against heartburn. H2 blocker treatment also allows healing of esophageal damage but is not very effective when there is a high degree of damage. It takes 30–45 minutes for these drugs to take effect, so they must be taken prior to an episode. Thus, they should be taken daily, usually two to four times per day for several weeks. Six to 12 weeks of standard-dose treatment relieves symptoms in about one-half the patients. Higher doses relieve symptoms in a greater fraction of the population, but at least 25% of heartburn sufferers are not helped by H2 blockers.

Proton-pump inhibitors also inhibit acid production by the stomach, but are much more effective than H2 blockers for some people. They are also more effective in aiding the healing process. Esophagitis is healed in about 90% of the patients undergoing proton-pump inhibitor treatment.

The long-term effects of inhibiting stomach acid production are unknown. Without the antiseptic effects of a consistently very acidic stomach environment, users of H2 blockers or proton-pump inhibitors may become more susceptible to bacterial and viral infection. Absorption of some drugs is also lowered by this less-acidic environment.

Prokinetic agents (also known as motility drugs) act on the LES, stimulating it to close more tightly, thereby keeping stomach contents out of the

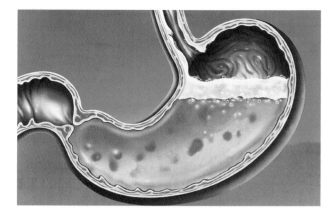

An illustration of foaming antacid on top of the contents of a human stomach. Heartburn is caused by a backflow of the stomach's acidic contents into the esophagus, causing inflammation and a sense of pain that can rise to the throat. *(Illustration by John Bavosi, Custom Medical Stock Photo. Reproduced by permission.)*

esophagus. It is not known how effectively these drugs promote healing. Some of the early motility drugs had serious neurological side effects, but a newer drug, cisapride, seems to act only on digestive system nerve connections.

Surgery

Fundoplication, a surgical procedure to increase pressure on the LES by stretching and wrapping the upper part of the stomach around the sphincter, is a treatment of last resort. About 10% of heartburn sufferers undergo this procedure. It is not always effective and its effectiveness may decrease over time, especially several years after surgery. Dr. Robert Marks and his colleagues at the University of Alabama reported in 1997 on the long-term outcome of this procedure. They found that 64% of the patients in their study who had fundoplication between 1992 and 1995 still suffered from heartburn and reported an impaired quality of life after the surgery.

However, **laparoscopy** (an examination of the interior of the abdomen by means of the laparoscope) now provides hope for better outcomes. Fundoplication performed with a laparoscope is less invasive. Five small incisions are required instead of one large incision. Patients recover faster, and it is likely that studies will show they suffer from fewer surgical complications.

Alternative treatment

Prevention, as outlined below, is a primary feature for heartburn management in alternative medicine and traditional medicine. Dietary adjustments can eliminate many causes of heartburn.

Herbal remedies include bananas, aloe vera gel, chamomile (*Matricaria recutita*), ginger (*Zingiber officinale*), and citrus juices, but there is little agreement here. For example, ginger, which seems to help some people, is claimed by other practitioners to *cause* heartburn and is thought to relax the LES. There are also many recommendations to *avoid* citrus juices, which are themselves acidic. Licorice (*Glycyrrhiza uralensis*) can help relieve the symptoms of heartburn by reestablishing balance in the acid output of the stomach.

Several homeopathic remedies are useful in treating heartburn symptoms. Among those most often recommended are *Nux vomica, Carbo vegetabilis*, and *Arsenicum album*. **Acupressure** and acupuncture may also be helpful in treating heartburn.

Sodium bicarbonate (baking soda) is an inexpensive alternative to use as an antacid. It reduces esophageal acidity immediately, but its effect is not long-lasting and should not be used by people on sodium-restricted **diets**.

Prognosis

The prognosis for people who get heartburn only occasionally or people without esophageal damage is excellent. The prognosis for people with esophageal damage who become involved in a treatment program that promotes healing is also excellent. The prognosis for anyone with esophageal **cancer** is very poor. There is a strong likelihood of a painful illness and a less than 5% chance of surviving more than five years.

Prevention

Given the lack of completely satisfactory treatments for heartburn or its consequences and the lack of a cure for esophageal cancer, prevention is of the utmost importance. Proponents of traditional *and* alternative medicine agree that people disposed to heartburn should:

- avoid eating large meals
- avoid alcohol, **caffeine**, fatty foods, fried foods, hot or spicy foods, chocolate, peppermint, and nicotine
- avoid drugs known to contribute to heartburn, such as nitrates (heart medications such as Isonate and Nitrocap), **calcium channel blockers** (e.g., Cardizem and Procardia), and anticholinergic drugs (e.g., Probanthine and Bentyl), and check with their doctors about any drugs they are taking

KEY TERMS

Barrett's syndrome—Also called Barrett's esophagus or Barrett's epithelia, this is a condition where the squamous epithelial cells that normally line the esophagus are replaced by thicker columnar epithelial cells.

Digestive enzymes—Molecules that catalyze the breakdown of large molecules (usually food) into smaller molecules.

Esophagitis—Inflammation of the esophagus.

Fundoplication—A surgical procedure that increases pressure on the LES by stretching and wrapping the upper part of the stomach around the sphincter.

Gastroesophageal reflux—The flow of stomach contents into the esophagus.

Hiatus hernia—A protrusion of part of the stomach through the diaphragm to a position next to the esophagus.

Metabolic—Refers to the chemical reactions in living things.

Mucus—Thick, viscous, gel-like material that functions to moisten and protect inner body surfaces.

Peristalsis—A sequence of muscle contractions that progressively squeeze one small section of the digestive tract and then the next to push food along the tract, something like pushing toothpaste out of its tube.

Scleroderma—An autoimmune disease with many consequences, including esophageal wall thickening.

Squamous epithelial cells—Thin, flat cells found in layers or sheets covering surfaces such as skin and the linings of blood vessels and esophagus.

Ulceration—An open break in surface tissue.

- avoid clothing that fits tightly around the abdomen
- control body weight
- wait about three hours after eating before going to bed or lying down
- elevate the head of the bed 6–9 inches to alleviate heartburn at night. This can be done with bricks under the bed or with a wedge designed for this purpose.

Preventing heartburn's switch to cancer begins with preventing heartburn in the first place. A study in Great Britain in 2004 also looked at using a combination of **aspirin** and an anti-ulcer drug to try to prevent Barrett's esophagus from forming in patients with long-term heartburn. Aspirin has been found in previous studies to reduce cases of esophageal cancer. However, since one of its side effects is an increased risk of stomach ulcers, the researchers were including an effective anti-ulcer drug for participants.

Resources

PERIODICALS

"Aspirin Trial Launched to Block Heartburn's Switch to Cancer." *Drug Week* January 23, 2004:188.

Bealfsky, Peter C., and William Halsey. "An Endoscopic View of a Wireless pH–Monitoring Capsule." *Ear, Nose and Throat Journal* April 2003: 254.

ORGANIZATIONS

The American College of Gastroenterology (ACG). PO Box 3099, Alexandria, VA 22302. (800) HRT-BURN. < http://www.healthtouch.com >.

The American Gastroenterological Association (AGA). 7910 Woodmont Ave., 7th Floor, Bethesda, MD 20814. (310) 654-2055. < http://www.gastro.org/index.html >.

American Society for Gastrointestinal Endoscopy. 13 Elm St., Manchester, MA 01944. (508) 526-8330. < http:// www.asge.org/doc/201 >.

National Digestive Diseases Information Clearinghouse. 2 Information Way, Bethesda, MD 20892-3570. (800) 891-5389. < http://www.niddk.nih.gov/health/ digest/nddic.htm >.

Lorraine Lica, PhD
Teresa G. Odle

Heat cramps *see* **Heat disorders**

Heat disorders

Definition

Heat disorders are a group of physically related illnesses caused by prolonged exposure to hot temperatures, restricted fluid intake, or failure of temperature regulation mechanisms of the body. Disorders of heat exposure include heat cramps, heat exhaustion, and heat **stroke** (also called sunstroke). Hyperthermia is the general name given to heat-related illnesses. The two most common forms of hyperthermia are heat exhaustion and heat stroke, which is especially dangerous and requires immediate medical attention.

Description

Heat disorders are harmful to people of all ages, but their severity is likely to increase as people age. Heat cramps in a 16-year-old may be heat exhaustion in a 45-year-old and heat stroke in a 65-year-old. The body's temperature regulating mechanisms rely on the thermal regulating centers in the brain. Through these complex centers, the body tries to adapt to high temperatures by adjusting the amount of salt in the perspiration. Salt helps the cells in body tissues retain water. In hot weather, a healthy body will lose enough water to cool the body while creating the lowest level of chemical imbalance. Regardless of extreme weather conditions, the healthy human body keeps a steady temperature of approximately 98.6 °F (37 °C). In hot weather, or during vigorous activity, the body perspires. As perspiration evaporates from the skin, the body is cooled. If the body loses too much salt and fluids, the symptoms of **dehydration** can occur.

Heat cramps

Heat cramps are the least severe of the heat-related illnesses. This heat disorder is often the first signal that the body is having difficulty with increased temperature. Individuals exposed to excessive heat should think of heat cramps as a warning sign to a potential heat-related emergency.

Heat exhaustion

Heat exhaustion is a more serious and complex condition than heat cramps. Heat exhaustion can result from prolonged exposure to hot temperatures, restricted fluid intake, or failure of temperature regulation mechanisms of the body. It often affects athletes, firefighters, construction workers, factory workers, and anyone who wears heavy clothing in hot humid weather.

Heat stroke

Heat exhaustion can develop rapidly into heat stroke. Heat stroke can be life threatening and because the percentage of victims dying from heat stroke is very high, immediate medical attention is critical when problems first begin. Heat stroke, like heat exhaustion, is also a result of prolonged exposure to hot temperatures, restricted fluid intake, or failure of temperature regulation mechanisms of the body. However, the severity of impact on the body is much greater with heat stroke.

Causes and symptoms

Heat cramps

Heat cramps are painful **muscle spasms** caused by the excessive loss of salts (electrolytes), due to heavy perspiration. The muscle tissue becomes less flexible, causing **pain**, difficult movement, and involuntary tightness. Heavy exertion in extreme heat, restricted fluid intake, or failure of temperature regulation mechanisms of the body may lead to heat cramps. This disorder occurs more often in the legs and abdomen than in other areas of the body. Individuals at higher risk are those working in extreme heat, elderly people, young children, people with health problems, and those who are unable to naturally and properly cool their bodies. Individuals with poor circulation and who take medications to reduce excess body fluids can be at risk when conditions are hot and humid.

Heat exhaustion

Heat exhaustion is caused by exposure to high heat and humidity for many hours, resulting in excessive loss of fluids and salts through heavy perspiration. The skin may appear cool, moist, and pale. The individual may complain of **headache** and nausea with a feeling of overall weakness and exhaustion. Dizziness, faintness, and mental confusion are often present, as is rapid and weak pulse. Breathing becomes fast and shallow. Fluid loss reduces blood volume and lowers blood pressure. Yellow or orange urine often is a result of inadequate fluid intake, along with associated intense thirst. Insufficient water and salt intake or a deficiency in the production of sweat place an individual at high risk for heat exhaustion.

Heat stroke

Heat stroke is caused by overexposure to extreme heat, resulting in a breakdown in the body's heat regulating mechanisms. The body's temperature reaches a dangerous level, as high as 106 °F (41.1 °C). An individual with heat stroke has a body temperature higher than 104 °F (40 °C). Other symptoms include mental confusion with possible combativeness and bizarre behavior, staggering, and faintness.

The pulse becomes strong and rapid (160–180 beats per minute) with the skin taking on a dry and flushed appearance. There is often very little perspiration. The individual can quickly lose consciousness or have convulsions. Before heat stroke, an individual suffers from heat exhaustion and the associated symptoms. When the body can no longer maintain a normal temperature, heat exhaustion becomes heat stroke.

Heat stroke is a life-threatening medical emergency that requires immediate initiation of life-saving measures.

Diagnosis

The diagnosis of heat cramps usually involves the observation of individual symptoms such as muscle cramping and thirst. Diagnosis of heat exhaustion or heat stroke, however, may require a physician to review the medical history, document symptoms, and obtain a blood pressure and temperature reading. The physician may also take blood and urine samples for further laboratory testing. A test to measure the body's electrolytes can also give valuable information about chemical imbalances caused by the heat-related illness.

Treatment

Heat cramps

The care of heat cramps includes placing the individual at rest in a cool environment, while giving cool water with a teaspoon of salt per quart, or a commercial sports drink. Usually rest and liquids are all that is needed for the patient to recover. Mild stretching and massaging of the muscle area follows once the condition improves. The individual should not take salt tablets, since this may actually worsen the condition. When the cramps stop, the person can usually start activity again if there are no other signs of illness. The individual needs to continue drinking fluids and should be watched carefully for further signs of heat-related illnesses.

Heat exhaustion

The individual suffering from heat exhaustion should stop all physical activity and move immediately to a cool place out of the sun, preferably a cool, air-conditioned location. She or he should then lay down with feet slightly elevated, remove or loosen clothing, and drink cold (but not iced), slightly salty water or commercial sports drink. Rest and replacement of fluids and salt is usually all the treatment that is needed, and hospitalization is rarely required. Following rehydration, the person usually recovers rapidly.

Heat stroke

Simply moving the individual afflicted with heat stroke to a cooler place is not enough to reverse the internal overheating. Emergency medical assistance

should be called immediately. While waiting for help to arrive, quick action to lower body temperature must take place. Treatment involves getting the victim to a cool place, loosening clothes or undressing the heat stroke victim, and allowing air to circulate around the body. The next important step is wrapping the individual in wet towels or clothing, and placing ice packs in areas with the greatest blood supply. These areas include the neck, under the arm and knees, and in the groin. Once the patient is under medical care, **cooling treatments** may continue as appropriate. The victim's body temperature will be monitored constantly to guard against overcooling. Breathing and heart rate will be monitored closely, and fluids and electrolytes will be replaced intravenously. Anti-convulsant drugs may be given. After severe heat stroke, bed rest may be recommended for several days.

Prognosis

Prompt treatment for heat cramps is usually very effective with the individual returning to activity thereafter. Treatment of heat exhaustion usually brings full recovery in one to two days. Heatstroke is a very serious condition and its outcome depends upon general health and age. Due to the high internal temperature of heat stroke, permanent damage to internal organs is possible.

Prevention

Because heat cramps, heat exhaustion, and heat stroke have a cascade effect on each other, the prevention of the onset of all heat disorders is similar. Avoid strenuous **exercise** when it is very hot. Individuals exposed to extreme heat conditions should drink plenty of fluids. Wearing light and loose-fitting clothing in hot weather is important, regardless of the activity. It is important to consume water often and not to wait until thirst develops. If perspiration is excessive, fluid intake should be increased. When urine output decreases, fluid intake should also increase. Eating lightly salted foods can help replace salts lost through perspiration. Ventilation in any working areas in warm weather must be adequate. This can be achieved as simply as opening a window or using an electric fan. Proper ventilation will promote adequate sweat evaporation to cool the skin. Sunblocks and **sunscreens** with a protection factor of 15 (SPF 15) can be very helpful when one is exposed to extreme direct sunlight.

Resources

OTHER

Griffith, H. Winter. "Complete Guide to Symptoms, Illness & Surgery." ThriveOnline. < http:// thriveonline.oxygen.com >.

Jeffrey P. Larson, RPT

Heat exhaustion *see* **Heat disorders**

Heat treatments

Definition

Heat treatments are applications of therapeutic thermal agents to specific body areas experiencing injury or dysfunction.

Purpose

The general purpose of a heat treatment is to increase the extensibility of soft tissues, remove toxins from cells, enhance blood flow, increase function of the tissue cells, encourage muscle relaxation, and help relieve **pain**. There are two types of heat treatments: superficial and deep. Superficial heat treatments apply heat to the outside of the body. Deep heat treatments direct heat toward specific inner tissues through ultrasound or by electric current. Heat treatments are beneficial prior to exercise, providing a warm-up effect to the soft tissues involved.

Precautions

Heat treatments should not be used on individuals with circulation problems, heat intolerance, or lack of

sensation in the affected area. Low blood circulation may contribute to heat-related injuries. Heat treatments also should not be used on individuals afflicted with heart, lung, or kidney diseases. Deep heat treatments should not be used on areas above the eye, heart, or on a pregnant patient. Deep heat treatments over areas with metal surgical implants should be avoided in case of rapid temperature increase and subsequent injury.

Description

There are four different ways to convey heat:

- Conduction is the transfer of heat between two objects in direct contact with each other.
- Conversion is the transition of one form of energy to heat.
- Radiation involves the transmission and absorption of electromagnetic waves to produce a heating effect.
- Convection occurs when a liquid or gas moves past a body part creating heat.

Hot packs, water bottles, and heating pads

Hot packs are a very common form of heat treatment utilizing conduction as a form of heat transfer. Moist heat packs are readily available in most hospitals, physical therapy centers, and athletic training rooms. Treatment temperature should not exceed 131 °F (55 °C). The pack is used over multiple layers of toweling to achieve a comfortable warming effect for approximately 30 minutes. More recently, several manufacturers have developed packs that may be warmed in a microwave over a specified amount of time prior to use.

Hot-water bottles are another form of superficial heat treatment. The bottles are filled half way with hot water between 115–125 °F (46.1–52 °C). Covered by a protective toweling, the hot-water bottle is placed on the treatment area and left until the water has cooled off.

Electrical heating pads continue to be used, however because of the need for an electrical outlet, safety and convenience become an issue.

Paraffin

Paraffin, a conductive form of superficial heat, is often used for heating uneven surfaces of the body such as the hands. It consists of melted paraffin wax and mineral oil. Paraffin placed in a small bath unit becomes solid at room temperature and is used as a liquid heat treatment when heated at 126–127.4 °F (52–53 °C). The most common form of paraffin application is called the dip and wax method. In this technique, the patient will dip eight to 12 times and then the extremity will be covered with a plastic bag and a towel for insulation. Most treatment sessions are about 20 minutes.

Hydrotherapy

Hydrotherapy is used in a form of heat treatment for many musculoskeletal disorders. The hydrotherapy tanks and pools are all generally set at warm temperatures, never exceeding 150°F (65.6°C). Because the patient often performs resistance exercises while in the water, higher water temperatures become a concern as the treatment becomes more physically draining. Because of this, many hydrotherapy baths are now being set at 95–110°F (35–43.3°C). There are also units available with moveable turbine jets, which provide a light massage effect. Hydrotherapy is helpful as a warm-up prior to **exercise**.

Fluidotherapy

Fluidotherapy is a form of heat treatment developed in the 1970s. It is a dry heat modality consisting of cellulose particles suspended in air. Units come in different sizes and some are restricted to only treating a hand or foot. The turbulence of the gas-solid mixture provides thermal contact with objects that are immersed in the medium. Temperatures of this treatment range from 110–123°F (43.3–50.5°C). Fluidotherapy allows the patient to exercise the limb during the treatment, and also massages the limb, increasing blood flow.

Ultrasound

Ultrasound heat treatments penetrate the body to provide relief to inner tissue. Ultrasound energy comes from the acoustic or sound spectrum and is undetectable to the human ear. By using conducting agents such as gel or mineral oil, the ultrasound transducer warms areas of the musculoskeletal system Some areas of the musculoskeletal system absorb ultrasound better that others. Muscle tissue and other connective tissue such as ligaments and tendons absorb this form of energy very well, however fat absorbs to a much lesser degree. Ultrasound has a relatively longlasting effect, continuing up to one hour.

Diathermy

Diathermy is another deep heat treatment. An electrode drum is used to apply heat to an affected area. It consists of a wire coil surrounded by dead space and other insulators such as a plastic housing. Plenty of toweling must be layered between the unit and the patient. This device is unique in that it utilizes the basis of a magnetic field on connective tissues. One advantage of diathermy over various other heat treatments is that fat does resist an electrical field, which is not the case with a magnetic field. It is found to be helpful with those experiencing chronic **low back pain** and **muscle spasms**. Prior to ultrasound technology, diathermy was a popular heat therapy of the 1940s–1960s.

Preparation

Before administering any form of heat treatment, heat sensitivity is accessed and the skin over the affected area is cleansed. When a patient is undergoing any form of heat treatment, supervision should always be present especially in the treatment of hydrotherapy.

Aftercare

Once the heat treatment has been completed, any symptoms of **dizziness** and **nausea** should be noted and documented along with any skin irritations or discoloring not present prior to the heat treatment. A one hour interval between treatments should be adhered to in order to avoid restriction of blood flow.

Risks

All heat treatments have the potential of tissue damage resulting from excessive temperatures. Proper insulation and treatment duration should be carefully administered for each method. Overexposure during a superficial heat treatment may result in redness, blisters, burns, or reduced blood circulation. During ultrasound therapy, excessive treatment over bony areas with little soft tissue (such as hand, feet, and elbow) can cause excessive heat resulting in pain and possible tissue damage. Exposure to the electrode drum during diathermy may produce hot spots.

Resources

ORGANIZATIONS

American Physical Therapy Association. 1111 North Fairfax St., Alexandria, Virginia 22314. (800) 999-2782. < https://www.apta.org >.

Jeffrey P. Larson, RPT

Heatstroke *see* **Heat disorders**

Heavy menstruation *see* **Dysfunctional uterine bleeding**

Heavy metal poisoning

Definition

Heavy metal **poisoning** is the toxic accumulation of heavy metals in the soft tissues of the body.

Description

Heavy metals are chemical elements that have a specific gravity (a measure of density) at least five times that of water. The heavy metals most often implicated in accidental human poisoning are lead, mercury, arsenic, and cadmium. More recently, thallium has gained some attention in the media as the poison used in several murder cases in the 1990s. Some heavy metals, such as zinc, copper, chromium, iron, and manganese, are required by the body in small amounts, but these same elements can be toxic in larger quantities.

Heavy metals may enter the body in food, water, or air, or by absorption through the skin. Once in the body, they compete with and displace essential **minerals** such as zinc, copper, magnesium, and calcium, and interfere with organ system function. People may come in contact with heavy metals in industrial work, pharmaceutical manufacturing, and agriculture. Children may be poisoned as a result of playing in contaminated soil. **Lead poisoning** in adults has been traced to the use of lead-based glazes on pottery vessels intended for use with food, and contamination of Ayurvedic and other imported herbal remedies. Arsenic and thallium have been mixed with food or beverages to attempt **suicide** or poison others.

Another form of mercury poisoning that is seen more and more frequently in the United States is self-injected mercury under the skin. Some boxers inject themselves with mercury in the belief that it adds muscle bulk. Metallic mercury is also used in folk medicine or religious rituals in various cultures. These practices increase the risk of mercury poisoning of children in these ethnic groups or subcultures.

Causes and symptoms

Symptoms will vary, depending on the nature and the quantity of the heavy metal ingested. Patients may complain of **nausea**, **vomiting**, **diarrhea**, stomach pain, **headache**, sweating, and a metallic taste in the mouth. Depending on the metal, there may be blue-black lines in the gum tissues. In severe cases, patients exhibit obvious impairment of cognitive, motor, and language skills. The expression "mad as a hatter" comes from the mercury poisoning prevalent in 17th-century France among hatmakers who soaked animal hides in a solution of mercuric nitrate to soften the hair.

Diagnosis

Heavy metal poisoning may be detected using blood and urine tests, hair and tissue analysis, or x ray. The diagnosis is often overlooked, however, because many of the early symptoms of heavy metal poisoning are nonspecific. The doctor should take a thorough patient history with particular emphasis on the patient's occupation.

In childhood, blood lead levels above 80 ug/dL generally indicate lead poisoning, however, significantly lower levels (>30 ug/dL) can cause **mental retardation** and other cognitive and behavioral problems in affected children. The Centers for Disease Control and Prevention considers a blood lead level of 10 ug/dL or higher in children a cause for concern. In adults, symptoms of lead poisoning are usually seen when blood lead levels exceed 80 ug/dL for a number of weeks.

Blood levels of mercury should not exceed 3.6 ug/dL, while urine levels should not exceed 15 ug/dL. Symptoms of mercury poisoning may be seen when mercury levels exceed 20 ug/dL in blood and 60 ug/dL in urine. Mercury levels in hair may be used to gauge the severity of chronic mercury exposure.

Since arsenic is rapidly cleared from the blood, blood arsenic levels may not be very useful in diagnosis. Arsenic in the urine (measured in a 24-hour collection following 48 hours without eating seafood) may exceed 50 ug/dL in people with arsenic poisoning. If acute arsenic or thallium poisoning is suspected, an x ray may reveal these substances in the abdomen (since both metals are opaque to x rays). Arsenic may also be detected in the hair and nails for months following exposure.

Cadmium toxicity is generally indicated when urine levels exceed 10 ug/dL of creatinine and blood levels exceed 5 ug/dL.

Thallium poisoning often causes hair loss (**alopecia**), **numbness**, and a burning sensation in the skin as well as nausea, vomiting, and **dizziness**. As little as 15–20 mg of thallium per kilogram of body weight is fatal in humans; however, smaller amounts can cause severe damage to the nervous system.

Treatment

When heavy metal poisoning is suspected, it is important to begin treatment as soon as possible to minimize long-term damage to the patient's nervous system and digestive tract. Heavy metal poisoning is considered a medical emergency, and the patient should be taken to a hospital emergency room.

The treatment for most heavy metal poisoning is chelation therapy. A chelating agent specific to the metal involved is given either orally, intramuscularly, or intravenously. The three most common chelating agents are calcium disodium edetate, dimercaprol (BAL), and penicillamine. The chelating agent encircles and binds to the metal in the body's tissues, forming a complex; that complex is then released from the tissue to travel in the bloodstream. The complex is filtered out of the blood by the kidneys and excreted in the urine. This process may be lengthy and painful, and typically requires hospitalization. Chelation therapy is effective in treating lead, mercury, and arsenic poisoning, but is not useful in treating cadmium poisoning. To date, no treatment has been proven effective for cadmium poisoning. Thallium poisoning is treated with a combination of Prussian blue (potassium ferric hexacyanoferrate) and a diuretic, because about 35% of it is excreted in the urine; however, if treatment is not started within 72 hours of ingesting the poisoning, damage to the patient's nervous system may be permanent.

In cases of acute mercury, arsenic, or thallium ingestion, vomiting may be induced. **Activated charcoal** may be given in cases of thallium poisoning. Washing out the stomach (gastric lavage) may also be useful. The patient may also require treatment such as intravenous fluids for such complications of poisoning as shock, anemia, and kidney failure.

Patients who have taken arsenic, thallium, or mercury in a suicide attempt will be seen by a psychiatrist as part of emergency treatment.

Prognosis

The chelation process can only halt further effects of the poisoning; it cannot reverse neurological damage already sustained.

Prevention

Because arsenic and thallium were commonly used in rat and insect poisons at one time, many countries have tried to lower the rate of accidental poisonings by banning the use of heavy metals in pest control products. Thallium was banned in the United States as a rodent poison in 1984. As a result, almost all recent cases of arsenic and thallium

---

KEY TERMS

Alopecia—Loss of hair.

Chelation—The process by which a molecule encircles and binds to a metal and removes it from tissue.

Heavy metal—One of 23 chemical elements that has a specific gravity (a measure of density) at least five times that of water.

Prussian blue—The common name of potassium ferric hexacyanoferrate, a compound approved in the United States for treatment of thallium poisoning. Prussian blue gets its name from the fact that it was first used by artists in 1704 as a dark blue pigment for oil paints. It has also been used in laundry bluing and fabric printing.

---

poisoning in the United States were deliberate rather than accidental.

Because exposure to heavy metals is often an occupational hazard, protective clothing and respirators should be provided and worn on the job. Protective clothing should then be left at the work site and not worn home, where it could carry toxic dust to family members. Industries are urged to reduce or replace the heavy metals in their processes wherever possible. Exposure to environmental sources of lead, including lead-based paints, plumbing fixtures, vehicle exhaust, and contaminated soil, should be reduced or eliminated.

People who use Ayurvedic or traditional Chinese herbal preparations as alternative treatments for various illnesses should purchase them only from reliable manufacturers.

Resources

BOOKS

Beers, Mark H., MD, and Robert Berkow, MD., editors. "Poisoning." Section 23, Chapter 307 In *The Merck Manual of Diagnosis and Therapy*. Whitehouse Station, NJ: Merck Research Laboratories, 2004.

Beers, Mark H., MD, and Robert Berkow, MD., editors. "Psychiatric Emergencies." Section 15, Chapter 194 In *The Merck Manual of Diagnosis and Therapy*. Whitehouse Station, NJ: Merck Research Laboratories, 2004.

Wilson, Billie A., Margaret T. Shannon, and Carolyn L. Stang. *Nurses Drug Guide 2000*. Stamford, CT: Appleton & Lange, 2000.

PERIODICALS

Boyarsky, Igor, DO, and Adrain D. Crisan, MD. "Toxicity, Thallium." *eMedicine* August 3, 2004. <http://www.emedicine.com/emerg/topic926.htm>.

Centers for Disease Control and Prevention (CDC). "Adult Blood Lead Epidemiology and Surveillance—United States, 2002." *Morbidity and Mortality Weekly Report* 53 (July 9, 2004): 578–582.

Counter, S. A., and L. H. Buchanan. "Mercury Exposure in Children: A Review." *Toxicology and Applied Pharmacology* 198 (July 15, 2004): 209–230.

Ferner, David J., MD. "Toxicity, Heavy Metals." *eMedicine* May 25, 2001. <http://www.emedicine.com/EMERG/topic237.htm>.

Prasad, V. L. "Subcutaneous Injection of Mercury: 'Warding Off Evil'." *Environmental Health Perspectives* 111 (September 2004): 1326–1328.

Schilling, U., R. Muck, and E. Heidemann. "Lead Poisoning after Ingestion of Ayurvedic Drugs." [in German] *Medizinische Klinik* 99 (August 15, 2004): 476–480.

Thompson, D. F., and E. D. Callen. "Soluble or Insoluble Prussian Blue for Radiocesium and Thallium Poisoning?" *Annals of Pharmacotherapy* 38 (September 2004): 1509–1514.

ORGANIZATIONS

American Society of Health-System Pharmacists (ASHP). 7272 Wisconsin Avenue, Bethesda, MD 20814. (301) 657-3000. <http://www.ashp.org>.

Centers for Disease Control and Prevention. 1600 Clifton Rd., NE, Atlanta, GA 30333. (800) 311-3435, (404) 639-3311. <http://www.cdc.gov>.

Food and Drug Administration. Office of Inquiry and Consumer Information. 5600 Fisher Lane, Room 12-A-40, Rockville, MD 20857. (301) 827-4420. <http://www.fda.gov/fdahomepage.html>.

National Institutes of Health. National Institute of Environmental Health Sciences Clearinghouse. EnviroHealth, 2605 Meridian Parkway, Suite 115, Durham, NC 27713. (919) 361-9408.

Bethany Thivierge
Rebecca J. Frey, PhD

Heel spurs

Definition

A heel spur is a bony projection on the sole (plantar) region of the heel bone (also known as the calcaneous). This condition may accompany or result from severe cases of inflammation to the structure called plantar fascia. This associated plantar fascia is a fibrous band of connective tissue on the sole of the foot, extending from the heel to the toes.

Description

Heel spurs are a common foot problem resulting from excess bone growth on the heel bone. The bone growth is usually located on the underside of the heel bone, extending forward to the toes. One explanation for this excess production of bone is a painful tearing of the plantar fascia connected between the toes and heel. This can result in either a heel spur or an inflammation of the plantar fascia, medically termed plantar fascitis. Because this condition is often correlated to a decrease in the arch of the foot, it is more prevalent after the age of six to eight years, when the arch is fully developed.

Causes and symptoms

One frequent cause of heel spurs is an abnormal motion and mal-alignment of the foot called pronation. For the foot to function properly, a certain degree of pronation is required. This motion is defined as an inward action of the foot, with dropping of the inside arch as one plants the heel and advances the weight distribution to the toes during walking. When foot pronation becomes extreme from the foot turning in and dropping beyond the normal limit, a condition known as excessive pronation creates a mechanical problem in the foot. In some cases the sole or bottom of the foot flattens and becomes unstable because of this excess pronation, especially during critical times of walking and athletic activities. The portion of the plantar fascia attached into the heel bone or calcaneous begins to stretch and pull away from the heel bone.

At the onset of this condition, **pain** and swelling become present, with discomfort particularly noted as pushing off with the toes occurs during walking. This movement of the foot stretches the fascia that is already irritated and inflamed. If this condition is allowed to continue, pain is noticed around the heel region because of the newly formed bone, in response to the **stress**. This results in the development of the heel spur. It is common among athletes and others who run and jump a significant amount.

An individual with the lower legs angulating inward, a condition called genu valgum or "knock knees," can have a tendency toward excessive pronation. As a result, this too can lead to a fallen arch resulting in plantar fascitis and heel spurs.

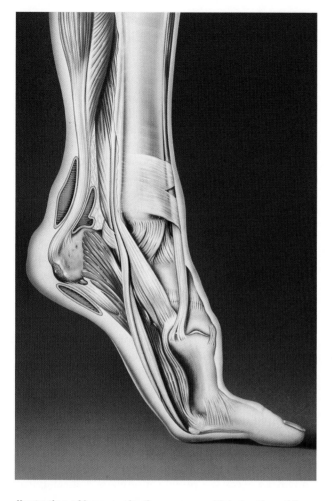

Ilustration of bony projection, a spur, which developed from chronic irritation. *(Photo Researchers. Reproduced by permission.)*

Women tend to have more genu valgum than men do. Heel spurs can also result from an abnormally high arch.

Other factors leading to heel spurs include a sudden increase in daily activities, an increase in weight, or a change of shoes. Dramatic increase in training intensity or duration may cause plantar fascitis. Shoes that are too flexible in the middle of the arch or shoes that bend before the toe joints will cause an increase in tension in the plantar fascia and possibly lead to heel spurs.

The pain this condition causes forces an individual to attempt walking on his or her toes or ball of the foot to avoid pressure on the heel spur. This can lead to other compensations during walking or running that in turn cause additional problems to the ankle, knee, hip, or back.

Diagnosis

A thorough medical history and physical exam by a physician is always necessary for the proper diagnosis of heel spurs and other foot conditions. X rays of the heel area are helpful, as excess bone production will be visible.

Treatment

Conservative

Heel spurs and plantar fascitis are usually controlled with conservative treatment. Early intervention includes stretching the calf muscles while avoiding re-injuring the plantar fascia. Decreasing or changing activities, losing excess weight, and improving the proper fitting of shoes are all important measures to decrease this common source of foot pain. Modification of footwear includes shoes with a raised heel and better arch support. Shoe orthotics recommended by a healthcare professional are often very helpful in conjunction with exercises to increase strength of the foot muscles and arch. The orthotic prevents excess pronation and lengthening of the plantar fascia and continued tearing of this structure. To aid in this reduction of inflammation, applying ice for 10–15 minutes after activities and use of anti-inflammatory medication can be helpful. Physical therapy can be beneficial with the use of heat modalities, such as ultrasound that creates a deep heat and reduces inflammation. If the pain caused by inflammation is constant, keeping the foot raised above the heart and/or compressed by wrapping with an ace bandage will help.

Corticosteroid injections are also frequently used to reduce pain and inflammation. Taping can help speed the healing process by protecting the fascia from reinjury, especially during stretching and walking.

Heel surgery

When chronic heel pain fails to respond to conservative treatment, surgical treatment may be necessary. Heel surgery can provide relief of pain and restore mobility. The type of procedure used is based on examination and usually consists of releasing the excessive tightness of the plantar fascia, called a plantar fascia release. Depending on the presence of excess bony build up, the procedure may or may not include removal of heel spurs. Similar to other surgical interventions, there are various modifications and surgical enhancements regarding surgery of the heel.

Alternative treatment

Acupuncture and accupressure have been used to address the pain of heel spurs, in addition to using friction massage to help break up scar tissue and delay onset of bony formations.

Prognosis

Usually, heel spurs are curable with conservative treatment. If not, heel spurs are curable with surgery. About 10% of those that continue to see a physician for plantar fascitis have it for more than a year. If there is limited success after approximately one year of conservative treatment, patients are often advised to have surgery.

Prevention

To prevent this condition, wearing shoes with proper arches and support is very important. Proper stretching is always a necessity, especially when there is an increase in activities or a change in running technique. It is not recommended to attempt working through the pain, as this can change a mild case of heel spurs and plantar fascitis into a long lasting and painful episode of this condition.

Resources

ORGANIZATIONS

American Orthopedic Foot and Ankle Society. 222 South Prospect, Park Ridge, IL 60068.

American Podiatry Medical Association. 9312 Old Georgetown Road, Bethesda, MD 20814.

Jeffrey P. Larson, RPT

Heimlich maneuver

Definition

The Heimlich maneuver is an emergency procedure for removing a foreign object lodged in the airway that is preventing a person from breathing.

Purpose

Every year about 3,000 adults die because they accidentally inhale rather than swallow food. The food gets stuck and blocks their trachea, making breathing impossible. **Death** follows rapidly unless the food or other foreign material can be displaced from the airway. This condition is so common it has been nicknamed the "cafe coronary."

In 1974 Dr. Henry Heimlich first described an emergency technique for expelling foreign material blocking the trachea. This technique, now called the Heimlich maneuver or abdominal thrusts, is simple enough that it can be performed immediately by anyone trained in the maneuver. The Heimlich maneuver is a standard part of all first aid courses.

The theory behind the Heimlich maneuver is that by compressing the abdomen below the level of the diaphragm, air is forced under pressure out of the lungs dislodging the obstruction in the trachea and bringing the foreign material back up into the mouth.

The Heimlich maneuver is used mainly when solid material like food, coins, vomit, or small toys are blocking the airway. There has been some controversy about whether the Heimlich maneuver is appropriate to use routinely on **near-drowning** victims. After several studies of the effectiveness of the Heimlich maneuver on reestablishing breathing in near-drowning victims, the American Red Cross and the American Heart Association both recommend that the Heimlich maneuver be used only as a last resort after traditional airway clearance techniques and **cardiopulmonary resuscitation (CPR)** have been tried repeatedly and failed or if it is clear that a solid foreign object is blocking the airway.

Precautions

Incorrect application of the Heimlich maneuver can damage the chest, ribs, and internal organs of the person on whom it is performed. People may also vomit after being treated with the Heimlich maneuver.

Description

The Heimlich maneuver can be performed on all people. Modifications are necessary if the **choking** victim is very obese, pregnant, a child, or an infant.

Indications that a person's airway is blocked include:

- The person can not speak or cry out.
- The person's face turns blue from lack of oxygen.
- The person desperately grabs at his or her throat.
- The person has a weak **cough**, and labored breathing produces a high-pitched noise.
- The person does all of the above, then becomes unconscious.

Performing the Heimlich maneuver on adults

To perform the Heimlich maneuver on a conscious adult, the rescuer stands behind the victim. The victim may either be sitting or standing. The rescuer makes a fist with one hand, and places it, thumb toward the victim, below the rib cage and above the waist. The rescuer encircles the victim's waist, placing his other hand on top of the fist.

In a series of 6–10 sharp and distinct thrusts upward and inward, the rescuer attempts to develop enough pressure to force the foreign object back up the trachea. If the maneuver fails, it is repeated. It is important not to give up if the first attempt fails. As the victim is deprived of oxygen, the muscles of the trachea relax slightly. Because of this loosening, it is possible that the foreign object may be expelled on a second or third attempt.

If the victim is unconscious, the rescuer should lay him or her on the floor, bend the chin forward, make sure the tongue is not blocking the airway, and feel in the mouth for **foreign objects**, being careful not to push any farther into the airway. The rescuer kneels astride the victim's thighs and places his fists between the bottom of the victim's breastbone and the navel. The rescuer then executes a series of 6–10 sharp compressions by pushing inward and upward.

After the abdominal thrusts, the rescuer repeats the process of lifting the chin, moving the tongue, feeling for and possibly removing the foreign material. If the airway is not clear, the rescuer repeats the abdominal thrusts as often as necessary. If the foreign object has been removed, but the victim is not breathing, the rescuer starts **CPR**.

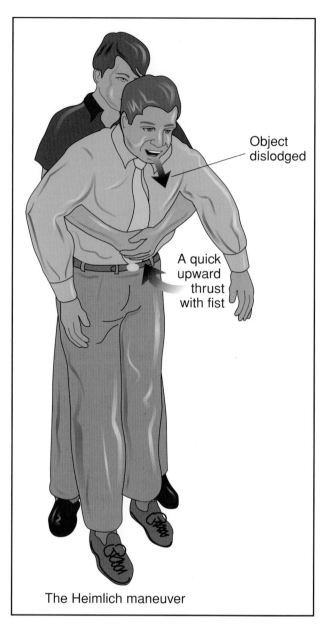

Object dislodged

A quick upward thrust with fist

The Heimlich maneuver

To perform the Heimlich maneuver on a conscious adult (as illustrated above), the rescuer stands behind the victim and encircles his waist. The rescuer makes a fist with one hand and places the other hand on top, positioned below the rib cage and above the waist. The rescuer then applies pressure by a series of upward and inward thrusts to force the foreign object back up the victim's trachea. (Illustration by Electronic Illustrators Group.)

Performing the Heimlich maneuver under special circumstances

OBVIOUSLY PREGNANT AND VERY OBESE PEOPLE. The main difference in performing the Heimlich maneuver on this group of people is in the placement of the fists. Instead of using abdominal thrusts, chest thrusts are used. The fists are placed against the middle of the breastbone, and the motion of the chest thrust is in and downward, rather than upward. If the victim is unconscious, the chest thrusts are similar to those used in CPR.

CHILDREN. The technique in children over one year of age is the same as in adults, except that the amount of force used is less than that used with adults in order to avoid damaging the child's ribs, breastbone, and internal organs.

INFANTS UNDER ONE YEAR OLD. The rescuer sits down and lays the infant along his or her forearm with the infant's face pointed toward the floor. The rescuer's hand supports the infant's head, and his or her forearm rests on his or her own thigh for additional support. Using the heel of the other hand, the rescuer administers four or five rapid blows to the infant's back between the shoulder blades.

After administering the back blows, the rescuer sandwiches the infant between his or her arms, and turns the infant over so that the infant is lying face up supported by the opposite arm. Using the free hand, the rescuer places the index and middle finger on the center of the breastbone and makes four sharp chest thrusts. This series of back blows and chest thrusts is alternated until the foreign object is expelled.

SELF-ADMINISTRATION OF THE HEIMLICH MANEUVER. To apply the Heimlich maneuver to oneself, one should make a fist with one hand and place it in the middle of the body at a spot above the navel and below the breastbone, then grasp the fist with the other hand and push sharply inward and upward. If this fails, the victim should press the upper abdomen over the back of a chair, edge of a table, porch railing or something similar, and thrust up and inward until the object is dislodged.

Preparation

Any lay person can be trained to perform the Heimlich maneuver. Knowing how may save someone's life. Before doing the maneuver, it is important to determine if the airway is completely blocked. If the person choking can talk or cry, Heimlich maneuver is not appropriate. If the airway is not completely blocked, the choking victim should be allowed to try to cough up the foreign object on his or her own.

Aftercare

Many people vomit after being treated with the Heimlich maneuver. Depending on the length and

---

KEY TERMS

Diaphragm—The thin layer of muscle that separates the chest cavity containing the lungs and heart from the abdominal cavity containing the intestines and digestive organs.

Trachea—The windpipe. A tube extending from below the voice box into the chest where it splits into two branches, the bronchi, that lead to each lung.

---

severity of the choking episode, the choking victim may need to be taken to a hospital emergency room.

Risks

Incorrectly applied, the Heimlich maneuver can break bones or damage internal organs. In infants, the rescuer should never attempt to sweep the baby's mouth without looking to remove foreign material. This is likely to push the material farther down the trachea.

Normal results

In many cases the foreign material is dislodged from the throat, and the choking victim suffers no permanent effects of the episode. If the foreign material is not removed, the person dies from lack of oxygen.

Resources

ORGANIZATIONS

American Heart Association. 7320 Greenville Ave. Dallas, TX 75231. (214) 373-6300. < http://www.americanheart.org >.

Tish Davidson, A.M.

Helicobacter pylori infection *see*
Helicobacteriosis

Helicobacteriosis

Definition

Helicobacteriosis refers to infection of the gastrointestinal tract with the bacteria, *Helicobacter pylori* (*H. pylori*). While there are other rarer strains of *Helicobacter* species that can infect humans, only

---

H. pylori has been convincingly shown to be a cause of disease in humans. The organism was first documented to cause injury to the stomach in 1983, by two researchers in Australia, who ingested the organism to prove their theory. Since then, *H. pylori* has been shown to be the main cause of ulcer disease, and has revolutionized the treatment of peptic ulcer disease. It also is believed to be linked to various cancers of the stomach.

Description

H. pylori is a gram-negative, spiral-shaped organism, that contains flagella (tail-like structures) and other properties. In addition to flagella, which help the organism to move around in the liquid mucous layer of the stomach, *H. pylori* also produces an enzyme called urease, that protects it from gastric acid present in the stomach. As the production of this enzyme is relatively unusual, new diagnostic tests have enabled rapid identification of the bacteria.

H. pylori also produces two other chemicals: a cytotoxin called vacA, and a protein known as cagA. Patients with ulcer disease are more likely to produce the cytotoxin (vacA). The cagA protein not only occurs frequently in ulcer disease but also in cancer. It is still not known how these substances enable *H. pylori* to cause disease.

Causes and symptoms

Infection with *H. pylori* is largely dependent on two factors; age and income status. The bacteria is acquired mainly in childhood, especially in areas of poor hygiene or overcrowding. *H. pylori* is two to three times more prevalent in developing, non-industrialized countries. In the United States for example, the organism is believed to be present in about one third of the population.

The exact way in which *H. pylori* gets passed from one individual to another is uncertain, but person to person transmission is most likely. In most cases, children are felt to be the source of spread. Reinfection of those who have been cured has been documented, especially in areas of overcrowding.

The bacteria is well adapted to survival within the stomach. Not only does it survive there for years, but once infection begins, a form of chronic inflammation (chronic **gastritis**) always develops. In most individuals, initial infection causes little or no symptoms; however, some individuals such as the original researchers who ingested the bacteria, wind up with abdominal **pain** and **nausea**.

In about 15% of infected persons, ulcer disease develops either in the stomach or duodenum. Why some develop ulcer disease and others do not remains unclear. Ulcer symptoms are characterized by upper abdominal pain that is typically of a burning or "gnawing" type, and usually is rapidly relieved by **antacids** or food.

Acid secretion increases in most patients with duodenal ulcers. This increase returns to normal once *H. pylori* is eliminated. It is now known that elimination of the bacteria will substantially decrease the risk of recurrent bouts of ulcer disease in the vast majority of patients. In fact, a 2003 report showed that by eradicating H. pylori, ulcer bleeding rarely recurs.

In the last decade it has been shown that *H. pylori* is not only the prime cause of ulcer disease of the stomach and duodenum, but is also strongly associated with various tumors of the stomach. Bacterial infection is nine times more common in patients with cancer of the stomach, and seven times more common in those with lymphoma of the stomach (tumor of the lymphatic tissue), called a MALT tumor. It is believed that the prolonged inflammation leads to changes in cell growth and tumors. Eliminating *H. pylori* can lead to regression of some tumors.

In addition to the above damage caused by *H. pylori*, some individuals lose normal gastric function, such as the ability to absorb vitamin B_{12}.

Diagnosis

There are basically two types of tests to identify infection: one group is "invasive" in that it involves the use of an endoscopy to obtain biopsy specimens for evaluation, while the other "noninvasive" methods depend on blood or breath samples. Invasive tests can be less accurate because of technical limitations: the biopsy may miss the area where the bacteria hides.

Invasive studies make use of tissue obtained by endoscopic biopsy to identify the organism. The bacteria can be searched for in pieces of biopsy tissue or grown (cultured) from the specimen. However, *H. pylori* is not easy to culture. Another method uses the bacteria's production of the enzyme urease. Biopsy specimens are placed on a card that changes color if urease is present. Results often are available within a few minutes, but can take up to 24 hours.

Noninvasive tests are of two types: blood tests and breath test. Blood tests measure antibodies to make a diagnosis accurately within minutes. This can be done immediately in the doctor's office. In addition,

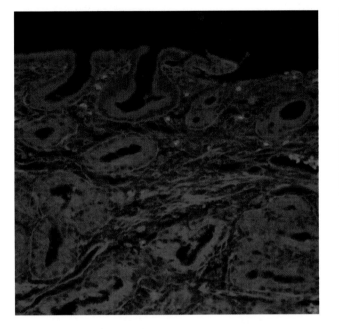

A light microscopic image of a stomach ulcer. Gastric and duodenal ulcers are usually caused by infection with the bacteria *Helicobacter pylori*. This bacterium is also believed to be a cause of various cancers of the stomach. *(Photograph by J.L. Carson, Custom Medical Stock Photo. Reproduced by permission.)*

antibody levels can be measured several months after treatment, to see if *H. pylori* has been eradicated.

The breath test uses radioactive or non-radioactive forms of a compound called urea, which the patient drinks. The method that uses a radioactive form urea is easier to perform, as the equipment is commonly available in x-ray departments. Radiation exposure is less than that of a chest x ray. The test that uses non-radioactive urea is safer for children. A 2003 study in Brazil showed that the urea breath test and H. pylori stool antigen test also worked well to detect the bacteria in children. The breath test is the best way to be sure of elimination of *H. pylori*. The test can be used within 30 days after treatment. This is an advantage over following antibody levels that take six months or longer to diminish.

Treatment

H. pylori peptic ulcers are treated with drugs to kill the bacteria, drugs to reduce stomach acid, and drugs to protect the lining of the stomach. The antibiotics most commonly used to kill the bacteria are: amoxicillin, clarithromycin, metronidazole, and tetracycline. Drugs used to reduce stomach acid may be histamine blockers or **proton pump inhibitors**. The most commonly used histamine blockers are:

cimetidine, famotidine, nizatidine, and ranitidine. The most commonly used proton pump inhibitors are: lansoprazole and omeprazole. The drug bismuth subsalicylate (a component of Pepto-Bismol) is used to protect the stomach lining.

The most common drug treatment is a two-week course of treatment called triple therapy. This treatment regimen involves taking two **antibiotics** to kill the bacteria and either an acid reducer or a stomach-lining shield. This therapy has been shown to kill the bacteria, reduce ulcer symptoms, and prevent ulcer recurrence in over 90% of patients.

The main drawback of triple therapy is that some patients find it difficult to follow because it often requires taking as many as 20 pills a day. The antibiotics also may cause unpleasant side effects that may make certain patients less likely to follow the treatment protocol. These side effects include: dark stools, **diarrhea**, **dizziness**, **headache**, a metallic taste in the mouth, nausea, **vomiting**, and yeast infections in women.

Prognosis

The elimination of *H. pylori* and cure of ulcer disease is now possible in more than 90% of those infected. The finding that most ulcers are due to an infectious agent has brought a dramatic change in treatment and outlook for those suffering from the disease. Some patients will wind up with repeated infection, but this is most common in overcrowded areas.

Prevention

Attempts to develop a vaccine to protect against infection may be worthwhile in areas where the *H. pylori* infection rate and occurrence of **cancer** of the stomach is high. Research has shown such a vaccine would likely be safe in humans, but a vaccine has yet to be fully identified and developed as of mid-2003.

Resources

PERIODICALS

"Urea Breath, Stool Antigen Tests Work Well to Detect H. Pylori in Children." *Health & Medicine Week* September 22, 2003: 315.
"Vaccination Against H. Pylori Is an Achievable Goal." *Drug Week* July 18, 2003: 153.
Worcester, Sharon. "Eradicating H. Pylori May Prevent Bleeding Ulcers: No [Histamine. Sub2] Blockers Needed." *Internal Medicine News* September 15, 2003: 33.

OTHER

"H. Pylori and Peptic Ulcer." National Institutes of Health. < http://www.niddk.nih.gov/health/digest/pubs/hpylori/hpylori.htm >.
"Management Strategies for Helicobacter pylori Seropositive Patients with Dyspepsia." < http://www.acponline.org/journals/annals/15feb97/treatcounsel.htm >.
"Moving closer to an ulcer vaccine." < http://www.msnbc.com/news/161712.asp > .
"Treating Stomach Ulcers and H. pylori Infection." < http://www.aafp.org/patientinfo/ulcers.html >.
"What Is Helicobacter pylori Infection?" Centers for Disease Control. < http://www.cdc.gov/ncidod/aip/aip_a2b.htm >.

Paul A. Johnson, Ed.M.
Teresa G. Odle

Hellerwork

Definition

Hellerwork is a system of bodywork that combines deep tissue massage, body movement education, and verbal dialogue. It is designed to realign the body's structure for overall health, improvement of posture, and reduction of physical and mental **stress**.

Purpose

Hellerwork improves posture and brings the body's natural structure into proper balance and alignment. This realignment can bring relief from general aches and pains; improve breathing; and relieve physical and mental stress. Hellerwork has also been used to treat such specific physical problems as chronic back, neck, shoulder, and joint **pain** as well as repetitive stress injuries, including **carpal tunnel syndrome**. Hellerwork is also used to treat and prevent athletic injuries.

Description

Origins

Joseph Heller (1940–) developed Hellerwork, a system of structural integration patterned after **Rolfing**. Although Heller received a degree in engineering and worked for NASA's Jet Propulsion Laboratory in Pasadena, CA, he became interested in humanistic psychology in the 1970s. He spent two years studying bioenergetics and **Gestalt therapy** as well as studying under architect and futurist Buckminster Fuller (1895–1983), flotation tank therapy developer John Lilly, family therapist Virginia Satir, and body movement pioneer **Judith Aston**.

During this period, he trained for six years with Dr. Ida P. Rolf (1896-1979), the founder of Rolfing, and became a certified Rolfer in 1972. After Heller developed his own system of bodywork, he founded Hellerwork in 1979 and established a training facility in Mt. Shasta, California, where he continues his work.

Hellerwork is based largely on the principles of Rolfing, in which the body's connective tissue is manipulated or massaged to realign and balance the body's structure. Because Heller believes that physical realignment is insufficient, however, he expanded his system to include movement education and verbal dialogue as well as deep tissue massage.

Connective tissue massage

The **massage therapy** aspect of Hellerwork is designed to release the tension that exists in the deep connective tissue, called fascia, and return it to a normal alignment. The fascia is plastic and highly adaptable; it can tighten and harden in response to the general effects of gravity on the body, other ongoing

JOSEPH HELLER(1940–)

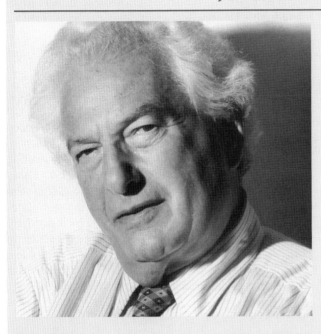

(AP/Wide World Photos. Reproduced by permission.)

Born in Poland, Joseph Heller attended school in Europe until age 16, when he immigrated to the United States. Living in Los Angeles, he attended the California Institute of Technology in Pasadena and graduated in 1962 with a degree in engineering. He worked for 10 years at the National Aeronautics and Space Administration's Jet Propulsion Laboratory (JPL) in Pasadena as an aerospace engineer. During his service at JPL, Heller became interested in humanistic psychology. After leaving JPL in 1972, he became director of Kairos, a center for human development in Los Angeles. He spent two years studying bioenergetics and gestalt. He also trained under Buckminster Fuller, flotation tank therapy developer John Lilly, self-esteem trainer Virginia Satir, and body movement pioneer Judith Aston.

He became a certified Rolfer in 1972 and spent the next six years studying structural integration under Rolfing founder Ida P. Rolf. He became the first president of the Rolf Institute in 1975. During his training with Rolf, Heller began developing his own system of bodywork. He left the institute in 1978 and moved to Northern California where he founded Hellerwork. He conducts classes and continues his work today at his headquarters, 406 Berry St., Mt. Shasta, CA 96067.

physical stresses, negative attitudes and emotions, and periodic physical traumas. One example of ongoing physical stress is carrying a briefcase, which pulls down the shoulder on one side of the body. Over time, the connective tissue becomes hard and stiff; the body becomes adapted to that position even when the person is not carrying a briefcase. In trying to adjust to the uneven weight distribution, the rest of the body becomes unbalanced and out of proper alignment.

Heller believes that as people age, more of these stress and trauma patterns become ingrained in the connective tissue, further throwing the body out of alignment. As stress accumulates, the body shortens and stiffens, a process commonly attributed to **aging**. Hellerwork seeks to recondition the body and make the connective tissue less rigid.

Movement education

The second component of Hellerwork, movement education, trains patients in the proper physical movements needed to keep the body balanced and correctly aligned. Movement education focuses on common actions, such as sitting, standing, and walking.

Hellerwork practitioners also teach better patterns of movement for activities that are specific to each individual, such as their job and favorite sports or social activities.

Verbal dialogue

Verbal dialogue is the third aspect of Hellerwork. It is designed to teach awareness of the relationships among emotions, life attitudes, and the body. Hellerwork practitioners believe that as patients become responsible for their attitudes, their body movements and patterns of self-expression improve. Dialogue focuses on the theme of each session and the area of the body that is worked on during that session.

Hellerwork consists of eleven 90-minute sessions costing about $90–100 each. The first three sessions focus on the surface layers of the fascia and on developmental issues of infancy and childhood. The next four sessions are the core sessions and work on the deep layers and on adolescent developmental issues. The final four treatments are the integrative sessions, and build upon all the previous ones, while also looking at questions of maturity.

KEY TERMS

Bioenergetics—A system of therapy that combines breathing and body exercises, psychological therapy, and the free expression of emotions to release blocked physical and psychic energy.

Bodywork—A term that covers a variety of therapies that include massage, realignment of the body, and similar techniques to treat deeply ingrained stresses and traumas carried in the tissues of the body.

Chronic—A disease or condition that progresses slowly but persists or reoccurs over time.

Fascia—The sheet of connective tissue that covers the body under the skin and envelops the muscles and various organs.

Gestalt therapy—A form of therapy that focuses on helping patients reconnect with their bodies and their feelings directly, as contrasted with verbal intellectual analysis.

Kinesiology—The study of the anatomy and physiology of body movement, particularly in relation to therapy.

Rolfing—A deep-tissue therapy that involves manipulating the body's fascia to realign and balance the body's structure.

Preparations

No advance preparations are required to begin Hellerwork treatment. The treatment is usually done on a massage table with the patient wearing only undergarments.

Precautions

Since Hellerwork involves vigorous deep tissue massage, it is often described as uncomfortable and sometimes painful, especially during the first several sessions. As it requires the use of hands, it may be a problem for people who do not like or are afraid of being touched. It is not recommended as a treatment for any disease or a chronic inflammatory condition such as arthritis, and can worsen such a condition. Anyone with a serious medical condition, including heart disease, diabetes, or respiratory problems, should consult a medical practitioner before undergoing Hellerwork.

Side effects

There are no reported serious side effects associated with Hellerwork when delivered by a certified practitioner to adults and juveniles.

Research and general acceptance

As most alternative or holistic treatments, there is little mainstream scientific research documenting the effectiveness of Hellerwork therapy. Since the deep tissue massage aspect of Hellerwork is similar to Rolfing, however, several scientific studies of Rolfing may be useful in evaluating Hellerwork. A 1988 study published in the *Journal of the American Physical Therapy Association* indicated that Rolfing stimulates the parasympathetic nervous system, which can help speed the recovery of damaged tissue. A 1997 article in *The Journal of Orthopaedic and Sports Physical Therapy* reported that Rolfing can provide effective and sustained pain relief from lower back problems.

Resources

BOOKS

Golten, Roger. *The Owner's Guide to the Body.* London: Thorsons, 1999.

Levine, Andrew S., and Valerie J. Levine. *The Bodywork and Massage Sourcebook.* Lincolnwood, IL: Lowell House, 1999.

ORGANIZATIONS

Hellerwork. 406 Berry St. Mt. Shasta, CA 96067. (530) 926-2500. < http://www.hellerwork.com >.

Ken R. Wells

HELLP syndrome *see* **Preeclampsia and eclampsia**

Hemangiomas *see* **Birthmarks**

Hematocrit

Definition

The hematocrit measures how much space in the blood is occupied by red blood cells. It is useful when evaluating a person for anemia.

Purpose

Blood is made up of red and white blood cells, and plasma. A decrease in the number or size of red cells also decreases the amount of space they occupy, resulting in a lower hematocrit. An increase in the number or size of red cells increases the amount of space they occupy, resulting in a higher hematocrit. **Thalassemia** is a condition which can cause an increased number of red blood cells but a decreased size and hematocrit.

The hematocrit is usually done on a person with symptoms of anemia. An anemic person has fewer or smaller than normal red cells. A low hematocrit, combined with other abnormal blood tests, confirms the diagnosis.

Some conditions, such as polycythemia, cause an overproduction of red blood cells, resulting in an increased hematocrit.

Transfusion decisions are based on the results of laboratory tests, including hematocrit. Transfusion is not considered if the hematocrit level is reasonable. The level differs for each person, depending on his or her clinical condition.

Description

Blood drawn from a fingerstick is often used for hematocrit testing. The blood fills a small tube, which is then spun in a small centrifuge. As the tube spins, the red blood cells go to the bottom of the tube, the white blood cells cover the red in a thin layer called the buffy coat, and the liquid plasma rises to the top. The spun tube is examined for the line that divides the red cells from the buffy coat and plasma. The height of the red cell column is measured as a percent of the total blood column. The higher the column of red cells, the higher the hematocrit.

The hematocrit test can also be done on an automated instrument as part of a complete blood count. It is also called Packed Red Cell Volume or Packed Cell Volume, or abbreviated as Hct or Crit. The test is covered by insurance when medically necessary. Results are usually available the same or following day.

Preparation

To collect the blood by fingerstick, a healthcare worker punctures a finger with a lancet and allows the blood to fill a small tube held to the puncture site.

Tests done on an automated instrument require 5–7 mL of blood. A healthcare worker ties a tourniquet on the person's upper arm, locates a vein in the inner elbow region, and inserts a needle into that vein. Vacuum action draws the blood through the needle into an attached tube. Collection of the sample takes only a few minutes.

KEY TERMS

Anemia—A condition where a person has fewer or smaller than normal red blood cells.

Hemoglobin—The percentage of space in blood occupied by red blood cells.

Aftercare

Discomfort or bruising may occur at the puncture site or the person may feel dizzy or faint. Pressure to the puncture site until the bleeding stops reduces bruising. Warm packs to the puncture site relieve discomfort.

Normal results

Normal values vary with age and sex. Adult male range is 42–52%, adult female 36–48%.

Abnormal results

Hematocrit values decrease when the size or number of red cells decrease. This is most common in anemia, but other conditions have similar effects: excessive bleeding, damaged cells due to a mechanical heart valve, **liver disease**, and cancers affecting the bone marrow. Additional tests, and the person's symptoms and medical history help distinguish these conditions or diagnose a specific type of anemia. Hematocrit values increase when the size or number of red cells increase, such as in polycythemia.

Fluid volume in the blood affects the hematocrit. Pregnant women have extra fluid, which dilutes the blood, decreasing the hematocrit. Dehydration concentrates the blood, increasing the hematocrit.

Nancy J. Nordenson

Hemiplegia *see* **Paralysis**

Hemochromatosis

Definition

Hemochromatosis is an inherited blood disorder that causes the body to retain excessive amounts of iron. This iron overload can lead to serious health consequences, most notably **cirrhosis** of the liver.

Description

Hemochromatosis is also known as iron overload, bronze diabetes, hereditary hemochromatosis and familial hemochromatosis. The inherited disorder causes increased absorption of intestinal iron, well beyond that needed to replace the body's loss of iron. Iron overload diseases afflict as many as 1.5 million persons in the United States. The most common of these, as well as one of the most common genetic disorders in the United States, is hereditary hemochromatosis. Men and women are equally affected by hemochromatosis, but women are diagnosed later in life because of blood loss from menstruation and **childbirth**. It most commonly appears in patients between the ages of 40–60 years, since it takes many years for the body to accumulate excessive iron. Symptoms appear later in females than in males—usually after **menopause**.

Hemochromatosis causes excess iron storage in several organs of the body including the liver, pancreas, endocrine glands, heart, skin, joints, and intestinal lining. The buildup of iron in these organs can lead to serious complications, including **heart failure**, **liver cancer**, and cirrhosis of the liver. It is estimated that about 5% of cirrhosis cases are caused by hereditary hemochromatosis.

Idiopathic pulmonary hemosiderosis, a disorder afflicting children and young adults, is a similar overload disorder characterized by abnormal accumulation of hemosiderin. Hemosiderin is a protein found in most tissues, especially the liver. It is produced by digestion of hematin, an iron-related substance.

Hemochromatosis is one of the most common genetic disorders in the United States. Approximately one in nine individuals have one abnormal hemochromatosis gene (11% of the population). Since everyone has two copies of each gene, these individuals have an abnormal *HFE* gene and a normal gene. They are called carriers. Between 1/200–1/400 individuals have two abnormal genes for hemochromatosis and no normal gene.

With most autosomal recessive conditions, an affected person's parents are carriers. If more than one family member has the condition, they are siblings. Hemochromatosis is so common, however, that families are seen in which both parents are affected, or one parent is affected and the other parent is a carrier. More than one generation may be affected, which is not usually seen in rare autosomal recessive conditions.

Causes and symptoms

Hereditary hemochromatosis is an autosomal recessive condition. This means that individuals with hemochromatosis have inherited an altered (mutated) gene from both of their parents. Affected individuals have two abnormal hemochromatosis genes and no normal hemochromatosis gene.

The gene that causes hemochromatosis has been identified, and the most common abnormalities of the gene have been described. The gene is on chromosome 6; it is called *HFE*. Scientists have not confirmed the function of the normal gene product; they do know that it interacts with the cell receptor for transferrin. Transferrin binds and transports iron in the blood.

Because it is an autosomal recessive condition, siblings of individuals who have hemochromatosis are at a 25% risk to also be affected. However, the likelihood that an individual will develop symptoms depends on which gene mutation he or she has as well as environmental factors. The two most common changes in the *HFE* gene are *C282Y* and *H63D*. The age at which symptoms begin is variable, even within the same family.

The symptoms of hemochromatosis include **fatigue**, weight loss, weakness, **shortness of breath**, heart **palpitations**, chronic abdominal **pain**, and impaired sexual performance. The patient may also show symptoms commonly connected with heart failure, diabetes or cirrhosis of the liver. Changes in the pigment of the skin may appear, such as grayness in certain areas, or a tanned or yellow (**jaundice**) appearance. The age of onset and initial symptoms vary.

Idiopathic pulmonary hemosiderosis may first, and only, appear as paleness of the skin. Sometimes, the patient will experience spitting of blood from the lungs or bronchial tubes.

Diagnosis

The most common diagnostic methods for hemochromatosis are blood studies of iron, genetic blood studies, **magnetic resonance imaging** (MRI), and **liver biopsy**. Blood studies of transferrin–iron saturation and ferritin concentration are often used to screen for iron overload. Ferritin is a protein that transports iron and liver enzymes. Additional studies are performed to confirm the diagnosis.

Blood studies used to confirm the diagnosis include additional iron studies and/or genetic blood studies. Genetic blood studies became available in the late 1990s. **Genetic testing** is a reliable method of diagnosis. However, in the year 2001 scientists and physicians are studying how accurately having a hemochromatosis mutation predicts whether a person will develop symptoms. Most individuals affected with hemochromatosis (87%) have two identifiable gene mutations; that is, genetic testing will confirm the diagnosis in most individuals. Genetic studies are also be used to determine whether the affected person's family members are at risk for hemochromatosis. The results of genetic testing are the same whether or not a person has developed symptoms.

MRI scans and/or liver biopsy may be necessary to confirm the diagnosis. MRI studies of the liver (or other iron absorbing organs), with quantitative assessment of iron concentration, may reveal abnormal iron deposits. For the liver biopsy, a thin needle is inserted into the liver while the patient is under **local anesthesia**. The needle will extract a small amount of liver tissue, which can be analyzed microscopically to measure its iron content and other signs of hemochromatosis. Diagnosis of idiopathic pulmonary hemosiderosis begins with blood tests and x-ray studies of the chest.

Treatment

Patients who show signs of iron overload will often be treated with **phlebotomy**. Phlebotomy is a procedure that involves drawing blood from the patient, just like **blood donation**. Its purpose as a treatment is to rid the body of excess iron storage. Patients may need these procedures one or two times a week for a year or more. Less frequent phlebotomy may be continued in subsequent years to keep excess iron from accumulating. Patients who cannot tolerate phlebotomy due to other medical problems can be treated with Desferal (desferrioxamine). Diet restrictions may also be prescribed to limit the amount of iron ingested. Complications from hemochromatosis, such as cirrhosis or diabetes, may also require treatment. Treatment for idiopathic pulmonary hemosiderosis is based on symptoms.

Diet restrictions may help lower the amount of iron in the body, but do not prevent or treat hemochromatosis. Individuals who are affected or who know they have two *C282Y* and/or *H63D* genes may reduce iron intake by avoiding iron and mineral supplements, excess vitamin C, and uncooked seafood. If a patient is symptomatic, he/she may be advised to abstain from drinking alcohol.

Prognosis

With early detection and treatment, the prognosis is usually good. All potential symptoms are prevented

if iron levels are kept within the normal range, which is possible if the diagnosis is made before an individual is symptomatic. If a patient is symptomatic but treated successfully before he/she develops liver cirrhosis, the patient's life expectancy is near normal. However, if left untreated, complications may arise which can be fatal. These include liver **cancer**, liver cirrhosis, **diabetes mellitus**, congestive heart failure, and difficulty depleting iron overload through phlebotomy. Liver biopsy can be helpful in determining prognosis of more severely affected individuals. Genetic testing may also be helpful, as variable severity has been noted in patients who have two *C282Y* genes compared to patients with two *H63D* genes or one of each. Men are two times more likely than women to develop severe complications. The prognosis for patients with idiopathic pulmonary hemosiderosis is fair, depending on detection and complications.

Prevention

Screening for hemochromatosis is cost effective, particularly for certain groups of people. Relatives of patients with hemochromatosis—including children, siblings, and parents—should be tested by the most appropriate method. The best screening method may be iron and ferritin studies or genetic testing. If the affected person's diagnosis has been confirmed by genetic testing, relatives may have genetic testing to determine whether or not they have the genetic changes present in the affected individual. Many medical groups oppose genetic testing of children. Relatives who are affected but do not have symptoms can reduce iron intake and/or begin phlebotomy prior to the onset of symptoms, possibly preventing ever becoming symptomatic.

In the winter of 2000, population screening for hereditary hemochromatosis is being widely debated. Many doctors and scientists want population screening because hemochromatosis is easily and cheaply treated, and quite common. Arguments against treatment include the range of symptoms seen (and not seen) with certain gene mutations, and the risk of discrimination in health and life insurance. Whether or not population screening becomes favored by a majority, the publicity is beneficial. Hemochromatisis is a common, easily and effectively treated condition. However, diagnosis may be difficult because the presenting symptoms are the same as those seen with many other medical problems. The screening debate has the positive effect of increasing awareness and suspicion of hemochromatisis. Increased knowledge leads to earlier diagnosis and treatment of symptomatic individuals, and increased testing of their asymptomatic at-risk relatives.

Resources

BOOKS

Barton, James C., and Corwin Q. Edwards, editors. *Hemochromatosis: Genetics, Pathophysiology, Diagnosis and Treatment*. Cambridge: Cambridge University Press, 2000.

PERIODICALS

Motulsky, A.G., and E. Beutler. "Population Screening for Hemochromatosis." *Annual Review of Public Health* 21 (2000): 65-79.

ORGANIZATIONS

American Hemochromatosis Society, Inc. 777 E. Atlantic Ave., PMB Z-363, Delray Beach, FL 33483-5352. (561) 266-9037 or (888) 655-IRON (4766). ahs@emi.net. < http://www.americanhs.org >.

American Liver Foundation. 1425 Pompton Ave., Cedar Grove, NJ 07009. (800) 223-0179. < http://www.liverfoundation.org >.

Hemochromatosis Foundation, Inc. PO Box 8569, Albany, NY 12208-0569. (518) 489-0972. s.kleiner@shiva.hunter.cuny.edu. < http://www.hemochromatosis.org >.

Iron Disorders Institute, Inc. PO Box 3021, Greenville, SC 29602. (864) 241-0111. irondis@aol.com. < http://www.irondisorders.org >.

Iron Overload Diseases Association, Inc. 433 Westwind Dr., North Palm Beach, FL 33408. (561) 840-8512. iod@ironoverload.org.

OTHER

"Hemochromatosis." *GeneClinics*. < http://www.geneclinics.org/profiles/hemochromatosis/ >.

Hemochromatosis Information Sheet. National Institute of Diabetes & Digestive & Kidney Diseases (NIDDK). < http://www.niddk.nih.gov/health/digest/pubs/hemochrom/hemochromatosis.htm >.

Hereditary Hemochromatosis. Lecture by Richard Fass, MD, hematologist, Advanced Oncology Associates, given April 25, 1999. < http://www.advancedoncology.org/listen.htm >.

Michelle Q. Bosworth, MS, CGC

Hemodialysis *see* **Dialysis, kidney**

Hemoglobin electrophoresis

Definition

Hemoglobin electrophoresis (also called Hgb electrophoresis), is a test that measures the different types of hemoglobin in the blood. The method used is called electrophoresis, a process that causes movement of particles in an electric field, resulting in formation of "bands" that separate toward one end or the other in the field.

Purpose

Hgb electrophoresis is performed when a disorder associated with abnormal hemoglobin (hemoglobinopathy) is suspected. The test is used primarily to diagnose diseases involving these abnormal forms of hemoglobin, such as sickle cell anemia and **thalassemia**.

Precautions

Blood transfusions within the previous 12 weeks may alter test results.

Description

Hemoglobin (Hgb) is comprised of many different types, the most common being A_1, A_2, F, S, and C.

Hgb A_1 is the major component of hemoglobin in the normal red blood cell. Hgb A_2 is a minor component of normal hemoglobin, comprising approximately 2–3% of the total.

Hgb F is the major hemoglobin component in the fetus, but usually exists only in minimal quantities in the normal adult. Levels of Hgb F greater than 2% in patients over three years of age are considered abnormal.

Hgb S is an abnormal form of hemoglobin associated with the disease of sickle cell anemia, which occurs predominantly in African-Americans. A distinguishing characteristic of sickle cell disease is the crescent-shaped red blood cell. Because the survival rate of this type of cell is limited, patients with **sickle cell disease** also have anemia.

Hgb C is another hemoglobin variant found in African Americans. Red blood cells containing Hgb C have a decreased life span and are more readily destroyed than normal red blood cells, resulting in mild to severe **hemolytic anemia**.

Each of the major hemoglobin types has an electrical charge of a different degree, so the most useful method for separating and measuring normal and abnormal hemoglobins is electrophoresis. This process involves subjecting hemoglobin components from dissolved red blood cells to an electric field. The components then move away from each other at different rates, and when separated form a series of distinctly pigmented bands. The bands are then compared with those of a normal sample. Each band can be further assessed as a percentage of the total hemoglobin, thus indicating the severity of any abnormality.

Preparation

This test requires a blood sample. No special preparation is needed before the test.

Risks

Risks for this test are minimal, but may include slight bleeding from the blood-drawing site, fainting or feeling lightheaded after venipuncture, or hematoma (blood accumulating under the puncture site).

Normal results

Normal reference values can vary by laboratory, but are generally within the following ranges.

Adults:

- Hgb A_1: 95–98%
- Hgb A_2: 2–3%
- Hgb F: 0.8–2.0%
- Hgb S: 0%
- Hgb C: 0%.

  Child (Hgb F):

- 6 months: 8%
- greater than 6 months: 1–2%
- newborn (Hgb F): 50–80%

> ## KEY TERMS
>
> **Hemoglobin C disease**—A disease of abnormal hemoglobin, occurring in 2–3% of African-Americans. Only those who have two genes for the disease develop anemia, which varies in severity. Symptoms include episodes of abdominal and joint pain, an enlarged spleen and mild jaundice.
>
> **Hemoglobin H disease**—A thalassemia-like syndrome causing moderate anemia and red blood cell abnormalities.
>
> **Heterozygous**—Two different genes controlling a specified inherited trait.
>
> **Homozygous**—Identical genes controlling a specified inherited trait.
>
> **Thalassemias**—The name for a group of inherited disorders resulting from an imbalance in the production of one of the four chains of amino acids that make up hemoglobin. Thalassemias are categorized according to the amino acid chain affected. The two main types are alpha-thalassemia and beta-thalassemia. The disorders are further characterized by the presence of one defective gene (thalassemia minor) or two defective genes (thalassemia major). Symptoms vary, but include anemia, jaundice, skin ulcers, gallstones, and an enlarged spleen.

Abnormal results

Abnormal reference values can vary by laboratory, but when they appear within these ranges, results are usually associated with the conditions that follow in parentheses.

Hgb A_2:

- 4–5.8% (β-thalassemia minor)
- under 2% (Hgb H disease)

  Hgb F:

- 2–5% (β-thalassemia minor)
- 10–90% (β-thalassemia major)
- 5–35% (Heterozygous hereditary persistence of fetal hemoglobin, or HPFH)
- 100% (Homozygous HPFH)
- 15% (Homozygous Hgb S)

  Homozygous Hgb S:

- 70–98% (Sickle cell disease).

Homozygous Hgb C:

• 90–98% (Hgb C disease)

Resources

BOOKS

Pagana, Kathleen Deska. *Mosby's Manual of Diagnostic and Laboratory Tests.* St. Louis: Mosby, Inc., 1998.

Janis O. Flores

Hemoglobin F test *see* **Fetal hemoglobin test**

Hemoglobin test

Definition

Hemoglobin is a protein inside red blood cells that carries oxygen throughout the body. A hemoglobin test reveals how much hemoglobin is in a person's blood, helping to diagnose and monitor anemia and **polycythemia vera**.

Purpose

A hemoglobin test is done when a person is ill or during a general **physical examination**. Good health requires an adequate amount of hemoglobin. The amount of oxygen in the body tissues depends on how much hemoglobin is in the red cells. Without enough hemoglobin, the tissues lack oxygen and the heart and lungs must work harder to try to compensate.

If the test indicates a "less than" or "greater than" normal amount of hemoglobin, the cause of the decrease or increase must be discovered. A low hemoglobin usually means the person has anemia. Anemia results from conditions that decrease the number or size of red cells, such as excessive bleeding, a dietary deficiency, destruction of cells because of a **transfusion** reaction or mechanical heart valve, or an abnormally formed hemoglobin.

A high hemoglobin may be caused by polycythemia vera, a disease in which too many red blood cells are made.

Hemoglobin levels also help determine if a person needs a blood transfusion. Usually a person's hemoglobin must be below 8 gm/dl before a transfusion is considered.

Description

Hemoglobin is made of heme, an iron compound, and globin, a protein. The iron gives blood its red color. Hemoglobin tests make use of this red color. A chemical is added to a sample of blood to make the red blood cells burst. When they burst, the red cells release hemoglobin into the surrounding fluid, coloring it clear red. By measuring the color using an instrument called a spectrophotometer, the amount of hemoglobin is determined.

Hemoglobin is often ordered as part of a complete blood count (CBC), a test that includes other blood cell measurements.

Some people inherit hemoglobin with an abnormal structure. These abnormal hemoglobins cause diseases, such as sickle cell or Hemoglobin C disease. Special tests, using a process called hemoglobin electrophoresis, identify abnormal hemoglobins.

Preparation

This test requires 5 mL of blood. A healthcare worker ties a tourniquet on the person's upper arm, locates a vein in the inner elbow region, and inserts a needle into that vein. Vacuum action draws the blood through the needle into an attached tube. Collection of the sample takes only a few minutes.

The person should avoid **smoking** before this test as smoking can increase hemoglobin levels.

Aftercare

Discomfort or bruising may occur at the puncture site or the person may feel dizzy or faint. Pressure to the puncture site until the bleeding stops reduces bruising. Warm packs to the puncture site relieve discomfort.

Normal results

Normal values vary with age and sex. Women generally have lower hemoglobin values than men. Men have 14.0–18.0 g/dL, while women have levels of 12.0–16.0 g/dL.

Abnormal results

A low hemoglobin usually indicates the person has anemia. Further tests are done to discover the cause and type of anemia. Dangerously low hemoglobin levels put a person at risk of a **heart attack**, congestive heart failure, or **stroke**.

KEY TERMS

Anemia—A condition characterized by a decrease in the size or number of red blood cells.

Hemoglobin—A protein inside red blood cells that carries oxygen to body tissues.

Polycythemia vera—A disease in which the bone marrow makes too many red blood cells.

A high hemoglobin indicates the body is making too many red cells. Further tests are done to see if this is caused by polycythemia vera, or as a reaction to illness, high altitudes, heart failure, or lung disease.

Fluid volume in the blood affects hemoglobin values. Pregnant women and people with cirrhosis have extra fluid, which dilutes the blood, decreasing the hemoglobin. **Dehydration** concentrates the blood, increasing the hemoglobin.

Resources

PERIODICALS

Hsia, Connie C. W. "Respiratory Function of Hemoglobin."*New England Journal of Medicine* 338 (January 1998): 239-247.

Nancy J. Nordenson

Hemoglobinopathies

Definition

Hemoglobinopathies are genetic (inherited) disorders of hemoglobin, the oxygen-carrying protein of the red blood cells.

Description

The hemoglobin molecule is composed of four separate polypeptide chains of amino acids, two alpha chains and two beta chains, as well as four iron-bearing heme groups that bind oxygen. The alpha chains are coded for by two similar genes on chromosome 16; the beta chains by a single gene on chromosome 11. Mutations and deletions in these genes cause one of the many hemoglobinopathies.

In general, hemoglobinopathies are divided into those in which the gene abnormality results in a qualitative change in the hemoglobin molecule and those in which the change is quantitative. Sickle cell anemia (**sickle cell disease**) is the prime example of the former, and the group of disorders known as the thalassemias constitute the latter. It has been estimated that one third of a million people worldwide are seriously affected by one of these genetic disorders.

Causes and symptoms

Sickle cell anemia (SSA), an autosomal recessive disorder more common in the Black population, is caused by a single mutation in the gene that codes for the beta polypeptide. Approximately 1/400 to 1/600 African-Americans are born with the disorder, and, one in ten is a carrier of one copy of the mutation. In certain parts of the African continent, the prevalence of the disease reaches one in fifty individuals.

The sickle cell mutation results in the substitution of the amino acid valine for glutamic acid in the sixth position of the beta polypeptide. In turn, this alters the conformation of the hemoglobin molecule and causes the red blood cells to assume a characteristic sickle shape under certain conditions. These sickle-shaped cells, no longer able to pass smoothly through small capillaries, can block the flow of blood. This obstruction results in symptoms including growth retardation, severe **pain** crises, tissue and organ damage, splenomegaly, and strokes. Individuals with SSA are anemic and prone to infections, particularly **pneumonia**, a significant cause of **death** in this group. Some or all of these symptoms are found in individuals who have the sickle mutation in both copies of their beta-globin gene. Persons with one abnormal gene and one normal gene are said to be carriers of the sickle cell trait. Carriers are unaffected because of the remaining normal copy of the gene.

The thalassemias are a diverse group of disorders characterized by the fact that the causative mutations result in a decrease in the amount of normal hemoglobin. Thalassemias are common in Mediterranean populations as well as in Africa, India, the Mideast, and Southeast Asia. The two main types of thalassemias are alpha-thalassemia due to mutations in the alpha polypeptide and beta-thalassemia resulting from beta chain mutations.

Since individuals possess a total of four genes for the alpha polypeptide (two genes on each of their two chromosomes 16), disease severity depends on how many of the four genes are abnormal. A defect in one or two of the genes has no clinical effect. Abnormalities of three results in a mild to moderately severe anemia (hemoglobin H disease) and splenomegaly. Loss of function of all four genes usually causes such severe oxygen deprivation that the affected fetus does not survive. A massive accumulation of fluid in the fetus (hydrops fetalis) results in **stillbirth** or neonatal death.

Beta thalassemias can range from mild and clinically insignificant (beta **thalassemia** minor) to severe and life-threatening (beta thalassemia major, also known as Cooley's anemia), depending on the exact nature of the gene mutation and whether one or both copies of the beta gene are affected. While the milder forms may only cause slight anemia, the more severe types result in growth retardation, skeletal changes, splenomegaly, vulnerability to infections, and death as early as the first decade of life.

Diagnosis

Many countries, including the United States, have made concerted efforts to screen for sickle cell anemia at birth because of the potential for beginning early treatment and counseling parents about their carrier status. Diagnosis is traditionally made by blood tests including **hemoglobin electrophoresis**. Similar tests are used to determine whether an individual is a sickle cell or thalassemia carrier. In certain populations with a high prevalence of one of the mutations, carrier testing is common. If both members of a couple are carriers of one of these conditions, it is possible through prenatal **genetic testing** to determine if the fetus will be affected, although the severity of the disease cannot always be predicted.

Treatment

Treatment of SSA has improved greatly in recent years with a resulting increase in life expectancy. The use of prophylactic (preventative) antibiotic therapy has been particularly successful. Other treatments include fluid therapy to prevent **dehydration**, oxygen supplementation, pain relievers, blood transfusions, and several different types of medications. Recent interest has focused on **bone marrow transplantation**, which has been successful in selected patients.

Since the clinically important thalassemias are characterized by severe anemia, the traditional treatment has been blood **transfusion**, but the multiple transfusions needed to sustain life lead to an iron overload throughout the tissues of the body and eventual destruction of the heart and other organs. For this reason, transfusion therapy must also include infusions of medications such as deferoxamine (desferroxamine) to rid the body of excess iron. **Phlebotomy** is another technique that has been used with some success to lower the concentration of iron in the patient's blood. As with sickle cell anemia, bone marrow therapy has been successful in some cases.

Until very recently, patients being treated with bone marrow transplants had to find a sibling or other closely related donor in order to avoid rejection of the transplant. Advances in the preparation of the transplanted cells, however, have made the use of bone marrow from unrelated donors (URD) an option for patients with hemoglobinopathies. As of 2003, the National Marrow Donor Program reports that about 40% of bone marrow transplants involve a patient in the United States receiving marrow from an international donor or an international patient receiving marrow from a donor in the United States.

Emphasis is also being placed on developing drugs that treat sickle cell anemia directly. The most promising of these drugs in the late 1990s is hydroxyurea, a drug that was originally designed for anticancer treatment. Hydroxyurea has been shown to reduce the frequency of painful crises and acute chest syndrome in adults, and to lessen the need for blood transfusions. Hydroxyurea seems to work by inducing a higher production of fetal hemoglobin. The major side effects of the drug include decreased production of platelets, red blood cells, and certain white blood cells. The effects of long-term hydroxyurea treatment are unknown; however, a nine-year follow-up study of 299 adults with frequent painful crises reported in 2003 that taking hydroxyurea was associated with a 40% reduction in mortality.

Another promising development for the treatment of hemoglobinopathies is **gene therapy**, which has interested researchers since the early 1990s. In late 2001, genetic scientists reported that they had designed a gene that might lead to a future treatment of sickle cell anemia. Although the gene had not been tested in humans, early results showed that the injected gene protected cells from sickling. As of 2003, experiments in gene therapy for sickle cell disease have been carried out in mice, using lentiviral vectors to transfer the corrective gene into the mouse's stem cells. This technique, however, has not yet been attempted in human subjects as of late 2003.

Prognosis

Hemoglobinopathies are life-long disorders. The prognosis depends upon the exact nature of the mutation, the availability of effective treatment, as well as the individual's compliance with therapies. Hemoglobinopathies significantly complicate **pregnancy**, and increase the risk of infant mortality.

KEY TERMS

Amino acids—Organic compounds that form the building blocks of protein. There are 20 different amino acids.

Autosomal recessive—A pattern of inheritance in which both copies of an autosomal gene must be abnormal for a genetic condition or disease to occur. An autosomal gene is a gene that is located on one of the autosomes or non-sex chromosomes. When both parents have one abnormal copy of the same gene, they have a 25% chance with each pregnancy that their offspring will have the disorder.

Hemoglobin—Protein-iron compound in the blood that carries oxygen to the cells and carries carbon dioxide away from the cells.

Hydroxyurea—A drug that has been shown to induce production of fetal hemoglobin. Fetal hemoglobin has a pair of gamma-globin molecules in place of the typical beta-globins of adult hemoglobin. Higher-than-normal levels of fetal hemoglobin can prevent sickling from occurring.

Phlebotomy—Drawing blood from a vein for diagnosis or treatment. Phlebotomy is sometimes used in the treatment of hemoglobinopathies to lower the iron concentration of the blood.

Sickle cell—A red blood cell that has assumed an elongated shape due to the presence of hemoglobin S.

Splenomegaly—Enlargement of the spleen.

Prevention

Because the hemoglobinopathies are inherited diseases, primary prevention involves carriers making reproductive decisions to prevent passage of the abnormal gene to their offspring. At present, most prevention is targeted toward the symptoms using treatments such as those described above.

Resources

BOOKS

Beers, Mark H., MD, and Robert Berkow, MD., editors. "Anemias Caused by Excessive Hemolysis: Sickle Cell Diseases." Section 11, Chapter 127 In *The Merck Manual of Diagnosis and Therapy*. Whitehouse Station, NJ: Merck Research Laboratories, 2004.

Beers, Mark H., MD, and Robert Berkow, MD., editors. "Pregnancy Complicated by Disease: Hemoglobinopathies." Section 18, Chapter 251 In *The Merck Manual of Diagnosis and Therapy*. Whitehouse Station, NJ: Merck Research Laboratories, 2004.

Behrman, Richard E., et al. *Nelson Textbook of Pediatrics*. 16th ed. Philadelphia, W. B. Saunders, 2000.

Jorde, Lynn B., et al. *Medical Genetics*. 2nd ed. New York: Mosby, 1999.

PERIODICALS

Davies, S. C., and A. Gilmore. "The Role of Hydroxyurea in the Management of Sickle Cell Disease." *Blood Reviews* 17 (June 2003): 99–109.

Koduri, P. R. "Iron in Sickle Cell Disease: A Review Why Less Is Better." *American Journal of Hematology* 73 (May 2003): 59–63.

Krishnamurti, L., S. Abel, M. Maiers, and S. Flesch. "Availability of Unrelated Donors for Hematopoietic Stem Cell Transplantation for Hemoglobinopathies." *Bone Marrow Transplantation* 31 (April 2003): 547–550.

Markham, M. J., R. Lottenberg, and M. Zumberg. "Role of Phlebotomy in the Management of Hemoglobin SC Disease: Case Report and Review of the Literature." *American Journal of Hematology* 73 (June 2003): 121–125.

Nienhuis, A. W., H. Hanawa, N. Sawai, et al. "Development of Gene Therapy for Hemoglobin Disorders." *Annals of the New York Academy of Science* 996 (May 2003): 101–111.

Olivieri, Nancy F. "The Beta-Thalassemias." *The New England Journal of Medicine* 341, no. 2 (July 1999): 99–109.

Steinberg, M. H., F. Barton, O. Castro, et al. "Effect of Hydroxyurea on Mortality and Morbidity in Adult Sickle Cell Anemia: Risks and Benefits up to 9 Years of Treatment." *Journal of the American Medical Association* 289 (April 2, 2003): 1645–1651.

ORGANIZATIONS

American Sickle Cell Anemia Association. < http://www.ascaa.org >.

National Marrow Donor Program (NMDP). Suite 500, 3001 Broadway Street Northeast, Minneapolis, MN 55413. (800) 627-7692. < http://www.marrow-donor.org >.

Sickle Cell Disease Association of America, Inc. 200 Corporate Point Suite 495, Culver City, CA 90230-8727. (800) 421-8453. Scdaa@sicklecelldisease.org. < http://sicklecelldisease.org/ >.

Sickle Cell Information Center. PO Box 109, Grady Memorial Hospital, 80 Bulter Street, SE, Atlanta, GA 30303. (404) 616- 3572. < http://www.emory.edu >.

Sallie Boineau Freeman, PhD
Rebecca J. Frey, PhD

Hemolytic anemia

Definition

Red blood cells have a normal life span of approximately 90–120 days, at which time the old cells are destroyed and replaced by the body's natural processes. Hemolytic anemia is a disorder in which the red blood cells are destroyed prematurely. The cells are broken down at a faster rate than the bone marrow can produce new cells. Hemoglobin, the component of red blood cells that carries oxygen, is released when these cells are destroyed.

Description

As a group, **anemias** (conditions in which the number of red blood cells or the amount of hemoglobin in them is below normal) are the most common blood disorders. Hemolytic anemias, which result from the increased destruction of red blood cells, are less common than anemias caused by excessive blood loss or by decreased hemoglobin or red cell production.

Since a number of factors can increase red blood cell destruction, hemolytic anemias are generally identified by the disorder that brings about the premature destruction. Those disorders are classified as either inherited or acquired. Inherited hemolytic anemias are caused by inborn defects in components of the red blood cells—the cell membrane, the enzymes, or the hemoglobin. Acquired hemolytic anemias are those that result from various other causes. With this type, red cells are produced normally, but are prematurely destroyed because of damage that occurs to them in the circulation.

Causes and symptoms

Inherited hemolytic anemias involve conditions that interfere with normal red blood cell production. Disorders that affect the red blood cell membrane include hereditary spherocytosis, in which the normally disk-shaped red cells become spherical, and hereditary elliptocytosis, in which the cells are oval, rather than disk-shaped. Other hereditary conditions that cause hemolytic anemia include disorders of the hemoglobin, such as sickle cell anemia and **thalassemia**, and red blood cell enzyme deficiencies, such as G6PD deficiency.

The causes of acquired hemolytic anemias vary, but the most common are responses to certain medications and infections. Medications may cause the body to develop antibodies that bind to the red blood cells and cause their destruction in the spleen. Immune hemolytic anemia most commonly involves antibodies that react against the red blood cells at body temperature (warm-antibody hemolytic anemia), which can cause premature destruction of the cells. About 20% of hemolytic anemias caused by warm antibodies come from diseases such as lymphocytic leukemia, 10% from an autoimmune disease, and others are drug-induced. Cold-antibody hemolytic anemia is a condition in which the antibodies react with the red blood cells at a temperature below that of normal body temperature. Red blood cells can also receive mechanical damage as they circulate through the blood vessels. Aneurysms, artificial heart valves, or very high blood pressure can cause the red cells to break up and release their contents. In addition, hemolytic anemia may be caused by a condition called **hypersplenism**, in which a large, overactive spleen rapidly destroys red blood cells.

Major symptoms of hemolytic anemias are similar to those for all anemias, including shortness of breath; noticeable increase in heart rate, especially with exertion; **fatigue**; pale appearance; and dark urine. A yellow tint, or **jaundice**, may be seen in the skin or eyes of hemolytic anemia patients. Examination may also show an enlarged spleen. A more emergent symptom of hemolytic anemia is **pain** in the upper abdomen. Severe anemia is indicated if there are signs of **heart failure** or an enlarged liver.

Diagnosis

In order to differentiate hemolytic anemia from others, physicians will examine the blood for the number of young red blood cells, since the number of young cells is increased in hemolytic anemia. The physician will also examine the abdominal area to check for spleen or liver enlargement. If the physician knows the duration of hemolysis, it may also help differentiate between types of anemia. There are a number of other indications that can be obtained from blood samples that will help a physician screen for hemolytic anemia. An antiglobulin (Coomb's) test may be performed as the initial screening exam after determining hemolysis. In the case of immune hemolytic anemia, a direct Coomb's test is almost always positive.

Treatment

Treatment will depend on the cause of the anemia, and may involve treatment of the underlying cause. If the hemolytic anemia was brought on by hereditary spherocytosis, the spleen may be removed. Corticosteroid medications, or adrenal steroids, may

KEY TERMS

Antibody—Antibodies are parts of the immune system which counteract or eliminate foreign substances or antigens.

Erythrocyte—The name for red blood cells or red blood corpuscles. These components of the blood are responsible for carrying oxygen to tissues and removing carbon dioxide from tissues.

Hemolysis—The process of breaking down of red blood cells. As the cells are destroyed, hemoglobin, the component of red blood cells which carries the oxygen, is liberated.

Thalassemia—One of a group of inherited blood disorders characterized by a defect in the metabolism of hemoglobin, or the portion of the red blood cells that transports oxygen throughout the blood stream.

be effective, especially in hemolytic anemia due to antibodies. If the cause of the disorder is a medication, the medication should be stopped. When anemia is severe in conditions such as sickle cell anemia and thalassemia, blood transfusions may be indicated.

Prognosis

Hemolytic anemias are seldom fatal. However, if left untreated, hemolytic anemia can lead to heart failure or liver complications.

Prevention

Hemolytic anemia due to inherited disorders can not be prevented. Acquired hemolytic anemia may be prevented if the underlying disorder is managed properly.

Resources

ORGANIZATIONS

American Autoimmune Related Diseases Association, Inc. *Focus: A quarterly newsletter of the AARDA.* Detroit, MI. (313) 371-8600. < http://www.aarda.org >.

The American Society of Hematology. 1200 19th Street NW, Suite 300, Washington, DC 20036-2422. (202) 857-1118. < http://www.hematology.org >.

National Heart, Lung and Blood Institute. PO Box 30105, Bethesda, MD 20824-0105. (301) 251-1222. < http://www.nhlbi.nih.gov >.

Teresa Odle

Hemolytic-uremic syndrome

Definition

Hemolytic-uremic syndrome (HUS) is a rare condition that affects mostly children under the age of 10, but also may affect the elderly as well as persons with other illnesses. HUS, which most commonly develops after a severe bowel infection with certain toxic strains of a bacteria, is characterized by destruction of red blood cells, damage to the lining of blood vessel walls, and in severe cases, kidney failure.

Description

Most cases of HUS occur after an infection in the digestive system that has been caused by toxin-producing strains of the bacterium *Escherichia coli.* About 75% of HUS cases in the United States are caused by the strain referred to as *E. coli* O157:H7, which is found in the intestinal tract of cattle, while the remaining cases are caused by non-O157 strains. Some children infected with *E. coli* O157:H7 will develop HUS. HUS also can follow respiratory infection episodes in young children. In the United States, there are about 20,000 infections and 250 deaths annually that are caused by *E. coli* O157:H7. HUS has also been known to occur in persons using drugs such as **oral contraceptives**, immunosuppressors, and antineoplastics, and in women during the postpartum period.

E. coli. O157:H7, first identified in 1982, and isolated with increasing frequency since then, is found in contaminated foods such as meat, dairy products, and juices. Infection with *E. coli.* O157:H7 causes severe **gastroenteritis**, which can include abdominal **pain**, **vomiting**, and bloody **diarrhea**. For most children, the vomiting and diarrhea stop within two to three days. However, about 5 to 10% of the children will develop HUS and will become pale, tired, and irritable. Toxins produced by the bacteria enter the blood stream, where they destroy red blood cells and platelets, which contribute to the clotting of blood. The damaged red blood cells and platelets clog tiny blood vessels in the kidneys, or form lesions to occur in the kidneys, making it difficult for the kidneys to remove wastes and extra fluid from the body, resulting in **hypertension**, fluid accumulation, and reduced production of urine.

Causes and symptoms

The most common way an *E. coli* O157:H7 infection is contracted is through the consumption of undercooked ground beef (e.g., eating hamburgers that are still pink inside). Healthy cattle carry *E. coli* within their intestines. During the slaughtering process, the meat can become contaminated with the *E. coli* from the intestines. When contaminated beef is ground up, the *E. coli* are spread throughout the meat. Additional ways to contract an *E. coli* infection include drinking contaminated water and unpasteurized milk and juices, eating contaminated fruits and vegetables, and working with cattle. The infection is also easily transmitted from an infected person to others in settings such as day care centers and nursing homes when improper sanitary practices are used.

Symptoms of an *E. coli* O157:H7 infection start about seven days after infection with the bacteria. The first symptom is sudden onset of severe abdominal cramps. After a few hours, watery diarrhea starts, causing loss of fluids and electrolytes (**dehydration**), which causes the person to feel tired and ill. The watery diarrhea lasts for about a day, and then changes to bright red bloody stools, as the infection causes sores to form in the intestines. The bloody diarrhea lasts for two to five days, with as many as ten bowel movements a day. Additional symptoms may include **nausea and vomiting**, without a **fever**, or with only a mild fever. After about five to ten days, HUS can develop, which is characterized by paleness, irritability, and **fatigue**, as well as reduced urine production.

Diagnosis

The diagnosis of an *E. coli* infection is made through a **stool culture**. The culture must be taken within the first 48 hours after the start of the bloody diarrhea. If a positive culture is obtained, the patient should be monitored for the development of HUS, with treatment initiated as required.

Children should not go to day care until they have had two negative stool cultures. Older people in nursing homes should stay in bed until two stool cultures are negative.

Treatment

Treatment of HUS is supportive, with particular attention to management of fluids and electrolytes. Treatment generally is provided in a hospital setting. Blood transfusions may be required. In about 50% of the cases, short term replacement of kidney function is required in the form of dialysis. Most patients will recover kidney function and be able to discontinue dialysis.

Some studies have shown that the use of **antibiotics** and antimotility agents during an *E. coli* infection

may worsen the course of the infection and should be avoided. However, other studies have been less definitive. Physicians should stay informed so that clinical practices matches medical advances on this aspect of treatment.

Alternative treatment

Persons with HUS must be under the care of health care professionals skilled in the treatment of HUS.

Prognosis

Ninety percent of children with HUS who receive careful supportive care survive the initial acute stages of the condition, with most having no long-term effects. However, between 10 and 30 percent of the survivors will have kidney damage that will lead to kidney failure immediately or within several years. These children with kidney failure require on-going dialysis to remove wastes and extra fluids from their bodies, or may require a kidney transplant.

Prevention

Prevention of HUS caused by ingestion of foods contaminated with *E. coli* O157:H7 and other toxin-producing bacteria is accomplished through practicing hygienic food preparation techniques, including adequate handwashing, cooking of meat thoroughly, defrosting meats safely, vigorous washing of fruits and vegetables, and handling leftovers properly. Irradiation of meat has been approved by the United States Food and Drug Administration and the United States Department of Agriculture in order to decrease bacterial contamination of consumer meat supplies.

Resources

OTHER

National Kidney and Urologic Diseases Information Clearinghouse. Fact Sheet: Hemolytic Uremic Syndrome. NIH Publication No. 99-4570. March 2000. <http:// www.niddk.nih.gov/health/kidney/summary/hus/>.

Judith Sims

Hemophilia

Definition

Hemophilia is a genetic disorder—usually inherited—of the mechanism of blood clotting. Depending on the degree of the disorder present in an individual, excess bleeding may occur only after specific, predictable events (such as surgery, dental procedures, or injury), or occur spontaneously, with no known initiating event.

Description

The normal mechanism for blood clotting is a complex series of events involving the interaction of the injured blood vessel, blood cells (called platelets), and over 20 different proteins which also circulate in the blood.

When a blood vessel is injured in a way that causes bleeding, platelets collect over the injured area, and form a temporary plug to prevent further bleeding. This temporary plug, however, is too disorganized to serve as a long-term solution, so a series of chemical events occur, resulting in the formation of a more reliable plug. The final plug involves tightly woven fibers of a material called fibrin. The production of fibrin requires the interaction of several chemicals, in particular a series of proteins called clotting factors. At least thirteen different clotting factors have been identified.

The clotting cascade, as it is usually called, is the series of events required to form the final fibrin clot. The cascade uses a technique called amplification to rapidly produce the proper sized fibrin clot from the small number of molecules initially activated by the injury.

In hemophilia, certain clotting factors are either decreased in quantity, absent, or improperly formed. Because the clotting cascade uses amplification to rapidly plug up a bleeding area, absence or inactivity of just one clotting factor can greatly increase **bleeding time**.

Hemophilia A is the most common type of bleeding disorder and involves decreased activity of factor VIII. There are three levels of factor VIII deficiency: severe, moderate, and mild. This classification is based on the percentage of normal factor VIII activity present:

- Individuals with less than 1% of normal factor VIII activity level have severe hemophilia. Half of all people with hemophilia A fall into this category. Such individuals frequently experience spontaneous bleeding, most frequently into their joints, skin, and muscles. Surgery or trauma can result in life-threatening hemorrhage, and must be carefully managed.

- Individuals with 1–5% of normal factor VIII activity level have moderate hemophilia, and are at risk for heavy bleeding after seemingly minor traumatic injury.

- Individuals with 5–40% of normal factor VIII activity level have mild hemophilia, and must prepare carefully for any surgery or dental procedures.

Individuals with hemophilia B have symptoms very similar to those of hemophilia A, but the deficient factor is factor IX. This type of hemophilia is also known as Christmas disease.

Hemophilia C is very rare, and much more mild than hemophilia A or B; it involves factor XI.

Hemophilia A affects between one in 5,000 to one in 10,000 males in most populations.

One recent study estimated the prevalence of hemophilia was 13.4 cases per 100,000 U.S. males (10.5 hemophilia A and 2.9 hemophilia B). By race/ethnicity, the prevalence was 13.2 cases/100,000 among white, 11.0 among African-American, and 11.5 among Hispanic males.

Causes and symptoms

Hemophilia A and B are both caused by a genetic defect present on the X chromosome. (Hemophilia C is inherited in a different fashion.) About 70% of all people with hemophilia A or B inherited the disease. The other 30% develop from a spontaneous genetic mutation.

The following concepts are important to understanding the inheritance of these diseases. All humans have two chromosomes determining their gender: females have XX, males have XY. Because the trait is carried only on the X chromosome, it is called "sex-linked." The chromosome's flawed unit is referred to as the gene.

Both factors VIII and IX are produced by a genetic defect of the X chromosome, so hemophilia

A and B are both sex-linked diseases. Because a female child always receives two X chromosomes, she nearly always will receive at least one normal X chromosome. Therefore, even if she receives one flawed X chromosome, she will still be capable of producing a sufficient quantity of factors VIII and IX to avoid the symptoms of hemophilia. Such a person who has one flawed chromosome, but does not actually suffer from the disease, is called a carrier. She carries the flaw that causes hemophilia and can pass it on to her offspring. If, however, she has a son who receives her flawed X chromosome, he will be unable to produce the right quantity of factors VIII or IX, and he will suffer some degree of hemophilia. (Males inherit one X and one Y chromosome, and therefore have only one X chromosome.)

In rare cases, a hemophiliac father and a carrier mother can pass on the right combination of parental chromosomes to result in a hemophiliac female child. This situation, however, is rare. The vast majority of people with either hemophilia A or B are male.

About 30% of all people with hemophilia A or B are the first member of their family to ever have the disease. These individuals have had the unfortunate occurrence of a spontaneous mutation; meaning that in their early development, some random genetic accident befell their X chromosome, resulting in the defect causing hemophilia A or B. Once such a spontaneous genetic mutation takes place, offspring of the affected person can inherit the newly created, flawed chromosome.

In the case of severe hemophilia, the first bleeding event usually occurs prior to eighteen months of age. In some babies, hemophilia is suspected immediately, when a routine **circumcision** (removal of the foreskin of the penis) results in unusually heavy bleeding. Toddlers are at particular risk, because they fall frequently, and may bleed into the soft tissue of their arms and legs. These small bleeds result in bruising and noticeable lumps, but don't usually need treatment. As a child becomes more active, bleeding may occur into the muscles; a much more painful and debilitating problem. These muscle bleeds result in **pain** and pressure on the nerves in the area of the bleed. Damage to nerves can cause **numbness** and decreased ability to use the injured limb.

Some of the most problematic and frequent bleeds occur into the joints, particularly into the knees and elbows. Repeated bleeding into joints can result in scarring within the joints and permanent deformities. Individuals may develop arthritis in joints that have suffered continued irritation from the presence of

blood. Mouth injuries can result in compression of the airway, and, therefore, can be life-threatening. A blow to the head, which might be totally insignificant in a normal individual, can result in bleeding into the skull and brain. Because the skull has no room for expansion, the hemophiliac individual is at risk for brain damage due to blood taking up space and exerting pressure on the delicate brain tissue.

People with hemophilia are at very high risk of hemorrhage (severe, heavy, uncontrollable bleeding) from injuries such as motor vehicle accidents and also from surgery.

Some other rare clotting disorders such as Von Willebrand disease present similar symptoms but are not usually called hemophilia.

Diagnosis

Various tests are available to measure, under very carefully controlled conditions, the length of time it takes to produce certain components of the final fibrin clot. Tests called assays can also determine the percentage of factors VIII and IX present compared to normal percentages. This information can help in demonstrating the type of hemophilia present, as well as the severity.

Individuals with a family history of hemophilia may benefit from genetic counseling before deciding to have a baby. Families with a positive history of hemophilia can also have tests done during a **pregnancy** to determine whether the fetus is a hemophiliac. The test called chorionic villous sampling examines proteins for the defects that lead to hemophilia. This test, which is associated with a 1% risk of miscarriage, can be performed at 10–14 weeks. The test called **amniocentesis** examines the DNA of fetal cells shed into the amniotic fluid for genetic mutations. Amniocentesis, which is associated with a one in 200 risk of miscarriage, is performed at 15–18 weeks gestation.

Treatment

The most important thing that individuals with hemophilia can do to prevent complications of this disease is to avoid injury. Those individuals who require dental work or any surgery may need to be pre-treated with an infusion of factor VIII to avoid hemorrhage. Also, hemophiliacs should be vaccinated against hepatitis. Medications or drugs that promote bleeding, such as aspirin, should be avoided.

Various types of factors VIII and IX are available to replace a patient's missing factors. These are administered intravenously (directly into the patient's veins

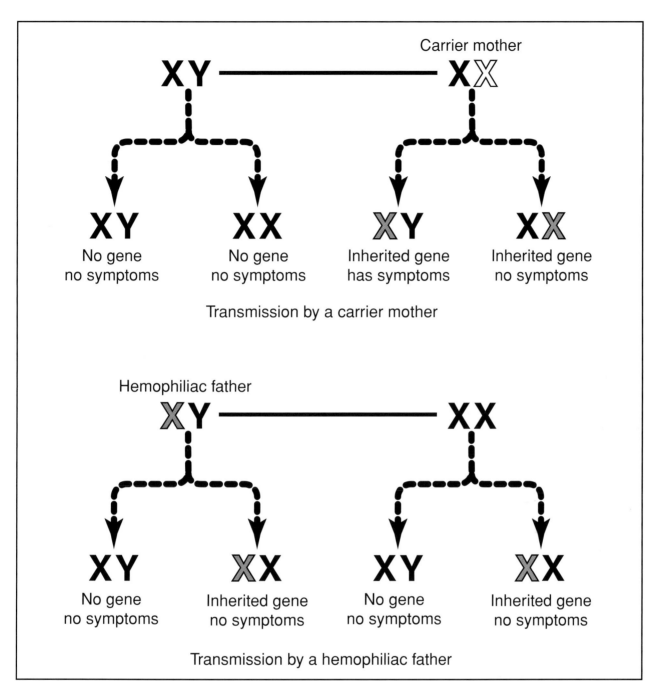

Carrier mother

XY ——————— X𝕏

XY — No gene no symptoms

XX — No gene no symptoms

XY — Inherited gene has symptoms

XX — Inherited gene no symptoms

Transmission by a carrier mother

Hemophiliac father

XY ——————— XX

XY — No gene no symptoms

XX — Inherited gene no symptoms

XY — No gene no symptoms

XX — Inherited gene no symptoms

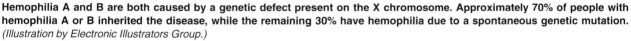

Transmission by a hemophiliac father

Hemophilia A and B are both caused by a genetic defect present on the X chromosome. Approximately 70% of people with hemophilia A or B inherited the disease, while the remaining 30% have hemophilia due to a spontaneous genetic mutation. *(Illustration by Electronic Illustrators Group.)*

by needle). These factor preparations may be obtained from a single donor, by pooling the donations of as many as thousands of donors, or by laboratory creation through highly advanced genetic techniques.

The frequency of treatment with factors depends on the severity of the individual patient's disease. Patients with relatively mild disease will only require

treatment in the event of injury, or to prepare for scheduled surgical or dental procedures. Patients with more severe disease will require regular treatment to avoid spontaneous bleeding.

While appropriate treatment of hemophilia can both decrease suffering and be life-saving, complications associated with treatment can also be quite

KEY TERMS

Amplification—A process by which something is made larger. In clotting, only a very few chemicals are released by the initial injury; they result in a cascade of chemical reactions which produces increasingly larger quantities of different chemicals, resulting in an appropriately-sized, strong fibrin clot.

Factors—Coagulation factors are substances in the blood, such as proteins and minerals, that are necessary for clotting. Each clotting substance is designated with roman numerals I through XIII.

Fibrin—The final substance created through the clotting cascade, which provides a strong, reliable plug to prevent further bleeding from the initial injury.

Hemorrhage—Very severe, massive bleeding that is difficult to control. Hemorrhage can occur in hemophiliacs after what would be a relatively minor injury to a person with normal clotting factors.

Mutation—A permanent change in the genetic material that may alter a trait or characteristic of an individual, or manifest as disease, and can be transmitted to offspring.

Platelets—Small disc-shaped structures that circulate in the blood stream and participate in blood clotting.

Trauma—Injury.

serious. About 20% of all patients with hemophilia A begin to produce chemicals in their bodies which rapidly destroy infused factor VIII. The presence of such a chemical may greatly hamper efforts to prevent or stop a major hemorrhage.

Individuals who receive factor prepared from pooled donor blood are at risk for serious infections that may be passed through blood. Hepatitis, a severe and potentially fatal viral liver infection, may be contracted from pooled factor preparations. Recently, a good deal of concern has been raised about the possibility of hemophiliacs contracting a fatal slow virus infection of the brain (**Creutzfeldt-Jakob disease**) from blood products. Unfortunately, pooled factor preparations in the early 1980s were contaminated with human immunodeficiency virus (HIV), the virus which causes **AIDS**. A large number of hemophiliacs were infected with HIV and some

statistics show that HIV is still the leading cause of **death** among hemophiliacs. Currently, careful methods of donor testing, as well as methods of inactivating viruses present in donated blood, have greatly lowered this risk.

The most exciting new treatments currently being researched involve efforts to transfer new genes to hemophiliacs. These new genes would have the ability to produce the missing factors. As yet, these techniques are not being performed on humans, but there is great hope that eventually this type of **gene therapy** will be available.

Prognosis

Prognosis is very difficult to generalize. Because there are so many variations in the severity of hemophilia, and because much of what befalls a hemophiliac patient will depend on issues such as physical activity level and accidental injuries, statistics on prognosis are not generally available.

Resources

BOOKS

Khoury, Muin J., Wylie Burke, and Elizabeth J. Thomson, editors. *Genetics and Public Health in the 21st Century: Using Genetic Information to Improve Health and Prevent Disease*. New York: Oxford University Press, 2000.

Resnick, Susan. *Blood Saga: Hemophilia, AIDS, and the Survival of a Community*. Berkeley: University of California Press, 1999.

PERIODICALS

Stephenson, J. "New Therapies Show Promise for Patients with Leukemia, Hemophilia, and Heart Disease." *JAMA* 285 (January 1, 2001): 153+.

ORGANIZATIONS

National Hemophilia Foundation. 116 West 32nd St., 11th Floor, New York, NY 10001. (800) 42-HANDI. < http://www.info@hemophilia.org>.

National Organization for Rare Disorders (NORD). PO Box 8923, New Fairfield, CT 06812-8923. (203) 746-6518 or (800) 999-6673. Fax: (203) 746-6481. < http://www.rarediseases.org >.

OTHER

March of Dimes. < www.modimes.org >.

National Organization for Rare Disorders. < www.rarediseases.org >.

Jennifer F. Wilson, MS

Hemophilus ducreyi infection *see* **Chancroid**

Hemophilus infections

Definition

Hemophilus infections, most of which are due to *Haemophilus influenzae* infections, are a group of contagious diseases that are caused by a gram-negative bacterium, and affect only humans. Some hemophilus infections are potentially fatal.

Description

H. influenzae is a common organism worldwide; it has been found in the nasal secretions of as many as 90% of healthy individuals in the general population. Hemophilus infections are characterized by acute inflammation with a discharge (exudate). They may affect almost any organ system, but are most common in the respiratory tract. The organism can be transmitted by person-to-person contact, or by contact with nasal discharges and other body fluids. Hemophilus infections in the United States are most likely to spread in the late winter or early spring.

The primary factor influencing the rate of infection is age; children between the ages of six months and four years are most vulnerable to *H. influenzae*. In previous years, about 50% of children would acquire a hemophilus infection before reaching one year of age; almost all children would develop one before age three. These figures are declining, however, as a result of the increasing use of hemophilus vaccines for children.

Adults are also susceptible to hemophilus diseases. *H. influenzae* **pneumonia** is a common nosocomial infection (illnesses contracted in hospitals). The rate of hemophilus infections in the adult population has increased over the past 40 years. The reasons for this change are unclear, but some researchers speculate that the overuse of **antibiotics** has led to the development of drug-resistant strains of *H. influenzae*. The risk factors for hemophilus infections among adults include:

- smoking
- alcoholism
- chronic lung disease
- old age
- living in a city or institutional housing with a large group of people
- poor **nutrition** and hygiene
- hIV infection, or other immune system disorder

Causes and symptoms

Hemophilus infections are primarily caused by *Haemophilus influenzae*, a gram-negative bacterium that is capable of spreading from the nasal tissues and upper airway, where it is usually found, to the chest, throat, or middle ear. The organism sometimes invades localized areas of tissue, producing **meningitis**, **infectious arthritis**, **conjunctivitis**, **cellulitis**, **epiglottitis**, or inflammation of the membrane surrounding the heart. The most serious infections are caused by a strain called *H. influenzae* b (Hib). Before routine **vaccination**, Hib was the most common cause of bacterial meningitis, and responsible for most of the cases of acquired mental retardation in the United States.

Hemophilus infections in children

BACTERIAL SEPSIS IN THE NEWBORN. Bacterial **sepsis** (sepsis is the presence of illness-causing microorganisms, or their poisons, in the blood) is a potentially fatal illness in newborn infants. The child may acquire the disease organism as it passes through the mother's birth canal, or from the hospital environment. *H. influenzae* can also produce inflammations of the eye (conjunctivitis) in newborn children. The signs of sepsis may include fever, crankiness, feeding problems, breathing difficulties, pale or mottled skin, or drowsiness. Premature birth is the most significant risk factor for hemophilus infections in newborns.

EPIGLOTTITIS. Epiglottitis is a potentially fatal hemophilus infection. Although children are more likely to develop epiglottitis, it can occur in adults as well. When the epiglottis (a piece of cartilage behind the tongue which protects the opening to the windpipe by opening and closing) is infected, it can swell to the point where it blocks the windpipe. The symptoms of epiglottitis include a sudden high **fever**, drooling, the feeling of an object stuck in the throat, and **stridor**. The epiglottis will look swollen and bright red if the doctor examines the patient's throat with a laryngoscope (a viewing device).

MENINGITIS. Meningitis caused by Hib is most common in children between nine months and four years of age. The child usually develops upper respiratory symptoms followed by fever, loss of appetite, vomiting, **headache**, and a stiff or sore neck or back. In severe cases, the child may have convulsions or go into **shock** or coma.

OTHER INFECTIONS. Hib is the second most common cause of middle ear infection and **sinusitis** in children. The symptoms of sinusitis include fever, **pain**, **bad breath**, and coughing. Children may also develop infectious arthritis from Hib. The joints most frequently affected are the large weight-bearing joints.

Hemophilus infections in adults

PNEUMONIA. Hib pneumonia is the most common hemophilus infection in adults. The symptoms include empyema (sputum containing pus), and fever. The hemophilus organism can usually be identified from sputum samples. Hib pneumonia is increasingly common in the elderly.

MENINGITIS. Meningitis caused by Hib can develop in adults as a complication of an ear infection or sinusitis. The symptoms are similar to those in children but are usually less severe in adults.

Diagnosis

The diagnosis is usually based on a combination of the patient's symptoms and the results of blood counts, cultures, or antigen detection tests.

Laboratory tests

Laboratory tests can be used to confirm the diagnosis of hemophilus infections. The bacterium can be grown on chocolate agar, or identified by blood cultures or Gram stain of body fluids. Antigen detection tests can be used to identify hemophilus infections in children. These tests include latex agglutination and electrophoresis.

Other laboratory findings that are associated with hemophilus infections include anemia (low red blood cell count), and a drop in the number of white blood cells in children with severe infections. Adults often show an abnormally high level of white blood cells; cell counts of 15,000–30,000/mm^3 are not unusual.

Treatment

Because some hemophilus infections are potentially fatal, treatment is started without waiting for the results of laboratory tests.

Medications

Hemophilus infections are treated with antibiotics. Patients who are severely ill are given ampicillin or a third-generation cephalosporin, such as cefotaxime or ceftriaxone, intravenously. Patients with milder infections are given oral antibiotics, including amoxicillin, cefaclor, erythromycin, or trimethoprim-sulfamethoxazole. Patients who are allergic to penicillin are usually given cefaclor or trimethoprim-sulfamethoxazole.

Patients with Hib strains that are resistant to ampicillin may be given chloramphenicol. Chloramphenicol is not a first-choice drug because of its side effects, including interference with bone marrow production of blood cells.

The duration of antibiotic treatment depends on the location and severity of the hemophilus infection. Adults with respiratory tract infections, or Hib pneumonia, are usually given a 10–14 day course of antibiotics. Meningitis is usually treated for 10–14 days, but a seven-day course of treatment with ceftriaxone appears to be sufficient for infants and children. Ear infections are treated for seven to 10 days.

Supportive care

Patients with serious hemophilus infections require bed rest and a humidified environment (such as a **croup** tent) if the respiratory tract is affected. Patients with epiglottitis frequently require intubation (insertion of a breathing tube) or a **tracheotomy** to keep the airway open. Patients with inflammation of the heart membrane, pneumonia, or arthritis may need surgical treatment to drain infected fluid from the chest cavity or inflamed joints.

Supportive care also includes monitoring of blood cell counts for patients using chloramphenicol, ampicillin, or other drugs that may affect production of blood cells by the bone marrow.

Prognosis

The most important factors in the prognosis are the severity of the infection and promptness of treatment. Untreated hemophilus infections—particularly meningitis, sepsis, and epiglottitis—have a high mortality rate. Bacterial sepsis of the newborn has a mortality rate between 13–50%. The prognosis is usually good for patients with mild infections who are treated without delay. Children who develop Hib arthritis sometimes have lasting problems with joint function.

Prevention

Hemophilus vaccines

There are three different vaccines for hemophilus infections used to immunize children in the United States: PRP-D, HBOC, and PRP-OMP. PRP-D is used only in children older than 15 months. HBOC is

KEY TERMS

Bacterium—A microscopic one-celled organism. *Haemophilus influenzae* is a specific bacterium.

Epiglottitis—Inflammation of the epiglottis. The epiglottis is a piece of cartilage behind the tongue that closes the opening to the windpipe when a person swallows. An inflamed epiglottis can swell and close off the windpipe, thus causing the patient to suffocate.

Exudate—A discharge produced by the body. Some exudates are caused by infections.

Gram-negative—A term that means that a bacterium will not retain the violet color when stained with Gram's dye. *Haemophilus influenzae* is a gram-negative bacterium.

Intubation—The insertion of a tube into the patient's airway to protect the airway from collapsing. Intubation is sometimes done as an emergency procedure for patients with epiglottitis.

Nosocomial—Contracted in a hospital. Pneumonia caused by *H. influenzae* is an example of a nosocomial infection.

Sepsis—Invasion of body tissues by disease organisms or their toxins. Sepsis may be either localized or generalized. *Haemophilus influenzae* can cause bacterial sepsis in newborns.

Stridor—A harsh or crowing breath sound caused by partial blockage of the patient's upper airway.

Tracheotomy—An emergency procedure in which the surgeon cuts directly through the patient's neck into the windpipe in order to keep the airway open.

administered to infants at two, four, and six months after birth, with a booster dose at 15–18 months. PRP-OMP is administered to infants at two and four months, with the third dose at the child's first birthday. All three vaccines are given by intramuscular injection. About 5% of children may develop fever or soreness in the area of the injection.

Other measures

Other preventive measures include isolating patients with respiratory hemophilus infections; treating appropriate contacts of infected patients with rifampin; maintaining careful standards of cleanliness in hospitals, including proper disposal of soiled tissues; and washing hands properly.

Resources

BOOKS

Chambers, Henry F. "Infectious Diseases: Bacterial & Chlamydial." In *Current Medical Diagnosis and Treatment, 1998*, edited by Stephen McPhee, et al., 37th ed. Stamford: Appleton & Lange, 1997.

Rebecca J. Frey, PhD

Hemophilus influenzae infections *see*
Hemophilus infections

▌Hemoptysis

Definition

Hemoptysis is the coughing up of blood or bloody sputum from the lungs or airway. It may be either self-limiting or recurrent. Massive hemoptysis is defined as 200–600 mL of blood coughed up within a period of 24 hours or less.

Description

Hemoptysis can range from small quantities of bloody sputum to life-threatening amounts of blood. The patient may or may not have chest **pain**.

Causes and symptoms

Hemoptysis can be caused by a range of disorders:

- Infections. These include **pneumonia**; **tuberculosis**; **aspergillosis**; and parasitic diseases, including ascariasis, **amebiasis**, and paragonimiasis.

- Tumors that erode blood vessel walls.

- Drug **abuse**. **Cocaine** can cause massive hemoptysis.

- Trauma. Chest injuries can cause bleeding into the lungs.

- Vascular disorders, including aneurysms, **pulmonary embolism**, and malformations of the blood vessels.

- Bronchitis. Its most common cause is long-term **smoking**.

- Foreign object(s) in the airway.

- Blood clotting disorders.

- Bleeding following such surgical procedures as bronchial biopsies and heart catheterization.

Diagnosis

The diagnosis of hemoptysis is complicated by the number of possible causes.

Patient history

It is important for the doctor to distinguish between blood from the lungs and blood coming from the nose, mouth, or digestive tract. Patients may aspirate, or breathe, blood from the nose or stomach into their lungs and **cough** it up. They may also swallow blood from the chest area and then vomit. The doctor will ask about stomach ulcers, repeated **vomiting**, **liver disease**, **alcoholism**, smoking, tuberculosis, mitral valve disease, or treatment with anticoagulant medications.

Physical examination

The doctor will examine the patient's nose, throat, mouth, and chest for bleeding from these areas and for signs of chest trauma. The doctor also listens to the patient's breathing and heartbeat for indications of heart abnormalities or lung disease.

Laboratory tests

Laboratory tests include blood tests to rule out clotting disorders, and to look for food particles or other evidence of blood from the stomach. Sputum can be tested for fungi, bacteria, or parasites.

X ray and bronchoscopy

Chest x rays and **bronchoscopy** are the most important studies for evaluating hemoptysis. They are used to evaluate the cause, location, and extent of the bleeding. The bronchoscope is a long, flexible tube used to identify tumors or remove **foreign objects**.

Imaging and other tests

Computed tomography scans (CT scans) are used to detect aneurysms and to confirm x-ray results. Ventilation-perfusion scanning is used to rule out pulmonary **embolism**. The doctor may also order an angiogram to rule out pulmonary embolism, or to locate a source of bleeding that could not be seen with the bronchoscope.

In spite of the number of diagnostic tests, the cause of hemoptysis cannot be determined in 20–30% of cases.

Treatment

Massive hemoptysis is a life-threatening emergency that requires treatment in an intensive care

---

KEY TERMS

Aneurysm—A sac formed by the dilation of the wall of an artery, vein, or heart; it is filled with clotted blood or fluid.

Angiography—A technique for imaging the blood vessels by injecting a substance that is opaque to x rays.

Aspergillosis—A lung infection caused by the mold *Aspergillus fumigatus.*

Intubation—The insertion of a tube into a body canal or hollow organ, as into the trachea or stomach.

Pulmonary embolism—The blocking of an artery in the lung by a blood clot.

---

unit. The patient will be intubated (the insertion of a tube to help breathing) to protect the airway, and to allow evaluation of the source of the bleeding. Patients with lung **cancer**, bleeding from an aneurysm (blood clot), or persistent traumatic bleeding require chest surgery.

Patients with tuberculosis, aspergillosis, or bacterial pneumonia are given **antibiotics**.

Foreign objects are removed with a bronchoscope.

If the cause cannot be determined, the patient is monitored for further developments.

Prognosis

The prognosis depends on the underlying cause. In cases of massive hemoptysis, the mortality rate is about 15%. The rate of bleeding, however, is not a useful predictor of the patient's chances for recovery.

Resources

BOOKS

Stauffer, John L. "Lung." In *Current Medical Diagnosis and Treatment, 1998,* edited by Stephen McPhee, et al., 37th ed. Stamford: Appleton & Lange, 1997.

Rebecca J. Frey, PhD

Hemorrhagic colitis *see* **Escherichia coli**

Hemorrhagic fever with renal syndrome *see* **Hantavirus infections**

Hemorrhagic fevers

Definition

Hemorrhagic fevers are caused by viruses that exist throughout the world. However, they are most common in tropical areas. Early symptoms, such as muscle aches and **fever**, can progress to a mild illness or to a more debilitating, potentially fatal disease. In severe cases, a prominent symptom is bleeding, or hemorrhaging, from orifices and internal organs.

Description

Although hemorrhagic fevers are regarded as emerging diseases, they probably have existed for many years. This designation isn't meant to imply that they are newly developing, but rather that human exposure to the causative viruses is increasing to the point of concern.

These viruses are maintained in nature in arthropod (insects, spiders and other invertebrates with external hard skeletons) or animal populations—so-called disease reservoirs. Individuals within these populations become infected with a virus but do not die from it. In many cases, they don't even develop symptoms. Then the viruses are transmitted from a reservoir population to humans by vectors—either members of the reservoir population or an intervening species, such as mosquitoes.

Hemorrhagic fevers are generally either endemic or linked to specific locations. If many people reside in an endemic area, the number of cases may soar. For example, dengue fever, a type of hemorrhagic fever, affects approximately 100 million people annually. A large percentage of those infected live in densely populated southeast Asia; an area in which the disease vector, a mosquito, thrives. Some hemorrhagic fevers are exceedingly rare, because people very infrequently encounter the virus. Marburg hemorrhagic fever, which has affected fewer than 40 people since its discovery in 1967, provides one such example. Fatality rates are also variable. In cases of dengue hemorrhagic fever–dengue **shock** syndrome, 1–5% of the victims perish. On the other end of the spectrum is Ebola, an African hemorrhagic fever, that kills 30–90% of those infected.

The onset of hemorrhagic fevers may be sudden or gradual, but all of them are linked by the potential for hemorrhaging. However, not all cases progress to this very serious symptom. Hemorrhaging may be attributable to the destruction of blood coagulating factors or to increased permeability of body tissues. The severity of bleeding ranges from petechiae, which are pinpoint hemorrhages under the skin surface, to distinct bleeding from such body orifices as the nose or vagina.

Causes and symptoms

The viruses that cause hemorrhagic fevers are found most commonly in tropical locations; however, some are found in cooler climates. Typical disease vectors include rodents, ticks, or mosquitoes, but person-to-person transmission in health care settings or through sexual contact can also occur.

Filoviruses

Ebola is the most famous of the Filoviridae, a virus family that also includes the Marburg virus. Ebola is endemic to Africa, particularly the Republic of the Congo and Sudan; the Marburg virus is found in sub-Saharan Africa. The natural reservoir of filoviruses is unknown. The incubation period, or time between infection and appearance of symptoms, is thought to last three to eight days, possibly longer.

Symptoms appear suddenly, and include severe headache, fever, chills, muscle aches, malaise, and appetite loss. These symptoms may be accompanied by nausea, **vomiting**, **diarrhea**, and abdominal **pain**. Victims become apathetic and disoriented. Severe bleeding commonly occurs from the gastrointestinal tract, nose and throat, and vagina. Other bleeding symptoms include petechiae and oozing from injection sites. Ebola is fatal in 30–90% of cases.

Arenaviruses

Viruses of the Arenaviridae family cause the Argentinian, Brazilian, Bolivian, and Venezuelan hemorrhagic fevers. Lassa fever, which occurs in west Africa, also arises from an arenavirus. Infected rodents, the natural reservoir, shed virus particles in their urine and saliva, which humans may inhale or otherwise come in contact with.

Fever, muscle aches, malaise, and appetite loss gradually appear one to two weeks after infection with the South American viruses. Initial symptoms are followed by **headache**, back pain, dizziness, and gastrointestinal upset. The face and chest appear flushed and the gums begin to bleed. In about 30% of cases, the disease progresses to bleeding under the skin and from the mucous membranes, and/or to effects on the nervous system, such as delirium, **coma**, and convulsions. Untreated, South American hemorrhagic fevers have a 10–30% fatality rate.

Lassa fever also begins gradually, following an 8–14 day incubation. Initial symptoms resemble those of the South American hemorrhagic fevers, followed by a **sore throat**, muscle and joint pain, severe headache, pain above the stomach, and a dry **cough**. The face and neck become swollen, and fluid may accumulate in the lungs. Bleeding occurs in 15–20% of infected individuals, mostly from the gums and nose. Overall, the fatality rate is lower than 2%, but hospitals may encounter 20% fatality rates, treating typically the most serious of cases.

Flaviviruses

The Flaviviridae family includes the viruses that cause yellow and dengue fevers.

Yellow fever occurs in tropical areas of the Americas and Africa and is transmitted from monkeys to humans by mosquitoes. The virus may produce a mild, possibly unnoticed illness, but some individuals are suddenly stricken with a fever, weakness, low back pain, muscle pain, **nausea**, and vomiting. This phase lasts one to seven days, after which the symptoms recede for one to two days. Symptoms then return with greater intensity, along with **jaundice**, **delirium**, seizures, stupor, and coma. Bleeding occurs from the mucous membranes and under the skin surface, and dark blood appears in stools and vomit.

Mosquitoes also transmit the dengue virus. **Dengue fever** is endemic in southeast Asia and areas of the Americas. Cases have also been reported in the Caribbean, Saudi Arabia, and northern Australia. In 2004 several cases were reported along the border between Texas and Mexico in the southwestern United States. This virus causes either the mild dengue fever or the more serious dengue hemorrhagic fever–dengue shock syndrome (DHF-DSS).

In children, dengue fever is characterized by a sore throat, runny nose, slight cough, and a fever lasting for a week or less. Older children and adults experience more severe symptoms: fever, headache, muscle and joint pain, loss of appetite, and a rash. The skin appears flushed, and intense pain occurs in the bones and limbs. After nearly a week, the fever subsides for one to two days before returning. Minor hemorrhaging, such as from the gums, or more serious gastrointestinal bleeding may occur.

DHF-DSS primarily affects children younger than 15 years. The symptoms initially resemble those of dengue fever in adults, without the bone and limb pain. As the fever begins to abate, the individual's condition worsens and hemorrhaging occurs from the nose, gums, and injection sites. Bleeding is also seen from the gastrointestinal, genitourinary, and respiratory tracts.

Bunyaviruses

The Bunyaviridae family includes several hundred viruses but only a few are responsible for hemorrhagic fevers in humans.

Rift Valley fever is caused by the phlebovirus, found in sub-Saharan Africa and the Nile delta. Natural reservoirs are wild and domestic animals, and transmission occurs through contact with infected animals or through mosquito bites. The incubation period lasts 3–12 days. Most cases of Rift Valley fever are mild and may be symptomless. If symptoms develop, they include fever, backache, muscle and joint pain, and headache. Hemorrhagic symptoms occur rarely; while **death**, which occurs in fewer than 3% of cases, is attributable to massive liver damage.

Crimean-Congo hemorrhagic fever is caused by nairovirus and occurs in central and southern Africa, Asia, Eurasia, and the Middle East. The virus is found in hares, birds, ticks, and domestic animals and may be transmitted by ticks or by contact with infected animals. The nairovirus incubation period is three to 12 days; after which an individual experiences fever, chills, headache, severe muscle pain, pain above the stomach, nausea, vomiting, and appetite loss. Bleeding under the skin and gastrointestinal and vaginal bleeding may develop in the most severe cases. Death rates range from 10% in southern Russia to 50% in parts of Asia.

Hemorrhagic fever with renal (kidney) syndrome is caused by the hantaviruses: Hantaan, Seoul, Puumala, and Dobrava. Hantaan virus occurs in northern Asia, the Far East, and the Balkans; Seoul virus is found worldwide; Puumala virus is found in Scandinavia and northern Europe; while Dobrava virus occurs in the Balkans. Wild rodents are the natural reservoirs and transmit the virus via their excrement or body fluids or through direct contact. Initial symptoms develop within 10–40 days and include fever, headache, muscle pain, and **dizziness**. Other symptoms are blurry vision, abdominal and back pain, nausea, and vomiting. High levels of protein in the urine signal kidney damage; hemorrhaging may also occur. Death rates range from 0–10%.

Diagnosis

Since the hemorrhagic fevers share symptoms with many other diseases, positive identification of the disease relies on evidence of the viruses in the bloodstream—such as detection of antigens and antibodies—or isolation of the virus from the body. Disruptions in the normal levels of bloodstream components may be helpful in determining some, but not all, hemorrhagic fevers.

Treatment

Lassa fever, and possibly other hemorrhagic fevers, respond to ribavirin, an antiviral medication. However, most of the hemorrhagic fever viruses can only be treated with supportive care. Interferon is not useful and may in fact complicate management. Such care centers around maintaining correct fluid and electrolyte balances in the body and protecting the patient against secondary infections. Heparin and vitamin K administration, coagulation factor replacement, and blood transfusions may be effective in lessening or stopping hemorrhage in some cases.

Some researchers are investigating the possibility of targeting tissue factor (TF) as a way of treating viral hemorrhagic fevers. TF is a protein that activates the coagulation process in these illnesses, and experimental models suggest that a blockade of tissue factor assists the body's immune response to hemorrhagic fever viruses.

Prognosis

Recovery from some hemorrhagic fevers is more certain than from others. The filoviruses are among the most lethal; fatality rates for Ebola range from 30–90%, while DHF-DSS cases result in a 1–5% fatality rate. Whether a case occurs during an epidemic or as an isolated case also has a bearing on the outcome. For example, isolated cases of yellow fever have a 5% mortality rate, but 20–50% of epidemic cases may be fatal.

Permanent disability can occur with some types of hemorrhagic fever. About 10% of severely ill Rift Valley fever victims suffer retina damage and may be permanently blind, and 25% of South American hemorrhagic fever victims suffer potentially permanent deafness.

Proper treatment is vital. In cases of DHF-DSS, fatality can be reduced from 40–50% to less than 2% with adequate medical care. For individuals who survive hemorrhagic fevers, prolonged convalescence is usually inevitable. However, survivors seem to gain lifelong immunity against the virus that made them ill.

KEY TERMS

Antibody—A molecule created by the body's immune system to combat a specific infectious agent, such as a virus or bacteria.

Antigen—A specific feature, such as a protein, on an infectious agent. Antibodies use this feature as a means of identifying infectious intruders.

Coagulating factors—Components within the blood that help form clots.

Endemic—Referring to a specific geographic area in which a disease may occur.

Hemorrhage—As a noun, this refers to the point at which blood is released. As a verb, this refers to bleeding.

Incubation—The time period between exposure to an infectious agent, such as a virus or bacteria, and the appearance of symptoms of illness.

Petechiae—Pinpoint hemorrhages that appear as reddish dots beneath the surface of the skin.

Reservoir—A population in which a virus is maintained without causing serious illness to the infected individuals.

Ribavirin—A drug that is used to combat viral infections.

Tissue factor—A glycoprotein involved in blood coagulation.

Vector—A member of the reservoir population or an intervening species that can transmit a virus to a susceptible victim. Mosquitoes are common vectors, as are ticks and rodents.

Prevention

Hemorrhagic fevers can be prevented through vector control and personal protection measures. Attempts have been made in urban and settled areas to destroy mosquito and rodent populations. In areas where such measures are impossible, individuals can use insect repellents, mosquito netting, and other methods to minimize exposure.

Vaccines have been developed against yellow fever, Argentinian hemorrhagic fever, and Crimean-Congo hemorrhagic fever. Vaccines against other hemorrhagic fevers are being researched. Another possible preventive measure is increasing the number of natural killer (NK) cells in the body. These cells appear to be an important innate source of protection against Ebola and other filoviruses.

Prevention of epidemics of hemorrhagic fevers has acquired a new importance in the early 2000s from concern that the causative viruses might be used as weapons of bioterrorism. These viruses can be transmitted in aerosol form as well as having a high mortality rate.

Resources

BOOKS

Beers, Mark H., MD, and Robert Berkow, MD., editors. "Viral Diseases." Section 13, Chapter 162 In *The Merck Manual of Diagnosis and Therapy*. Whitehouse Station, NJ: Merck Research Laboratories, 2004.

PERIODICALS

Izadi, S., K. H. Naieni, S. R. Madjdzadeh, and A. Nadim. "Crimean-Congo Hemorrhagic Fever in Sistan and Baluchestan Province of Iran, A Case-Control Study on Epidemiological Characteristics." *International Journal of Infectious Diseases* 8 (September 2004): 299–306.

Mahanty, S., and M. Bray. "Pathogenesis of Filoviral Haemorrhagic Fevers." *Lancet Infectious Diseases* 4 (August 2004): 487–498.

Ruf, W. "Emerging Roles of Tissue Factor in Viral Hemorrhagic Fever." *Trends in Immunology* 25 (September 2004): 461–464.

Salvaggio, M. R., and J. W. Baddley. "Other Viral Bioweapons: Ebola and Marburg Hemorrhagic Fever." *Dermatologic Clinics* 22 (July 2004): 291–302.

Setlick, R. F., D. Ouellette, J. Morgan, et al. "Pulmonary Hemorrhage Syndrome Associated with an Autochthonous Case of Dengue Hemorrhagic Fever." *Southern Medical Journal* 97 (July 2004): 688–691.

Warfield, K. L., J. G. Perkins, D. L. Swenson, et al. "Role of Natural Killer Cells in Innate Protection against Lethal Ebola Virus Infection." *Journal of Experimental Medicine* 200 (July 19, 2004): 169–179.

ORGANIZATIONS

Centers for Disease Control and Prevention. 1600 Clifton Rd., NE, Atlanta, GA 30333. (800) 311-3435, (404) 639-3311. < http://www.cdc.gov >.

Infectious Diseases Society of America (IDSA). 66 Canal Center Plaza, Suite 600, Alexandria, VA 22314. (703) 299-0200. Fax: (703) 299-0204. < http://www.idsociety.org >.

World Health Organization (WHO). < http://www.who.int/en/ >.

OTHER

Centers for Disease Control and Prevention, Special Pathogens Branch. "Ebola Hemorrhagic Fever," August 23, 2004. < http://www.cdc.gov/ncidod/dvrd/spb/mnpages/dispages/ebola.htm >.

Centers for Disease Control and Prevention, Special Pathogens Branch. "Marburg Hemorrhagic Fever," August 23, 2004. < http://www.cdc.gov/ncidod/dvrd/spb/mnpages/dispages/marburg.htm >.

Julia Barrett
Rebecca J. Frey, PhD

Hemorrhoids

Definition

Hemorrhoids are enlarged veins in the anus or lower rectum. They often go unnoticed and usually clear up after a few days, but can cause long-lasting discomfort, bleeding and be excruciatingly painful. Effective medical treatments are available, however.

Description

Hemorrhoids (also called piles) can be divided into two kinds, internal and external. Internal hemorrhoids lie inside the anus or lower rectum, beneath the anal or rectal lining. External hemorrhoids lie outside the anal opening. Both kinds can be present at the same time.

Hemorrhoids are a very common medical complaint. More than 75% of Americans have hemorrhoids at some point in their lives, typically after age 30. Pregnant women often develop hemorrhoids, but the condition usually clears up after childbirth. Men are more likely than women to suffer from hemorrhoids that require professional medical treatment.

Causes and symptoms

Precisely why hemorrhoids develop is unknown. Researchers have identified a number of reasons to explain hemorrhoidal swelling, including the simple fact that people's upright posture places a lot of pressure on the anal and rectal veins. Aging, obesity, **pregnancy**, chronic constipation or **diarrhea**, excessive use of **enemas** or **laxatives**, straining during bowel movements, and spending too much time on the toilet are considered contributing factors. Heredity may also play a part in some cases. There is no reason to believe that hemorrhoids are caused by jobs requiring, for instance, heavy lifting or long hours of sitting,

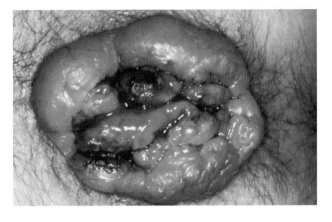

Clinical photo of a thrombosed external hemorrhoid. *(Custom Medical Stock Photo. Reproduced by permission.)*

although activities of that kind may make existing hemorrhoids worse.

The commonest symptom of internal hemorrhoids is bright red blood in the toilet bowl or on one's feces or toilet paper. When hemorrhoids remain inside the anus they are almost never painful, but they can prolapse (protrude outside the anus) and become irritated and sore. Sometimes, prolapsed hemorrhoids move back into the anal canal on their own or can be pushed back in, but at other times they remain permanently outside the anus until treated by a doctor.

Small external hemorrhoids usually do not produce symptoms. Larger ones, however, can be painful and interfere with cleaning the anal area after a bowel movement. When, as sometimes happens, a blood clot forms in an external hemorrhoid (creating what is called a thrombosed hemorrhoid), the skin around the anus becomes inflamed and a very painful lump develops. On rare occasions the clot will begin to bleed after a few days and leave blood on the underwear. A thrombosed hemorrhoid will not cause an **embolism**.

Diagnosis

Diagnosis begins with a visual examination of the anus, followed by an internal examination during which the doctor carefully inserts a gloved and lubricated finger into the anus. The doctor may also use an anoscope, a small tube that allows him or her to see into the anal canal. Under some circumstances the doctor may wish to check for other problems by using a sigmoidoscope or colonoscope, a flexible instrument that allows inspection of the lower colon (in the case of the sigmoidoscope) or the entire colon (in the case of the colonoscope).

Treatment

Hemorrhoids can often be effectively dealt with by dietary and lifestyle changes. Softening the feces and avoiding **constipation** by adding fiber to one's diet is important, because hard feces lead to straining during defecation. Fruit, leafy vegetables, and whole-grain breads and cereals are good sources of fiber, as are bulk laxatives and fiber supplements such as Metamucil or Citrucel. Exercising, losing excess weight, and drinking six to eight glasses a day of water or another liquid (not alcohol) also helps. Soap or toilet paper that is perfumed may irritate the anal area and should be avoided, as should excessive cleaning, rubbing, or wiping of that area. Reading in the bathroom is also considered a bad idea, because it adds to the time one spends on the toilet and may increase the strain placed on the anal and rectal veins. After each bowel movement, wiping with a moistened tissue or pad sold for that purpose helps lessen irritation. Hemorrhoid **pain** is often eased by sitting in a tub of warm water for about 10 or 15 minutes two to four times a day (**sitz bath**). A cool compress or ice pack to reduce swelling is also recommended (the ice pack should be wrapped in a cloth or towel to prevent direct contact with the skin). Many people find that over-the-counter hemorrhoid creams and foams bring relief, but these medications do not make hemorrhoids disappear.

When painful hemorrhoids do not respond to home-based remedies, professional medical treatment is necessary. The choice of treatment depends on the type of hemorrhoid, what medical equipment is available, and other considerations.

Rubber band ligation is probably the most widely used of the many treatments for internal hemorrhoids (and the least costly for the patient). This procedure is performed in the office of a family doctor or specialist, or in a hospital on an outpatient basis. An applicator is used to place one or two small rubber bands around the base of the hemorrhoid, cutting off its blood supply. After three to 10 days in the bands, the hemorrhoid falls off, leaving a sore that heals in a week or two. Because internal hemorrhoids are located in a part of the anus that does not sense pain, anesthetic is unnecessary and the procedure is painless in most cases. Although there can be minor discomfort and bleeding for a few days after the bands are applied, complications are rare and most people are soon able to return to work and other activities. If more than one hemorrhoid exists or if banding is not entirely effective the first time (as occasionally happens), the procedure may need to be repeated a few weeks later. After five years, 15–20% of patients experience a recurrence of

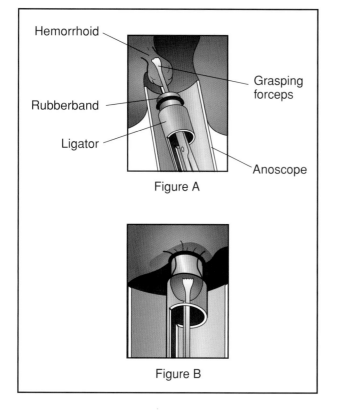

Figure A

Figure B

Rubber band ligation is probably the most widely used treatment for internal hemorrhoids. An applicator is used to place one or two small rubber bands around the base of the hemorrhoid, cutting off its blood supply (figures A and B). After 3-10 days, the rubber bands and the hemorrhoid fall off, leaving a scab which disappears within a week or two. *(Illustration by Electronic Illustrators Group.)*

internal hemorrhoids, but in most cases all that is needed is another banding.

External hemorrhoids, and some prolapsed internal hemorrhoids, are removed by conventional surgery in a hospital. Depending on the circumstances, this requires a local, regional, or general anesthetic. Surgery does cause a fair amount of discomfort, but an overnight hospital stay is usually not necessary. Full healing takes two to four weeks, but most people are able to resume normal activities at the end of a week. Hemorrhoids rarely return after surgery.

Alternative treatment

Like mainstream practitioners, alternative practitioners **stress** the importance of a high-fiber diet. To prevent hemorrhoids by strengthening the veins of the anus, rectum, and colon, they recommend blackberries, blueberries, cherries, vitamin C, butcher's broom (*Ruscus aculeatus*), and flavonoids (plant pigments

found in fruit and fruit products, tea, and soy). Herbal teas, ointments, and suppositories, and other kinds of herbal preparations, are suggested for reducing discomfort and eliminating hemorrhoids. In particular, pilewort (*Ranunculusficaria*), applied in an ointment or taken as a tea, can reduce the pain of external hemorrhoids. **Acupuncture**, **acupressure**, **aromatherapy**, and homeopathy are also used to treat hemorrhoids.

Prognosis

Hemorrhoids do not cause **cancer** and are rarely dangerous or life threatening. Most clear up after a few days without professional medical treatment. However, because colorectal cancer and other digestive system diseases can cause anal bleeding and other hemorrhoid-like symptoms, people should always consult a doctor when those symptoms occur.

Prevention

A high-fiber diet and the other lifestyle changes recommended for coping with existing hemorrhoids also help to prevent hemorrhoids. Not straining during bowel movements is essential.

Resources

ORGANIZATIONS

National Digestive Diseases Information Clearinghouse. 2 Information Way, Bethesda, MD 20892-3570. (800) 891-5389. < http://www.niddk.nih.gov/health/digest/nddic.htm >.

Howard Baker

Henoch-Schönlein purpura *see* **Allergic purpura**

Hepatic carcinoma *see* **Liver cancer, primary**

Hepatic encephalopathy *see* **Liver encephalopathy**

Hepatitis-associated antigen (HAA) test *see* **Hepatitis virus tests**

Hepatitis A

Definition

Hepatitis A is an inflammation of the liver caused by a virus, the hepatitis A virus (HAV). It varies in severity, running an acute course, generally starting within two to six weeks after contact with the virus, and lasting no longer than two or three months. HAV may occur in single cases after contact with an infected relative or sex partner. Alternately, epidemics may develop when food or drinking water is contaminated by the feces of an infected person.

Description

Hepatitis A was previously known as infectious hepatitis because it spread relatively easily from those infected to close household contacts. Once the infection ends, there is no lasting, chronic phase of illness. However it is not uncommon to have a second episode of symptoms about a month after the first; this is called a relapse, but it is not clear that the virus persists when symptoms recur. Both children and adults may be infected by HAV. Children are the chief victims, but very often have no more than a flu-like illness or no symptoms at all (so-called "subclinical" infection),

whereas adults are far likelier to have more severe symptoms.

Epidemics of HAV infection can infect dozens and even hundreds (or, on rare occasions, thousands) of persons. In the public's mind, outbreaks of hepatitis A usually are linked with the eating of contaminated food at a restaurant. It is true that food-handlers, who may themselves have no symptoms, can start an alarming, widespread epidemic. Many types of food can be infected by sewage containing HAV, but shellfish, such as clams and oysters, are common culprits.

Apart from contaminated food and water, certain groups are at increased risk of getting infectious hepatitis:

- Children at day care centers make up an estimated 14–40% of all cases of HAV infection in the United States. Changing diapers transmits infection through fecal-oral contact. Toys and other objects may remain contaminated for some time. Often a child without symptoms brings the infection home to siblings and parents.

- Troops living under crowded conditions at military camps or in the field. During World War II there were an estimated five million cases in German soldiers and civilians.

- Anyone living in heavily populated and squalid conditions, such as the very poor and those placed in refugee or prisoner-of-war camps.

- Homosexual men are increasingly at risk of HAV infection from oral-anal sexual contact.

- Travelers visiting an area where hepatitis A is common are at risk of becoming ill.

Causes and symptoms

The time from exposure to HAV and the onset of symptoms ranges from two to seven weeks and averages about a month. The virus is passed in the feces, especially late during this incubation period, before symptoms first appear. Infected persons are most contagious starting a week or so before symptoms develop, and remain so up until the time **jaundice** (yellowing of the skin) is noted.

Often the first symptoms to appear are **fatigue**, aching all over, **nausea**, and a loss of appetite. Those who like drinking coffee and **smoking** cigarettes may lose their taste for them. Mild **fever** is common; it seldom is higher than 101 °F (38.3 °C). The liver often enlarges, causing **pain** or tenderness in the right upper part of the abdomen. Jaundice then develops, typically lasting seven to ten days. Many patients do

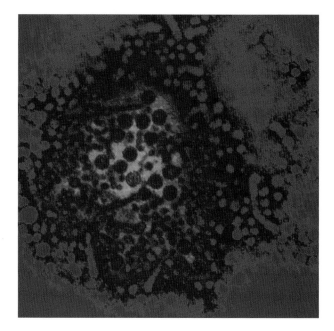

Hepatitis A virus magnified 225,000 times. *(Custom Medical Stock Photo. Reproduced by permission.)*

not visit the doctor until their skin turns yellow. As many as three out of four children have no symptoms of HAV infection, but about 85% of adults will have symptoms. Besides jaundice, the commonest are abdominal pain, loss of appetite, and feeling generally poorly.

Special situations

An occasional patient with hepatitis A will remain jaundiced for a month, two months or even longer, but eventually the jaundice will pass. Very rarely, a patient will develop such severe hepatitis that the liver fails. HAV infection causes about 100 deaths each year in the United States. In developed countries, a pregnant woman who contracts hepatitis A can be expected to do well although a different form of viral hepatitis (**hepatitis E**) can cause severe infection in pregnant women. In developing countries, however, the infection may prove fatal, probably because **nutrition** is not adequate.

Diagnosis

The early, flu-like symptoms and jaundice, as well as rapid recovery, suggest infectious hepatitis without special tests being done. If there is any question, a specialist in gastrointestinal disorders or infectious diseases can confirm the diagnosis—the detection of a specific antibody, called hepatitis A IgM antibody, that develops when HAV is present in the body. This test always registers positive when a patient has symptoms, and should continue to register positive for four to six months. However, hepatitis A IgM antibody will persist lifelong in the blood and is protective against reinfection.

Treatment

Once symptoms appear, no **antibiotics** or other medicines will shorten the course of infectious hepatitis. Patients should rest in bed as needed, take a healthy diet, and avoid drinking alcohol and/or any medications that could further damage the liver. If a patient feels well it is all right to return to school or work even if some jaundice remains.

Prognosis

Most patients with acute hepatitis, even when severe, begin feeling better in two to three weeks, and recover completely in four to eight weeks. After recovering from hepatitis A, a person no longer carries the virus and remains immune for life. In the United States, serious complications are infrequent and deaths are very rare. In the United States, as many as 75% of adults over 50 years of age will have blood test evidence of previous hepatitis A.

Prevention

The single best way to keep from spreading hepatitis A infection is to wash the hands carefully after using the toilet. Those who are infected should not share items that might carry infection. Special care should be taken to avoid transmitting infection to a sex partner. Travelers should avoid water and ice if unsure of their purity, or they can boil water for one minute before drinking it. All foods eaten should be packaged, well cooked or, in the case of fresh fruit, peeled.

If exposure is a possibility, infection may be prevented by an injection of a serum fraction containing antibody against HAV. This material, called immune serum globulin (ISG), is 90% protective even when injected after exposure—providing it is given within two weeks. Anyone living with an infected patient should receive ISG. For long-term protection, a killed virus hepatitis A vaccine became available in 1995. More than 95% of those vaccinated will develop an adequate amount of anti-HAV antibody. Those who should consider being vaccinated include healthcare professionals, those working at day care and similar facilities, frequent travelers to areas with poor sanitation, those with any form of chronic **liver disease**, and those who are very sexually active. Starting in 2000, routine immunization with the hepatitis A vaccine was recommended for children born in states where the rate of hepatitis A was two or more times the national average (Alaska, Arizona, California, Idaho, Nevada, New Mexico, Oklahoma, Oregon, South Dakota, Utah, and Washington) and suggested in states where the rate was 1.5 times the national average (Arkansas, Colorado, Missouri, Montana, Texas and Wyoming).

Larry I. Lutwick, MD

Hepatitis, alcoholic

Definition

Alcoholic hepatitis is an inflammation of the liver caused by alcohol.

Description

Irritation, be it from toxins or infections, causes a similar response in body organs. The response is known as inflammation and consists of:

- an increase in the blood to the affected organ
- redness and swelling of the organ
- influx of immune agents like white blood cells and their arsenal of chemical weapons
- **pain**

As the acute process subsides, there is either healing or lingering activity. Lingering activity—chronic disease—has a milder presentation with similar ingredients. Healing often takes the form of scarring, wherein normal functioning tissue is replaced by tough, fibrous, and non-productive scar. Both chronic disease and healing can happen simultaneously, so that scar tissue progressively replaces normal tissue. This leads to cirrhosis, a liver so scarred it is unable to do its job adequately.

Alcohol can cause either an acute or a chronic disease in the liver. The acute disease can be severe, even fatal, and can bring with it hemolysis–blood cell destruction. Alcohol can also cause a third type of liver disease, fatty liver, in which the continuous action of alcohol turns the liver to useless fat. This condition eventually progresses to **cirrhosis** if the **poisoning** continues.

Causes and symptoms

Inflammation of the liver can be caused by a great variety of agents—poisons, drugs, viruses, bacteria, protozoa, and even larger organisms like worms. Alcohol is a poison if taken in more than modest amounts. It favors destroying stomach lining, liver, heart muscle, and brain tissue. The liver is a primary target because alcohol travels to the liver after leaving the intestines. Those who drink enough to get alcohol poisoning have a tendency to be undernourished, since alcohol provides ample calories but little **nutrition**. It is suspected that both the alcohol and the poor nutrition produce alcoholic hepatitis.

Diagnosis

Hepatitis of all kinds causes notable discomfort, loss of appetite, **nausea**, pain in the liver, and usually **jaundice** (turning yellow). Blood test abnormalities are unmistakably those of hepatitis, but selecting from so many the precise cause may take additional diagnostic work.

Treatment

As with all poisonings, removal of the offending agent is primary. There is no specific treatment for

KEY TERMS

Cirrhosis—Disruption of normal liver structure and function caused by any type of chronic disease such as hepatitis and alcohol abuse.

Fatty liver—An abnormal amount of fat tissue in the liver caused by alcohol abuse.

Hemolysis—Disintegration of read blood cells.

Protozoa—One celled microscopic organisms like amoeba.

alcohol poisoning. General supportive measures must see the patient through until the liver has healed by itself. In the case of fulminant (sudden and severe) disease, the liver may be completely destroyed and have to be replaced by a transplant.

Prognosis

The liver is robust. It can heal without scarring after one or a few episodes of hepatitis that resolve without lingering. It can, moreover, regrow from a fragment of its former self, provided there is not disease or poison still inhibiting it.

Prevention

Alcohol is lethal in many ways when ingested in excess. Research suggests that the maximum healthy dose of alcohol per day is roughly one pure ounce—the amount in two cocktails, two glasses of wine, or two beers.

Resources

ORGANIZATIONS

American Liver Foundation. 1425 Pompton Ave., Cedar Grove, NJ 07009. (800) 223-0179. < http:// www.liverfoundation.org >.
Local chapters of Alcoholics Anonymous.

J. Ricker Polsdorfer, MD

Hepatitis, autoimmune

Definition

A form of liver inflammation in which the body's immune system attacks liver cells.

Description

Autoimmunity causes the body's defense mechanisms to turn against itself. Many of the tissues in the body can be the target of such an attack. While one tissue type predominates, others may be involved in a general misdirection of immune activity, perhaps because the specific target antigen is present in differing quantities in each of the affected tissues. There seem to be hereditary causes for autoimmunity, since these diseases tend to run in families and have genetic markers. Among the more common diseases believed to fall within this category are **rheumatoid arthritis**, **systemic lupus erythematosus**, **multiple sclerosis**, and **psoriasis**.

The process of autoimmune disease is very similar to infectious disease and allergy, so that great caution is observed in placing a disorder in this class. Germs were found to cause several diseases originally thought to be autoimmune. Allergens cause others. Many more may be uncovered. Autoimmunity is often believed to originate with a virus infection. A chemical in the virus resembles a body chemical so closely that the immune system attacks both.

Autoimmune hepatitis is similiar to viral hepatitis, a disease of the liver. It can be an acute disease that kills over a third of its victims within six months, it can persist for years, or it can return periodically. Some patients develop **cirrhosis** of the liver which, over time, causes the liver to cease functioning.

Causes and symptoms

Symptoms of autoimmune hepatitis resemble those of other types of hepatitis. Patients who develop autoimmune hepatitis experience **pain** under the right ribs, **fatigue** and general discomfort, loss of appetite, **nausea**, sometimes **vomiting** and **jaundice**. In addition, other parts of the body may be involved and contribute their own symptoms.

Diagnosis

Extensive laboratory testing may be required to differentiate this disease from viral hepatitis. The distinction may not even be made during the initial episode. There are certain markers of autoimmune disease in the blood that can lead to the correct diagnosis if they are sought. In advanced or chronic cases a **liver biopsy** may be necessary.

Treatment

Autoimmune hepatitis is among the few types of hepatitis that can be treated effectively. Since treatment itself introduces problems in at least 20%

of patients, it is reserved for the more severe cases. Up to 80% of patients improve with cortisone treatment, although a cure is unlikely. Another drug—azathioprine—is sometimes used concurrently. Treatment continues for over a year and may be restarted during a relapse. At least half the patients relapse at some point, and most will still continue to have progressive liver scarring.

If the liver fails, transplant is the only recourse.

Prognosis

In spite of treatment autoimmune hepatitis can re-erupt at any time, and may continue to damage and scar the liver. The rate of progression varies considerably from patient to patient.

Resources

ORGANIZATIONS

American Liver Foundation. 1425 Pompton Ave., Cedar Grove, NJ 07009. (800) 223-0179. < http://www.liverfoundation.org >.

J. Ricker Polsdorfer, MD

Hepatitis B

Definition

Hepatitis B is a potentially serious form of liver inflammation due to infection by the hepatitis B virus (HBV). It occurs in both rapidly developing (acute) and long-lasting (chronic) forms, and is one of the most common chronic infectious diseases worldwide. An effective vaccine is available that will prevent the disease in those who are later exposed.

Description

Commonly called "serum hepatitis," hepatitis B ranges from mild to severe. Some people who are infected by HBV develop no symptoms and are totally unaware of the fact, but they may carry HBV in their blood and pass the infection on to others. In its chronic form, HBV infection may destroy the liver through a scarring process, called **cirrhosis**, or it may lead to **cancer** of the liver.

When a person is infected by HBV, the virus enters the bloodstream and body fluids, and is able to pass through tiny breaks in the skin, mouth, or the male or female genital area. There are several ways of getting the infection:

- During birth, a mother with hepatitis B may pass HBV on to her infant.

- Contact with infected blood is a common means of transmitting hepatitis B. One way this may happen is by being stuck with a needle. Both health care workers and those who inject drugs into their veins are at risk in this way.

- Having sex with a person infected by HBV is an important risk factor (especially anal sex).

Although there are many ways of passing on HBV, the virus actually is not very easily transmitted. There is no need to worry that casual contact, such as shaking hands, will expose one to hepatitis B. There is no reason not to share a workplace or even a restroom with an infected person.

More than 300 million persons throughout the world are infected by HBV. While most who become chronic carriers of the virus live in Asia and Africa, there are no fewer than 1.5 million carriers in the United States. Because carriers represent a constant threat of transmitting the infection, the risk of hepatitis B is always highest where there are many carriers. Such areas are said to be endemic for hepatitis B. When infants or young children living in an endemic area are infected, their chance of becoming a chronic hepatitis B carrier is at least 90%. This probably is because their bodies are not able to make the substances (antibodies) that destroy the virus. In contrast, no more than 5% of infected teenagers and adults develop chronic infection.

Causes and symptoms

With the exception of HBV, all the common viruses that cause hepatitis are known as RNA viruses because they contain ribonucleic acid or RNA as their genetic material. HBV is the only deoxyribonucleic acid or DNA virus that is a major cause of hepatitis. HBV is made up of several fragments, called antigens, that stimulate the body's immune system to produce the antibodies that can neutralize or even destroy the infecting virus. It is, in fact, the immune reaction, not the virus, that seems to cause the liver inflammation.

Acute hepatitis B

In the United States, a majority of acute HBV infections occur in teenagers and young adults. Half of these youth never develop symptoms, and only about 20%—or one in five infected patients—develop severe symptoms and yellowing of the skin (**jaundice**). Jaundice occurs when the infected liver is unable to get rid of certain colored substances, or pigments, as it normally does. The remaining 30% of patients have only "flu-like" symptoms and will probably not even be diagnosed as having hepatitis unless certain tests are done.

The most commom symptoms of acute hepatitis B are loss of appetite, **nausea**, generally feeling poorly, and **pain** or tenderness in the right upper part of the abdomen (where the liver is located). Compared to patients with **hepatitis A** or C, those with HBV infection are less able to continue their usual activities and require more time resting in bed.

Occasionally patients with HBV infection will develop joint swelling and pain (arthritis) as well as **hives** or a skin rash before jaundice appears. The joint symptoms usually last no longer than three to seven days.

Typically the symptoms of acute hepatitis B do not persist longer than two or three months. If they continue for four months, the patient has an abnormally long-lasting acute infection. In a small number of patients—probably fewer than 3%—the infection keeps getting worse as the liver cells die off. Jaundice deepens, and patients may bleed easily when the levels of coagulation factors (normally made by the liver) decrease. Large amounts of fluid collect in the abdomen and beneath the skin (**edema**). The least common outcome of acute HBV infection, seen in fewer than 1% of patients, is fulminant hepatitis, when the liver fails entirely. Only about half of these patients can be expected to live.

Chronic hepatitis B

HBV infection lasting longer than six months is said to be chronic. After this time it is much less likely for the infection to disappear. Not all carriers of the virus develop chronic **liver disease**; in fact, a majority have no symptoms. But, about one in every four HBV carriers develop liver disease that gets worse over time,

as the liver becomes more and more scarred and less able to carry out its normal functions. A badly scarred liver is called cirrhosis. Patients are likely to have an enlarged liver and spleen, as well as tiny clusters of abnormal blood vessels in the skin that resemble spiders.

The most serious complication of chronic HBV infection is **liver cancer**. Worldwide this is the most common cancer to occur in men. Nevertheless, the overall chance that liver cancer will develop at any time in a patient's life is probably much lower than 10%. Patients with chronic hepatitis B who drink or smoke are more likely to develop liver cancer. It is not unusual for a person to simultaneously have both HBV infection and infection by HIV (human **immuno-deficiency** virus, the cause of **AIDS**). A study released in 2003 reported that men infected with both HIV and HBV were more likely to die from liver disease than people infected with just one of the diseases.

Diagnosis

Hepatitis B is diagnosed by detecting one of the viral antigens—called hepatitis B surface antigen (HBsAg)—in the blood. Later in the acute disease, HBsAg may no longer be present, in which case a test for antibodies to a different antigen—hepatitis B core antigen—is used. If HBsAg can be detected in the blood for longer than six months, chronic hepatitis B is diagnosed. A number of tests can be done to learn how well, or poorly, the liver is working. They include blood clotting tests and tests for enzymes that are found in abnormally high amounts when any form of hepatitis is present.

Treatment

In the past, there was no treatment available for hepatitis B. But developments have been made in recent years on drugs that suppress the virus and its symptoms. In early 2003, a drug called adefovir was reported as an effective treatment. Another drug called tenofovir was demonstrated as effective in patients infected with both hepatitis B and HIV. Two studies also reported on the effectiveness of a drug called Preveon, which was more expensive than others. Patients also should rest in bed as needed, continue to eat a healthy diet, and avoid alcohol. Any non-critical surgery should be postponed.

Prognosis

Each year an estimated 150,000 persons in the United States get hepatitis B. More than 10,000 will

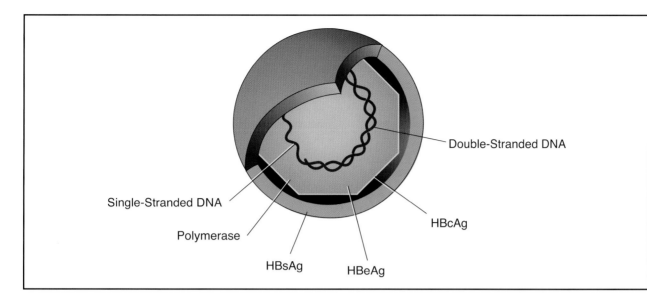

Single-Stranded DNA

Polymerase

HBsAg

HBeAg

Double-Stranded DNA

HBcAg

Hepatitis B virus (HBV) is composed of an inner protein core and an outer protein capsule. The outer capsule contains the hepatitis B surface antigen (HBsAg). The inner core contains HBV core antigen (HBcAg) and hepatitis B e-antigen (HBeAg). This cell also contains polymerase, which catalyzes the formation of the cell's DNA. HBV is the only hepatitis-causing virus that has DNA, instead of RNA. *(Illustration by Electronic Illustrators Group.)*

require hospital care, and as many as 5,000 will die from complications of the infection. About 90% of all those infected will have acute disease only. A large majority of these patients will recover within three months. It is the remaining 10%, with chronic infection, who account for most serious complications and deaths from HBV infection. In the United States, perhaps only 2% of all those who are infected will become chronically ill. The course of chronic HBV infection in any particular patient is unpredictable. Some patients who do well at first may later develop serious complications. Even when no symptoms of liver disease develop, chronic carriers remain a threat to others by serving as a source of infection.

Prevention

The best way to prevent any form of viral hepatitis is to avoid contact with blood and other body fluids of infected individuals. The use of condoms during sex also is advisable.

If a person is exposed to hepatitis B, a serum preparation containing a high level of antibody against HBV may prevent infection if given within three to seven days of exposure. Babies born of a mother with HBV should receive the vaccine within 24 hours. An effective and safe vaccine is available that reliably prevents hepatitis B. **Vaccination** is suggested for most infants and for children aged 10 and younger whose parents are from a place where hepatitis B is

common. Teenagers not vaccinated as children and all adults at risk of exposure also should be vaccinated against hepatitis B. Three doses are recommended.

Those at increased risk of getting hepatitis B, and who therefore should be vaccinated, include:

- household contacts of a person carrying HBV

- healthcare workers who often come in contact with patients' blood or other body fluids

- patients with **kidney disease** who periodically undergo hemodialysis

- homosexual men who are sexually active, and heterosexuals who have multiple sex partners

- persons coming from areas where HBV infection is a major problem

- prisoners and others living in crowded institutions

- drug abusers who use needles to inject drugs into their veins

Studies released in 2003 showed increased risk of nonresponse to hepatitis B vaccines among adults over age 30. This may be related to age-associated changes in the immune system.

Resources

PERIODICALS

"Antiviral Effective Against Hepatitis B Virus in HIV-coinfected." *Virus Weekly* January 28, 2003: 16.

Bauer, Jeff. "Co-infection with Hepatitis B and HIV Increases Men's Risks of Death from Liver Disease." *RN* March 2003: 97.

Elliott, William T. "Warfarin Effectively Prevents Venous Thromboembolism (Pharmacology Watch)." *Critical Care Alert* April 2003.

"Hepatitis B Vaccine Loses Effectiveness in Older Adults." *Vaccine Weekly* January 29, 2003: 23.

ORGANIZATIONS

Hepatitis B Foundation. 101 Greenwood Ave., Suite 570, Jenkintown, PA 19046. (215) 884-8786. <info@hepb.org>.

David A. Cramer, MD
Teresa G. Odle

Hepatitis C

Definition

Hepatitis C is a form of liver inflammation that causes primarily a long-lasting (chronic) disease. Acute (newly developed) hepatitis C is rarely observed as the early disease is generally quite mild. Spread mainly by contact with infected blood, the hepatitis C virus (HCV) causes most cases of viral liver infection not due to the A and B hepatitis viruses. In fact, before other viral types were found, hepatitis C was referred to as "non-A, non-B hepatitis." It is not a new infection, just newly diagnosable and has been widely present in the U.S. population for decades.

Description

HCV is a blood-borne virus that is and always was the major cause of "transfusion hepatitis," which can develop in patients who are given blood or most blood products except for gamma-globulin. The existence of a third hepatitis virus (besides the A and B viruses) became clear in 1974, but HCV was first identified in 1989. Thereafter, tests were devised to detect the virus in blood units before transfusing them. As a result, since the early 1990s transfused blood is less commonly the cause of hepatitis C.

The hepatitis C form of hepatitis is generally mild in its early, acute stage, but it is much likelier than **hepatitis B** (85% as compared to 10%) to produce chronic **liver disease**. Therefore, more than two of every three persons who are infected by HCV may continue to have the virus in their blood and so become carriers, who can transmit the infection to others.

The most common way of transmitting hepatitis C is when blood containing the virus enters another person's circulation through a break in the skin or the mucosa (inner lining) of the mouth or genitals. HCV also can be passed (although uncommonly) from an infected mother to the infant she is carrying. (The risk of infection from breast milk is very low.) Also, HCV can be rarely spread through sexual intercourse. Usually, however, the sexual contacts of chronic carriers of hepatitis C are not infected.

Those at increased risk of developing hepatitis C include:

- healthcare workers who come in contact with infected blood from a cut or bruise, or from a device or instrument that has been infected ("contaminated")

- persons who inject illicit drugs into their veins and skin, especially if they share needles and syringes with other users

- anyone who gets a tattoo or has his or her skin pierced with an infected needle

- persons with **hemophilia** (who because they bleed very easily may require large amounts of blood and blood products over time)

- patients with **kidney disease** who have periodic dialysis—a treatment that rids their blood of toxic substances—and often requires the patient to have blood transfusions

About one-fourth of patients with hepatitis C do not belong to any of these high-risk groups. Although blood **transfusion** is a much less common cause of HCV infection than in earlier years, cases still occur. Also, sexual transmission is possible, and may take place with either heterosexual or homosexual behavior.

Causes and symptoms

More than half of all patients who develop hepatitis C have no symptoms or signs of liver disease. Some, however, may have a minor illness with flu-like symptoms. Any form of hepatitis may keep the liver from eliminating certain colored (pigmented) substances as it normally does. These pigments collect in the skin, turning it yellow, and also may cause yellowing of the whites of the eyes. About one in four patients with hepatitis C will develop this yellowing of the skin called jaundice (or yellow **jaundice**). Some patients lose their appetite and frequently feel tired. Patients may also feel nauseous or even vomit.

In most patients, HCV can still be found in the blood six months after the start of acute infection, and these patients are considered to be carriers. If the virus persists for one year, it is very unlikely to disappear. About 20% of chronic carriers develop **cirrhosis** (scarring) of the liver when the virus damages or destroys large numbers of liver cells, which are then replaced by scar tissue. Cirrhosis may develop only after a long period of time (as long as 20 years) and often even more has passed. Most (four in five) patients will not develop cirrhosis and instead have a mild, chronic form of infection called chronic persistent hepatitis and when they die, will die with, not of, the infection.

Patients with chronic HCV infection are at risk of developing certain very serious complications:

• Patients with hepatitis C who develop cirrhosis may go on to have liver cancer—called hepatocellular carcinoma. Patients with liver cancer have an average life expectancy measured in months unless the tumor is totally removed.

• Patients also are at risk of developing a combination of joint **pain**, weakness, and areas of bleeding into the skin. The kidneys and brain also may be affected. Perhaps 5% of patients with chronic HCV infection develop this condition, called cryoglobulinemia.

• Patients with porphyria (metabolic disturbances characterized by extreme sensitivity to light) develop blisters in areas of their skin that are exposed to sunlight. The skin also may be easily bruised, and, in time, can become discolored.

Diagnosis

Hepatitis C should be suspected if a patient develops jaundice and reports recent contact with the blood of a person who may have been infected. There is a blood test to detect HCV IgG antibody, a substance that the body makes to combat HCV. Care is required, as the test often does not show positive for up to two to three months after infection. Also, the test only shows whether a person has ever been infected by HCV, not whether the virus is still present. A less available and more expensive test measuring HCV RNA (the viral gene) can be found in early infection before the antibody is measurable. Simpler blood tests can be done to show how much jaundice-causing pigment is in a patient's blood, or to measure the levels of certain proteins made by the liver. High levels of these "liver enzymes" (called ALT and AST) indicate that the liver is inflamed. Rising levels could suggest that the infection is getting worse.

Treatment

Patients who fail to recover promptly may be advised to see a specialist in gastrointestinal disorders (which include liver disease) or infectious diseases. A balanced diet with little fat is best, and patients should limit their alcohol intake, or, better, avoid alcohol altogether. Any medication that can cause liver damage should be avoided. The amount of time in bed depends on how poorly a particular patient feels.

A natural body protein, interferon alpha, now can be made in large amounts by genetic engineering, and improves the outlook for many patients who have chronic hepatitis C. The protein can lessen the symptoms of infection and improve liver function. Not all patients respond, however, and others get less benefit the longer they take interferon. **Fever** and flu-like symptoms are frequent side effects of this treatment. Using a high dose for six months, nearly half of patients have responded positively. Half the patients who do respond well will relapse after the drug is stopped. A newer medication called ribavirin is now commonly used with interferon and, if tolerated, does increase response rates. A newer form of interferon, called pegylated interferon, is also being used for treatment. Because of the problems with treatment, many people have sought alternative medications such as milk thistle or certain Asian herbs.

When hepatitis destroys most or all of the liver, the only hope may be a liver transplant. Unfortunately the new liver usually becomes infected by HCV. On the other hand, total liver failure is less frequent than in patients with hepatitis B.

Prognosis

In roughly one-fifth of patients who develop hepatitis C, the acute infection will subside, and they will recover completely within four to eight weeks and

KEY TERMS

Antibody—A substance formed in the body in response to a foreign body, such as a virus, which can attack and destroy the invading foreign body or virus.

Carrier—A person who, after recovering from a viral infection, continues to "carry" the virus in the blood and can pass it on to others who then may develop infection.

Contamination—Passage of an infectious organism, such as a virus, from an infected person to an object such as a needle, which then, when used, may pass infection to another person.

Hepatocellular carcinoma—A dangerous cancer of the liver that may develop in patients who have had hepatitis, sometimes as long as 20 or 30 years earlier.

Porphyria—Any of a group of disturbances of porphyrin metabolism characterized by excess pophyrins (various biologically active compounds with a distinct structure) in the urine and by extreme sensitivity to light.

have no later problems. Other patients face two risks: they themselves may develop chronic liver infection and possibly serious complications such as **liver cancer**, and, also, they will continue carrying the virus and may pass it on to others. The overall risk of developing cirrhosis, or liver scarring, is about 15% of all patients infected by HCV. Acute liver failure is less frequent in patients with chronic hepatitis C than in those with other forms of hepatitis.

Prevention

No vaccine has yet been developed to prevent hepatitis C in persons exposed to the virus. In addition, there is no role of gamma-globulin in the prevention of the infection. There are, however, many ways in which infection may be avoided:

- Those who inject drugs should never share needles, syringes, swabs, spoons, or anything else that comes in contact with bodily fluids. They should always use clean equipment.

- Hands should be washed before and after contact with another person's blood or if the skin is penetrated.

- The sharing of personal items should be avoided, particularly those that can puncture the skin or inside of the mouth, such as razors, nail files and scissors, and even toothbrushes.

- Condoms should be used for either vaginal or oral sex.

If a person does develop hepatitis C, its spread may be prevented by:

- not donating blood

- not sharing personal items with others

- wiping up any spilled blood while using gloves, household bleach, and disposable paper towels

- carefully covering any cut or wound with a bandaid or dressing

- practicing safe sex, especially during the acute phase of the infection

Larry I. Lutwick, MD

Hepatitis D

Definition

Hepatitis D (or delta, the Greek letter "D"), is a form of liver inflammation that occurs only in patients who also are infected by the **hepatitis B** virus. Infection by the hepatitis delta virus (HDV) either occurs at the same time as hepatitis B develops, or develops later when infection by hepatitis B virus (HBV) has entered the chronic (long-lasting) stage.

Description

Delta hepatitis can be quite severe, but it is seen only in patients already infected by HBV. In the late 1970s, Italian physicians discovered that some patients with hepatitis B had another type of infectious agent in their liver cells. Later the new virus—HDV—was confirmed by experimentally infecting chimpanzees. When both viruses are present, acute infection tends to be more severe. Furthermore, patients with both infections are likelier than those with HBV alone to develop chronic **liver disease**, and, when it occurs, it is more severe.

About 300 million persons worldwide carry HBV. Of them, at least 5% probably also have delta hepatitis. In North America HDV infection appears to be less frequent: 4% of all patients with acute hepatitis B have HDV infection. The delta virus causes an estimated 2% of all cases of acute viral hepatitis in the United States. The rate of HDV infection varies widely in different parts of the world; it is a very serious infection in some countries and quite mild in others. Chronic delta hepatitis is a more serious disease than either chronic hepatitis B alone or **hepatitis C**.

Certain individuals—the same ones who are at increased risk of developing hepatitis B—are the prime candidates to be infected by HDV. For example:

- Not infrequently, HDV infection occurs in patients with chronic HBV infection who also have **hemophilia**, a bleeding disease. These patients are at risk because they require large amounts of transfused blood and blood products that may contain HDV.

- In some areas, one-fourth to one-half of patients with chronic HBV infection who inject themselves with illicit drugs become infected by HDV as well. Drug abusers who share contaminated needles are likely to infect one another.

- Patients who get HBV infection by sexual contact may also be infected by HDV, although the delta virus is less often spread in this way than is HBV itself. Between 10–25% of homosexual men with chronic HBV infection harbor the delta virus.

- Like hepatitis B, HDV infection may develop in healthcare workers who are victims of a needle stick, and it also can be spread within households when personal items such as a razor or toothbrush are shared.

Causes and symptoms

The delta virus is a small and incomplete viral particle. Perhaps this is why it cannot cause infection on its own. Its companion virus, HBV, actually forms a covering over the HDV particle. In chronically ill patients (those whose virus persists longer than six months), the combined viruses cause inflammation throughout the liver and eventually destroy the liver cells, which are then replaced by scar tissue. This scarring is called **cirrhosis**.

When HBV and HDV infections develop at the same time, a condition called coinfection, recovery is the rule. Only 2–5% of patients become chronic carriers (have the virus remain in their blood more than six months after infection). It may be that HDV actually keeps HBV from reproducing as rapidly as it would if it were alone, so chronic infection is less likely.

When HBV infection occurs first and is followed by HDV infection, the condition is called superinfection. This is a more serious situation. Between half and two-thirds of patients with superinfection develop severe acute hepatitis. Once the liver cells contain large numbers of HBV viruses, HDV tends to reproduce more actively. Massive infection and liver failure are more common in superinfection. The risk of **liver cancer**, however, is no greater than from hepatitis B alone.

As with other forms of hepatitis, the earliest symptoms are **nausea**, loss of appetite, joint pains, and tiredness. There may be **fever** (not marked) and an enlarged liver may cause discomfort or actual **pain** in the right upper part of the abdomen. Later, **jaundice** (a yellowing of the skin and whites of the eyes that occurs when the liver is no longer able to eliminate certain pigmented substances) may develop.

Diagnosis

HDV infection may be diagnosed by detecting the antibody against the virus. Unfortunately this test cannot detect acute coinfection or superinfection as early as when symptoms first develop. Antibody against HDV usually is found no sooner than 30 days after symptoms appear. Until recently, the virus itself could only be identified by testing a small sample of liver tissue. Scientists now are developing a blood test for HDV that should make diagnosis faster and easier. When HDV is present, liver enzymes (proteins made by the liver) are present in abnormally high amounts. In some patients with coinfection, the enzyme levels peak twice, once when HBV infection starts and again at the time of HDV infection.

Treatment

As in any form of hepatitis, patients in the acute stage should rest in bed as needed, eat a balanced diet, and avoid alcohol. Alpha-interferon, the natural body substance which helps control hepatitis C, has generally not been found helpful in treating hepatitis D. If the liver is largely destroyed and has stopped functioning, **liver transplantation** is an option. Even when the procedure is successful, disease often recurs and cirrhosis may actually develop more rapidly than before.

Prognosis

A large majority of patients with coinfection of HBV and HDV recover from an episode of acute hepatitis. However, about two-thirds of patients chronically infected by HDV go on to develop cirrhosis of the liver. In one long-term study, just over half of patients who became carriers of HDV had moderate or severe liver disease, and one-fourth of them died. If very severe liver failure develops, the chance of

KEY TERMS

Alpha-interferon—A natural body substance that now can be made in large quantities and is an effective treatment for some types of viral inflammatory disease, including hepatitis C.

Antibody—A substance formed in the body in response to an invading microorganism, such as a virus, which can attack and destroy the invading virus.

Coinfection—Invasion of the body by two viruses at about the same time.

Hemophilia—A bleeding disease that may call for the transfusion of large amounts of blood and blood products.

Superinfection—Infection by a second virus after a previous infection by a different virus has become well established.

a patient surviving is no better than 50%. A liver transplant may improve this figure to 70%. When transplantation is done for cirrhosis, rather than for liver failure, nearly 90% of patients live five years or longer. The major concern with transplantation is infection of the transplanted liver; this may occur in as many as 40% of transplant patients.

When a child with viral hepatitis develops cirrhosis, HDV infection is commonly responsible. A woman who develops delta hepatitis while pregnant will do as well as if she were not pregnant; and there is no increased risk that the newborn will be malformed in any way.

Prevention

The vaccine against hepatitis B also prevents delta hepatitis, since it cannot occur unless HBV infection is present. Hopefully, a vaccine can be developed that will keep delta infection from developing in chronic HBV carriers. However, if a person already has HBV infection, any exposure to blood should be strictly avoided. A high level of sexual activity with multiple partners is also a risk factor for delta hepatitis.

Resources

ORGANIZATIONS

American Liver Foundation. 1425 Pompton Ave., Cedar Grove, NJ 07009. (800) 223-0179. < http:// www.liverfoundation.org >.

David A. Cramer, MD

Hepatitis, drug-induced

Definition

Inflammation of the liver due to an adverse reaction with a drug.

Description

The liver is a very important organ to the body. It is a large internal organ weighing more than three pounds in the average adult. It performs over 100 functions including formation of bile, detoxification of harmful substances, vitamin storage and metabolism of carbohydrates, fats and proteins. Serious complications could arise when the liver becomes inflamed due to hepatitis when it is not able to perform these tasks. A virus most often causes hepatitis but certain drugs can also induce it.

Drug-induced hepatitis (also called toxic hepatitis) occurs in eight in every 10,000 people because the liver reacts abnormally during drug exposure, leading to liver damage. This pathology causes the liver not to function properly and the symptoms can begin to be seen. Women tend to be affected almost twice as often as men. Older people are more prone to this type of hepatitis because their bodies aren't able to repair themselves as fast as younger people. Drugs that can be associated with drug-induced hepatitis include acetaminophen, vitamin A, and PTU (a drug treatment for **tuberculosis**).

Causes and symptoms

There are three general types of drug-induced hepatitis: toxic, metabolic idiosyncrasy and immunologic idiosyncrasy. With toxic hepatitis liver damage as the result of a drug complication with hepatotoxins happens to everyone who takes that particular drug. On the other hand, hepatitis resulting from a metabolic or immunologic idiosyncrasy only happens to certain people, those predisposed to particular idiosyncrasy.

In patients with a metabolic idiosyncrasy the person metabolizes the drug differently than most people causing a harmful by-product that damages the liver. A metabolic idiosyncrasy is seen in 0.1-2% of people and it is complicated by use of alcohol.

With an immunologic idiosyncrasy the patient's body recognizes the metabolized drug by-products as foreign. This leads to the destruction of liver cells containing the by-product via the immune system

KEY TERMS

Hepatitis—General inflammation of the liver.

Hepatomegaly—General swelling of the liver.

Hepatotoxin—A substance that is toxic to the liver.

Idiosyncrasy—A defect in that particular pathway resulting in an abnormality.

resulting in hepatitis. An immunologic idiosyncrasy is seen in less than one person per 10,000 (0.01%) people and is more than twice as common in women.

The symptoms of drug-induced hepatitis are similar to viral hepatitis. Drug induced hepatitis tends to be acute. If it is not caught soon enough the damage could be permanent resulting in chronic hepatitis. Some of the common symptoms are:

- nausea

- vomiting

- headache

- anorexia

- jaundice

- clay color stools

- dark urine

- hepatomegaly

Diagnosis

Diagnosis is typically made through a physical exam along with a patient history to identify any possible hepatotoxins. Blood tests are usually done as well. An increased white blood cell count is typical.

Treatment

There isn't any specific treatment other than immediate discontinuance of the causative agent. Rest during the acute phase of the disease is vital along with the intake of fluids to maintain hydration.

Prognosis

Usually the symptoms will go away after the drug has been eliminated due to the liver repairing itself. A full recovery is typically expected unless it wasn't treated quickly resulting in more liver damage being done than normal.

Prevention

If there is a history of liver damage certain medications should not be taken. Doctors will be familiar with these.

Resources

BOOKS

Feldman, Sleisenger, and Scharschmidt. "Liver Diseases Caused by Drugs, Anesthetics, and Toxins." In *Gastrointestinal and Liver Disease.* Philadelphia: W.B. Saunders Company, 2001, pp.1232-1237.

Holmes, Nancy H. "Hepatobiliary Disorders." In *Diseases.* Pennsylvania: Springhouse Corporation, 2001, pp.744-53.

PERIODICALS

Hautekeete, Horsmans, Van Waeyenberge, Demanet, Henrion, Verbist, Brenard, Sempoux, Michielsen, Yap, Rahier, and Geubel. "HLA Association of Amoxicillin-Clavulanate—Induced Hepatitis." *Gastroenterology* November 1999: 1181-86.

Thomas Scott Eagan
Ronald Watson, PhD

Hepatitis E

Definition

The hepatitis E virus (HEV) is a common cause of hepatitis that is transmitted via the intestinal tract, and is not caused by the **hepatitis A** virus. Spread most often by contaminated drinking water, HEV infection occurs mainly in developing countries.

Description

Hepatitis E is also known as epidemic non-A, non-B hepatitis. Like hepatitis A, it is an acute and short-lived illness that can sometimes cause liver failure. HEV, discovered in 1987, is spread by the fecal-oral route. It is constantly present (endemic) in countries where human waste is allowed to get into drinking water without first being purified. Large outbreaks (epidemics) have occurred in Asian and South American countries where there is poor sanitation. In the United States and Canada no outbreaks have been reported, but persons traveling to an endemic region may return with HEV.

Causes and symptoms

There are at least two strains of HEV, one found in Asia and another in Mexico. The virus may start dividing in the gastrointestinal tract, but it grows mostly in the liver. After an incubation period (the time from when a person is first infected by a virus until the appearance of the earliest symptoms) of two to eight weeks, infected persons develop **fever**, may feel nauseous, lose their appetite, and often have discomfort or actual **pain** in the right upper part of the abdomen where the liver is located. Some develop yellowing of the skin and the whites of the eyes (**jaundice**). Most often the illness is mild and disappears within a few weeks with no lasting effects. Children younger than 14 years and persons over age 50 seldom have jaundice or show other clinical signs of hepatitis.

Hepatitis E never becomes a chronic (long-lasting) illness, but on rare occasions the acute illness damages and destroys so many liver cells that the liver can no longer function. This is called fulminant liver failure, and may cause **death**. Pregnant women are at much higher risk of dying from fulminant liver failure; this increased risk is not true of any other type of viral hepatitis. The great majority of patients who recover from acute infection do not continue to carry HEV and cannot pass on the infection to others.

Diagnosis

HEV can be found by microscopically examining a stool sample, but this is not a reliable test, as the virus often dies when stored for a short time. Like other hepatitis viruses, HEV stimulates the body's immune system to produce a substance called an antibody, which can swallow up and destroy the virus. Blood tests can determine elevated antibody levels, which indicate the presence of HEV virus in the body. Unfortunately, such antibody blood tests are not widely available.

Treatment

There is no way of effectively treating the symptoms of any acute hepatitis, including hepatitis E. During acute infection, a patient should take a balanced diet and rest in bed as needed.

Prognosis

In the United States hepatitis E is not a fatal illness, but elsewhere about 1–2% of those infected

---

KEY TERMS

Antibody—A substance made by the body's immune system in response to an invading virus, the antibodies then attack and destroy the virus.

Incubation period—The time from when a person is first infected by a virus until the appearance of the earliest symptoms.

Jaundice—Yellowing of the skin that occurs when pigments normally eliminated by the liver collect in high amounts in the blood.

Sanitation—The process of keeping drinking water, foods, or any anything else with which people come into contact free of microorganisms such as viruses.

Vaccine—A substance prepared from a weakened or killed virus which, when injected, stimulates the immune system to produce antibodies that can prevent infection by the natural virus.

---

die of advanced liver failure. In pregnant women the death rate is as high as 20%. It is not clear whether having hepatitis E once guarantees against future HEV infection.

Prevention

Most attempts to use blood serum containing HEV antibody to prevent hepatitis in those exposed to HEV have failed. Hopefully, this approach can be made to work so that pregnant women living in endemic areas can be protected. No vaccine is available, though several are being tested. It also is possible that effective anti-viral drugs will be found. The best ways to prevent hepatitis E are to provide safe drinking water and take precautions to use sterilized water and beverages when traveling.

Resources

ORGANIZATIONS

American Liver Foundation. 1425 Pompton Ave., Cedar Grove, NJ 07009. (800) 223-0179. < http://www.liverfoundation.org >.

OTHER

King, J. W. *Bug Bytes*. Louisiana State University Medical Center. < http://www.ccm.lsumc.edu/bugbytes >.

David A. Cramer, MD

Hepatitis G

Definition

Hepatitis G is a newly discovered form of liver inflammation caused by hepatitis G virus (HGV), a distant relative of the **hepatitis C** virus.

Description

HGV, also called hepatitis GB virus, was first described early in 1996. Little is known about the frequency of HGV infection, the nature of the illness, or how to prevent it. What is known is that transfused blood containing HGV has caused some cases of hepatitis. For this reason, patients with **hemophilia** and other bleeding conditions who require large amounts of blood or blood products are at risk of hepatitis G. HGV has been identified in between 1–2% of blood donors in the United States. Also at risk are patients with **kidney disease** who have blood exchange by hemodialysis, and those who inject drugs into their veins. It is possible that an infected mother can pass on the virus to her newborn infant. Sexual transmission also is a possibility.

Often patients with hepatitis G are infected at the same time by the **hepatitis B** or C virus, or both. In about three of every thousand patients with acute viral hepatitis, HGV is the only virus present. There is some indication that patients with hepatitis G may continue to carry the virus in their blood for many years, and so might be a source of infection in others.

Causes and symptoms

Some researchers believe that there may be a group of GB viruses, rather than just one. Others remain doubtful that HGV actually causes illness. If it does, the type of acute or chronic (long-lasting) illness that results is not clear. When diagnosed, acute HGV infection has usually been mild and brief. There is no evidence of serious complications, but it is possible that, like other hepatitis viruses, HGV can cause severe liver damage resulting in liver failure. The virus has been identified in as many as 20% of patients with long-lasting viral hepatitis, some of whom also have hepatitis C.

Diagnosis

The only method of detecting HGV is a complex and costly DNA test that is not widely available.

KEY TERMS

Antibody—A substance made by the body's immune system in response to an invading virus; antibodies then attack and destroy the virus.

Hemophilia—A bleeding disorder that often makes it necessary to give patients dozens or even hundreds of units of blood and blood products over time.

Efforts are under way, however, to develop a test for the HGV antibody, which is formed in response to invasion by the virus. Once antibody is present, however, the virus itself generally has disappeared, making the test too late to be of use.

Treatment

There is no specific treatment for any form of acute hepatitis. Patients should rest in bed as needed, avoid alcohol, and be sure to eat a balanced diet.

Prognosis

What little is known about the course of hepatitis G suggests that illness is mild and does not last long. When more patients have been followed up after the acute phase, it will become clear whether HGV can cause severe liver damage.

Prevention

Since hepatitis G is a blood-borne infection, prevention relies on avoiding any possible contact with contaminated blood. Drug users should not share needles, syringes, or other equipment.

Resources

ORGANIZATIONS

American Liver Foundation. 1425 Pompton Ave., Cedar Grove, NJ 07009. (800) 223-0179. < http://www.liverfoundation.org >.

David A. Cramer, MD

Hepatitis virus studies *see* **Hepatitis virus tests**

Hepatitis virus tests

Definition

Viral hepatitis is any type of liver inflammation caused by a viral infection. The three most common viruses now recognized to cause **liver disease** are hepatitis A, **hepatitis B**, and hepatitis non-A, non-B (also called hepatitis C). Several other types have been recognized: **hepatitis D**, **hepatitis E**, and the recently identified **hepatitis G**. A seventh type (hepatitis F) is suspected but not yet confirmed.

Purpose

The different types of viral hepatitis produce similar symptoms, but they differ in terms of transmission, course of treatment, prognosis, and carrier status. When the clinical history of a patient is insufficient for differentiation, hepatitis virus tests are used as an aid in diagnosis and in monitoring the course of the disease. These tests are based primarily on antigen-antibody reactions—an antigen being a protein foreign to the body, and an antibody another type of protein manufactured by lymphocytes (a type of white blood cell) to neutralize the antigen.

Description

There are five major types of viral hepatitis. The diseases, along with the antigen-antibody tests available to aid in diagnosis, are described below.

Hepatitis A

Commonly called infectious hepatitis, this is caused by the **hepatitis A** virus (HAV). It is usually a mild disease, most often spread by food and water contamination, but sometimes through sexual contact. Immunologic tests are not commercially available for the HAV antigen, but two types of antibodies to HAV can be detected. IgM antibody (anti-HAV/IgM), appears approximately three to four weeks after exposure and returns to normal within several months. IgG (anti-HAV/IgG) appears approximately two weeks after the IgM begins to increase and remains positive. Acute hepatitis is suspected if IgM is elevated; conversely, if IgG is elevated without IgM, a convalescent stage of HAV is presumed. IgG antibody can remain detectable for decades after infection.

Hepatitis B

Commonly known as serum hepatitis, this is caused by the hepatitis B virus (HBV). The disease can be mild or severe, and it can be acute (of limited duration) or chronic (ongoing). It is usually spread by sexual contact with another infected person, through contact with infected blood, by intravenous drug use, or from mother to child at birth.

HBV, also called the Dane particle, is composed of an inner protein core surrounded by an outer protein capsule. The outer capsule contains the hepatitis B surface antigen (HBsAg), formerly called the Australia antigen. The inner core contains HBV core antigen (HBcAg), and the hepatitis B e-antigen (HBeAg). Antibodies to these antigens are called anti-HBs, anti-HBc, and anti-HBe. Testing for these antigens and antibodies is as follows:

- Hepatitis B surface antigen (HBsAg). This is the first test for hepatitis B to become abnormal. HBsAg begins to elevate before the onset of clinical symptoms, peaks during the first week of symptoms, and usually disappears by the time the accompanying **jaundice** (yellowing of the skin and other tissues) begins to subside. HBsAg indicates an active HBV infection. A person is considered to be a carrier if this antigen persists in the blood for six or more months.

- Hepatitis B surface antibody (anti-HBs). This appears approximately one month after the disappearance of the HBsAg, signaling the end of the acute infection period. Anti-HBs is the antibody that demonstrates immunity after administration of the hepatitis B vaccine. Its presence also indicates immunity to subsequent infection.

- Hepatitis B core antigen (HBcAg). No tests are commercially available to detect this antigen.

- Hepatitis B core antibody (anti-HBc). This appears just before acute hepatitis develops and remains elevated (although it slowly declines) for years. It is also present in chronic hepatitis. The hepatitis B core antibody is elevated during the time lag between the disappearance of the hepatitis B surface antigen and the appearance of the hepatitis B surface antibody in an interval called the "window." During this time, the hepatitis B core antibody is the only detectable marker of a recent hepatitis B infection.

- Hepatitis B e-antigen (HBeAg). This is more useful as an index of infection than for diagnostic purposes. The presence of this antigen correlates with early and active disease, as well as with high infectivity in patients with acute HBV infection. When HBeAg levels persist in the blood, the development of chronic HBV infection is suspected.

- Hepatitis B e-antibody (anti-HBe). In the bloodstream, this indicates a reduced risk of infectivity in patients who have previously been HBeAg positive. Chronic hepatitis B surface antigen carriers can be positive for either HBeAg or anti-HBe, but are less infectious when anti-HBe is present. Antibody to e antigen can persist for years, but usually disappears earlier than anti-HBs or anti-HBc.

Hepatitis C

Previously known as non-A, non-B hepatitis, this disease is primarily caused by the hepatitis C virus (HCV). It is generally mild, but more likely than hepatitis B to lead to chronic liver disease, possible liver failure, and the eventual need for transplant. Chronic carrier states develop in more than 80% of patients, and chronic liver disease is a major problem. As many as 20% of patients with chronic **hepatitis C** will develop liver failure or liver cancer. HCV is spread through sexual contact, as well as through sharing drug needles, although nearly half of infections can't be traced as to origin.

Hepatitis C is detected by HCV serology (tests on blood sera). A specific type of assay called enzyme-linked immunosorbent assay (ELISA) was developed to detect antibody to hepatitis C for diagnostic purposes, as well as for screening blood donors. Most cases of post-transfusion non-A, non-B hepatitis are caused by HCV, but application of this test has virtually eliminated post-transfusion hepatitis. An HCV viral titer to detect HCV RNA in the blood is now available, and recently, IgM anti-HCV core is proving to be a useful acute marker for HCV infection.

Hepatitis D

Also called delta hepatitis, this is caused by the hepatitis D virus (HDV). The disease occurs only in those who have HBV in the blood from a past or simultaneously occurring infection. Experts believe transmission may occur through sexual contact, but further research is needed to confirm that. Most cases occur among those who are frequently exposed to blood and blood products. Many cases also occur among drug users who share contaminated needles. Hepatitis D virus (HDV) antigen can be detected by radioimmunoassay within a few days after infection, together with IgM and total antibodies to HDV.

Hepatitis E

Caused by the hepatitis E virus (HEV), this is actually another type of non-A, non-B hepatitis. The virus is most often spread through fecally contaminated water, but the role of person-to-person transmission is unclear. This form of hepatitis is quite rare in the United States. There are currently no antigen or antibody tests widely available to accurately detect HEV.

Preparation

Hepatitis virus tests require a blood sample. It is not necessary for the patient to withhold food or fluids before any of these tests, unless requested to do so by the physician.

Risks

Risks for these tests are minimal for the patient, but may include slight bleeding from the blood-drawing site, **fainting** or feeling lightheaded after venipuncture, or hematoma (blood accumulating under the puncture site).

Normal results

Reference ranges for the antigen/antibody tests are as follows:

- hepatitis A antibody, IgM: Negative
- hepatitis B core antibody: Negative
- hepatitis B e antibody: Negative
- hepatitis B e-antigen: Negative
- hepatitis B surface antibody: Varies with clinical circumstance (Note: As the presence of anti-HBs indicates past infection with resolution of previous hepatitis B infection, or **vaccination** against hepatitis B, additional patient history may be necessary for diagnosis.)
- hepatitis B surface antigen: Negative
- hepatitis C serology: Negative
- hepatitis D serology: Negative.

Abnormal results

Hepatitis A: A single positive anti-HAV test may indicate previous exposure to the virus, but due to the antibody persisting so long in the bloodstream, only evidence of a rising anti-HAV titer confirms hepatitis A. Determining recent infection rests on identifying the antibody as IgM (associated with recent infection). A negative anti-HAV test rules out hepatitis A.

Hepatitis B: High levels of HBsAg that continue for three or more months after onset of acute infection suggest development of chronic hepatitis or carrier status. Detection of anti-HBs signals late convalescence or recovery from infection. This antibody remains in the blood to provide immunity to reinfection.

Hepatitis C (non-A, non-B hepatitis): Anti-HBc develops after exposure to hepatitis B. As an early indicator of acute infection, antibody (IgM) to core antigen (anti-HBc IgM) is rarely detected in chronic infection, so it is useful in distinguishing acute from chronic infection, and hepatitis B from non-A, non-B.

Resources

BOOKS

Pagana, Kathleen Deska. *Mosby's Manual of Diagnosticand Laboratory Tests*. St. Louis: Mosby, Inc., 1998.

Janis O. Flores

Hepatobiliary scan *see* **Gallbladder nuclear medicine scan**

Hepatocellular carcinoma *see* **Liver cancer, primary**

Hepatolenticular degeneration *see* **Wilson's disease**

Hepatoma *see* **Liver cancer, primary**

Herbal medicine *see* **Herbalism, western**

▌Herbalism, traditional Chinese

Definition

Chinese herbalism is one of the major components of traditional Chinese medicine (TCM), or Oriental medicine (OM). In TCM, herbs are often used in conjunction with other techniques, such as **acupuncture** or massage. Chinese herbalism is a holistic medical system, meaning that it looks at treating a patient as a whole person, looking at the mental and spiritual health, as well as the physical health, of the individual. Illness is seen as a disharmony or imbalance among these aspects of the individual. Chinese herbalism has been practiced for over 4,000 years.

One of the earliest and certainly the most important Chinese herbal text is the *Huang Ti Nei Ching*, or *Yellow Emperor's Classic of Internal Medicine*. It is believed to be authored by Huang Ti during his reign over China, which started about 2697 B.C. Since that time, herbal practices have been more extensively documented and refined. In modern China, traditional Chinese herbalism is taught alongside conventional Western pharmacology. Chinese herbal remedies have been used in the West only relatively recently, over the past two decades. These remedies are more gentle and natural that conventional medicines. In addition, they have fewer unpleasant side effects. Individuals with chronic disorders in particular are increasingly drawn to the holistic aspect of Chinese herbalism and TCM in general.

Purpose

Because it is a safe, inexpensive solution to health problems of all kinds, Chinese herbalism is very popular in China. In recent years, herbalism has been modernized with the introduction of quality control. For example, herbs are subjected to absorption spectrometry to determine levels of heavy metals found in some. Because they are standardized, Chinese herbs are safer for self-treatment. This puts the individual, not the physician, in charge of the individual's health; that is a basic goal of Chinese herbalism.

Chinese herbalism offers unique advice regarding what foods can help and what can hinder, and an herbalist can help an individual discover what he is allergic to. In addition, Chinese herbs stimulate the immune system and provide beneficial nutrients, aside from their role in curing illness.

At M.D. Anderson Hospital in Texas, medical research has confirmed that patients undergoing **chemotherapy** were shown to have an improved degree of immune function when they took the tonic herb astragulus (*huang qi*). (It is well known that chemotherapy suppresses the immune system.) Research also showed that T-cell and macrophage activity and interferon production was increased in patients using the Chinese herbs ganoderma, lentinus, and polyporous, helping the body fight cancer cells. Agents also found in ganoderma were found to inhibit platelet aggregation and thrombocyte formation, which would be helpful to counter circulation and heart problems.

An ingredient of ginseng was found to promote adrenal function, which would give the herb properties of enhancing many hormone functions in the body.

Description

Origins

HISTORICAL BACKGROUND. Traditional Chinese medicine originated in the region of eastern Asia that today includes China, Tibet, Vietnam, Korea, and Japan. Tribal shamans and holy men who lived as

Five Popular Chinese Herbs Used In The U.S.	
Herb	**Purpose**
Astragalus (huang chi)	Builds immune systemp offsets side effects of chemotherapy and radiation treatments
Don Quai (dang qui)	Stimulates the production of red blood cells and bone marrow; increases cardiovascular endurance; regulates menstrual disorders
Ginseng (ren shen)	Increases physical stamina; general tonic
Reishi mushroom (ling zhi)	Eliminates toxins; increases physical stamina
Schisandra (wu wei zu)	Prevents fluid loss, e.g., excessive sweating, runny nose, incontinence

hermits in the mountains of China as early as 3500 B.C. practiced what was called the "Way of Long Life." This regimen included a diet based on herbs and other plants; kung-fu exercises; and special breathing techniques that were thought to improve vitality and life expectancy.

After the Han dynasty, the next great age of Chinese medicine was under the Tang emperors, who ruled from A.D. 608 to 906. The first Tang emperor established China's first medical school in A.D. 629 Under the Song (A.D.) 960–1279 and Ming (A.D. 1368–1644) dynasties, new medical schools were established, their curricula and qualifying examinations were standardized, and the traditional herbal prescriptions were written down and collected into encyclopedias. One important difference between the development of medicine in China and in the West is the greater interest in the West in surgical procedures and techniques.

PHILOSOPHICAL BACKGROUND: THE COSMIC AND NATURAL ORDER. In Taoist thought, the Tao, or universal first principle, generated a duality of opposing principles that underlie all the patterns of nature. These principles, yin and yang, are mutually dependent as well as polar opposites. They are basic concepts in traditional Chinese medicine. Yin represents everything that is cold, moist, dim, passive, slow, heavy, and moving downward or inward; while yang represents heat, dryness, brightness, activity, rapidity, lightness, and upward or outward motion. Both forces are equally necessary in nature and in human well-being, and neither force can exist without the other. The dynamic interaction of these two principles is reflected in the cycles of the seasons, the human life cycle, and other natural phenomena. One objective of traditional Chinese medicine is to keep yin and yang in harmonious balance within a person.

In addition to yin and yang, Taoist teachers also believed that the Tao produced a third force, primordial energy or qi (also spelled chi or ki). The interplay between yin, yang, and qi gave rise to the Five Elements of water, metal, earth, wood, and fire. These entities are all reflected in the structure and functioning of the human body.

THE HUMAN BEING. Traditional Chinese physicians did not learn about the structures of the human body from dissection because they thought that cutting open a body insulted the person's ancestors. Instead they built up an understanding of the location and functions of the major organs over centuries of observation, and then correlated them with the principles of yin, yang, qi, and the Five Elements. Thus wood is related to the liver (yin) and the gall bladder (yang); fire to the heart (yin) and the small intestine (yang); earth to the spleen (yin) and the stomach (yang); metal to the lungs (yin) and the large intestine (yang); and water to the kidneys (yin) and the bladder (yang). The Chinese also believed that the body contains Five Essential Substances, which include blood, spirit, vital essence (a principle of growth and development produced by the body from qi and blood), Fluids (all body fluids other than blood, such as saliva, spinal fluid, sweat, etc.), and qi.

Chinese herbal treatment differs from **Western herbalism** in several respects. In Chinese practice, several different herbs may be used, according to each plant's effect on the individual's Qi and the Five Elements. There are many formulas used within traditional Chinese medicine to treat certain common imbalance patterns. These formulas can be modified to fit specific individuals more closely.

A traditional Chinese herbal formula typically contains four classes of ingredients, arranged in a hierarchical order: a chief (the principal ingredient, chosen for the patient's specific illness); a deputy (to reinforce the chief's action or treat a coexisting condition); an assistant (to counteract side effects of the first two ingredients); and an envoy (to harmonize all the other ingredients and convey them to the parts of the body that they are to treat).

Methods of diagnosis

A Chinese herbalist will not prescribe a particular herb on the strength of symptoms only, but will take into consideration the physical condition, emotional health, and mental state of the patient. He or she may look at the condition of the patient's hair, skin, and tongue, as well as the appearance of the eyes, lips, and general complexion. The practitioner then listens to the sounds the body makes when breathing. He or she may smell the breath, body odor, or sputum in diagnosis.

TCM practitioners take an extensive medical history of a patient. He or she may ask about dietary habits, lifestyle, and sleep patterns. The patient will be questioned about chief medical complaints, as well as on his or her particular emotional state and sexual practices.

Chinese herbalists employ touch as a diagnostic tool. They may palpate the body or use light massage to assess the patient's physical health. Another chief component of Chinese medical diagnosis is pulse diagnosis, or sphygmology. This is a very refined art that takes practitioners years to master. Some practitioners can detect 12 different pulse points that correspond to the 12 major organs in Chinese medicine. There are over 30 pulse qualities that practitioners are able to detect on each point. The strength, speed, quality, and rhythm of the pulse, to name a few, will be determined before a diagnosis is given.

Herbs

Chinese herbs may be used alone or in combination. Relatively few are used alone for medicinal purposes. Practitioners believe that illness can be effectively treated by combining herbs based on their various characteristics and the patient's overall health. Every herb has four basic healing properties: nature, taste, affinity, and effect.

An herb's nature is described according to its yin or yang characteristics. Yang, or warming, herbs treat cold deficiencies. They are frequently used in the treatment of the upper respiratory tract, skin, or extremities. Yin, or cooling, herbs, treat hot excess conditions. They are most often used to treat internal conditions and problems with organs. Herbs can also be neutral in nature.

An herb's taste does not refer to its flavor, but to its effect on qi, blood, fluids, and phlegm. Sour herbs have a concentrating action. They are prescribed to treat bodily excess conditions, such as **diarrhea**, and concentrate qi. Bitter herbs have an eliminating or moving downward action. They are used to treat coughs, **constipation**, and heart problems. Sweet or bland herbs have a harmonizing action. They are used as restorative herbs and to treat **pain**. Spicy herbs have a stimulating action. They are prescribed to improve blood and qi circulation. Salty herbs have a softening action. They are used to treat constipation and other digestion problems.

An herb's affinity describes its action on a specific bodily Organ. (Note that Chinese medicine does not have the anatomical correlation for organ names. They correspond more closely to the organ's function.) Sour herbs have an affinity for the Liver and Gallbladder. Bitter herbs act on the Heart and Small Intestine. Sweet and bland herbs affect the Stomach and Spleen. Spicy herbs have an affinity for Lungs and Large Intestine, whereas salty herbs act on the Kidneys and Bladder.

Chinese herbs are lastly classified according to their specific actions, which are divided into four effects. Herbs that dispel are used to treat an accumulation, sluggishness, or spasm by relaxing or redistributing. Herbs with an astringent action are used to consolidate or restrain a condition characterized by discharge or excessive elimination. Herbs that purge treat an obstruction or "poison" by encouraging elimination and **detoxification**. Tonifying herbs nourish, support, and calm where there is a deficiency.

Treatment of diabetes

The incidence of diabetes has increased quite dramatically in recent years, especially in the United States, where in general people take less **exercise**, and food is taken in greater quantity with a general reduction in quality. This has lead to a scramble to find new solutions to the problem, and many researchers have focused their interest on Chinese herbal remedies. In the search for more effective and more convenient treatments, the alkaloid berberine has come under close scrutiny for its many uses, among them the treatment of diabetes. In trials, rats given a mixture of berberine and alloxan showed less likelihood of incurring a rise in blood sugar. Patients suffering from type II diabetes who were given between 300 and 600 mg of berberine daily for between one and three months, showed a reduction in blood sugar levels, when taken in conjunction with a controlled diet.

Treatment of AIDS and cancer

Independent researchers are investigating indications that Chinese herbalism can reduce the toxicity of chemotherapy and other medications, in addition to stimulating immune responses.

Preparations

Those who are unfamiliar with Chinese herbs and their uses should consult a practitioner before starting any treatment. Once a remedy is prescribed, it may be found at Oriental markets or health food stores. The

KEY TERMS

Absorption spectrometry—A scientific procedure to determine chemical makeup of samples.

Interferon—A substance proved to be necessary in the body to help fight cancer cells.

Immune function—The body's defense system against bacteria, viruses and fungi, and any malfunction of the organism.

Pharmaco-dynamics—The study of the relationships and interactions of herbs.

Platelet aggregation—The clumping together of blood cells, possibly forming a clot.

Thrombocyte—Another name for platelet.

remedies used in Chinese herbalism are standardized and sold prepared for use, with instructions for dosage. A Chinese herbalist may prescribe herbs to be made into tea, or taken as capsules.

Precautions

When treating a patient, the herbalist will aim to gently "nudge" the system into shape, rather than producing any immediate reaction. A return to health, therefore, may take time, and it is important that the patient realizes the principle of the treatment. Some practitioners estimate that treatment will take a month for every year that a chronic condition has existed. The advantage of the slow pace is that if there is a bad reaction to any herb, which is rare, it will be mild because the treatment itself is gentle.

As with most naturopathic therapies, Chinese herbal remedies work best when taken in conjunction with a healthy lifestyle and program of exercise.

Side effects

Some Chinese herbs are incompatible with certain prescription drugs, certain foods, or should not be taken during **pregnancy**. To be certain, a Chinese herbalist should be consulted.

Research and general acceptance

At present, there is renewed interest in the West in traditional Chinese medicine and Chinese herbalism. Of the 700 herbal remedies used by traditional Chinese practitioners, over 100 have been tested and found effective by the standards of Western science. Several

United States agencies, including the National Institutes of Health, the Office of Alternative Medicine, and the Food and Drug Administration are currently investigating Chinese herbal medicine as well as acupuncture and *Tui na* massage. In general, however, Western studies of Chinese medicine focus on the effects of traditional treatments and the reasons for those effects, thus attempting to fit traditional Chinese medicine within the Western framework of precise physical measurements and scientific hypotheses.

Resources

ORGANIZATIONS

The California Association of Acupuncture and Oriental Medicine. < http://www.CAAOM.ORG/medicine/overview.htm >.

For help with herbs and a list of practitioners. < http://www.craneherb.com >.

Institute of Chinese Materia Medica. China Academy of Traditional Chinese Medicine. *Beijing, 100700.*

National Center for Complementary and Alternative Medicine. < http://nccam.nih.gov/nccam >.

Patricia Skinner

Herbalism, Western

Definition

Western herbalism is a form of the healing arts that draws from herbal traditions of Europe and the Americas, and that emphasizes the study and use of European and Native American herbs in the treatment and prevention of illness. Western herbalism is based on physicians' and herbalists' clinical experience and traditional knowledge of medicinal plant remedies preserved by oral tradition and in written records over thousands of years. Western herbalism, like the much older system of **traditional Chinese medicine**, relies on the synergistic and curative properties of the plant to treat symptoms and disease and maintain health.

Western herbalism is based upon pharmacognosy, the study of natural products. Pharmocognosy includes the identification, extraction methods, and applications of specific plant constituents responsible for specific therapeutic actions, such as the use of digoxin from Digitalis leaf for **heart failure**. These constituents are extracted, purified and studied in vitro, in vivo, and in clinical research. They may be concentrated to deliver standardized, set doses. Sometimes, the natural constituent can be synthesized in the lab, or changed and patented. Practitioners may choose to use fresh medicinal plants, simple extracts, or standardized extracts.

In standardized extracts, a specific quantity of a constituent is called a marker compound, and it may or may not be the active constituent(s) in the plant medicine. There are preparations with standardized active constituent quantities, and preparations with greater emphasis on quality of crude plant material and traditional preparation methodology than on finalized total quantity of marker compounds. The preference between the two for precision dosing is philosophical, practical and variable. When using plant extracts in which the active constituents and their cofactors are well established, or the therapeutic and lethal dose are close, standardized products are often preferred. When using plant extracts whose active constituents remain obscure, or the active constituents when purified produce weaker therapeutic results or more undesirable side effects, the products produced under good manufacturing processes and according to the traditional *National Formulary U. S. Dispensatory* or *U. S. Pharmacopeia* are preferred.

Purpose

The benefits of botanical medicine may be subtle or dramatic, depending on the remedy used and the symptom or problem being addressed. Herbal remedies usually have a much slower effect than pharmaceutical drugs. Some herbal remedies have a cumulative effect and work slowly over time to restore balance, and others are indicated for short-term treatment of acute symptoms. When compared to the pharmaceutical drugs, herbal remedies prepared from the whole plant have relatively few side effects. This is due to the complex chemistry and synergistic action of the full range of phytochemicals present in the whole plant, and the relatively lower concentrations. They are generally safe when used in properly designated therapeutic dosages, and less costly than the isolated chemicals or synthetic prescription drugs available from western pharmaceutical corporations.

Description

Origins

Over 2,500 years ago Hippocrates wrote, "In medicine one must pay attention not to plausible theorizing but to experience and reason together." This Greek physician and herbalist from the fourth century B.C. is considered the father of western medicine. He stressed the importance of diet, water quality, climate, and social environment in the development of disease. Hippocrates believed in treating the whole person, rather than merely isolating and treating symptoms. He recognized the innate capacity of the body to heal itself, and emphasized the importance of keen observation in the medical practice. He recommended simple herbal remedies to assist the body in restoring health.

Ancient Greek medicine around the fifth century B.C. was a fertile ground for contrasting philosophies and religions. Greek physicians were influenced by the accumulated medical knowledge from Egypt, Persia, and Babylon. Medical advances flourished and practitioners and scholars were free to study and practice without religious and secular constraints. In the fourth century B.C., Theophrastus wrote the *Historia Plantarum*, considered to be the founding text in the science of botany.

During the first century A.D. Dioscorides, a Greek physician who traveled with the Roman legions, produced five medical texts. His herbal text, known as the *De Materia Medica* is considered to be among the most influential of all western herbal texts. It became a standard reference for practitioners for the next 1,500 years. This influential book also included information on medicinal herbs and treatments that had been used for centuries in Indian **Ayurvedic medicine**. Galen of Pergamon, who also lived in the first century A.D., was a Roman physician and student of anatomy and physiology. He authored a recipe book containing 130 antidotes and medicinal preparations. These elaborate mixtures, known as galenicals, sometimes included up to one hundred herbs and other substances. This complex approach to herbal medicine was a dramatic change from the simple remedies recommended by Hippocrates and employed by traditional folk healers. Galen developed a rigid system of medicine in which the physician, with his specialized knowledge of complex medical formulas, was considered the ultimate authority in matters of health care. The Galenic system, relying on theory and scholarship rather than observation, persisted throughout the Middle Ages. The galenical compounds, along with bloodletting, and purging, were among the drastic techniques practiced by the medical professionals during those times; however, traditional herbal healers persisted outside the mainstream medical system.

During the eighth century a medical school was established in Salerno, Italy, where the herbal knowledge accumulated by Arab physicians was preserved. The Arabian Muslims conducted extensive research on medicinal herbs found in Europe, Persia, India, and the Far East. Arab businessmen opened the first herbal pharmacies early in the ninth century. The *Leech Book of Bald*, the work of a Christian monk, was compiled in the tenth century. It preserved important medical writings that had survived from the work of physicians in ancient Greece and Rome.

The Middle Ages in Europe were a time of widespread **death** by plagues and pestilence. The Black **Plague** of 1348, particularly, and other health catastrophes in later years, claimed so many lives that survivors began to lose faith in the dominant Galenic medical system. Fortunately, the knowledge of traditional herbal medicine had not been lost. Medieval monks who cultivated extensive medicinal gardens on the monastery grounds, also patiently copied the ancient herbal and medical texts. Folk medicine as practiced in Europe by traditional healers persisted, even though many women herbalists were persecuted as witches and enemies of the Catholic church and their herbal arts were suppressed.

The growing spice trade and explorations to the New World introduced exotic plants, and a whole new realm of botanical medicines became available to Europeans. Following the invention of the printing press in the fifteenth century, a large number of herbal texts, also simply called herbals, became available for popular use. Among them were the beautifully illustrated works of the German botanists Otto Brunfels and Leonhard Fuchs published in 1530, and the Dutch herbal of Belgian physician Rembert Dodoens, a popular work that was later reproduced in English. In 1597, the physician and gardener John Gerard published one of the most famous of the English herbals, still in print today. Gerard's herbal, known as *The Herball or General Historie of Plantes* was not an original work. Much of the content was taken from the translated text of his Belgian predecessor Dodoens. Gerard did, however, include descriptions of some of the more than one thousand species of rare and exotic plants and English flora from his own garden.

The correspondence of astrology with herbs was taught by Arab physicians who regarded astrology as a science helpful in the selection of medicines and in the treatment of diseases. This approach to western herbalism was particularly evident in the herbal texts published in the sixteenth and seventeenth centuries. One of the most popular and controversial English herbals is *The English Physician Enlarged* published in 1653. The author, Nicholas Culpeper, was an apothecary by trade. He also published a translation of the Latin language *London Pharmacopoeia* into

English. Culpeper was a nonconformist in loyalist England, and was determined to make medical knowledge more accessible to the apothecaries, the tradesmen who prescribed most of the herbal remedies. Culpeper's herbal was criticized by the medical establishment for its mix of magic and astrology with botanical medicine, but it became one of the most popular compendiums of botanical medicine of its day. Culpeper also accepted the so-called "Doctrine of Signatures," practiced by medieval monks in their medicinal gardens. This theory teaches that the appearance of plants is the clue to their curative powers. Plants were chosen for treatment of particular medical conditions based on their associations with the four natural elements and with a planet or sign. The place where the plant grows, its dominant physical feature, and the smell and taste of an herb determined the plant's signature. Culpeper's herbal is still in print in facsimile copies, and some pharmocognosists and herbalists in the twenty-first century voice the same criticisms that Culpeper's early critics did.

European colonists brought their herbal knowledge and plant specimens to settlements in North America where they learned from the indigenous Americans how to make use of numerous nutritive and medicinal plants, native to the New World. Many European medicinal plants escaped cultivation from the early settlements and have become naturalized throughout North America. The first record of Native American herbalism is found in the manuscript of the native Mexican Indian physician, Juan Badianus published in 1552. The American Folk tradition of herbalism developed as a blend of traditional European medicine and Native American herbalism. The pioneer necessity for self-reliance contributed to the perseverance of folk medicine well into the twentieth century.

In Europe in the seventeenth century, the alchemist Paracelsus changed the direction of western medicine with the introduction of chemical and mineral medicines. He was the son of a Swiss chemist and physician. Paracelsus began to apply chemicals, such as arsenic, mercury, sulfur, iron, and copper sulfate to treat disease. His chemical approach to the treatment of disease was a forerunner to the reliance in the twentieth century on chemical medicine as the orthodox treatment prescribed in mainstream medical practice.

The nineteenth and twentieth centuries brought a renewed interest in the practice of western herbalism and the development of natural therapies and health care systems that ran counter to the mainstream methods of combating disease symptoms with synthetic pharmaceuticals.

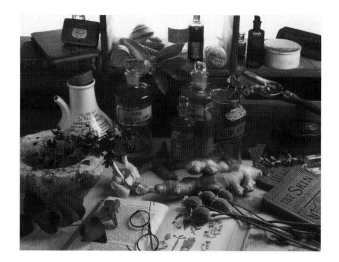

A selection of Western herbal medical equipment and traditional herbs, including foxglove (upper right), ginger (center right), and periwinkle (lower left). *(Photo Researchers, Inc. Reproduced by permission.)*

In the late eighteenth century, the German physician **Samuel Hahnemann** developed a system of medicine known as homeopathy. This approach to healing embraces the philosophy of "like cures like." Homeopathy uses extremely diluted solutions of herbs, animal products, and chemicals that are believed to hold a "trace memory" or energetic imprint of the substance used. Homeopathic remedies are used to amplify the patient's symptoms with remedies that would act to produce the same symptom in a healthy person. Homeopathy holds that the symptoms of illness are evidence of the body's natural process of healing and eliminating the cause of the disease.

In 1895, the European medical system known as Naturopathy was introduced to the North America. Like homeopathy, this medical approach is based on the Hippocratic idea of eliminating disease by assisting the body's natural healing abilities. The naturopath uses nontoxic methods to assist the body's natural healing processes, including **nutritional supplements**, herbal remedies, proper diet, and **exercise** to restore health.

Western herbalism is regaining popularity at a time when the world is assaulted by the **stress** of overpopulation and development that threatens the natural biodiversity necessary for these valuable medicinal plants to survive. The American herb market is growing rapidly and increasing numbers of individuals are choosing alternative therapies over the mainstream allopathic western medicine. It is projected that by the year 2002 consumers will spend more than seven billion dollars a year on herbal products.

An estimated 2,400 acres of native plant habitat are lost to development every day. As much as 29% of all plant life in North America is in danger of extinction, including some of the most important native medicinal plants, according to the 1997 World Conservation Union Red List of Threatened Plants.

Though research into the efficacy and safety of traditional herbal remedies is increasing, it has been limited by the high costs of clinical studies and laboratory research, and by the fact that whole plants and their constituents are not generally patentable (therefore, there is no drug profit after market introduction). Outside the United States, herbalism has successfully combined with conventional medicine, and in some countries is fully integrated into the nations' health care systems. At the beginning of the twenty-first century, 80% of the world's population continues to rely on herbal treatments. The World Health Organization, an agency of the United Nations, promotes traditional herbal medicine for treatment of many local health problems, particularly in the third world where it is affordable and already well-integrated into the cultural fabric.

In the United States, the re-emergence in interest in holistic approaches to health care is evident. Citizens are demanding access to effective, safe, low-cost, natural medicine. Legislative and societal change is needed, however, before natural therapies can be fully integrated into the orthodox allopathic health care system and provide citizens with a wide range of choices for treatment. If the current trend continues, U. S. citizens will benefit from a choice among a variety of safe and effective medical treatments.

Herbs are generally defined as any plant or plant part that may be used for medicinal, nutritional, culinary, or other beneficial purposes. The active constituents of plants (if known) may be found in varying amounts in the root, stem, leaf, flower, and fruit, etc. of the plant. Herbs may be classified into many different categories. Some western herbalists categorize herbal remedies according to their strength, action, and characteristics. Categories may include sedatives, stimulants, **laxatives**, febrifuges (to reduce **fever**), and many others. One system of classification is based on a principle in traditional Chinese medicine that categorizes herbs into four classes: tonics, specifics, heroics, or cleansers and protectors. Within these broad classifications are the numerous medicinal actions of the whole herb which may be due to a specific chemical or combination of chemicals in the plant.

- Tonics. Herbs in this classification are also known as alteratives in western herbalism. They are generally mild in their action and act slowly in the body, providing gentle stimulation and **nutrition** to specific organs and systems. Tonic herbs act over time to strengthen and nourish the whole body. These herbs are generally safe and may be used regularly, even in large quantities. These tonic herbs are known as "superior" remedies in traditional Chinese medicine. The therapeutic dose of tonic remedies is far removed from the possible toxic dose. American ginseng is an example of a tonic herb.

- Specifics. Herbs in this classification are strong and specific in their therapeutic action. They are generally used for short periods of time in smaller dosages to treat acute conditions. Herbs classified as specifics are not used beyond the therapeutic treatment period. **Echinacea** is a specific herb.

- Heroic. These herbs offer high potency but are potentially toxic, and should not be used in self-treatment. Because the therapeutic dosage may be close to the lethal dosage, these herbs are presented cautiously and closely monitored or avoided by trained clinicians. They should not be used continuously or without expert supervision. Poke (*Phytolacca americana*) is an example of a heroic remedy.

- Cleansers and protectors. These herbs, plants, and plant tissues remove wastes and pollutants, while minimally affecting regular body processes. An example of a cleanser is pectin. Pectins are the water soluble substances that bind cell walls in plant tissues, and some believe that they help remove heavy metals and environmental toxins from the body.

Preparations

Herbal preparations are commercially available in a variety of forms including tablets or capsules, tinctures, teas, fluid extracts, douches, washes, suppositories, dried herbs, and many other forms. The medicinal properties of herbs are extracted from the fresh or dried plant parts by the use of solvents appropriate to the particular herb. Alcohol, oil, water, vinegar, glycerin, and propylene glycol are some of the solvents used to extract and concentrate the medicinal properties. Steam distillation and cold-pressing techniques are used to extract the essential oils. The quality of any herbal remedy and the potency of the phytochemicals found in the herb depends greatly on the conditions of weather and soil where the herb was grown, the timing and care in harvesting, and the manner of preparation and storage.

KEY TERMS

In vitro—A biological reaction occurring in a laboratory apparatus.

In vivo—Occurring in a living organism.

Phyto-, as in phytochemical, phytomedicinal, and phytotherapy—Meaning, or pertaining to, a plant or plants.

Wildcrafting—Gathering of herbs or other natural materials.

Precautions

Herbal remedies prepared by infusion, decoction, or alcohol tincture from the appropriate plant part, such as the leaf, root, or flower are generally safe when ingested in properly designated therapeutic dosages. However, many herbs have specific contraindications for use when certain medical conditions are present. Not all herbal remedies may be safely administered to infants or small children. Many herbs are not safe for use by pregnant or lactating women. Some herbs are toxic, even deadly, in large amounts, and there is little research on the chronic toxicity that may result from prolonged use. Herbal remedies are sold in the United States as dietary supplements and are not regulated for content or efficacy. Self-diagnosis and treatment with botanical medicinals may be risky. A consultation with a clinical herbalist, Naturopathic physician, or certified clinical herbalist is prudent before undertaking a course of treatment.

Essential oils are highly concentrated and should not be ingested as a general rule. They should also be diluted in water or in a non-toxic carrier oil before application to the skin to prevent **contact dermatitis** or photo-sensitization. The toxicity of the concentrated essential oil varies depending on the chemical constituents of the herb.

The American Professor of Pharmacognosy, Varro E. Tyler, believes that "herbal chaos" prevails in the United States with regard to herbs and phytomedicinals. In part he blames the herb producers and marketers of crude herbs and remedies for what he terms unproven hyperbolic, poor quality control, deceptive labeling, resistance to standardization of dosage forms, and continued sale of herbs determined to be harmful.

Side effects

Herbs have a variety of complex phytochemicals that act on the body as a whole or on specific organs and systems. Some of these chemical constituents are mild and safe, even in large doses. Other herbs contain chemicals that act more strongly and may be toxic in large doses or when taken continuously. **Drug interactions** are possible with certain herbs when combined with certain pharmaceutical drugs. Some herbs are tonic in a small amount and toxic in larger dosages.

Research and general acceptance

Western herbalism is experiencing a revival of popular and professional interest. The number of training schools and qualified herbal practitioners is growing to meet the demand. Western herbalism is incorporated into the medical practice of licensed Naturopathic doctors, who receive special training in clinical herbalism. Folk herbalists, heir to the continuing oral traditions passed from generation to generation in many rural areas, as well as amateur, self-taught herbalists, keep the practice of botanical medicine alive at the grassroots level. Traditional western herbalism relies on traditional use and materia medica, folk wisdom, and recent clinical research and advances in the extraction processes. These advances provide increased quality control on the concentration and potency of the active ingredients. Western physicians, educated in allopathic medicine, typically receive no training in the use of herbs. These doctors rely on pharmaceutical drugs for their patients, and some cite the following reasons for continuing to do so: lack of standardized dosages, lack of quality control in the preparation of herbal medicinals, and the dearth of clinical research verifying the safety and effectiveness of many traditional herbal remedies.

Herbalism is widely practiced throughout Europe, particularly in England, France, Italy, and Germany where phytomedicinals are available in prescription form and as over-the-counter remedies. In Germany, plant medicines are regulated by a special government body known as the Commission E. In the United States, however, despite increasing popularity, traditional herbalism is not integrated into the allopathic medical system. Phytomedicinals are sold as dietary supplements rather than being adequately researched and recognized as safe and effective drugs. The Dietary Supplement Health and Education Act of 1994 circumvented a U. S. Food and Drug Administration (FDA) effort to effectively remove botanicals from the marketplace and implement regulations restricting sale. Massive popular outcry against the proposed regulations on the sale of herbs and phytomedicinals resulted in this Congressional action. In 2000, U.S. President Bill Clinton, by executive order, created the White House Commission on Alternative Medicine in an effort to hold alternative medicine therapies "to the same standard of scientific rigor as more traditional health care interventions." That Commission is charged with recommending federal guidelines and legislation regarding the use of alternative medical therapies in the twenty-first century.

Resources

PERIODICALS

Deneen, Sally, with Rembert, Tracey. "Uprooted, The Worldwide Plant Crisis Is Accelerating." *E Magazine* July-August 1999: 36-40.

Liebmann, Richard, N.D. "United Plant Savers—Planting the Future." *PanGaia* 22 (Winter 1999-2000): 23- 26.

ORGANIZATIONS

National Center for the Preservation of Medicinal Herbs. 3350 Beech Grove Road, Rutland, Ohio 45775. (740)742- 4401.

United Plant Savers. P.O. Box 98, East Barre, Vermont 05649. (802) 479-9825. < http://www.plantsavers.org >.

OTHER

Hobbs, Christopher. "Specific and Tonic Immune Herbs: Exploring a Practical System of Western Herbalism." Health World. < http://www.healthy.net >.

Oracle Tree New Age Mall. "Western Medical Astrology: A Brief History." < http://ww.oracletree.com/ avalonphysics/wesmedas.html >.

Wicke, Roger, Ph.D. "A World History of Herbology and Herbalism: Oppressed Arts." Rocky Mountain Herbal Institute. < http://www.rmhiherbalorg/a/ f.ahrl.hist.html >.

Clare Hanrahan

Herbs *see* **Echinacea; Ginkgo biloba; Ginseng; Saw palmetto; St. John's wort**

Hereditary cerebral hemorrhage with amyloidosis *see* **Cerebral amyloid angiopathy**

Hereditary chorea *see* **Huntington's disease**

Hereditary fructose intolerance

Definition

Hereditary fructose intolerance is an inherited condition where the body does not produce the chemical needed to break down fructose (fruit sugar).

Description

Fructose is a sugar found naturally in fruits, vegetables, honey, and table sugar. Fructose intolerance is a disorder caused by the body's inability to produce an enzyme called aldolase B (also called fructose 1-phosphate aldolase) that is necessary for absorption of fructose. The undigested fructose collects in the liver and kidneys, eventually causing liver and kidney failure. One person in about 20,000 is born with this disorder. It is reported more frequently in the United States and Northern European countries than in other parts of the world. It occurs with equal frequency in males and females.

Causes and symptoms

Fructose intolerance is an inherited disorder passed on to children through their parents' genes. Both the mother and father have the gene that causes the condition, but may not have symptoms of fructose intolerance themselves. (This is called an autosomal recessive pattern of inheritance.) The disorder will not be apparent until the infant is fed formula, juice, fruits, or baby foods that contain fructose. Initial symptoms include **vomiting**, **dehydration**, and unexplained **fever**. Other symptoms include extreme thirst and excessive urination and sweating. There will also be a loss of appetite and a failure to grow. **Tremors** and seizures caused by low blood sugar can occur. The liver becomes swollen and the patient becomes jaundiced with yellowing of the eyes and skin. Left untreated, this condition can lead to **coma** and **death**.

Diagnosis

Urine tests can be used to detect fructose sugar in the urine. Blood tests can also be used to detect *hyperbilirubinemia* and high levels of liver enzymes in the blood. A **liver biopsy** may be performed to test for levels of enzymes present and to evaluate the extent of damage to the liver. A fructose-loading test where a dose of fructose is given to the patient in a well-controlled hospital or clinical setting may also be used to confirm fructose intolerance. Both the biopsy and the loading test can be very risky, particularly in infants that are already sick.

Treatment

Once diagnosed, fructose intolerance can be successfully treated by eliminating fructose from the diet. Patients usually respond within three to four weeks and can make a complete recovery if fructose-containing foods are avoided. Early recognition and treatment of the disease is important to avoid damage to the liver, kidneys, and small intestine.

KEY TERMS

Aldolase B—Also called fructose 1-phosphate aldolase, this chemical is produced in the liver, kidneys, and brain. It is needed for the breakdown of fructose, a sugar found in fruits, vegetables, honey, and other sweeteners.

Hyperbilirubinemia—A condition where there is a high level of bilirubin in the blood. Bilirubin is a natural by-product of the breakdown of red blood cells, however, a high level of bilirubin may indicate a problem with the liver.

Liver biopsy—A surgical procedure where a small piece of the liver is cut out for examination. A needle or narrow tube may be inserted either directly through the skin and muscle or through a small incision and passed into the liver for collection of a sample of liver tissue.

Prognosis

If the condition is not recognized and the diet is not well controlled, death can occur in infants or young children. With a well-controlled diet, the child can develop normally.

Prevention

Carriers of the gene for hereditary fructose intolerance can be identified through DNA analysis. Anyone who is known to carry the disease or who has the disease in his or her family can benefit from **genetic counseling**. Since this is a hereditary disorder, there is currently no known way to prevent it other than assisting at-risk individuals with family planning and reproductive decisions.

Resources

ORGANIZATIONS

National Institutes of Health. National Institute of Diabetes, Digestive and Kidney Diseases. Building 31, Room 9A04, 31 Center Drive, Bethesda, MD 20892-2560. (301) 496-3583.

OTHER

"What Is Hereditary Fructose Intolerance?" Hereditary Fructose Intolerance & Aldolase Homepage. <http://www.bu.edu/aldolase>.

Altha Roberts Edgren

Hereditary hemorrhagic telangiectasia

Definition

Hereditary hemorrhagic telangiectasia is an inherited condition characterized by abnormal blood vessels which are delicate and prone to bleeding. Hereditary hemorrhagic telangiectasia is also known as Rendu-Osler-Weber disease.

Description

The term telangiectasia refers to a spot formed, usually on the skin, by a dilated capillary or terminal artery. In hereditary hemorrhagic telangiectasia these spots occur because the blood vessel is fragile and bleeds easily. The bleeding may appear as small, red or reddish-violet spots on the face, lips, inside the mouth and nose or the tips of the fingers and toes. Other small telangiectasias may occur in the digestive tract.

Unlike **hemophilia**, where bleeding is caused by an ineffective clotting mechanism in the blood, bleeding in hereditary hemorrhagic telangiectasia is caused by fragile blood vessels. However, like hemophilia, bleeding may be extensive and can occur without warning.

Causes and symptoms

Hereditary hemorrhagic telangiectasia, an autosomal dominant inherited disorder, occurs in one in 50,000 people.

Recurrent nosebleeds are a nearly universal symptom in this condition. Usually the nosebleeds begin in childhood and become worse with age. The skin changes begin at **puberty**, and the condition becomes progressively worse until about 40 years of age, when it stabilizes.

Diagnosis

The physician will look for red spots on all areas of the skin, but especially on the upper half of the body, and in the mouth and nose and under the tongue.

Treatment

There is no specific treatment for hereditary hemorrhagic telangiectasia. The bleeding resulting from the condition can be stopped by applying compresses or direct pressure to the area. If necessary, a laser can be used to destroy the vessel. In severe cases, the leaking artery can be plugged or covered with a graft from normal tissue.

KEY TERMS

Autosomal dominant—A pattern of inheritance in which the dominant gene on any non-sex chromosome carries the defect.

Chromosome—A threadlike structure in the cell which transmits genetic information.

Prognosis

In most people, recurrent bleeding results in an iron deficiency. It is usually necessary to take iron supplements.

Prevention

Hereditary hemorrhagic telangiectasia is an inherited disorder and cannot be prevented.

Resources

ORGANIZATIONS

American Medical Association. 515 N. State St., Chicago, IL 60612. (312) 464-5000. < http://www.ama-assn.org >.
Association of Birth Defect Children. 3526 Emerywood Lane, Orlando, FL, 32806. (305) 859-2821.

Dorothy Elinor Stonely

Hereditary hyperuricemia see **Lesch-Nyhan syndrome**

Hereditary spinocerebellar ataxia see **Friedreich's ataxia**

Hermaphroditism see **Intersex states**

Hernia

Definition

Hernia is a general term used to describe a bulge or protrusion of an organ through the structure or muscle that usually contains it.

Description

There are many different types of hernias. The most familiar type are those that occur in the abdomen, in which part of the intestines protrude through the abdominal wall. This may occur in different areas and, depending on the location, the hernia is given a different name.

An inguinal hernia appears as a bulge in the groin and may come and go depending on the position of the person or their level of physical activity. It can occur with or without **pain**. In men, the protrusion may descend into the scrotum. Inguinal hernias account for 80% of all hernias and are more common in men.

Femoral hernias are similar to inguinal hernias but appear as a bulge slightly lower. They are more common in women due to the strain of **pregnancy**.

A ventral hernia is also called an incisional hernia because it generally occurs as a bulge in the abdomen at the site of an old surgical scar. It is caused by thinning or stretching of the scar tissue, and occurs more frequently in people who are obese or pregnant.

An umbilical hernia appears as a soft bulge at the navel (umbilicus). It is caused by a weakening of the area or an imperfect closure of the area in infants. This type of hernia is more common in women due to pregnancy, and in Chinese and black infants. Some umbilical hernias in infants disappear without treatment within the first year.

A hiatal or diaphragmatic hernia is different from abdominal hernias in that it is not visible on the outside of the body. With a hiatal hernia, the stomach bulges upward through the muscle that separates the chest from the abdomen (the diaphragm). This type of hernia occurs more often in women than in men, and it is treated differently from other types of hernias.

Causes and symptoms

Most hernias result from a weakness in the abdominal wall that either develops or that an infant is born with (congenital). Any increase in pressure in the abdomen, such as coughing, straining, heavy lifting, or pregnancy, can be a considered causative factor in developing an abdominal hernia. **Obesity** or recent excessive weight loss, as well as **aging** and previous surgery, are also risk factors.

Most abdominal hernias appear suddenly when the abdominal muscles are strained. The person may feel tenderness, a slight burning sensation, or a feeling of heaviness in the bulge. It may be possible for the person to push the hernia back into place with gentle pressure, or the hernia may disappear by itself when the person reclines. Being able to push the hernia back is called reducing it. On the other hand, some hernias cannot be pushed back into place, and are termed incarcerated or irreducible.

A hiatal hernia may also be caused by obesity, pregnancy, aging, or previous surgery. About 50% of all people with hiatal hernias do not have any symptoms. If symptoms exist they will include **heartburn**, usually 30–60 minutes following a meal. There may be some mid chest pain due to gastric acid from the stomach being pushed up into the esophagus. The pain and heartburn are usually worse when lying down. Frequent belching and feelings of abdominal fullness may also be present.

Diagnosis

Generally, abdominal hernias need to be seen and felt to be diagnosed. Usually the hernia will increase in size with an increase in abdominal pressure, so the doctor may ask the person to cough while he or she feels the area. Once a diagnosis of an abdominal hernia is made, the doctor will usually send the person to a surgeon for a consultation. Surgery provides the only cure for a hernia through the abdominal wall.

With a hiatal hernia, the diagnosis is based on the symptoms reported by the person. The doctor may then order tests to confirm the diagnosis. If a barium swallow is ordered, the person drinks a chalky white barium solution, which will help any protrusion through the diaphragm show up on the x ray that follows. Currently, a diagnosis of hiatal hernia is more frequently made by endoscopy. This procedure is done by a gastroenterologist (a specialist in digestive diseases). During an endoscopy the person is given an intravenous sedative and a small tube is inserted through the mouth, then into the esophagus and stomach where the doctor can visualize the hernia. The procedure takes about 30 minutes and usually causes no discomfort. It is done on an outpatient basis.

Treatment

Once an abdominal hernia occurs it tends to increase in size. Some patients with abdominal hernias wait and watch for a while prior to choosing surgery. In these cases, they must avoid strenuous physical activity such as heavy lifting or straining with **constipation**. They may also wear a truss, which is a support worn like a belt to keep a small hernia from protruding. People can tell if their hernia is getting worse if they develop severe constant pain, **nausea and vomiting**, or if the bulge does not return to normal when lying down or when they try to gently push it back in place. In these cases they should consult with their doctor immediately. But, ultimately, surgery is the treatment in almost all cases.

There are risks to not repairing a hernia surgically. Left untreated, a hernia may become incarcerated,

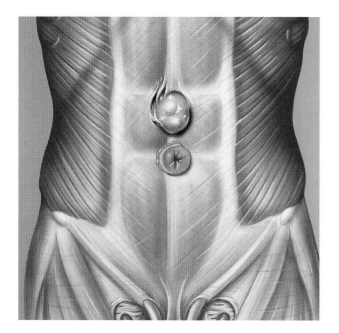

An illustration of an epigastric (abdominal) hernia in an adult male. The torso is shown with its skin removed. Epigastric hernia is caused commonly by a congenital weakness in muscles of the central upper abdomen; the intestine bulges out through the muscle at a point between the navel and breastbone. *(Photograph by John Bavosi, Photo Researchers, Inc. Reproduced by permission.)*

which means it can no longer be reduced or pushed back into place. With an incarcerated hernia the intestines become trapped outside the abdomen. This could lead to a blockage in the intestine. If it is severe enough it may cut off the blood supply to the intestine and part of the intestine might actually die.

When the blood supply is cut off, the hernia is termed "strangulated." Because of the risk of tissue death (necrosis) and **gangrene**, and because the hernia can block food from moving through the bowel, a strangulated hernia is a medical emergency requiring immediate surgery. Repairing a hernia before it becomes incarcerated or strangulated is much safer than waiting until complications develop.

Surgical repair of a hernia is called a herniorrhaphy. The surgeon will push the bulging part of the intestine back into place and sew the overlying muscle back together. When the muscle is not strong enough, the surgeon may reinforce it with a synthetic mesh.

Surgery can be done on an outpatient basis. It usually takes 30 minutes in children and 60 minutes in adults. It can be done under either local or **general anesthesia** and is frequently done with a laparoscope. In this type of surgery, a tube that allows visualization of the abdominal cavity is inserted through a small puncture wound. Several small punctures are made to allow surgical instruments to be inserted. This type of surgery avoids a larger incision.

A hiatal hernia is treated differently. Medical treatment is preferred. Treatments include:

- avoiding reclining after meals
- avoiding spicy foods, acidic foods, alcohol, and tobacco
- eating small, frequent, bland meals
- eating a high-fiber diet.

There are also several types of medications that help to manage the symptoms of a hiatal hernia. **Antacids** are used to neutralize gastric acid and decrease heartburn. Drugs that reduce the amount of acid produced in the stomach (H2 blockers) are also used. This class of drugs includes famotidine (sold under the name Pepcid), cimetidine (Tagamet), and ranitidine (Zantac). Omeprazole (Prilosec) is not an H2 blocker, but is another drug that suppresses gastric acid secretion and is used for hiatal hernias. Another option may be metoclopramide (Reglan), a drug that increases the tone of the muscle around the esophagus and causes the stomach to empty more quickly.

Alternative treatment

There are alternative therapies for hiatal hernia. Visceral manipulation, done by a trained therapist, can help replace the stomach to its proper positioning. Other options in addition to H2 blockers are available to help regulate stomach acid production and balance. One of them, deglycyrrhizinated licorice (DGL), helps balance stomach acid by improving the protective substances that line the stomach and intestines and by improving blood supply to these tissues. DGL does not interrupt the normal function of stomach acid.

As with traditional therapy, dietary modifications are important. Small, frequent meals will keep pressure down on the esophageal sphincter. Also, raising the head of the bed several inches with blocks or books can help with both the quality and quantity of sleep.

Prognosis

Abdominal hernias generally do not recur in children but can recur in up to 10% of adult patients. Surgery is considered the only cure, and the prognosis is excellent if the hernia is corrected before it becomes strangulated.

Hiatal hernias are treated successfully with medication and diet modifications 85% of the time.

KEY TERMS

Endoscopy—A diagnostic procedure in which a tube is inserted through the mouth, into the esophagus and stomach. It is used to visualize various digestive disorders, including hiatal hernias.

Herniorrhaphy—Surgical repair of a hernia.

Incarcerated hernia—A hernia that can not be reduced, or pushed back into place inside the intestinal wall.

Reducible hernia—A hernia that can be gently pushed back into place or that disappears when the person lies down.

Strangulated hernia—A hernia that is so tightly incarcerated outside the abdominal wall that the intestine is blocked and the blood supply to that part of the intestine is cut off.

The prognosis remains excellent even if surgery is required in adults who are in otherwise good health.

Prevention

Some hernias can be prevented by maintaining a reasonable weight, avoiding heavy lifting and constipation, and following a moderate **exercise** program to maintain good abdominal muscle tone.

Resources

BOOKS

Bare, Brenda G., and Suzanne C. Smeltzer. *Brunner and Suddarth's Textbook of Medical-Surgical Nursing.* 8th ed. Philadelphia: Lippincott-Raven Publishers, 1996.

Joyce S. Siok, RN

Hernia repair

Definition

Hernia repair is a surgical procedure to return an organ that protrudes through a weak area of muscle to its original position.

Purpose

Hernias occur when a weakness in the wall of the abdomen allows an organ, usually the intestines, to bulge out of place. Hernias may result from a genetic predisposition toward this weakness. They can also be the result of weakening the muscle through improper **exercise** or poor lifting techniques. Both children and adults get hernias. Some are painful, while others are not.

There are three levels of hernias. An uncomplicated hernia is one where the intestines bulge into the peritoneum (the membrane lining the abdomen), but they can still be manipulated back into the body (although they don't stay in place without corrective surgery). This is termed a reducible hernia.

If the intestines bulge through the hernia defect and become trapped, this is called an incarcerated hernia. If the blood supply to an incarcerated hernia is shut off, the hernia is called a strangulated hernia. Strangulated hernias can result in **gangrene**.

Both incarcerated and strangulated hernias are medical emergencies and require emergency surgery to correct. For this reason, doctors generally recommend the repair of an uncomplicated hernia, even if it causes no discomfort to the patient.

Precautions

Hernia repair can be performed under local, regional, or **general anesthesia**. The choice depends on the age and health of the patient and the type of hernia. Generally hernia repair is very safe surgery, but—as with any surgery—the risk of complications increases if the patient smokes, is obese, is very young or very old, uses alcohol heavily, or uses illicit drugs.

Description

Hernia repairs are performed in a hospital or outpatient surgical facility by a general surgeon. Depending on the patient's age, health, and the type of hernia, patients may be able to go home the same day or may remain hospitalized for up to three to five days.

There are two types of hernia repair. A herniorrhaphy is used for simpler hernias. The intestines are returned to their proper place and the defect in the abdominal wall is mended. A hernioplasty is used for larger hernias. In this procedure, plastic or steel mesh is added to the abdominal wall to repair and reinforce the weak spot.

There are five kinds of common hernia repairs. They are named for the part of the body closest to the hernia, or bulge.

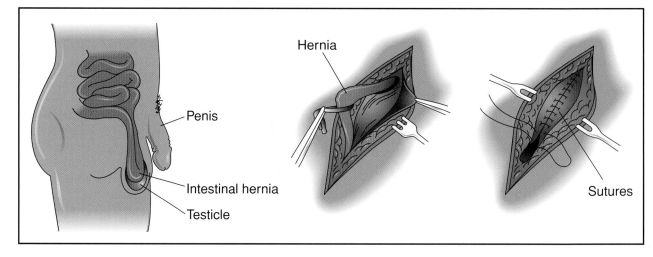

In this inguinal hernia repair, an incision is made in the abdomen. The hernia is located, and the intestines are returned to the abdomen. The abdominal wall is then sutured together to close any space and reinforce the weak area. *(Illustration by Electronic Illustrators Group.)*

Femoral hernia repair

This procedure repairs a hernia that occurs in the groin where the thigh meets the abdomen. It is called a femoral hernia repair because it is near the spot where the femoral artery and vein pass from the leg into the trunk of the body. Sometimes this type of hernia creates a noticeable bulge.

An incision is made in the groin area. The tissues are separated from the hernia sac, and the intestines are returned to the abdomen. The area is often reinforced with webbing before it is sewn shut. The skin is closed with sutures or metal clips that can be removed in about one week.

Inguinal hernia repair

Inguinal hernia repair closes a weakness in the abdominal wall that is near the inguinal canal, the spot where the testes descend from the body into the scrotum. This type of hernia occurs in about two percent of adult males.

An incision is made in the abdomen, then the hernia is located and repaired. The surgeon must be alert not to injure the spermatic cord, the testes, or the blood supply to the testes. If the hernia is small, it is simply repaired. If it is large, the area is reinforced with mesh to prevent a recurrence. External skin sutures can be removed in about a week. Patients should not resume sexual activity until being cleared by their doctor.

Umbilical hernia repair

This procedure repairs a hernia that occurs when the intestines bulge through the abdomen wall near the navel. Umbilical hernias are most common in infants.

An incision is made near the navel. The hernia is located and the intestines are returned to the abdomen. The peritoneum is closed, then the large abdominal muscle is pulled over the weak spot in such a way as to reinforce the area. External sutures or skin clips can be removed in about 10 days.

Incisional hernia repair

Incisional hernias occur most frequently at the site of a scar from earlier abdominal surgery. Once again, the abdomen is opened and the intestines returned to their proper place. The area is reinforced with mesh, and the abdominal wall is reconstructed to prevent another hernia from developing. External sutures can be removed in about a week.

Hiatal hernia

A hiatal hernia repair is slightly different from the other hernias described here, because it corrects a weakness or opening in the diaphragm, the muscle that separates the chest cavity from the abdominal cavity. This surgery is done to prevent the stomach from shifting up into the chest cavity and to prevent the stomach from spilling gastric juices into the esophagus, causing **pain** and scarring.

An incision is made in the abdomen or chest, and the hole or weakness in the diaphragm is located and repaired. The top of the stomach is wrapped around the bottom of the esophagus, and they are sutured together to hold the stomach in place. Sometimes the

KEY TERMS

Endoscopy—A procedure in which an instrument containing a camera is inserted into the gastrointestinal tract so that the doctor can visually inspect the gastrointestinal system.

Gangrene—Death and decay of body tissue because the blood supply is cut off. Tissues that have died in this way must be surgically removed.

Peritoneum—The transparent membrane lining the abdominal cavity that holds organs such as the intestines in place.

vagus nerve is cut in order to decrease the amount of acid the stomach produces. External sutures can be removed in about one week. This type of hernia repair often requires a longer hospital stay than the other types, although techniques are being improved that reduce invasiveness of the surgery and the length of the hospital stay.

Preparation

Before the operation, the patient will have blood and urine collected for testing. X rays are taken of the affected area. In a hiatal hernia, an endoscopy (a visual inspection of the organs) is done.

Patients should meet with the anesthesiologist before the operation to discuss any medications or conditions that might affect the administration of anesthesia. Patients may be asked to temporarily discontinue certain medications. The day of the operation, patients should not eat or drink anything. They may be given an enema to clear the bowels.

Aftercare

Patients should eat a clear liquid diet until the gastrointestinal tract begins functioning again. Normally this is a short period of time. After that, they are free to eat a healthy, well-balanced diet of their choice. They may bathe normally, using a gentle, unscented soap. An antibiotic ointment may be prescribed for the incision. After the operation, a hard ridge will form along the incision line. With time, this ridge softens and becomes less noticeable. Patients who remain in the hospital will have blood drawn for follow-up studies.

Patients should begin easy activities, such as walking, as soon as they are comfortable, but should avoid strenuous exercise for four to six weeks, and especially avoid heavy lifting. Learning and practicing proper lifting techniques is an important part of patient education after the operation. Patients may be given a laxative or stool softener so that they will not strain to have bowel movements. They should discuss with their doctor when to resume driving and sexual activity.

Risks

As with any surgery, there exists the possibility of excessive bleeding and infection after the surgery. In inguinal and femoral hernia repair, a slight risk of damage to the testicles or their blood supply exists for male patients. Accidental damage may be caused to the intestinal tract, but generally complications are few.

Normal results

The outcome of surgery depends on the age and health of the patient and on the type of hernia. Although most hernias can be repaired without complications, hernias recur in 10–20% of people who have had hernia surgery.

Resources

OTHER

"Hernia Repair." *ThriveOnline.*
    < http://thriveonline.oxygen.com >.

Tish Davidson, A.M.

Herniated disk

Definition

Disk herniation is a rupture of fibrocartilagenous material (annulus fibrosis) that surrounds the intervertebral disk. This rupture involves the release of the disk's center portion containing a gelatinous substance called the nucleus pulposus. Pressure from the vertebrae above and below may cause the nucleus pulposus to be forced outward, placing pressure on a spinal nerve and causing considerable **pain** and damage to the nerve. This condition most frequently occurs in the lumbar region and is also commonly called herniated nucleus pulposus, prolapsed disk, ruptured intervertebral disk, or slipped disk.

Description

The spinal column is made up of 26 vertebrae that are joined together and permit forward and backward bending, side bending, and rotation of the spine. Five distinct regions comprise the spinal column, including the cervical (neck) region, thoracic (chest) region, lumbar (low back) region, sacral and coccygeal (tailbone) region. The cervical region consists of seven vertebrae, the thoracic region includes 12 vertebrae, and the lumbar region contains five vertebrae. The sacrum is composed of five fused vertebrae, which are connected to four fused vertebrae forming the coccyx. Intervertebral disks lie between each adjacent vertebra.

Each disk is composed of a gelatinous material in the center, called the nucleus pulposus, surrounded by rings of a fiberous tissue (annulus fibrosus). In disk herniation, an intervertebral disk's central portion herniates or slips through the surrounding annulus fibrosus into the spinal canal, putting pressure on a nerve root. Disk herniation most commonly affects the lumbar region between the fifth lumbar vertebra and the first sacral vertebra. However, disk herniation can also occur in the cervical spine. The incidence of cervical disk herniation is most common between the fifth and sixth cervical vertebrae. The second most common area for cervical disk herniation occurs between the sixth and seventh cervical vertebrae. Disk herniation is less common in the thoracic region.

Predisposing factors associated with disk herniation include age, gender, and work environment. The peak age for occurrence of disk herniation is between 20–45 years of age. Studies have shown that males are more commonly affected than females in lumbar disk herniation by a 3:2 ratio. Prolonged exposure to a bent-forward work posture is correlated with an increased incidence of disk herniation.

There are four classifications of disk pathology:

- A protrusion may occur where a disk bulges without rupturing the annulus fibrosis.

- The disk may prolapse where the nucleus pulposus migrates to the outermost fibers of the annulus fibrosis.

- There may be a disk extrusion, which is the case if the annulus fibrosis perforates and material of the nucleus moves into the epidural space.

- The sequestrated disk may occur as fragments from the annulus fibrosis and nucleus pulposus are outside the disk proper.

Causes and symptoms

Any direct, forceful, and vertical pressure on the lumbar disks can cause the disk to push its fluid contents into the vertebral body. Herniated nucleus pulposus may occur suddenly from lifting, twisting, or direct injury, or it can occur gradually from degenerative changes with episodes of intensifying symptoms. The annulus may also become weakened over time, allowing stretching or tearing and leading to a disk herniation. Depending on the location of the herniation, the herniated material can also press directly on nerve roots or on the spinal cord, causing a shock-like pain (sciatica) down the legs, weakness, **numbness**, or problems with bowels, bladder, or sexual function.

Diagnosis

Several radiographic tests are useful for confirming a diagnosis of disk herniation and locating the source of pain. These tests also help the surgeon indicate the extent of the surgery needed to fully decompress the nerve. X rays show structural changes of the lumbar spine. Myelography is a special x ray of the spine in which a dye or air is injected into the patient's spinal canal. The patient lies strapped to a table as the table tilts in various directions and spot x rays are taken. X rays showing a narrowed dye column in the intervertebral disk area indicate possible disk herniation.

Computed tomography scan (CT or CAT scans) exhibit the details of pathology necessary to obtain consistently good surgical results. Magnetic resonance imaging (MRI) analysis of the disks can accurately detect the early stages of disk aging and degeneration. Electomyograms (EMGs) measure the electrical activity of the muscle contractions and possibly show evidence of nerve damage. An EMG is a powerful tool for assessing muscle **fatigue** associated with muscle impairment with **low back pain**.

Treatment

Drugs

Unless serious neurologic symptoms occur, herniated disks can initially be treated with pain medication and up to 48 hours of bed rest. There is no proven benefit from resting more than 48 hours. Patients are then encouraged to gradually increase their activity. Pain medications, including antiinflammatories, muscle relaxers, or in severe cases, **narcotics**, may be continued if needed.

Epidural steroid injections have been used to decrease pain by injecting an antiinflammatory drug,

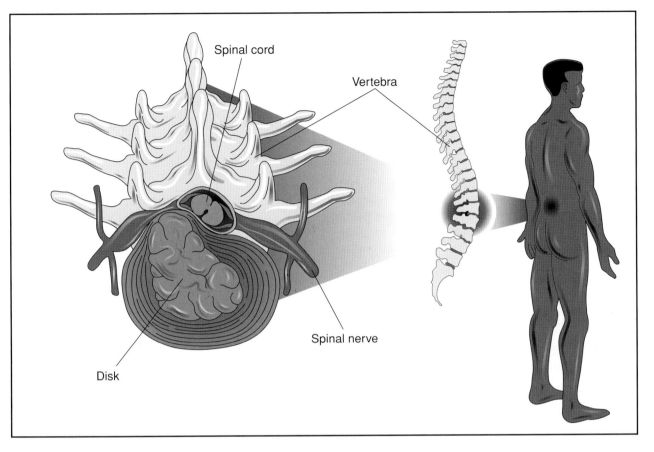

Spinal cord

Vertebra

Spinal nerve

Disk

A herniated disk refers to the rupture of fibrocartilagenous material, called the annulus fibrosis, that surrounds the intervertebral disk. When this occurs, pressure from the vertebrae above and below may force the disk's center portion, a gel-like substance, outward, placing additional pressure on the spinal nerve and causing pain and damage to the nerve. *(Illustration by Electronic Illustrators Group.)*

usually a corticosteroid, around the nerve root to reduce inflammation and edema (swelling). This partly relieves the pressure on the nerve root as well as resolves the inflammation.

Physical therapy

Physical therapists are skilled in treating acute back pain caused by the disk herniation. The physical therapist can provide noninvasive therapies, such as ultrasound or diathermy to project heat deep into the tissues of the back or administer manual therapy, if mobility of the spine is impaired. They may help improve posture and develop an exercise program for recovery and long-term protection. Appropriate **exercise** can help take pressure off inflamed nerve structures, while improving overall posture and flexibility. **Traction** can be used to try to decrease pressure on the disk. A lumbar support can be helpful for a herniated disk at this level as a temporary measure to reduce pain and improve posture.

Surgery

Surgery is often appropriate for conditions that do not improve with the usual treatment. In this event, a strong, flexible spine is important for a quick recovery after surgery. There are several surgical approaches to treating a herniated disk, including the classic discectomy, microdiscectomy, or percutanteous discectomy. The basic differences among these procedures are the size of the incision, how the disk is reached surgically, and how much of the disk is removed.

Discectomy is the surgical removal of the portion of the disk that is putting pressure on a nerve causing the back pain. In the classic disectomy, the surgeon first enters through the skin and then removes a bony portion of the vertebra called the lamina, hence the term laminectomy. The surgeon removes the disk material that is pressing on a nerve. Rarely is the entire lamina or disk entirely removed. Often, only one side is removed and the surgical procedure is termed hemi-laminectomy.

In microdiscectomy, through the use of an operating microscope, the surgeon removes the offending bone or disk tissue until the nerve is free from compression or stretch. This procedure is possible using **local anesthesia**. Microsurgery techniques vary and have several advantages over the standard discectomy, such as a smaller incision, less trauma to the musculature and nerves, and easier identification of structures by viewing into the disk space through microscope magnification.

Percutaneous disk excision is performed on an outpatient basis, is less expensive than other surgical procedures, and does not require a **general anesthesia**. The purpose of percutaneous disk excision is to reduce the volume of the affected disk indirectly by partial removal of the nucleus pulposus, leaving all the structures important to stability practically unaffected. In this procedure, large incisions are avoided by inserting devices that have cutting and suction capability. Suction is applied and the disk is sliced and aspirated.

Arthroscopic microdiscectomy is similar to percutaneous discectomy, however it incorporates modified arthroscopic instruments, including scopes and suction devices. A suction irrigation of saline solution is established through two entry sites. A video discoscope is introduced from one site and the deflecting instruments from the opposite side. In this way, the surgeon is able to search and extract the nuclear fragments under direct visualization.

Laser disk decompression is performed using similar means as percutaneous excision and arthroscopic microdiscectomy, however laser energy is used to remove the disk tissue. Here, laser energy is percutaneously introduced through a needle to vaporize a small volume of nucleus pulposus, thereby dropping the pressure of the disk and decompressing the involved neural tissues. One disadvantage of this procedure is the high initial cost of the laser equipment. It is important to realize that only a very small percentage of people with herniated lumbar disks go on to require surgery. Further, surgery should be followed by appropriate **rehabilitation** to decrease the chance of reinjury.

Chemonucleolysis

Chemonucleolysis is an alternative to surgical excision. Chymopapain, a purified enzyme derived from the papaya plant, is injected percutaneously into the disk space to reduce the size of the herniated disks. It hydrolyses proteins, thereby decreasing water-binding capacity, when injected into the nucleus pulposus inner disk material. The reduction in size of the disk relieves pressure on the nerve root.

Spinal fusion

Spinal fusion is the process by which bone grafts harvested from the iliac crest (thick border of the ilium located on the pelvis) are placed between the intervertebral bodies after the disk material is removed. This approach is used when there is a need to reestablish the normal bony relationship between the vertebrae. A total discectomy may be needed in some cases because lumbar spinal fusion can help prevent recurrent lumbar disk herniation at a particular level.

Alternative treatment

Acupuncture involves the use of fine needles inserted along the pathway of the pain to move energy locally and relieve the pain. An acupuncturist determines the location of the nerves affected by the herniated disk and positions the needles appropriately. Massage therapists may also provide short-term relief from a herniated disk. Following manual examination and x-ray diagnosis, **chiropractic** treatment usually includes manipulation to correct muscle and joint malfunctions, while care is taken not to place an additional strain on the injured disk. If a full trial of conservative therapy fails, or if neurologic problems (weakness, bowel or bladder problems, and sensory loss) develop, the next step is usually evaluation by an orthopedic surgeon.

Prognosis

Only 5–10% of patients with unrelenting **sciatica** and neurological involvement, leading to chronic pain of the lumbar spine, need to have a surgical procedure performed. This strongly suggests that many patients with herniated disks at the lumbar level respond well to conservative treatment. For those patients who do require surgery for lumbar disk herniation, the reviewed procedures of nerve root decompression caused by disk herniation is favorable. Results of studies varied from 60–90% success rates. Disk surgery has progressively evolved in the direction of decreasing invasiveness. Each surgical procedure is not without possible complications, which can lead to chronic low back pain and restricted lifestyle.

Prevention

Proper exercises to strengthen the lower back and abdominal muscles are key in preventing excess **stress** and compressive forces on lumbar disks. Good posture will help prevent problems on cervical, thoracic, and lumbar disks. A good flexibility program is critical for prevention of muscle and spasm that can cause an increase in compressive forces on disks at any level. Proper lifting of heavy objects is important for all muscles and levels of the individual disks. Good posture in sitting, standing, and lying down is helpful for the spine. Losing weight, if needed, can prevent weakness and unnecessary stress on the disks caused by obesity. Choosing proper footwear may also be helpful to reduce the impact forces to the lumbar disks while walking on hard surfaces. Wearing special back support devices may be helpful if heavy lifting is required with combinations of twisting.

Resources

OTHER
"Back Pain." Healthtouch Online Page. < http://www.healthtouch.com >.

Jeffrey P. Larson, RPT

Hernioplasty *see* **Hernia repair**

Herniorrhaphy *see* **Hernia repair**

Herpes *see* **Cold sore**

Herpes encephalitis *see* **Encephalitis**

Herpes genitalis *see* **Genital herpes**

Herpes simplex *see* **Cold sore**

Herpes simplex type 2 *see* **Genital herpes**

Herpes type 2 *see* **Genital herpes**

Herpes zoster infection *see* **Shingles**

Heterotopic transplant *see* **Liver transplantation**

Heterotropia *see* **Strabismus**

HFRS *see* **Hantavirus infections**

Hiccups

Definition

Hiccups are the result of an involuntary, spasmodic contraction of the diaphragm followed by the closing of the throat.

Description

Hiccups are one of the most common, but thankfully mildest, disorders to which humans are prey. Virtually everyone experiences them at some point, but they rarely last long or require a doctor's care. Occasionally, a bout of hiccups will last longer than two days, earning it the name "persistent hiccups." Very few people will experience intractable hiccups, in which hiccups last longer than one month.

A hiccup involves the coordinated action of the diaphragm and the muscles that close off the windpipe (trachea). The diaphragm is a dome-shaped muscle separating the chest and abdomen, normally responsible for expanding the chest cavity for inhalation. Sensation from the diaphragm travels to the spinal cord through the phrenic nerve and the vagus nerve, which pass through the chest cavity and the neck. Within the spinal cord, nerve fibers from the brain monitor sensory information and adjust the outgoing messages that control contraction. These messages travel along the phrenic nerve.

Irritation of any of the nerves involved in this loop can cause the diaphragm to undergo involuntary contraction, or spasm, pulling air into the lungs. When this occurs, it triggers a reflex in the throat muscles. Less than a tenth of a second afterward, the trachea is closed off, making the characteristic "hic" sound.

Causes and symptoms

Hiccups can be caused by central nervous system disorders, injury or irritation to the phrenic and vagus nerves, and toxic or metabolic disorders affecting the central or peripheral nervous systems. They may be of unknown cause or may be a symptom of psychological **stress**. Hiccups often occur after drinking carbonated beverages or alcohol. They may also follow overeating or rapid temperature changes.

Persistent or intractable hiccups may be caused by any condition which irritates or damages the relevant nerves, including:

- overstretching of the neck
- laryngitis
- heartburn (gastroesophageal reflux)
- irritation of the eardrum (which is innervated by the vagus nerve)
- general anesthesia
- surgery
- bloating
- tumor
- infection
- diabetes

Diagnosis

Hiccups are diagnosed by observation, and by hearing the characteristic sound. Diagnosing the cause of intractable hiccups may require imaging studies, blood tests, pH monitoring in the esophagus, and other tests.

Treatment

Most cases of hiccups will disappear on their own. Home remedies which interrupt or override the spasmodic nerve circuitry are often effective. Such remedies include:

- holding one's breath for as long as possible
- breathing into a paper bag
- swallowing a spoonful of sugar
- bending forward from the waist and drinking water from the wrong side of a glass

Treating any underlying disorder will usually cure the associated hiccups. Chlorpromazine (Thorazine) relieves intractable hiccups in 80% of cases. Metoclopramide (Reglan), carbamazepam, valproic acid (Depakene), and phenobarbital are also used. As a last resort, surgery to block the phrenic nerve may be performed, although it may lead to significant impairment of respiration.

Prognosis

Most cases of hiccups last no longer than several hours, with or without treatment.

KEY TERMS

Nerve—Fibers that carry sensory information, movement stimuli, or both from the brain and spinal cord to other parts of the body and back again. Some nerves, including the vagus nerve, innervate distantly separated parts of the body.

Prevention

Some cases of hiccups can be avoided by drinking in moderation, avoiding very hot or very cold food, and avoiding cold showers. Carbonated beverages when drunk through a straw deliver more gas to the stomach than when sipped from a container; therefore, avoid using straws.

Resources

BOOKS

Hurst, J. Willis. *Medicine for the Practicing Physician.* Stamford: Appleton & Lange, 1988.

Richard Robinson

High-altitude sickness *see* **Altitude sickness**

High blood phosphate level *see* **Phosphorus imbalance**

High blood pressure *see* **Pulmonary hypertension**

High calcium blood level *see* **Hypercalcemia**

High cholesterol *see* **Cholesterol, high**

High potassium blood level *see* **Hyperkalemia**

High-risk pregnancy

Definition

A high risk **pregnancy** is one in which some condition puts the mother, the developing fetus, or both at higher-than-normal risk for complications during or after the pregnancy and birth.

Description

A pregnancy can be considered a high-risk pregnancy for a variety of reasons. Factors can be divided into maternal and fetal. Maternal factors include age (younger than age 15, older than age 35); weight (pre-pregnancy weight under 100 lb or obesity); height (under five feet); history of complications during previous pregnancies (including stillbirth, fetal loss, preterm labor and/or delivery, small-for-gestational age baby, large baby, pre-eclampsia or **eclampsia**); more than five previous pregnancies; bleeding during the third trimester; abnormalities of the reproductive tract; **uterine fibroids**; **hypertension**; Rh incompatability; **gestational diabetes**; infections of the vagina and/or cervix; kidney infection; **fever**; acute surgical emergency (appendicitis, gallbladder disease, bowel obstruction); post-term pregnancy; pre-existing chronic illness (such as asthma, autoimmune disease, **cancer**, sickle cell anemia, **tuberculosis**, herpes, **AIDS**, heart disease, kidney disease, **Crohn's disease**, ulcerative colitis, diabetes). Fetal factors include exposure to infection (especially herpes simplex, viral hepatitis, **mumps**, **rubella**, varicella, **syphilis**, **toxoplasmosis**, and infections caused by coxsackievirus); exposure to damaging medications (especially phenytoin, **folic acid** antagonists, lithium, streptomycin, tetracycline, thalidomide, and warfarin); exposure to addictive substances (cigarette **smoking**, alcohol intake, and illicit or abused drugs). A pregnancy is also considered high-risk when prenatal tests indicate that the baby has a serious health problem (for example, a heart defect). In such cases, the mother will need special tests, and possibly medication, to carry the baby safely through to delivery. Furthermore, certain maternal or fetal problems may prompt a physician to deliver a baby early, or to choose a surgical delivery (cesarean section) rather than a vaginal delivery.

Most women will see one healthcare provider during pregnancy, either an obstetrician, a midwife, or a nurse practitioner. Women who have a medical problem may need to see a medical specialist as well. Women diagnosed with a high-risk pregnancy may also need the expert advice and care of a perinatologist. A perinatologist is a medical doctor (obstetrician) who specializes in the care of women who are at high risk for having problems during pregnancy. Perinatologists care for women who have pre-existing medical problems as well as women who develop complications during pregnancy.

Diagnosis

A woman with a high-risk pregnancy will need closer monitoring than the average pregnant woman. Such monitoring may include more frequent visits with the primary caregiver, tests to monitor the medical problem, blood tests to check the levels of medication, **amniocentesis**, serial ultrasound examination, and fetal monitoring. These tests are designed to track the original condition, survey for complications, verify that the fetus is growing adequately, and make decisions regarding whether labor may need to be induced to allow for early delivery of the fetus.

Treatment

Treatment varies widely with the type of disease, the effect that pregnancy has on the disease, and the effect that the disease has on pregnancy. Additional tests may help determine the need for changes in medication or additional treatment.

Prognosis

The prognosis depends in large part on the specific medical condition. Some medical conditions make it difficult to get pregnant and lead to a higher risk of problems in the baby. An example of this type of condition is thyroid disease. In thyroid disease, the thyroid gland (located in the neck) may produce too much or too little thyroid hormone. Abnormal levels of thyroid hormone can cause problems in pregnancy and affect the health of the baby. Fortunately, thyroid disease can be treated with medication. As long as the level of thyroid hormone is controlled throughout pregnancy, there should be no problems for mother or baby.

There are many medical conditions that usually do not interfere with pregnancy, but are themselves affected by pregnancy. This group includes **asthma**, epilepsy, and ulcerative colitis. For example, some women with **ulcerative colitis** experience a worsening of their symptoms during pregnancy, while others will have no change or may get better during pregnancy. The same is true of asthma; some women notice that their asthma symptoms are better during pregnancy, some find their asthma worse, and some women notice no change in symptoms during pregnancy. No one understands why this is so, but due to this unpredictability, all women with chronic illnesses should be monitored carefully throughout pregnancy.

There is also a group of medical conditions that can have a major impact on pregnancy. Women with lupus (disease caused by alterations in the immune system that result in inflammation of connective tissue and organs) or **kidney disease** face real risks during pregnancy. Pregnancy can cause their symptoms to worsen significantly and can lead to serious illness. Because these diseases can affect the mother's ability to supply oxygen and nutrients to the baby through the placenta, they can cause problems for the baby as well. These babies may not be able to grow and gain weight properly (**intrauterine growth retardation**). There is also an increased risk of **stillbirth**.

Diabetes is a medical condition that is both affected by pregnancy and affects pregnancy. Diabetes can lead to miscarriages, **birth defects**, and stillbirths. When a woman monitors her blood sugar carefully and treats high levels with insulin, the risk of these negative outcomes drops a great deal. Unfortunately, pregnancy makes diabetes much harder to control. In general, blood sugar and the need for insulin to control it rise throughout pregnancy.

Most medical conditions do not lead to complications in pregnancy. With frequent visits to healthcare providers, and careful attention to medication, women with medical problems usually enjoy healthy, successful pregnancies. There are a few medical conditions that can cause health risks to both mother and baby during pregnancy. Women with these medical problems should consider these risks before deciding to become pregnant. Many of these women will benefit from the care of a perinatologist during pregnancy. Only rarely (in the case of severe heart disease, for example) are the risks to the mother so high that she should not consider pregnancy at all.

Prevention

A pre-pregnancy visit with a healthcare provider is especially important for a woman who has a medical problem. The doctor will discuss how women with this condition usually fare during pregnancy. For some diseases (such as lupus), pregnancy can mean increased risk of health problems for mother and baby.

Sometimes, the medication a woman needs to control a medical condition can cause problems for the baby. There may be another medication available that is safer for use in pregnancy. In some cases there is no other medication, and a woman must weigh the risks to the baby when deciding whether or not to become pregnant.

A woman who has not had a pre-pregnancy visit should contact a healthcare provider as soon as she learns she is pregnant. Often, the provider will schedule the first prenatal visit within a day or two, instead of waiting until eight to 10 weeks of pregnancy. This is because certain medical conditions can increase the risk of **miscarriage**. The provider will want to be sure

---

KEY TERMS

Gestational diabetes—Diabetes of pregnancy leading to increased levels of blood sugar. Unlike diabetes mellitus, gestational diabetes is caused by pregnancy and goes away when pregnancy ends. Like diabetes mellitus, gestational diabetes is treated with a special diet and insulin, if necessary.

Preeclampsia—A disease that only affects pregnant women. The most common signs and symptoms are increased blood pressure, swelling in the hands and feet, and abnormal results on special blood and urine tests.

Premature labor—Labor beginning before 36 weeks of pregnancy.

---

that any medication is adjusted properly to increase the chance of having a successful pregnancy.

Resources

BOOKS

Beers, Mark H., et al., editors. "High-Risk Pregnancies." In *The Merck Manual of Diagnosis and Therapy*. Rahway, NJ: Merck Research Laboratories, 2004.

Rosalyn Carson-DeWitt, MD

High sodium blood level *see* **Hypernatremia**

Hindu medicine *see* **Ayurvedic medicine**

Hip bath *see* **Sitz bath**

Hip replacement *see* **Joint replacement**

Hirschsprung's disease

Definition

Hirschsprung's disease, also known as congenital megacolon or aganglionic megacolon, is an abnormality in which certain nerve fibers are absent in segments of the bowel, resulting in severe bowel obstruction. It was first identified in 1886 by a physician named Harold Hirschsprung.

Description

Hirschsprung's disease is caused when certain nerve cells (called parasympathetic ganglion cells) in the wall of the large intestine (colon) do not develop before birth. Without these nerves, the affected segment of the colon lacks the ability to relax and move bowel contents along. This causes a constriction and as a result, the bowel above the constricted area dilates due to stool becoming trapped, producing megacolon (dilation of the colon). The disease can affect varying lengths of bowel segment, most often involving the region around the rectum. In up to 10% of children, however, the entire colon and part of the small intestine are involved. This condition is known as total colonic aganglionosis, or TCA.

Hirschsprung's disease occurs once in every 5,000 live births, and it is about four times more common in males than females. Between 4% and 50% of siblings are also afflicted. The wide range for recurrence is due to the fact that the recurrence risk depends on the gender of the affected individual in the family (i.e., if a female is affected, the recurrence risk is higher) and the length of the aganglionic segment of the colon (i.e., the longer the segment that is affected, the higher the recurrence risk).

Causes and symptoms

Hirschsprung's disease occurs early in fetal development when, for unknown reasons, there is either failure of nerve cell development, failure of nerve cell migration, or arrest in nerve cell development in a segment of the bowel. The absence of these nerve fibers, which help control the movement of bowel contents, is what results in intestinal obstruction accompanied by other symptoms.

There is a genetic basis to Hirschsprung's disease, and it is believed that it may be caused by different genetic factors in different subsets of families. Proof that genetic factors contribute to Hirschprung's disease is that it is known to run in families, and it has been seen in association with some chromosome abnormalities. For example, about 10% of children with the disease have Down syndrome (the most common chromosomal abnormality). Molecular diagnostic techniques have identified many genes that cause susceptibility to Hirschsprung's disease. As of the early 2000s, a total of six genes have been identified: the RET gene, the glial cell line-derived neurotrophic factor gene, the endothelin-B receptor gene, endothelin converting enzyme, the endothelin-3 gene, and the Sry-related transcription factor SOX10. Mutations that inactivate the RET gene are the most frequent, occurring in 50% of familial cases (cases which run in families) and 15–20% of sporadic (non-familial) cases. Mutations in these genes do not cause the disease, but they make the chance of developing it more likely. Mutations in other genes or environmental factors are required to develop the disease, and these other factors are not understood. As of 2004, at least three chromosomes are known to be involved: 13q22, 21q22, and 10q. Hirschsprung's disease has also been reported in association with abnormal forms of chromosome 18.

For persons with a **ganglion** growth beyond the sigmoid segment of the colon, the inheritance pattern is autosomal dominant with reduced penetrance (risk closer to 50%). For persons with smaller segments involved, the inheritance pattern is multifactorial (caused by an interaction of more than one gene and environmental factors, risk lower than 50%) or autosomal recessive (one disease gene inherited from each parent, risk closer to 25%) with low penetrance.

The initial symptom is usually severe, continuous **constipation**. A newborn may fail to pass meconium (the first stool) within 24 hours of birth, may repeatedly vomit yellow- or green-colored bile and may have a distended (swollen, uncomfortable) abdomen. Occasionally, infants may have only mild or intermittent constipation, often with **diarrhea**.

While two-thirds of cases are diagnosed in the first three months of life, Hirschsprung's disease may also be diagnosed later in infancy or childhood. Occasionally, even adults are diagnosed with a variation of the disease. In older infants, symptoms and signs may include anorexia (lack of appetite or inability to eat), lack of the urge to move the bowels or empty the rectum on **physical examination**, distended abdomen, and a mass in the colon that can be felt by the physician during examination. It should be suspected in older children with abnormal bowel habits, especially a history of constipation dating back to infancy and ribbon-like stools.

Occasionally, the presenting symptom may be a severe intestinal infection called enterocolitis, which is life-threatening. The symptoms are usually explosive, watery stools and fever in a very ill-appearing infant. It is important to diagnose the condition before the intestinal obstruction causes an overgrowth of bacteria that evolves into a medical emergency. Enterocolitis can lead to severe diarrhea and massive fluid loss, which can cause **death** from **dehydration** unless surgery is done immediately to relieve the obstruction.

Hirschsprung's disease sometimes occurs in children with other disorders of the autonomic nervous system, such as congenital central hypoventilation syndrome, a breathing disorder. Other syndromes associated with Hirschsprung disease include congenital deafness and Waardenburg syndrome, a genetic disorder characterized by facial abnormalities and the loss of normal pigmentation in the hair, skin, and the iris of the eye.

Diagnosis

Hirschsprung's disease in the newborn must be distinguished from other causes of intestinal obstruction. The diagnosis is suspected by the child's medical history and physical examination, especially the rectal exam. The diagnosis is confirmed by a barium enema x ray, which shows a picture of the bowel. The x ray will indicate if a segment of bowel is constricted, causing dilation and obstruction. A biopsy of rectal tissue will reveal the absence of the nerve fibers. Adults may also undergo manometry, a balloon study (device used to enlarge the anus for the procedure) of internal anal sphincter pressure and relaxation.

Treatment

Hirschsprung's disease is treated surgically. The goal is to remove the diseased, nonfunctioning segment of the bowel and restore bowel function. This is often done in two stages. The first stage relieves the intestinal obstruction by performing a **colostomy**. This is the creation of an opening in the abdomen (stoma) through which bowel contents can be discharged into a waste bag. When the child's weight, age, or condition is deemed appropriate, surgeons close the stoma, remove the diseased portion of bowel, and perform a "pull-through" procedure, which repairs the colon by connecting functional bowel to the anus. The pull-through operation usually establishes fairly normal bowel function.

Children with total colonic aganglionosis occasionally fail to benefit from a pull-through procedure. One option in treating these patients is the construction of an ileoanal S-pouch.

The surgeon may recommend a permanent **ostomy** if the child has **Down syndrome** in addition to Hirschsprung disease, as these children usually have more difficulty with bowel control.

Prognosis

Overall, prognosis is very good. Most infants with Hirschsprung's disease achieve good bowel control after surgery, but a small percentage of children may have lingering problems with soilage or constipation. These infants are also at higher risk for an overgrowth of bacteria in the intestines, including subsequent

---

KEY TERMS

Anus—The opening at the end of the intestine that carries waste out of the body

Barium enema x ray—A procedure that involves the administration of barium into the intestines by a tube inserted into the rectum. Barium is a chalky substance that enhances the visualization of the gastrointestinal tract on x ray.

Colostomy—The creation of an artificial opening into the colon through the skin for the purpose of removing bodily waste. Colostomies are usually required because key portions of the intestine have been removed.

Enterocolitis—Severe inflammation of the intestines that affects the intestinal lining, muscle, nerves and blood vessels.

Manometry—A balloon study of internal anal sphincter pressure and relaxation.

Meconium—The first waste products to be discharged from the body in a newborn infant, usually greenish in color and consisting of mucus, bile and so forth.

Megacolon—Dilation of the colon.

Parasympathetic ganglion cell—Type of nerve cell normally found in the wall of the colon.

---

episodes of enterocolitis, and should be closely followed by a physician. Mortality from enterocolitis or surgical complications in infancy is 25–30%.

Prevention

Hirschsprung's disease is a congenital abnormality that has no known means of prevention. It is important to diagnose the condition early in order to prevent the development of enterocolitis. Genetic counseling can be offered to a couple with a previous child with the disease or to an affected individual considering pregnancy to discuss recurrence risks and treatment options. Prenatal diagnosis is not available as of the early 2000s.

Resources

BOOKS

Beers, Mark H., MD, and Robert Berkow, MD., editors. "Congenital Anomalies." Section 19, Chapter 261 In *The Merck Manual of Diagnosis and Therapy.* Whitehouse Station, NJ: Merck Research Laboratories, 2004.

PERIODICALS

Chen, M. L., and T. G. Keens. "Congenital Central Hypoventilation Syndrome: Not Just Another Rare Disorder." *Paediatric Respiratory Reviews* 5 (September 2004): 182–189.

Lal, D. R., P. F. Nichol, B. A. Harms, et al. "Ileo-Anal S-Pouch Reconstruction in Patients with Total Colonic Aganglionosis after Failed Pull-Through Procedure." *Journal of Pediatric Surgery* 39 (July 2004): e7–e9.

Martucciello, G., et al. "Pathogenesis of Hirschprung's Disease." *Journal of Pediatric Surgery* 35 (2000): 1017–1025.

Munnes, M., et al. "Familial Form of Hirschprung Disease: Nucleotide Sequence Studies Reveal Point Mutations in the RET Proto-oncogene in Two of Six Families But Not in Other Candidate Genes." *American Journal of Medical Genetics* 94 (2000): 19–27.

Neville, Holly, MD, and Charles S. Cox, Jr., MD. "Hirschsprung Disease." *eMedicine* July15, 2003. < http://www.emedicine.com/ped/topic1010.htm > .

Prabhakara, K., H. E. Wyandt, X. L. Huang, et al. "Recurrent Proximal 18p Monosomy and 18q Trisomy in a Family with a Maternal Pericentric Inversion of Chromosome 18." *Annales de génétique* 47 (July-September 2004): 297–303.

ORGANIZATIONS

American Pseudo-Obstruction & Hirschsprung's Society. 158 Pleasant St., North Andover, MA 01845. (978)685-4477.

National Organization for Rare Disorders (NORD). 55 Kenosia Avenue, P. O. Box 1968, Danbury, CT 06813-1968. (203) 744-0100. Fax: (203) 798-2291. < http://www.rarediseases.org >.

Pull-thru Network. 316 Thomas St., Bessemer, AL 35020. (205) 428-5953.

Amy Vance, MS, CGC
Rebecca J. Frey, PhD

Hirsutism

Definition

Excessive growth of facial or body hair in women is called hirsutism.

Description

Hirsutism is not a disease. The condition usually develops during **puberty** and becomes more pronounced as the years go by. However, an inherited tendency, over-production of male hormones (androgens), medication, or disease, can cause it to appear at any age.

Women who have hirsutism usually have irregular menstrual cycles. They sometimes have small breasts and deep voices, and their muscles and genitals may become larger than women without the condition.

Types of hirsutism

Idiopathic hirsutism is probably hereditary, because there is usually a family history of the disorder. Women with idiopathic hirsutism have normal menstrual cycles and no evidence of any of the conditions associated with secondary hirsutism.

Secondary hirsutism is most often associated with polycystic ovary syndrome (an inherited hormonal disorder characterized by menstrual irregularities, biochemical abnormalities, and **obesity**). This type of hirsutism may also be caused by:

- malfunctions of the pituitary or adrenal glands
- use of male hormones or **minoxidil** (Loniten), a drug used to widen blood vessels
- adrenal or ovarian tumors.

Causes and symptoms

Hirsutism is rarely caused by a serious underlying disorder. **Pregnancy** occasionally stimulates its development. Hirsutism triggered by tumors is very unusual.

Hair follicles usually become enlarged, and the hairs themselves become larger and darker. A woman whose hirsutism is caused by an increase in male hormones has a pattern of hair growth similar to that of a man. A woman whose hirsutism is not hormone-related has long, fine hairs on her face, arms, chest, and back.

Diagnosis

Diagnosis is based on a family history of hirsutism, a personal history of menstrual irregularities, and masculine traits. Laboratory tests are not needed to assess the status of patients whose menstrual cycles are normal and who have mild, gradually progressing hirsutism.

A family physician or endocrinologist may order blood tests to measure hormone levels in women with long-standing menstrual problems or more severe hirsutism. **Computed tomography scans** (CT scans) are sometimes performed to evaluate diseases of the adrenal glands. Additional diagnostic procedures may be used to confirm or rule out underlying diseases or disorders.

Treatment

Primary hirsutism can be treated mechanically. Mechanical treatment involves bleaching or physically removing unwanted hair by:

- cutting
- electrolysis
- shaving
- tweezing
- waxing
- using hair-removing creams (depilatories)

Low-dose dexamethasone (a synthetic adrenocortical steroid), birth-control pills, or medications that suppress male hormones (for example, spironolactone) may be prescribed for patients whose condition stems from high androgen levels.

Treatment of secondary hirsutism is determined by the underlying cause of the condition.

Prognosis

Birth-control pills alone cause this condition to stabilize in one of every two patients and to improve in one of every 10.

When spironolactone (Aldactone) is prescribed to suppress hair growth, 70% of patients experience improvement within six months. When women also take birth-control pills, menstrual cycles become regular and hair growth is suppressed even more.

Resources

ORGANIZATIONS

American Society for Reproductive Medicine. 1209 Montgomery Highway, Birmingham, AL 35216-2809. (205) 978-5000. < http://www.asrm.com >.

Maureen Haggerty

Hispanic American health *see* **Minority health**

Histamine *see* **Antiulcer drugs**

Histamine headache *see* **Cluster headache**

Histiocytosis X

Definition

Histiocytosis X is a generic term that refers to an increase in the number of histiocytes, a type of white blood cell, that act as scavengers to remove foreign material from the blood and tissues. Since recent research demonstrated Langerhan cell involvement as well as histiocytes, this led to a proposal that the term Langerhans Cell Histiocytosis (LCH) be used in place of histiocytosis X. Either term refers to three separate illnesses (listed in order of increasing severity): eosinophilic granuloma, Hand-Schuller-Christian disease and Letterer-Siwe disease.

Description

Epidermal (skin) Langerhans cells (a form of dendritic cell) accumulate with other immune cells in various parts of the body and cause damage by the release of chemicals. Normally, Langerhans cells recognize foreign material, including bacteria, and stimulate the immune system to react to them. Langerhans cells are usually found in skin, lymph nodes, lungs, and the gastrointestinal tract. Under abnormal conditions these cells affect skin, bone, and the pituitary gland as well as the lungs, intestines, liver, spleen, bone marrow, and brain. Therefore, the disease is not confined to areas where Langerhans cells are normally found. The disease is more common in children than adults and tends to be most severe in very young children.

Histiocytosis X or LCH is a family of related conditions characterized by a distinct inflammatory and proliferative process but differs from each other in which parts of the body are involved. The least severe of the histiocytosis X/LCH family is eosinophilic granuloma. Approximately 60–80% of all diagnosed cases are in this classification, which usually occurs in children aged 5–10 years. The bones are involved 50–75% of the time, which includes the skull or mandible, and the long bones. If the bone marrow is involved, anemia can result. With skull involvement, growths can occur behind the eyes, bulging them forward. One recent case study involved swelling of the eyes caused by histiocytosis in a three-year-old girl. The lungs are involved less than 10% of the time, and this involvement signals the worst prognosis.

Next in severity is Hand-Schuller-Christian disease, a chronic, scattered form of histiocytosis. It occurs most commonly from the age of one to three years and is a slowly progressive disease that affects the softened areas of the skull, other flat bones, the eyes, and skin.

Letterer-Siwe disease is the acute form of this series of diseases. It is generally found from the time of birth to one year of age. It causes an enlarged liver, bruising and skin lesions, anemia, enlarged lymph glands, other organ involvement, and extensive skull lesions.

Causes and symptoms

This is a rare disorder affecting approximately 1 in 200,000 children or adults each year. The International Histiocyte Society formed a registry in 2000 that has registered a total of 274 adults from 13 countries as of 2003. Because histiocytic disorders are so rare, little research has been done to determine their cause. Over time, histiocytosis may lessen in its assault on the body but there are still problems from damage to the tissues. There are no apparent inheritance patterns in these diseases with the exception of a form involving the lymphatic system; of the 274 adults in the international registry, only one came from a family with a history of the disease.

The symptoms of histiocytosis are caused by substances called cytokines and prostaglandins, which are normally produced by histiocytes and act as messengers between cells. When these chemicals are produced in excess amounts and in the wrong places, they cause tissue swelling and abnormal growth. Thus, symptoms may include painful lumps in the skull and limbs as well as **rashes** on the skin. General symptoms may include: poor appetite, failure to gain weight, recurrent **fever**, and irritability. Symptoms from other possible sites of involvement include:

- gums: swelling, usually without significant discomfort
- ear: chronic discharge
- liver or spleen: abdominal discomfort or swelling
- pituitary: This gland at the base of the brain is affected at some stage in approximately 20%–30% of children causing a disturbance in water balance to produce thirst and frequent urination.
- eyes: Due to the bony disease, behind-the-eye bulging may occur (exophthalmos)
- lungs: breathing problems

Diagnosis

The diagnosis can be made only by performing a biopsy, that is, taking a tissue sample under anesthesia from a site in the patient thought to be involved. Blood and urine tests, chest and other x rays, **magnetic resonance imaging** (MRI) and **computed tomography scans** (CAT scans) (to check the extent of involvement), and

possibly bone marrow or breathing tests may be required to confirm the diagnosis.

Treatment

Although this disease is not **cancer**, most patients diagnosed with it are treated in cancer clinics. There are two reasons for this:

- Historically, cancer specialists treated it before the cause was known.
- The treatment requires the use of drugs typically required to treat cancer.

Any cancer drugs utilized are usually given in smaller doses, which diminishes the severity of their side effects. **Radiation therapy** is rarely used, and special drugs may be prescribed for skin symptoms. If there is only one organ affected, steroids may be injected locally, or a drug called indomethacin may be used. Indomethacin is an anti-inflammatory medication

KEY TERMS

Anemia—Abnormally low level of red blood cells in the blood.

Biopsy—Surgical removal of tissue for examination.

CT or CAT—Computed tomography, a radiologic imaging that uses computer processing to generate an image of tissue density in slices through the patient's body.

Cytokines—The term used to include all protein messengers that regulate immune responses.

Dendritic—Branched like a tree.

Eosinophils—A leukocyte with coarse, round granules present.

Epidermal—The outermost layer of the skin.

Inflammatory—A localized protective response of the body caused by injury or destruction of tissues.

MRI—Magnetic resonance imaging, a noninvasive nuclear procedure that uses electromagnetic energy to create images of structures inside the body.

Pituitary gland—The master gland located in the middle of the head that controls the endocrine glands and affects most bodily functions.

Prostaglandins—A group of nine naturally occurring chemicals in the body that affect smooth muscles.

Serous—Thin and watery, like serum.

that may achieve a similar response with less severe side effects.

Prognosis

The disease fluctuates markedly. If only one system is involved, the disease often resolves by itself. Multisystem disease usually needs treatment although it may disappear spontaneously. The disease is not normally fatal unless organs vital to life are damaged. In general, the younger the child at diagnosis and the more organs involved, the poorer the outlook. If the condition resolves, there could still be long-term complications because of the damage done while the disease was active.

Resources

BOOKS

Beers, Mark H., MD, and Robert Berkow, MD., editors. "Histiocytic Syndromes." Section 11, Chapter 137 In *The Merck Manual of Diagnosis and Therapy*. Whitehouse Station, NJ: Merck Research Laboratories, 2004.

Behrman, Richard E., Robert Kliegman, and Hal B. Jenson, editors.*Nelson Textbook of Pediatrics*. Philadelphia: W. B. Saunders, 2000.

PERIODICALS

Arico, M., M. Girschikofsky, T. Genereau, et al. "Langerhans Cell Histiocytosis in Adults. Report from the International Registry of the Histiocyte Society." *European Journal of Cancer* 39 (November 2003): 2341–2348.

Eckhardt, A., and A. Schulze. "Maxillofacial Manifestations of Langerhans Cell Histiocytosis: A Clinical and Therapeutic Analysis of 10 Patients." *Oral Oncology* 39 (October 2003): 687–694.

Kobyahsi, M., O. Yamamoto, Y. Suenaga, and M. Asahi. "Electron Microscopic Study of Langerhans Cell Histiocytosis." *Journal ofDermatology* July 27, 2000: 453–7.

Levy, J., T. Monos, J.Kapelushnik, et al. "Langerhans Cell Histiocytosis with Periorbital Cellulitis." *American Journal of Ophthalmology* 136 (November 2003): 939 942.

ORGANIZATIONS

Histiocytosis Association of America. 302 North Broadway, Pitman, NJ 08071. (800) 548–2758 (USA and Canada). < http://www.histio.org >.

OTHER

"Immunity Disorders." *NurseMinerva*. June 26, 2001. < http://nurseminerva.co.uk/immunity.htm >.

Linda K. Bennington, CNS
Rebecca J. Frey, PhD

Histoplasmosis

Definition

Histoplasmosis is an infectious disease caused by inhaling the microscopic spores of the fungus *Histoplasma capsulatum*. The disease exists in three forms. Acute or primary histoplasmosis causes flu-like symptoms. Most people who are infected recover without medical intervention. Chronic histoplasmosis affects the lungs and can be fatal. Disseminated histoplasmosis affects many organ systems in the body and is often fatal, especially to people with acquired **immunodeficiency** syndrome (**AIDS**).

Description

Histoplasmosis is an airborne infection. The spores that cause this disease are found in soil that has been contaminated with bird or bat droppings. In the United States, the disease is most common in eastern and midwestern states and is widespread in the upper Mississippi, Ohio, Missouri, and St. Lawrence river valleys. Sometimes histoplasmosis is called Ohio Valley disease, Central Mississippi River Valley disease, Appalachian Mountain disease, Darling's disease, or *Histoplasma capsulatum* infection.

Anyone can get histoplasmosis, but people who come in contact with bird and bat excrement are more likely to be infected. This includes farmers, gardeners, bridge inspectors and painters, roofers, chimney cleaners, demolition and construction workers, people installing or servicing heating and air conditioning units, people restoring old or abandoned buildings, and people who explore caves.

The very young and the elderly, especially if they have a pre-existing lung disease or are heavy smokers, are more likely to develop symptoms that are more severe. People who have a weakened immune system, either from diseases such as AIDS or leukemia, or as the result of medications they take (**corticosteroids**, **chemotherapy** drugs), are more likely to develop chronic or disseminated histoplasmosis.

Causes and symptoms

When the spores of *H. capsulatum* are inhaled, they lodge in the lungs where they divide and cause lesions. This is known as acute or primary histoplasmosis. It is not contagious.

Many otherwise healthy people show no symptoms of infection at all. When symptoms do occur, they appear 3–17 days after exposure (average time is 10 days).

The symptoms are usually mild and resemble those of a cold or flu; **fever**, dry cough, enlarged lymph glands, tiredness, and a general feeling of ill health. A small number of people develop bronchopneumonia. About 95% of people who are infected either experience no symptoms or have symptoms that clear up spontaneously. These people then have partial immunity to re-infection.

In some people, the spores that cause the disease continue to live in the lungs. In about 5% of people who are infected, usually those with chronic lung disease, diabetes mellitus, or weakened immune systems, the disease progresses to chronic histoplasmosis. This can take months or years. Symptoms of chronic histoplasmosis resemble those of **tuberculosis**. Cavities form in the lung tissue, parts of the lung may collapse, and the lungs fill with fluid. Chronic histoplasmosis is a serious disease that can result in death.

The rarest form of histoplasmosis is disseminated histoplasmosis. Disseminated histoplasmosis is seen almost exclusively in patients with AIDS or other immune defects. In disseminated histoplasmosis the infection may move to the spleen, liver, bone marrow, or adrenal glands. Symptoms include a worsening of those found in chronic histoplasmosis, as well as weight loss, **diarrhea**, the development of open sores in the mouth and nose, and enlargement of the spleen, liver, and adrenal gland.

Diagnosis

A simple skin test similar to that given for tuberculosis will tell if a person has previously been infected by the fungus *H. capsulatum*. Chest x rays often show lung damage caused by the fungus, but do not lead to a definitive diagnosis because the damage caused by other diseases has a similar appearance on the x ray. Diagnosis of chronic or disseminated histoplasmosis can be made by culturing a sample of sputum or other body fluids in the laboratory to isolate the fungus. The urine, blood serum, washings from the lungs, or cerebrospinal fluid can all be tested for the presence of an antigen produced in response to the infection. Most cases of primary histoplasmosis go undiagnosed.

Treatment

Acute primary histoplasmosis generally requires no treatment other than rest. Non-prescription drugs such as **acetaminophen** (Tylenol) may be used to treat **pain** and relieve fever. Avoiding smoke and using a cool air humidifier may ease chest pain.

Patients with an intact immune system who develop chronic histoplasmosis are treated with the drug ketoconazole (Nizoral) or amphotericin B (Fungizone). Patients with suppressed immune systems are treated with amphotericin B, which is given intravenously. Because of its potentially toxic side effects, hospitalization is often required. The patient may also receive other drugs to minimize the side effects of the amphotericin B.

Patients with AIDS must continue to take the drug itraconazole (Sporonox) orally for the rest of their lives in order to prevent a relapse. If the patient can not tolerate itraconazole, the drug fluconazole (Diflucan) can be substituted.

Alternative treatment

In non-immunocompromised patients, alternative therapies can be very successful. Alternative treatment for fungal infections focuses on creating an environment where the fungus cannot survive. This is accomplished by maintaining good health and eating a diet low in dairy products, sugars, including honey and fruit juice, and foods like beer that contain yeast. This is complemented by a diet high in raw food. Supplements of antioxidant **vitamins** C, E, and A, along with B complex, may also be added to the diet. *Lactobacillus acidophilus* and *Bifidobacteria* will replenish the good bacteria in the intestines. Antifungal herbs, like garlic, can be consumed in relatively large does and for an extended period of time in order to be most effective.

Prognosis

Most people recover from primary histoplasmosis in a few weeks without medical intervention. Patients with chronic histoplasmosis who are treated with antifungal drugs generally recover rapidly if they do not have an underlying serious disease. When left untreated, or if serious disease is present, histoplasmosis can be fatal.

AIDS patients with disseminated histoplasmosis vary in their response to amphotericin B, depending on their general health and how well they tolerate the side effects of the drug. Treatment often suppresses the infection temporarily, but patients with AIDS are always in danger of a relapse and must continue to take medication for the rest of their lives to keep the infection at bay. New combinations of therapies and new drugs are constantly being evaluated, making hard statistics on prognosis difficult to come by. AIDS patients have problems with multiple opportunistic infections, making it difficult to isolate **death** rates due to any one particular fungal infection.

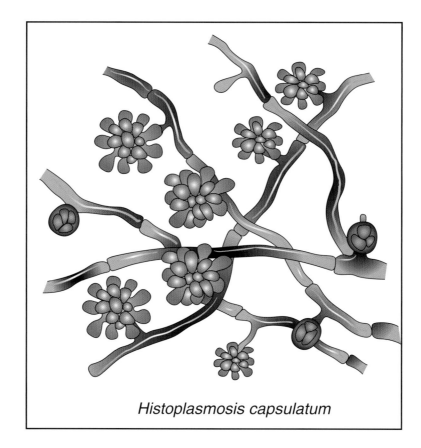

Histoplasmosis capsulatum

Histoplasma capsulatum. If a person inhales the spores of this fungus, they may contract histoplasmosis, an infectious disease which can exist in three forms: acute or primary histoplasmosis, which causes flu-like symptoms; chronic histoplasmosis, which affects the lungs and can be fatal; and disseminated histoplasmosis, which can affect multiple body systems and is often fatal. *(Illustration by Electronic Illustrators Group.)*

KEY TERMS

Acidophilus—The bacteria *Lactobacillus acidophilus,* usually found in yogurt.

Adrenal gland—A pair of organs located above the kidneys. The outer tissue of the gland produces the hormones epinephrine (adrenaline) and norepinephrine, while the inner tissue produces several steroid hormones.

Antigen—A foreign protein to which the body reacts by making antibodies.

Bifidobacteria—A group of bacteria normally present in the intestine. Commercial supplements are available.

Corticosteroids—A group of hormones produced naturally by the adrenal gland or manufactured synthetically. They are often used to treat inflammation. Examples include cortisone and prednisone.

Prevention

Since the spores of *H. capsulatum* are so widespread, it is almost impossible to prevent exposure in endemic areas. Dust suppression measures when working with contaminated soil may help limit exposure. Individuals who are at risk of developing the more severe forms of the disease should avoid situations where they will be exposed to bat and bird droppings.

Resources

ORGANIZATIONS

American Lung Association. 1740 Broadway, New York, NY 10019. (800) 586-4872. < http://www.lungusa.org >.

Histoplasmosis: Protecting Workers at Risk. Centers for Disease Control and Prevention. < http://www.cdc.gov/niosh/97146eng.html >.

National Center for Infectious Diseases. Atlanta, Georgia. (404) 639-3158. < http://www.cdc.gov/ncidod/ncid/ncid.htm >.

National Institute for Occupational Safety and Health. Cincinnati, Ohio. (800) 356-4674.

OTHER

Histoplasmosis: Protecting Workers at Risk. Centers for Disease Control and Prevention. < http://www.cdc.gov/niosh/97146eng.html >.

Tish Davidson, A.M.

HIV infection *see* **AIDS**

Hives

Definition

Hives is an allergic skin reaction causing localized redness, swelling, and **itching**.

Description

Hives is a reaction of the body's immune system that causes areas of the skin to swell, itch, and become reddened (wheals). When the reaction is limited to small areas of the skin, it is called "urticaria." Involvement of larger areas, such as whole sections of a limb, is called "angioedema."

Causes and symptoms

Causes

Hives is an allergic reaction. The body's immune system is normally responsible for protection from foreign invaders. When it becomes sensitized to normally harmless substances, the resulting reaction is called an allergy. An attack of hives is set off when such a substance, called an allergen, is ingested, inhaled, or otherwise contacted. It interacts with immune cells called mast cells, which reside in the skin, airways, and digestive system. When mast cells encounter an allergen, they release histamine and other chemicals, both locally and into the bloodstream. These chemicals cause blood vessels to become more porous, allowing fluid to accumulate in tissue and leading to the swollen and reddish appearance of hives. Some of the chemicals released sensitize pain nerve endings, causing the affected area to become itchy and sensitive.

A wide variety of substances may cause hives in sensitive people, including foods, drugs, and insect bites or stings. Common culprits include:

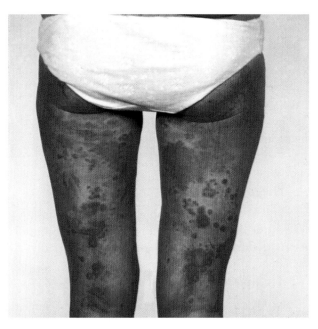

Hives on the back of a young woman's legs. The accompanying inflammation develops as an allergic reaction which ranges in size from small spots to patches measuring several inches across. *(Photograph by John Radcliffe, Custom Medical Stock Photo. Reproduced by permission.)*

- nuts, especially peanuts, walnuts, and Brazil nuts
- fish, mollusks, and shellfish
- eggs
- wheat
- milk
- strawberries
- food additives and preservatives
- penicillin or other **antibiotics**
- flu vaccines
- tetanus toxoid vaccine
- gamma globulin
- bee, wasp, and hornet stings
- bites of mosquitoes, fleas, and scabies

Symptoms

Urticaria is characterized by redness, swelling, and itching of small areas of the skin. These patches usually grow and recede in less than a day, but may be replaced by hives in other locations. Angioedema is characterized by more diffuse swelling. Swelling of the airways may cause **wheezing** and respiratory distress. In severe cases, airway obstruction may occur.

Resources

PERIODICALS

Kirn, F. Timothy. "Desloratadine Improves Urticaria in Clinical Setting." *Skin & Allergy News* September 2004: 41.

Richard Robinson
Teresa G. Odle

HLA-B27 antigen test *see* **Tissue typing**

HLA test *see* **Human leukocyte antigen test**

HMG-CoA reductase inhibitors *see* **Cholesterol-reducing drugs**

Hodgkin's disease

Hodgkin's disease is a rare lymphoma, a **cancer** of the lymphatic system.

Hodgkin's disease, or Hodgkin's lymphoma, was first described in 1832 by Thomas Hodgkin, a British physician. Hodgkin clearly differentiated between this disease and the much more common non-Hodgkin's lymphomas. Prior to 1970, few individuals survived Hodgkin's disease. Now, however, the majority of individuals with this cancer can be cured.

The lymphatic system is part of the body's immune system, for fighting disease, and a part of the blood-producing system. It includes the lymph vessels and nodes, and the spleen, bone marrow, and thymus. The narrow lymphatic vessels carry lymphatic fluid from throughout the body. The lymph nodes are small organs that filter the lymphatic fluid and trap foreign substances, including viruses, bacteria, and cancer cells. The spleen, in the upper left abdomen, removes old cells and debris from the blood. The bone marrow, the tissue inside the bones, produces new red and white blood cells.

Lymphocytes are white blood cells that recognize and destroy disease-causing organisms. Lymphocytes are produced in the lymph nodes, spleen, and bone marrow. They circulate throughout the body in the blood and lymphatic fluid. Clusters of immune cells also exist in major organs.

Hodgkin's disease is a type of lymphoma in which antibody-producing cells of the lymphatic system begin to grow abnormally. It usually begins in a lymph node and progresses slowly, in a fairly

---

KEY TERMS

Allergen—A substance capable of producing an immediate type of hypersensitivity, or allergy.

Wheal—A smooth, slightly elevated area on the body surface, which is redder or paler than the surrounding skin.

Diagnosis

Hives are easily diagnosed by visual inspection. The cause of hives is usually apparent, but may require a careful medical history in some cases.

Treatment

Mild cases of hives are treated with **antihistamines**, such as diphenhydramine (Benadryl) or desloratadine (Clarinex). Clarinex is non-sedating, meaning it will not make patients drowsy. More severe cases may require oral **corticosteroids**, such as prednisone. Topical corticosteroids are not effective. Airway swelling may require emergency injection of epinephrine (adrenaline).

Alternative treatment

An alternative practitioner will try to determine what allergic substance is causing the reaction and help the patient eliminate or minimize its effects. To deal with the symptoms of hives, an oatmeal bath may help to relieve itching. Chickweed (*Stellaria media*), applied as a poultice (crushed or chopped herbs applied directly to the skin) or added to bath water, may also help relieve itching. Several homeopathic remedies, including *Urtica urens* and *Apis* (*Apis mellifica*), may help relieve the itch, redness, or swelling associated with hives.

Prognosis

Most cases of hives clear up within one to seven days without treatment, providing the cause (allergen) is found and avoided.

Prevention

Preventing hives depends on avoiding the allergen causing them. Analysis of new items in the diet or new drugs taken may reveal the likely source of the reaction. Chronic hives may be aggravated by **stress**, caffeine, alcohol, or tobacco; avoiding these may reduce the frequency of reactions.

DOROTHY MENDENHALL
(1874–1964)

Dorothy Reed Mendenhall, the last of three children, was born September 22, 1874, in Columbus, Ohio, to William Pratt Reed, a shoe manufacturer, and Grace Kimball Reed, both of whom had descended from English settlers who came to America in the seventeenth century. Mendenhall attended Smith College and obtained a baccalaureate degree. Although she initially contemplated a career in journalism, Mendenhall's interest in medicine was inspired by a biology course she attended.

Dorothy Reed Mendenhall was a well-respected researcher, obstetrician, and pioneer in methods of childbirth. She was the first to discover that Hodgkin's disease was not a form of tuberculosis, as had been thought. This finding received international acclaim. As a result of her work, the cell type characteristic of Hodgkin's disease bears her name. The loss of her first child due to poor obstetrics changed her research career to a lifelong effort to reduce infant mortality rates. Mendenhall's efforts paid off with standards being set for weight and height for children ages birth to six and also in programs that stressed the health of both the mother and child in the birthing process.

predictable way, spreading via the lymphatic vessels from one group of lymph nodes to the next. Sometimes it invades organs that are adjacent to the lymph nodes. If the cancer cells spread to the blood, the disease can reach almost any site in the body. Advanced cases of Hodgkin's disease may involve the spleen, liver, bone marrow, and lungs.

There are different subtypes of Hodgkin's disease:

- nodular sclerosis (30–60% of cases)
- mixed cellularity (20–40% of cases)
- lymphocyte predominant (5–10% of cases)
- lymphocyte depleted (less than 5% of cases)
- unclassified

The American Cancer Society estimates that there will be 7,400 new cases of Hodgkin's disease in the United States in 2001—3,500 in females and 3,900 in males. It is estimated that 700 men and 600 women in the United States will die of the disease in 2001.

Hodgkin's disease can occur at any age. However, the majority of cases develop in early adulthood (ages 15–40) and late adulthood (after age 55). Approximately 10–15% of cases are in children under age 17. It is more common in boys than in girls under the age of 10. The disease is very rare in children under five.

The cause of Hodgkin's disease is not known. It is suspected that some interaction between an individual's genetic makeup, environmental exposures, and infectious agents may be responsible. Immune system deficiencies also may be involved.

Early symptoms of Hodgkin's disease may be similar to those of the flu:

- fevers, night sweats, chills
- **fatigue**
- loss of appetite
- weight loss
- itching
- pain after drinking alcoholic beverages
- swelling of one or more lymph nodes

Sudden or emergency symptoms of Hodgkin's disease include:

- sudden high fever
- loss of bladder and/or bowel control
- numbness in the arms and legs and a loss of strength

As lymph nodes swell, they may push on other structures, causing a variety of symptoms:

- pain due to pressure on nerve roots
- loss of function in muscle groups served by compressed nerves
- coughing or **shortness of breath** due to compression of the windpipe and/or airways, by swollen lymph nodes in the chest
- kidney failure from compression of the ureters, the tubes that carry urine from the kidneys to the bladder
- swelling in the face, neck, or legs, due to pressure on veins
- paralysis in the legs due to pressure on the spinal cord

As Hodgkin's disease progresses, the immune system becomes less effective at fighting infection. Thus, patients with Hodgkin's lymphoma become more susceptible to both common infections caused by bacteria and unusual (opportunistic) infections. Later symptoms of Hodgkin's disease include the formation of tumors.

Significantly, as many as 75% of individuals with Hodgkin's disease do not have any typical symptoms.

As with many forms of cancer, diagnosis of Hodgkin's disease has two major components.

- identification of Hodgkin's lymphoma as the cause of the patient's disease

- staging of the disease to determine how far the cancer has spread

The initial diagnosis of Hodgkin's disease often results from abnormalities in a **chest x ray** that was performed because of nonspecific symptoms. The physician then takes a medical history to check for the presence of symptoms and conducts a complete **physical examination**.

The size, tenderness, firmness, and location of swollen lymph nodes are determined and correlated with any signs of infection. In particular, lymph nodes that do not shrink after treatment with **antibiotics** may be a cause for concern. The lymph nodes that are most often affected by Hodgkin's disease include those of the neck, above the collarbone, under the arms, and in the chest above the diaphragm.

Diagnosis of Hodgkin's disease requires either the removal of an entire enlarged lymph node (an excisional biopsy) or an incisional biopsy, in which only a small part of a large tumor is removed. If the node is near the skin, the biopsy is performed with a local anesthetic. However, if it is inside the chest or abdomen, **general anesthesia** is required.

The sample of biopsied tissue is examined under a microscope. Giant cells called Reed-Sternberg cells must be present to confirm a diagnosis of Hodgkin's disease. These cells, which usually contain two or more nuclei, are named for the two pathologists who discovered them. Normal cells have only one nucleus (the organelle within the cell that contains the genetic material). Affected lymph nodes may contain only a few Reed-Sternberg cells and they may be difficult to recognize. Characteristics of other types of cells in the biopsied tissue help to diagnose the subtype of Hodgkin's disease.

A fine needle aspiration (FNA) biopsy, in which a thin needle and syringe are used to remove a small amount of fluid and bits of tissue from a tumor, has the advantage of not requiring surgery. An FNA may be performed prior to an excisional or incisional biopsy, to check for infection or for the spread of cancer from another organ. However an FNA biopsy does not provide enough tissue to diagnose Hodgkin's disease.

Occasionally, additional biopsies are required to diagnose Hodgkin's disease. In rare instances, other tests, that detect certain substances on the surfaces of cancer cells or changes in the DNA of cells, are used to distinguish Hodgkin's disease from non-Hodgkin's lymphoma.

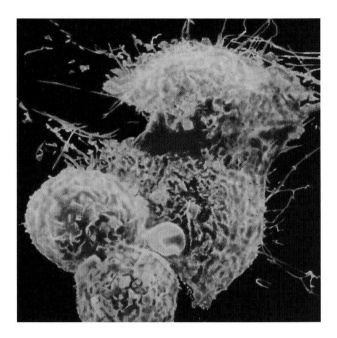

A scanning electron micrograph (SEM) image of dividing Hodgkin's cells from the pleural effusions (abnormal accumulations of fluid in the lungs) of a 55-year-old male patient. *(Photograph by Dr. Andrejs Liepins, Photo Researchers, Inc. Reproduced by permission.)*

Staging is very important in Hodgkin's disease. This is because the cancer usually spreads in a predictable pattern, without skipping sets of lymph nodes until late in the progression of the disease.

Imaging of the abdomen, chest, and pelvis is used to identify areas of enlarged lymph nodes and abnormalities in the spleen or other organs. Computerized axial tomography (CT or CAT) scans use a rotating x-ray beam to obtain pictures. Magnetic resonance imaging (MRI) uses magnetic fields and radio waves to produce images of the body. Chest x rays also may be taken. These images will reveal rounded lumps called nodules in the affected lymph nodes and other organs.

Another imaging technique for Hodgkin's disease is a gallium scan, in which the radioactive element gallium is injected into a vein. The cancer cells take up the gallium and a special camera that detects the gallium is used to determine the location and size of tumors. Gallium scans are used when Hodgkin's disease is in the chest and may be hard to detect by other methods. Gallium scans also are used to monitor progress during treatment.

A lymphangiogram, a radiograph of the lymphatic vessels, involves injecting a dye into a lymphatic vessel in the foot. Tracking of the dye locates the disease in the abdomen and pelvis. This method is used less frequently and is usually not used with children.

Positron emission tomography (PET) scans are an extremely accurate method for staging Hodgkin's disease. A very low dose of radioactive glucose, a sugar, is injected into the body. The glucose travels to metabolically active sites, including cancerous regions that require large amounts of glucose. The PET scan detects the radioactivity and produces images of the entire body that distinguish between cancerous and non-cancerous tissues.

Anemia (a low red-blood-cell count), fevers, or night sweats are indications that Hodgkin's disease may be in the bone marrow. In these cases, a bone-marrow biopsy, in which a large needle is used to remove a narrow, cylindrical piece of bone, may be necessary to determine the spread of the cancer. Alternatively, an aspiration, in which a needle is used to remove small bits of bone marrow, may be used. The marrow usually is removed from the back of the hip or other large bone.

Sometimes further staging, called pathological staging or a staging laparotomy, is used for Hodgkin's disease. In this operation, a surgeon checks the abdominal lymph nodes and other organs for cancer and removes small pieces of tissue. A pathologist examines the tissue samples for Hodgkin's disease cells. Usually the spleen is removed (a **splenectomy**) during the laparotomy. The splenectomy helps with staging Hodgkin's disease, as well as removing a disease site.

All of the available treatments for Hodgkin's disease have serious side effects, both short and long-term. However, with accurate staging, physicians and patients often can choose the minimum treatment that will cure the disease. The staging system for Hodgkin's disease is the Ann Arbor Staging Classification, also called the Cotswold System or the Revised Ann Arbor System.

Hodgkin's disease is divided into four stages, with additional substages:

- Stage I: The disease is confined to one lymph node area
- Stage IE: The disease extends from the one lymph node area to adjacent regions
- Stage II: The disease is in two or more lymph node areas on one side of the diaphragm (the muscle below the lungs)
- Stage IIE: The disease extends to adjacent regions of at least one of these nodes

- Stage III: The disease is in lymph node areas on both sides of the diaphragm
- Stage IIIE/IIISE: The disease extends into adjacent areas or organs (IIIE) and/or the spleen (IIISE)
- Stage IV: The disease has spread from the lymphatic system to one or more other organs, such as the bone marrow or liver

Treatment for Hodgkin's disease depends both on the stage of the disease and whether or not symptoms are present. Stages are labeled with an A if no symptoms are present. If symptoms are present, the stage is labeled with a B. These symptoms include:

- loss of more than 10% of body weight over the previous six months
- fevers above 100 (37.70 C) degrees F
- drenching night sweats

Radiation therapy and/or **chemotherapy** (drug therapy) are the standard treatments for Hodgkin's disease. If the disease is confined to one area of the body, radiotherapy is usually used. This treatment, with x rays or other high-energy rays, also is used when the disease is in bulky areas such as the chest, where chemotherapeutic drugs cannot reach all of the cancer. External-beam radiation, a focused beam from an external machine, is used to irradiate only the affected lymph nodes. This procedure is called involved field radiation.

More advanced stages of Hodgkin's disease may be treated with mantle field radiation, in which the lymph nodes of the neck, chest, and underarms are irradiated. Inverted Y field radiation is used to irradiate the spleen and the lymph nodes in the upper abdomen and pelvis. Total nodal irradiation includes both mantle field and inverted Y field radiation.

Since external-beam radiation damages healthy tissue near the cancer cells, the temporary side effects of radiotherapy can include sunburn-like skin damage, fatigue, **nausea**, and **diarrhea**. Other temporary side effects may include a sore throat and difficulty swallowing. Long-term side effects depend on the dose and the location of the radiation and the age of the patient. Since radiation of the ovaries causes permanent sterility (the inability to have offspring), the ovaries of girls and young women are protected during radiotherapy. Sometimes the ovaries are surgically moved from the region to be irradiated.

If the Hodgkin's disease has progressed to additional lymph nodes or other organs, or if there is a recurrence of the disease within two years of radiation treatment, chemotherapy is used.

Chemotherapy utilizes a combination of drugs, each of which kills cancer cells in a different way. The most common chemotherapy regimens for Hodgkin's disease are MOPP (either mechlorethamine or methotrexate with Oncovin, procarbazine, prednisone) and ABVD (Adriamycin or doxorubicin, bleomycin, vincristine, dacarbazine). Each of these consists of four different drugs. ABVD is used more frequently than MOPP because it has fewer severe side effects. However MOPP is used for individuals who are at risk for heart failure. The chemotherapeutic drugs may be injected into a vein or muscle, or taken orally, as a pill or liquid.

Children who are sexually mature when they develop Hodgkin's disease, and whose muscle and bone mass are almost completely developed, usually receive the same treatment as adults. Younger children usually are treated with chemotherapy, since radiation will adversely affect bone and muscle growth. However, radiation may be used in low dosages, in combination with chemotherapy. The chemotherapy for children with Hodgkin's disease usually includes more drugs than ABVD and MOPP.

The side effects of chemotherapy for Hodgkin's disease depend on the dose of drugs and the length of time they are taken. Since these drugs target rapidly dividing cancer cells, they also affect normal cells that grow rapidly. These include the cells of the bone marrow, the linings of the mouth and intestines, and hair follicles. Damage to bone marrow leads to lower white blood cell counts and lower resistance to infection. It also leads to lower red blood cell counts, which can result in fatigue and easy bleeding and bruising. Damage to intestinal cells leads to a loss of appetite, nausea, and **vomiting**. Mouth sores and hair loss also are common side effects of chemotherapy. These side effects disappear when the chemotherapy is discontinued. Some drugs can reduce or prevent the **nausea and vomiting**.

Chemotherapy for Hodgkin's disease may lead to long-term complications. The drugs may damage the heart, lungs, kidneys, and liver. In children, growth may be impeded. Some chemotherapy can cause sterility, so men may choose to have their sperm frozen prior to treatment. Women may stop ovulating and menstruating during chemotherapy. This may or may not be permanent.

Treatment for higher-stage Hodgkin's disease often involves a combination of radiotherapy and chemotherapy. Following three or four chemotherapy regimens, involved field radiation may be directed at the most affected areas of the body. The long-term side effects often are more severe when radiation and chemotherapy are used in combination.

The development of a second type of cancer is the most serious risk from radiation and chemotherapy treatment for Hodgkin's disease. In particular, there is a risk of developing leukemia, **breast cancer**, bone cancer, or thyroid cancer. Chemotherapy, particularly MOPP, or chemotherapy in conjunction with radiotherapy, significantly increases the risk for leukemia.

Following treatment, the original diagnostic tests for Hodgkin's disease are repeated, to determine whether all traces of the cancer have been eliminated and to check for long-term side effects of treatment. In resistant Hodgkin's disease, some cancer cells remain following treatment. If the cancer continues to spread during treatment, it is called progressive Hodgkin's disease. If the disease returns after treatment, it is known as recurrent Hodgkin's disease. It may recur in the area where it first started or elsewhere in the body. It may recur immediately after treatment or many years later.

Additional treatment is necessary with these types of Hodgkin's disease. If the initial treatment was radiation therapy alone, chemotherapy may be used, or vice versa. Chemotherapy with different drugs, or higher doses, may be used to treat recurrent Hodgkin's. However, radiation to the same area is never repeated.

An autologous bone marrow and/or a peripheral blood **stem cell transplantation** (PBSCT) often is recommended for treating resistant or recurrent Hodgkin's disease, particularly if the disease recurs within a few months of a chemotherapy-induced remission. These transplants are autologous because they utilize the individual's own cells. The patient's bone marrow cells or peripheral blood stem cells (immature bone marrow cells found in the blood) are collected and frozen prior to high-dosage chemotherapy, which destroys bone marrow cells. A procedure called leukapheresis is used to collect the stem cells. Following the high-dosage chemotherapy, and possibly radiation, the bone marrow cells or stem cells are reinjected into the individual.

Most complementary therapies for Hodgkin's disease are designed to stimulate the immune system to destroy cancer cells and repair normal cells that have been damaged by treatment. These therapies are used in conjunction with standard treatment.

Immunologic therapies, also known as immunotherapies, biological therapies, or biological response modifier therapies, utilize substances that are produced by the immune system. These include interferon (an immune system protein), monoclonal antibodies

KEY TERMS

Antibody—An immune system protein that recognizes a specific foreign molecule.

Biopsy—The removal of a small sample of tissue for examination under a microscope; used for the diagnosis of cancer and to check for infection.

Bone marrow—Tissue inside the bones that produce red and white blood cells.

Chemotherapy—Treatment with various combinations of chemicals or drugs, particularly for the treatment of cancer.

Epstein-Barr virus (EBV)—Very common virus that infects immune cells and can cause mononucleosis.

Interferon—A potent immune-defense protein produced by viral-infected cells; used as an anti-cancer and anti-viral drug.

Interleukins—A family of potent immune-defense molecules; used in various medical therapies.

Laparotomy—A surgical incision of the abdomen.

Leukapheresis—A technique that uses a machine to remove stem cells from the blood; the cells are frozen and then returned to the patient following treatment that has destroyed the bone marrow.

Lymph nodes—Small round glands, located throughout the body and containing lymphocytes that remove foreign organisms and debris from the lymphatic fluid.

Lymphatic system—The vessels, lymph nodes, and organs, including the bone marrow, spleen, and thymus, that produce and carry white blood cells to fight disease.

Lymphocyte—White blood cells that produce antibodies and other agents for fighting disease.

PBSCT—Peripheral blood stem cell transplant; a method for replacing blood-forming cells that are destroyed by cancer treatment.

Radiotherapy—Disease treatment involving exposure to x rays or other types of radiation.

Reed-Sternberg cells—An abnormal lymphocyte that is characteristic of Hodgkin's disease.

Spleen—An organ of the lymphatic system, on the left side of the abdomen near the stomach; it produces and stores lymphocytes, filters the blood, and destroys old blood cells.

Splenectomy—Surgical removal of the spleen.

Staging—The use of various diagnostic methods to accurately determine the extent of disease; used to select the appropriate type and amount of treatment and to predict the outcome of treatment.

Stem cells—The cells from which all blood cells are derived.

Thymus—An organ of the lymphatic system, located behind the breast bone, that produces the T lymphocytes of the immune system.

Thyroid—A gland in the throat that produces hormones that regulate growth and metabolism.

(specially engineered antibodies), colony-stimulating (growth) factors (such as filgrastim), and vaccines. Many immunotherapies for Hodgkin's disease are experimental and available only through clinical trials. These biological agents may have side effects.

Coenzyme Q10 (CoQ10) and polysaccharide K (PSK) are being evaluated for their ability to stimulate the immune system and protect healthy tissue, as well as possible anti-cancer activities. Camphor, also known as 714-X, green tea, and hoxsey (which is a mixture of a number of substances), have been promoted as immune system enhancers. However there is no evidence that they are effective against Hodgkin's disease. Hoxsey, in particular, can produce serious side effects.

Hodgkin's disease, particularly in children, is one of the most curable forms of cancer. Approximately 90% of individuals are cured of the disease with chemotherapy and/or radiation.

The one-year relative survival rate following treatment for Hodgkin's disease is 93%. Relative survival rates do not include individuals who die of causes other than Hodgkin's disease. The percentage of individuals who have not died of Hodgkin's disease within five years of diagnosis is 90–95% for those with stage I or stage II disease. The figure is 85–90% for those diagnosed with stage III Hodgkin's and approximately 80% for those diagnosed with stage IV disease. The 15-year relative survival rate is 63%. Approximately 75% of children are alive and cancer free 20 years after the original diagnosis of Hodgkin's.

Acute myelocytic leukemia, a very serious cancer, may develop in as many as 2–6% of individuals receiving certain types of treatment for Hodgkin's disease. Women under the age of 30 who are treated with radiation to the chest have a much higher risk for developing breast cancer. Both men and women are at higher risk for developing lung or thyroid cancers as a result of chest irradiation.

Individuals with the type of Hodgkin's disease known as nodular lymphocytic predominance have a 2% chance of developing non-Hodgkin's lymphoma. Apparently, this is a result of the Hodgkin's disease itself and not the treatment.

Rosalyn Carson-DeWitt, MD
Margaret Alic, Ph.D.

Holistic medicine

Definition

Holistic medicine is a term used to describe therapies that attempt to treat the patient as a whole person. That is, instead of treating an illness, as in orthodox allopathy, holistic medicine looks at an individual's overall physical, mental, spiritual, and emotional well-being before recommending treatment. A practitioner with a holistic approach treats the symptoms of illness as well as looking for the underlying cause of the illness. Holistic medicine also attempts to prevent illness by placing a greater emphasis on optimizing health. The body's systems are seen as interdependent parts of the person's whole being. Its natural state is one of health, and an illness or disease is an imbalance in the body's systems. Holistic therapies tend to emphasize proper nutrition and avoidance of substances—such as chemicals—that pollute the body. Their techniques are non-invasive.

Some of the world's health systems that are holistic in nature include **naturopathic medicine**, homeopathy, and traditional Chinese medicine. Many alternative or natural therapies have a holistic approach, although that is not always the case. The term complementary medicine is used to refer to the use of both allopathic and holistic treatments. It is more often used in Great Britain, but is gaining acceptance in the United States.

There are no limits to the range of diseases and disorders that can be treated in a holistic way, as the principle of holistic healing is to balance the body, mind, spirit, and emotions so that the person's whole being functions smoothly. When an individual seeks holistic treatment for a particular illness or condition, other health problems improve without direct treatment, due to improvement in the performance of the immune system, which is one of the goals of holistic medicine.

Origins

The concept of holistic medicine is not new. In the 4th century B.C., Socrates warned that treating one part of the body only would not have good results. Hippocrates considered that many factors contribute to the health or otherwise of a human being, weather, **nutrition**, emotional factors, and in our time, a host of different sources of pollution can interfere with health. And of course, holistic medicine existed even before ancient Greece in some ancient healing traditions, such as those from India and China, which date back over 5,000 years. However, the term "holistic" only became part of everyday language in the 1970s, when Westerners began seeking an alternative to allopathic medicine.

Interestingly, it was only at the beginning of the twentieth century that the principles of holistic medicine fell out of favor in Western societies, with the advent of major advances in what we now call allopathic medicine. Paradoxically, many discoveries of the twentieth century have only served to confirm many natural medicine theories. In many cases, researchers have set out to debunk holistic medicine, only to find that their research confirms it, as has been the case, for example, with many herbal remedies.

Purpose

Many people are now turning to holistic medicine, often when suffering from chronic ailments that have not been successfully treated by allopathic means. Although many wonderful advances and discoveries have been made in modern medicine, surgery and drugs alone have a very poor record for producing optimal health because they are designed to attack illness. Holistic medicine is particularly helpful in treating chronic illnesses and maintaining health through proper nutrition and **stress** management.

Description

There are a number of therapies that come under the umbrella of "holistic medicine." They all use basically the same principles, promoting not only physical health, but also mental, emotional, and spiritual health. Most emphasize quality nutrition. Refined foods typically eaten in modern America contain chemical additives and preservatives, are high in fat, cholesterol, and sugars, and promote disease. Alternative nutritionists counter that by recommending whole foods whenever possible and minimizing the amount of meat—especially red meat—that is consumed. Many alternative therapies promote vegetarianism as a method of **detoxification**.

ANDREW WEIL (1942–)

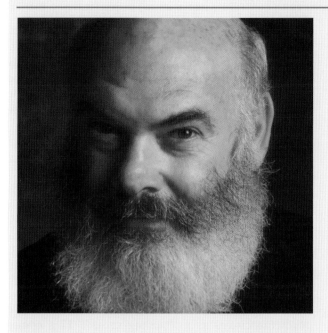

(Photograph by M. Greenberg. Gamma Liaison. Reproduced by permission.)

Dr. Andrew Weil, a Harvard-educated physician, adds credibility and expertise to the natural healing methods he espouses in his best-selling books, on his Internet Web site, in his talk show appearances, and in his popular audio CD of music and **meditation**. Weil's *Spontaneous Healing* spent more than a year on the best-seller list, and his 1997 book, *Eight Weeks to Optimum Health*, also was

a runaway best-seller. Perhaps the best-known proponent of naturalistic healing methods, Weil has been trying to establish a field he calls integrative medicine. He is director of Tucson's Center for Integrative Medicine, which he founded in 1993. In 1997, he began training doctors in the discipline at the University of Arizona, where he teaches.

After getting his bachelor's degree in botany from Harvard University, Weil applied for admission to Harvard Medical School in 1964. During his second year, he led a group of students who argued they could succeed better studying on their own than going to classes; in fact, the group got higher scores on their final exams than their classmates. After graduating from Harvard Medical School, he volunteered at the notorious counter-cultural Haight-Asbury Free Clinic in San Francisco, CA. Later in 1969, Weil got a job in Washington, DC, with the National Institute of Mental Health's Drug Studies Division. From 1971 to 1975, he traveled extensively in South America and Africa, soaking up information about medicinal plants, **shamanism**, and natural healing techniques. He never returned to the practice of conventional medicine.

His approach to alternative medicine is eclectic, mingling traditional medicine with herbal therapy, **acupuncture**, **homeopathy**, **chiropractic**, hypnotism, cranial manipulation, and other alternative healing methods. Though his books discuss the benefits of everything from healing touch to herbal cures, Weil doesn't dismiss the benefits of standard Western medicine when appropriate.

The aim of holistic medicine is to bring all areas of an individual's life, and most particularly the energy flowing through the body, back into harmony. Ultimately, of course, only the patient can be responsible for this, for no practitioner can make the necessary adjustments to diet and lifestyle to achieve health. The practice of holistic medicine does not rule out the practice of allopathic medicine; the two can complement each other.

A properly balanced holistic health regimen, which takes into consideration all aspects of human health and includes noninvasive and nonpharmaceutical healing methods, can often completely eradicate even acute health conditions safely. If a patient is being treated with allopathic medicine, holistic therapies may at least support the body during treatment, and alleviate the symptoms that often come with drug treatments and surgery. In addition, holistic therapies aim at the underlying source of the illness, to prevent recurrence.

Here are some of the major holistic therapies:

- herbal medicine
- homeopathy
- naturopathic medicine
- **traditional Chinese medicine**
- Ayurvedic medicine
- nutritional therapies
- **chiropractic**
- stress reduction
- psychotherapy
- massage

Because holistic medicine aims to treat the whole person, holistic practitioners sometimes may advise treatment from more than one type of practitioner. This is to ensure that all aspects of health are addressed. Some practitioners also specialize in more than one therapy, and so may be able to offer more comprehensive assistance.

Preparations

How to choose a holistic practitioner

- How did you hear of this therapist? A personal referral can sometimes be more reliable than a professional one. What do other professionals say about this therapist? What qualifications, board certification, or affiliations does this practitioner have?

- How do you feel personally about this practitioner? Do you feel comfortable in his/her office and with his/her staff? Is your sense of well being increased? Are you kept waiting for appointments?

- Do you have confidence in this practitioner, does he/she respect you as a person? Does he/she show an interest in your family, lifestyle, and diet? Are various treatment options explained to you?

- Is your personal dignity respected?

- Do you feel that this practitioner is sensitive to your feelings and fears regarding treatment?

- Is this practitioner a good advertisement for his/her profession? Signs of stress or ill health may mean that you would be better off choosing another practitioner.

- Do you feel that you are rushed into decisions, or do you feel that you are allowed time to make an informed choice regarding treatment?

- Are future health goals outlined for you? And do you feel that the practitioner is taking your progress seriously?

- Do you feel unconditionally accepted by this practitioner?

- Would you send your loved ones to this practitioner?

If you answered yes to all the above, then you have found a suitable practitioner. The cost of treatment by a holistic therapist varies widely, depending on the level of qualification and the discipline, so it is best to discuss how much treatment can be expected to cost with a practitioner before beginning a course. Some forms of holistic treatment may be covered by health insurance.

Precautions

Many people who try holistic therapies focus on one area of their health only, often detoxification and nutrition. However, practitioners stress that it is only when all areas of a person's potential well being are

tackled that total health and happiness can be achieved. They stress that the spiritual and emotional health contribute just as much as physical and mental health to a person's overall state of well-being.

When seeking treatment from a holistic practitioner, it is important to ensure that they are properly qualified. Credentials and reputation should always be checked. In addition, it is important that allopathic physicians and alternative physicians communicate about a patient's care.

Side effects

One of the main advantages of holistic therapies is that they have few side effects when used correctly. If a reputable practitioner is chosen, and guidelines are adhered to, the worst that typically happens is that when lifestyle is changed, and fresh nutrients are provided, the body begins to eliminate toxins that may have accumulated in the cells over a lifetime.

Often this results in what is known in alternative medicine circles as a "healing crisis." This comes about when the cells eliminate poisons into the blood stream all at the same time, throwing the system into a state of toxic overload until it can clear the "backlog." Symptoms such as **nausea**, headaches, or sensitivities to noise and other stimulations may be experienced.

The answer to most otherwise healthy patients is often just to lie quietly in a darkened room and take herbal teas. However, in the case of someone who has a serious illness, such as arthritis, colitis, diabetes, or **cancer**, (the list is much longer than this), it is strongly advised that they seek the help of a qualified practitioner. Therapists can help patients achieve detoxification in a way that causes the least stress to their bodies.

Research and general acceptance

Traditionally, holistic medicine, in all its different forms, has been regarded with mistrust and skepticism on the part of the allopathic medical profession. This situation is gradually changing. As of the year 2000, many insurance companies will provide for some form of alternative, or complementary treatment.

In addition, many allopathic physicians, recognizing the role alternative medicine can play in overall health and well being, are actually referring patients to reputable practitioners, particularly chiropractic and relaxation therapists, for help with a varied range of complaints.

Training and certification

Holistic or alternative medicine practitioners are usually affiliated with an organization in their field. Training varies tremendously with the category, and ranges from no qualifications at all—experience only—to holding a Ph.D. from an accredited university. Again, credentials and memberships should be checked by prospective patients.

An excellent source for qualified practitioners is the American Board of Holistic Medicine, (AHBM), which was incorporated in 1996. Also, the American Holistic Medicine Association has a comprehensive list of practitioners in all types of therapies across the United States, which they call "the holistic doctor finder." However, they stress that it is the responsibility of the patient to check each practitioner's credentials prior to treatment.

The ABHM has established the core curriculum upon which board certification for holistic medicine will be based. It includes the following twelve categories:

Body

Physical and environmental health
- nutritional medicine
- exercise medicine
- environmental medicine

Mind

Mental and emotional health
- behavioral medicine

Spirit

Spiritual health
- spiritual attunement
- social health

The six specialized areas:
- biomolecular diagnosis and therapy
- botanical medicine
- energy medicine
- ethno-medicine—including traditional Chinese medicine, Ayurveda, and Native American medicine
- homeopathy
- manual medicine

Founded in 1978 for the purpose of uniting practitioners of holistic medicine, membership of the AHMA is open to licensed medical doctors (MDs)

and doctors of osteopathic medicine (DOs) from every specialty, and to medical students studying for those degrees. Associate membership is open to health care practitioners who are certified, registered or licensed in the state in which they practice. The mission of the AHMA is to support practitioners in their personal and professional development as healers, and to educate physicians about holistic medicine.

Resources

ORGANIZATIONS

American Holistic Medicine Association. 4101 Lake Boone Trail, Suite 201, Raleigh, NC 27607. < http://www.holisticmedicine.org/index.html >.
Holistic medicine Website. < http://www.holisticmed.com/whatis.html >.

Patricia Skinner

Holter monitoring

Definition

Holter monitoring is continuous monitoring of the electrical activity of a patient's heart muscle (**electrocardiography**) for 24 hours, using a special portable device called a Holter monitor. Patients wear the Holter monitor while carrying out their usual daily activities.

Purpose

Holter monitoring is used to help determine whether someone has an otherwise undetected heart disease, such as abnormal heart rhythm (cardiac arrhythmia), or inadequate blood flow through the heart. Specifically, it can detect abnormal electrical activity in the heart that may occur randomly or only under certain circumstances, such as during sleep or periods of physical activity or **stress**, which may or may not be picked up by standard, short-term electrocardiography performed in a doctor's office.

Traditionally, an **exercise** stress test has been used to screen people for "silent" heart disease (heart disease with none of the usual symptoms). However, an exercise **stress test** is not completely foolproof, often producing false negative results (indicating no heart disease when heart disease is actually present) and false positives (indicating heart disease when there is none). Furthermore, some people cannot undergo exercise stress testing because of other medical conditions, such as arthritis.

Holter monitoring, also known as ambulatory or 24-hour electrocardiography, offers an alternate means of testing people for heart disease. By monitoring electrocardiographic activity throughout the day, Holter monitoring can uncover heart problems that occur during the patient's everyday activities. It can also help to recognize any activities that may be causing the heart problems. And it can define and correlate symptoms that may be caused by irregularities of the heart.

Precautions

Holter monitoring is an extremely safe procedure and no special precautions are required.

Description

The technician affixes electrodes on the surface of the skin at specific areas of the patient's chest, using adhesive patches with special gel that conducts electrical impulses. Typically, electrodes are placed under each collarbone and each bottom rib, and several electrodes are placed across the chest in a rough outline of the heart. The electrodes are attached to a portable electrocardiographic device called a Holter monitor, which records the electrical activity of the heart over 24–48 hours. The device is worn over the patient's shoulder or attached to a belt around the waist.

The Holter monitor records the continuous electrical activity throughout the course of the day, while the patient carries out his or her daily activities. During this time, the patient also keeps a detailed log or diary, recording his or her various activities, such as exercise, eating, sleeping, straining, breathing too hard (hyperventilating), and any stressful situations. The patient also notes the time and circumstances of any symptoms–especially chest pain, dizziness, **shortness of breath**, heart palpitations, and any other signs of heart trouble. Some Holter monitors allow patients to record their symptoms electronically, highlighting the portion of the electrocardiogram recorded while the symptoms are occurring.

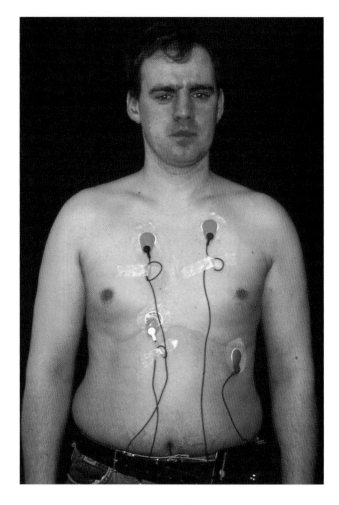

A male patient wears electrodes attached to his chest, which is connected to a Holter monitor at his waist. *(Photograph by Dr. P. Marazzi, Photo Researchers, Inc. Reproduced by permission.)*

After 24–48 hours, the Holter monitor is removed. A computer-assisted analysis is performed on the electrocardiographic recording, and the doctor compares the recording against the patient's log to see if there is any correlation between electrocardiographic abnormalities and any of the patient's activities or symptoms. The physician makes a final interpretation.

Preparation

In the doctor's office, electrodes are attached to the patient's chest. In some cases, the patient's chest hair may have to be shaved to facilitate attaching the electrodes. The patient then begins carrying the monitor on a shoulder harness, in a pocket, or on the belt while carrying out his or her usual daily routine. The patient should inform the doctor of any drugs he or she may be taking, because certain drugs can alter heart rhythms and may affect the results of the test.

Aftercare

The patient returns to the doctor's office to have the monitor and electrodes removed. No special measures need to be taken following Holter monitoring. The test results are usually available within a few days after the monitor is removed.

Risks

There are no known risks associated with Holter monitoring. The main complaint that people have with Holter monitoring is that the monitor may be cumbersome and interfere with certain activities, especially sleeping. Bathing and showering are not allowed during the study.

Normal results

A normal Holter monitoring test shows relatively normal electrical activity in the heart around the clock and no evidence of silent **ischemia** (deprivation of oxygen-rich blood).

Abnormal results

An abnormal result on Holter monitoring may indicate ischemia to the heart muscle or heart rhythm disturbances. Abnormalities are especially likely to show up during periods of stress or heavy activity, but sometimes serious abnormalities are recorded while the patient is sleeping.

Resources

ORGANIZATIONS

American Heart Association. 7320 Greenville Ave. Dallas, TX 75231. (214) 373-6300. < http://www.americanheart.org >.

National Heart, Lung and Blood Institute. PO Box 30105, Bethesda, MD 20824-0105. (301) 251-1222. < http://www.nhlbi.nih.gov >.

Robert Scott Dinsmoor

Holtzman ink blot test

Definition

The Holtzman Inkblot Technique (HIT) is a projective personality assessment test for persons ages five and up.

Purpose

The HIT is used to assess the personality structure of a test subject. It is sometimes used as a diagnostic tool in assessing **schizophrenia**, depression, **addiction**, and character disorders.

Precautions

Psychometric testing requires a clinically trained examiner. The HIT should be administered and interpreted by a trained psychologist, psychiatrist, or appropriately trained mental health professional.

Some consider projective tests to be less reliable than objective personality tests. If the examiner is not well-trained in psychometric evaluation, subjective interpretations may affect the outcome of the test.

Description

The HIT, developed by psychologist Wayne Holtzman and colleagues, was introduced in 1961. The test was designed to overcome some of the deficiencies of its famous predecessor, the Rorschach Inkblot Test.

Unlike the Rorschach, the Holtzman is a standardized measurement with clearly defined objective scoring criteria. The HIT consists of 45 inkblots. The test administrator, or examiner, has a stack of 47 cards with inkblots (45 test cards and 2 practice cards) face down in front of him or her. The examiner hands each card to the subject and asks the test subject what he or she sees in the inkblot. Only one response per inkblot is requested. Occasionally, the examiner may ask the test subject to clarify or elaborate on a response. The Administration of the HIT typically takes 50–80 minutes. The HIT is then scored against 22 personality-related characteristics.

The HIT can also be administered in a group setting. In group testing, 30–45 inkblots are projected onto a screen and test subjects provide written responses to each inkblot.

The 1997 Medicare reimbursement rate for psychological and neuropsychological testing is $58.35 an

KEY TERMS

Projective personality assessment—A test in which the subject is asked to interpret ambiguous stimuli, such as an inkblot. The subject's responses provide insight into his or her thought processes.

Standardization—The process of determining established norms and procedures for a test to act as a standard reference point for future test results.

hour. Billing time typically includes test administration, scoring and interpretation, and reporting. Many insurance plans cover all or a portion of diagnostic psychological testing.

Normal results

Because of the complexity of the scoring process and the projective nature of the test, results for the HIT should only be interpreted by a clinically trained psychologist, psychiatrist, or appropriately trained mental health professional.

Resources

ORGANIZATIONS

American Psychological Association (APA). 750 First St. NE, Washington, DC 20002-4242. (202) 336-5700. < ttp://www.apa.org >.

Paula Anne Ford-Martin

Homeopathic medicine

Definition

Homeopathy, or homeopathic medicine, is a holistic system of treatment that originated in the late eighteenth century. The name homeopathy is derived from two Greek words that mean "like disease." The system is based on the idea that substances that produce symptoms of sickness in healthy people will have a curative effect when given in very dilute quantities to sick people who exhibit those same symptoms. Homeopathic remedies are believed to stimulate the body's own healing processes. Homeopaths use the term "allopathy," or "different than disease," to describe the use of drugs used in conventional medicine to oppose or counteract the symptom being treated.

Purpose

Homeopathic physicians seek to cure their patients on the physical, mental and emotional levels, and each treatment is tailored to a patient's individual needs. Homeopathy is generally a safe treatment, as it uses medicines in extremely diluted quantities, and there are usually minimal side effects. Its non-toxicity makes it a good choice for the treatment of children. Another benefit of homeopathy is the cost of treatments; homeopathic remedies are inexpensive, often a fraction of the cost of conventional drugs.

Homeopathic treatment has been shown effective in treating many conditions. Colds and flu may be effectively treated with aconite and bryonia. Influenza suffers in a double-blind study found that they were twice as likely to recover in 48 hours when they took homeopathic remedies. Studies have been published in British medical journals confirming the efficacy of homeopathic treatment for rheumatoid arthritis. Homeopathic remedies are effective in treating infections, circulatory problems, respiratory problems, heart disease, depression and nervous disorders, migraine headaches, **allergies**, arthritis, and diabetes. Homeopathy is a good treatment to explore for acute and chronic illnesses, particularly if these are found in the early stages and where there is not severe damage. Homeopathy can be used to assist the healing process after surgery or **chemotherapy**.

Description

Origins

Homeopathy was founded by German physician **Samuel Hahnemann** (1755–1843), who was much disturbed by the medical system of his time, believing that its cures were crude and some of its strong drugs and treatments did more harm than good to patients. Hahnemann performed experiments on himself using Peruvian bark, which contains quinine, a **malaria** remedy. He concluded that in a healthy person, quinine creates the same symptoms as malaria, including fevers and chills, which is the reason why it is effective as a remedy. He then began to analyze the remedies available in nature by what he called provings. Provings of homeopathic remedies are still compiled by dosing healthy adults with various substances and documenting the results, in terms of the dose needed to produce the symptoms and the length of the dose's effectiveness. The provings are collected in large homeopathic references called *materia medica* or materials of medicine.

SAMUEL HAHNEMANN (1755–1843)

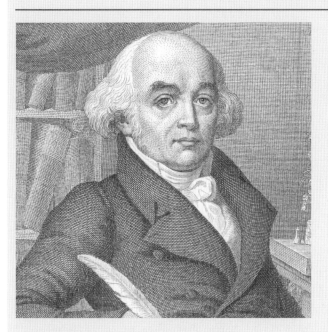

(Corbis Corporation. Reproduced by permission.)

Samuel Christian Hahnemann created and developed the system called homeopathy. It is also known as *similia similibus curentor* or like cures like. Although his new methods initially met with ridicule and criticism, by the time of his death they were accepted the world over as a result of the great success he had with his new cure.

Hahnemann was born in Meissen, Saxony (now part of Germany) into a financially challenged middle class family. His parents initially educated him at home, where his father taught him never to accept anything he learned without first questioning it. He graduated as a physician at Erlangen in 1779 after studying at Leipzig and Vienna. He was also fluent in English, German, Italian, French, Greek, Arabic, Latin and Hebrew.

At age 27 he married his first wife, Johanna Henriette Kuchler, the daughter of an apothecary, with whom he had 11 children.

Living in poverty, Hahnemann began practicing medicine in 1781 and translating scientific texts to supplement his income. However, disillusioned with medicine, he eventually gave it up entirely.

He discovered the concept of homeopathy when considering the effect of quinine on malaria, and went on to cure soldiers and then sufferers of a typhus epidemic with astounding success. He documented his discoveries in the *Organon*, a treatise on his work. Homeopathy also proved its worth in 1831 when there was an outbreak of cholera. Hahnemann used homeopathic treatment with a 96% success rate, compared to the 41% of allopathic medicine. He also wrote his *Materia Medica Pura.*

In 1834, Hahnemann met his second wife, Marie Melanie d'Hervilly. Despite a great difference in age, they were happily married until his death in Paris on July 2, 1843, at the age of 88.

Hahnemann formulated these principles of homeopathy:

- Law of Similars (like cures like)
- Law of the Infinitesimal Dose (The more diluted a remedy is, the more potent it is.)
- illness is specific to the individual

Hahnemann's Law of Similars was based on thinking that dated back to Hippocrates in the fourth century B.C. It is the same thinking that provided the basis for vaccinations created by Edward Jenner and Louis Pasteur. These vaccines provoke a reaction in the individual that protects against the actual disease. Allergy treatments work the same way. By exposing a person to minute quantities of the allergen, the person's tolerance levels are elevated.

The Law of the Infinitesimal Dose has always caused controversy among those outside the field of homeopathy. Hahnemann contended that as he diluted his remedies with water and alcohol and succussed, or shook, them, the remedies actually worked more effectively. In fact, diluted homeopathic remedies may have no chemical trace of the original substance. Practitioners believe that the electromagnetic energy of the original substance is retained in the dilution, but toxic side effects of the remedy are not. It is this electrochemical "message" that stimulates the body to heal itself.

Homeopathic practitioners believe that illness is specific to an individual. In other words, two people with severe headaches may not receive the same remedies. The practitioner will ask the patient questions about lifestyle, dietary habits, and personality traits, as well as specific questions about the nature of the **headache** and when it occurs. This information gathering is called profiling or case-taking.

In the early 1900s, homeopathy was popular in America, with over 15 percent of all doctors being homeopathic. There were 22 major homeopathic

Homeopathic Remedies That Work

Name	Description
Aconite	Commonly known as monkshood, aconite is highly toxic. A nontoxic, diluted extract of aconite is used in homeopathy to treat symptoms similar to that of poison.
Allium cepa	Commonly known as red onion, homeopathic physicians use a dilute extract of red onion to treat symptoms similar to that of red onion—watery eyes, burning, etc.
Apis	Commonly known as the honeybee, apis as a homeopathic remedy is made from the body of the bee. It is used to treat symptoms similar to that of a bee sting—redness, swelling, etc.
Arnica	Commonly known as the mountain daisy, arnica is used by homeopathic physicians to treat bruises, sprains, and strains.
Arsenicum album	Also known as ars alb, arsenicum album is a diluted form of arsenic, a metallic poison. It is used by homeopathic physicians to treat symptoms similar to the effects of arsenic poisoning—dehydration, burning pain, etc.
Belladonna	Commonly known as deadly knightshade, belladonna is used in homeopathy to treat symptoms of dry mouth, nausea, delirium, etc.
Bryonia	Commonly known as wild hops, bryonia is used in homeopathy to treat vomiting, diarrhea, inflammation, etc.
Calcarea carbonica	Also known as calcium carbonate or calc carb, it is used in homeopathy to treat symptoms of exhaustion, depression, and anxiety.
Cantharis	Commonly known as Spanish fly, cantharis is used in homeopathy to treat conditions with symptoms of abdominal cramps, vomiting, diarrhea, convulsions, etc.
Chamomilla	Derived from German chamomile, it is used in homeopathy to treat irritability, impatience, etc. It is most often prescribed to children.
Ferrum phosphoricum	Also known as ferrum phos or iron phosphate, it is used to treat symptoms of low energy and anemia.
Gelsemium	Also known as yellow jasmine, it is used to treat conditions that effect vision, balance, though, and locomotion.
Hepar sulphuris	Derived from the inner layer of oyster shells, hepar sulphuris is used to treat infection.
Hypericum	Commonly known as St. John's wort, hypericum is used to treated nerve damage.
Ignatia	Derived from seeds of a plant, this homeopathic remedy is prescribed to treat conditions with symptoms such as headache, cramping, and tremors.
Ipecac	Ipecac induces vomiting and causes gastrointestinal distress. Homeopaths prescribe it to treat similar symptoms.
Kali bichromicum	Commonly known as potassium bichromate, kali bichromicum is a poison used also in textile dyes, wood stain, etc. Homeopaths use it to treat localized pain.
Lachesis	Derived from the venom of the bushmaster snake, this homeopathic remedy is used to treat conditions that cause the same symptoms as the venom itself.
Ledum	Also known as marsh tea, ledum is used to treat infections, most often from animal bites, stings, cuts, etc.
Lycopodium	Commonly known as club moss, lycopodium is used to treat diarrhea, digestive upset, etc.
Mercurius vivus	Also known as quicksilver, it is used to treat symptoms of sweats, shaking, nausea, etc.
Natrum muriaticum	Commonly known as salt, it is used to treat conditions that cause excessive thirst and salt cravings.
Nux vomica	It is used to treat symptoms caused by overeating and too much caffeine or alcohol.
Phosphorus	It is used to treat symptoms of excessive thirst, fatigue, and nervousness.
[Continued]	

Homeopathic Remedies That Work [Continued]

Name	Description
Pulsatilla	It is used to treat conditions that are accompanied by discharge, such as bedwetting, sinusitis, etc.
Rhus toxicodendron	Commonly known as poison ivy, homeopaths use it to treat conditions with symptoms of fever, swollen glands, and restlessness.
Ruta	It is used to treat conditions with bruising, such as tennis elbow, sciatica, etc.
Sepia	Sepia is the discharge used by the cuttlefish to disappear from a predator. Homeopaths use sepia to treat symptoms of apathy and weakness.
Silica	Also called flint, silica is used by homeopaths to treat conditions that cause weakness, sweating, and sensitivity to cold.
Sulphur	It is used to treat conditions with symptoms of itching, burning pains, and odor.

medical schools, including Boston University and the University of Michigan. However, with the formation of the American Medical Association, which restricted and closed down alternative practices, homeopathy declined for half a century. When the 1960s invigorated back-to-nature trends and distrust of artificial drugs and treatments, homeopathy began to grow again dramatically through the next decades. In 1993, *The New England Journal of Medicine* reported that 2.5 million Americans used homeopathic remedies and 800,000 patients visited homeopaths in 1990, and it has continued to grow. Homeopathy is much more popular in Europe than in the United States. French pharmacies are required to make homeopathic remedies available along with conventional medications. Homeopathic hospitals and clinics are part of the national health system in Britain. It is also practiced in India and Israel, among other countries.

A visit to a homeopath can be a different experience than a visit to a regular physician. Surveys have shown that homeopathic doctors spend much more time during initial consultations than conventional doctors spend. This is because a homeopath does a complete case-taking to get a complete picture of a person's general health and lifestyle, as well as particular symptoms, on the physical, mental and emotional levels. Some symptoms can be so subtle that the patient is not always completely aware of them, and the doctor must spend time getting to know the patient.

The initial visit often includes a long questionnaire about a patient's medical and family history, and then a long interview with the doctor, who prompts the patient with many questions. Sometimes a homeopathic doctor will use lab tests to establish a patient's general level of health. The initial interview usually lasts between one and two hours.

The purpose of homeopathy is the restoration of the body to homeostasis, or healthy balance, which is its natural state. The symptoms of a disease are regarded as the body's own defensive attempt to correct its imbalance, rather than as enemies to be defeated. Because a homeopath regards symptoms as positive evidence of the body's inner intelligence, he or she will prescribe a remedy designed to stimulate this internal curative process, rather than suppress the symptoms.

In homeopathy, the curative process extends beyond the relief of immediate symptoms of illness. Healing may come in many stages, as the practitioner treats layers of symptoms that are remnants of traumas or chronic disease in the patient's past. This is part of Hering's Laws of Cure, named for Constantine Hering, the father of homeopathy in America. Hering believed that healing starts from the deepest parts of the body to the extremities, and from the upper parts of the body to the lower parts. Hering's Laws also state that homeopaths should treat disease symptoms in reverse chronological order, from the most recent to the oldest, restoring health in stages. Sometimes, the patient may feel worse before feeling better. This is called a healing crisis.

When prescribing a remedy, homeopaths will match a patient's symptoms with the proper remedy in a repertory or *materia medica* that has been compiled throughout the history of homeopathy. Classical homeopaths prescribe only one remedy at a time. However, it is becoming more common, especially in Europe, to use combination formulas of several remedies for the treatment of some combinations of symptoms.

The cost of homeopathic care can vary. The cost of visits will be comparable to conventional medicine, with initial visits ranging from $50 to $300. Non-M.D. homeopaths can charge from $50 to $250. Follow-up visits are less, at about $35 to $100. Homeopathic medicine is significantly cheaper than pharmaceuticals, and most remedies cost between $2 and $10. Some doctors provide remedies without charge. Homeopaths rarely use lab tests, which reduces the cost of treatment further. In general, homeopathy is much more economical than conventional medicine. In 1991, the French government did a study on the cost of homeopathic medicine, and found that it costs half as much to treat patients, considering all costs involved.

KEY TERMS

Aggravation—Temporary increase in symptoms due to homeopathic remedy.

Antidote—Substance which cancels the effect of homeopathic remedies

Homeopath—A homeopathic physician.

Proving—Case study of the effect of a homeopathic medicine.

Repertory—Reference manual of homeopathic remedies.

Vital force—Innate wisdom and energy of the body.

When homeopaths are licensed professionals, most insurance companies will pay for their fees. Consumers should consult their insurance policies to determine individual regulations. Insurance usually will not cover homeopathic medicine, because it is sold over-the-counter.

Precautions

Although homeopathic remedies sometimes use substances that are toxic, they are diluted and prescribed in non-toxic doses. Remedies should be prescribed by a homeopathic practitioner. Those preparing to take homeopathic remedies should also avoid taking *antidotes*, substances which homeopathic doctors believe cancel the effects of their remedies. These substances include alcohol, coffee, prescription drugs, peppermint (in toothpaste and mouthwash), camphor (in salves and lotions), and very spicy foods. Homeopathic medicine should also be handled with care, and should not be touched with the hands or fingers, which can contaminate it.

Side effects

A homeopathic *aggravation* sometimes occurs during initial treatment with homeopathic remedies. This means that symptoms can temporarily worsen during the process of healing. Although this is usually mild, the aggravation can sometimes be severe. Homeopaths see aggravation as a positive sign that the remedy is a good match for the patient's symptoms. The healing crisis, which happens when the patient is undergoing treatment for layers of symptoms, may also cause the patient to feel worse before feeling better. Some patients can experience emotional disturbances like weeping or depression, if suppressed emotional problems led to the illness in the first place.

Research and general acceptance

Since the early 1900s, when the American Medical Association and pharmacists waged a battle against it, homeopathy has been neglected and sometimes ridiculed by mainstream medicine. Aside from politics, part of the reason for this is that there are some aspects of homeopathy which have not been completely explained scientifically. For instance, homeopaths have found that the more they dilute and succuss a remedy, the greater effect it seems to have on the body. Some homeopathic remedies are so diluted that not even a single molecule of the active agent remains in a solution, yet it still works; studies have demonstrated this paradox, yet can't explain it. Also, homeopathy puts an emphasis on analyzing symptoms and then applying remedies to these symptoms, rather than working by classifying diseases. Thus, some people with the same disease may require different homeopathic medicines and treatments. Furthermore, conventional medicine strives to find out how medicines work in the body before they use them; homeopathy is less concerned with the intricate biochemistry involved than with whether a remedy ultimately works and heals holistically. For all these reasons, conventional medicine claims that homeopathy is not scientific, but homeopaths are quick to reply that homeopathy has been scientifically developed and studied for centuries, with much documentation and success.

There continue to be many studies that affirm the effectiveness of homeopathic treatments. Among the most celebrated, the *British Medical Journal* in 1991 published a large analysis of homeopathic treatments that were given over the course of 25 years. This project involved over 100 studies of patients with problems ranging from vascular diseases, respiratory problems, infections, stomach problems, allergies, recovery from surgeries, arthritis, trauma, psychological problems, diabetes, and others. The study found improvement with homeopathic treatment in most categories of problems, and concluded that the evidence was "sufficient for establishing homeopathy as a regular treatment for certain indications."

Resources

PERIODICALS

Homeopathy Today. 801 N. Fairfax St. #306, Alexandria, VA 22314. (703) 548-7790.
Similimum. P.O. Box 69565, Portland, OR 97201. (503) 795-0579.

OTHER

Ayurvedic Institute. < http://www.ayurveda.com > .
National Center for Homeopathy. < http://www.healthy. net/nch > .
North American Society of Homeopaths. < http://www.homeopathy.org > .

Homeopathic medicine, acute prescribing

Definition

Acute homeopathic prescribing is that part of homeopathy that treats illness which has an abrupt onset and needs immediate attention. In homeopathic medicine, acute refers primarily to the speed of onset and self-limiting character of the disorder rather than its seriousness. Colds, **influenza**, sore throats, insect stings, cuts, **bruises**, **vomiting**, **diarrhea**, **fever**, muscle aches, and short-term insomnia are all examples of conditions that are treated by acute prescribing. The remedies given in acute homeopathic prescribing are intended to stimulate the body's internal ability to heal itself; they do not kill germs or suppress symptoms. Acute prescribing can be done—within limits—by patients at home, as well as by homeopathic practitioners. Study courses, self-treatment guides, and homeopathic home medicine kits are now available by mail order from homeopathic pharmacies and educational services.

Purpose

Homeopathic physicians seek to cure their patients on physical, mental, and emotional levels, and each treatment is tailored to a patient's individual needs. Homeopathy is generally a safe treatment, as it uses medicines in extremely diluted quantities, and there are usually minimal side effects. Its non-toxicity makes it a good choice for the treatment of children. Another benefit of homeopathy is the cost of treatments; homeopathic remedies are inexpensive, often a fraction of the cost of conventional drugs.

Acute homeopathic prescribing is thought to benefit a wide range of ailments. These include **altitude sickness**, Bell's palsy, the **common cold**, **allergies**, coughing, **dengue fever**, dysentery, earaches, migraine headaches, fever, **food poisoning**, grief, influenza, **motion sickness**, shock, sore throat, surgical complications, and reactions to vaccinations and drug therapy. Acute remedies may also be prescribed to treat insect stings, animal bites, and problems related to poison oak and poison ivy. It may be further employed in treating injuries including black eyes, **burns**, bruises, concussions, cuts, damaged tendons and ligaments, **dislocations**, **fractures**, herniated discs, nosebleeds, puncture **wounds**, **sprains**, and **strains**.

Description

Origins

Homeopathy is a gentle, painless, holistic system of healing developed during the 1790s by Samuel Hahnemann, a German physician. Experimenting on himself with the anti-malarial drug quinine, Hahnemann noticed that large doses of the medicine actually caused malaria-like symptoms, while smaller doses cured the symptoms. From this, he advanced his concept of *Similia similibus curentur*, or "let like be cured with like." Hahnemann then developed an extensive system of medicine based on this concept. He named it homeopathy, from the Greek words *homoios* (the same) and *pathos* (suffering).

Homeopathic remedies are almost always made from natural materials—plant, animal, or mineral substances—that have been treated to form mother tinctures or nonsoluble powders. Liquid extracts are then potentized, or increased in power, by a series of dilutions and succussions, or shakings. It is thought that succussion is necessary to transfer the energy of the natural substance to the solution. In addition, the potency of the remedy is regarded as increasing with each dilution. After the tincture has been diluted to the prescribed potency, the resulting solution is added to a bottle of sucrose/lactose tablets, which are stored in a cool, dark place. If the remedy is not soluble in water, it is ground to a fine powder and triturated with powdered lactose to achieve the desired potency.

Proponents of homeopathy over the years have included Louisa May Alcott, Charles Dickens, Benjamin Disraeli, Johann Wolfgang Goethe, Nathaniel Hawthorne, William James, Henry Wadsworth Longfellow, Pope Pius X, John D. Rockefeller, Harriet Beecher Stowe, William Thackeray, Daniel Webster, and W. B. Yeats. England's Royal Family has employed homeopathic practitioners since the 1830s.

Homeopathic prescribing differs in general from allopathic medicine in its tailoring of remedies to the patient's overall personality type and totality of symptoms, rather than to the disease. Whereas a conventional physician would prescribe the same medication

or treatment regimen to all patients with the common cold, for example, a homeopathic practitioner would ask detailed questions about each patient's symptoms and the modalities, or factors, that make them better or worse. As a result, the homeopath might prescribe six different remedies for six different patients with the same illness. In acute prescribing homeopathy, consultations are more brief compared to constitutional homeopathic prescribing. A typical patient might spend just 10–15 minutes with the practitioner, compared to more than an hour for constitutional prescribing.

Homeopathic classification of symptoms

Homeopathic practitioners use the word symptom in a more inclusive fashion than traditional medicine. In homeopathy, symptoms include any change that the patient experiences during the illness, including changes in emotional or mental patterns.

Homeopaths classify symptoms according to a hierarchy of four categories for purposes of acute prescribing:

- Peculiar symptoms. These are symptoms unique to the individual that do not occur in most persons with the acute disease. Homeopaths make note of peculiar symptoms because they often help to determine the remedy.

- Mental and emotional symptoms. These are important general symptoms that inform the homeopath about the patient's total experience of the disorder.

- Other general symptoms. These are physical symptoms felt throughout the patient's body, such as tiredness, changes in appetite, or restlessness.

- Particular symptoms. Particular symptoms are localized in the body; they include such symptoms as **nausea**, skin **rashes**, **headache**, etc.

During homeopathic case-taking, the practitioner will evaluate the intensity of the patient's symptoms, assess their depth within the patient's body, note any peculiar symptoms, evaluate the modalities of each symptom, and make a list of key symptoms to guide the selection of the proper medicine.

Homeopathic remedies

There are several hundred homeopathic remedies. Homeopathic medicines are usually formulated from diluted or triturated natural substances, including plants, **minerals**, or even venom from snakes or stinging insects. Some remedies may be given in a spray, ointment, or cream, but the most common forms of administration are liquid dilutions and two sizes of pellets, or cylindrical tablets (for triturated remedies). A dose consists of one drop of liquid; 10–20 small pellets; or 1–3 large pellets. Since the remedies are so dilute, the exact size of the dose is not of primary importance. The frequency of dosing is considered critical, however; patients are advised not to take further doses until the first has completed its effect.

Homeopathic remedies can be kept indefinitely with proper handling. Proper handling includes storing the remedies in the original bottles and discarding them if they become contaminated by sunlight or other intense light; temperatures over 100 °F (37.8 °C); vapors from camphor, mothballs, or perfume; or from other homeopathic remedies being opened in the same room at the same time.

Preparations

Case-taking

The first step in acute prescribing is a lengthy interview with the patient, known as case-taking. In addition to noting the character, location, and severity of the patient's symptoms, the homeopath will ask about their modalities. The modalities are the circumstances or factors (e.g., weather, time of day, body position, behavior or activity, etc.) that make the symptoms either better or worse. Case-taking can be done by the patient or a family member as well as by a homeopath.

Selection and administration of a remedy

The choice of a specific remedy is guided by the patient's total symptom profile rather than by the illness. Homeopathic remedies are prescribed according to the law of similars, which holds that a substance that produces specific symptoms in healthy people cures those symptoms in sick people when given in highly diluted forms. For example, a patient with influenza who is irritable, headachy, and suffering from joint or muscle pains is likely to be given *bryonia* (wild hops), because this plant extract would cause this symptom cluster in a healthy individual.

Patients are instructed to avoid touching homeopathic medicines with their fingers. The dose can be poured onto a piece of white paper or the bottle's cap and tipped directly into the mouth. Homeopathic remedies are not taken with water; patients should not eat or drink anything for 15–20 minutes before or after taking the dose.

Precautions

Homeopathic acute prescribing is not recommended for the treatment of chronic conditions requiring constitutional prescribing, for severe infections requiring antibiotic treatment, or for conditions requiring major surgery. It is also not recommended for the treatment of mental health problems.

Persons who are treating themselves with homeopathic remedies should follow professional guidelines regarding the limitations of home treatment. Most homeopathic home treatment guides include necessary information regarding symptoms and disorders that require professional attention.

Homeopathic remedies may lose their potency if used at the same time as other products. Some homeopathic practitioners recommend the avoidance of mint and mentholated products (toothpastes, candies, chewing gum, mouth rinses), as well as camphor and camphorated products (including eucalyptus and Tiger Balm), patchouli and other essential oils, moth balls, strong perfumes, aftershaves, scented soaps, **stress**, x rays, coffee, nicotine, recreational drugs (**marijuana**) and certain therapeutic drugs (most notably cortisone and prednisone) during treatment. Patients are also advised to avoid electric blankets and dental work, as these are thought to adversely affect homeopathic therapy. Homeopathic remedies should never be placed near magnets.

Practitioners caution that high-potency preparations should be used only under the supervision of a homeopathic practitioner.

Side effects

Homeopathic medicines are so diluted that sometimes no trace of the original substance can be detected. These medicines are therefore considered non-toxic and generally free of harmful side effects. There may, however, be individual reactions to **homeopathic medicine**.

An intensified healing response may occur as treatment begins, which causes symptoms to worsen, but the phenomenon is temporary. In some patients, old symptoms may re-appear from past conditions from which recovery was not complete. Such phenomena are taken as positive indications that the healing process has commenced.

Research and general acceptance

As Samuel Hahnemann's healing system grew in popularity during the 1800s, it quickly attracted vehement opposition from the medical and apothecary professions. Since the early 1900s, when the American Medical Association and pharmacists waged a battle against it, homeopathy has been neglected and sometimes ridiculed by mainstream medicine. Aside from politics, part of the reason for this is that there are some aspects of homeopathy which have not been completely explained scientifically. For instance, homeopaths have found that the more they dilute and succuss a remedy, the greater effect it seems to have on the body. Some homeopathic remedies are so diluted that not even a single molecule of the active agent remains in a solution, yet homeopaths maintain it still works; some studies have demonstrated this paradox, yet cannot explain it. Also, homeopathy puts an emphasis on analyzing symptoms and then applying remedies to these symptoms, rather than working by classifying diseases. Thus, some people with the same disease may require different homeopathic medicines and treatments. Furthermore, conventional medicine strives to find out how medicines work in the body before they use them; homeopathy is less concerned with the intricate biochemistry involved than with whether a remedy ultimately works and heals holistically. For all these reasons, conventional medicine claims that homeopathy is not scientific, but homeopaths are quick to reply that homeopathy has been scientifically developed and studied for centuries, with much documentation and success.

There continue to be many studies that affirm the effectiveness of homeopathic treatments. Among the most celebrated, the *British Medical Journal* in 1991 published a large analysis of homeopathic treatments that were given over the course of 25 years. This project involved over 100 studies of patients with problems ranging from vascular diseases, respiratory problems, infections, stomach problems, allergies, recovery from surgeries, arthritis, trauma, psychological problems, diabetes, and others. The study found improvement with homeopathic treatment in most categories of problems, and concluded that the evidence was "sufficient for establishing homeopathy as a regular treatment for certain indications."

In the United Kingdom and other countries where homeopathy is especially popular, some medical doctors incorporate aspects of acute prescribing homeopathy into their practices. Countries in which homeopathy is popular include France, India, Pakistan, Sri Lanka, Brazil, and Argentina. Large homeopathic hospitals exist in London and

KEY TERMS

Acute prescribing—Homeopathic treatment for self-limiting illnesses with abrupt onset.

Allopathy—Conventional medical treatment of disease symptoms that uses substances or techniques to oppose or suppress the symptoms.

Law of similars—The basic principle of homeopathic medicine that governs the selection of a specific remedy. It holds that a substance of natural origin that produces certain symptoms in a healthy person will cure those same symptoms in a sick person.

Modalities—The factors and circumstances that cause a patient's symptoms to improve or worsen.

Mother tincture—The first stage in the preparation of a homeopathic remedy, made by soaking a plant, animal, or mineral product in a solution of alcohol.

Potentization—The process of increasing the power of homeopathic preparations by successive dilutions and succussions of a mother tincture.

Succussion—The act of shaking diluted homeopathic remedies as part of the process of potentization.

Trituration—The process of diluting a nonsoluble substance for homeopathic use by grinding it to a fine powder and mixing it with lactose powder.

Glasgow, and homeopathic medical centers can be found in India and South America.

Resources

BOOKS
Strohecker, James. *Alternative Medicine: The Definitive Guide.* Tiburon, Calif.: Future Medicine Publishing, Inc., 1999.

ORGANIZATIONS
The American Institute of Homeopathy. 1585 Glencoe, Denver, CO 80220. (303) 898-5477.

Council for Homeopathic Certification. P.O. Box 157, Corte Madera, CA 94976.

International Foundation for Homeopathy. 2366 Eastlake Avenue East, #301, Seattle, WA 98102. (425) 776-4147.

National Center for Homeopathy. 801 North Fairfax Street, Suite 306, Alexandria, VA 22134. (703) 548-7790.

North American Society of Homeopaths. 10700 Old County Rd. 15, #350, Minneapolis, MN 55441. (612) 593-9458.

Homeopathic medicine, constitutional prescribing

Definition

Constitutional homeopathic prescribing, also called classical prescribing, is a holistic system of medicine that has been practiced for more than 200 years. Unlike acute homeopathic prescribing, constitutional prescribing refers to the selection and administration of homeopathic preparations over a period of time for treatment related to what practitioners call miasmic disorders, those caused by an inherited predisposition to a disease. The term miasm comes from a Greek word meaning stain or pollution. As in acute prescribing, constitutional prescribing is holistic in that it is intended to treat the patient on the emotional and spiritual levels of his or her being as well as the physical. Constitutional prescribing is also aimed at eventual cure of the patient, not just suppression or relief of immediate symptoms.

Purpose

Homeopathic physicians seek to cure their patients on physical, mental, and emotional levels, and each treatment is tailored to a patient's individual needs. Homeopathy is generally a safe treatment, as it uses medicines in extremely diluted quantities, and there are usually minimal side effects. Its non-toxicity makes it a good choice for the treatment of children. Another benefit of homeopathy is the cost of treatments; homeopathic remedies are inexpensive, often a fraction of the cost of conventional drugs.

Classical homeopathy has been used to treat a wide range of diseases and conditions, most of which tend to be long-term. These include: alcoholism, allergies, **anxiety**, arthritis, asthma, bladder conditions, chronic fatigue syndrome, depression, drug dependencies, gastrointestinal problems, Gulf War sickness, **headache**, hearing problems, herpes, hypersensitivity, immune disorders, **insomnia**, joint problems, kidney conditions, liver problems, **Lyme disease**, lower back problems, **malaria**, **menopause**, menstrual problems, migraine, **multiple sclerosis**, **paralysis**, **phobias**, **shingles**, sinus problems, skin disorders, repetitive **stress** injury, rheumatism, vertigo, vision problems, and yeast infections.

Description

Origins

Homeopathy was developed during the 1790s by **Samuel Hahnemann**, a German physician.

Experimenting on himself with the anti-malarial drug quinine, Hahnemann noticed that large doses of the medicine actually caused malaria-like symptoms, while smaller doses cured the symptoms. From this, he advanced his concept of *Similia similibus curentur*, or "let like be cured with like." Hahnemann then developed an extensive system of medicine based on this concept. He named it homeopathy, from the Greek words *homoios* (the same) and *pathos* (suffering).

There are several hundred homeopathic remedies. They are almost always made from natural materials—plant, animal, or mineral substances—that have been treated to form mother tinctures or nonsoluble powders. Liquid extracts are then potentized, or increased in power, by a series of dilutions and succussions, or shakings. It is thought that succussion is necessary to transfer the energy of the natural substance to the solution. In addition, the potency of the remedy is regarded as increasing with each dilution. After the tincture has been diluted to the prescribed potency, the resulting solution is added to a bottle of sucrose/lactose tablets, which are stored in a cool, dark place. If the remedy is not soluble in water, it is ground to a fine powder and triturated with powdered lactose to achieve the desired potency.

Proponents of homeopathy over the years have included Louisa May Alcott, Charles Dickens, Benjamin Disraeli, Johann Wolfgang Goethe, Nathaniel Hawthorne, William James, Henry Wadsworth Longfellow, Pope Pius X, John D. Rockefeller, Harriet Beecher Stowe, William Thackeray, Daniel Webster, and W. B. Yeats. England's Royal Family has employed homeopathic practitioners since the 1830s.

Constitutional prescribing is based on the patient's symptom profile and specific aspects of homeopathic theory.

Homeopathic classification of symptoms

Homeopathic practitioners use the word symptom in a more inclusive fashion than traditional medicine. In homeopathy, symptoms include any change that the patient experiences during the illness, including changes in emotional or mental patterns.

Homeopaths classify symptoms according to a hierarchy of four categories:

• Peculiar symptoms. These are symptoms unique to the individual that do not occur in most persons. Homeopaths make note of peculiar symptoms because they often help to determine the remedy.

- Mental and emotional symptoms. These are important general symptoms that inform the homeopath about the patient's total experience of the disorder.

- Other general symptoms. These are physical symptoms felt throughout the patient's body, such as tiredness, changes in appetite, or restlessness.

- Particular symptoms. Particular symptoms are localized in the body; they include such symptoms as **nausea**, skin **rashes**, or headaches.

Miasms

Homeopaths regard the patient's symptom profile as a systemic manifestation of an underlying chronic disorder called a miasm. Miasms are serious disturbances of what homeopaths call the patient's vital force that are inherited from parents at the time of conception. Hahnemann believed that the parents' basic lifestyle, their emotional condition and habitual diet, and even the atmospheric conditions at the time of conception would affect the number and severity of miasms passed on to the child. Hahnemann himself distinguished three miasms: the psoric, which he considered the most universal source of chronic disease in humans; the syphilitic; and the sycotic, which he attributed to **gonorrhea**. Later homeopaths identified two additional miasms, the cancernic and the tuberculinic. The remaining major source of miasms is allopathic medicine. It is thought that specific allopathic treatments—particularly **smallpox** vaccinations, cortisone preparations, major tranquilizers, and antibiotics—can produce additional layers of miasms in the patient's constitution. Constitutional prescribing evaluates the person's current state or miasmic picture, and selects a remedy intended to correct or balance that state. The homeopath may prescribe a different remedy for each miasmic layer over time, but gives only one remedy at a time directed at the person's current state. The basic principle governing the prescription of each successive remedy is the law of similars, or "like cures like."

Hering's laws of cure

The homeopathic laws of cure were outlined by Constantine Hering, a student of Hahnemann who came to the United States in the 1830s. Hering enunciated three laws or principles of the patterns of healing that are used by homeopaths to evaluate the effectiveness of specific remedies and the overall progress of constitutional prescribing:

- Healing progresses from the deepest parts of the organism to the external parts. Homeopaths consider the person's mental and emotional dimensions,

together with the brain, heart, and other vital organs, as a person's deepest parts. The skin, hands, and feet are considered the external parts.

- Symptoms appear or disappear in the reverse of their chronological order of appearance. In terms of constitutional treatment, this law means that miasms acquired later in life will resolve before earlier ones.

- Healing proceeds from the upper to the lower parts of the body.

Healing crises

Homeopaths use Hering's laws to explain the appearance of so-called healing crises, or aggravations, in the course of homeopathic treatment. It is not unusual for patients to experience temporary worsening of certain symptoms after taking their first doses of homeopathic treatment. For example, a person might notice that arthritic pains in the shoulders are better but that the hands feel worse. Hering's third law would indicate that the remedy is working because the symptoms are moving downward in the body. In constitutional prescribing, a remedy that removes one of the patient's miasmic layers will then allow the symptoms of an older miasm to emerge. Thus the patient may find that a physical disease is followed by a different set of physical problems or by emotional symptoms.

Preparations

The most important aspects of preparation for constitutional prescribing are the taking of a complete patient history and careful patient education.

Case-taking

Homeopathic case-taking for constitutional prescribing is similar to that for acute prescribing, but more in-depth. The initial interview generally takes one to two hours. The practitioner is concerned with recording the totality of the patient's symptoms and the modalities that influence their severity. Also included are general characteristics about the patient and his or her lifestyle choices. For example, a practitioner might ask the patient if he or she likes being outside or is generally hot or cold. There is also an emphasis on the patient's lifetime medical history, particularly records of allopathic treatments.

Patient education

Homeopaths regard patients as equal partners in the process of recovery. They will take the time to explain the theories underlying constitutional prescribing to the patient as well as taking the history. Patient education is especially important in constitutional prescribing in order to emphasize the need for patience with the slowness of results and length of treatment, and to minimize the possibility of self-treatment with allopathic drugs if the patient has a healing crisis.

Homeopathic remedies

In constitutional prescribing, one dose of the selected remedy is given. Patients then wait two to six weeks before following up with the homeopath, while the body begins the healing process. At the follow-up visit, the remedy may be repeated, or a different remedy prescribed. The preparation, selection, administration, and storage of remedies for constitutional prescribing are the same as for acute prescribing. These procedures are described more fully in the article on acute prescribing.

Precautions

Constitutional homeopathic prescribing is not appropriate for diseases or health crises requiring emergency treatment, whether medical, surgical, or psychiatric. In addition, constitutional prescribing should not be self-administered. Although home treatment kits of homeopathic remedies are available for acute self-limited disorders, the knowledge of homeopathic theory and practice required for constitutional evaluation is beyond the scope of most patients.

Patients are instructed to avoid touching homeopathic medicines with their fingers. The dose can be poured onto a piece of white paper or the bottle's cap and tipped directly into the mouth. Homeopathic remedies are not taken with water; patients should not eat or drink anything for 15–20 minutes before or after taking the dose.

Homeopathic remedies may lose their potency if used at the same time as other products. Some homeopathic practitioners recommend the avoidance of mint and mentholated products (toothpastes, candies, chewing gum, mouth rinses), as well as camphor and camphorated products (including eucalyptus and Tiger Balm), patchouli and other essential oils, moth balls, strong perfumes, aftershaves, scented soaps, stress, x rays, coffee, nicotine, recreational drugs (marijuana) and certain therapeutic drugs (most notably cortisone and prednisone) during treatment. Patients are also advised to avoid electric blankets and dental work, as these are thought to adversely affect homeopathic therapy. Homeopathic remedies should never be placed near magnets.

Side effects

Homeopathic medicines are so diluted that sometimes no trace of the original substance can be detected. These medicines are therefore considered non-toxic and generally free of harmful side effects. The primary risks to the patient from constitutional homeopathic treatment are the symptoms of the healing crisis and individual reactions to **homeopathic medicine**. The complexity of constitutional prescribing requires homeopaths to have detailed knowledge of the *materia medica* and the repertories, and to take careful and extensive case notes.

An intensified healing response may occur as treatment begins, which causes symptoms to worsen, but the phenomenon is temporary. In some patients, old symptoms may re-appear from past conditions from which recovery was not complete. Such phenomena are taken as positive indications that the healing process has commenced.

Research and general acceptance

As Samuel Hahnemann's healing system grew in popularity during the 1800s, it quickly attracted vehement opposition from the medical and apothecary professions. Since the early 1900s, when the American Medical Association and pharmacists waged a battle against it, homeopathy has been neglected and sometimes ridiculed by mainstream medicine. Aside from politics, part of the reason for this is that there are some aspects of homeopathy which have not been completely explained scientifically. For instance, homeopaths have found that the more they dilute and succuss a remedy, the greater effect it seems to have on the body. Some homeopathic remedies are so diluted that not even a single molecule of the active agent remains in a solution, yet homeopaths maintain it still works; some studies have demonstrated this paradox, yet cannot explain it. Also, homeopathy puts an emphasis on analyzing symptoms and then applying remedies to these symptoms, rather than working by classifying diseases. Thus, some people with the same disease may require different homeopathic medicines and treatments. Furthermore, conventional medicine strives to find out how medicines work in the body before they use them; homeopathy is less concerned with the intricate biochemistry involved than with whether a remedy ultimately works and heals holistically. For all these reasons, conventional medicine claims that homeopathy is not scientific, but homeopaths are quick to reply that homeopathy has been scientifically developed and studied for centuries, with much documentation and success.

KEY TERMS

Aggravation—Another term used by homeopaths for the healing crisis.

Allopathy—Conventional medical treatment of disease symptoms that uses substances or techniques to oppose or suppress the symptoms.

Constitutional prescribing—Homeopathic treatment for long-term or chronic disorders related to inherited predispositions to certain types of illnesses.

Healing crisis—A temporary worsening of the patient's symptoms during successive stages of homeopathic treatment.

Law of similars—The basic principle of homeopathic medicine that governs the selection of a specific remedy. It holds that a substance of natural origin that produces certain symptoms in a healthy person will cure those same symptoms in a sick person.

Laws of cure—A set of three rules used by homeopaths to assess the progress of a patient's recovery.

Materia medica—In homeopathy, reference books compiled from provings of the various natural remedies.

Miasm—In homeopathic theory, a general weakness or predisposition to chronic disease that is transmitted down the generational chain.

Modalities—The factors and circumstances that cause a patient's symptoms to improve or worsen, including weather, time of day, effects of food, and similar factors.

Repertories—Homeopathic reference books consisting of descriptions of symptoms. The process of selecting a homeopathic remedy from the patient's symptom profile is called repertorizing.

There continue to be many studies that affirm the effectiveness of homeopathic treatments. Among the most celebrated, the *British Medical Journal* in 1991 published a large analysis of homeopathic treatments that were given over the course of 25 years. This project involved over 100 studies of patients with problems ranging from vascular diseases, respiratory problems, infections, stomach problems, **allergies**, recovery from surgeries, arthritis, trauma, psychological problems, diabetes, and others. The study found improvement with homeopathic treatment in most

categories of problems, and concluded that the evidence was "sufficient for establishing homeopathy as a regular treatment for certain indications."

In the United Kingdom and other countries where homeopathy is especially popular, some medical doctors incorporate aspects of acute prescribing homeopathy into their practices. Countries in which homeopathy is popular include France, India, Pakistan, Sri Lanka, Brazil, and Argentina. Large homeopathic hospitals exist in London and Glasgow, and homeopathic medical centers can be found in India and South America.

Resources

BOOKS

Strohecker, James. *Alternative Medicine: The DefinitiveGuide*. Tiburon, Calif.: Future Medicine Publishing, Inc.,1999.

ORGANIZATIONS

American Institute of Homeopathy. 1585 Glencoe, Denver, CO 80220. (303) 898-5477.

Council for Homeopathic Certification. P.O. Box 157, Corte Madera, CA 94976.

International Foundation for Homeopathy. 2366 Eastlake Avenue East, #301, Seattle, WA 98102. (425) 776-4147.

National Center for Homeopathy. 801 North Fairfax Street, Suite 306, Alexandria, VA 22134. (703) 548-7790.

North American Society of Homeopaths. 10700 Old County Rd. 15, #350, Minneapolis, MN 55441. (612) 593-9458.

Homocysteine

Definition

Homocysteine is a naturally occurring amino acid found in blood plasma. High levels of homocysteine in the blood are believed to increase the chance of heart disease, **stroke**, **Alzheimer's disease**, and **osteoporosis**.

Description

Homocysteine is a sulfur-containing amino acid that occurs naturally in all humans. It is broken down in the body through two metabolic pathways. The chemical changes that must occur to break down homocysteine require the presence of **folic acid** (also called folate) and **vitamins** B^6 and B^{12}. The level of homocysteine in the blood is influenced by the presence of these substances.

Homocystinuria is a rare genetic disorder that occurs in about one in every 200,000 individuals. This congenital metabolic disorder causes large amounts of homocysteine to be excreted in the urine. Homocystinuria is associated **mental retardation** and the development of heart disease before age 30.

In the late 1960s, doctors documented that individuals with homocystinuria developed narrowing of the arteries at a very early age, sometimes even in childhood. Although homocystinuria is rare, this finding stimulated research on whether people who did not have homocystinuria but who did have unusually high levels of homocysteine in their blood were at greater risk of developing heart disease or stroke.

Many risk factors, including family history of heart disease, **smoking**, **obesity**, lack of **exercise**, diabetes, high levels of low-density lipoprotein cholesterol (LDL or "bad" cholesterol), low levels of high-density lipoprotein cholesterol (HDL or "good" cholesterol), and high blood pressure have been documented to increase the risk of stroke and heart disease. With so many other risk factors, it has been difficult to determine whether high levels of homocysteine are an independent risk factor for the development these diseases. However, a substantial number of controlled, well-designed, and well-documented studies have shown that individuals who have high levels of homocysteine in the blood are at increased risk of developing blocked blood vessels, a condition known as occlusive arterial disease or at risk to worsen **atherosclerosis** ("hardening of the arteries").

In the 2000s, studies also suggested that high levels of homocysteine were associated with poorer mental functioning, leading to ongoing investigations into the role of homocysteine in Alzheimer's disease. Additional studies have also suggested that high levels of homocysteine can lead to osteoporosis and an increased risk of broken bones in the elderly. As of 2005, homocysteine was being tested in half a dozen clinical trials to determine its role in these and several other conditions. Information on clinical trials that are enrolling patients can be found on-line at < http://www.clinicaltrials.gov >.

Causes and symptoms

Homocysteine is thought to irritate the lining of the blood vessels causing them to become scarred, hardened, and narrowed. This increases the work the heart must do, leading to heart disease. High levels of homocysteine also cause increased blood clotting. **Blood clots** can decrease or block the flow of blood through blood vessels, resulting in strokes and heart

attacks. If and how homocysteine directly plays a role in osteoporosis and Alzheimer's disease is not clear as of 2005.

The level of homocysteine in the blood naturally varies with age, gender, diet, hereditary factors, and general health, but it is estimated that 5–10% of the population has homocysteine levels that are considered high. With the exception of rare individuals who have congenital homocystinuria, people with high blood levels of homocysteine do not have any obvious signs or symptoms.

Diagnosis

The American Heart Association and the American College of Cardiology do not recommend routine screening of homocysteine levels, but they do recommend screening as part of a cardiac risk assessment for individuals who have a family history of **coronary artery disease** but no obvious symptoms of heart disease. The level of homocysteine in the blood can be measured with a simple blood test that is often, but not always, done after **fasting**. Homocysteine levels of 12 mmol/L are considered normal and levels below 10 mmol/L are considered desirable.

Treatment

Lowering homocysteine blood levels is linked to increasing the intake of folic acid and vitamins B_6 and B_{12}. The healthiest way to increase intake is by eating more foods that are high in these substances. Good sources of folic acid, vitamin B_6 and B_{12} include green leafy vegetables, fortified breakfast cereals, lentils, chickpeas, asparagus, spinach, and most beans. Taking a daily multivitamin is also a way to increase the levels of these substances. However, megadoses of folic acid, vitamin B_6 and B_{12} are not recommended. Individuals should discuss dosage with their doctor before beginning any supplements. It is important to note that a direct link between increased intake of folic acid, vitamin B_6, and vitamin B_{12} and decreased incidence stroke and **heart attack** has not been proved. However, one study published in the *Journal of the American Medical Association* found that women whose folic acid levels were in the lowest 25% were 69% more likely to die of coronary problems than women whose folic acid levels were in the top 25%.

Individuals with homocystinuria are treated with the drug betaine (Cystadane). This is a powder dissolved in water, juice, or milk and drunk usually twice a day with meals. This drug is not normally used

KEY TERMS

Alzheimer's disease—A degenerative brain disease of unknown origin that is a common cause of dementia in older individuals.

Amino acid—A nitrogen-containing building block of protein molecules.

Androgens—Male sex hormones.

Congenital—Present at birth.

Osteoporosis—Loss of minerals from the bones, causing bones to break more easily.

Plasma—The liquid part of the blood in which cells are suspended.

simply to lower high levels of homocysteine in the absence of congenital disease.

Prognosis

Individuals who increase the folic acid, vitamin B_6 and B_{12} in their diet are expected to see a decrease in blood levels of homocysteine and as a result decrease their risk of heart disease and stroke.

Prevention

Certain drugs are suspected of increasing the level of homocysteine in the blood. People using these drugs should discuss with their doctor the advisability of increasing their intake of folic acid, vitamin B_6, and vitamin B_{12}. These drugs include:

- lipid-lowering drugs such as fenofibrate (Tricor) and bezafibrate (Bezalip)
- metformin (Glucophage), a drug to modify insulin resistance
- anti-epileptic drugs such as phenobarbital, phenytoin (Dilantin), primidone (Mysoline) and carbamazepine (Tegretol)
- levadopa (Sinemet) for treatment of Parkinson's disease
- methotrexate (Rheumatrex, Trexall) for treatment of **cancer**, **psoriasis**, **rheumatoid arthritis**, and systemic lupus erythematosus
- androgen treatment
- nitrous oxide ("laughing gas"), a mild anesthetic

Resources

BOOKS

McCully, Kilmer S. *The Homocysteine Revolution.* 2nd ed. New York: McGraw Hill 1999.

PERIODICALS

McLean, Robert R., et al. "Homocysteine as a Predictive Factor for Hip Fracture in Older Persons." *New England Journal of Medicine*, 350 (May 13, 2004): 2042–49 [cited 23 March 2005]. < http://content.nejm.org/cgi/content/abstract/350/20/2042 >.

Morey, Sharon S. "Practice Guidelines: AHA and ACC Outline Approaches to Coronary Disease Risk Assessment." *American Family Physician*, 61, no. 8 (April 15, 2000): 2534–44 [cited March 23, 2005]. < http://www.aafp.org/afp/2000415/practice.html >.

ORGANIZATIONS

American Heart Association. 7272 Greenville Ave., Dallas, TX 75231. (800)242-8721. < http://www.americanheart.org >.

OTHER

Homocysteine.net, May 10, 2004. [cited March 23, 2005]. < http://www.homocysteine.net >

Tish Davidson, A.M.

Hong Kong flu *see* **Influenza**

Hookworm disease

Definition

Hookworm disease is an illness caused by one of two types of S-shaped worms that infect the intestine of humans (the worm's host).

Description

Two types of hookworm are responsible for hookworm disease in humans. *Necator americanus* and *Ancylostoma duodenale* have similar life cycles and similar methods of causing illness. The adult worm of both *Necator americanus* and *Ancylostoma duodenale* is about 10 mm long, pinkish-white in color, and curved into an S-shape or double hook.

Both types of hookworm have similar life cycles. The females produce about 10,000–20,000 eggs per day. These eggs are passed out of the host's body in feces. The eggs enter the soil, where they incubate. After about 48 hours, the immature larval form hatches out of the eggs. These larvae take about six weeks to develop into the mature larval form that is capable of causing human infection. If exposed to human skin at this point (usually bare feet walking in the dirt or bare hands digging in the dirt), the larvae will bore through the skin and ride through the lymph circulation to the right side of the heart. The larvae are then pumped into

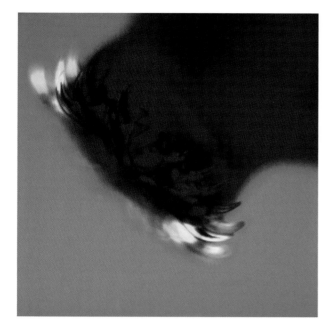

A **micrograph image of the head of the hookworm** *Ancylostoma spp. (Photo Researchers, Inc. Reproduced by permission.)*

the lungs. There they bore into the tiny air sacs (alveoli) of the lungs. Their presence within the lungs usually causes enough irritation to produce coughing. The larvae are coughed up into the throat and mouth, and are then swallowed and passed into the small intestine. It is within the intestine that they develop into the adult worm, producing illness in their human host.

Ancylostoma duodenale is found primarily in the Mediterranean, the Middle East, and throughout Asia. *Necator americanus* is common in tropical areas including Asia, parts of the Americas, and throughout Africa. Research suggests that at least 25% of all people in the world have hookworm disease. In the United States, 700,000 people are believed to be infected with hookworms at any given time.

Causes and symptoms

Hookworms cause trouble for their human host when the worms attach their mouths to the lining of the small intestine and suck the person's blood.

An itchy, slightly raised rash called "ground itch" may appear around the area where the larvae first bored through the skin. The skin in this area may become red and swollen. This lasts for several days and commonly occurs between the toes.

When the larvae are in the lungs, the patient may have a **fever**, **cough**, and some **wheezing**. Some people, however, have none of these symptoms.

Once established within the intestine, the adult worms can cause abdominal **pain**, decreased appetite, **diarrhea**, and weight loss. Most importantly, the worms suck between 0.03–0.2 ml of blood per day. When a worm moves from one area of the intestine to another, it detaches its mouth from the intestinal lining, leaving an irritated area that may continue to bleed for some time. This results in even further blood loss. A single adult worm can live for up to 14 years in a patient's intestine. Over time, the patient's blood loss may be very significant. Anemia is the most serious complication of hookworm disease, progressing over months or years. Children are particularly harmed by such anemia, and can suffer from heart problems, mental retardation, slowed growth, and delayed sexual development. In infants, hookworm disease can be deadly.

Diagnosis

Diagnosis of hookworm disease involves collecting a stool sample for examination under a microscope. Hookworm eggs have a characteristic appearance. Counting the eggs in a specific amount of feces allows the healthcare provider to estimate the severity of the infection.

Treatment

Minor infections are often left untreated, especially in areas where hookworm is very common. If treatment is required, the doctor will prescribe a three-day dose of medication. One to two weeks later, another stool sample will be taken to see if the infection is still present.

Anemia is treated with iron supplements. In severe cases, blood **transfusion** may be necessary. Two medications, pyrantel pamoate and mebendazole, are frequently used with good results.

Prognosis

The prognosis for patients with hookworm disease is generally good. However, reinfection rates are extremely high in countries with poor sanitation.

Prevention

Prevention of hookworm disease involves improving sanitation and avoiding contact with soil in areas with high rates of hookworm infection. Children should be required to wear shoes when playing outside in such areas, and people who are gardening should wear gloves.

Resources

ORGANIZATIONS

Centers for Disease Control and Prevention. 1600 Clifton Rd., NE, Atlanta, GA 30333. (800) 311-3435, (404) 639-3311. <http://www.cdc.gov>.

Rosalyn Carson-DeWitt, MD

Hormone replacement therapy

Definition

Hormone replacement therapy (HRT) is the use of synthetic or natural female hormones to make up for the decline or lack of natural hormones produced in a woman's body. HRT is sometimes referred to as estrogen replacement therapy (ERT), because the first medications that were used in the 1960s for female hormone replacement were estrogen compounds.

Estrogens

In order to understand how HRT works and the controversies surrounding it, women should know that there are different types of estrogen medications commonly prescribed in the United States and Europe. These drugs are given in a variety of prescription strengths and methods of administration. There are at present three estrogen compounds used in Western countries. Only the first two are readily available in the United States.

- Estrone. Estrone is the form of estrogen present in women after **menopause**. It is available as tablets under the brand name Ogen. The most commonly prescribed estrogen in the United States, Premarin, is a so-called conjugated estrogen that is a mixture of estrone and other estrogens.

- Estradiol. This is the form of estrogen naturally present in perimenopausal women. It is available as tablets (Estrace), skin patches (Estraderm), or vaginal creams (Estrace).

- Estriol. Estriol is a weaker form of estrogen produced by the breakdown of other forms of estrogen in the body. This is the form of estrogen most commonly given in Europe, under the brand name Estriol. It is the only form that is thought not to cause **cancer**.

In addition to pills taken by mouth, skin patches, and vaginal creams, estrogen preparations can be given by injection or by pellets implanted under the skin. Estrogen implants, however, are used less and less frequently.

Progestins

Most HRT programs include progestin treatment with estrogen compounds. Progestins—sometimes called progestogens—are synthetic forms of progesterone that are given to reduce the possibility that estrogen by itself will cause cancer of the uterus. Progestins are commonly prescribed under the brand names Provera and **Depo-Provera**. Other common brand names are Norlutate, Norlutin, and Aygestin.

Estrogen/testosterone combinations

Women's ovaries secrete small amounts of a male sex hormone (testosterone) throughout their lives. Women who have had both ovaries removed by surgery are sometimes given testosterone along with estrogen as part of HRT. Combinations of these hormones are available as tablets under the brand name Estratest or as vaginal creams. Women who cannot take estrogens can use 1% testosterone cream alone for problems with vaginal soreness.

Estrogen/tranquilizer combinations

There are several medications that combine estrogen with a tranquilizer like chlordiazepoxide (sold under the trade name Menrium) or meprobamate (sold under the trade name PMB). Many doctors warn against these combination drugs because the tranquilizers can be habit-forming.

Purpose

Hormone replacement therapy has been prescribed for two primary purposes: preventive treatment against **osteoporosis** and heart disease; and relief of physical symptoms associated with menopause.

Menopausal symptoms

Women in midlife enter a stage of development called menopause, when their menstrual periods become irregular and finally stop. The early phase of this transition is called the perimenopause. In the United States, the average age at menopause is presently 50 or 51, but some women begin menopause as early as 40 and others as late as 55. It can take as long as 10 years for a woman to complete the process. Women who have had their ovaries removed surgically are said to have undergone surgical menopause.

Doctors have not always agreed on definitions of menopause. Some use age as the baseline. Others define menopause as the point when a woman has had no menstrual periods for a full calendar year. Still others define menopause as the end of ovulation. It is not always clear, however, when a woman has had her last period or when she has stopped ovulating. In addition, women who take **oral contraceptives** can have breakthrough bleeding long after they have stopped ovulating. As a result, some doctors now measure the level of follicle-stimulating hormone (FSH) in a woman's blood to estimate whether the woman has entered menopause. During perimenopause, the FSH levels in a woman's blood rise as her body attempts to stimulate the release of ripe ova. An FSH level over 40 is considered an indicator of menopause.

During the menopausal transition, the levels of estrogen in the woman's body drop. The lowered estrogen level is responsible for a group of symptoms that include hot flashes (or flushes), weight gain, changes in skin texture, mood swings, heart **palpitations**, sleep disturbances, a need to urinate more frequently, and loss of sexual desire. The estrogen that is given in HRT has been shown to eliminate hot flashes, night sweats, lack of vaginal lubrication, and urinary tract problems. HRT will not prevent weight gain or wrinkles. It also does not cure depression in most women.

Preventive care

HRT has been recommended by some doctors to protect women against two serious midlife health problems, including osteoporosis and heart disease.

While clinical trials have continued to demonstrate HRT's effectiveness in preventing osteoporosis, women must weigh the risk of the therapy with the benefits. The trials also showed that HRT actually increased rather than decreased risk of heart disease.

OSTEOPOROSIS. Osteoporosis is a disorder in which the bones become more brittle and more easily fractured. It is a particular problem for postmenopausal women because the lower levels of estrogen in the blood lead to weakening of the bone. About 25% of Caucasian women will develop severe osteoporosis; Asian women have a slightly lower risk level; Latino and African American women are least at risk.

In addition to race, there are other factors that put some women at higher risk of developing osteoporosis. Women in any of the following groups should take bone loss into account when considering HRT:

- family history of osteoporosis
- menopause before age 40
- kidney disease and dialysis
- thin body build or being underweight
- history of colitis, **Crohn's disease**, or chronic **diarrhea**
- thyroid medications
- childlessness
- chronic use of **antacids**
- lack of **exercise**
- poor food choices, including high salt intake, lack of vitamin D, high **caffeine** consumption, and low calcium intake
- **smoking** and alcohol **abuse**
- cortisone therapy

HEART DISEASE. Heart disease is a major health concern of women in midlife. It is the leading cause of **death** in women over 60. The primary disorders of the circulatory system in postmenopausal women are **stroke**, **hypertension**, and **coronary artery disease**. While doctors once believed that HRT helped decrease heart disease and stroke among postmenopausal women, a major clinical trial discovered the opposite to be true. In 2002, the Women's Health Initiative (WHI) stopped giving HRT to the women enrolled in the study because of adverse effects. Among these effects was a 29% increase in coronary heart disease and 41% increase in stroke in postmenopausal women taking HRT.

Other major factors that are known to increase the risk of heart disease include:

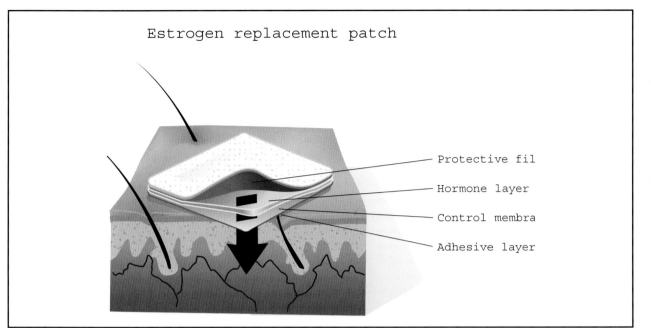

Estrogen replacement patch

— Protective fil

— Hormone layer

— Control membra

— Adhesive layer

Estrogen replacement patches adhere to a patient's skin and slowly administer estrogen to the body. *(Illustration by Argosy Inc.)*

- history of smoking
- being overweight
- high-fat **diets**
- alcohol abuse
- family history of heart disease
- high blood pressure
- high blood cholesterol levels
- diabetes.

Less important risk factors include being African American, having a sedentary lifestyle, undergoing menopause before age 45, and having high levels of family- or job-related **stress**.

Precautions

Medical conditions

The findings of the WHI presented new problems for the women relying on hormones to ease their transition to menopause and postmenopausal years and for doctors prescribing HRT. The combination of estrogen and progesterone also was found to increase risk of invasive **breast cancer** by 26%, which was the reason researchers halted the study. In addition, while some clinicians have thought that HRT helped delay **dementia** (a disorder of the mind that affects memory and perception), the

WHI also found that combined estrogen/progesterone increased the risk of probable dementia in women age 65 and older. Physicians and women were advised not to panic about HRT, however. Short-term use of the therapy may not produce these risks. Women have been advised to meet with their physicians and weigh the benefits against the risks on an individual basis.

Certain groups of women should not use HRT. They include women with:

- breast cancer
- cancer of the uterus
- heart disease
- abnormal vaginal bleeding that has not been diagnosed
- high blood pressure that rises when HRT is used
- liver disease
- **gallstones** or diseases of the gallbladder

Drug interactions

HRT can interact with other prescription medications that a woman may be taking. Women who are taking **corticosteroids**, drugs to slow the clotting of blood (anticoagulants), and rifampin should ask their doctor about possible interactions.

Combining estrogens with certain other medicines can cause liver damage. Among the drugs that may cause liver damage when taken with estrogens are:

- acetaminophen (Tylenol), when used in high doses over long periods

- anabolic steroids such as nandrolone (Anabolin) or oxymetholone (Anadrol)

- medicine for infections

- antiseizure medicines such as divalproex (Depakote), valproic acid (Depakene), or phenytoin (Dilantin)

- antianxiety drugs, including chlorpromazine (Thorazine), prochlorperazine (Compazine), and thioridazine (Mellaril).

In addition, estrogens may interfere with the effects of bromocriptine (Parlodel), used to treat Parkinson's disease and other conditions; they may also increase the chance of toxic side effects when taken with cyclosporine (Sandimmune), a drug that helps prevent organ transplant rejection.

Description

HRT medications come in several different forms, including tablets, stick-on patches, injections, and creams that are worn inside the vagina. The form prescribed depends on the purpose of the hormone replacement therapy. Women who want relief from vaginal dryness, for example, would be given a cream or vaginal ring. Women using HRT to relieve hot flashes or to prevent osteoporosis and heart disease often prefer oral medications or patches. All HRT medications used in the United States are available only with a doctor's prescription.

HRT treatment regimens

One of the complications of HRT is the number of treatment options, including combinations of types of estrogen; dosage levels; forms of administration; and whether or not progestins are used with the estrogen to offset the risk of uterine cancer. This variety, however, means that a woman who wants to use HRT while minimizing side effects can try different forms of medication or dosage schedules when she consults her doctor. It is vital, however, for women to follow their doctor's directions exactly and not change dosages themselves.

At present, women who are taking a combination of estrogens and progestins are placed on one of three dosage schedules:

- Estrogen pills taken daily from the first through the 25th day of each month, with a progestin pill taken daily during the last 10–14 days of the cycle. Both

drugs are then stopped for the next five to six days to allow the uterus to shed its lining.

- Estrogen pills taken on a daily basis with low-dose progestin pills, also on a daily basis. Both medications are taken continuously with no days off.

- Estrogen pills and low-dose progestins taken on a daily basis for five days each week, with both medications stopped on the last two days of each week.

TIMING AND LENGTH OF TREATMENT. One of the disagreements about HRT concerns the best time to begin using it. Some doctors think that women should begin using HRT while they are still in perimenopause. Others think that there is no harm in a woman's waiting to decide. Either way, the question of timing means that a woman should keep track of changes in her periods and other signs of perimenopause so that her doctor can evaluate her readiness for HRT.

The other question of timing concerns length of treatment. Some women use HRT only as long as they need it to relieve the symptoms of menopause. Others regard it as a lifetime commitment because of concerns about osteoporosis. One study found that the average length of time that women stay on HRT is 23 months. Information from the WHI released in 2002 and 2003 would indicate that long-term HRT use produced too many risks for the expected benefits.

UNWANTED SIDE EFFECTS. In addition to the identified health risks mentioned above, much of the disagreement about unwanted side effects from HRT concerns the role of progestins in the estrogen/progestin combinations that are commonly prescribed. Many women who find that estrogen relieves hot flashes and other symptoms of menopause have the opposite experience with progestin. Progestin frequently causes moodiness, depression, sore breasts, weight gain, and severe headaches.

Other treatment approaches

Women who are uncertain about HRT, or who should not take estrogens, should know about other treatment options, such as natural progesterone. Progestins, which are synthetic hormones, were developed because natural progesterone cannot be absorbed in the body when taken in pill form. A new technique called micronization has made it possible for women to take natural progesterone by mouth. Many women prefer this form of hormone because it lacks the side effects of the synthetic progestins even though it is somewhat more expensive. The most common form of natural progesterone is called Prometrium. which is available by prescription only. Another form of natural progesterone consists of the hormone suspended in vitamin E oil. It is absorbed through the skin and is available without a prescription.

Alternative therapies also are available. Many mainstream as well as alternative practitioners recommend changes in diet and **nutrition** as helpful during menopause. Women who limit their intake of fats and salts, increase their use of fresh fruits and vegetables, quit smoking, and drink only in moderation often find that these dietary changes help them feel better. Naturopaths typically recommend vitamin and mineral supplements for general well-being as well as for relief from hot flashes and leg cramps. In addition, herbal teas and tonics are helpful to some women in treating water retention, **insomnia**, **constipation**, or moodiness.

Women who find menopause emotionally stressful because of negative social attitudes toward older women are often helped by **meditation**, **biofeedback**, therapeutic massage, and other relaxation techniques. **Yoga** and **tai chi** provide physical exercise as well as **stress reduction**. Exercise is an important safeguard against osteoporosis.

Preparation

Women who are considering HRT should visit their doctor for a series of tests to make sure that they do not have any serious health disorders. They should have a Pap smear and breast examination to rule out cancer. They also should have a **urinalysis**, a **bone density test**, and blood tests to measure their red blood cell level, blood sugar level, cholesterol level, and liver and thyroid function.

In addition to these tests, most doctors will also give a progesterone challenge test. It consists of doses of progesterone given over a 10-day period to see if the woman is still producing her own estrogen. If she bleeds at the end of the test, she is still producing estrogen.

Aftercare

Aftercare is a very important part of HRT. Women who are taking HRT will need to see their doctor more frequently. At a minimum, they should be checked twice a year with a blood pressure test and breast examination. They should have a complete physical on a yearly basis. Any abnormal bleeding must be reported to the doctor as soon as it occurs. The doctor will need to order a tissue biopsy or dilation and curettage (D & C) in order to rule out cancer of the uterus.

Women who are taking HRT and decide to stop should taper their dosage over a period of several months rather than discontinuing abruptly. A gradual reduction minimizes the possibility of hot flashes and other side effects.

KEY TERMS

Dilation and curettage (D & C)—A surgical procedure in which the patient's cervix is widened (dilated) and the endometrium is scraped with a scoop-shaped instrument (curette).

Estrogen—The primary sex hormone that controls normal sexual development in females. During the menstrual cycle, estrogen helps prepare the body for possible pregnancy.

Follicle-stimulating hormone (FSH)—A hormone produced by the pituitary gland that stimulates the follicles in the ovaries to swell and release ripe ova. Doctors sometimes use its levels in a woman's blood to evaluate whether she is in menopause.

Hormone—A substance secreted by an endocrine gland that is carried by blood or other body fluids to its target tissues or organs.

Hot flash—A warm or hot sensation on the face, neck and upper body, sometimes accompanied by flushing and sweating. Some women refer to hot flashes as hot flushes.

Osteoporosis—A bone disorder in which the bones become brittle, porous, and easily broken. It is a major health concern for postmenopausal women.

Ovary—The female sex gland that produces eggs and female reproductive hormones.

Ovulation—The cyclical process of egg maturation and release from the ovary.

Progesterone—A female hormone produced by the ovary. It functions to prepare the lining of the uterus to receive a fertilized ovum.

Progesterone challenge test—A test that is given to see if a woman is still secreting estrogen. It consists of doses of progesterone given over a 10-day period.

Progestin—Synthetic progesterone available as an oral medication.

Testosterone—A male sex hormone that is sometimes given as part of HRT to women whose ovaries have been removed. Testosterone helps with problems of sexual desire.

Uterus—The hollow organ in women in which fertilized eggs develop during pregnancy. The uterus is sometimes called the womb.

Risks

The short-term risks associated with HRT include a range of physical side effects. Common side effects include fluid retention, bloating, weight gain, sore breasts, leg cramps, vaginal discharges, migraine headaches, hair loss, **nausea and vomiting**, **acne**, depression, **shortness of breath**, and **dizziness**. Potentially serious side effects include tissue growths in the uterus (fibroids), gallstones, **thrombophlebitis**, **hypoglycemia**, abnormal growth (hyperplasia) of uterine tissue, thyroid disorders, high blood pressure, and cancer.

Long-term risks should be discussed with a woman's physicians before considering hormone replacement therapy. Identified risks for combined (estrogen plus progestin) HRT use include increased incidence of invasive breast cancer, stroke, heart disease, and **pulmonary embolism**.

Normal results

Normal results of HRT include relief of hot flashes, night sweats, vaginal dryness, and urinary symptoms associated with menopause.

Resources

BOOKS

Goldman, Lee, et al, editors. *Cecil Textbook of Medicine.* 21st ed. W. B. Saunders, 2000.

Goroll, Alan H. *Primary Care Medicine.* 4th ed. Lippincott Williams & Wilkins, 2000.

PERIODICALS

Doering, Paul L. "Treatment of Menopause Post-WHI: What Now?" *Drug Topics* April 21, 2003: 85.

Elliott, William T. "HRT, Estrogen, and Postmenopausal Women: Year-old WHI Study Continues to Raise Questions." *Critical Care Alert* July 2003: 1.

OTHER

Menopausal Hormone Replacement Therapy. Fact sheet. National Cancer Institute. < http://rex.nci.nih.gov >.

Laith Farid Gulli, M.D.
Teresa G. Odle

Hospital-acquired infections

Definition

A hospital-acquired infection is usually one that first appears three days after a patient is admitted to a hospital or other health care facility. Infections acquired in a hospital are also called nosocomial infections.

Description

About 5–10% of patients admitted to hospitals in the United States develop a nosocomial infection. The Centers for Disease Control and Prevention (CDC) estimate that more than two million patients develop hospital-acquired infections in the United States each year. About 90,000 of these patients die as a result of their infections. Hospital-acquired infections usually are related to a procedure or treatment used to diagnose or treat the patient's illness or injury. About 25% of these infections can be prevented by healthcare workers taking proper precautions when caring for patients.

Hospital-acquired infections can be caused by bacteria, viruses, fungi, or parasites. These microorganisms may already be present in the patient's body or may come from the environment, contaminated hospital equipment, health care workers, or other patients. Depending on the causal agents involved, an infection may start in any part of the body. A localized infection is limited to a specific part of the body and has local symptoms. For example, if a surgical wound in the abdomen becomes infected, the area of the wound becomes red, hot, and painful. A generalized infection is one that enters the bloodstream and causes general systemic symptoms such as **fever**, chills, low blood pressure, or mental confusion.

Hospital-acquired infections may develop from surgical procedures, catheters placed in the urinary tract or blood vessels, or from material from the nose or mouth that is inhaled into the lungs. The most common types of hospital-acquired infections are urinary tract infections (UTIs), pneumonia, and surgical wound infections.

Causes and symptoms

All hospitalized patients are susceptible to contracting a nosocomial infection. Some patients are at greater risk than others—young children, the elderly, and persons with compromised immune systems are more likely to get an infection. Other risk factors for getting a hospital-acquired infection are a long hospital stay, the use of indwelling catheters, failure of healthcare workers to wash their hands, and overuse of **antibiotics**.

Any type of invasive procedure can expose a patient to the possibility of infection. Common causes of hospital-acquired infections include:

- urinary bladder catheterization
- respiratory procedures
- surgery and **wounds**
- intravenous (IV) procedures

Urinary tract infection (UTI) is the most common type of hospital-acquired infection. Most hospital-acquired UTIs happen after urinary catheterization. Catheterization is the placement of a catheter through the urethra into the urinary bladder. This procedure is done to empty urine from the bladder, relieve pressure in the bladder, measure urine in the bladder, put medicine into the bladder, or for other medical reasons.

The healthy urinary bladder is sterile, which means it doesn't have any bacteria or other microorganisms in it. There may be bacteria in or around the urethra but they normally cannot enter the bladder. A catheter can pick up bacteria from the urethra and allow them into the bladder, causing an infection to start.

Bacteria from the intestinal tract are the most common type to cause UTIs. Patients with poorly functioning immune systems or who are taking antibiotics are also at risk for infection by a fungus called *Candida*.

Pneumonia is the second most common type of hospital-acquired infection. Bacteria and other microorganisms are easily brought into the throat by respiratory procedures commonly done in the hospital. The microorganisms come from contaminated equipment or the hands of health care workers. Some of these procedures are respiratory intubation, suctioning of material from the throat and mouth, and mechanical ventilation. The introduced microorganisms quickly colonize the throat area. This means that they grow and form a colony, but do not yet cause an infection. Once the throat is colonized, it is easy for a patient to inhale the microorganisms into the lungs.

Patients who cannot **cough** or gag very well are most likely to inhale colonized microorganisms into their lungs. Some respiratory procedures can keep patients from gagging or coughing. Patients who are sedated or who lose consciousness may also be unable to cough or gag. The inhaled microorganisms grow in the lungs and cause an infection that can lead to pneumonia.

Surgical procedures increase a patient's risk of getting an infection in the hospital. Surgery directly invades the patient's body, giving bacteria a way into normally sterile parts of the body. An infection can be acquired from contaminated surgical equipment or from healthcare workers. Following surgery, the surgical wound can become infected. Other wounds from trauma, burns, and ulcers may also become infected.

Many hospitalized patients need a steady supply of medications or nutrients delivered to their bloodstream. An intravenous (IV) catheter is placed in a vein and the medication or other substance is infused into the vein. Bacteria transmitted from the surroundings, contaminated equipment, or healthcare workers' hands can invade the site where the catheter is inserted. A local infection may develop in the skin around the catheter. The bacteria also can enter the blood through the vein and cause a generalized infection. The longer a catheter is in place, the greater the risk of infection.

Other hospital procedures that put patients at risk for nosocomial infection are gastrointestinal procedures, obstetric procedures, and kidney dialysis.

Fever is often the first sign of infection. Other symptoms and signs of infection are rapid breathing, mental confusion, low blood pressure, reduced urine output, and a high white blood cell count.

Patients with a UTI may have **pain** when urinating and blood in the urine. Symptoms of pneumonia may include difficulty breathing and coughing. A localized infection causes swelling, redness, and tenderness at the site of infection.

Diagnosis

An infection is suspected any time a hospitalized patient develops a fever that cannot be explained by a known illness. Some patients, especially the elderly, may not develop a fever. In these patients, the first signs of infection may be rapid breathing or mental confusion.

Diagnosis of a hospital-acquired infection is based on:

- symptoms and signs of infection
- examination of wounds and catheter entry sites
- review of procedures that might have led to infection
- laboratory test results

A complete **physical examination** is conducted in order to locate symptoms and signs of infection. Wounds and the skin where catheters have been placed are examined for redness, swelling, or the presence of pus or an **abscess**. The physician reviews the patient's record of procedures performed in the hospital to determine if any posed a risk for infection.

Laboratory tests are done to look for signs of infection. A complete **blood count** can reveal if the white blood cell count is high. White blood cells are immune system cells that increase in numbers in response to an infection. White blood cells or blood may be present in the urine when there is a UTI.

Cultures of blood, urine, sputum, other body fluids, or tissue are done to look for infectious microorganisms. If an infection is present, it is necessary to identify the microorganism so the patient can be treated with the correct medication. A sample of the fluid or tissue is placed in a special medium that bacteria will grow in. Other tests can also be done on blood and body fluids to look for and identify bacteria, fungi, viruses, or other microorganisms responsible for an infection.

If a patient has symptoms suggestive of pneumonia, a chest x ray is done to look for infiltrates of white blood cells and other inflammatory substances in the lung tissue. Samples of sputum can be studied with a microscope or cultured to look for bacteria or fungi.

Treatment

Once the source of the infection is identified, the patient is treated with antibiotics or other medication that kills the responsible microorganism. Many different antibiotics are available that are effective against different bacteria. Some common antibiotics are penicillin, **cephalosporins**, **tetracyclines**, and erythromycin. More and more commonly, some types of bacteria are becoming resistant to the standard antibiotic treatments. When this happens, a different, more powerful antibiotic must be used. Two strong antibiotics that have been effective against resistant bacteria are vancomycin and imipenem, although some bacteria are developing resistance to these antibiotics as well.

Fungal infections are treated with antifungal medications. Examples of these are amphotericin B, nystatin, ketoconazole, itraconazole, and fluconazole.

A number of **antiviral drugs** have been developed that slow the growth or reproduction of viruses. Acyclovir, ganciclovir, foscarnet, and amantadine are examples of antiviral medications.

Prognosis

Hospital-acquired infections are serious illnesses that cause **death** in about 1% of cases. Rapid diagnosis and identification of the responsible microorganism is necessary, so treatment can be started as soon as possible.

Prevention

Hospitals and other healthcare facilities have developed extensive **infection control** programs to

prevent nosocomial infections. These programs focus on identifying high risk procedures and other possible sources of infection. High risk procedures such as **urinary catheterization** should be performed only when necessary and catheters should be left in for as little time as possible. Medical instruments and equipment must be properly sterilized to ensure they are not contaminated. Frequent handwashing by healthcare workers and visitors is necessary to avoid passing infectious microorganisms to hospitalized patients. In 2003, the Joint Commission on Accreditation of Healthcare Organizations (JCAHO) announced it would make prevention of nosocomial infections a major goal in 2004 and the coming years. JCAHO, the body that inspects hospitals for quality and accredits them accordingly, issued an alert stating that hospital-acquired infections are seriously underreported. The problem has become more serious for hospitals to address as many bacteria are becoming resistant to antibiotics.

Antibiotics should be used only when necessary. Use of antibiotics creates favorable conditions for infection with the fungal organism *Candida*. Overuse of antibiotics is also responsible for the development of bacteria that are resistant to antibiotics.

Resources

PERIODICALS

Burke, John P. "Infection Control—A Problem for Patient Safety." *The New England Journal of Medicine* February 13, 2003: 651–656.

"Hospital-Acquired Infections are Being Underreported."
RN March 2003: 16.
"Nosocomial Infection (From the Editor)." *Health Care Food & Nutrition Focus* June 2003: 2.

Toni Rizzo
Teresa G. Odle

Hot-spot imaging *see* **Technetium heart scan**

HRT *see* **Hormone replacement therapy**

HTLV-1 associated myelopathy *see* **Tropical spastic paraparesis**

HTLV-1 infection *see* **Tropical spastic paraparesis**

Human-potential movement

Definition

The human-potential movement is a term used for humanistic psychotherapies that first became popular in the 1960s and early 1970s. The movement emphasized the development of individuals through such techniques as encounter groups, sensitivity training, and primal therapy. Although the human-potential movement and humanistic therapy are sometimes used as synonyms, in reality, humanistic therapy preceded the human-potential movement and provided the movement's theoretical base. Humanistic therapy flourished in the 1940s and 1950s. Its theorists were mostly psychologists rather than medical doctors. They included Gordon Allport, Abraham Maslow, Everett Shostrom, Carl Rogers, and Fritz Perls.

The human-potential movement and humanistic therapy is distinguished by the following emphases:

- A concern for what is uniquely human rather than what humans share with other animals.

- A focus on each person's open-ended growth rather than reshaping individuals to fit society's demands.

- An interest in the here-and-now rather than in a person's childhood history or supposed unconscious conflicts.

- A holistic approach concerned with all levels of human being and functioning—not just the intellectual—including creative and spiritual functioning.

- A focus on psychological health rather than disturbance.

Purpose

The purpose of humanistic therapy is to allow a person to make full use of his or her personal capacities leading to self-actualization. Self-actualization requires the integration of all the components of one's unique personality. These elements or components of personality include the physical, emotional, intellectual, behavioral, and spiritual. The marks of a self-actualized person are maturity, self-awareness, and authenticity. Humanistic therapists think that most people—not only those with obvious problems—can benefit from opportunities for self-development. Humanistic therapy uses both individual and group approaches.

Precautions

Psychotic patients, substance abusers, and persons with severe **personality disorders** or disorders of impulse control may not be appropriate for treatment with humanistic methods.

Description

Humanistic approaches to individual treatment usually follow the same format as other forms of outpatient counseling. Therapists may be medical doctors, nurses, psychologists, social workers, or clergy. Humanistic group treatment formats are flexible, and a wide range of treatment methods are used, ranging from encounter groups and therapy groups to assertiveness training and consciousness-raising groups. In addition, the humanistic tradition has fostered the publication of self-help books for people interested in psychological self-improvement.

Risks

The chief risks include the reinforcement of self-centered tendencies in some patients and the dangers resulting from encounter groups led by persons without adequate training. Poorly led encounter groups can be traumatic to persons with low tolerance for confrontation or "uncovering" of private issues.

Normal results

The anticipated outcome of humanistic therapy is a greater degree of personal wholeness, self-acceptance, and exploration of one's potential. In group treatment, participants are expected to grow in interpersonal empathy and relationship skills. However, there have been few controlled studies to determine the reasonableness of these expectations.

KEY TERMS

Encounter group—A form of humanistic therapy in which participants meet with a trained leader to increase self-awareness and social skills through emotional sharing and confrontation.

Humanistic therapy—An approach to psychotherapy that emphasizes human uniqueness, positive qualities, and individual potential. It is sometimes used as a synonym for the human potential movement.

Primal therapy—A form of humanistic therapy that originated in the 1970s. Participants were encouraged to relive painful events and release feelings through screaming or crying rather than analysis.

Sensitivity training—A form of humanistic group therapy that began in the 1950s. Members participated in unstructured discussions in order to improve understanding of themselves and others.

Resources

BOOKS

Severin, Frank T. "Humanistic Psychology." In *The Encyclopedia of Psychiatry, Psychology, and Psychoanalysis*, edited by Benjamin B. Wolman. New York: Henry Holt and Co., 1996.

Rebecca J. Frey, PhD

Human bite infections

Definition

Human bite infections are potentially serious infections caused by rapid growth of bacteria in broken skin.

Description

Bites—animal and human—are responsible for about 1% of visits to emergency rooms. Bite injuries are more common during the summer months.

Closed-fist injury

In adults, the most common form of human bite is the closed-fist injury, sometimes called the "fight bite." These injuries result from the breaking of the skin over the knuckle joint when a person's fist strikes someone's teeth during a fight.

Causes and symptoms

In children, bite infections result either from accidents during play or from fighting. Most infected bites in adults result from fighting.

The infection itself can be caused by a number of bacteria that live in the human mouth. These include streptococci, staphylococci, anaerobic organisms, and *Eikenella corrodens*. Infections that begin less than 24 hours after the injury are usually produced by a mixture of organisms and can cause a necrotizing infection (causing the death of a specific area of tissue), in which tissue is rapidly destroyed. If a bite is infected, the skin will be sore, red, swollen, and warm to the touch.

Diagnosis

In most cases the diagnosis is made by an emergency room physician on the basis of the patient's history.

Because the human mouth contains a variety of bacteria, the physician will order a laboratory culture to choose the most effective antibiotic.

Treatment

Treatment involves surgical attention as well as medications. Because bites cause puncturing and tearing of skin rather than clean-edged cuts, they must be carefully cleansed. The doctor will wash the wound with water under high pressure and debride it. **Debridement** is the removal of dead tissue and **foreign objects** from a wound to prevent infection. If the bite is a closed-fist injury, the doctor will look for torn tendons or damage to the spaces between the joints. Examination includes x rays to check for bone **fractures** or foreign objects in the wound.

Doctors do not usually suture a bite wound because the connective tissues and other structures in the hand form many small closed spaces that make it easy for infection to spread. Emergency room doctors often consult surgical specialists if a patient has a deep closed-fist injury or one that appears already infected.

The doctor will make sure that the patient is immunized against **tetanus**, which is routine procedure for any open wound. A study released in June 2004 showed that routine use of **antibiotics** for human bites may not be necessary, as physicians try to minimize overuse of antibiotics. Superficial **wounds** in low-risk areas may no longer need antibiotic treatment, but more serious human bites to high-risk areas such as the hands should be treated with antibiotics to prevent serious infection. Patients with closed-fist injuries

KEY TERMS

Closed-fist injury—A hand wound caused when the skin of the fist is torn open by contact with teeth.

Debridement—The surgical removal of dead tissue and/or foreign bodies from a wound or cut.

"Fight bite"—Another name for closed-fist injury.

Necrotizing—Causing the death of a specific area of tissue. Human bites frequently cause necrotizing infections.

may need inpatient treatment in addition to an intravenous antibiotic.

Prognosis

The prognosis depends on the location of the bite and whether it was caused by a child or an adult. Bites caused by children rarely become infected because they are usually shallow. Between 15–30% of bites caused by adults become infected, with a higher rate for closed-fist injuries.

Prevention

Prevention of human bite infections depends upon prompt treatment of any bite caused by a human being, particularly a closed-fist injury.

Resources

PERIODICALS

"Do All Human Bite Wounds Need Antibiotics?" *Emergency Medicine Alert* June 2004: 3.

Rebecca J. Frey, PhD
Teresa G. Odle

Human chorionic gonadotropin *see*
Infertility drugs

Human chorionic gonadotropin pregnancy test

Definition

The most common test of **pregnancy** involves the detection of a hormone known as human chorionic gonadotropin (hCG) in a sample of blood or urine.

Purpose

To determine whether or not a woman is pregnant.

Description

Shortly after a woman's egg is fertilized by her male partner's sperm and is implanted in the lining or the womb (uterus), a placenta begins to form. This organ will help nourish the developing new life. The placenta produces hCG, whose presence, along with other hormones, helps maintain the early stages of pregnancy. Because hCG is produced only by placental tissue and the hormone can be found in the blood or urine of a pregnant woman, it has become a convenient chemical test of pregnancy.

After implantation, the level of detectable hCG rises very rapidly, approximately doubling in quantity every two days until a peak is reached between the sixth and eighth week. Over the next ten or more weeks, the quantity of hCG slowly decreases. After this point, a much lower level is sustained for the duration of the pregnancy. Detectable levels of this hormone may even persist for a month or two after delivery.

Blood tests for hCG are the most sensitive and can detect a pregnancy earlier than urine tests. Blood tests for hCG can also distinguish normal pregnancies from impending miscarriages or pregnancies that occur outside of the uterus (ectopic pregnancies).

If a woman misses her menstrual period and wants to know if she may be pregnant, she can purchase one of many home pregnancy test kits that are currently available. Although each of these products may look slightly different and provide a different set of directions for use, each one detects the presence of hCG. This indicator contains chemical components called antibodies that are sensitive to a certain quantity of this hormone.

Precautions

Although home pregnancy tests may be advertised as having an accuracy of 97% or better, studies indicate that, in practice, pregnancy tests performed in the home may incorrectly indicate that a woman is not pregnant (a false positive result) between 25–50% of the time. Studies also indicate that the false negative results usually result from failing to follow the package directions or testing too soon after a missed menstrual period. Waiting a few days

KEY TERMS

Ectopic pregnancy—A pregnancy that develops outside of the mother's uterus. Ectopic pregnancies often cause severe pain in the lower abdomen and are potentially life-threatening because of the massive blood loss that may occur as the developing embryo/fetus ruptures and damages the tissues in which it has implanted.

Embryo—In humans, the developing individual from the time of implantation to about the end of the second month after conception. From the third month to the point of delivery, the individual is called a fetus.

Hormone—A chemical produced by a specific organ or tissue of the body that is released into the bloodstream in order to exert an effect in another part of the body.

Human chorionic gonadotropin (hCG)—A hormone produced by the placenta of a developing pregnancy.

Hydatidiform mole—A rare, generally benign grape-like mass that grows in the uterus from the remains of an abnormally developed embryo and surrounding tissue. In extremely rare cases, the mole develops into a choriocarcinoma, a malignant tumor whose cells can invade the wall of the uterus.

Implantation—The attachment of the fertilized egg or embryo to the wall of the uterus.

Menstrual cycle—A hormonally regulated series of monthly events that occur during the reproductive years of the human female to ensure that the proper internal environment exists for fertilization, implantation, and development of a baby. Each month, a mature egg is released from the follicle of an ovary. If an egg is released, fertilized, and implanted, the lining of the uterus continues to build. If fertilization and/or implantation does not occur, the egg and all of the excess uterine lining are shed from the body during menstruation.

Miscarriage—Loss of the embryo or fetus and other products of pregnancy before the middle of the second trimester. Often, early in a pregnancy, if the condition of the baby and/or the mother's uterus is not compatible with sustaining life, the pregnancy stops, and the contents of the uterus are expelled. For this reason, miscarriage is also referred to as spontaneous abortion.

Placenta—The organ that unites the developing new life (first called an embryo and later a fetus) to the mother's uterus. The placenta produces hCG, among other hormones, to help maintain the pregnancy. After delivery, the placenta, known at this point as afterbirth, is expelled.

after the missed period was expected can increase the accuracy of the test. Blood and urine tests performed by a laboratory are from 97–100% accurate in detecting pregnancy.

Preparation

Generally, no preparation is required for a pregnancy test given in a doctor's office.

Home pregnancy test kits can be divided into two basic types. One type involves the use of a wand-like device that a woman must place into her urine stream for a brief period of time. The other type of kit involves the use of a cup, a dropper, and a wand or stick with a small well. The cup is used to collect the urine, and the dropper is used to transfer a specific number of drops into the well. Results are displayed by a color change. It's important to follow the package directions very carefully (the techniques vary from brand to brand) and to read the results in the time specified.

Aftercare

No special care is required after a urine test for hCG. Women who feel faint or who continue to bleed after a blood test should be observed until the condition goes away.

Risks

Tests for hCG levels pose no direct risk to a woman's health. The main risk with a home pregnancy test is a false negative result, which may be lessened by following the manufacturer's instructions carefully and waiting at least several days after the expected menstrual period to test. A false negative result can cause a delay in seeking prenatal care, which can pose a risk to both the woman and the baby.

Abnormal results

In most cases, a positive result is an indication of pregnancy. However, false positive results may also occur. If a pregnancy test is performed within a month or two of a recent birth or **miscarriage**, it is possible to test positive for pregnancy since hCG may still be detected in a woman's urine. Sometimes positive pregnancy tests provide clues of an early miscarriage that might have otherwise gone unrecognized because it occurred before or just after a missed period. An **ectopic pregnancy** (one in which an embryo implants outside the uterus), certain types of masses (such as an ovarian tumor or a **hydatidiform mole**), and the use of some fertility drugs that contain hCG are among other possibilities behind false positive results.

Normal results

A woman should notify her physician immediately if her home pregnancy test is positive. Pregnancy can then be confirmed with hCG urine or blood tests taken in the doctor's office and evaluated by laboratory personnel. If performed accurately, home pregnancy tests have been found to be highly reliable. However, the versions of these tests performed by qualified laboratory technologists are considered to be definitive. Often, such a test will produce positive results before a woman experiences symptoms or before a doctor's exam reveals signs of pregnancy.

Resources

PERIODICALS

Bastian, L. A., et al. "Is This Patient Pregnant?" *The Journal of the American Medical Association* 278, no. 7: 586-591.

Peredy, T. R., and R. D. Powers. "Bedside Diagnostic Testing of Body Fluids." *American Journal of Emergency Medicine* 15, no. 4: 404-405.

Betty Mishkin

Human herpes *see* **Roseola**

Human leukocyte antigen test

Definition

The human leukocyte antigen test, also known as HLA, is a test that detects antigens (genetic markers) on white blood cells. There are four types of human leukocyte antigens: HLA-A, HLA-B, HLA-C, and HLA-D.

Purpose

The HLA test is used to provide evidence of tissue compatibility typing of tissue recipients and donors. It is also an aid in **genetic counseling** and in paternity testing.

Precautions

This test may have to be postponed if the patient has recently undergone a **transfusion**.

Description

Human leukocyte antigen (leukocyte is the name for white blood cell, while antigen refers to a genetic marker) is a substance that is located on the surface of white blood cells. This substance plays an important role in the body's immune response.

Because the HLA antigens are essential to immunity, identification aids in determination of the degree of tissue compatibility between transplant recipients and donors. Testing is done to diminish the likelihood of rejection after transplant, and to avoid graft-versus-host disease (GVHD) following major organ or **bone marrow transplantation**. It should be noted that risk of GVHD exists even when the donor and recipient share major antigens. As an example, it was recently discovered that a mismatch of HA-1 (a minor antigen) was a cause of GVHD in bone marrow grafts from otherwise HLA-identical donors.

HLA can aid in paternity exclusion testing, a highly specialized area of forensic medicine. To resolve cases of disputed paternity, a man who demonstrates a phenotype (two haplotypes: one from the father and one from the mother) with no haplotype or antigen pair identical to one of the child's is excluded as the father. Conversely, a man who has one haplotype identical to one of the child's may be the father (the probability varies with the appearance of that particular haplotype in the population). Because of the issues involved, this type of testing is referred to experts.

Certain HLA types have been linked to diseases, such as **rheumatoid arthritis**, **multiple sclerosis**, serum lupus erythematosus, and other **autoimmune disorders**. By themselves, however, none of the HLA types are considered definitive. Because the clinical significance of many of the marker antigens has not yet been well defined, definitive diagnosis of disease is obtained by the use of more specific tests.

Preparation

The HLA test requires a blood sample. There is no need for the patient to be **fasting** (having nothing to eat or drink) before the test.

Risks

Risks for this test are minimal, but may include slight bleeding from the blood-drawing site, **fainting** or feeling lightheaded after venipuncture, or hematoma (blood accumulating under the puncture site).

Normal results

Identification of specific leukocyte antigens, HLA-A, HLA-B, HLA-C and HLA-D.

Abnormal results

ncompatible groups between organ donors and recipients may cause unsuccessful tissue transplantation.

Certain diseases have a strong association with certain types of HLAs, which may aid in genetic counseling. For example, Hashimoto's **thyroiditis** (an autoimmune disorder involving underproduction by the thyroid gland) is associated with HLA-DR5, while B8 and Dw3 are allied with Graves' disease (another autoimmune disorder, but with overproduction by the thyroid gland). Hereditary **hemochromatosis** (too much iron in the blood) is associated with HLA-A3,

B7, and B14. HLA-A3 is found in approximately 70% of patients with hemochromatosis, but as is the case with other HLA-associated disorders, the expense of HLA typing favors use of other tests. In cases of suspected hemochromatosis, for example, diagnosis is better aided by two tests called transferrin saturation and serum ferritin.

Resources

BOOKS

Pagana, Kathleen Deska. *Mosby's Manual of Diagnostic and Laboratory Tests.* St. Louis: Mosby, Inc., 1998.

Janis O. Flores

Humanistic therapy *see* **Gestalt therapy; Human-potential movement**

Humpback *see* **Kyphosis**

Hunchback *see* **Kyphosis**

Hunter's syndrome *see* **Mucopolysaccharidoses**

Huntington disease

Definition

Huntington disease (HD) is a progressive neurodegenerative disease causing uncontrolled physical movements and mental deterioration. The disease was discovered by George Sumner Huntington (1850–1916), an Ohio doctor who first described the hereditary movement disorder in 1872.

Description

Huntington disease is also called Huntington chorea or hereditary chorea. The word chorea comes from the Greek word for "dance" and refers to the involuntary movements of the patient's feet, lower arms, and face that develop as the disease progresses. It is occasionally referred to as "Woody Guthrie's disease" for the American folk singer who died from it. Huntington disease (HD) causes progressive loss of cells in areas of the brain responsible for certain aspects of movement control and mental abilities. A person with HD gradually develops abnormal movements and changes in cognition (thinking), behavior and personality.

The onset of symptoms of HD usually occurs between the ages of 30 and 50; although in 10% of cases, onset is in late childhood or early adolescence. Approximately 30,000 people in the United States are affected by HD, with another 150,000 at risk for developing this disorder. The frequency of HD is 4–7 cases per 100,000 persons.

Causes and symptoms

Huntington disease is caused by a defect in the HD gene (an inherited unit which contains a code for a protein), which is located on the short arm of chromosome 4. The gene codes for a protein called huntingtin, whose function is not known as of early 2005. The nucleotide codes (building blocks of genes arranged in a specific code which chemically forms into proteins), contain CAG repeats (40 or more of these repeat sequences). The extra building blocks in the huntingtin gene cause the protein that is made from it to contain an extra section as well. It is currently thought that this extra protein section, or portion, interacts with other proteins in brain cells where it occurs, and that this interaction ultimately leads to cell death.

The HD gene is a dominant gene, meaning that only one copy of it is needed to develop the disease. HD affects both males and females. The gene may be inherited from either parent, who will also be affected by the disease. A parent with the HD gene has a 50% chance of passing it on to each offspring. The chances of passing on the HD gene are not affected by the results of previous pregnancies.

The symptoms of HD fall into three categories: motor or movement symptoms; personality and behavioral changes; and cognitive decline. The severity and rate of progression of each type of symptom can vary from person to person.

Early motor symptoms include restlessness, twitching and a desire to move about. Handwriting may become less controlled, and coordination may decline. Later symptoms include:

- dystonia, or sustained abnormal postures, including facial grimaces, a twisted neck, or an arched back

- chorea, in which involuntary jerking, twisting or writhing motions become pronounced

- slowness of voluntary movements, inability to regulate the speed or force of movements, inability to initiate movement and slowed reactions

- difficulty speaking and swallowing due to involvement of the throat muscles

- localized or generalized weakness and impaired balance ability

- rigidity, especially in late-stage disease

Personality and behavioral changes include depression, irritability, **anxiety** and apathy. The person with HD may become impulsive, aggressive or socially withdrawn.

Cognitive changes include loss of ability to plan and execute routine tasks, slowed thought, and impaired or inappropriate judgment. Short-term memory loss usually occurs, although long-term memory is usually not affected. The person with late-stage HD usually retains knowledge of his environment and recognizes family members or other loved ones, despite severe cognitive decline.

Diagnosis

Diagnosis of HD begins with a detailed medical history, and a thorough physical and neurological examination. The family's medical history is very important. **Magnetic resonance imaging** (MRI) or computed tomography scan (CT scan) imaging may be performed to look for degeneration in the basal ganglia and cortex, the brain regions most affected in HD.

Physicians have recently developed a Uniform Huntington's Disease Rating Scale, or UHDRS, to assess a patient's symptoms and the speed of progression of the disease.

A genetic test is available for confirmation of the clinical diagnosis. In this test, a small blood sample is taken, and DNA from it is analyzed to determine the CAG repeat number. A person with a repeat number of 30 or below will not develop HD. A person with a repeat number between 35 and 40 may not develop the disease within their normal lifespan. A person with a very high number of repeats (70 or above) is likely to develop the juvenile-onset form. An important part of **genetic testing** is extensive **genetic counseling**.

Prenatal testing is available. A person at risk for HD (a child of an affected person) may obtain fetal testing without determining whether she herself carries the gene. This test, also called a linkage test, examines the pattern of DNA near the gene in both parent and fetus, but does not analyze for the triple nucleotide repeat (CAG). If the DNA patterns do not match, the fetus can be assumed not to have inherited the HD gene, even if present in the parent. A pattern match indicates the fetus probably has the same genetic makeup of the at-risk parent.

Treatment

There is no cure for HD, nor any treatment that can slow the rate of progression. Treatment is aimed at reducing the disability caused by the motor impairments, and treating behavioral and emotional symptoms.

Physical therapy is used to maintain strength and compensate for lost strength and balance. Stretching and range of motion exercises help minimize contracture, or muscle shortening, a result of weakness and disuse. The physical therapist also advises on the use of mobility aids such as walkers or wheelchairs.

Motor symptoms may be treated with drugs, although some studies suggest that anti-chorea treatment rarely improves function. Chorea (movements caused by abnormal muscle contractions) can be suppressed with drugs that deplete dopamine, an important brain chemical regulating movement. As HD progresses, natural dopamine levels fall, leading to loss of chorea and an increase in rigidity and movement slowness. Treatment with L-dopa (which resupplies dopamine) may be of some value. Frequent reassessment of the effectiveness and appropriateness of any drug therapy is necessary.

Occupational therapy is used to design compensatory strategies for lost abilities in the activities of daily living, such as eating, dressing, and grooming. The occupational therapist advises on modifications to the home that improve safety, accessibility, and comfort.

Difficulty swallowing may be lessened by preparation of softer foods, blending food in an electric blender, and taking care to eat slowly and carefully. Use of a straw for all liquids can help. The potential for **choking** on food is a concern, especially late in the disease progression. Caregivers should learn the use of the **Heimlich maneuver**. In addition, passage of food into the airways increases the risk for **pneumonia**. A gastric feeding tube may be needed, if swallowing becomes too difficult or dangerous.

Speech difficulties may be partially compensated by using picture boards or other augmentative communication devices. Loss of cognitive ability affects both speech production and understanding. A speech-language pathologist can work with the family to develop simplified and more directed communication strategies, including speaking slowly, using simple words, and repeating sentences exactly.

Early behavioral changes, including depression and anxiety, may respond to drug therapy. Maintaining a calm, familiar, and secure environment is useful as the disease progresses. Support groups for both patients and caregivers form an important part of treatment.

Experimental transplant of fetal brain tissue has been attempted in a few HD patients. Early results show some promise, but further trials are needed to establish the effectiveness of this treatment.

Tetrabenazine (Nitoman), a drug that has been considered investigational in the United States, appears to benefit some patients with HD by controlling the involuntary movements of chorea. It works by lowering the levels of dopamine and other neurotransmitters in the brain. The Food and Drug Administration (FDA) granted tetrabenazine fast-track and orphan drug status in the United States as of 2004. It is not yet manufactured in the United States but can be obtained from the United Kingdom.

In 2004 the Food and Drug Administration (FDA) also approved deep brain stimulation (DBS) as an acceptable treatment for HD and other **movement disorders**. In DBS, the surgeon implants a battery-operated medical device called a neurostimulator, which delivers electrical impulses to the areas of the brain that govern movement. In the case of Huntington's patients, the part of the brain that is targeted is a structure called the globus pallidus. It is thought that DBS works by increasing the flow of blood to this area. A group of Canadian researchers reported in 2004 that some patients with HD are better able to control their movements after DBS of the globus pallidus.

Psychotherapy is often recommended for individuals who know themselves to be at risk for the disease. Some persons want to know their risk status while others prefer not to be tested. Psychotherapy may be useful in helping at-risk persons decide about testing as well as coping with the results of the test.

Prognosis

The person with Huntington disease may be able to maintain a job for several years after diagnosis, despite the increase in disability. Loss of cognitive functions and increase in motor and behavioral symptoms eventually prevent the person with HD from continuing employment. Ultimately, severe motor symptoms prevent mobility. Death usually occurs between 10 and 30 years after disease onset, typically as the result of pneumonia or a fall. Progressive weakness of respiratory and swallowing muscles leads to increased risk of respiratory infection and choking, the most common causes of death. Future research in this area is currently focusing on nerve cell transplantation.

Basal ganglia—A structure at the base of the brain composed of four groups of nerve cells, responsible for body movements and coordination.

Chorea—Brief and purposeless involuntary movements of the lower arms, feet, and face.

Chromosome—The structures that carry genetic information. Chromosomes are located within every cell, and are responsible for directing the development and functioning of all the cells in the body. The normal number is 46 (23 pairs).

Cortex—The part of the brain responsible for thought, memory, and sensory perception.

Dystonia—A movement disorder characterized by sustained muscle contractions that result in writhing or twisting movements and unsual body postures.

Globus pallidus—A pale-colored spherical structure within the basal ganglia. Deep brain stimulation of this area is helpful in controlling the chorea of some patients with HD.

Huntingtin—A protein of unknown function encoded by the HD gene. The repeated CAG sequence in a defective HD gene causes the body to produce an abnormal form of huntingtin. It is not yet known why the abnormal form of huntingtin affects only certain regions of the brain.

Orphan drug—A term for a drug that treats a rare disease, defined by the Food and Drug Administration (FDA) as one that affects fewer than 200,000 Americans. The FDA has an Office of Orphan Products Development (OOPD), which offers grants to researchers to develop these products.

Tetrabenazine—A drug given to control chorea that appears to benefit HD patients.

Resources

BOOKS

Beers, Mark H., MD, and Robert Berkow, MD., editors. "Disorders of Movement." Section 14, Chapter 179 In *The Merck Manual of Diagnosis and Therapy*. Whitehouse Station, NJ: Merck Research Laboratories, 2004.

PERIODICALS

Montgomery, E. B., Jr. "Deep Brain Stimulation for Hyperkinetic Disorders." *Neurosurgical Focus* 17 (July 15, 2004): E1.

Moro, E., A. E. Lang, A. P. Strafella, et al. "Bilateral Globus Pallidus Stimulation for Huntington's Disease." *Annals of Neurology* 56 (August 2004): 290–294.

Revilla, Fredy J., MD, and Jaime Grutzendler, MD. "Huntington Disease." *eMedicine* November 3, 2004. < http://www.emedicine.com/NEURO/ topic81.htm >.

Richartz, E. R., and C. Frank. "A Psychodynamic Approach in Counselling Vulnerable Persons for Chorea Huntington—A Case Report." [in German] *Psychiatrische Praxis* 31 (July 2004): 255–258.

Seneca, S., D. Fagnart, K. Keymolen, et al. "Early-Onset Huntington Disease: A Neuronal Degeneration Syndrome." *European Journal of Pediatrics* 26 (August 2004): e-pub.

ORGANIZATIONS

Huntington Disease Society of America. 140 W. 22nd St. New York, NY 10011. (800) 345-HDSA.

National Institute of Neurological Disorders and Stroke (NINDS). NIH Neurological Institute, P. O. Box 5801, Bethesda, MD 20824. (800) 352-9424 or (301) 496-5751. < http://www.ninds.nih.gov >.

National Organization for Rare Disorders (NORD). 55 Kenosia Avenue, P. O. Box 1968, Danbury, CT 06813-1968. (203) 744-0100. Fax: (203) 798-2291. < http://www.rarediseases.org >.

United States Food and Drug Administration (FDA). 5600 Fishers Lane, Rockville, MD 20857-0001. (888) INFO-FDA. < http://www.fda.gov >.

OTHER

Food and Drug Administration (FDA). "Grants Awarded by the OOPD Program." < http://www.fda.gov/ orphan/grants/previous.htm >.

National Institute of Neurological Disorders and Stroke (NINDS). "Huntington's Disease: Hope Through Research." NIH Publication No. 98-49. Bethesda, MD: NINDS, 2005. < http://www.ninds.nih.gov/disorders/ huntington/detail_huntington.htm >.

National Institute of Neurological Disorders and Stroke (NINDS). "NINDS Deep Brain Stimulation for Parkinson's Disease Information Page." Bethesda, MD: NINDS, 2004. < http://www.ninds.nih.gov/ disorders/deep_brain_stimulation/ deep_brain_stimulation.htm >.

Laith Farid Gulli, M.D.
Rebecca J. Frey, PhD

Huntington's chorea *see* **Huntington's disease**

Hurler's syndrome *see* **Mucopolysaccharidoses**

HUS *see* **Hemolytic-uremic syndrome**

Hyaline *see* **Respiratory distress syndrome**

Hydatid *see* **Echinococcosis**

Hydatidiform mole

Definition

A hydatidiform mole is a relatively rare condition in which tissue around a fertilized egg that normally would have developed into the placenta instead develops as an abnormal cluster of cells. (This is also called a molar pregnancy.) This grapelike mass forms inside of the uterus after fertilization instead of a normal embryo. A hydatidiform mole triggers a positive **pregnancy** test and in some cases can become cancerous.

Description

A hydatidiform mole ("hydatid" means "drop of water" and "mole" means "spot") occurs in about 1 out of every 1,500 (1/1,500) pregnancies in the United States. In some parts of Asia, however, the incidence may be as high as 1 in 200 (1/200). Molar pregnancies are most likely to occur in younger and older women (especially over age 45) than in those between ages 20–40. About 1–2% of the time a woman who has had a molar pregnancy will have a second one.

A molar pregnancy occurs when cells of the chorionic villi (tiny projections that attach the placenta to the lining of the uterus) don't develop correctly. Instead, they turn into watery clusters that can't support a growing baby. A partial molar pregnancy includes an abnormal embryo (a fertilized egg that has begun to grow) that does not survive. In a compete molar pregnancy there is a small cluster of clear blisters or pouches that don't contain an embryo.

If not removed, about 15% of **moles** can become cancerous. They burrow into the wall of the uterus and cause serious bleeding. Another 5% will develop into fast-growing cancers called choriocarcinomas. Some of these tumors spread very quickly outside the uterus in other parts of the body. Fortunately, **cancer** developing from these moles is rare and highly curable.

Causes and symptoms

The cause of hydatidiform mole is unclear; some experts believe it is caused by problems with the chromosomes (the structures inside cells that contain genetic information) in either the egg or sperm, or both. It may be associated with poor **nutrition**, or a problem with the ovaries or the uterus. A mole sometimes can develop from placental tissue that is left behind in the uterus after a **miscarriage** or **childbirth**.

Women with a hydatidiform mole will have a positive pregnancy test and often believe they have a normal pregnancy for the first three or four months. However, in these cases the uterus will grow abnormally fast. By the end of the third month, if not earlier, the woman will experience vaginal bleeding ranging from scant spotting to excessive bleeding. She may have **hyperthyroidism** (overproduction of **thyroid hormones** causing symptoms such as weight loss, increased appetite, and intolerance to heat). Sometimes, the grapelike cluster of cells itself will be shed with the blood during this time. Other symptoms may include severe **nausea and vomiting** and high blood pressure. As the pregnancy progresses, the fetus will not move and there will be no fetal heartbeat.

Diagnosis

The physician may not suspect a molar pregnancy until after the third month or later, when the absence of a fetal heartbeat together with bleeding and severe nausea and vomiting indicates something is amiss.

First, the physician will examine the woman's abdomen, feeling for any strange lumps or abnormalities in the uterus. A tubal pregnancy, which can be life threatening if not treated, will be ruled out. Then the physician will check the levels of human chorionic gonadotropin (hCG), a hormone that is normally produced by a placenta or a mole. Abnormally high levels of hCG together with the symptoms of vaginal bleeding, lack of fetal heartbeat, and an unusually large uterus all indicate a molar pregnancy. An ultrasound of the uterus to make sure there is no living fetus will confirm the diagnosis.

Treatment

It is extremely important to make sure that all of the mole is removed from the uterus, since it is possible that the tissue is potentially cancerous. Often, the tissue is naturally expelled by the fourth month of pregnancy. In some instances, the physician will give the woman a drug called oxytocin to trigger the release of the mole that is not spontaneously aborted.

If this does not happen, however, a vacuum aspiration can be performed to remove the mole. In a procedure similar to a **dilatation and curettage** (D & C), a woman is given an anesthetic (to deaden feeling during the procedure), her cervix (the structure at the bottom of the uterus) is dilated and the contents of the uterus is gently suctioned out. After the mole has been mostly removed, gentle scraping of the uterus lining is usually performed.

If the woman is older and does not want any more children, the uterus can be surgically removed (**hysterectomy**) instead of a vacuum aspiration because of the higher risk of cancerous moles in this age group.

Because of the cancer risk, the physician will continue to monitor the patient for at least two months after the end of a molar pregnancy. Since invasive disease is usually signaled by high levels of hCG that don't go down after the pregnancy has ended, the woman's hCG levels will be checked every two weeks. If the levels don't return to normal by that time, the mole may have become cancerous.

If the hCG level is normal, the woman's hCG will be tested each month for six months, and then every two months for a year.

If the mole has become cancerous, treatment includes removal of the cancerous issue and **chemotherapy**. If the cancer has spread to other parts of the body, radiation will be added. Specific treatment depends on how advanced the cancer is.

Women should make sure not to become pregnant within a year after hCG levels have returned to normal. If a woman were to become pregnant sooner than that, it would be difficult to tell whether the resulting high levels of hCG were caused by the pregnancy or a cancer from the mole.

Prognosis

A woman with a molar pregnancy often goes through the same emotions and sense of loss as does a woman who has a miscarriage. Most of the time, she truly believed she was pregnant and now has suffered a loss of the baby she thought she was carrying. In addition, there is the added worry that the tissue left behind could become cancerous.

In the unlikely case that the mole is cancerous the cure rate is almost 100%. As long as the uterus was not removed, it would still be possible to have a child at a later time.

Resources

BOOKS

Carlson, Karen J., Stephanie A. Eisenstat, and Terra Ziporyn. *The Harvard Guide to Women's Health.* Cambridge, MA: Harvard University Press, 1996.

Carol A. Turkington

Hydrocelectomy

Definition

Hydrocelectomy is a surgical procedure to remove a hydrocele. A hydrocele is collected fluid in the membrane surrounding the testes.

Purpose

Hydrocelectomy is performed to relieve the **pain** or reoccurrence of a hydrocele. Normally, hydroceles are not very painful. They tend to be a soft swelling in the membrane surrounding the testes. As the hydrocele grows, the scrotum gets larger. Hydroceles do not damage the testes. The main symptom is scrotal swelling. There are two types of hydroceles depending on how they form. One type is seen in children, generally shortly after birth. It is caused by a failure of the processus vaginalis to close. Usually, surgery isn't used to treat hydrocele until after two years of age because the processus vaginalis frequently closes by itself if given extra time. In adults, hydroceles develop slowly. Most hydroceles develop because of blocked lymphatic flow. Hydroceles also develop after infection, injury, or local **cancer** tumors. Generally, hydroceles are treated by aspiration of the collected fluid. To do this, a needle is inserted into the scrotum and directed toward the hydrocele. Once there, as much fluid as possible is removed. Hydroceles can reoccur. Rarely, hydroceles grow larger and cause pain. Surgery is used to remove large or painful hydroceles. It is also the recommended procedure to remove hydroceles that reoccur after aspiration. Hydroceles are distinguished from other testicular problems by transillumination and **scrotal ultrasound** examinations.

Precautions

No special precautions are required for hydrocelectomy. It is typically performed on an outpatient basis.

activities may be delayed for up to six weeks. The hydrocele does not grow back.

Abnormal results

Swelling that lasts for several months is sometimes a complication of hydrocelectomy. Infection can also occur.

Resources

BOOKS

Way, Lawrence W., editor. *Current Surgical Diagnosis and Treatment*. 10th ed. Stamford: Appleton & Lange, 1994.

KEY TERMS

Aspiration—The process of removing fluids or gases from the body by suction.

Hernia—The protrusion of an organ or tissue through a wall that normally contains it.

Hydrocele—An accumulation of fluid in the membrane surrounding the testes (tunica vaginalis testis).

Description

Aspiration of the fluid in a hydrocele is usually successful. However, aspiration may be only a temporary solution because of the potential that the hydrocele will reoccur. Generally, surgical repair of a hydrocele will eliminate the hydrocele. The extent of the surgery depends on whether other factors are present. If the hydrocele is uncomplicated, an incision is made in the scrotum. The hydrocele is cut out, removing the tissues involved in the hydrocele. If there are complications present, such as a **hernia**, an incision is made in the inguinal (groin) area. This approach allows repair of hernias and other complicating factors at the same time. Patients are placed under **general anesthesia** for these operations.

Preparation

A physician or nurse will explain the procedure and, in some cases, the need for a temporary drain to be inserted. The drain lessens the chance of infection and prevents fluid build-up.

Aftercare

Following surgery, the patient usually only needs a follow-up examination several weeks after the surgery to examine the incision and to check for signs of infection.

Risks

There is a slight risk of infection and internal hemorrhage as well as a chance of excessive bleeding from the surgical incision.

Normal results

There may be swelling of the scrotum for up to a month. The patient is able to resume most activities within 7–10 days, although heavy lifting and sexual

Hydrocephalus

Definition

Hydrocephalus is an abnormal expansion of cavities (ventricles) within the brain that is caused by the accumulation of cerebrospinal fluid. Hydrocephalus comes from two Greek words: *hydros* means water and *cephalus* means head.

There are two main varieties of hydrocephalus: congenital and acquired. An obstruction of the cerebral aqueduct (aqueductal stenosis) is the most frequent cause of congenital hydrocephalus. Acquired hydrocephalus may result from spina bifida, intraventricular hemorrhage, **meningitis**, head trauma, tumors, and cysts.

Description

Hydrocephalus is the result of an imbalance between the formation and drainage of cerebrospinal fluid (CSF). Approximately 500 milliliters (about a pint) of CSF is formed within the brain each day, by epidermal cells in structures collectively called the choroid plexus. These cells line chambers called ventricles that are located within the brain. There are four ventricles in a human brain. Once formed, CSF usually circulates among all the ventricles before it is absorbed and returned to the circulatory system. The normal adult volume of circulating CSF is 150 ml. The CSF turn-over rate is more than three times per day. Because production is independent of absorption, reduced absorption causes CSF to accumulate within the ventricles.

There are three different types of hydrocephalus. In the most common variety, reduced absorption occurs when one or more passages connecting the ventricles become blocked. This prevents the movement of CSF to its drainage sites in the subarachnoid space just inside the skull. This type of hydrocephalus is called "noncommunicating." In a second type, a reduction in the absorption rate is caused by damage to the absorptive tissue. This variety is called "communicating hydrocephalus."

Both of these types lead to an elevation of the CSF pressure within the brain. This increased pressure pushes aside the soft tissues of the brain. This squeezes and distorts them. This process also results in damage to these tissues. In infants whose skull bones have not yet fused, the intracranial pressure is partly relieved by expansion of the skull, so that symptoms may not be as dramatic. Both types of elevated-pressure hydrocephalus may occur from infancy to adulthood.

A third type of hydrocephalus, called "normal pressure hydrocephalus," is marked by ventricle enlargement without an apparent increase in CSF pressure. This type affects mainly the elderly.

Hydrocephalus has a variety of causes including:

- congenital brain defects
- hemorrhage, either into the ventricles or the subarachnoid space
- infection of the central nervous system (**syphilis**, herpes, meningitis, **encephalitis**, or mumps)
- tumor

Hydrocephalus is believed to occur in approximately one to two of every 1,000 live births. The incidence of adult onset hydrocephalus is not known. There is no known way to prevent hydrocephalus.

Causes and symptoms

Hydrocephalus that is congenital (present at birth) is thought to be caused by a complex interaction of genetic and environmental factors. Aqueductal stenosis, an obstruction of the cerebral aqueduct, is the most frequent cause of congenital hydrocephalus. As of 2001, the genetic factors are not well understood. According to the British Association for **Spina Bifida** and Hydrocephalus, in very rare circumstances, hydrocephalus is due to hereditary factors, which might affect future generations.

Signs and symptoms of elevated-pressure hydrocephalus include:

- headache
- nausea and **vomiting**, especially in the morning

- lethargy
- disturbances in walking (gait)
- double vision
- subtle difficulties in learning and memory
- delay in children achieving developmental milestones

Irritability is the most common sign of hydrocephalus in infants. If this is not treated, it may lead to lethargy. Bulging of the fontanelles, or the soft spots between the skull bones, may also be an early sign. When hydrocephalus occurs in infants, fusion of the skull bones is prevented. This leads to abnormal expansion of the skull.

Symptoms of normal pressure hydrocephalus include **dementia**, gait abnormalities, and incontinence (involuntary urination or bowel movements).

Diagnosis

Imaging studies—x ray, computed tomography scan (CT scan), ultrasound, and especially **magnetic resonance imaging** (MRI)—are used to assess the presence and location of obstructions, as well as changes in brain tissue that have occurred as a result of the hydrocephalus. Lumbar puncture (spinal tap) may be performed to aid in determining the cause when infection is suspected.

Treatment

The primary method of treatment for both elevated and normal pressure hydrocephalus is surgical installation of a shunt. A shunt is a tube connecting the ventricles of the brain to an alternative drainage site, usually the abdominal cavity. A shunt contains a one-way valve to prevent reverse flow of fluid. In some cases of non-communicating hydrocephalus, a direct connection can be made between one of the ventricles and the subarachnoid space, allowing drainage without a shunt.

Installation of a shunt requires lifelong monitoring by the recipient or family members for signs of recurring hydrocephalus due to obstruction or failure of the shunt. Other than monitoring, no other management activity is usually required.

Some drugs may postpone the need for surgery by inhibiting the production of CSF. These include acetazolamide and furosemide. Other drugs that are used to delay surgery include glycerol, digoxin, and isosorbide.

Some cases of elevated pressure hydrocephalus may be avoided by preventing or treating the

KEY TERMS

Cerebral ventricles—Spaces in the brain that are located between portions of the brain and filled with cerebrospinal fluid.

Cerebrospinal fluid—Fluid that circulates throughout the cerebral ventricles and around the spinal cord within the spinal canal.

Choroid plexus—Specialized cells located in the ventricles of the brain that produce cerebrospinal fluid.

Fontanelle—One of several "soft spots" on the skull where the developing bones of the skull have yet to fuse.

Shunt—A small tube placed in a ventricle of the brain to direct cerebrospinal fluid away from the blockage into another part of the body.

Stenosis—The constricting or narrowing of an opening or passageway.

Subarachnoid space—The space between two membranes surrounding the brain, the arachnoid and pia mater.

infectious diseases which precede them. Prenatal diagnosis of congenital brain malformation is often possible, offering the option of family planning.

Prognosis

The prognosis for elevated-pressure hydrocephalus depends on a wide variety of factors, including the cause, age of onset, and the timing of surgery. Studies indicate that about half of all children who receive appropriate treatment and follow-up will develop IQs greater than 85. Those with hydrocephalus at birth do better than those with later onset due to meningitis. For individuals with normal pressure hydrocephalus, approximately half will benefit by the installation of a shunt.

Resources

BOOKS

Toporek, Chuck, and Kellie Robinson. *Hydrocephalus: A Guide for Patients, Families & Friends.* Cambridge, Mass.: O'Reilly &Associates, 1999.

PERIODICALS

"Hydrocephalus." *Review of Optometry* 137, no. 8 (August 15, 2000): 56A.

ORGANIZATIONS

Association for Spina Bifida and Hydrocephalus. 42 Park Rd., Peterborough, PE1 2UQ. UK 0173 355 5988. Fax: 017 3355 5985. postmaster@asbah.org. < http:// www.asbah.demon.co.uk >.

Hydrocephalus Foundation, Inc., (HyFI). 910 Rear Broadway, Saugus, MA 01906. (781) 942-1161. HyFI1@netscape.net. < http:// www.hydrocephalus.org >.

OTHER

"Hydrocephalus." *American Association of Neurological Surgeons/Congress of Neurological Surgeons.* < http://www.neurosurgery.org/pubpages/patres/ hydrobroch.html >.

"Hydrocephalus." *Institute for Neurology and Neurosurgery.* Beth Israel Medical Center, New York, NY. < http://nyneurosurgery.org/child/hydrocephalus/ hydrocephalus.htm >.

"Hydrocephalus." National Library of Medicine. *MEDLINEplus.* < http://www.nlm.nih.gov/ medlineplus/hydrocephalus.html >.

L. Fleming Fallon, MD, PhD, DrPH

Hydrochlorothiazide *see* **Diuretics**

Hydrocodone *see* **Analgesics, opioid**

Hydrogen peroxide *see* **Antiseptics**

Hydronephrosis

Definition

Hydronephrosis is the swelling of the kidneys when urine flow is obstructed in any of part of the urinary tract. Swelling of the ureter, which always accompanies hydronephrosis, is called hydroureter. Hydronephrosis implies that a ureter and the renal pelvis (the connection of the ureter to the kidney) are overfilled with urine.

Description

The kidneys filter urine out of the blood as a waste product. It collects in the renal pelvis and flows down the ureters into the bladder. The ureters are not simple tubes, but muscular passages that actively propel urine into the bladder. At their lower end is a valve (the ureterovesical junction) that prevents urine from flowing backward into the ureter. The bladder stores urine. The prostate gland surrounds the bladder outlet in males. Urine then flows through the urethra and out of the body as a waste product.

Because the urinary tract is closed save for the one opening at the bottom, urine cannot escape. Instead, the parts distend. Rupture is rare unless there is violent trauma like an automobile accident.

Obstructed flow anywhere along the drainage route can cause swelling of the upper urinary tract, but if the obstruction is below the bladder, the uretero-vesical valve will protect the upper tract to a certain extent. Even then, with no place to go, the urine will back up all the way to its source. Eventually, the back pressure causes kidney function to deteriorate.

Obstruction need not be complete for problems to arise. Intermittent or partial obstruction is far more common than complete blockage, allowing time for the parts to enlarge gradually. Furthermore, if a ure-terovesical valve is absent or incompetent, the pressure generated by bladder emptying will force urine backward into the ureter and kidney, causing dilation even without mechanical obstruction.

Causes and symptoms

Causes are numerous. Various congenital deformities of the ureter may sooner or later produce back pressure. **Kidney stones** are a common cause. They form in the renal pelvis and become lodged in the kidney, usually at the ureterovesical junction. In older men, the continued growth of the prostate gland leads commonly to restricted urine flow out of the bladder. **Prostate cancer**, and **cancer** anywhere else along the urine pathways, can obstruct flow. **Pregnancy** normally causes ureteral obstruction from the pressure of the enlarged uterus (womb) on the ureters.

Symptoms relate to the passage of urine. Sometimes, urine may be difficult to pass, irregular, or uncontrolled. **Pain** from distension of the structures is present. Blood in the urine may be visible, but it is usually microscopic.

In all cases where bodily fluids cannot flow freely, infection is inevitable. Symptoms of urinary infection may include:

- painful, burning urine
- cloudy urine
- pain in the back, flank, or groin
- fever, sweats, chills, and generalized discomfort

Patients often mistake a serious urinary infection for the flu.

Diagnosis

If the bladder is significantly distended, it can be felt through the abdomen. An analysis of the urine may reveal blood (if there is a stone), infection, or chemical changes suggesting kidney damage. Blood tests may also detect a decrease in kidney function.

All urinary obstructions will undergo imaging of some sort. Beginning with standard x rays to look for stones, radiologists, physicians specializing in the use of radiant energy for diagnostic purposes, will select from a wide array of tests. Ultrasound is simple, inexpensive, and very useful for these conditions. Standard x rays can be enhanced with contrast agents in several ways. If the kidneys are functioning, they will filter an x ray dye out of the blood and concentrate it in the urine, giving excellent pictures and also an assessment of kidney function. For better images of the lower urinary tract, contrast agents can be instilled from below. This is usually done with a cystoscope placed in the bladder. Through the cystoscope, a small tube can be threaded into the ureter through the ureterovesical valve, allowing dye to be injected all the way up to the kidney. CT and MRI scanning provide miraculous detail, more than is often needed for this condition.

Treatment

The obstruction must be relieved, even if it is partial or functional, as in the case of reflux from the bladder. If not, the kidney will ultimately be damaged, infection will appear, or both. The task may be as simple as placing a catheter through a restricting prostate or as complicated as removing a cancerous bladder and rebuilding a new one with a piece of bowel. In some cases, a badly damaged kidney may have to be removed.

Alternative treatment

Catheters or other urinary diversions may be better for weak or ill patients who cannot tolerate more extensive procedures. There is support using botanical medicine that can help the patient using a catheter avoid infections. Consultation with a trained health care practitioner is necessary.

Prognosis

After relief of the obstruction, a kidney may react with a brief flood of urine, but if the obstruction has been of short duration, normal kidney function will return. If one kidney is destroyed, the other will compensate for the lost organ.

Prevention

Kidney stones can be prevented by dietary changes and medication. Prompt evaluation of infections and urinary complaints will usually detect problems early enough to prevent long-term complications.

Resources

ORGANIZATIONS

American Association of Kidney Patients. 100 S. Ashley Dr., #280, Tampa, FL 33602. (800) 749-2257. < http://www.aakp.org >.

American Kidney Foundation. 6110 Executive Boulevard, #1010, Rockville, MD 20852. (800) 638-8299.

National Kidney Foundation. 30 East 33rd St., New York, NY 10016. (800) 622-9010. < http://www.kidney.org >.

J. Ricker Polsdorfer, MD

Hydrotherapy

Definition

Hydrotherapy, or water therapy, is the use of water (hot, cold, steam, or ice) to relieve discomfort and promote physical well-being.

Purpose

Hydrotherapy can soothe sore or inflamed muscles and joints, rehabilitate injured limbs, lower fevers, soothe headaches, promote relaxation, treat **burns** and frostbite, ease labor pains, and clear up skin problems. The temperature of water used affects the therapeutic

properties of the treatment. Hot water is chosen for its relaxing properties. It is also thought to stimulate the immune system. Tepid water can also be used for stress reduction, and may be particularly relaxing in hot weather. Cold water is selected to reduce inflammation. Alternating hot and cold water can stimulate the circulatory system and improve the immune system. Adding herbs and essential oils to water can enhance its therapeutic value. Steam is frequently used as a carrier for essential oils that are inhaled to treat respiratory problems.

Since the late 1990s, hydrotherapy has been used in critical care units to treat a variety of serious conditions, including such disorders of the nervous system as **Guillain-Barré syndrome**.

Description

Origins

The therapeutic use of water has a long history. Ruins of an ancient bath were unearthed in Pakistan and date as far back as 4500 B.C. Bathhouses were an essential part of ancient Roman culture. The use of steam, baths, and aromatic massage to promote well being is documented since the first century. Roman physicians Galen and Celsus wrote of treating patients with warm and cold baths in order to prevent disease.

By the seventeenth and eighteenth centuries, bathhouses were extremely popular with the public throughout Europe. Public bathhouses made their first American appearance in the mid 1700s.

In the early nineteenth century, Sebastien Kneipp, a Bavarian priest and proponent of water healing, began treating his parishioners with cold water applications after he himself was cured of tuberculosis through the same methods. Kneipp wrote extensively on the subject, and opened a series of hydrotherapy clinics known as the Kneipp clinics, which are still in operation today. Around the same time in Austria, Vincenz Priessnitz was treating patients with baths, packs, and showers of cold spring water. Priessnitz also opened a spa that treated over 1,500 patients in its first year of operation, and became a model for physicians and other specialists to learn the techniques of hydrotherapy.

Water can be used therapeutically in a number of ways. Common forms of hydrotherapy include:

- Whirlpools, jacuzzis, and hot tubs. These soaking tubs use jet streams to massage the body. They are frequently used by physical therapists to help injured patients regain muscle strength and to soothe joint and muscle **pain**. Some midwives and obstetricians also approve of the use of hot tubs to soothe the pain of labor.

- Pools and Hubbard tanks. Physical therapists and **rehabilitation** specialists may prescribe underwater pool exercises as a low-impact method of rebuilding muscle strength in injured patients. The buoyancy experienced during pool immersion also helps ease pain in conditions such as arthritis.

- Baths. Tepid baths are prescribed to reduce a **fever**. Baths are also one of the oldest forms of relaxation therapy. Aromatherapists often recommend adding essential oils of lavender (*Lavandula angustifolia*) to a warm to hot bath to promote relaxation and **stress reduction**. Adding Epsom salts (magnesium sulfate) or Dead Sea salts to a bath can also promote relaxation and soothe rheumatism and arthritis.

- Showers. Showers are often prescribed to stimulate the circulation. Water jets from a shower head are also used to massage sore muscles. In addition, showering hydrotherapy has been shown to be preferable to immersion hydrotherapy for treating burn patients.

- Moist compresses. Cold, moist compresses can reduce swelling and inflammation of an injury. They can also be used to cool a fever and treat a headache. Hot or warm compresses are useful for soothing muscle aches and treating abscesses.

- Steam treatments and saunas. Steam rooms and saunas are recommended to open the skin pores and cleanse the body of toxins. Steam inhalation is prescribed to treat respiratory infections. Adding botanicals to the steam bath can increase its therapeutic value.

- Internal hydrotherapy. **Colonic irrigation** is an enema that is designed to cleanse the entire bowel. Proponents of the therapy say it can cure a number of digestive problems. Douching, another form of internal hydrotherapy, directs a stream of water into the vagina for cleansing purposes. The water may or may not contain medications or other substances. Douches can be self-administered with kits available at most drug stores.

Preparations

Because of the expense of the equipment and the expertise required to administer effective treatment, hydrotherapy with pools, whirlpools, Hubbard tanks, and saunas is best taken in a professional healthcare facility, and/or under the supervision of a healthcare professional. However, baths, steam inhalation treatments, and compresses can be easily administered at home.

Bath preparations

Warm to hot bath water should be used for relaxation purposes, and a tepid bath is recommended for reducing fevers. Herbs can greatly enhance the therapeutic value of the bath for a variety of illnesses and minor discomforts.

Herbs for the bath can be added to the bath in two ways—as essential oils or whole herbs and flowers. Whole herbs and flowers can be placed in a muslin or cheesecloth bag that is tied at the top to make an herbal bath bag. The herbal bath bag is then soaked in the warm tub, and can remain there throughout the bath. When using essential oils, add five to 10 drops of oil to a full tub. Oils can be combined to enhance their therapeutic value. Marjoram (*Origanum marjorana*) is good for relieving sore muscles; juniper (*Juniperus communis*) is recommended as a detoxifying agent for the treatment of arthritis; lavender, ylang ylang (*Conanga odorata*), and chamomile (*Chamaemelum nobilis*) are recommended for stress relief; cypress (*Cupressus sempervirens*), yarrow (*Achillea millefolium*), geranium (*Pelargonium graveolens*), clary sage (*Savlia sclaria*), and myrtle (*Myrtus communis*) can promote healing of **hemorrhoids**; and spike lavender and juniper (*Juniperus communis*) are recommended for rheumatism.

To prepare salts for the bath, add one or two handfuls of epsom salts or Dead Sea salts to boiling water until they are dissolved, and then add them to the tub.

A **sitz bath**, or hip bath, can also be taken at home to treat hemorrhoids and promote healing of an **episiotomy**. There is special apparatus available for taking a seated sitz bath, but it can also be taken in a regular tub partially filled with warm water.

Steam inhalation

Steam inhalation treatments can be easily administered with a bowl of steaming water and a large towel. For colds and other conditions with nasal congestion, aromatherapists recommend adding five drops of an essential oil that has decongestant properties, such as peppermint (*Mentha piperita*) and eucalyptus blue gum (*Eucalyptus globulus*). Oils that act as **expectorants**, such as myrtle (*Myrtus communis*) or rosemary (*Rosmarinus officinalis*), can also be used. After the oil is added, the individual should lean over the bowl of water and place the towel over head to trap the steam. After approximately three minutes of inhaling the steam, with eyes closed, the towel can be removed.

Other herbs and essential oils that can be beneficial in steam inhalation include:

- tea tree oil (*Melaleuca alternaifolia*) for **bronchitis** and sinus infections

- sandalwood (*Santalum album*), virginian cedarwood (*Juniperus virginiana*), and frankincense (*Boswellia carteri*) for sore throat

- lavender (*Lavandula angustifolia*) and thyme (*Thymus vulgaris*) for cough

Compresses

A cold compress is prepared by soaking a cloth or cotton pad in cold water and then applying it to the area of injury or distress. When the cloth reaches room

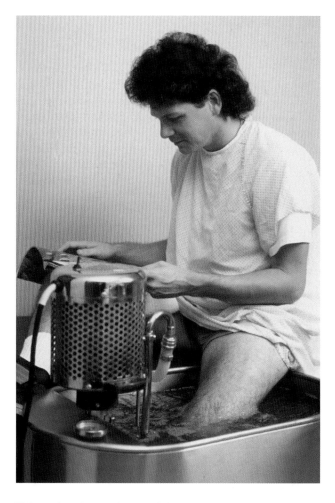

This patient is treating his injured left leg with a whirlpool bath. *(Custom Medical Stock Photo. Reproduced by permission.)*

temperature, it should be resoaked and reapplied. Applying gentle pressure to the compress with the hand may be useful. Cold compresses are generally used to reduce swelling, minimize bruising, and to treat headaches and **sprains**.

Warm or hot compresses are used to treat abscesses and muscle aches. A warm compress is prepared in the same manner as a cold compress, except steaming water is used to wet the cloth instead of cold water. Warm compresses should be refreshed and reapplied after they cool to room temperature.

Essential oils may be added to moist compresses to increase the therapeutic value of the treatment. Peppermint, a cooling oil, is especially effective when added to cold compresses. To add oils to compresses, place five drops of the oil into the bowl of water the compress is to be soaked in. Never apply essential oils directly to a cloth, as they may irritate the skin in undiluted form.

Precautions

Individuals with **paralysis**, **frostbite**, or other conditions that impair the nerve endings and cause reduced sensation should only take hydrotherapy treatments under the guidance of a trained hydrotherapist, physical therapist, or other appropriate healthcare professional. Because these individuals cannot accurately sense temperature changes in the water, they run the risk of being seriously burned without proper supervision. Diabetics and people with hypertension should also consult their healthcare professional before using hot tubs or other heat hydrotherapies.

Hot tubs, jacuzzis, and pools can become breeding grounds for bacteria and other infectious organisms if they are not cleaned regularly, maintained properly, kept at the appropriate temperatures, and treated with the proper chemicals. Individuals should check with their healthcare provider to ensure that the hydrotherapy equipment they are using is sanitary. Those who are using hot tubs and other hydrotherapy equipment in their homes should follow the directions for use and maintenance provided by the original equipment manufacturer.

Certain essential oils should not be used by pregnant or nursing women or by people with specific illnesses or physical conditions. Individuals suffering from any chronic or acute health condition should inform their healthcare provider before starting treatment with any essential oil.

Essential oils such as cinnamon leaf, juniper, lemon, eucalyptus blue gum, peppermint, and thyme can be extremely irritating to the skin if applied in full concentration. Oils used in hydrotherapy should always be diluted in water before they are applied to the skin. Individuals should never apply essential oils directly to the skin unless directed to do so by a trained healthcare professional and/or aromatherapist.

Colonic irrigation should only be performed by a healthcare professional. Pregnant women should never douche, as the practice can introduce bacteria into the vagina and uterus. They should also avoid using hot tubs without the consent of their healthcare provider.

The vagina is self-cleansing, and douches have been known to upset the balance of vaginal pH and flora, promoting vaginitis and other infections. Some studies have linked excessive vaginal douching to increased incidence of pelvic inflammatory disease (PID).

Side effects

Most forms of hydrotherapy are well tolerated. There is a risk of allergic reaction (also known as

---

> ### KEY TERMS
>
> **Contact dermatitis**—Skin irritation as a result of contact with a foreign substance.
>
> **Episiotomy**—An incision made in the perineum during labor to assist in delivery and to avoid abnormal tearing of the perineum.
>
> **Essential oil**—A volatile oil extracted from the leaves, fruit, flowers, roots, or other components of a plant and used in aromatherapy, perfumes, and foods and beverages.
>
> **Hubbard tank**—A large water tank or tub used for underwater exercises.

---

contact dermatitis) for some patients using essential oils and herbs in their bath water. These individuals may want to test for allergic sensitization to herbs by performing a skin patch test (i.e., rubbing a small amount of diluted herb on the inside of their elbow and observing the spot for redness and irritation). People who experience an allergic reaction to an essential oil should discontinue its use and contact their healthcare professional for further guidance.

The most serious possible side effect of hydrotherapy is overheating, which may occur when an individual spends too much time in a hot tub or jacuzzi. However, when properly supervised, this is a minimal risk.

Research and general acceptance

Hydrotherapy treatments are used by both allopathic and complementary medicine to treat a wide variety of discomforts and disorders. Not as well accepted are invasive hydrotherapy techniques, such as colonic irrigation, **enemas**, and douching. These internal cleansing techniques can actually harm an individual by upsetting the natural balance of the digestive tract and the vagina. Most conventional medical professionals agree that vaginal douches are not necessary to promote hygiene in most women, and can actually do more harm than good.

Resources

BOOKS

Chaitow, Leon. *Hydrotherapy: Water Therapy for Health and Beauty*. Boston, MA: Element Books, 1999.

Pelletier, Dr. Kenneth R. *The Best Alternative Medicine, Part I: Naturopathic Medicine*. New York: Simon and Schuster, 2002.

PERIODICALS

Baird, Carol L. "First-Line Treatment for Osteoarthritis: Part 2: Nonpharmacologic Interventions and Evaluation." *Orthopaedic Nursing* 20 (November-December 2001): 13–20.

Barker, K. L., H. Dawes, P. Hansford, and D. Shamley. "Perceived and Measured Levels of Exertion of Patients with Chronic Back Pain Exercising in a Hydrotherapy Pool." *Archives of Physical Medicine and Rehabilitation* 84 (September 2003): 1319–1323.

Cider, A., M. Schaufelberger, K. S. Sunnerhagen, and B. Andersson. "Hydrotherapy—A New Approach to Improve Function in the Older Patient with Chronic Heart Failure." *European Journal of Heart Failure* 5 (August 2003): 527–535.

Johnson, Kate. "Hydrotherapy Greatly Eases Delivery Stress, Pain." *OB GYN News* 34 (November 1999): 27.

Keegan, L. "Therapies to Reduce Stress and Anxiety." *Critical Care Nursing Clinics of North America* 15 (September 2003): 321–327.

Mayhall, C. G. "The Epidemiology of Burn Wound Infections: Then and Now." *Clinical Infectious Diseases* 37 (August 15, 2003): 543–550.

Molter, N. C. "Creating a Healing Environment for Critical Care." *Critical Care Nursing Clinics of North America* 15 (September 2003): 295–304.

Taylor, S. "The Ventilated Patient Undergoing Hydrotherapy: A Case Study." *Australian Critical Care* 16 (August 2003): 111–115.

ORGANIZATIONS

The American Association of Naturopathic Physicians. 8201 Greensboro Drive, Suite 300, McLean, Virginia 22102. (206) 298-0126. < http://naturopathic.org >.

Canadian Naturopathic Association/Association canadienne de naturopathie. 1255 Sheppard Avenue East at Leslie, North York, ON M2K 1E2. (800) 551-4381 or (416) 496-8633. < http://www.naturopathicassoc.ca >.

Paula Anne Ford-Martin
Rebecca J. Frey, PhD

Hydroxzine *see* **Anti-itch drugs**

Hyperactivity *see* **Attention-deficit/ Hyperactivity disorder (ADHD)**

Hyperaldosteronism

Definition

Hyperaldosteronism is a disorder which is defined by the body's overproduction of aldosterone, a hormone that controls sodium and potassium levels in the blood. Its overproduction leads to retention of salt and loss of potassium, which leads to **hypertension** (high blood pressure).

Description

Also known as Conn's syndrome, primary aldosteronism, and secondary aldosteronism, this disorder takes several forms. It often begins with a tumor that produces aldosterone. In fact, approximately 60–70% of the cases of primary aldosteronism result from tumors in the adrenal gland area. Aldosterone is normally produced by the adrenal cortex, or the outer portion of the gland that rests on top of each kidney. Primary aldosteronism is due to adenoma, a typically benign tumor in which the cells form to act as glands or cause the glands on which they rest to overproduce. It can cause a number of problems, most notably hypertension. In secondary aldosteronism, factors outside the adrenal gland may cause overproduction of aldosterone, or overproduction of renin, an enzyme stored in the kidney area that stimulates aldosterone and raises blood pressure. Obstructive renal artery disease may also cause hypertension from elevated renin stimulating aldosterone. **Oral contraceptives** have been known to increase the secretion of aldosterone in some patients. This disorder is more common in women.

Causes and symptoms

Hyperaldosteronism is most often caused by the invasion of adenoma. Other adrenal cancers and hyperplasia, or the increase in the bulk of an organ due to increased cell production, may also cause hyperaldosteronism. Those diseases and factors influencing the adrenal and kidney functions may lead to secondary aldosteronism. The primary symptom of hyperaldosteronism is moderate hypertension, or high blood pressure. In addition, a patient may experience **orthostatic hypotension**, or reduced blood pressure when a person stands after lying down. **Constipation**, muscle weakness (sometimes to the point of **periodic paralysis**), excessive urination, excessive thirst, headache, and personality changes are also possible symptoms. Some patients will show no obvious symptoms.

Diagnosis

Screening tests can be conducted to pinpoint a diagnosis of hyperaldosteronism. If a patient is taking drugs to reduce high blood pressure, the physician may order these drugs stopped for a time period before conducting tests, since these drugs will affect results.

Blood and urine tests may be conducted to check for levels of aldosterone, potassium levels, or renin activity. A computed tomography scan (CT scan) may be ordered to detect tumors as small as five to seven mm. These combined tests approach 95% accuracy for detecting aldosterone-producing adenoma. Laboratory findings recording blood pressure, **edema**, and aldosterone and plasma renin activity can help the physician differentiate between primary aldosteronism and secondary aldosteronism.

Treatment

Once the physician has made a diagnosis of hyperaldosteronism, the adrenal glands should be checked for possible adenomas. This can be done through imaging or with a surgical dissection of the gland. Surgical or ablative treatment will vary depending on the number of tumors found. Since more than 60% of hyperaldosteronism cases are caused by these tumors, treatment of the tumors will help eliminate the resulting high blood pressure in many patients. Some patients will receive **antihypertensive drugs**, like calcium channel blockers, to control high blood pressure. The use of **diuretics** can help control hypertension by reducing volume. Potassium levels should be considered in the type of diuretic ordered and the levels should be checked throughout treatment. The most widely used drug for treatment of hyperaldosteronism is spironolactone. This drug helps control aldosterone, but should not be prescribed for some patients, especially those with certain kidney diseases. Spironolactone has several possible adverse effects, depending on the dosage. In all cases of hyperaldosteronism, the treatment should be carefully based on the specific type or underlying cause of the disorder.

Alternative treatment

Patients may choose to work with their physician or alternative provider to control hypertension with diet, **stress reduction** (including massage, meditation, **biofeedback**, and yoga), and other remedies. Blood pressure elevation needs to be controlled and monitored by frequent blood pressure measurements. There is no alternative treatment known for the underlying adenoma.

Prognosis

Hyperaldosteronism carries with it all the possible complications of high blood pressure, including thickening of arterial walls and a higher risk of angina,

KEY TERMS

Ablative—Used to describe a procedure involving removal of a tissue or body part, or destruction of its function.

Adenoma—A growth of cells, usually a benign tumor, that forms a gland or gland-like substance. These tumors can secrete hormones or cause changes in hormone production in nearby glands.

Adrenal—Refers to the glands which sit on top of each kidney and that secrete various hormones.

Antihypertensive—Used to describe drugs or treatments designed to control hypertension, or high blood pressure.

Diuretic—A substance or drug that is taken to promote the formation and release of urine. In the treatment of high blood pressure, diuretics can help reduce the overall fluid volume in the body.

Renal—Relating to the kidney. The renal artery is one of two branches of the large blood vessel in the stomach area that serves the kidneys, ureters (tubes that carry urine from the kidney to the bladder) and adrenal glands.

kidney failure, **stroke**, or heart attack. Another possible, and less reversible complication than hypertension, is kidney damage. When primary aldosteronism is caused by a solitary adenoma, the prognosis is good. Once this tumor is removed, blood pressure will drop, and 70% of these patients have full remission. Patients whose hyperaldosteronism results from adrenal hyperplasia will remain hypertensive. However, in up to 70% of patients, blood pressure can be reduced somewhat with drug therapy. Many patients will be faced with the prospect of controlling their hypertension for the remainder of their lives.

Prevention

There is no known prevention for most causes of hyperaldosteronism.

Resources

ORGANIZATIONS

American Heart Association. 7320 Greenville Ave. Dallas, TX 75231. (214) 373-6300. < http://www.americanheart.org >.

American Society of Hypertension. 515 Madison Ave., Suite 1212, New York, NY 10022. (212) 644-0650. < http://www.ash-us.org >.

National Heart, Lung and Blood Institute. PO Box 30105, Bethesda, MD 20824-0105. (301) 251-1222. < http://www.nhlbi.nih.gov >.

OTHER

Hypertension Network. < http://www.bloodpressure.com >.

Teresa Odle

Hyperbaric Chamber

Definition

A hyperbaric chamber is a room that allows an individual to breathe 100% pure oxygen at greater than 1 standard atmosphere of pressure.

Purpose

Hyperbaric chambers are used to deliver hyperbaric **oxygen therapy** (HBOT). HBOT was developed to treat underwater divers suffering from **decompression sickness** (the bends). It has since been approved by the Undersea and Hyperbaric Medical Society for 13 conditions including:

- air or gas embolism
- carbon monoxide (CO) **poisoning**
- smoke inhalation
- gas **gangrene** caused by certain bacteria
- decompression sickness
- radiation tissue damage
- thermal burns
- non-healing skin grafts
- crush injuries
- wounds that fail to heal through conventional treatment
- serious blood loss
- intracranial abscess.

Although hyperbaric therapy has become increasingly popular for other uses, especially in sports medicine, its use is controversial. Terrell Owens of the Philadelphia Eagles used HBOT for an ankle injury prior to playing in the Super Bowl in 2005, but medical professionals questioned the appropriateness of this treatment.

Precautions

Individuals who have lung disease including **asthma**, **emphysema**, obstructive lung disease, or any condition in which air is trapped in the lungs, are poor candidates for this therapy and should discuss the relative benefits and drawbacks of HBOT with their doctor. Individuals who have had chest surgery or who have had a central venous catheter implanted are also at higher risk for complications. People with seizure disorders should be carefully monitored, as this treatment may increase the risk and severity of seizures. People with colds or clogged ears may want to wait to undergo HBOT, as they may experience difficulties with pressure equalization that can cause damage to the middle or inner ear. HBOT in **pregnancy** is controversial. Individuals with diabetes may need to adjust their glucose and insulin balance, since HBOT slows the absorption of insulin.

Description

At normal atmospheric pressure, oxygen binds with a molecule in red blood cells called hemoglobin. The oxygen is carried through the body to tissues where it is needed as the blood circulates. Under normal conditions, almost all (about 97%) of the available hemoglobin carries oxygen. Increasing the atmospheric pressure does little to increase the oxygen-carrying capacity of the blood. However, under normal conditions, only a small amount of oxygen is dissolved in the fluid that carries the red blood cells (blood plasma). Increasing the atmospheric pressure to two to three times normal and breathing 100% oxygen forces more oxygen to dissolve into the blood plasma. In this way, hyperbaric chambers increase the amount of oxygen circulating in the body. This can promote healing in areas that are not receiving adequate oxygen. The extra oxygen can also help to cure certain infections caused by anerobic bacteria that can live only in the absence of oxygen.

There are two types of hyperbaric chambers—monoplace and multiplace. Monoplace chambers accommodate a single person. The patient enters the chamber, then it is closed and the pressure is increased. The advantages of a monoplace chamber are that the patient does not have to wear a mask or a hood to receive the oxygen and the treatment regimen is designed specifically for each individual. The major disadvantages are that the patient is inaccessible to the staff during treatment should an emergency arise, and the pure oxygen atmosphere creates an increased fire hazard. In multiplace chambers, several patients use the same chamber simultaneously. Each person is given oxygen through a face mask or hood, but all patients receive the same treatment. A staff member remains in the chamber throughout the procedure.

Hyperbaric chambers can be associated with hospitals, but are increasingly part of free-standing clinics. Insurance may cover the cost of treatment for approved indications such as **carbon monoxide poisoning**, but may reject payment for uses that are considered experimental or controversial. The American Board of Medical Specialists certifies physician competency in the undersea medicine, including the use of hyperbaric chambers. The Baromedical Nurses Association offers three levels of certification for hyperbaric nurses, and the National Board of Hyperbaric Medicine Technology certifies hyperbaric technicians. Individuals considering hyperbaric therapy should seek facilities run by health care providers credentialed by these organizations.

Preparation

No special preparation is needed to use a hyperbaric chamber other than educating patients about what to expect during treatment.

Aftercare

After HBOT is complete, a period of decompression in the chamber is required until the pressure in the chamber is equal to the pressure outside. Serious complications can occur if decompression occurs suddenly.

Risks

Hyperbaric chambers, because of their use of 100% oxygen, present a potential fire risk. In addition, although hyperbaric oxygen therapy is very safe when used correctly, complications can occur. Oxygen poisoning, also called oxygen toxicity, can occur when an individual is exposed to high doses of oxygen for a prolonged period. Excess oxygen causes chemical changes in the body that negatively affect cells and metabolic processes. Symptoms of oxygen poisoning include **nausea**, **vomiting**, dry **cough**, seizures, chest **pain**, sweating, muscle twitching, ringing of the ears, **hallucinations**, **dizziness**, **shortness of breath** and a decreased level of consciousness.

Other complications can occur as the result of increased pressure within the chamber. These include pain and bloody discharge from congested sinuses, ear pain, rupture of the eardrum, and bleeding from the ear if the Eustachian tube that connects the ear to the back of the throat is clogged and pressure on either

---

> **KEY TERMS**
>
> **Embolism**—An obstruction in a blood vessel, often caused by gas or a blood clot.
>
> **Eustachian tube**—A tube of cartilage that connects the middle ear to the back of the throat. Its purpose is to equalize the pressure on either side of the eardrum.

side of the eardrum is not equalized. Teeth that are infected or have been repaired may become painful or explode if gas is trapped within them. A few individuals develop **pneumothorax**. This is a serious condition where air is trapped between the lungs and the chest cavity.

Normal results

HBOT is expected to promote healing and improve the health of individuals with conditions for which it is approved.

Abnormal results

Under some conditions HBOT fails to cause improvement or complications occur.

Resources

ORGANIZATION

Undersea and Hyperbaric Medicine Society. 10531 Metropolitan Avenue, Kensington, MD 20895. 310-942-7804. < www.uhns.0rg > .

OTHER

Moder, Cheryl. *Hyperbaric Oxygen Therapy: Where Medicine Meets the Deep Blue Sea,* 20 February 2005 [cited 20 February 2005]. < http://www.emedicine.com/plastic/topic526.htm >.

Neumeister, Michael. *Hyperbaric Oxygen Therapy,* 11 November 2004 [cited 16 February 2005]. < http://www.emedicine.com/plastic/topic526.htm >.

Prince, Mark. *Hyperbaric Oxygen,* 27 October 2004 [cited 16 February 2005]. < http://www.emedicine.com/ent/topic733.htm >.

Tish Davidson, A. M.

Hyperbaric oxygenation *see* **Oxygen/ozone therapy**

Hyperbilirubinemia *see* **Neonatal jaundice**

Hypercalcemia

Definition

Hypercalcemia is an abnormally high level of calcium in the blood, usually more than 10.5 milligrams per deciliter of blood.

Description

Calcium plays an important role in the development and maintenance of bones in the body. It is also needed in tooth formation and is important in other body functions. Normally, the body maintains a balance between the amount of calcium in food sources and the calcium already available in the body's tissues. The balance can be upset if excess amounts of calcium are eaten or if the body is unable to process the mineral because of disease.

Calcium is one of the most important and most abundant **minerals** in the human body. Dairy products are the major source of calcium. Eggs, green leafy vegetables, broccoli, legumes, nuts, and whole grains provide smaller amounts. Only about 10–30% of the calcium in food is absorbed into the body. Most calcium is found in combination with other dietary components and must be broken down by the digestive system before it can be used. Calcium is absorbed into the body in the small intestine. Its absorption is influenced by such factors as the amount of vitamin D hormone available to aid the process and the levels of calcium already present in the body. As much as 99% of the body's calcium is stored in bone tissue. A healthy person experiences a constant turnover of calcium as bone tissue is built and reshaped. The remaining 1% of the body's calcium circulates in the blood and other body fluids. Circulating calcium plays an important role in the control of many body functions, such as blood clotting, transmission of nerve impulses, muscle contraction, and other metabolic activities. In the bloodstream, calcium maintains a constant balance with another mineral, phosphate.

Two main control agents are vital in maintaining calcium levels, vitamin D hormone and parathyroid hormone. A hormone is a chemical substance that is formed in one organ or part of the body and carried in the blood to another organ. It can alter the function, and sometimes the structure, of one or more organs.

- Parathyroid hormone (PTH). The four parathyroid glands are endocrine glands located next to the thyroid gland in the neck. A gland is a cell or group of cells that produces a material substance (secretion). When the level of calcium circulating in the blood drops, the parathyroid gland releases its hormone. PTH then acts in three ways to restore the normal blood calcium level. It stimulates the absorption of more calcium in the intestine; it takes more calcium from the bone tissue, and it causes the kidneys to excrete more phosphate.

- Vitamin D hormone. This hormone works with parathyroid hormone to control calcium absorption and affects the deposit of calcium and phosphate in the bone tissue.

The kidneys also help to control calcium levels. Healthy kidneys can increase calcium excretion almost fivefold to maintain normal concentrations in the body. Hypercalcemia can occur when the concentration of calcium overwhelms the ability of the kidneys to maintain balance.

Causes and symptoms

Causes of hypercalcemia

Many different conditions can cause hypercalcemia; the most common are **hyperparathyroidism** and **cancer**.

PRIMARY HYPERPARATHYROIDISM. Primary hyperparathyroidism is the excessive secretion of parathyroid hormone by one or more of the parathyroid glands. It is the most common cause of hypercalcemia in the general population. Women have this condition more frequently than men do, and it is more common in older people. It can appear thirty or more years after radiation treatments to the neck. Ninety percent of the cases of primary hyperparathyroidism are caused by a non-malignant growth on the gland.

Hyperparathyroidism can also occur as part of a rare hereditary disease called multiple endocrine neoplasia. In this disease, tumors develop on the parathyroid gland.

CANCER. People with cancer often have hypercalcemia. In fact, it is the most common life-threatening metabolic disorder associated with cancer. Ten to twenty percent of all persons with cancer have hypercalcemia. Cancers of the breast, lung, head and neck, and kidney are frequently associated with hypercalcemia. It also occurs frequently in association with certain cancers of the blood, particularly malignant myeloma. It is seen most often in patients with tumors of the lung (25–35%) and breast (20–40%), according to the National Cancer Institute. Cancer causes hypercalcemia in two ways. When a tumor grows into the bone, it destroys bony tissue (osteolysis). When the bone is not involved, factors secreted by cancer cells can increase calcium levels (humoral hypercalcemia of malignancy). The two mechanisms may operate at the same time.

Because immobility causes an increase in the loss of calcium from bone, cancer patients who are weak and spend most of their time in bed are more prone to hypercalcemia. Cancer patients are often dehydrated because they take in inadequate amounts of food and fluids and often suffer from **nausea and vomiting**. **Dehydration** reduces the ability of the kidneys to remove excess calcium from the body. Hormones and **diuretics** that increase the amount of fluid released by the body can also trigger hypercalcemia.

OTHER CAUSES. Other conditions can cause hypercalcemia. Excessive intake of vitamin D increases intestinal absorption of calcium. During therapy for peptic ulcers, abnormally high amounts of calcium **antacids** are sometimes taken. Over use of antacids can cause milk-alkali syndrome and hypercalcemia. Diseases such as Paget's, in which bone is destroyed or reabsorbed, can also cause hypercalcemia. As in cancer or **paralysis** of the arms and legs, any condition in which the patient is immobilized for long periods of time can lead to hypercalcemia due to bone loss.

Common symptoms

Many patients with mild hypercalcemia have no symptoms and the condition is discovered during routine laboratory screening. Gastrointestinal symptoms include loss of appetite, nausea, vomiting, **constipation**, and abdominal **pain**. There may be a blockage in the bowel. If the kidneys are involved, the individual will have to urinate frequently during both the day and night and will be very thirsty. As the calcium levels rise, the symptoms become more serious. Stones may form in the kidneys and waste products can build up. Blood pressure rises. The heart rhythm may change. Muscles become increasingly weak. The individual may experience mood swings, confusion, **psychosis**, and eventually, **coma** and **death**.

Diagnosis

High levels of calcium in the blood are a good indication of hypercalcemia, but these levels may fluctuate. Calcium levels are influenced by other compounds in the blood that may combine with calcium. Higher calcium and lower phosphate levels may suggest primary hyperparathyroidism. The blood levels of protein (serum albumin) and parathyroid hormone (PTH) are also measured in the diagnosis of hypercalcemia. Too much PTH in the blood may indicate primary hyperparathyroidism. Levels of calcium and phosphate in the urine should also be measured. The medical history and physical condition of the individual must be taken into consideration, especially in the early stages of hypercalcemia when symptoms are mild.

Treatment

The treatment of hypercalcemia depends on how high the calcium level is and what is causing the elevation. Hypercalcemia can be life-threatening and rapid reduction may be necessary. If the patient has normal kidney function, fluids can be given by vein (intravenously) to clear the excess calcium. The amount of fluid taken in and eliminated must be carefully monitored. If the patient's kidneys are not working well, acute hemodyalysis is probably the safest and most effective method to reduce dangerous calcium levels. In this procedure, blood is circulated through tubes made of semi-permeable membranes against a special solution that filters out unwanted substances before returning the blood to the body.

Drugs such as furosemide, called loop diuretics, can be given after adequate fluid intake is established. These drugs inhibit calcium reabsorption in the kidneys and promote urine production. Drugs that inhibit bone loss, such as calcitonin, biphosphates, and plicamycin, are helpful in achieving long-term control. Phosphate pills help lower high calcium levels caused by a deficiency in phosphate. Anti-inflammatory agents such as steroids are helpful with some cancers and toxic levels of vitamin D.

Treatment of the underlying cause of the hypercalcemia will also correct the imbalance. Hyperparathyroidism is usually treated by surgical removal of one or more of the parathyroid glands and any tissue, other than the glands themselves, that is producing excessive amounts of the hormone.

The hypercalcemia caused by cancer is difficult to treat without controlling the cancer. Symptoms can be alleviated with fluids and drug therapy as outlined above.

Prognosis

Surgery to remove the parathyroid glands and any misplaced tissue that is producing excessive amounts of hormone succeeds in about 90% of all cases. Outcome is also influenced by whether any damage to the kidneys can be reversed.

Mild hypercalcemia can be controlled through good fluid intake and the use of effective drugs.

Hypercalcemia generally develops as a late complication of cancer and the expected outlook is grim without effective anticancer therapy.

Prevention

People with cancer who are at risk of developing hypercalcemia should be familiar with early symptoms and know when to see a doctor. Good fluid intake (up to four quarts of liquid a day if possible), controlling nausea and vomiting, paying attention to fevers, and keeping physically active as much as possible can help prevent problems. Dietary calcium restriction is not necessary because hypercalcemia reduces absorption of calcium in the intestine.

Resources

OTHER

"Hypercalcemia." *National Cancer Institute Page.* < http://www.nci.nih.gov >.

Karen Ericson, RN

Hypercholesterolemia

Definition

Hypercholesterolemia refers to levels of cholesterol in the blood that are higher than normal.

Description

Cholesterol circulates in the blood stream. It is an essential molecule for the human body. Cholesterol is a molecule from which hormones and steroids are made. It is also used to maintain nerve cells. Between 75 and 80% of the cholesterol that circulates in a person's bloodstream is made in that person's liver. The remainder is acquired from outside sources. Cholesterol is found in animal sources of food. It is not found in plants.

Normal blood cholesterol level is a number derived by laboratory analysis. A normal or desirable cholesterol level is defined as less than 200 mg of cholesterol per deciliter of blood (mg/dL). Blood cholesterol is considered to be borderline when it is in the range of 200 to 239 mg/dL. Elevated cholesterol level is 240 mg/dL or above. Elevated blood cholesterol is considered to be hypercholesterolemia.

Cholesterol has been divided into two major categories: low-density lipoprotein (LDL), the so-called "bad" cholesterol, and high-density lipoprotein (HDL), the so-called "good" cholesterol. Diet, **exercise**, **smoking**, alcohol, and certain illnesses can affect the levels of both types of cholesterol. Eating a high fat diet will increase one's level of LDL cholesterol. Exercising and reducing one's weight will both increase HDL cholesterol and lower LDL cholesterol.

The most common cause of elevated serum cholesterol is eating foods that are rich in saturated fats or contain high levels of cholesterol. Elevated cholesterol also can be caused by an underlying disease that raises blood cholesterol levels such as **diabetes mellitus**, **kidney disease**, **liver disease**, or **hypothyroidism**. It also can be caused by an inherited disorder in which cholesterol is not metabolized properly by the body.

Obesity, which generally results from eating a diet high in fat, also can lead to elevated cholesterol levels in the blood. This is because obesity itself leads the body to produce excessive amounts of cholesterol.

Hypercholesterolemia increases the risk of heart disease. Elevated levels of circulating cholesterol cause deposits to form inside blood vessels. These deposits, called plaque, are composed of fats deposited from the bloodstream. When the deposits become sufficiently large, they block blood vessels and decrease the flow of blood. These deposits result in a disease process called **atherosclerosis**, which can cause **blood clots** to form that will ultimately stop blood flow. If this happens in the arteries supplying the heart, a **heart attack** will occur. If it happens in the brain, the result is a **stroke** where a portion of brain tissue dies. Atherosclerosis causes more deaths from heart disease than any other single condition. Heart disease has been the leading cause of **death** in the United States for the past half century.

There is a syndrome called familial hypercholesterolemia. Affected persons have consistently high levels of LDL. This leads to early clogging of the coronary arteries. In turn this leads to a heart attack. Among affected males, a first heart attack typically occurs in their 40s to 50s. Approximately 85% of men with this disorder have experienced a heart attack by the time they reach 60 years of age. The incidence of heart attacks among women with this disorder also is increased. However, it is delayed 10 years compared to men. The incidence of familial hypercholesterolemia is seven out of 1,000 people.

Causes and symptoms

Hypercholesterolemia is silent. There are no symptoms that are obvious to the naked eye. It is diagnosed by a blood test or after a heart attack or stroke occurs.

Diagnosis

Hypercholesterolemia is diagnosed by using a blood test. A blood specimen is obtained after the patient does not eat or drink anything (except water) for 12 hours. The **fasting** is done to measure the LDL and HDL cholesterol, which can only be determined accurately in a fasting state. Some experts agree that an acceptable limit for LDL cholesterol as 130 mg/dL, though the National Cholesterol Education Program Adult Treatment Panel III recommended a goal of less than 100mg/dL. Total cholesterol of under 200 mg/dL is thought to be an acceptable range.

Treatment

If an individual's cholesterol is elevated, discussions with a physician should be scheduled to determine what course of treatment may be needed. Initial treatment for hypercholesterolemia usually requires dietary changes to reduce the intake of total fat, saturated fat, and cholesterol. Most health care professionals will recommend that a person's weight and height be proportionate. In addition to diet, guidelines recommend exercise to help bring weight and cholesterol to acceptable levels. Further, experts counsel persons with elevated blood cholesterol levels to increase their intake of soluble fiber. Sources of soluble fiber include bran, foods containing whole grains and other sources of indigestible fiber such as lignin. Physicians also recommend that patients with **high cholesterol** stop smoking as part of first-line therapy for hypercholesterolemia.

The reason for treating elevated cholesterol is to reduce an individual's risk of complications. If a diet low in cholesterol and saturated fats doesn't significantly reduce a person's cholesterol level, medication may be required. For every 1 percent reduction in cholesterol level, the risk of heart disease is reduced by 2 percent. It also is possible to partially reverse atherosclerosis that has already occurred by aggressively lowering cholesterol levels with diet and medications.

Prescription drugs are available to help lower cholesterol levels in the blood. These may be used as first-line therapy in high-risk patients or after about three months of dietary and lifestyle therapy. Cholestyramine, cholestipol, lovastatin, simvastatin, pravastatin, fluvaststin, rosuvastatin, and gemfibrazol are some of the drugs approved for use in the United States. The most often prescribed group of drugs are the statins, which also have been shown in some studies to reduce risk of depression and **dementia**.

Alternative treatment

There are advocates of treatment using **vitamins, minerals** and antioxidant substances in relatively high amounts. These amounts generally exceed those provided by the Food and Drug Administration in its Minimum Daily Requirements (MDR). Advocates of such therapies also emphasize increased levels of exercise, attaining an ideal body weight and increasing levels of fiber in one's diet.

Some people have advocated the use of garlic, soy and isoflavones to lower serum cholesterol levels. In 2003, enriched green tea was found to be an effective addition to a low-fat diet for lowering LDL cholesterol in adults.

Prognosis

The prognos is in direct proportion to serum cholesterol levels. People with hypercholesterolemia are at high risk of dying from heart disease.

Many studies have looked at the relationship between elevated cholesterol levels, increased risk for heart attack and death. In one investigation of relatively young males who had no known heart disease, cholesterol levels were measured and participants were followed for six years. During this time, all heart attacks and deaths that occurred among participants were recorded. As serum cholesterol levels increased, so did the risk of experiencing a fatal heart attack. The risk of a fatal heart attack was approximately five times higher among persons having cholesterol levels of 300 mg/dL or more compared to those with cholesterol levels below 200 mg/dL.

The Framingham Heart Study is an ongoing research effort. Cholesterol levels, smoking habits, heart attack rates, and deaths in the population of an entire town have been recorded for over 40 years. After 30 years, more than 85% of persons with cholesterol levels of 180 mg/dL or less were still alive; almost a third of those with cholesterol levels greater than 260 mg/dL had died.

Prevention

Experts suggest the following steps to maintain serum cholesterol within normal limits: an important component is to maintain a normal weight for height and to reduce one's weight if it is inappropriate for height. Changing dietary habits by reducing the amount of fat and cholesterol consumed is advised. Doctors recommend avoiding smoking by not starting or quitting if currently a smoker. Increasing levels of fiber in the diet by including foods such as beans, raw fruits, whole grains and vegetables is receommended. It is important to exercise on a regular basis. Aerobic exercise is especially helpful in reducing serum cholesterol levels.

People from families with a strong history of early heart attacks should be evaluated with a lipid screen. Proper diet, exercise and the use of effective drugs can reduce serum lipid levels.

Nutrition and cardiac experts offer the following suggestions:

- purchasing low-fat or fat-free dairy products such as milk, cheese, sour cream, and yogurt
- eating lean red meats, chicken without skin, and fish
- reducing consumption of foods high in saturated fat such as french fries

---

KEY TERMS

Atherosclerosis—A disease process whereby plaques of fatty substances are deposited inside arteries, reducing the inside diameter of the vessels and eventually causing damage to the tissues located beyond the site of the blockage.

Coronary artery—One of five vessels that supply blood to the heart.

Deciliter (dL)—100 cubic centimeters (cc).

High density lipoprotein (HDL)—A fraction of total serum lipids, the so called "good" cholesterol.

Low density lipoprotein (LDL)—A fraction of total serum lipids, the so called "bad" cholesterol.

- avoid foods that are rich sources of cholesterol such as eggs, liver, cheese, and bacon
- eating smaller servings
- keeping a food journal and writing down everything eaten each day
- prepare food by microwaving, boiling, broiling, or baking food instead of frying
- trimming the fat from meat before cooking it.

Resources

BOOKS

Braunwald, Eugene, Douglas Zipes, and Perter Libby. *Heart Disease: A Textbook of Cardiovascular Medicine*. 6th ed. Philadelphia: Saunders, 2001.

Foody, J.M, and Eugene Braunwald. *Preventive Cardiology: Strategies for the Prevention and Treatment of Coronary Artery Disease*. Totowa, NJ: Humana Press, 2001.

Hiatt, William R. "Atheroclerotic peripheral arterial disease." In *Cecil Textbook of Medicine*, edited by Lee Goldman and J. Claude Bennett, 21st ed. Philadelphia: W.B. Saunders, 2000, pp. 357-362.

Hiatt, William R., Judith Regensteiner, and Alan T. Hirsch. *Peripheral Arterial Disease Handbook*. Boca Raton, FL: CRC Press, 2001.

Silver, Malcom, and Schoen Gottlieb. *Cardiovascular Pathology*. 3rd ed. Boston, Churchill Livingstone, 2001.

PERIODICALS

Aronow, Wilbert S. "Hypercholesterolemia: The Evidence Supports Use of Statins." *Geriatrics* August 2003: 18.

"Cholesterol-lowering Effect of Green Tea." *Nutraceuticals International* September 2003.

Jackson, P.R. "Cholesterol-lowering Therapy for Smokers." *The Lancet* 357, no. 9260 (2001): 960–961.

"Link to Cholesterol Drugs Disputed." *Cardiovascular Week* September 29, 2003: 73.

Mechcatie, Elizabeth. "FDA Okays Rosuvastatin for Hypercholeterolemia: Most Potent Statin to Date." *Internal Medicine News* September 1, 2003: 30–31.

Shamir R., A. Lerner, and E. A. Fisher. "Hypercholesterolemia in Children." *Israel Medical Association Journal* 2, no. 10 (2000): 767–771.

ORGANIZATIONS

American Heart Association, National Center. 7272 Greenville Avenue, Dallas, Texas 75231. (877) 242-4277. < http://www.americanheart.org >.

American Medical Association. 515 N. State Street, Chicago, IL 60610. (312) 464-5000. < http://www.ama-assn.org/ >.

American Society of Nuclear Cardiology. 9111 Old Georgetown Road, Bethesda, MD 20814-1699. (301) 493-2360. Fax: (301) 493-2376, < http://www.asnc.org >.

OTHER

American Academy of Family Practice: < http://www.aafp.org/afp/20000201/675.html >.

American Heart Association. < http://www.american-heart.org/Scientific/pubs/hyperchol/ >.

Merck Manual. < http://www.merck.com/pubs/mmanual/section2/chapter15/15c.htm >.

National Library of Medicine: < http://www.nlm.nih.gov/medlineplus/ency/article/000403.htm >.

L. Fleming Fallon, Jr., MD, DrPH
Teresa G. Odle

Hypercoagulation disorders

Definition

Hypercoagulation disorders (or hypercoagulable states or disorders) have the opposite effect of the more common **coagulation disorders**. In hypercoagulation, there is an increased tendency for clotting of the blood, which may put a patient at risk for obstruction of veins and arteries (phlebitis or pulmonary embolism).

Description

In normal hemostasis, or the stoppage of bleeding, clots form at the site of the blood vessel's injury. The difference between that sort of clotting and the clotting present in hypercoagulation is that these clots develop in circulating blood.

This disorder can cause clots throughout the body's blood vessels, sometimes creating a condition known as thrombosis. Thrombosis can lead to infarction, or death of tissue, as a result of blocked blood supply to the tissue. However, hypercoagulability does not always lead to thrombosis. In **pregnancy**, and other hypercoagulable states, the incidence of thrombosis is higher than that of the general population, but is still under 10%. However, in association with certain genetic disorders, hypercoagulation disorders may be more likely to lead to thrombosis. Hypercoagulation disorders may also be known as hyperhomocystinemia, antithrombin III deficiency, factor V leyden, and protein C or protein S deficiency.

Causes and symptoms

Hypercoagulation disorders may be acquired or hereditary. Some of the genetic disorders that lead to hypercoagulation are abnormal clotting factor V, variations in fibrinogen, and deficiencies in proteins C and S. Other body system diseases may also lead to these disorders, including diabetes, sickle cell anemia, congenital heart disease, lupus, **thalassemia**, polycythemia rubra vera, and others. Antithrombin III deficiency is a hereditary hypercoagulation disorder that affects both sexes. Symptoms include obstruction of a blood vessel by a clot (thromboembolic disease), vein inflammation (phlebitis), and ulcers of the lower parts of the legs. The role of proteins C and S is a complex one. In order for coagulation to occur, platelets (small, round fragments in the blood) help contract blood vessels to lessen blood loss and also to help plug damaged blood vessels. However, the conversion of platelets into actual clots is a complicated web involving proteins that are identified clotting factors. The factors are carried in the plasma, or liquid portion of the blood. Proteins C and S are two of the clotting factors that are present in the plasma to help regulate or activate parts of the clotting process. Protein C is considered an anticoagulant. Mutation defects in the proteins may decrease their concentrations in the blood, and may or may not affect their resulting anticoagulant activity. Factor V is an unstable clotting factor also present in plasma. Abnormal factor V resists the changes that normally occur through the influence of protein C, which can also lead to hypercoagulability. Prothrombin, a glycoprotein that converts to thrombin in the early stage of the clotting process, is affected by the presence of these proteins, as well as other clotting factors.

Diagnosis

The diagnosis of hypercoagulation disorders is completed with a combination of **physical examination**, medical history, and blood tests. An accurate medical history is important to determine possible symptoms

KEY TERMS

Antithrombin—Any substance that counters the effect of thrombin, an enzyme that converts fibrinogen into fibrin, leading to blood coagulation.

Congenital—Refers to a condition or disorder present at birth.

Hemostasis—The arrest of bleeding.

Heparin—An anticoagulant, or blood clot "dissolver."

Polycythemia—A condition characterized by an overabundance of red blood cells.

Thalassemia—One of a group of inherited blood disorders characterized by a defect in the metabolism of hemoglobin, or the portion of the red blood cells that transports oxygen throughout the blood stream.

Thrombosis—Formation of a clot in the blood that either blocks, or partially blocks, a blood vessel. The thrombus may lead to infarction, or death of tissue due to a blocked blood supply.

and causes of hypercoagulation disorders. There are a number of blood tests that can determine the presence or absence of proteins, clotting factors, and platelet counts in the blood. Among the tests used to detect hypercoagulation is the Antithrombin III assay. Protein C and Protein S concentrations can be diagnosed with immunoassay or plasma antigen level tests.

Treatment

Coumadin and heparin anticoagulants may be administered to reduce the clotting effects and maintain fluidity in the blood. Heparin is an anticoagulant that prevents thrombus formation and is used primarily for liver and lung clots.

Prognosis

The prognosis for patients with hypercoagulation disorders varies depending on the severity of the clotting and thrombosis. If undetected and untreated, thrombosis could lead to recurrent thrombosis and **pulmonary embolism**, a potentially fatal problem.

Prevention

Hereditary hypercoagulation disorders may not be prevented. Genetic and blood testing may help determine a person's tendency to develop these disorders.

Resources

ORGANIZATIONS

National Heart, Lung and Blood Institute. PO Box 30105, Bethesda, MD 20824-0105. (301) 251-1222. < http://www.nhlbi.nih.gov >.

National Hemophilia Foundation. 116 West 32nd St., 11th Floor, New York, NY 10001. 800-424-2634. < http://www.hemophilia.org/home.htm >.

Teresa Odle

Hyperemesis gravidarum

Definition

Hyperemesis gravidarum means excessive **vomiting** during **pregnancy**.

Description

In pregnant women, **nausea and vomiting** (morning sickness) are common, affecting up to 80% of pregnancies. Hyperemesis, or extreme nausea and excessive vomiting, occur in about 1% of pregnancies. This condition causes uncontrollable vomiting, severe dehydration, and weight loss for the mother. However, hyperemesis gravidarum rarely causes problems for the unborn baby.

Causes and symptoms

The cause of nausea and vomiting during pregnancy is unknown but may be related to the level of certain hormones produced during pregnancy. Hyperemesis is seen more often in first pregnancies and multiple pregnancies (twins, triplets, etc.). The main symptom of hyperemesis is severe vomiting, which causes **dehydration** and weight loss.

Diagnosis

Although many women with morning sickness feel like they are vomiting everything they eat, they continue to gain weight and are not dehydrated; they do not have hyperemesis gravidarum. Women with this condition will start to show signs of starvation, including weight loss. **Physical examination** and laboratory tests of blood and urine samples will be used to help diagnose the condition. One of the most common tests used to help diagnosis and monitor hyperemesis gravidarum is a test for ketones in the urine. Excessive ketones in the urine (ketonuria) indicate that the body is not using carbohydrates from food as fuel and is inadequately trying to break down fat as fuel. Ketonuria is a sign that the body is beginning to operate in **starvation** mode.

Treatment

Hospitalization is often required. Intravenous fluids with substances that help the body conduct nerve signals (electrolytes) may be given to correct the dehydration and excessive acid in the blood (acidosis). Anti-nausea or sedative medications may be given by injection to stop the vomiting. In some cases, oral medication may be prescribed to control the nausea and vomiting while food is reintroduced. If food cannot be tolerated at all, intravenous nutritional supplements may be necessary. Injections of vitamin B$_6$, in particular, may help overcome nutritional deficiencies that often occur.

Alternative treatment

The severe vomiting associated with hyperemesis gravidarum requires medical attention. Milder episodes of nausea or vomiting may be reduced with deep breathing and relaxation exercises. The use of herbal remedies should be done with extreme caution during pregnancy, especially in the first trimester. Natural remedies to reduce nausea include a teaspoon of cider vinegar in a cup of warm water, or tea made from anise (*Pinpinella anisum*), fennel seed (*Foeniculum vulgare*), red raspberry (*Rubus idaeus*), or ginger (*Zingiber officinale*). Wristbands can be positioned over **acupressure** points on both wrists. **Aromatherapy** with lavender, rose, or chamomile can be soothing, as can smelling ground ginger. Homeopathic remedies—which use extremely diluted solutions as treatments—can be safe and effective for controlling symptoms in some women.

Prognosis

In virtually all cases, the pregnancy can continue to the successful delivery of a healthy baby.

Prevention

Although there is no evidence that hyperemesis gravidarum can be prevented, vomiting during pregnancy sometimes may be lessened. Maintaining a

---

KEY TERMS

Ketonuria—The presence of large amount of ketones in the urine. These byproducts of inadequate breakdown of nutrients indicate that the body is in starvation.

---

healthy diet, getting adequate sleep, and controlling **stress** may contribute to prevention or improvement of symptoms. Several strategies may help lessen the nausea and vomiting. Eating dry foods and limiting fluid intake may also be helpful. Small meals should be eaten frequently throughout the day, with a protein snack at night. Eating soda crackers before rising from bed in the morning may help prevent early morning nausea. Iron supplements may cause nausea and can be eliminated until the nausea is controlled. Sitting upright for 45 minutes after meals may also help.

Resources

OTHER

Levy, B. T., and P. L. Brown. "Nausea and Vomiting in Pregnancy." *The Virtual Hospital Page.* University of Iowa. < http://www.vh.org >.
"Natural Remedies During Pregnancy: Frequently Asked Questions." *Childbirth.Org.* < http://www.childbirth.org/articles/remedy.html >.

Altha Roberts Edgren

Hyperhidrosis

Definition

Hyperhidrosis is a disorder marked by excessive sweating. It usually begins at **puberty** and affects the palms, soles, and armpits.

Description

Sweating is the body's way of cooling itself and is a normal response to a hot environment or intense **exercise**. However, excessive sweating unrelated to these conditions can be a problem for some people. Those with constantly moist hands may feel uncomfortable shaking hands or touching, while others with sweaty armpits and feet may have to contend with the unpleasant odor that results from the bacterial breakdown of sweat and cellular debris (bromhidrosis). People with hyperhidrosis often must change their clothes at least once a day, and their shoes can be ruined by the excess moisture. Hyperhidrosis may also contribute to such skin diseases as **athlete's foot** (tinea pedis) and **contact dermatitis**.

In addition to excessive sweat production, the texture and color of the skin itself may be affected by hyperhidrosis. The skin may turn pink or bluish white. Severe hyperhidrosis of the soles of the feet may produce cracks, fissures, and scaling of the skin.

Hyperhidrosis in general and axillary hyperhidrosis (excessive sweating in the armpits) in particular are more common in the general population than was previously thought. A group of dermatologists in Virginia reported in 2004 that 2.8% of the United States population, or about 7.8 million persons, have hyperhidrosis. Of this group, slightly more than half (4 million persons) have axillary hyperhidrosis. One-third of the latter group, or about 1.3 million persons, find that the condition significantly interferes with daily activities and is barely tolerable. Only 38%, however, had ever discussed their excessive sweating with their doctor.

Causes and symptoms

There are three basic forms of hyperhidrosis: emotionally induced; localized; and generalized. Emotionally induced hyperhidrosis typically affects the palms of the hands, soles of the feet, and the armpits. Localized hyperhidrosis typically affects the palms, armpits, groin, face, and the area below the breasts in women, while generalized hyperhidrosis may affect the entire body.

Hyperhidrosis may be either idiopathic (of unknown cause) or secondary to **fever**, metabolic disorders, **alcoholism**, **menopause**, **Hodgkin's disease**, **tuberculosis**, various types of **cancer**, or the use of certain medications. The medications most commonly associated with hyperhidrosis are propranolol, venlafaxine, **tricyclic antidepressants**, pilocarpine, and physostigmine.

Most cases of hyperhidrosis begin during childhood or adolescence. Hyperhidrosis that begins in adult life should prompt the doctor to look for a systemic illness, medication side effect, or metabolic disorder.

Hyperhidrosis affects both sexes equally and may occur in any age group. People of any race may be affected; however, for some reason unknown as of the early 2000s, Japanese are affected 20 times more frequently than members of other ethnic groups.

Diagnosis

Hyperhidrosis is diagnosed by patient report and a **physical examination**. In many cases the physician can directly observe the excessive sweating.

The doctor may also perform an iodine starch test, which involves spraying the affected areas of the patient's body with a mixture of 500 g of water-soluble starch and 1 g iodine crystals. Areas of the skin producing sweat will turn black.

The doctor will order other laboratory or imaging tests if he or she suspects that the sweating is associated with another disease or disorder.

Treatment

Most over-the-counter antiperspirants are not strong enough to effectively prevent hyperhidrosis. To treat the disorder, doctors usually prescribe 20% aluminum chloride hexahydrate solution (Drysol), which the patient applies at night to the affected areas that are then wrapped in a plastic film until morning. Drysol works by blocking the sweat pores. Formaldehyde- and glutaraldehyde-based solutions can also be prescribed; however, formaldehyde may trigger an allergic reaction and glutaraldehyde can stain the skin (for this reason it is primarily applied to the soles). Anticholinergic drugs may also be given. These drugs include such medications as propantheline, oxybutynin, and benztropine.

Injections of botulinum toxin (Botox) given under the skin work well for some patients. Botox works to stop the excessive sweating by preventing the transmission of nerve impulses to the sweat glands. These injections must be repeated every 4–12 months, however.

In addition, an electrical device that emits low-voltage current can be held against the skin to reduce sweating. These treatments are usually conducted in a doctor's office on a daily basis for several weeks, followed by weekly visits. Dermatologists also recommend that patients wear clothing made of natural or absorbent fabrics also may help, avoid high-buttoned collars, use talc or cornstarch, and keep underarms shaved.

The only permanent cure for hyperhidrosis of the palms is a surgical procedure known as a **sympathectomy**. To treat severe excessive sweating, a surgeon can remove a portion of the nerve near the top of the spine that controls palm sweat. However, not very many neurosurgeons in the United States will perform the procedure, because it often results in compensatory sweating in other regions of the body. Alternatively,

KEY TERMS

Anticholinergic drugs—Drugs that block the action of the neurotransmitter acetylcholine.

Axilla (plural, axillae)—The medical term for the armpit.

Bromhidrosis—Bacterial breakdown of sweat and cellular debris resulting in a foul odor.

Contact dermatitis—Skin inflammation that occurs when the skin is exposed to a substance originating outside of the body.

Idiopathic—Of spontaneous origin or unknown cause. Many cases of hyperhidrosis are idiopathic.

Sympathectomy—Surgical cutting or interruption of any of the pathways in the sympathetic nervous system. It may be performed to control hyperhidrosis that does not respond to medications.

Sympathetic nervous system—The part of the nervous system that originates in the lumbar and thoracic portions of the spinal cord. It regulates involuntary reactions to stress, including sweating as well as heart rate, breathing rate, and digestive secretions.

Tinea pedis—Fungal infection of the feet of the skin characterized by dry, scaly lesions.

it is possible to surgically remove the sweat gland-bearing skin of the armpits, but this is a major procedure that may require skin grafts.

More recently, **liposuction** under the armpits has been successfuly used to treat hyperhydrosis in this region of the body. The liposuction removes some of the excess sweat glands responsible for axillary hyperhidrosis. The procedure also has the advantage of leaving smaller **scars** and being less disruptive of the overlying skin.

Prognosis

Hyperhidrosis is not associated with increased mortality; it primarily affects the patient's quality of life rather than longevity. While the condition cannot be cured without radical surgery, it can usually be controlled effectively.

Resources

BOOKS

Beers, Mark H., MD, and Robert Berkow, MD., editors. "Disorders of Sweating." Section 10, Chapter 124 In

The Merck Manual of Diagnosis and Therapy. Whitehouse Station, NJ: Merck Research Laboratories, 2004.

PERIODICALS

Altman, Rachel, MD, George Kihiczak, MD, and Robert Schwartz, MD. "Hyperhidrosis." *eMedicine* August 18, 2004. < http://www.emedicine.com/derm/topic893.htm >.

Licht, P. B., and H. K. Pilegaard. "Severity of Compensatory Sweating after Thoracoscopic Sympathectomy." *Annals of Thoracic Surgery* 78 (August 2004): 427–431.

Strutton, D. R., J. W. Kowalski, D. A. Glaser, and P. E. Stang. "US Prevalence of Hyperhidrosis and Impact on Individuals with Axillary Hyperhidrosis: Results from a National Survey." *Journal of the American Academy of Dermatology* 51 (August 2004): 241–248.

ORGANIZATIONS

American Academy of Dermatology (AAD). P. O. Box 4014, Schaumburg, IL 60168-4014. (847) 330-0230. < http://www.aad.org >.

Carol A. Turkington
Rebecca J. Frey, PhD

Hyperhomocystinemia *see* **Hypercoagulation disorders**

Hypericum perforatum see **St. Johns wort**

Hyperkalemia

Definition

The normal concentration of potassium in the serum is in the range of 3.5 to 5.0 mM. Hyperkalemia refers to serum or plasma levels of potassium ions above 5.0 mM. The concentration of potassium is often expressed in units of milliequivalents per liter (mEq/L), rather than in units of millimolarity (mM). Both units mean the same thing when applied to concentrations of potassium ions.

Description

A normal adult who weighs about 70 kg contains a total of about 3.6 moles of potassium ions in the body. Most of this potassium (about 98%) occurs inside various cells and organs, where its concentration is about 150 mM. This level is in contrast to the much lower concentration found in the blood serum, where only about 0.4% of the body's potassium resides. Hyperkalemia can be caused by an overall excess of body potassium, or by a shift from inside to outside cells. For example, hyperkalemia can be caused by the sudden release of potassium ions from muscle into the surrounding fluids.

In a normal person, hyperkalemia from too much potassium in the diet is prevented by at least three types of regulatory processes. First, various cells and organs act to prevent hyperkalemia by taking up potassium from the blood. It is also prevented by the action of the kidneys, which excrete potassium into the urine. A third protective mechanism is **vomiting**. Consumption of a large dose of potassium ions, such as potassium chloride, induces a vomiting reflex to expel most of the potassium before it can be absorbed.

Causes and symptoms

Hyperkalemia can occur from a variety of causes, including the consumption of too much of a potassium salt; the failure of the kidneys to normally excrete potassium ions into the urine; the leakage of potassium from cells and tissues into the bloodstream; and from acidosis. The most common cause of hyperkalemia is kidney (or renal) disease, which accounts for about three quarters of all cases. Kidney function is measured by the glomerular filtration rate, the rate at which each kidney performs its continual processing and cleansing of blood. The normal glomerular filtration rate is about 100 ml/min. If the kidney is damaged so that the glomerular filtration rate is only 5 ml/min or less, hyperkalemia may result, especially if high-potassium foods are consumed. The elderly are at particular risk, since many regulatory functions of the body do not work well in this population. Elderly patients who are being treated with certain drugs for high blood pressure, such as spironolactone (Aldactone) and triamterene (Dyazide), must especially be monitored for possible hyperkalemia, as these medications promote the retention of potassium by the kidneys.

Hyperkalemia can also be caused by a disease of the adrenal gland called **Addison's disease**. The adrenal gland produces the hormone aldosterone that promotes the excretion of potassium into the urine by the kidney.

Hyperkalemia can also result from injury to muscle or other tissues. Since most of the potassium in the body is contained in muscle, a severe trauma that crushes muscle cells results in an immediate increase in the concentration of potassium in the blood. Hyperkalemia may also result from severe **burns** or infections.

Acidic blood plasma, or acidosis, is an occasional cause of hyperkalemia. Acidosis, which occurs in a number of diseases, is defined as an increase in the concentration of hydrogen ions in the bloodstream. In the body's attempt to correct the situation, hydrogen is taken up by muscle cells out of the blood in an exchange mechanism involving the transfer of potassium ions into the bloodstream. This can abnormally elevate the plasma's concentration of potassium ions. When acidosis is the cause of hyperkalemia, treating the patient for acidosis has two benefits: a reversal of both the acidosis and the hyperkalemia.

Symptoms of hyperkalemia include abnormalities in the behavior of the heart. Heart abnormalities of mild hyperkalemia (5.0 to 6.5 mM potassium) can be detected by an electrocardiogram (ECG or EKG). With severe hyperkalemia (over 8.0 mM potassium), the heart may beat at a dangerously rapid rate (fibrillation) or stop beating entirely (cardiac arrest). Patients with moderate or severe hyperkalemia may also develop nervous symptoms such as **tingling** of the skin, **numbness** of the hands or feet, weakness, or a flaccid **paralysis**, which is characteristic of both hyperkalemia and **hypokalemia** (low plasma potassium).

Diagnosis

Hyperkalemia can be measured by acquiring a sample of blood, preparing blood serum, and using a potassium sensitive electrode for measuring the concentration of potassium ions. Alternatively, atomic absorption spectroscopy can be used for measuring potassium. Since high or low potassium levels result in abnormalities in heart function, the electrocardiogram is usually the method of choice for the diagnosis of both hyperkalemia and hypokalemia.

Treatment

Insulin injections are used to treat hyperkalemia in emergency situations. Insulin is a hormone well known for its ability to stimulate the entry of sugar (glucose) into cells. It also provokes the uptake of potassium ions by cells, decreasing potassium ion concentration in the blood. When insulin is used to treat hyperkalemia, glucose is also injected. Serum potassium levels begin to decline within 30 to 60 minutes and remain low for several hours. In non-emergency situations, hyperkalemia can be treated with a low potassium diet. If this does not succeed, the patient can be given a special resin to bind potassium ions. One such resin, sodium polystyrene sulfonate (Kayexalate), remains in the intestines, where it absorbs potassium and forms a complex of resin and potassium. Eventually this complex is excreted in the feces. A typical dose of resin is 15 grams, taken one to four times per day. The correction of hyperkalemia with resin treatment takes at least 24 hours.

Prognosis

The prognosis for specifically correcting hyperkalemia is excellent. However, hyperkalemia is usually caused by kidney failure, an often irreversible and eventually fatal condition.

Prevention

Healthy people are not at risk for hyperkalemia. Patients with renal disease and those on certain diuretic medications must be monitored to prevent its occurrence.

Resources

PERIODICALS

Greenberg, A. "Hyperkalemia: treatment options." *Seminars in Nephrology* 18 (1998): 46-57.

Tom Brody, PhD

Hyperkinetic disorder *see* **Attention-deficit/ Hyperactivity disorder (ADHD)**

Hyperlipemia *see* **Hyperlipoproteinemia**

Hyperlipidemia *see* **Hyperlipoproteinemia**

Hyperlipoproteinemia

Definition

Hyperlipoproteinemia occurs when there is too much lipid (fat) in the blood. Shorter terms that mean the same thing are hyperlipidemia and hyperlipemia. Dyslipidemia refers to a redistribution of cholesterol from one place to another that increases the risk of vascular disease without increasing the total amount of cholesterol. When more precise terms are needed, hypercholesterolemia and hypertriglyceridemia are used.

Description

It is commonly known that oil and water do not mix unless another substance like a detergent is added. Yet the body needs to transport both lipids (fats) and water-based blood within a single circulatory system. There must be a way to mix the two, so that essential fatty nutrients can be transported in the blood and so that fatty waste products can be carried away from tissues. The solution is to combine the lipids with protein to form water-soluble packages that can be transported in the blood.

These packages of fats are called lipoproteins. They are a complex mixture of triglycerides, cholesterol, phospholipids and special proteins. Some of these chemicals are fatty nutrients absorbed from the intestines on their way to being made part of the body. Cholesterol is a waste product on its way out of the body through the liver, the bile, and ultimately the bowel for excretion. The proteins and phospholipids make the packages water-soluble.

There are five different sizes of these chemical packages. Each package needs all four chemicals in it to hold everything in solution. They differ in how much of each they contain. If blood serum is spun very rapidly in an ultracentrifuge, these five packages will layer out according to their density. They have, therefore, been named according to their densities— high-density lipoproteins (HDL), low-density lipoproteins (LDL), intermediate-density lipoproteins (IDL), very low density lipoproteins (VLDL), and chylomicrons. Only the HDLs and the LDLs will be discussed in the rest of this article.

If there is not enough detergent in the laundry, the oily stains will remain in the clothes. In the same way, if the balance of chemicals in these packages is not right, cholesterol will stay in tissues rather than being excreted from the body. What is even worse, if the chemical composition of these packages changes, the cholesterol can fall out of the blood and stay where it lands. On the other hand, a different change in the balance can remove cholesterol from tissues where there is too much. This appears to be exactly what is going on in **atherosclerosis**. The lesions contain lots of cholesterol.

The LDLs are overloaded with cholesterol. A minor change in the other chemicals in this package will leave cholesterol behind. The HDLs have a third to a half as much cholesterol. They seem to be able to pick up cholesterol left behind by the LDLs. It seems that atherosclerosis begins with tiny tears at stressed places in the walls of the arteries. Low density lipoproteins from the blood enter these tears, where their chemistry changes enough to leave cholesterol behind. The cholesterol causes irritation; the body responds with inflammation; damage and scarring follow. Eventually the artery gets so diseased blood cannot flow through it. Strokes and heart attacks are the result.

But if there are lots of HDLs in the blood, the cholesterol is rapidly picked up and not allowed to cause problems. Women before **menopause** have estrogen (the female hormone), which encourages the formation of HDLs. This is the reason they have so little vascular disease, and why they rapidly catch up to men after menopause, when estrogen levels fall. Replacement of estrogen after menopause has been prescribed to for protection through the later years. However, in 2003, the Women's Health Initiative, a large clinical trial involving postmenopausal women, was halted in July 2002 because of the many detrimental effects of combined estrogen and progesterone therapy (called **hormone replacement therapy**). Among the effects was increased risk of heart disease, sometimes within the first year of use.

Cholesterol is the root of the problem, but like any other root it cannot just be eliminated. Ninety percent of the cholesterol in the body is created there as a waste product of necessary processes. The solution lies in getting it out to the body without clogging the arteries.

Of course the story is much more complex. The body has dozens of chemical processes that make up, break down, and reconfigure all these chemicals. It is these processes that are the targets of intervention in the effort to cure vascular disease.

Diseases

Near the dawn of concern over cholesterol and vascular disease a family of hereditary diseases was identified, all of which produced abnormal quantities of blood fats. These diseases were called dyslipoproteinemias and came in both too many and too little varieties. The hyperlipoproteinemias found their way into five categories, depending on which chemical was in excess.

- Type 1 has a pure elevation of triglycerides in the chylomicron fraction. These people sometimes get **pancreatitis** and abdominal pains, but they do not seem to have an increase in vascular disease.
- Type 2 appears in two distinct genetic patterns and a third category, which is by far the most important

kind, because everyone is at risk for it. All Type 2s have elevated cholesterol. Some have elevated triglycerides also. The familial (genetic) versions of Type 2 often develop xanthomas, which are yellow fatty deposits under the skin of the knuckles, elbows, buttocks or heels. They also may have xanthelasmas, smaller yellow patches on the eyelids.

- Type 3 appears in one in 10,000 people and elevates both triglycerides and cholesterol with consequent vascular disease. In 2003, researchers discovered the molecular mechanism that contributes to high triglycerides in those with this type of hyperlipopoproteinemia.
- Type 4 elevates only triglycerides and does not increase the risk of vascular disease.
- Type 5 is similar to Type 1.
- Dyslipidemia refers to a normal amount of cholesterol that is mostly in LDLs, where it causes problems.

All but Type 2 are rare and of interest primarily because they give insight into the chemistry of blood fats.

In addition to the above genetic causes of blood fat disorders, a number of acquired conditions can raise lipoprotein levels.

- Diabetes mellitus, because it alters the way the body handles its energy needs, and also affects the way it handles fats. The result is elevated triglycerides and reduced HDL cholesterol. This effect is amplified by **obesity**.
- Hypothyroidism is a common cause of lipid abnormalities. The thyroid hormone affects the rate of many chemical processes in the body, including the clearing of fats from the blood. The consequence usually is an elevation of cholesterol.
- Kidney disease affects the blood's proteins and consequently the composition of the fat packages. It usually raises the LDLs.
- Liver disease, depending on its stage and severity, can raise or lower any of the blood fats.
- Alcohol raises triglycerides. In moderate amounts (if they are very moderate) it raises HDLs and can be beneficial.
- Cigarette **smoking** lowers HDL cholesterol, as does malnutrition and obesity.

Certain medications elevate blood fat levels. Because some of these medications are used to treat heart disease, it has been necessary to reevaluate their usefulness:

- Thiazides, water pills used to treat high blood pressure, can raise both cholesterol and triglycerides.

- Beta-blockers, another class of medication used to treat high blood pressure, cortisone-like drugs, and estrogen can raise triglycerides.

- Progesterone, the **pregnancy** hormone, raises cholesterol.

Not all of these effects are necessarily bad, nor are they necessarily even significant. For instance, estrogen is clearly beneficial. Each effect must be considered in the overall goal of treatment.

Causes and symptoms

A combination of heredity and diet is responsible for the majority of fat disorders. It is not so much the cholesterol in the diet that is the problem, because that accounts for only 10% of the body's store. It is the other fats in the diet that alter the way the body handles its cholesterol. There is a convincing relation between fats in the diet and the incidence of atherosclerosis. The guilty fats are mostly the animal fats, but palm and coconut oil also are harmful. These fats are called saturated fats for the chemical reason that most of their carbon atoms have as many hydrogen atoms attached as they can accommodate. More important than the kind of fat is the amount of fat. For many people, fat is half of their diet. One-fifth to one-fourth is a much healthier fraction, the rest of the diet being made up of complex carbohydrates and protein.

This disease is silent for decades, until the first episode of heart disease or **stroke**.

Diagnosis

It would be easier if simple cholesterol and triglyceride tests were all it took to assess the risk of atherosclerosis. But the important information is which package the cholesterol is in—the LDLs or the HDLs. That takes a more elaborate testing process. To complicate matters further, the amount of fats in the blood varies greatly in relation to the last meal—how long ago it was and what kind of food was eaten. A true estimate of the risk comes from several tests several weeks apart, each done after at least twelve hours of **fasting**.

Treatment

Diet and lifestyle change are the primary focus for most cholesterol problems. It is a mistake to think that a pill will reverse the effects of a bad diet, obesity, smoking, excess alcohol, stress, and inactivity. Reducing the amount of fat in the diet by at least half is the most important move to make. Much of the food eaten to satisfy a "sweet tooth" is higher in fat than in sugar. A switch away from saturated fats is the next step, but the rush to polyunsaturated fats was ill-conceived. These, particularly the hydrogenated fats in margarine, have problems of their own. They raise the risk of **cancer** and are considered more dangerous than animal fat by many experts. Theory supports population studies that suggest monounsaturated olive oil may be the healthiest of all.

There was a tremendous push at the end of the 20th century to use lipid-lowering medications. The most popular and most expensive agents, the "statins," hinder the body's production of cholesterol and sometimes damage the liver as a side effect. Their full name is 3-hydroxy-3-methylglutaryl-coemzyme A *(HMG-CoA)* reductase inhibitors. Their generic names are cervistatin, fluvastatin, lovastatin, pravastatin, simvastatin, and the newest and most powerful to date, rosuvastatin. Studies show that these drugs lower cholesterol. Only recently, though, has any evidence appeared that this affects health and longevity. Earlier studies showed, in fact, an increased **death** rate among users of the first class of lipid-altering agents—the fibric acid derivatives. The chain of events connecting raised HDL and lowered LDL cholesterol to longer, healthier lives is still to be forged.

High-tech methods of rapidly reducing very high blood fat levels are performed for those rare disorders that require it. There are resins that bind cholesterol in the intestines. They taste awful, feel like glue and routinely cause gas, bloating, and **constipation**. For acute cases, there is a filtering system that takes fats directly out of the blood.

Niacin (nicotinic acid) lowers cholesterol effectively and was the first medication proven to improve overall life expectancy. It also can be liver toxic, and the usual formulation causes a hot flash in many people. This can be overcome by taking a couple of aspirins 30 minutes before the niacin, or by taking a special preparation called "flush free," "inositol-bound" or inositol hexanicotinate.

Alternative treatment

Omega-3 oil is a special kind found mostly in certain kinds of fish. It is beneficial in lowering cholesterol. An herbal alternative called guggulipid, *Commiphora mukul*, an extract of an Indian plant, has been touted as working the same way as the expensive and liver toxic cholesterol-lowering medications. However, a 2003 clinical trial found that the supplement did not meet these claims. In fact, guggul did not lower total cholesterol, LDL cholesterol, or triglycerides. Most patients tolerated the supplement, but some developed a hypersensitivity rash.

To lower cholesterol, **naturopathic medicine**, **traditional Chinese medicine**, and ayurvedic medicine may be considered. Some herbal therapies include alfalfa (*Medicago sativa*), Asian ginseng (*Panax ginseng*), and fenugreek (*Trigonella foenum-graecum*). Garlic (*Allium sativum*) and onions are also reported to have cholesterol-lowering effects. In naturopathic medicine, the liver is considered to be an organ that needs cleansing and rebalancing. The liver often is treated with a botanical formula that will act as a bitter to stimulate bile flow in the liver. Before initiating alternative therapies, medical consultation is strongly advised.

Prognosis

The prognosis is good for Type 1 hyperlipoproteinemia with treatment; without treatment, death may result. For Type 2 the prognosis is poor even with treatment. The prognosis for type 3 is good when the prescribed diet is strictly followed. For types 4 and 5 the prognosis is uncertain, due to the risk of developing premature **coronary artery disease** and pancreatitis, respectively.

Prevention

Genetic inheritance cannot be changed, but its effects may be modified with proper treatment. Family members of an individual with hyperlipoproteinemia should consider having their blood lipids assessed. The sooner any problems are identified, the better the chances of limiting or preventing the associated health risks. Anyone with a family history of disorders leading to hyperlipoproteinemia also may benefit from genetic testing and counseling to assist them in making reproductive decisions.

Resources

PERIODICALS

Brunk, Doug. "Three Studies Further Confirm Ill Effects of HRT: Heart Disease Risk Rises First Year of Use: Continuing Analysis of WHI Data." *Family Practice News* 33, no. 17 (September 1, 2003): 1–2.

Dowhower Karpa, Kelly. "New Statin Said to be More Powerful than Others." *Drug Topics* 147, no. 17 (September 1, 2003): 27.

"Herbal Extract Not Effective in Treating High Cholesterol." *Drug Week* August 29, 2003: 197.

Kyperos, Kyriakos E., et al. "Molecular Mechanisms of Type III Hyperlipoproteinemia: the Contribution of the Carboxy-terminal Domain of ApoE Can Account for the Dyslipidemia that is Associated With the E2/E2 Phenotype." *Biochemistry* 42, no. 33 (August 26, 2003): 9841–9853.

ORGANIZATIONS

Inherited High Cholesterol Foundation. 410 Chipeta Way, Room 167, Salt Lake City, UT 84104. (888) 244-2465.

J. Ricker Polsdorfer, MD
Teresa G. Odle

Hypermagnesemia *see* **Magnesium imbalance**

Hypermenorrhea *see* **Dysfunctional uterine bleeding**

Hypermetropia *see* **Hyperopia**

Hypernatremia

Definition

The normal concentration of sodium in the blood plasma is 136–145 mM. Hypernatremia is defined as a serum sodium level over 145 mM. Severe hypernatremia, with serum sodium above 152 mM, can result in seizures and **death**.

Description

Sodium is an atom, or ion, that carries a single positive charge. The sodium ion may be abbreviated as Na$^+$ or as simply Na. Sodium can occur as a salt in a crystalline solid. Sodium chloride (NaCl), sodium phosphate (Na$_2$HPO$_4$) and sodium bicarbonate (NaHCO$_3$) are commonly occurring salts. These salts can be dissolved in water or in juices of various foods. Dissolving involves the complete separation of ions, such as sodium and chloride in common table salt (NaCl).

About 40% of the body's sodium is contained in bone. Approximately 2–5% occurs within organs and cells and the remaining 55% is in blood plasma and other extracellular fluids. The amount of sodium in blood plasma is typically 140 mM, a much higher amount than is found in intracellular sodium (about 5 mM). This asymmetric distribution of sodium ions is essential for human life. It makes possible proper nerve conduction, the passage of various nutrients into cells, and the maintenance of blood pressure.

The body continually regulates its handling of sodium. When dietary sodium is too high or low, the intestines and kidneys respond to adjust concentrations to normal. During the course of a day, the intestines absorb dietary sodium while the kidneys excrete a nearly equal amount of sodium into the urine. If a low sodium diet is consumed, the intestines increase their efficiency of sodium absorption, and the kidneys reduce its release into urine.

The concentration of sodium in the blood plasma depends on two things: the total amount of sodium and water in arteries, veins, and capillaries (the circulatory system). The body uses separate mechanisms to regulate sodium and water, but they work together to correct blood pressure when it is too high or too low. Too high a concentration of sodium, or hypernatremia, can be corrected either by decreasing sodium or by increasing body water. The existence of separate mechanisms that regulate sodium concentration account for the fact that there are numerous diseases that can cause hypernatremia, including diseases of the kidney, pituitary gland, and hypothalamus.

Causes and symptoms

Vasopressin, also called anti-diuretic hormone, is made by the hypothalamus and released by the pituitary gland into the bloodstream. There it travels to the kidney where it reduces the release of water into the urine. With less vasopressin production, the body fails to conserve water, and the result is a trend toward higher plasma sodium concentrations. Hypernatremia may occur in diabetes insipidus, a disease that causes excessive urine production. (It is not the same disease as **diabetes mellitus**, a disease resulting from impaired insulin production.) The defect involves either the failure of the hypothalamus to make vasopressin or the failure of the kidney to respond to vasopressin. In either case, the kidney is able to conserve and regulate the body's sodium levels, but is unable to conserve and retain the body's water. Hypernatremia does not occur in **diabetes insipidus** if the patient is able to drink enough water to keep up with urinary loss, which may be as high as 10 liters per day.

Hypernatremia may occur in unconscious (or comatose) patients due to the inability to drink water. Water is continually lost by evaporation from the lungs and in the urine. If the patient is not given water via infusion, the sodium concentration in the blood may increase and hypernatremia could develop. Hypernatremia can also occur in rare diseases in which the thirst impulse is impaired.

Hypernatremia can also occur accidentally in the hospital when patients are infused with solutions containing sodium, such as sodium bicarbonate for the treatment of acidosis (acidic blood). It can also be accidentally induced with sodium chloride infusions, especially in elderly patients with impaired kidney function.

Hypernatremia can cause neurological damage due to shrinkage of brain cells. Neurological symptoms include confusion, **coma**, **paralysis** of the lung muscles, and death. The severity of the symptoms is related to how rapidly the hypernatremia developed. Hypernatremia that comes on rapidly does not allow the cells of the brain time to adapt to their new high-sodium environment. Hypernatremia is especially dangerous for children and the elderly.

Diagnosis

Hypernatremia is diagnosed by acquiring a blood sample, preparing plasma, and using a sodium-sensitive electrode for measuring the concentration of sodium ions.

Treatment

Hypernatremia is treated with infusions of a solution of water containing 0.9% sodium chloride (0.9 grams NaCl/100 ml water), which is the normal concentration of sodium chloride in the blood plasma. The infusion is performed over many hours or days to prevent abrupt and dangerous changes in brain cell volume. In emergencies, such as when hypernatremia is causing neurological symptoms, infusions may be conducted with salt solutions containing 0.45% sodium chloride, which is half the normal physiologic level.

Prognosis

The prognosis for treating hypernatremia is excellent, except if neurological symptoms are severe or if overly rapid attempts are made to treat and reverse the condition.

Prevention

Hypernatremia occurs only in unusual circumstances that are not normally under a person's control.

Resources

PERIODICALS

Fried, L. F., and P. M. Palevsky. "Hyponatremia and hypernatremia." *Medical Clinics of North America* 81 (1997): 585-609.

Tom Brody, PhD

Hypernephroma *see* **Kidney cancer**

Hyperopia

Definition

Hyperopia (farsightedness) is the condition of the eye where incoming rays of light reach the retina before they converge into a focused image.

Description

When light goes through transparent but dense material like the materials of the eye's lens system (the lens and cornea), its velocity decreases. If the surface of the dense material is not perpendicular to the incoming light, as is the case with the curved surfaces on lenses and corneas, the direction of the light changes. The greater the curvature of the lens system, the greater the change in the direction of the light.

When parallel light rays from an object go through the lens system of the eye, they are bent so they converge at a point some distance behind the lens. With perfect vision this point of convergence, where the light rays are focused, is on the retina. This happens when the cumulative curvature of the lens plus cornea and the distance from the lens to the retina are just right for each other. The condition where the point of focus of parallel light rays from an object is behind the retina is called hyperopia. This condition exists when the combined curvature of the lens and cornea is insufficient (e.g., flatter than needed for the length of the eyeball). This condition can be equivalently described by saying hyperopia exists when the eyeball is too short for the curvature of its lens system.

There is a connection between the focusing of the lens of the eye (accommodation) and convergence of the eyes (the two eyes turning in to point at a close object). The best example is during reading. The lens accommodates to make the close-up material clear and the eyes turn in to look at the print and keep it single. Because of this connection between accommodation and convergence, if the lens needs to accommodate to focus for distance (to bring the image back onto the retina) the eyes may appear to turn in even when looking at the distance. This can cause a condition known as accommodative esotropia in children. The eyes turn in and the cause is accommodation because of hyperopia.

Causes and symptoms

Babies are generally born slightly hyperopic. This tends to decrease with age. There is normal variation in eyeball length and curvature of the lens and cornea. Some combinations of these variables give rise to eyes where the cornea is too flat for the distance between the cornea and the retina. If the hyperopia is not too severe the lens may be able to accommodate and bring the image back onto the retina. This would result in clear distance vision, but the constant focusing might result in headaches or eyestrain. If the lens cannot accommodate for the full amount of the hyperopia the distance image would be blurry.

If the eyes are focusing for distance and now the person is looking at a near object, the eyes need to accommodate further. This may result in blurry near objects or headaches during near work.

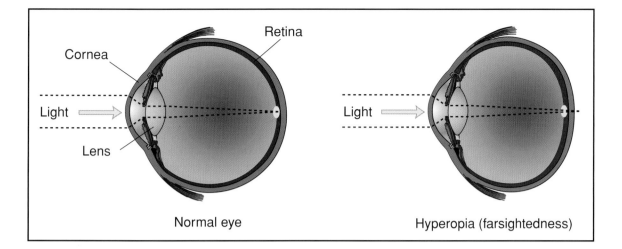

Hyperopia, or farsightedness, is a condition of the eye where incoming rays of light impinge on the retina before converging into a focused image, resulting in difficulty seeing nearby objects clearly. *(Illustration by Electronic Illustrators Group.)*

Depending upon the amount of hyperopia, symptoms can range from none to clear distance vision but blurry near vision, to blurry distance and near vision. Headaches and eyestrain may also occur, particularly when doing near tasks. An eye turned in (esotropia) may be a result of hyperopia, particularly in children. However, because a turned eye may be a result of more serious causes it is very important to have it checked out.

Diagnosis

Because it is possible to have good visual acuity with some degree of hyperopia it is important to relax accommodation before the eye exam. This is done with the use of eyedrops and is called a cycloplegic exam or cycloplegic refraction. The drops relax the accommodation (thus making reading blurry until the drops wear off). Patients will usually be asked to have someone drive them home because of the blurriness. The doctor can then determine the patient's visual status with a hand-held instrument called a retinoscope and/or have the patient read from an eye chart while placing different lenses in front of the patient's eyes. Refractive error is measured in units called diopters (D).

Treatment

The usual treatment for hyperopia is corrective lenses (spectacles or contact lenses).

Different surgical methods to correct hyperopia are under investigation. One approach is to implant

corrective contact lenses behind the patient's iris. The first experimental implantable contact lenses were implanted in 1997. Another approach is to surgically increase the curvature of the eye's existing cornea or lens. Although there have been many reports of success using different kinds of lasers to increase corneal curvature, as of 1998 there are still problems with stability and predictability. The introduction of light-activated biologic tissue glue in 1997 holds promise for improvements in those areas.

Prognosis

The prognosis for fully corrected vision is excellent for patients with low to moderate amounts of hyperopia. Patients with very high hyperopia (+10.00D or more) may not achieve full correction. Moreover, surgery to correct hyperopia will probably be perfected and approved in the near future.

Hyperopia increases the chances of chronic **glaucoma**, but vision loss from glaucoma is preventable.

Prevention

Hyperopia is usually present at birth, and there is no known way to prevent it.

Resources

ORGANIZATIONS

American Academy of Ophthalmology. 655 Beach Street, PO Box 7424, San Francisco, CA 94120-7424. <http://www.eyenet.org>.

American Optometric Association. 243 North Lindbergh Blvd., St. Louis, MO 63141. (314) 991-4100. <http://www.aoanet.org>.

OTHER

Edmiston, Dave. "Hyperopia." Lasikpatient.org. <http://www.lasikpatient.org>.

Lorraine Lica, PhD

Hyperparathyroidism

Definition

Parathyroid glands are four pea-sized glands located just behind the thyroid gland in the front of the neck. The function of parathyroid glands is to produce a hormone called parathyroid hormone (parathormone), which helps regulate calcium and phosphate in the body. Hyperparathyroidism is the overproduction of this hormone.

Description

Thyroid glands and parathyroid glands, despite their similar name and proximity, are entirely separate, and each produces hormones with different functions. Hyperparathyroidism may be primary or secondary. It most often occurs in those over age 30, and most commonly in patients 50 to 60 years old. It rarely occurs in children or the elderly. Women are affected by the disease up to three times more often than men. It is estimated that 28 of every 100,000 people in the United States will develop hyperparathyroidism each year.

Normally, parathyroid glands produce the parathormone as calcium levels drop and lower to meet the demands of a growing skeleton, **pregnancy**, or **lactation**. However, when one or more parathyroid glands malfunctions, it can lead to overproduction of the hormone and elevated calcium level in the blood. Therefore, a common result of hyperparathyroidism is **hypercalcemia**, or an abnormally high level of calcium in the blood. Primary hyperparathyroidism occurs as a malfunction of one of the glands, usually as a result of a benign tumor, called adenoma. Secondary hyperparathyroidism occurs as the result of a metabolic abnormality outside the parathyroid glands, which causes a resistance to the function of the parathyroid hormones. Primary hyperparathyroidism is one of the most common endocrine disorders, led only by diabetes and **hyperthyroidism**.

Causes and symptoms

Often, there are no obvious symptoms or suspicion of hyperparathyroidism, and it is first diagnosed when a patient is discovered to be hypercalcemic during a routine blood chemistry profile. Patients may believe they have felt fine, but realize improvements in sleep, irritability, and memory following treatment. When symptoms are present, they may include development of gastric ulcers or **pancreatitis** because high calcium levels can cause inflammation and **pain** in the linings of the stomach and pancreas.

Most of the symptoms of hyperparathyroidism are those present as a result of hypercalcemia, such as **kidney stones**, **osteoporosis**, or bone degradation resulting from the bones giving up calcium. Muscle weakness, central nervous system disturbances such as depression, psychomotor and personality disturbances, and rarely, even **coma** can occur. Patients may also experience **heartburn**, **nausea**, **constipation**, or abdominal pain. In secondary hyperparathyroidism, patients may show signs of calcium imbalance such as deformities of the long bones. Symptoms of the underlying disease may also be present.

Most commonly, hyperparathyroidism occurs as the result of a single adenoma, or benign tumor, in one of the parathyroid glands. About 90% of all cases of hyperparathyroidism are caused by an adenoma. The tumors are seldom cancerous. They will grow to a much larger size than the parathyroid glands, often to the size of a walnut. Genetic disorders or multiple endocrine tumors can also cause a parathyroid gland to enlarge and oversecrete hormone. In 10% or fewer of patients with primary hyperparathyroidism, there is enlargement of all four parathyroid glands. This condition is called parathyroid hyperplasia.

Diagnosis

Diagnosis of hyperparathyroidism is most often made when a blood test (radioimmunoassay) reveals high levels of parathyroid hormone and calcium. A blood test that specifically measures the amount of parathyroid hormone has made diagnosis simpler. X-ray examinations may be performed to look for areas of diffuse bone demineralization, bone cysts, outer bone absorption and erosion of the long bones of the fingers and toes. Hypercalcemia is mild or intermittent in some patients, but is an excellent indicator of primary hyperparathyroidism. Dual energy x-ray absorptiometry (DEXA or DXA), a tool used to diagnose and measure osteoporosis, is used to show reduction in bone mass for primary hyperparathryroidism patients. Once a diagnosis of hyperparathyroidism is reached, the physician will probably order further tests to evaluate complications. For example, abdominal radiographs might reveal kidney stones.

For secondary hyperparathyroidism, normal or slightly decreased calcium levels in the blood and variable phosphorous levels may be visible. Patient history of familial **kidney disease** or convulsive disorders may suggest a diagnosis of secondary hyperparathyroidism. Other tests may reveal a disease or disorder, which is causing the secondary hyperparathyroidism.

Treatment

Hyperparathyroidism cases will usually be referred to an endocrinologist, a physician specializing in hormonal problems, or a nephrologist, who specializes in kidney and mineral disorders.

Patients with mild cases of hyperparathyroidism may not need immediate treatment if they have only slight elevations in blood calcium level and normal kidneys and bones. These patients should be regularly checked, probably as often as every six months, by **physical examination** and measurement of kidney function and calcium levels. A bone densitometry measurement should be performed every one or two years. After several years with no worsened symptoms, the length of time between exams may be increased.

KEY TERMS

Demineralization—A loss or decrease of minerals in the bones.

Endocrine—Glands and hormone secretions in the body circulation.

Phosphate—An organic compound necessary for mineralization of bone and other key cellular processes.

Patients with more advanced hyperparathyroidism will usually have all or half of the affected parathyroid gland or glands surgically removed. This surgery is relatively safe and effective. The primary risks are those associated with **general anesthesia**. There are some instances when the surgery can be performed with the patient under regional, or cervical block, anesthesia. Often studies such as ultrasonography prior to surgery help pinpoint the affected areas.

Alternative treatment

Forcing fluids and reducing intake of calcium-rich foods can help decrease calcium levels prior to surgery or if surgery is not necessary.

Prognosis

Removal of the enlarged parathyroid gland or glands cures the disease 95% of the time and relief of bone pain may occur in as few as three days. In up to 5% of patients undergoing surgery, chronically low calcium levels may result, and these patients will require calcium supplement or vitamin D treatment. Damage to the kidneys as a result of hyperparathyroidism is often irreversible. Prognosis is generally good, however complications of hyperparathyroidism such as osteoporosis, bone **fractures**, kidney stones, peptic ulcers, pancreatitis, and nervous system difficulties may worsen prognosis.

Prevention

Secondary hyperparathyroidism may be prevented by early treatment of the disease causing it. Early recognition and treatment of hyperparathyroidism may prevent hypercalcemia. Since the cause of primary hyperparathyroidism, or the adenoma which causes parathyroid enlargement, is largely unknown, there are not prescribed prevention methods.

Resources

ORGANIZATIONS

Osteoporosis and Related Bone Diseases—National Resource Center. 1150 17th S. NW, Ste. 500, Washington, DC 20036. (800) 624-2663.

Paget Foundation. 200 Varick St., Ste. 1004. New York, NY 10014-4810. (800) 23-PAGET.

OTHER

"Endocrine Disorder and Endocrine Surgery." Endocrine Web Page. < http://www.endocrineweb.com >.

Teresa Odle

Hyperpigmentation

Definition

Hyperpigmentation is the increase in the natural color of the skin.

Description

Melanin, a brown pigment manufactured by certain cells in the skin called melanocytes, is responsible for skin color. Melanin production is stimulated by a pituitary hormone called melanocyte stimulating hormone (MSH). Other pigments appear in the skin much less often.

Causes and symptoms

Darkened spots on the skin come in several varieties. The most ominous is **malignant melanoma**, a very aggressive cancer that begins as an innocent mole. The majority of **moles** (nevus), however, are and remain benign (harmless). The average person has several dozen, and certain people with a hereditary excess may have hundreds. Freckles, age spots, and cafe au lait spots, known as ephelides, are always flat and not as dark. Cafe au lait spots are seen mostly in people with another hereditary disorder called neurofibromatosis. "Port wine stains" are congenital dark red blotches on the skin. Other common dark colorations on the skin are called keratosis and consist of locally overgrown layers of skin that are dark primarily because there is more tissue than normal. A few of these turn into skin cancers of a much less dangerous kind than melanoma.

Darkened regions of the skin occur as a result of abnormal tanning when the skin is sensitive to sunlight. Several diseases and many drugs can cause **photosensitivity**. Among the common drugs responsible for this uncommon reaction are birth control pills, **antibiotics (sulfonamides** and **tetracyclines), diuretics**, nonsteroidal anti-inflammatory drugs (NSAID), **pain** relievers, and some psychoactive medications. Some of the same drugs may also cause patches of discolored skin known as localized drug reactions and representing an allergy to that drug. Sunlight darkens an abnormal chemical in the skin of patients with porphyria cutanea tarda. Several endocrine diseases, some cancers, and several drugs abnormally stimulate melanocytes, usually through an overproduction of MSH. Arsenic **poisoning** and Addison's disease are among these causes. A condition known as acanthosis nigricans is a velvety darkening of skin in folded areas (arm pits, groin, and neck) that can signal a **cancer** or hormone imbalance.

Of particular note is a condition called melasma (dark pigmentation of the skin), caused by the female hormone estrogen. Normal in **pregnancy**, this brownish discoloration of the face can also happen with birth control pills that contain estrogen.

Overall darkening of the skin may be due to pigmented chemicals in the skin. Silver, gold, and iron each have a characteristic color when visible in the skin. Several drugs and body chemicals, like bilirubin, can end up as deposits in the skin and discolor it.

There are a number of other rare entities that color the skin, each in its own peculiar way. Among these are strange syndromes that seem to be birth defects and vitamin and nutritional deficiencies.

Diagnosis

The pattern of discoloration is immediately visible to the trained dermatologist, a physician specializing in skin diseases, and may be all that is required to name and characterize the discoloration. Many of these pigment changes are signs of internal disease that must be identified. Pigmentation changes may also be caused by medication, and the drug responsible for the reaction must be identified and removed.

Treatment

Skin sensitive to sunlight must be protected by shade or **sunscreens** with an SPF of 15 or greater. Skin cancers must be, and unsightly benign lesions may be, surgically removed. **Laser surgery** is an effective removal technique for many localized lesions.

KEY TERMS

Addison's disease—A degenerative disease that is characterized by weight loss, low blood pressure, extreme weakness, and dark brown pigmentation of the skin.

Dermatologist—A physician specializing in the study of skin conditions and diseases

Diuretic—A cause of increased urine flow.

Keratosis—A skin disease characterized by an overgrowth of skin, which usually appears discolored.

Lesion—Any localized abnormality.

Melasma—Dark pigmentation of the skin.

Neurofibromatosis—Otherwise known as von Recklinghausen's disease, consists of pigmented skin spots and numerous soft tumors all over the body.

Nevus—Birthmark or mole.

NSAID—Nonsteroidal anti-inflammatory drugs—aspirin, ibuprofen, naproxen, and many others.

Porphyria cutanea tarda—An inherited disease that results in the overproduction of porphyrins.

Syndrome—Common features of a disease or features that appear together often enough to suggest they may represent a single, as yet unknown, disease entity.

Because it spreads so rapidly, melanoma should be immediately removed, as well as some of the surrounding tissue to prevent regrowth.

Prevention

Sunlight is the leading cause of dark spots on the skin, so shade and sunscreens are necessary preventive strategies, especially in people who burn easily.

Resources

PERIODICALS

Bernstein L. J., et al. "The Short- and Long-term Side Effects of Carbon Dioxide Laser Resurfacing." *Dermatologic Surgery* 23 (July 1997): 519-525.

J. Ricker Polsdorfer, MD

Hyperprolactation *see* **Galactorrhea**

Hypersensitivity pneumonitis

Definition

Hypersensitivity pneumonitis refers to an inflammation of the lungs caused by repeated breathing in of a foreign substance, such an organic dust, a fungus, or a mold. The body's immune system reacts to these substances, called antigens, by forming antibodies, molecules that attack the invading antigen and try to destroy it. The combination of antigen and antibody produces acute inflammation, or pneumonitis (a hypersensitivity reaction), which later can develop into chronic lung disease that impairs the lungs' ability to take oxygen from the air and eliminate carbon dioxide.

Description

Hypersensitivity pneumonitis (HP) is sometimes called "allergic alveolitis." "Allergic" refers to the antigen-antibody reaction, and "alveolitis" means an inflammation of the tiny air sacs in the lungs where oxygen and CO_2 are exchanged, the alveoli. It also is known as "extrinsic" allergic alveolitis, meaning that the antigen that sets up the allergic reaction (also called an allergen) comes from the outside. Most of the antigens that cause this disease come from plant or animal proteins or microorganisms, and many of those affected are exposed either at work or in the course of some hobby or other activity. The first known type of HP, farmer's lung, is caused by antigens from tiny microorganisms living on moldy hay. An example of disease connected with a hobby is pigeon breeder's lung, caused by inhaling protein material from bird droppings or feathers. After a time, very little of the allergenic material is needed to set off a reaction in the lungs.

Roughly one in every 10,000 persons develops some form of HP. A mysterious aspect of this condition is that, even though many persons may be exposed to a particular antigen, only a small number of them will develop the disease. Genetic differences may determine who becomes ill; this remains unclear. Probably between 5% and 15% of all persons who are regularly exposed to organic materials develop HP. Most of those who do get it do *not* smoke (**smoking** may create the type of cells that take up antigens and neutralize them). The amount of antigen is an important factor in whether HP will develop and what form it will take. Sudden heavy exposure can produce symptoms in a matter of hours, whereas mild but frequent exposures tend to produce a long-lasting, "smoldering" illness. HP may be more likely to develop in persons exposed to polluted air or industrial fumes.

Typical changes occur in the lungs of persons with HP. In the acute stage, large numbers of inflammatory cells are found throughout the lungs and the air sacs may be filled by a thick fluid mixed with these cells. In the subacute stage, disease extends into the small breathing tubes, or bronchioles, and the inflammatory cells collect into tiny granules called granulomas. Finally, in the chronic stage of HP, the previously inflamed parts of the lungs become scarred and unable to function, as in **pulmonary fibrosis**.

Causes and symptoms

A number of different types of HP are known, since a wide range of allergens may produce an allergic reaction in the lungs. Many of them produce similar symptoms and abnormal physical findings, but some have their own typical features. Some of the more common forms are:

- Farmer's lung. Can affect any farmer who works with wet hay or other moldy dust. Small farmers who have to directly thresh and handle their hay are most at risk, as are those living in cold and humid areas where damp weather is common.

- Pigeon breeder's lung. Also called "bird fancier's lung," it is second to farmer's lung as the best known type of HP. A substance has been found in pigeon droppings that may cause the allergic reaction, but there may be more than one such substance. Besides pigeons, the disorder may follow exposure to ducks, geese, pheasants, and even canaries. Parakeets produce an especially severe form of disease. Most patients are middle-aged women, who usually care for birds either at home or on bird breeding farms.

- Bagassosis. Caused by bagasse, a substance produced when juice is extracted from sugar cane and is used in making paper and explosives. A fungus is probably responsible. Young and middle-aged men who work in the sugar industry are at risk.

- Byssinosis. A similar condition affecting workers who inhale dust from cotton, flax, or hemp.

- Humidifier lung. An acute form of HP caused by inhaling actinomycetes, the same organisms that cause farmer's lung, which grow in contaminated humidifier vents, air conditioners, heating systems, and even saunas.

- Other antigens. HP has been seen in persons working with detergents, silicone, mushrooms, cheese, wood dust, maple bark, coffee, and furs.

In the acute stage, patients with HP begin coughing, develop **fever**, and note tightness in the chest as well as extreme tiredness and aching, four to eight hours after the most recent exposure. Most patients are well aware of the connection between their work (or an activity) and their symptoms. After a time, patients may have trouble breathing. They also may lose their appetite, lose weight, and generally feel ill. Finally, in the chronic stage, the patient will have increasing trouble breathing and may sometimes wheeze. With advanced disease, the skin may appear bluish (because too little oxygen is getting into the blood). When the physician listens to the patient's chest with a stethoscope, there may be crackling sounds or loud **wheezing**. In the late stages, club-shaped fingertips are a sign that the patient has not been getting enough oxygen for an extended period of time.

Diagnosis

No single test can make a definite diagnosis of HP. The key is to relate some specific exposure or activity to episodes of symptoms. The **chest x ray** may be normal in the acute stage, but later may show a hazy appearance that looks like "ground glass." There may be linear or rounded shadows in the central parts of the lungs. Studies of lung function in the acute stage typically show abnormally small lung volume. The ability to breathe at a fast rate is impaired. Blood from an artery typically has a low level of oxygen. Later, when the lungs have begun to scar, the airways (breathing tubes) are obstructed and the rate of air flow is reduced.

Some experts believe that skin testing can help diagnose HP and show which particular antigen is causing the symptoms. Small amounts of several suspect antigens are injected just beneath the surface of the skin, usually on the arm or back, and the reactions compared to that caused by injecting a harmless salt solution. Another diagnostic test is to place a thin tube into the airways, inject a small amount of fluid, and draw it back up (bronchoalveolar lavage). A very large number of cells called lymphocytes is typical of HP, and mast cells, which are part of the immune system, may also be seen. Rarely, a tissue sample (biopsy) of lung tissue may be taken through a tube placed in the airways and examined under a microscope. Finally, a patient may be "challenged" by actually inhaling a particular antigen in the form of an aerosol and noting whether lung function suddenly becomes worse. This test is usually not necessary.

KEY TERMS

Allergen—An outside substance, such as dust or a mold, that, when inhaled, sets off an allregic (hypersensitivity) reaction in the lungs.

Fibrosis—A result of long-standing inflammatory disease in which normal tissue is replaced by scar tissue that is functionally useless.

Granuloma—A collection of inflammatory cells forming a microscopic lesion, many of which are scattered throughout the lung tissue in patients who have had numerous acute episodes of HP.

Hypersensitivity—After the body's immune system attacks an outside invader (such as organic dust or a fungus) many times, exposure to even a tiny amount of this allergen can provoke a strong inflammatory response.

Pneumonitis—Inflammation of the lung tissues.

Steroid—A natural body substance may be given orally or by injection, and serves to dampen or even halt inflammation anywhere in the body, including the lungs.

Treatment

Treatment of HP requires identifying the offending antigen and avoiding further exposure. Although it may sometimes be necessary for a patient to find a totally different type of work, often it is possible to simply perform different duties or switch to a work site where exposure is minimal. In some cases, (like pigeon breeder's lung), wearing a mask can prevent exposure. If acute symptoms are severe, the patient may be treated with a steroid hormone for two to six weeks. This often suppresses the inflammatory response and allows the lungs a chance to recover. In the chronic stage, steroid treatment can delay further damage to the lungs and help preserve their function.

Prognosis

In general, most of the symptoms of HP disappear when the patient is no longer exposed to the causative allergen. The actual chances of complete recovery depend in part on what form of HP is present. Older patients and those exposed repeatedly for long periods after initially developing symptoms tend to have a poorer long-term outlook. The worst outcome is that long repeated episodes of exposure will cause chronic lung inflammation, scar the lungs, and permanently make them unable to properly provide oxygen to the blood. Rarely, a patient will become permanently disabled.

Prevention

It is often not possible to prevent initial episodes of HP, because there is no way of predicting which individuals (such as farmers) will have an allergic reaction to a particular allergen. Once the connection is made between a type of exposure and definite hypersensitivity symptoms, prevention of further episodes is simple as long as further exposure can be avoided.

Exactly how to avoid exposure depends on a person's work or activities and what he or she is reacting to. People with farmer's lung can dry hay thoroughly before storing it. For pigeon breeder's lung (and many other types of HP), a mask can be worn. In many industrial settings, it is possible to take precautions that will limit the amount of allergen that workers will inhale. If it is not possible to avoid exposure altogether, exposure can be timed and strictly minimized.

Resources

ORGANIZATIONS

American Lung Association. 1740 Broadway, New York, NY 10019. (800) 586-4872. < http://www.lungusa.org >.

Asthma and Allergy Foundation of America. 1233 20th Street, NW, Suite 402, Washington, DC 20036. (800) 727-8462. < http://www.aafa.org >.

David A. Cramer, MD

Hypersomnia *see* **Sleep disorders**

Hypersplenism

Definition

Hypersplenism is a type of disorder which causes the spleen to rapidly and prematurely destroy blood cells.

Description

The spleen is located in the upper left area of the abdomen. One of this organ's major functions is to remove blood cells from the body's bloodstream. In hypersplenism, its normal function accelerates, and it begins to automatically remove cells that may still be normal in function. Sometimes, the spleen will temporarily hold onto up to 90% of the body's platelets and 45% of the red blood cells. Hypersplenism may occur as a primary disease, leading to other complications, or as a secondary disease, resulting from an underlying disease or disorder. Hypersplenism is sometimes referred to as enlarged spleen (splenomegaly). An enlarged spleen is one of the symptoms of hypersplenism. What differentiates hypersplenism is its premature destruction of blood cells.

Causes and symptoms

Hypersplenism may be caused by a variety of disorders. Sometimes, it is brought on by a problem within the spleen itself and is referred to as primary hypersplenism. Secondary hypersplenism results from another disease such as chronic **malaria**, **rheumatoid arthritis**, **tuberculosis**, or **polycythemia vera**, a blood disorder. Spleen disorders in general are almost always secondary in nature. Hypersplenism may also be caused by tumors.

Symptoms of hypersplenism include easy bruising, easy contracting of bacterial diseases, fever, weakness, heart palpitations, and ulcerations of the mouth, legs and feet. Individuals may also bleed unexpectedly and heavily from the nose or other mucous membranes, and from the gastrointestinal or urinary tracts. Most patients will develop an enlarged spleen, anemia, leukopenia, or abnormally low white blood cell counts, or **thrombocytopenia**, a deficiency of circulating platelets in the blood. Other symptoms may be present that reflect the underlying disease that has caused hypersplenism.

An enlarged spleen can be caused by a variety of diseases, including **hemolytic anemia**, liver **cirrhosis**, leukemia, malignant lymphoma and other infections and inflammatory diseases. Splenomegaly occurs in about 10% of **systemic lupus erythematosus** patients. Sometimes, it is caused by recent viral infection, such as mononucleosis. An enlarged spleen may cause pain in the upper left side of the abdomen and a premature feeling of fullness at meals.

Diagnosis

Diagnosis of hypersplenism begins with review of symptoms and patient history, and careful feeling (palpation) of the spleen. Sometimes, a physician can feel an enlarged spleen. X-ray studies, such as ultrasound and computed tomography scan (CT scan), may help diagnose an enlarged spleen and possible underlying causes, such as tumors. Blood tests indicate decreases in white blood cells, red blood cells, or platelets. Another test measures red blood cells in the liver and spleen after injection of a radioactive substance,

and indicates areas where the spleen is holding on to large numbers of red cells or is destroying them.

Enlarged spleens are diagnosed using a combination of patient history, **physical examination**, including palpation of the spleen, if possible, and diagnostic tests. A history of **fever** and systemic symptoms may be present because of infection, malaria, or an inflammatory disorder. A complete **blood count** is taken to check counts of young red blood cells. Liver function tests, CT scans, and ultrasound exams can also help to detect an enlarged spleen.

Treatment

In secondary hypersplenism, the underlying disease must be treated to prevent further sequestration or destruction of blood cells, and possible spleen enlargement. Those therapies will be tried prior to removal of the spleen (**splenectomy**), which is avoided if possible. In severe cases, the spleen must be removed. Splenectomy will correct the effects of low blood cell concentrations in the blood.

Prognosis

Prognosis depends on the underlying cause and progression of the disease. Left untreated, spleen enlargement can lead to serious complications. Hypersplenism can also lead to complications due to decreased blood cell counts.

Prevention

Some of the underlying causes of hypersplenism or enlarged spleen can be prevented, such as certain forms of anemia and cirrhosis of the liver due to alcohol. In other cases, the hypersplenism may not be preventable, as it is a complication to an underlying disorder.

Resources

ORGANIZATIONS

American Liver Foundation. 1425 Pompton Ave., Cedar Grove, NJ 07009. (800) 223-0179. < http:// www.liverfoundation.org >.

American Society of Hematology. 1200 19th Street NW, Suite 300, Washington, DC 20036-2422. (202) 857-1118. < http://www.hematology.org >.

National Heart, Lung and Blood Institute. PO Box 30105, Bethesda, MD 20824-0105. (301) 251-1222. < http:// www.nhlbi.nih.gov >.

Teresa Norris, RN

Hypertension

Definition

Hypertension is high blood pressure. Blood pressure is the force of blood pushing against the walls of arteries as it flows through them. Arteries are the blood vessels that carry oxygenated blood from the heart to the body's tissues.

Description

As blood flows through arteries it pushes against the inside of the artery walls. The more pressure the blood exerts on the artery walls, the higher the blood pressure will be. The size of small arteries also affects the blood pressure. When the muscular walls of arteries are relaxed, or dilated, the pressure of the blood flowing through them is lower than when the artery walls narrow, or constrict.

Blood pressure is highest when the heart beats to push blood out into the arteries. When the heart relaxes to fill with blood again, the pressure is at its lowest point. Blood pressure when the heart beats is called systolic pressure. Blood pressure when the heart is at rest is called diastolic pressure. When blood pressure is measured, the systolic pressure is stated first and the diastolic pressure second. Blood pressure is measured in millimeters of mercury (mm Hg). For example, if a person's systolic pressure is 120 and diastolic pressure is 80, it is written as 120/80 mm Hg. The American Heart Association has long considred blood pressure less than 140 over 90 normal for adults. However, the National Heart, Lung, and Blood Institute in Bethesda, Maryland released new clinical guidelines for blood pressure in 2003, lowering the standard normal readings. A normal reading was lowered to less than 120 over less than 80.

Hypertension is a major health problem, especially because it has no symptoms. Many people have hypertension without knowing it. In the United States, about 50 million people age six and older have high blood pressure. Hypertension is more common in men than women and in people over the age of 65 than in younger persons. More than half of all Americans over the age of 65 have hypertension. It also is more common in African-Americans than in white Americans.

Hypertension is serious because people with the condition have a higher risk for heart disease and other medical problems than people with normal blood pressure. Serious complications can be avoided by getting regular blood pressure checks and treating hypertension as soon as it is diagnosed.

If left untreated, hypertension can lead to the following medical conditions:

- arteriosclerosis, also called **atherosclerosis**

- **heart attack**

- **stroke**

- enlarged heart

- kidney damage.

Arteriosclerosis is hardening of the arteries. The walls of arteries have a layer of muscle and elastic tissue that makes them flexible and able to dilate and constrict as blood flows through them. High blood pressure can make the artery walls thicken and harden. When artery walls thicken, the inside of the blood vessel narrows. Cholesterol and fats are more likely to build up on the walls of damaged arteries, making them even narrower. **Blood clots** also can get trapped in narrowed arteries, blocking the flow of blood.

Arteries narrowed by arteriosclerosis may not deliver enough blood to organs and other tissues.

Reduced or blocked blood flow to the heart can cause a heart attack. If an artery to the brain is blocked, a stroke can result.

Hypertension makes the heart work harder to pump blood through the body. The extra workload can make the heart muscle thicken and stretch. When the heart becomes too enlarged it cannot pump enough blood. If the hypertension is not treated, the heart may fail.

The kidneys remove the body's wastes from the blood. If hypertension thickens the arteries to the kidneys, less waste can be filtered from the blood. As the condition worsens, the kidneys fail and wastes build up in the blood. Dialysis or a kidney transplant are needed when the kidneys fail. About 25% of people who receive **kidney dialysis** have kidney failure caused by hypertension.

Causes and symptoms

Many different actions or situations can normally raise blood pressure. Physical activity can temporarily raise blood pressure. Stressful situations can make blood pressure go up. When the **stress** goes away, blood pressure usually returns to normal. These temporary increases in blood pressure are not considered hypertension. A diagnosis of hypertension is made only when a person has multiple high blood pressure readings over a period of time.

The cause of hypertension is not known in 90 to 95 percent of the people who have it. Hypertension without a known cause is called primary or essential hypertension.

When a person has hypertension caused by another medical condition, it is called secondary hypertension. Secondary hypertension can be caused by a number of different illnesses. Many people with kidney disorders have secondary hypertension. The kidneys regulate the balance of salt and water in the body. If the kidneys cannot rid the body of excess salt and water, blood pressure goes up. Kidney infections, a narrowing of the arteries that carry blood to the kidneys, called **renal artery stenosis**, and other kidney disorders can disturb the salt and water balance.

Cushing's syndrome and tumors of the pituitary and adrenal glands often increase levels of the adrenal gland hormones cortisol, adrenalin, and aldosterone, which can cause hypertension. Other conditions that can cause hypertension are blood vessel diseases, thyroid gland disorders, some prescribed drugs, **alcoholism**, and **pregnancy**.

Even though the cause of most hypertension is not known, some people have risk factors that give them a greater chance of getting hypertension. Many of these risk factors can be changed to lower the chance of developing hypertension or as part of a treatment program to lower blood pressure.

Risk factors for hypertension include:

- age over 60
- male sex
- race
- heredity
- salt sensitivity
- obesity
- inactive lifestyle
- heavy alcohol consumption
- use of **oral contraceptives**

Some risk factors for getting hypertension can be changed, while others cannot. Age, male sex, and race are risk factors that a person can't do anything about. Some people inherit a tendency to get hypertension. People with family members who have hypertension are more likely to develop it than those whose relatives are not hypertensive. People with these risk factors can avoid or eliminate the other risk factors to lower their chance of developing hypertension. A 2003 report found that the rise in incidence of high blood pressure among children is most likely due to an increase in the number of overweight and obese children and adolescents.

Diagnosis

Because hypertension doesn't cause symptoms, it is important to have blood pressure checked regularly. Blood pressure is measured with an instrument called a sphygmomanometer. A cloth-covered rubber cuff is wrapped around the upper arm and inflated. When the cuff is inflated, an artery in the arm is squeezed to momentarily stop the flow of blood. Then, the air is let out of the cuff while a stethoscope placed over the artery is used to detect the sound of the blood spurting back through the artery. This first sound is the systolic pressure, the pressure when the heart beats. The last sound heard as the rest of the air is released is the diastolic pressure, the pressure between heart beats. Both sounds are recorded on the mercury gauge on the sphygmomanometer.

Normal blood pressure is defined by a range of values. Blood pressure lower than 120/80 mm Hg is considered normal. A number of factors such as **pain**, stress or anxiety can cause a temporary increase in blood pressure. For this reason, hypertension is not diagnosed on one high blood pressure reading. If a blood pressure reading is 120/80 or higher for the first time, the physician will have the person return for another blood pressure check. Diagnosis of hypertension usually is made based on two or more readings after the first visit.

Systolic hypertension of the elderly is common and is diagnosed when the diastolic pressure is normal or low, but the systolic is elevated, e.g.170/70 mm Hg. This condition usually co-exists with hardening of the arteries (atherosclerosis).

Blood pressure measurements are classified in stages, according to severity:

- normal blood pressure: less than less than 120/80 mm Hg

- pre-hypertension: 120–129/80–89 mm Hg

- Stage 1 hypertension: 140–159/90–99 mm Hg

- Stage 2 hypertension: at or greater than 160–179/ 100–109 mm Hg

A typical **physical examination** to evaluate hypertension includes:

- medical and family history

- physical examination

- ophthalmoscopy: Examination of the blood vessels in the eye

- **chest x ray**

- electrocardiograph (ECG)

- blood and urine tests.

The medical and family history help the physician determine if the patient has any conditions or disorders that might contribute to or cause the hypertension. A family history of hypertension might suggest a genetic predisposition for hypertension.

The physical exam may include several blood pressure readings at different times and in different positions. The physician uses a stethoscope to listen to sounds made by the heart and blood flowing through the arteries. The pulse, reflexes, and height and weight are checked and recorded. Internal organs are palpated, or felt, to determine if they are enlarged.

Because hypertension can cause damage to the blood vessels in the eyes, the eyes may be checked with a instrument called an ophthalmoscope. The physician will look for thickening, narrowing, or hemorrhages in the blood vessels.

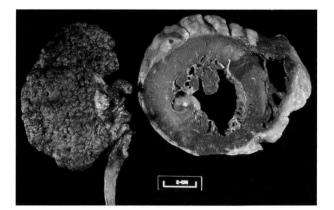

The effects of hypertension on the heart and kidney. Hypertension has caused renal atrophy and scarring, and left ventricular hypertrophy in the sectioned heart (at right). (Photograph by Dr. E. Walker, Photo Researchers, Inc. Reproduced by permission.)

A chest x ray can detect an enlarged heart, other vascular (heart) abnormalities, or lung disease.

An electrocardiogram (ECG) measures the electrical activity of the heart. It can detect if the heart muscle is enlarged and if there is damage to the heart muscle from blocked arteries.

Urine and blood tests may be done to evaluate health and to detect the presence of disorders that might cause hypertension.

Treatment

There is no cure for primary hypertension, but blood pressure can almost always be lowered with the correct treatment. The goal of treatment is to lower blood pressure to levels that will prevent heart disease and other complications of hypertension. In secondary hypertension, the disease that is responsible for the hypertension is treated in addition to the hypertension itself. Successful treatment of the underlying disorder may cure the secondary hypertension.

Guidelines advise that clinicians work with patients to agree on blood pressure goals and develop a treatment plan for the individual patient. Actual combinations of medications and lifestyle changes will vary from one person to the next. Treatment to lower blood pressure may include changes in diet, getting regular exercise, and taking antihypertensive medications. Patients falling into the pre-hypertension range who don't have damage to the heart or kidneys often are advised to make needed lifestyle changes only. A 2003 report of a clinical trial showed that adults with elevated blood pressures lowered them as mush as 38% by making lifestyle changes and participating in the DASH diet, which encourages eating more fruit and vegetables.

Lifestyle changes that may reduce blood pressure by about 5 to 10 mm Hg include:

- reducing salt intake
- reducing fat intake
- losing weight
- getting regular **exercise**
- quitting **smoking**
- reducing alcohol consumption
- managing stress

Patients whose blood pressure falls into the Stage 1 hypertension range may be advised to take antihypertensive medication. Numerous drugs have been developed to treat hypertension. The choice of medication will depend on the stage of hypertension, side effects, other medical conditions the patient may have, and other medicines the patient is taking.

If treatment with a single medicine fails to lower blood pressure enough, a different medicine may be tried or another medicine may be added to the first. Patients with more severe hypertension may initially be given a combination of medicines to control their hypertension. Combining antihypertensive medicines with different types of action often controls blood pressure with smaller doses of each drug than would be needed for just one.

Antihypertensive medicines fall into several classes of drugs:

- **diuretics**
- beta-blockers
- **calcium channel blockers**
- angiotensin converting enzyme inhibitors (ACE inhibitors)
- alpha-blockers
- alpha-beta blockers
- **vasodilators**
- peripheral acting adrenergic antagonists
- centrally acting agonists

Diuretics help the kidneys eliminate excess salt and water from the body's tissues and the blood. This helps reduce the swelling caused by fluid buildup in the tissues. The reduction of fluid dilates the walls of arteries and lowers blood pressure. New guidelines released in 2003 suggest diuretics as the first drug of choice for most patients with high blood pressure and as part of any multi-drug combination.

Beta-blockers lower blood pressure by acting on the nervous system to slow the heart rate and reduce the force of the heart's contraction. They are used with caution in patients with heart failure, **asthma**, diabetes, or circulation problems in the hands and feet.

Calcium channel blockers block the entry of calcium into muscle cells in artery walls. Muscle cells need calcium to constrict, so reducing their calcium keeps them more relaxed and lowers blood pressure.

ACE inhibitors block the production of substances that constrict blood vessels. They also help reduce the build-up of water and salt in the tissues. They often are given to patients with heart failure, **kidney disease**, or diabetes. ACE inhibitors may be used together with diuretics.

Alpha-blockers act on the nervous system to dilate arteries and reduce the force of the heart's contractions.

Alpha-beta blockers combine the actions of alpha and beta blockers.

Vasodilators act directly on arteries to relax their walls so blood can move more easily through them. They lower blood pressure rapidly and are injected in hypertensive emergencies when patients have dangerously high blood pressure.

Peripheral acting adrenergic antagonists act on the nervous system to relax arteries and reduce the force of the heart's contractions. They usually are prescribed together with a diuretic. Peripheral acting adrenergic antagonists can cause slowed mental function and lethargy.

Centrally acting agonists also act on the nervous system to relax arteries and slow the heart rate. They are usually used with other antihypertensive medicines.

Prognosis

There is no cure for hypertension. However, it can be well controlled with the proper treatment. Therapy with a combination of lifestyle changes and antihypertensive medicines usually can keep blood pressure at levels that will not cause damage to the heart or other organs. The key to avoiding serious complications of hypertension is to detect and treat it before damage occurs. Because antihypertensive medicines control blood pressure, but do not cure it, patients must continue taking the medications to maintain reduced blood pressure levels and avoid complications.

KEY TERMS

Arteries—Blood vessels that carry blood to organs and other tissues of the body.

Arteriosclerosis—Hardening and thickening of artery walls.

Cushing's syndrome—A disorder in which too much of the adrenal hormone, cortisol, is produced; it may be caused by a pituitary or adrenal gland tumor.

Diastolic blood pressure—Blood pressure when the heart is resting between beats.

Hypertension—High blood pressure.

Renal artery stenosis—Disorder in which the arteries that supply blood to the kidneys constrict.

Sphygmomanometer—An instrument used to measure blood pressure.

Systolic blood pressure—Blood pressure when the heart contracts (beats).

Vasodilator—Any drug that relaxes blood vessel walls.

Ventricle—One of the two lower chambers of the heart.

Prevention

Prevention of hypertension centers on avoiding or eliminating known risk factors. Even persons at risk because of age, race, or sex or those who have an inherited risk can lower their chance of developing hypertension.

The risk of developing hypertension can be reduced by making the same changes recommended for treating hypertension:

- reducing salt intake
- reducing fat intake
- losing weight
- getting regular exercise
- quitting smoking
- reducing alcohol consumption
- managing stress

Resources

PERIODICALS

McNamara, Damian. "Obesity Behind Rise in Incidence of Primary Hypertension." *Family Practice News* April 1, 2003: 45-51.

McNamara, Damian. "Trial Shows Efficacy of Lifestyle Changes for BP: More Intensive Than Typical Office Visit." *Family Practice News* July 1, 2003: 1-2.

"New BP Guidelines Establish Diagnosis of Pre-hypertension: Level Seeks to Identify At-risk Individuals Early." *Case Management Advisor* July 2003: S1.

"New Hypertension Guidelines: JNC-7." *Clinical Cardiology Alert* July 2003: 54-63.

ORGANIZATIONS

American Heart Association. 7320 Greenville Ave. Dallas, TX 75231. (214) 373-6300. < http://www.americanheart.org >.

National Heart, Lung and Blood Institute. PO Box 30105, Bethesda, MD 20824-0105. (301) 251-1222. < http://www.nhlbi.nih.gov >.

Texas Heart Institute. Heart Information Service. PO Box 20345, Houston, TX 77225-0345. < http://www.tmc.edu/thi >.

Toni Rizzo
Teresa G. Odle

Hyperthermia *see* **Fever**

Hyperthyroidism

Definition

Hyperthyroidism is the overproduction of thyroid hormones by an overactive thyroid.

Description

Located in the front of the neck, the thyroid gland produces the hormones thyroxine (T_4) and triiodothyronine (T_3) that regulate the body's metabolic rate by helping to form protein ribonucleic acid (RNA) and increasing oxygen absorption in every cell. In turn, the production of these hormones are controlled by thyroid-stimulating hormone (TSH) that is produced by the pituitary gland. When production of the thyroid hormones increases despite the level of TSH being produced, hyperthyroidism occurs. The excessive amount of **thyroid hormones** in the blood increases the body's metabolism, creating both mental and physical symptoms.

The term hyperthyroidism covers any disease which results in overabundance of thyroid hormone. Other names for hyperthyroidism, or specific diseases within the category, include Graves' disease, diffuse toxic **goiter**, Basedow's disease, Parry's disease, and thyrotoxicosis. The disease is 10 times more common in women than in men, and the annual incidence of hyperthyroidism in the United States is about one per 1,000 women. Although it occurs at all ages, hyperthyroidism is most likely to occur after the age of 15. There is a form of hyperthyroidism called Neonatal Grave's disease, which occurs in infants born of mothers with Graves' disease. Occult hyperthyroidism may occur in patients over 65 and is characterized by a distinct lack of typical symptoms. Diffuse toxic goiter occurs in as many as 80% of patients with hyperthyroidism.

Causes and symptoms

Hyperthyroidism is often associated with the body's production of autoantibodies in the blood which cause the thyroid to grow and secrete excess thyroid hormone. This condition, as well as other forms of hyperthyroidism, may be inherited. Regardless of the cause, hyperthyroidism produces the same symptoms, including weight loss with increased appetite, **shortness of breath** and **fatigue**, intolerance to heat, heart **palpitations**, increased frequency of bowel movements, weak muscles, **tremors**, **anxiety**, and difficulty sleeping. Women may also notice decreased menstrual flow and irregular menstrual cycles.

Patients with Graves' disease often have a goiter (visible enlargement of the thyroid gland), although as many as 10% do not. These patients may also have bulging eyes. Thyroid storm, a serious form of hyperthyroidism, may show up as sudden and acute symptoms, some of which mimic typical hyperthyroidism, as well as the addition of fever, substantial weakness, extreme restlessness, confusion, emotional swings or **psychosis**, and perhaps even **coma**.

Diagnosis

Physicians will look for physical signs and symptoms indicated by patient history. On inspection, the physician may note symptoms such as a goiter or eye bulging. Other symptoms or family history may be clues to a diagnosis of hyperthyroidism. An elevated body temperature (basal body temperature) above 98.6 °F (37 °C) may be an indication of a heightened metabolic rate (basal metabolic rate) and hyperthyroidism. A simple blood test can be performed to determine the amount of thyroid hormone in the patient's blood. The diagnosis is usually straightforward with this combination of clinical history, physical examination, and routine blood hormone tests. Radioimmunoassay, or a test to show concentrations of thyroid hormones with the use of a radioisotope

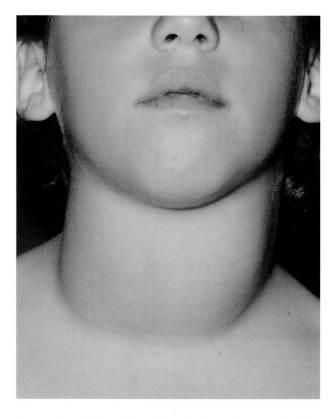

A symptom of hyperthyroidism is the enlargement of the thyroid gland. *(Photograph by Lester V. Bergman, Corbis Images. Reproduced by permission.)*

mixed with fluid samples, helps confirm the diagnosis. A thyroid scan is a nuclear medicine procedure involving injection of a radioisotope dye which will tag the thyroid and help produce a clear image of inflammation or involvement of the entire thyroid. Other tests can determine thyroid function and thyroid-stimulating hormone levels. Ultrasonography, computed tomography scans (CT scan), and magnetic resonance imaging (MRI) may provide visual confirmation of a diagnosis or help to determine the extent of involvement.

Treatment

Treatment will depend on the specific disease and individual circumstances such as age, severity of disease, and other conditions affecting a patient's health.

Antithyroid drugs

Antithyroid drugs are often administered to help the patient's body cease overproduction of thyroid hormones. This medication may work for young adults, pregnant women, and others. Women who are pregnant should be treated with the lowest dose required to maintain thyroid function in order to minimize the risk of **hypothyroidism** in the infant.

Radioactive iodine

Radioactive iodine is often prescribed to damage cells that make thyroid hormone. The cells need iodine to make the hormone, so they will absorb any iodine found in the body. The patient may take an iodine capsule daily for several weeks, resulting in the eventual shrinkage of the thyroid in size, reduced hormone production and a return to normal blood levels. Some patients may receive a single larger oral dose of radioactive iodine to treat the disease more quickly. This should only be done for patients who are not of reproductive age or are not planning to have children, since a large amount can concentrate in the reproductive organs (gonads).

Surgery

Some patients may undergo surgery to treat hyperthyroidism. Most commonly, patients treated with **thyroidectomy**, in the form of partial or total removal of the thyroid, suffer from large goiter and have suffered relapses, even after repeated attempts to address the disease through drug therapy. Some patients may be candidates for surgery because they were not good candidates for iodine therapy, or refused iodine administration. Patients receiving thyroidectomy or iodine therapy must be carefully monitored for years to watch for signs of hypothyroidism, or insufficient production of thyroid hormones, which can occur as a complication of thyroid production suppression.

Alternative treatment

Consumption of foods such as broccoli, brussel sprouts, cabbage, cauliflower, kale, rutabagas, spinach, turnips, peaches, and pears can help naturally suppress thyroid hormone production. Caffeinated drinks and dairy products should be avoided. Under the supervision of a trained physician, high dosages of certain vitamin/mineral combinations can help alleviate hyperthyroidism.

Prognosis

Hyperthyroidism is generally treatable and carries a good prognosis. Most patients lead normal lives with proper treatment. Thyroid storm, however, can be life-

> **KEY TERMS**
>
> **Goiter**—Chronic enlargement of the thyroid gland.
>
> **Gonads**—Organs that produce sex cells—the ovaries and testes.
>
> **Palpitations**—Rapid and forceful heartbeat.
>
> **Radioisotope**—A chemical tagged with radioactive compounds that is injected during a nuclear medicine procedure to highlight organ or tissue.
>
> **Thyroidectomy**—Removal of the thyroid gland.

threatening and can lead to heart, liver, or kidney failure.

Prevention

There are no known prevention methods for hyperthyroidism, since its causes are either inherited or not completely understood. The best prevention tactic is knowledge of family history and close attention to symptoms and signs of the disease. Careful attention to prescribed therapy can prevent complications of the disease.

Resources

ORGANIZATIONS
Thyroid Foundation of America. 350 Ruth Sleeper Hall - RSL 350, Parkman St., Boston, MA. 02114. (800) 832-8321. <http://www.clark.net/pub/tfa>.

OTHER
"Endocrine Disorder and Endocrine Surgery." *Endocrine Web Page.* <http://www.endocrineweb.com>.

Teresa Odle

Hypertrophic cardiomyopathy
Definition

Cardiomyopathy is an ongoing disease process that damages the muscle wall of the lower chambers of the heart. Hypertrophic cardiomyopathy is a form of cardiomyopathy in which the walls of the heart's chambers thicken abnormally. Other names for hypertrophic cardiomyopathy are idiopathic hypertrophic subaortic stenosis and asymmetrical septal hypertrophy.

Description

Hypertrophic cardiomyopathy usually appears in young people, often in athletes. For this reason it is sometimes called athletic heart muscle disease. However, people of any age can develop hypertrophic cardiomyopathy. Often there are no symptoms of hypertrophic cardiomyopathy. Sudden **death** can occur, caused by a heart arrhythmia. The American Heart Association reports that 36% of young athletes who die suddenly have probable or definite hypertrophic cardiomyopathy.

Hypertrophic cardiomyopathy is the result of abnormal growth of the heart muscle cells. The wall between the heart's chambers (the septum) may become so thickened that it blocks the flow of blood through the lower left chamber (left ventricle). The thickened wall may push on the heart valve between the two left heart chambers (mitral valve), making it leaky. The thickened muscle walls also prevent the heart from stretching as much as it should to fill with blood.

Causes and symptoms

The cause of hypertrophic cardiomyopathy is not known. In about one-half of cases, the disease is inherited. An abnormal gene has been identified in these patients. In cases that are not hereditary, a gene that was normal at birth may later become abnormal.

Often people with hypertrophic cardiomyopathy have no symptoms. Unfortunately, the first sign of the condition may be sudden death caused by an abnormal heart rhythm. When symptoms do appear, they include **shortness of breath** on exertion, **dizziness**, **fainting**, **fatigue**, and chest **pain**.

Diagnosis

The diagnosis is based on the patient's symptoms (if any), a complete **physical examination**, and tests that detect abnormalities of the heart chambers. Usually, there is an abnormal heart murmur that worsens with the Valsalva maneuver. The electrocardiogram (ECG), which provides a record of electrical changes in the heart muscle during the heartbeat, also is typically abnormal.

Sometimes, a routine **chest x ray** may show that the heart is enlarged. **Echocardiography**, a procedure that produces images of the heart's structure, is

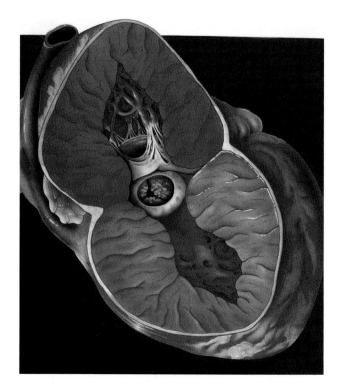

This illustration shows hypertrophic muscle in the heart. The abnormally thick wall of muscle prevents the chambers from stretching to fill up with blood, making the heart less efficient. The extra tissue may also push on the heart valve (center), causing it to leak. (Illustration by Bryson Biomedical Illustrations, Custom Medical Stock Photo. Reproduced by permission.)

usually done. These images can show if the heart wall is thickened and if there are any abnormalities of the heart valves.

Treatment

Treatment of hypertrophic cardiomyopathy usually consists of taking medicines and restricting strenuous **exercise**. Drugs called beta blockers and **calcium channel blockers** are usually prescribed. **Beta blockers** reduce the force of the heart's contractions. Calcium channel blockers can help improve the flexibility of the heart muscle walls, allowing them to stretch more. Antiarrhythmic drugs may also be given to prevent abnormal heart rhythms.

Patients with hypertrophic cardiomyopathy are also told to avoid strenuous exercise to reduce the risk of passing out or sudden death.

In some cases, if the medications do not help relieve symptoms, surgery may help. In an operation called myotomy-myectomy a piece of the septum is removed to improve blood flow through the heart chamber.

KEY TERMS

Arrhythmias—Abnormal heartbeat.

Calcium channel blocker—A drug that relaxes blood vessels and lowers blood pressure.

Mitral valve—The heart valve that controls blood flow between the heart's left upper chamber (atrium) and left lower chamber (ventricle).

Septum—The muscular wall dividing the left and right heart chambers.

Ventricles—The two lower chambers of the heart.

Some patients have **pacemakers** and/or defibrillators implanted to help control the heart rate and rhythm. Pacemakers and defibrillators provide electrical impulses to the heart, which can return the heart beat to a normal rhythm.

If these treatment methods fail and a patient develops heart failure, a heart transplant may be necessary.

Prognosis

Some people with hypertrophic cardiomyopathy may not have obstructed blood flow and may never experience symptoms. Others may only experience mild symptoms. With treatment, symptoms may improve. In some patients, the disease may progress to **heart failure**.

Prevention

While hypertrophic cardiomyopathy cannot be prevented, precautionary measures may prevent sudden deaths. Anyone planning to take part in a program of strenuous competitive exercise should have a checkup by a physician first. A physical examination before athletic participation can usually, but not always, detect conditions like hypertrophic cardiomyopathy. Anyone who experiences symptoms of shortness of breath, tiredness, or fainting with exercise should see a physician.

Resources

ORGANIZATIONS

American Heart Association. 7320 Greenville Ave. Dallas, TX 75231. (214) 373-6300. <http://www.americanheart.org>.

National Heart, Lung and Blood Institute. PO Box 30105, Bethesda, MD 20824-0105. (301) 251-1222. <http://www.nhlbi.nih.gov>.

Texas Heart Institute. Heart Information Service. PO Box 20345, Houston, TX 77225-0345. <http://www.tmc.edu/thi>.

Toni Rizzo

Hypervitaminosis *see* **Vitamin toxicity**

Hyphema

Definition

A hyphema is an accumulation of blood in the front (anterior) chamber of the eye. It is usually caused by blunt eye trauma.

Description

The anterior chamber (AC) is located behind the front of the eye. The AC is filled with a fluid called aqueous humor. This fluid helps form a cushion for the eye and provides an important route for nutrient and waste transport. Contusive forces from high velocity projectiles (approximately 34% of emergency room cases) such as a rock, crab apples, ice balls, badminton birds, and bungee cords can tear local blood vessels in the eye. Blunt impact from a basketball or racketball accounts for about 62% of cases. Tearing a small blood vessel can cause seepage of blood into a visible layer portion of the AC, causing the affected person to have red eye.

Causes and symptoms

Hyphema is caused by blunt, projectile, or explosion (about 4% of cases) injuries. These injuries cause a local blood vessel in the eye to tear, filling the front portion of the AC with blood. The initial complaint is a dramatic decrease in vision that eventually gets better as blood seeps towards the back of the eye. Patients will have extreme pain, an increase in intraocular pressure (the pressure inside the eye), and **nausea**. Patients usually will show a red eye and a recent history of trauma. Patients are vulnerable to more bleeding three to five days post injury.

Diagnosis

All persons with hyphema must be examined by an ophthalmologist (a physician who specializes in the medical and surgical care of the eye). Usually the clinician will use an ophthalmoscope to visualize

Microhyphema—Small bleed in the anterior chamber of the eye.

Ophthalmologist—A physician with specialized training in the medical and surgical treatment of eye diseases.

Optic Nerve—A cranial nerve that carries visual impulses to the brain for processing

the internal structures and damage. In some cases there may be small microscopic bleeds that may form clots (microhyphema) and require specialized instrumentation (a slit lamp) for visualization.

Treatment

Bloodthinners, such as **aspirin** and nonsteroidal anti-inflammatory drugs, should be avoided. In most cases the affected person can be medically managed on an outpatient basis. The eye should be shielded, but not patched. The patient should be placed at bed rest with the head elevated 45°. This position allows blood to leave the AC allowing for better vision. Several studies suggest administering medications (aminocaproic acid) that stabilize clot formation, reducing the possibility of increased bleeding.

Prognosis

The outcome depends on the severity of the trauma. Most cases progress well with conservative treatment. Some cases may develop an increase in the pressure within the eye (glaucoma). If this develops the hyphema must be surgically removed by an ophthalmologist. In patients who have a preexisting blood disorder, surgical evacuation should be considered to prevent damage to the optic nerve (the nerve that transmits impulses for processing in the brain).

Prevention

The American Academy of Ophthalmology recommends special eyewear made of polycarbonate lenses when at risk of eye injury. This type of lens has sufficient impact resistance.

Resources

BOOKS

Behrman, Richard E., et al, editors. *Nelson Textbook of Pediatrics*. 16th ed. W. B. Saunders Company, 2000.

Yanoff, Myron, et al, editors. *Ophthalmology*. Mosby International Ltd., 1999.

Laith Farid Gulli, M.D.

Hypnosis *see* **Hypnotherapy**

Hypnotherapy

Definition

Hypnotherapy is the treatment of a variety of health conditions by hypnotism or by inducing prolonged sleep.

Pioneers in this field, such as James Braid and James Esdaile discovered that hypnosis could be used to successfully anesthetize patients for surgeries. James Braid accidentally discovered that one of his patients began to enter a hypnotic state while staring at a fixed light as he waited for his **eye examination** to begin. Since mesmerism had fallen out of favor, Braid coined the term hypnotism, which is derived from the Greek word for sleep. Braid also used the techniques of monotony, rhythm, and imitation to assist in inducing a hypnotic state. As of 2000, these techniques are still in use.

Around 1900, there were very few preoperative anesthetic drugs available. Patients were naturally apprehensive when facing surgery. One out of four hundred patients would die, not from the surgical procedure, but from the anesthesia. Dr. Henry Munro was one of the first physicians to use hypnotherapy to alleviate patient fears about having surgery. He would get his patients into a hypnotic state and discuss their fears with them, telling them they would feel a lot better following surgery. Ether was the most common anesthetic at that time, and Dr. Munro found that he was able to perform surgery using only about 10% of the usual amount of ether.

Purpose

Hypnotherapy is used in a number of fields including psychotherapy, surgery, dentistry, research, and medicine. Hypnotherapy is commonly used as an alternative treatment for a wide range of health conditions, including weight control, pain management, and **smoking** cessation. It is also used to control **pain** in a variety of conditions such as **headache**, facial **neuralgia**, arthritis, **burns**, musculoskeletal disorders, childbirth, and many more. Hypnotherapy is being used in place of anesthesia, particularly in patients who prove to be allergic to anesthetic drugs, for surgeries such as hysterectomies, cesarean sections, certain cardiovascular procedures, **thyroidectomy**, and others. Dentistry is using hypnotherapy with success on patients who are allergic to all types of novocaine drugs. Hypnotherapy is also useful in helping patients overcome **phobias**.

Hypnotherapy is used for nonmedical patients as well as those who wish to overcome bad habits. Hypnotherapy has been shown to help those who suffer from performance **anxiety**, such as in sports, and speaking in public. In academic applications, it has also been shown to help with learning, participating in the classroom, concentrating, studying, focusing attention span, improving memory, and helping remove mental blocks about particular subjects.

In more general areas, hypnotherapy has been found to be beneficial for problems such as motivation, procrastination, decision making, personal achievement and development, job performance, buried or repressed memories, relaxation, and stress management.

Description

Origins

Hypnotherapy is thought to date back to the healing practices of ancient Greece and Egypt. Many religions such as Judaism, Christianity, Islam, and others have attributed trance-like behavior to spiritual or divine possession.

Austrian physician, Franz Mesmer (1734–1815), is credited with being the first person to scientifically investigate the idea of hypnotherapy, in 1779, to treat a variety of health conditions. Mesmer studied medicine at the University of Vienna and received his medical degree in 1766. Mesmer is believed to have been the first doctor to understand the relationship of psychological trauma to illness. He induced a trance-like state, which became known as mesmerism, in his patients to successfully treat nervous disorders. These techniques became the foundation for modern-day hypnotherapy.

Mesmer's original interest was in the effect of celestial bodies on human lives. He later became interested in the effects of magnetism, and found that magnets could have tremendous healing effects on the human body. Mesmer believed that the human body contained a magnetic fluid that promoted health and well being. It was thought that any blockage to the normal flow of this magnetic fluid would result in illness, and that the use of the mesmerism technique could restore the normal flow.

Mesmer performed his technique by passing his hands up and down the patient's body. The technique was supposed to transmit magnetic fluid from his hands to the bodies of his patients. During this time period, there was no clear delineation between health conditions that were physical or psychological in nature. Although Mesmer did not realize it at that time, his treatments were most effective for those conditions that were primarily psychosomatic.

Mesmer's technique appeared to be quite successful in the treatment of his patients, but he was the subject of scorn and ridicule from the medical profession. Because of all the controversy surrounding mesmerism, and because Mesmer's personality was quite eccentric, a commission was convened to investigate his techniques and procedures. A very distinguished panel of investigators included Benjamin Franklin, the French chemist Antoine-Laurent Lavoisier, and physician Jacques Guillotin. The commission acknowledged that patients did seem to obtain noticeable relief from their conditions, but the whole idea was dismissed as being medical quackery.

It took more than two hundred years for hypnotherapy to become incorporated into medical treatment. In 1955, the British Medical Association approved the use of hypnotherapy as a valid medical treatment, with the American Medical Association (AMA) giving its approval in 1958.

Hypnotherapy involves achieving a psychological state of awareness that is different from the ordinary state of consciousness. While in a hypnotic state, a variety of phenomena can occur. These phenomena include alterations in memory, heightened susceptibility to suggestion, paralysis, sweating, and blushing. All of these changes can be produced or removed in the hypnotic state. Many studies have shown that roughly 90% of the population is capable of being hypnotized.

This state of awareness can be achieved by relaxing the body, focusing on breathing, and shifting attention away from the external environment. In this state, the patient has a heightened receptivity to suggestion. The usual procedure for inducing a hypnotic trance in another person is by direct command repeated in a soothing, monotonous tone of voice.

Preparations

Ideally, the following conditions should be present to successfully achieve a state of hypnosis:

- willingness to be hypnotized

- rapport between the patient or client and the hypnotherapist

- a comfortable environment that is conducive to relaxation

Precautions

Hypnotherapy can have negative outcomes. When used as entertainment, people have been hypnotized to say or do things that would normally embarrass them. There have been instances where people already dangerously close to psychological breakdown have been pushed into an emotional crisis during what was supposed to be a harmless demonstration of hypnosis. A statement from the World Hypnosis Organization (WHO) warns against performing hypnosis on patients suffering from **psychosis**, organic psychiatric conditions, or antisocial **personality disorders**. Because there are no standard licensing requirements, in the wrong hands, there is a risk that the hypnotist will have difficulty in controlling or ending a hypnotic state that has been induced in the patient.

There is a commonly held belief that a person cannot be coerced into doing things that they would not normally do while under hypnosis. The hynotherapist should take care however, not to give suggestions during hypnosis that are contrary to the patient's moral code.

Many religions do not condone the practice of hypnotherapy. Leaders of the Jehovah's Witnesses and Christian Science religions oppose the use of hypnotherapy and advise their members to avoid it completely, whether for entertainment or therapy. The Church of Jesus Christ of Latter-Day Saints approves it for medical purposes, but cautions members against allowing themselves to be hypnotized for entertainment or demonstration purposes.

In 1985, The AMA convened a commission that warned against using hypnotherapy to aid in recollection of events. The commission cited studies that showed the possibility of hypnotic recall resulting on confabulation or an artificial sense of certainty about the course of events. As a result, many states limit or prohibit testimony of hypnotized witnesses or victims.

Side effects

Experiments have been conducted to determine any side effects of hypnotherapy. Some subjects have reported side effects such as headache, stiff neck, drowsiness, cognitive distortion or confusion, **dizziness**, and anxiety. However, most of these effects cleared up within several hours of the hypnotherapy session.

Research and general acceptance

Research on the effectiveness of hypnotherapy on a variety of medical conditions is extensive. In one study, the use of hypnotherapy did not seem to alter the core symptoms in the treatment of attention-deficit hyperactivity disorder (ADHD); however, it did seem to be useful in managing the associated symptoms including sleep disturbances and tics.

Hypnotherapy is being studied in children who have common, chronic problems and to aid in relieving pain. Children are particularly good candidates for hypnotherapy because their lack of worldly experience enables them to move easily between the rational world and their imagination. Studies with children have shown responses to hypnotherapy ranging from diminished pain and anxiety during a number of medical procedures, a 50% range in reduction of symptoms or a complete resolution of a medical condition, and a reduction in use of anti-nausea medication and vomiting during **chemotherapy** for childhood cancers.

The use of hypnotherapy with **cancer** patients is another area being investigated. A meta-analysis of 116 studies showed very positive results of using hypnotherapy with cancer patients. Ninety-two percent showed a positive effect on depression; 93% showed a positive effect on physical well-being; 81% showed a positive effect on vomiting; and 92% showed a positive effect on pain.

Resources

PERIODICALS

Baumgaertel, Anna. "Attention-Deficit/Hyperactivity Disorder:Alternative and Controversial Treatments for Attention-Deficit/Hyperactivity Disorder." *Pediatric Clinics of North America* October 1999.

Margolis, Clorinda G. "Hypnotic Trance: The Old and the New." *Primary Care Clinics in Office Practice.*

Newell, Sallie, and Rob W. Sanson-Fisher. "Australian on Bologists' self-reported knowledge and attitudes about non-traditional therapies used by cancer patients." *Medical Journal of Australia* February 7, 2000.

ORGANIZATIONS

American Board of Hypnotherapy. 16842 Von Karman Avenue, Suite 476, Irvine, CA 92714. < http://www.hypnosis.com >.

American Psychotherapy & Medical Hypnosis Association. 210 S. Sierra, Reno, NV 89501. < http://members.xoom.com/Hypnosis >.

American Society of Clinical Hypnosis. 200 E. Devon Avenue, Des Plaines, IL 60018.

International Council for Medical and Clinical Therapists. 7361 McWhorter Place, Suite 300, Annandale, VA 22003-5469. < http://www.ultradepth.com/ICMCT.htm >.

International Medical and Dental Hypnotherapy Association. 4110 Edgeland, Suite 800, Royal Oak, MI 48073-2285. < http://www.infinityinst.com >.

National Board for Hypnotherapy and Hypnotic Anaesthesiology. 7841 West Ludlow Drive, Suite A, Peoria, AZ 85381. < http://www.nbha-medicine.com/index.html >.

National Guild of Hypnotists. PO Box 308, Merrimack, NH. < http://www.ngh.net >.

Society for Clinical and Experimental Hypnosis. 6728 Old McLean Village Drive, McLean, VA 22101.

World Hypnosis Organization, Inc. 2521 W. Montrose Avenue, Chicago, IL 60618. < http://www.worldhypnosis.org/about.html >.

Kim A. Sharp, M.Ln.

Hypocalcemia

Definition

Hypocalcemia, a low bood calcium level, occurs when the concentration of free calcium ions in the blood falls below 4.0 mg/dL (dL = one tenth of a liter). The normal concentration of free calcium ions in the blood serum is 4.0–6.0 mg/dL.

Description

Calcium is an important mineral for maintaining human helath. It is not only a component of bones and teeth, but is also essential for normal blood clotting and necessary for normal muscle and nerve functions. The calcium ion (Ca^{2+}) has two positive charges. In bone, calcium ions occur as a complex with phosphate to form crystals of calcium phosphate. In the bloodstream, calcium ions also occur in complexes, and here calcium is found combined with proteins and various nutrients. However, in the bloodstream, calcium also occurs in a free form. Normally, about 47% of the calcium in the blood plasma is free, while 53% occurs in a complexed form. Although all of the calcium in the bloodstream serves a useful purpose, it is only the concentration of free calcium ions which has a direct influence on the functioning of our nerves and muscles. For this reason, the measurement of the concentration of free calcium is more important, in the diagnosis of disease, than measuring the level of total calcium or of complexed calcium. The level of total calcium in the blood serum is normally 8.5–10.5 mg/dL, while the level of free calcium is normally 4–5 mg/dl.

Causes and symptoms

Hypocalcemia can be caused by **hypoparathyroidism**, by failure to produce 1,25-dihydroxyvitamin D, by low levels of plasma magnesium, or by failure to get adequate amounts of calcium or vitamin D in the diet. Hypoparathyroidism involves the failure of the parathyroid gland to make parathyroid hormone. Parathyroid hormone controls and maintains plasma calcium levels. The hormone exerts its effect on the kidneys, where it triggers the synthesis of 1,25-dihydroxyvitamin D. Thus, hypocalcemia can be independently caused by damage to the parathyroid gland or to the kidneys. 1,25-Dihydroxyvitamin D stimulates the uptake of calcium from the diet and the mobilization of calcium from the bone. Bone mobilization means the natural process by which the body dissolves part of the bone in the skeleton in order to maintain or raise the levels of plasma calcium ions.

Low plasma magnesium levels (hypomagnesia) can result in hypocalcemia. Hypomagnesemia can occur with **alcoholism** or with diseases characterized by an inability to properly absorb fat. Magnesium is required for parathyroid hormone to play its part in maintaining plasma calcium levels. For this reason, any disease that results in lowered plasma magnesium levels may also cause hypocalcemia.

Hypocalcimia may also result from the consumption of toxic levels of phosphate. Phosphate is a constituent of certain enema formulas. An enema is a solution that is used to cleanse the intestines via a hose inserted into the rectum. Cases of hypocalcemia have been documented where people swallowed enema formulas, or where an enema has been administered to an infant.

Symptoms of severe hypocalcemia include **numbness** or **tingling** around the mouth or in the feet and hands, as well as in **muscle spasms** in the face, feet, and hands. Hypocalcemia can also result in depression, memory loss, or **hallucinations**. Severe hypocalcemia occurs when serum free calcium is under 3 mg/dL. Chronic and moderate hypocalcemia can result in **cataracts** (damage to the eyes). In this case, the term "chronic" means lasting one year or longer.

Diagnosis

Hypocalcemia is diagnosed by acquiring a sample of blood serum and measuring the concentraton of free calcium using a calcium-sensitive electrode. Hypocalcemia has several causes, and hence a full diagnosis requires assessment of health of the parathyroid gland, kidneys, and of plasma magnesium concentration.

Treatment

The method chosen for treatment depends on the exact cause and on the severity of the hypocalcemia. Severe hypocalcemia requires injection of calcium ions, usually in the form of calcium gluconate. Oral calcium supplements are prescribed for long term treatment (non-emergency) of hypocalcemia. The oral supplements may take the form of calcium carbonate, calcium chloride, calcium lactate, or calcium gluconate. Where hypocalcemia results from kidney failure, treatment includes injections of 1,25-dihydroxyvitamin D. Oral vitamin D supplements can increase gastrointestinal absorption of calcium. Where hypocalcemia results from hypoparathyroidism, treatment may include oral calcium, 1,25-dihydroxyvitamin D, or other drugs. Where low serum magnesium levels occur, concurrently with hypocalcemia, the magnesium deficiency must be corrected to effectively treat the hypocalcemia.

Prognosis

The prognosis for correcting hypocalcemia is excellent. However, the eye damage that may result from chronic hypocalcemia cannot be reversed.

Prevention

The first, and most obvious, way to help prevent hypocalcemia is to ensure that adequate amounts of calcium and vitamin D are consumed each day, either in the diet or as supplements. The hypocalcemia that may occur with damage to the parathyroid gland or to the kidneys cannot be prevented. Hypocalcemia resulting from overuse of **enemas** can be prevented by reducing enema usage. Hypocalcemia resulting from magnesium deficiency tends to occur in chronic alcoholics, and this type of hypocalcemia can be prevented by reducing alcohol consumption and increasing the intake of healthful food.

Resources

BOOKS

Brody, Tom. *Nutritional Biochemistry.* San Diego:Academic Press, 1998.

Tom Brody, PhD

Hypochondriac *see* **Hypochondriasis**

Hypochondriasis

Definition

Hypochondriasis is a mental disorder characterized by excessive fear of or preoccupation with a serious illness, despite medical testing and reassurance to the contrary. It was formerly called hypochondriacal neurosis.

Description

Although hypochondriasis is often considered a disorder that primarily affects adults, it is now increasingly recognized in children and adolescents. In addition, hypochondriasis may develop in elderly people without previous histories of health-related fears. The disorder accounts for about 5% of psychiatric patients and is equally common in men and women.

Causes and symptoms

The causes of hypochondriasis are not precisely known. Children may have physical symptoms that resemble or mimic those of other family members. In adults, hypochondriasis may sometimes reflect a self-centered character structure or a wish to be taken care of by others; it may also have been copied from a parent's behavior. In elderly people, hypochondriasis may be associated with depression or grief. It may also involve biologically based hypersensitivity to internal stimuli.

Most hypochondriacs are worried about being physically sick, although some express fear of insanity. The symptoms reported can range from general descriptions of a specific illness to unusual complaints. In many instances the symptoms reflect intensified awareness of ordinary body functions, such as heartbeat, breathing, or stomach noises. It is important to understand that a hypochondriac's symptoms are not "in the head" in the sense of being delusional. The symptoms are real, but the patient misinterprets bodily functions and attributes them to a serious or even lethal cause.

Diagnosis

The diagnosis is often complicated by the patient's detailed understanding of symptoms and medical terminology from previous contacts with doctors. If a new doctor suspects hypochondriasis, he or she will usually order a complete medical workup in order to rule out physical disease.

Psychological evaluation is also necessary to rule out other disorders that involve feelings of **anxiety** or complaints of physical illness. These disorders include depression, **panic disorder**, and **schizophrenia** with somatic (physical) **delusions**. The following features are characteristic of hypochondriasis:

- The patient is not psychotic (out of touch with reality or hallucinating).
- The patient gets upset or blames the doctor when told there is "nothing wrong," or that there is a psychological basis for the problem.
- There is a correlation between episodes of hypochondriacal behavior and stressful periods in the patient's life.
- The behavior has lasted at least six months.

Evaluation of children and adolescents with hypochondriasis should include the possibility of **abuse** by family members.

Treatment

The goal of therapy is to help the patient (and family) live with the symptoms and to modify thinking and behavior that reinforces hypochondriacal symptoms. This treatment orientation is called supportive, as distinct from insight-oriented, because hypochondriacs usually resist psychological interpretations of their symptoms. Supportive treatment may include medications to relieve anxiety. Some clinicians look carefully for "masked" depression and treat with antidepressants.

Follow-up care includes regular physical checkups, because about 30% of patients with hypochondriasis will eventually develop a serious physical illness. The physician also tries to prevent unnecessary medical testing and "doctor shopping" on the patient's part.

Prognosis

From 33–50% of patients with hypochondriasis can expect significant improvement from the current methods of treatment.

Resources

BOOKS

Eisendrath, Stuart J. "Psychiatric Disorders." In *Current Medical Diagnosis and Treatment, 1998*, edited by Stephen McPhee, et al., 37th ed. Stamford: Appleton & Lange, 1997.

Rebecca J. Frey, PhD

Hypoesthesias *see* **Numbness and tingling**

Hypoglycemia

Definition

The condition called hypoglycemia is literally translated as low blood sugar. Hypoglycemia occurs when blood sugar (or blood glucose) concentrations fall below a level necessary to properly support the body's need for energy and stability throughout its cells.

Description

Carbohydrates are the main dietary source of the glucose that is manufactured in the liver and absorbed into the bloodstream to fuel the body's cells and organs. Glucose concentration is controlled by hormones, primarily insulin and glucagon. Glucose concentration also is controlled by epinephrine (adrenalin) and norepinephrine, as well as growth hormone. If these regulators are not working properly, levels of blood sugar can become either excessive (as in hyperglycemia) or inadequate (as in hypoglycemia). If a person has a blood sugar level of 50 mg/dl or less, he or she is considered hypoglycemic, although glucose levels vary widely from one person to another.

Hypoglycemia can occur in several ways.

Drug-induced hypoglycemia

Drug-induced hypoglycemia, a complication of diabetes, is the most commonly seen and most dangerous form of hypoglycemia.

Hypoglycemia occurs most often in diabetics who must inject insulin periodically to lower their blood sugar. While other diabetics also are vulnerable to low blood sugar episodes, they have a lower risk of a serious outcome than insulin-dependant diabetics. Unless recognized and treated immediately, severe hypoglycemia in the insulin-dependent diabetic can lead to generalized convulsions followed by **amnesia** and unconsciousness. Death, though rare, is a possible outcome.

In insulin-dependent diabetics, hypoglycemia known as an insulin reaction or insulin shock can be caused by several factors. These include overmedicating with manufactured insulin, missing or delaying a meal, eating too little food for the amount of insulin taken, exercising too strenuously, drinking too much alcohol, or any combination of these factors.

Ideopathic or reactive hypoglycemia

Ideopathic or reactive hypoglycemia (also called postprandial hypoglycemia) occurs when some people eat. A number of reasons for this reaction have been proposed, but no single cause has been identified.

In some cases, this form of hypoglycemia appears to be associated with malfunctions or diseases of the liver, pituitary, adrenals, liver, or pancreas. These conditions are unrelated to diabetes. Children intolerant of a natural sugar (fructose) or who have inherited defects that affect digestion also may experience hypoglycemic attacks. Some children with a negative reaction to aspirin also experience reactive hypoglycemia. It sometimes occurs among people with an intolerance to the sugar found in milk (galactose), and it also often begins before diabetes strikes later on.

Fasting hypoglycemia

Fasting hypoglycemia sometimes occurs after long periods without food, but it also happens occasionally following strenuous **exercise**, such as running in a marathon.

Other factors sometimes associated with hypoglycemia include:

- pregnancy
- a weakened immune system
- a poor diet high in simple carbohydrates
- prolonged use of drugs, including antibiotics
- chronic physical or mental **stress**
- heartbeat irregularities (arrhythmias)
- **allergies**
- breast **cancer**
- high blood pressure treated with beta-blocker medications (after strenuous exercise)
- upper gastrointestinal tract surgery.

Causes and symptoms

When carbohydrates are eaten, they are converted to glucose that goes into the bloodstream and is distributed throughout the body. Simultaneously, a combination of chemicals that regulate how our body's cells absorb that sugar is released from the liver, pancreas, and adrenal glands. These chemical regulators include insulin, glucagon, epinephrine (adrenalin), and norepinephrine. The mixture of these regulators released following digestion of carbohydrates is never the same, since the amount of carbohydrates that are eaten is never the same.

Interactions among the regulators are complicated. Any abnormalities in the effectiveness of any one of the regulators can reduce or increase the body's absorption of glucose. Gastrointestinal enzymes such as amylase and lactase that break down carbohydrates may not be functioning properly. These abnormalities may produce hyperglycemia or hypoglycemia, and can be detected when the level of glucose in the blood is measured.

Cell sensitivity to these regulators can be changed in many ways. Over time, a person's stress level, exercise patterns, advancing age, and dietary habits influence cellular sensitivity. For example, a diet consistently overly rich in carbohydrates increases insulin requirements over time. Eventually, cells can become less receptive to the effects of the regulating chemicals, which can lead to glucose intolerance.

Diet is both a major factor in producing hypoglycemia as well as the primary method for controlling it. **Diets** typical of western cultures contain excess carbohydrates, especially in the form of simple carbohydrates such as sweeteners, which are more easily converted to sugar. In poorer parts of the world, the typical diet contains even higher levels of carbohydrates. Fewer dairy products and meats are eaten, and grains, vegetables, and fruits are consumed. This dietary trend is balanced, however, since people in these cultures eat smaller meals and usually use carbohydrates more efficiently through physical labor.

Early symptoms of severe hypoglycemia, particularly in the drug-induced type of hypoglycemia, resemble an extreme **shock** reaction. Symptoms include:

- cold and pale skin
- numbness around the mouth
- apprehension
- heart **palpitations**
- emotional outbursts
- hand tremors
- mental cloudiness
- dilated pupils
- sweating
- fainting

Mild attacks, however, are more common in reactive hypoglycemia and are characterized by extreme tiredness. Patients first lose their alertness, then their muscle strength and coordination. Thinking grows fuzzy, and finally the patient becomes so tired that he or she becomes "zombie-like," awake but not functioning. Sometimes the patient will actually fall asleep. Unplanned naps are typical of the chronic hypoglycemic patient, particularly following meals.

Additional symptoms of reactive hypoglycemia include headaches, double vision, staggering or inability to walk, a craving for salt and/or sweets, abdominal distress, premenstrual tension, chronic colitis, allergies, ringing in the ears, unusual patterns in the frequency of urination, skin eruptions and inflammations, **pain** in the neck and shoulder muscles, memory problems, and sudden and excessive sweating.

Unfortunately, a number of these symptoms mimic those of other conditions. For example, the depression, **insomnia**, irritability, lack of concentration, crying spells, **phobias**, forgetfulness, confusion, unsocial behavior, and suicidal tendencies commonly seen in nervous system and psychiatric disorders also may be hypoglycemic symptoms. It is very important that anyone with symptoms that may suggest reactive hypoglycemia see a doctor.

Because all of its possible symptoms are not likely to be seen in any one person at a specific time, diagnosing hypoglycemia can be difficult. One or more of its many symptoms may be due to another illness. Symptoms may persist in a variety of forms for long periods of time. Symptoms also can change over time within the same person. Some of the factors that can influence symptoms include physical or mental activities, physical or mental state, the amount of time passed since the last meal, the amount and quality of sleep, and exercise patterns.

Diagnosis

Drug-induced hypoglycemia

Once diabetes is diagnosed, the patient then monitors his or her blood sugar level with a portable machine called a glucometer. The diabetic places a small blood sample on a test strip that the machine can read. If the test reveals that the blood sugar level is too low, the diabetic can make a correction by eating or drinking an additional carbohydrate.

Reactive hypoglycemia

Reactive hypoglycemia only can be diagnosed by a doctor. Symptoms usually improve after the patient has gone on an appropriate diet. Reactive hypoglycemia was diagnosed more frequently 10–20 years ago than today. Studies have shown that most people suffering from its symptoms test normal for blood sugar, leading many doctors to suggest that actual cases of reactive hypoglycemia are quite rare. Some doctors think that people with hypoglycemic symptoms may be particularly sensitive to the body's normal postmeal release of the hormone epinephrine, or are actually suffering from some other physical or mental problem. Other doctors believe reactive hypoglycemia actually is the early onset of diabetes that occurs after a number of years. There continues to be disagreement about the cause of reactive hypoglycemia.

A common test to diagnose hypoglycemia is the extended oral glucose tolerance test. Following an overnight fast, a concentrated solution of glucose is drunk and blood samples are taken hourly for five to six hours. Though this test remains helpful in early identification of diabetes, its use in diagnosing chronic reactive hypoglycemia has lost favor because it can trigger hypoglycemic symptoms in people with otherwise normal glucose readings. Some doctors now recommend that blood sugar be tested at the actual time a person experiences hypoglycemic symptoms.

Treatment

Treatment of the immediate symptoms of hypoglycemia can include eating sugar. For example, a patient can eat a piece of candy, drink milk, or drink fruit juice. Glucose tablets can be used by patients, especially those who are diabetic. Effective treatment of hypoglycemia over time requires the patient to follow a modified diet. Patients usually are encouraged to eat small, but frequent, meals throughout the day, avoiding excess simple sugars (including alcohol), fats, and fruit drinks. Those patients with severe hypoglycemia may require fast-acting glucagon injections that can stabilize their blood sugar within approximately 15 minutes.

Alternative treatment

A holistic approach to reactive hypoglycemia is based on the belief that a number of factors may create the condition. Among them are heredity, the effects of other illnesses, emotional stress, too much or too little exercise, bad lighting, poor diet, and environmental pollution. Therefore, a number of alternative methods have been proposed as useful in treating the condition. Homeopathy, **acupuncture**, and **applied kinesiology**, for example, have been used, as have herbal remedies. One of the herbal remedies commonly suggested for hypoglycemia is a decoction (an extract made by boiling) of gentian (*Gentiana lutea*). It should be drunk warm 15–30 minutes before a meal. Gentian is believed to help stimulate the endocrine (hormone-producing) glands.

In addition to the dietary modifications recommended above, people with hypoglycemia may benefit from supplementing their diet with chromium, which is believed to help improve blood sugar levels. Chromium is found in whole grain breads and cereals, cheese, molasses, lean meats, and brewer's yeast. Hypoglycemics should avoid alcohol, **caffeine**, and cigarette smoke, since these substances can cause significant swings in blood sugar levels.

Prevention

Drug-induced hypoglycemia

Preventing hypoglycemic insulin reactions in diabetics requires taking glucose readings through frequent blood sampling. Insulin then can be regulated based on those readings. Continuous glucose monitoring sensors have been developed to help diabetics remain more aware of possible hypoglycemic episodes. These monitors even can check for episodes while the patient sleeps, when many will experience severe hypoglycemia but not know it. Those who don't pay attention to severe hypoglycemia events or who have had previous severe hypoglycemia are the most likely to have future severe hypoglycemia. An audible alert can let the patient know immediately that he or she needs to take care of his or her blood sugar level. Continuous monitoring has proved particularly helpful in pediatric patients with Type 1 diabetes.

Maintaining proper diet also is a factor. Programmable insulin pumps implanted under the skin have proven useful in reducing the incidence of hypoglycemic episodes for insulin-dependent diabetics. As of late 1997, clinical studies continue to seek additional ways to control diabetes and drug-induced hypoglycemia. Tests of a substance called pramlintide indicate that it may help improve glycemic control in diabetics.

Reactive hypoglycemia

The onset of reactive hypoglycemia can be avoided or at least delayed by following the same kind of diet used to control it. While not as restrictive as the diet diabetics must follow to keep tight control over their disease, it is quite similar.

There are a variety of diet recommendations for the reactive hypoglycemic. Patients should:

- avoiding overeating
- never skipping breakfast
- including protein in all meals and snacks, preferably from sources low in fat, such as the white meat of chicken or turkey, most fish, soy products, or skim milk
- restricting intake of fats (particularly saturated fats, such as animal fats), and avoiding refined sugars and processed foods
- being aware of the differences between some vegetables, such as potatoes and carrots. These vegetables have a higher sugar content than others (like squash and broccoli). Patients should be aware of these differences and note any reactions they have to them.
- being aware of differences found in grain products. White flour is a carbohydrate that is rapidly absorbed into the bloodstream, while oats take much longer to break down in the body.
- keeping a "food diary." Until the diet is stabilized, a patient should note what and how much he/she eats and drinks at every meal. If symptoms appear following a meal or snack, patients should note them and look for patterns.

KEY TERMS

Adrenal glands—Two organs that sit atop the kidneys; these glands make and release hormones such as epinephrine.

Epinephrine—Also called adrenalin, a secretion of the adrenal glands (along with norepinephrine) that helps the liver release glucose and limits the release of insulin. Norepinephrine is both a hormone and a neurotransmitter, a substance that transmits nerve signals.

Fructose—A type of natural sugar found in many fruits, vegetables, and in honey.

Glucagon—A hormone produced in the pancreas that raises the level of glucose in the blood. An injectable form of glucagon, which can be bought in a drug store, is sometimes used to treat insulin shock.

Postprandial—After eating or after a meal.

• eat fresh fruits, but restrict the amount they eat at one time. Patients should remember to eat a source of protein whenever they eat high sources of carbohydrate like fruit. Apples make particularly good snacks because, of all fruits, the carbohydrate in apples is digested most slowly.

• following a diet that is high in fiber. Fruit is a good source of fiber, as are oatmeal and oat bran. Fiber slows the buildup of sugar in the blood during digestion.

A doctor can recommend a proper diet, and there are many cookbooks available for diabetics. Recipes found in such books are equally effective in helping to control hypoglycemia.

Prognosis

Like diabetes, there is no cure for reactive hypoglycemia, only ways to control it. While some chronic cases will continue through life (rarely is there complete remission of the condition), others will develop into type II (age onset) diabetes. Hypoglycemia appears to have a higher-than-average incidence in families where there has been a history of hypoglycemia or diabetes among their members, but whether hypoglycemia is a controllable warning of oncoming diabetes has not yet been determined by clinical research.

A condition known as hypoglycemia unawareness can develop in those who do not control their blood glucose, particularly in people with Type 1 diabetes.

These people may lose notice of the automatic warning symptoms of hypoglycemia that normally occur as their bodies become so used to frequent periods of hypoglycemia. It is not a permanent event, but can be treated by careful avoidance of hypoglycemia for about two weeks.

Resources

BOOKS

Ruggiero, Roberta. *The Do's and Don'ts of Low Blood Sugar.* Hollywood, FL: Frederick Fell Publishers.

PERIODICALS

Brauker, James, et al. "Use of Continuous Glucose Monitoring Alerts to Better Predict, Prevent and Treat Postprandial Hyperglycemia." *Diabetes* June 2003: 90-91.

Gertzman, Jerilyn, et al. "Severity of Hypoglycemia and Hypoglycemia Unawareness Are Associated with the Extent of Unsuspected Nocturnal Hypoglycemia." *Diabetes* June 2003:146-151.

Kumar, Rajeev, and Miles Fisher. "Impaired Hypoglycemia Awareness: Are we Aware?" *Diabetes and Primary Care* Summer 2004: 33–38.

Ludvigsson, Johnny, and Ragnar Hanas. "Continuous Subcutaneous Glucose Monitoring Improved Metabolic Control in Pediatric Patients With Type 1 Diabetes: A Controlled Crossover Study." *Pediatrics* May 2003: 933-936.

ORGANIZATIONS

Hypoglycemia Association, Inc. 18008 New Hampshire Ave., PO Box 165, Ashton, MD 20861-0165.

National Hypoglycemia Association, Inc. PO Box 120, Ridgewood, NJ 07451. (201) 670-1189.

Martin W. Dodge, PhD
Teresa G. Odle

Hypogonadism

Definition

Hypogonadism is the condition more prevalent in males in which the production of sex hormones and germ cells are inadequate.

Description

Gonads are the organs of sexual differentiation—in the female, they are ovaries; in the male, the testes. Along with producing eggs and sperm, they produce sex hormones that generate all the differences between men and women. If they produce too little sex hormone, then either the growth of the sexual organs or their function is impaired.

The gonads are not independent in their function, however. They are closely controlled by the pituitary gland. The pituitary hormones are the same for males and females, but the gonadal hormones are different. Men produce mostly androgens, and women produce mostly estrogens. These two hormones regulate the development of the embryo, determining whether it is a male or a female. They also direct the adolescent maturation of sex organs into their adult form. Further, they sustain those organs and their function throughout the reproductive years. The effects of estrogen reach beyond that to sustain bone strength and protect the cardiovascular system from degenerative disease.

Hormones can be inadequate during or after each stage of development—embryonic and adolescent. During each stage, inadequate hormone stimulation will prevent normal development. After each stage, a decrease in hormone stimulation will result in failed function and perhaps some shrinkage. The organs affected principally by sex hormones are the male and female genitals, both internal and external, and the female breasts. Body hair, fat deposition, bone and muscle growth, and some brain functions are also influenced.

Causes and symptoms

Sex is determined at the moment of conception by sex chromosomes. Females have two X chromosomes, while males have one X and one Y chromosome. If the male sperm with the Y chromosome fertilizes an egg, the baby will be male. This is true throughout the animal kingdom. Genetic defects sometimes result in changes in the chromosomes. If sex chromosomes are involved, there is a change in the development of sexual characteristics.

Female is the default sex of the embryo, so most of the sex organ deficits at birth occur in boys. Some, but not all, are due to inadequate androgen stimulation. The penis may be small, the testicles undescended (cryptorchidism) or various degrees of "feminization" of the genitals may be present.

After birth, sexual development does not occur until **puberty**. Hypogonadism most often shows up as an abnormality in boys during puberty. Again, not every defect is due to inadequate hormones. Some are due to too much of the wrong ones. Kallmann's syndrome is a birth defect in the brain that prevents release of hormones and appears as failure of male puberty. Some boys have adequate amounts of androgen in their system but fail to respond to them, a condition known as androgen resistance.

KEY TERMS

Biopsy—Surgical removal of pieces of tissue for examination.

Embryo—Refers to life before birth, specifically the first two months after conception.

Fetus—The unborn person or animal, still in the womb.

Hypothalamus—Part of the brain just above the pituitary that stimulates pituitary gland function.

Ionizing radiation—X rays. Diagnostic x rays are too weak to do damage under normal circumstances, but x rays used to treat cancer must be used with great care.

Undescended testicle—A testicle that is still in the groin and has not made its way into the scrotum.

Female problems in puberty are not caused by too little estrogen. Even female reproductive problems are rarely related to a simple lack of hormones, but rather to complex cycling rhythms gone wrong. All the problems with too little hormone happen during **menopause**, which is a normal hypogonadism.

A number of adverse events can damage the gonads and result in decreased hormone levels. The childhood disease **mumps**, if acquired after puberty, can infect and destroy the testicles—a disease called viral **orchitis**. Ionizing radiation and **chemotherapy**, trauma, several drugs (spironolactone, a diuretic and ketoconazole, an antifungal agent), alcohol, **marijuana**, heroin, **methadone**, and environmental toxins can all damage testicles and decrease their hormone production. Severe diseases in the liver or kidneys, certain infections, sickle cell anemia, and some cancers also affect gonads. To treat some male cancers, it is necessary to remove the testicles, thereby preventing the androgens from stimulating **cancer** growth. This procedure, still called castration or *orchiectomy*, removes androgen stimulation from the whole body.

For several reasons the pituitary can fail. It happens rarely after **pregnancy**. It used to be removed to treat advanced breast or **prostate cancer**. Sometimes the pituitary develops a tumor that destroys it. Failure of the pituitary is called **hypopituitarism** and, of course, leaves the gonads with no stimulation to produce hormones.

Besides the tissue changes generated by hormone stimulation, the only other symptoms relate to sexual desire and function. Libido is enhanced by testosterone, and male sexual performance requires androgens. The role of female hormones in female sexual activity is less clear, although hormones strengthen tissues and promote healthy secretions, facilitating sexual activity.

Diagnosis

Presently, there are accurate blood tests for most of the hormones in the body, including those from the pituitary and even some from the hypothalamus. Chromosomes can be analyzed, and gonads can, but rarely are, biopsied.

Treatment

Replacement of missing body chemicals is much easier than suppressing excesses. Estrogen replacement is recommended for nearly all women after menopause for its many beneficial effects. Estrogen can be taken by mouth, injection, or skin patch. It is strongly recommended that the other female hormone, progesterone, be taken as well, because it prevents overgrowth of uterine lining and uterine cancer. Testosterone replacement is available for males who are deficient.

Resources

BOOKS

Carr, Bruce R., and Karen D. Bradshaw. "Disorders of the Ovary and Female Reproductive Tract." In *Harrison's Principles of Internal Medicine*, edited by Anthony S. Fauci, et al. New York: McGraw-Hill, 1998.

J. Ricker Polsdorfer, MD

Hypokalemia

Definition

Hypokalemia is a condition of below normal levels of potassium in the blood serum. Potassium, a necessary electrolyte, facilitates nerve impulse conduction and the contraction of skeletal and smooth muscles, including the heart. It also facilitates cell membrane function and proper enzyme activity. Levels must be kept in a proper (homeostatic) balance for the maintenance of health. The normal concentration of potassium in the serum is in the range of 3.5–5.0 mM. Hypokalemia means serum or plasma levels of potassium ions that fall below 3.5 mM. (Potassium concentrations are often expressed in units of milliequivalents per liter [mEq/L], rather than in units of

millimolarity [mM], however, both units are identical and mean the same thing when applied to concentrations of potassium ions.)

Hypokalemia can result from two general causes: either from an overall depletion in the body's potassium or from excessive uptake of potassium by muscle from surrounding fluids.

Description

A normal adult weighing about 154 lbs (70 kg) has about 3.6 moles of potassium ions in his body. Most of this potassium (about 98%) occurs inside various cells and organs, where normal concentration are about 150 mM. Blood serum concentrations are much lower—only about 0.4% of the body's potassium is found in blood serum. As noted above, hypokalemia can be caused by the sudden uptake of potassium ions from the bloodstream by muscle or other organs or by an overall depletion of the body's potassium. Hypokalemia due to overall depletion tends to be a chronic phenomenon, while hypokalemia due to a shift in location tends to be a temporary disorder.

Causes and symptoms

Hypokalemia is most commonly caused by the use of **diuretics**. Diuretics are drugs that increase the excretion of water and salts in the urine. Diuretics are used to treat a number of medical conditions, including **hypertension** (high blood pressure), congestive heart failure, **liver disease**, and **kidney disease**. However, diuretic treatment can have the side effect of producing hypokalemia. In fact, the most common cause of hypokalemia in the elderly is the use of diuretics. The use of furosemide and thiazide, two commonly used diuretic drugs, can lead to hypokalemia. In contrast, spironolactone and triamterene are diuretics that do not provoke hypokalemia.

Other commons causes of hypokalemia are excessive **diarrhea** or **vomiting**. Diarrhea and vomiting can be produced by infections of the gastrointestinal tract. Due to a variety of organisms, including bacteria, protozoa, and viruses, diarrhea is a major world health problem. It is responsible for about a quarter of the 10 million infant deaths that occur each year. Although nearly all of these deaths occur in the poorer parts of Asia and Africa, diarrheal diseases are a leading cause of infant **death** in the United States. Diarrhea results in various abnormalities, such as dehydration (loss in body water), **hyponatremia** (low sodium level in the blood), and hypokalemia.

Because of the need for potassium to control muscle action, hypokalemia can cause the heart to stop beating. Young infants are especially at risk for death from this cause, especially where severe diarrhea continues for two weeks or longer. Diarrhea due to laxative **abuse** is an occasional cause of hypokalemia in the adolescent or adult. Enema abuse is a related cause of hypokalemia. Laxative abuse is especially difficult to diagnose and treat, because patients usually deny the practice. Up to 20% of persons complaining of chronic diarrhea practice laxative abuse. Laxative abuse is often part of eating disorders, such as anorexia nervosa or **bulimia nervosa**. Hypokalemia that occurs with these eating disorders may be life-threatening.

Surprisingly, the potassium loss that accompanies vomiting is only partly due to loss of potassium from the vomit. Vomiting also has the effect of provoking an increase in potassium loss in the urine. Vomiting expels acid from the mouth, and this loss of acid results in alkalization of the blood. (Alkalization of the blood means that the pH of the blood increases slightly.) An increased blood pH has a direct effect on the kidneys. Alkaline blood provokes the kidneys to release excessive amounts of potassium in the urine. So, severe and continual vomiting can cause excessive losses of potassium from the body and hypokalemia.

A third general cause of hypokalemia is prolonged fasting and **starvation**. In most people, after three weeks of **fasting**, blood serum potassium levels will decline to below 3.0 mM and result in severe hypokalemia. However, in some persons, serum potassium may be naturally maintained at about 3.0 mM, even after 100 days of fasting. During fasting, muscle is naturally broken down, and the muscle protein is converted to sugar (glucose) to supply to the brain the glucose which is essential for its functioning. Other organs are able to survive with a mixed supply of fat and glucose. The potassium within the muscle cell is released during the gradual process of muscle breakdown that occurs with starvation, and this can help counteract the trend to hypokalemia during starvation. Eating an unbalanced diet does not cause hypokalemia because most foods, such as fruits (especially bananas, oranges, and melons), vegetables, meat, milk, and cheese, are good sources of potassium. Only foods such as butter, margarine, vegetable oil, soda water, jelly beans, and hard candies are extremely poor in potassium.

Alcoholism occasionally results in hypokalemia. About one half of alcoholics hospitalized for withdrawal symptoms experience hypokalemia. The hypokalemia of alcoholics occurs for a variety of reasons, usually poor **nutrition**, vomiting, and diarrhea. Hypokalemia can also be caused by hyperaldosteronism; Cushing's syndrome; hereditary kidney defects such as Liddle's syndrome, Bartter's syndrom, and Franconi's syndrome; and eating too much licorice.

Symptoms

Mild hypokalemia usually results in no symptoms, while moderate hypokalemia results in confusion, disorientation, weakness, and discomfort of muscles. On occasion, moderate hypokalemia causes cramps during **exercise**. Another symptom of moderate hypokalemia is a discomfort in the legs that is experienced while sitting still. The patient may experience an annoying feeling that can be relieved by shifting the positions of the legs or by stomping the feet on the floor. Severe hypokalemia results in extreme weakness of the body and, on occasion, in **paralysis**. The paralysis that occurs is "flaccid paralysis," or limpness. Paralysis of the muscles of the lungs results in death. Another dangerous result of severe hypokalemia is abnormal heart beat (arrhythmia) that can lead to death from cardiac arrest (cessation of heart beat). Moderate hypokalemia may be defined as serum potassium between 2.5 and 3.0 mM, while severe hypokalemia is defined as serum potassium under 2.5 mM.

Diagnosis

Hypokalemia can be measured by acquiring a sample of blood, preparing blood serum, and using a potassium sensitive electrode for measuring the concentration of potassium ions. Atomic absorption spectroscopy can also be used to measure the potassium ions. Since hypokalemia results in abnormalities in heart behavior, the electrocardiogram is usually used in the diagnosis of hypokalemia. The diagnosis of the cause of hypokalemia can be helped by measuring the potassium content of the urine. Where urinary potassium is under 25 mmoles per day, it means that the patient has experienced excessive losses of potassium due to diarrhea. The urinary potassium test is useful in cases where the patient is denying the practice of laxative or enema abuse. In contrast, where hypokalemia is due to the use of diuretic drugs, the content of potassium in the urine will be high—over 40 mmoles per day.

Treatment

In emergency situations, when severe hypokalemia is suspected, the patient should be put on a cardiac monitor, and respiratory status should be assessed. If laboratory test results show potassium levels below 2.5 mM, intravenous potassium should be given. In less urgent cases, potassium can be given orally in the pill form. Potassium supplements take the form of pills

KEY TERMS

Diuretics—A class of drugs that cause the kidneys to excrete excess sodium, water, and potassium.

pH—The unit of acid content is pH. The blood plasma normally has a pH of 7.35–7.45. Acidic blood has a pH value slightly less than pH 7.35. Alkaline blood has a pH value slightly greater than pH 7.45.

Potassium—An electrolyte necessary to proper functioning of the body.

containing potassium chloride (KCl), potassium bicarbonate (KHCO$_3$), and potassium acetate. Oral potassium chloride is the safest and most effective treatment for hypokalemia. Generally, the consumption of 40–80 mmoles of KCl per day is sufficient to correct the hypokalemia that results from diuretic therapy. For many people taking diuretics, potassium supplements are not necessary as long as they eat a balanced diet containing foods rich in potassium.

Prognosis

The prognosis for correcting hypokalemia is excellent. However, in emergency situations, where potassium is administered intravenously, the physician must be careful not to give too much potassium. The administration of potassium at high levels, or at a high rate, can lead to abnormally high levels of serum potassium.

Prevention

Hypokalemia is not a concern for healthy persons, since potassium is present in a great variety of foods. For patients taking diuretics, however, the American Dietetic Association recommends use of a high potassium diet. The American Dietetic Association states that if hypokalemia has already occurred, use of the high potassium diet alone may not reverse hypokalemia. Useful components of a high potassium diet include bananas, tomatoes, cantaloupes, figs, raisins, kidney beans, potatoes, and milk.

Resources

BOOKS

Brody, Tom. *Nutritional Biochemistry*. San Diego:Academic Press, 1998.

Tom Brody, PhD

Hypolipoproteinemia

Definition

Hypolipoproteinemia (or hypolipidemia) is the lack of fat in the blood.

Description

Although quite rare, hypolipoproteinemia is a serious condition. Blood absorbs fat from food in the intestine and transports it as a combined package with proteins and other chemicals like cholesterol. Much of the fat goes straight into the liver for processing. The cholesterol, a waste product, ends up in the bile. The proteins act as vessels, carrying the other chemicals around. These packages of fat, cholesterol, and proteins are called lipoproteins.

Causes and symptoms

Low blood fats can be the result of several diseases, or they can be a primary genetic disease with other associated abnormalities.

- **Malnutrition** is a lack of food, including fats, in the diet.

- Malabsorption is the inability of the bowel to absorb food, causing malnutrition.

- Anemia (too few red blood cells) and **hyperthyroidism** (too much thyroid hormone) also reduce blood fats.

- Rare genetic conditions called hypobetalipoproteinemia and abetalipoproteinemia cause malabsorption plus nerve, eye, and skin problems in early childhood.

- Tangier disease, causes only the cholesterol to be low. It also produces nerve and eye problems in children.

Symptoms are associated more closely with the cause rather than the actual low blood fats.

Diagnosis

Blood studies of the various fat particles help identify both the low and high fat diseases. These tests are often done after an overnight fast to prevent interference from fat just being absorbed from food. Fats and proteins are grouped together and described by density—high-density lipoproteins (HDL), low-density lipoproteins (LDL), and very low-density lipoproteins (VLDL). There are also much bigger particles called chylomicrons. Each contain different proportions of cholesterol, fats, and protein.

Treatment

Supplemental vitamin E helps children with the betalipoprotein deficiencies. There is no known treatment for Tangier disease. Treatment of the causes of the other forms of low blood fats reverses the condition.

Resources

BOOKS

Ginsberg, Henry N., and Ira J. Goldberg. "Disorders Of Lipoprotein Metabolism." In *Harrison's Principles of Internal Medicine*, edited by Anthony S. Fauci, et al. New York: McGraw-Hill, 1997.

J. Ricker Polsdorfer, MD

Hypomagnesemia *see* **Magnesium imbalance**

Hyponatremia

Definition

The normal concentration of sodium in the blood plasma is 136–145 mM. Hyponatremia occurs when sodium falls below 130 mM. Plasma sodium levels of 125 mM or less are dangerous and can result in seizures and **coma**.

Description

Sodium is an atom, or ion, that carries a single positive charge. The sodium ion may be abbreviated as Na^+ or as simply Na. Sodium can occur as a salt in a crystalline solid. Sodium chloride (NaCl), sodium phosphate (Na_2HPO_4) and sodium bicarbonate ($NaHCO_3$) are commonly occurring salts. These salts can be dissolved in water or in juices of various foods. Dissolving involves the complete separation of ions, such as sodium and chloride in common table salt (NaCl).

About 40% of the body's sodium is contained in bone. Approximately 2–5% occurs within organs and cells and the remaining 55% is in blood plasma and other extracellular fluids. The amount of sodium in blood plasma is typically 140 mM, a much higher amount than is found in intracellular sodium (about 5 mM). This asymmetric distribution of sodium ions is essential for human life. It makes possible proper nerve conduction, the passage of various nutrients into cells, and the maintenance of blood pressure.

The body continually regulates its handling of sodium. When dietary sodium is too high or low, the intestines and kidneys respond to adjust concentrations to normal. During the course of a day, the intestines absorb dietary sodium while the kidneys excrete a nearly equal amount of sodium into the urine. If a low sodium diet is consumed, the intestines increase their efficiency of sodium absorption, and the kidneys reduce its release into urine.

The concentration of sodium in the blood plasma depends on two things: the total amount of sodium and water in arteries, veins, and capillaries (the circulatory system). The body uses separate mechanisms to regulate sodium and water, but they work together to correct blood pressure when it is too high or too low. Too low a concentration of sodium, or hyponatremia, can be corrected either by increasing sodium or by decreasing body water. The existence of separate mechanisms that regulate sodium concentration account for the fact that there are numerous diseases that can cause hyponatremia, including diseases of the kidney, pituitary gland, and hypothalamus.

Causes and symptoms

Hyponatremia can be caused by abnormal consumption or excretion of dietary sodium or water and by diseases that impair the body's ability to regulate them. Maintenance of a low salt diet for many months or excessive sweat loss during a race on a hot day can present a challenge to the body to conserve adequate sodium levels. While these conditions alone are not likely to cause hyponatremia, it can occur under special circumstances. For example, hyponatremia often occurs in patients taking diuretic drugs who maintain a low sodium diet. This is especially of concern in elderly patients, who have a reduced ability to regulate the concentrations of various nutrients in the bloodstream. Diuretic drugs that frequently cause hyponatremia include furosemide (Lasix), bumetanide (Bumex), and most commonly, the thiazides. Diuretics enhance the excretion of sodium into the urine, with the goal of correcting high blood pressure. However, too much sodium excretion can result in hyponatremia. Usually only mild hyponatremia occurs in patients taking **diuretics**, but when combined with a low sodium diet or with the excessive drinking of water, severe hyponatremia can develop.

Severe and prolonged **diarrhea** can also cause hyponatremia. Severe diarrhea, causing the daily output of 8–10 liters of fluid from the large intestines, results in the loss of large amounts of water, sodium, and various nutrients. Some diarrheal diseases release particularly large quantities of sodium and are therefore most likely to cause hyponatremia.

Drinking excess water sometimes causes hyponatremia, because the absorption of water into the bloodstream can dilute the sodium in the blood. This cause of hyponatremia is rare, but has been found in psychotic patients who compulsively drink more than 20 liters of water per day. Excessive drinking of beer, which is mainly water and low in sodium, can also produce hyponatremia when combined with a poor diet.

Marathon running, under certain conditions, leads to hyponatremia. Races of 25–50 miles can result in the loss of great quantities (8 to 10 liters) of sweat, which contains both sodium and water. Studies show that about 30% of marathon runners experience mild hyponatremia during a race. But runners who consume only pure water during a race can develop severe hyponatremia because the drinking water dilutes the sodium in the bloodstream. Such runners may experience neurological disorders as a result of the severe hyponatremia and require emergency treatment.

Hyponatremia also develops from disorders in organs that control the body's regulation of sodium or water. The adrenal gland secretes a hormone called aldosterone that travels to the kidney, where it causes the kidney to retain sodium by not excreting it into the urine. **Addison's disease** causes hyponatremia as a result of low levels of aldosterone due to damage to the adrenal gland. The hypothalamus and pituitary gland are also involved in sodium regulation by making and releasing vasopressin, known as anti-diuretic hormone, into the bloodstream. Like aldosterone, vasopressin acts in the kidney, but it causes it to reduce the amount of water released into urine. With more vasopressin production, the body conserves water, resulting in a lower concentration of plasma sodium. Certain types of **cancer** cells produce vasopressin, leading to hyponatremia.

KEY TERMS

Blood plasma and serum—Blood plasma, or plasma, is prepared by obtaining a sample of blood and removing the blood cells. The red blood cells and white blood cells are removed by spinning with a centrifuge. Chemicals are added to prevent the blood's natural tendency to clot. If these chemicals include sodium, than a false measurement of plasma sodium content will result. Serum is prepared by obtaining a blood sample, allowing formation of the blood clot, and removing the clot using a centrifuge. Both plasma and serum are light yellow in color.

Symptoms of moderate hyponatremia include tiredness, disorientation, **headache**, **muscle cramps**, and **nausea**. Severe hyponatremia can lead to seizures and coma. These neurological symptoms are thought to result from the movement of water into brain cells, causing them to swell and disrupt their functioning.

In most cases of hyponatremia, doctors are primarily concerned with discovering the underlying disease causing the decline in plasma sodium levels. **Death** that occurs during hyponatremia is usually due to other features of the disease rather than to the hyponatremia itself.

Diagnosis

Hyponatremia is diagnosed by acquiring a blood sample, preparing plasma, and using a sodium-sensitive electrode for measuring the concentration of sodium ions. Unless the cause is obvious, a variety of tests are subsequently run to determine if sodium was lost from the urine, diarrhea, or from **vomiting**. Tests are also used to determine abnormalities in aldosterone or vasopressin levels. The patient's diet and use of diuretics must also be considered.

Treatment

Severe hyponatremia can be treated by infusing a solution of 5% sodium chloride in water into the bloodstream. Moderate hyponatremia due to use of diuretics or an abnormal increase in vasopressin is often treated by instructions to drink less water each day. Hyponatremia due to adrenal gland insufficiency is treated with hormone injections.

Prognosis

Hyponatremia is just one manifestation of a variety of disorders. While hyponatremia can easily be corrected, the prognosis for the underlying condition that causes it varies.

Prevention

Patients who take diuretic medications must be checked regularly for the development of hyponatremia.

Resources

PERIODICALS

Fried, L. F., and P. M. Palevsky. "Hyponatremia and Hypernatremia." *Medical Clinics of North America* 81 (1997): 585-609.

Tom Brody, PhD

Hypoparathyroidism

Definition

Hypoparathyroidism is the result of a decrease in production of parathyroid hormones by the parathyroid glands located behind the thyroid glands in the neck. The result is a low level of calcium in the blood.

Description

Parathyroid glands consist of four pea-shaped glands located on the back and side of the thyroid gland. The gland produces parathyroid hormone which, along with vitamin D and calcitonin, are important for the regulation of the calcium level in the body. Hypoparathyroidism affects both males and females of all ages.

Causes and symptoms

The accidental removal of the parathyroid glands during neck surgery is the most frequent cause of hypoparathyroidism. Complications of surgery on the parathyroid glands is another common cause of this disorder. There is the possibility of autoimmune genetic disorders causing hypoparathyroidism such as Hashimoto's **thyroiditis**, **pernicious anemia**, and **Addison's disease**. The destruction of the gland by radiation is a rare cause of hypoparathyroidism. Occasionally, the parathyroids are absent at birth causing low calcium levels and possible convulsions in the newborn. Symptoms in the advanced and continuous stages of hypoparathyroidism include splitting of the nails, inadequate tooth development and **mental retardation** in children, and seizures.

Abnormal low levels of calcium result in irritability of nerves, causing **numbness and tingling** of the hands and feet, with painful-cramp like muscle spasms known as tetany. Laryngeal spasms may also occur causing respiratory obstruction.

Diagnosis

Diagnostic measures begin with the individual's own observation of symptoms. A thorough medical history and **physical examination** by a physician is always required for an accurate diagnosis. The general practitioner may refer the individual to an endocrinologist, a medical specialist who studies the function of the parathyroid glands as well as other hormone producing glands. Laboratory studies include blood and urine tests to help determine phosphate and calcium levels. X rays are useful to determine any abnormalities in bone density associated with abnormal calcium levels. These autoimmune disorders may accompany hypoparathyroidism, but are not an actual cause of it.

Treatment

In the event of severe **muscle spasms**, hospitalization may be warranted for calcium injections. Raising carbon-dioxide levels in the blood, which can decrease muscle spasms, may be achieved in immediate situations by placing a paper bag over the mouth and blowing into it to "reuse" each breath. It is critical to obtain timely periodic laboratory tests to check calcium levels. A high calcium, low-phosphorous diet may be of significance and is directed by the physician or dietitian.

Prognosis

Presently hypoparathyroidism is considered incurable. The disorder requires lifelong replacement therapy to control symptoms. Medical research however, continues to search for a cure.

Prevention

There are no specific preventive measures for hypoparathyroidism. However, careful surgical techniques are critical to reduce the risk of damage to the gland during surgery.

KEY TERMS

Addison's disease—A disease caused by partial or total failure of adrenocortical (relating to, or derived from the adrenal gland) function, which is characterized by a bronze-like pigmentation of the skin and mucous membranes, anemia, weakness, and low blood pressure.

Autoimmunity—A condition by which the body's defense mechanism attacks itself.

Calcitonin—A hormone produced by the thyroid gland in human beings that lowers plasma calcium and phosphate levels without increasing calcium accumulation.

Hashimoto's thyroiditis—The self destruction of the thyroid cells from an autoimmune disorder.

Hormones—A substance produced by one tissue and conveyed by the bloodstream to another to affect physiological activity, such as growth or metabolism.

Pernicious anemia—A severe anemia most often affecting older adults, caused by failure of the stomach to absorb vitamin B12 and characterized by abnormally large red blood cells, gastrointestinal disturbances, and lesions of the spinal cord.

Resources

ORGANIZATIONS

American Medical Association. 515 N. State St., Chicago, IL 60612. (312) 464-5000. <http://www.ama-assn.org>.

Jeffrey P. Larson, RPT

Hypophysectomy

Definition

Hypophysectomy or hypophysis is the removal of the pituitary gland.

Purpose

The pituitary gland is in the middle of the head. Removing this master gland is a drastic step that was taken in the extreme circumstance of two cancers that had escaped all other forms of treatment. Cancers of the female breast and male prostate grow faster in the presence of sex hormones. It used to be that sex hormones could be suppressed only by removing their source, the glands that made them. After the gonads were removed, some cancers continued to grow, so other stimulants to their growth had to removed. At this point, some **cancer** specialists turned to the pituitary.

With the development of new therapeutic agents and methods, especially new ways to manipulate hormones without removing their source, this type of endocrine surgery has been largely relegated to history. However, tumors develop in the pituitary gland that require removal. Here, the idea is to remove the tumor but partially preserve the gland.

Description

There are several surgical approaches to the pituitary. The surgeon will choose the best one for the specific procedure. The pituitary lies directly behind the nose, and access through the nose or the sinuses is often the best approach. Opening the skull and lifting the frontal lobe of the brain will expose the delicate neck of the pituitary gland. This approach works best if tumors have extended above the pituitary fossa (the cavity in which the gland lies).

Newer surgical methods using technology have made other approaches possible. Stereotaxis is a three-dimensional aiming technique using x rays or scans for guidance. Instruments can be placed in the brain with pinpoint accuracy through tiny holes in the skull. These instruments can then manipulate brain tissue, either to destroy it or remove it. Stereotaxis is also used to direct radiation with similar precision using a gamma knife. Access to some brain lesions can be gained through the blood vessels using tiny tubes and wires guided by x rays.

Preparation

Pituitary surgery is performed by neurosurgeons deep inside the skull. All the patient can do to prepare is keep as healthy as possible and trust that the surgeon will do his usual excellent job. Informed surgical consent is important so that the patient is fully confident of the need for surgery and the expected outcome.

Aftercare

Routine post-operative care is required. In addition, pituitary function will be assessed.

Risks

The risks of surgery are multiple. Procedures are painstakingly selected to minimize risk and maximize benefit. Unique to surgery on the pituitary is the risk of

KEY TERMS

Endocrine system—Group of glands and parts of glands that control metabolic activity. Pituitary, thyroid, adrenals, ovaries, and testes are all part of the endocrine system.

Hormone—A chemical made in one place that has effects in distant places in the body. Hormone production is usually triggered by the pituitary gland.

destroying the entire gland and leaving the entire endocrine system without guidance. This used to be the whole purpose of hypophysectomy. After the procedure, the endocrinologist, a physician specializing in the study and care of the endocrine system, would provide the patient with all the hormones needed. Patients with no pituitary function did and still do quite well because of the available hormone replacements.

Normal results

Complete removal of the pituitary was the goal for cancer treatment. Today, removal of tumors with preservation of the gland is the goal.

Abnormal results

Tumors may not be completely removed, due to their attachment to vital structures.

Resources

BOOKS

Biller, Beverly M. K., and Gilbert H. Daniels. "Neuroendocrine Regulation and Diseases of the Anterior Pituitary and Hypothalamus." In *Harrison's Principles of Internal Medicine*, edited by Anthony S. Fauci, et al. New York: McGraw-Hill, 1997.

J. Ricker Polsdorfer, MD

Hypopigmentation *see* **Albinism; Vitiligo**

Hypopituitarism

Definition

Hypopituitarism is loss of function in an endocrine gland due to failure of the pituitary gland to secrete hormones which stimulate that gland's function. The pituitary gland is located at the base of the brain. Patients diagnosed with hypopituitarism may be deficient in one single hormone, several hormones, or have complete pituitary failure.

Description

The pituitary is a pea-sized gland located at the base of the brain, and surrounded by bone. The hypothalamus, another endocrine organ in the brain, controls the function of the pituitary gland by providing "hormonal orders." In turn, the pituitary gland regulates the many hormones that control various functions and organs within the body. The posterior pituitary acts as a sort of storage area for the hypothalamus and passes on hormones that control function of the muscles and kidneys. The anterior pituitary produces its own hormones which help to regulate several endocrine functions.

In hypopituitarism, something interferes with the production and release of these hormones, thus affecting the function of the target gland. Commonly affected hormones may include:

Gonadotropin deficiency

Gonadotropin deficiency involves two distinct hormones affecting the reproductive system. Luteinizing hormone (LH) stimulates the testes in men and the ovaries in women. This deficiency can affect fertility in men and women and menstruation in women. Follicle-stimulating hormone (FSH) has similar effects to LH.

Thyroid stimulating hormone deficiency

Thyroid stimulating hormone (TSH) is involved in stimulation of the thyroid gland. A lack of stimulation in the gland leads to **hypothyroidism**.

Adrenocorticotopic hormone deficiency

Also known as corticotropin, adrenocorticotopic hormone (ACTH) stimulates the adrenal gland to produce a hormone similar to cortisone, called cortisol. The loss of this hormone can lead to serious problems.

Growth hormone deficiency

Growth hormone (GH) regulates the body's growth. Patients who lose supply of this hormone before physical maturity will suffer impaired growth. Loss of the hormone can also affect adults.

Other hormone deficiencies

Prolactin stimulates the female breast to produce milk. A hormone produced by the posterior pituitary, antidiuretic hormone (ADH), controls the function of the kidneys. When this hormone is deficient, **diabetes insipidus** can result. However, patients with hypopituitarism rarely suffer ADH deficiency, unless the hypopituitarism is the result of hypothalamus disease.

Multiple hormone deficiencies

Deficiency of a single pituitary hormone occurs less commonly than deficiency of more than one hormone. Sometimes referred to as progressive pituitary hormone deficiency or partial hypopituitarism, there is usually a predictable order of hormone loss. Generally, growth hormone is lost first, then luteinizing hormone deficiency follows. The loss of follicle-stimulating hormone, thyroid stimulating hormone and adrenocorticotopic hormones follow much later. The progressive loss of pituitary hormone secretion is usually a slow process, which can occur over a period of months or years. Hypopituitarism does occasionally start suddenly with rapid onset of symptoms.

Panhypopituitarism

This condition represents the loss of all hormones released by the anterior pituitary gland. Panhypopituitarism is also known as complete pituitary failure.

Causes and symptoms

There are three major mechanisms which lead to the development of hypopituitarism. The first involves decreased release of hypothalamic hormones that stimulate pituitary function. The cause of decreased hypothalamic function may be congenital or acquired through interference such as tumors, inflammation, infection, mass lesions or interruption of blood supply. A second category of causes is any event or mass which interrupts the delivery of hormones from the hypothalamus. These may include particular tumors and aneurysms. Damage to the pituitary stalk from injury or surgery can also lead to hypopituitarism.

The third cause of hypopituitarism is damage to the pituitary gland cells. Destroyed cells can not produce the pituitary hormones that would normally be secreted by the gland. Cells may be destroyed by a number of tumors and diseases. Hypopituitarism is often caused by tumors, the most common of which is pituitary adenoma.

Symptoms of hypopituitarism vary with the affected hormones and severity of deficiency.

Frequently, patients have had years of symptoms that were nonspecific until a major illness or stress occurred. Overall symptoms may include **fatigue**, sensitivity to cold, weakness, decreased appetite, weight loss and abdominal **pain**. Low blood pressure, **headache** and visual disturbances are other associated symptoms.

Gonadotropin deficiency

Symptoms specific to this hormone deficiency include decreased interest in sex for women and **infertility** in women and men. Women may also have premature cessation of menstruation, hot flashes, vaginal dryness and pain during intercourse. Women who are postmenopausal will not have obvious symptoms such as these and may first present with headache or loss of vision. Men may also suffer sexual dysfunction as a result of gonadotropin deficiency. In acquired gonadotropin deficiency, both men and women may notice loss of body hair.

Thyroid stimulating hormone deficiency

Intolerance to cold, fatigue, weight gain, **constipation** and pale, waxy and dry skin indicate thyroid hormone deficiency.

Adrenocorticotopic hormone deficiency

Symptoms of ACTH deficiency include fatigue, weakness, weight loss and low blood pressure. **Nausea**, pale skin and loss of pubic and armpit hair in women may also indicate deficiency of ACTH.

Growth hormone deficiency

In children, growth hormone deficiency will result in short stature and growth retardation. Symptoms such as **obesity** and skin wrinkling may or may not show in adults and normal release of growth hormone normally declines with age.

Other hormone deficiencies

Prolactin deficiency is rare and is the result of partial or generalized anterior pituitary failure. When present, the symptom is absence of milk production in women. There are no known symptoms for men. ADH deficiency may produce symptoms of diabetes insipidus, such as excessive thirst and frequent urination.

Multiple hormone deficiencies

Patients with multiple hormone deficiencies will show symptoms of one or more specific hormone deficiencies or some of the generalized symptoms listed above.

Panhypopituitarism

The absence of any pituitary function should show symptoms of one or all of the specific hormone deficiencies. In addition to those symptoms, patients may have dry, pale skin that is finely textured. The face may appear finely wrinkled and contain a disinterested expression.

Diagnosis

Once the diagnosis of a single hormone deficiency is made, it is strongly recommended that tests for other hormone deficiencies be conducted.

Gonadotropin deficiency

The detection of low levels of gonadotropin can be accomplished through simple blood tests which measure luteinizing hormone and follicle-stimulating hormone, simultaneously with gonadal steroid levels. The combination of results can indicate to a physician if the cause of decreased hormone levels or function belongs to hypopituitarism or some sort of primary gonadal failure. Diagnosis will vary among men and women.

Thyroid stimulating hormone deficiency

Laboratory tests measuring thyroid function can help determine a diagnosis of TSH deficiency. The commonly used tests are T4 and TSH measurement done simultaneously to determine the reserve, or pool, of thyroid-stimulating hormone.

Adrenocorticotopic hormone deficiency

An insulin tolerance test may be given to determine if cortisol levels rise when **hypoglycemia** is induced. If they do not rise, there is insufficient reserve of cortisol, indicating an ACTH deficiency. If the insulin tolerance test is not safe for a particular patient, a glucagon test offers similar results. A CRH (corticotropin-releasing hormone) test may also be given. It involves injection of CRH to measure, through regularly drawn blood samples, a resulting rise in ACTH and cortisol. Other tests which stimulate ACTH may be ordered.

Growth hormone deficiency

Growth hormone deficiency is measured through the use of insulin-like growth factor I tests, which measure growth factors that are dependent on growth hormones. Sleep and **exercise** studies may also be used to test for growth hormone deficiency, since these activities are known to stimulate growth hormone secretion. Several drugs also induce secretion of growth hormone and may be given to measure hormone response. The standard test for growth hormone deficiency is the insulin-induced hypoglycemia test. This test does carry some risk from the induced hypoglycemia. Other tests include an arginine infusion test, clonidine test and growth-hormone releasing hormone test.

Other hormone deficiencies

If a test calculates normal levels of prolactin, deficiency of the hormone is eliminated as a diagnosis. A TRH (thyrotropin-releasing hormone) simulation test can determine prolactin levels. A number of tests are available to detect ADH levels and to determine diagnosis of diabetes insipidus.

Multiple and general hypopituitarism tests

Physicians should be aware that nonspecific symptoms can indicate deficiency of one or more hormones and should conduct a thorough clinical history. In general, diagnosis of hypopituitarism can be accomplished with a combination of dynamic tests and simple blood tests, as well as imaging exams. Most of these tests can be conducted in an outpatient lab or radiology facility. **Magnetic resonance imaging** (MRI) exams with gadolinium contrast enhancement are preferred imaging exams to study the region of the hypothalamus and pituitary gland. When MRI is not available, a properly conducted computed tomography scan (CT scan) exam can take its place. These exams can demonstrate a tumor or other mass, which may be interfering with pituitary function.

Panhypopituitarism

The insulin-induced hypoglycemia, or insulin tolerance test, which is used to determine specific hormone deficiencies, is an excellent test to diagnose panhypopituitarism. This test can reveal levels of growth hormone, ACTH (cortisol) and prolactin deficiency. The presence of insufficient levels of all of these hormones is a good indication of complete pituitary failure. Imaging studies and clinical history are also important.

Treatment

Treatment differs widely, depending on the age and sex of the patient, severity of the deficiency, the number of hormones involved, and even the underlying cause of the hypopituitarism. Immediate hormone replacement is generally administered to replace the specific deficient hormone. Patient education is encouraged to help patients manage the impact of their hormone deficiency on daily life. For instance, certain illnesses, accidents or surgical procedures may have adverse complications due to hypopituitarism.

Gonadotropin deficiency

Replacement of gonadal steroids is common treatment for LH and FSH deficiency. Estrogen for women and testosterone for men will be prescribed in the lowest effective dosage possible, since there can be complications to this therapy. To correct women's loss of libido, small doses of androgens may be prescribed. To restore fertility in men, regular hormone injections may be required. Male and female patients whose hypopituitarism results from hypothalamic disease may be successfully treated with a hypothalamic releasing hormone (GnRH), which can restore gonadal function and fertility.

Thyroid stimulating hormone deficiency

In patients who have hypothyroidism, the function of the adrenal glands will be tested and treated with steroids before administering thyroid hormone replacement.

Adrenocorticotopic hormone deficiency

Hydrocortisone or cortisone in divided doses may be given to replace this hormone deficiency. Most patients require 20 mg or less of hydrocortisone per day.

Growth hormone deficiency

It is essential to treat children suffering from growth hormone deficiency. The effectiveness of growth hormone therapy in adults, particularly elderly adults, is not as well documented. It is thought to help restore normal muscle to fat ratios. Growth hormone is an expensive and cautiously prescribed treatment.

Treatment of multiple deficiencies and panhypopituitarism

The treatment of hypopituitarism is usually very straightforward, but must normally continue for the remainder of the patient's life. Some patients may receive treatment with GnRH, the hypothalamic hormone. In most cases, treatment will be based on the specific deficiency demonstrated. Patients with hypopituitarism should be followed regularly to measure treatment effectiveness and to avoid overtreatment with

---

KEY TERMS

Adenoma—A benign (not threatening or cancerous) tumor that originates in a gland.

Androgen—A hormone that usually stimulates the sex hormones of the male.

Congenital—Present at birth.

Diabetes insipidus—A disorder originating in the pituitary gland which is characterized by excessive thirst and urination.

Endocrine—Refers to the system of internal secretion of substances into the body system from glands.

Hypoglycemia—Abnormal decrease of sugar in the blood.

Hypothyroidism—Deficient activity of the thyroid gland and resulting loss of energy.

---

hormone therapy. If the cause of the disorder is a tumor or lesion, radiation or surgical removal are treatment options. Successful removal may reverse the hypopituitarism. However, even after removal of the mass, hormone replacement therapy may still be necessary.

Prognosis

The prognosis for most patients with hypopituitarism is excellent. As long as therapy is continued, many experience normal life spans. However, hypopituitarism is usually a permanent condition and prognosis depends on the primary cause of the disorder. It can be potentially life threatening, particularly when acute hypopituitarism occurs as a result of a large pituitary tumor. Morbidity from the disease has increased, although the cause is not known. It is possible that increased morbidity and **death** are due to overtreatment with hormones. Any time that recovery of pituitary function can occur is preferred to lifelong hormone therapy.

Prevention

There is no known prevention of hypopituitarism, except for prevention of damage to the pituitary/hypothalamic area from injury.

Resources

ORGANIZATIONS

Alliance for Genetic Support Groups. 35 Wisconsin Circle, Suite 440. Chevy Chase, MD 20815-7015. < http://www.medhelp.org/geneticalliance >.

Human Growth Foundation. 997 Glen Cove Ave., Glen Head, NY 11545. (800) 451-6434. < http://www.hgfound.org >.

OTHER

HealthAnswers.com < http://www.healthanswers.com >.

Teresa Norris, RN

Hypoplastic anemia *see* **Aplastic anemia**

Hypospadias and epispadias

Definition

Hypospadias is a congenital defect, primarily of males, in which the urethra opens on the underside (ventrum) of the penis. It is one of the most common congenital abnormalities in the United States, occurring in about one of every 125 live male births. The corresponding defect in females is an opening of the urethra into the vagina and is rare.

Epispadias (also called bladder exstrophy) is a congenital defect of males in which the urethra opens on the upper surface (dorsum) of the penis. The corresponding defect in females is a fissure in the upper wall of the urethra and is quite rare.

Description

In a male, the external opening of the urinary tract (external meatus) is normally located at the tip of the penis. In a female, it is normally located between the clitoris and the vagina.

In males with hypospadias, the urethra opens on the inferior surface or underside of the penis. In females with hypospadias, the urethra opens into the cavity of the vagina.

In males with epispadias, the urethra opens on the superior surface or upper side of the penis. In females with epispadias, there is a crack or fissure in the wall of the urethra and out of the body through an opening in the skin above the clitoris.

During the embryological development of males, a groove of tissue folds inward and then fuses to form a tube that becomes the urethra. Hypospadias occurs when the tube does not form or does not fuse completely. Epispadias is due to a defect in the tissue that folds inward to form the urethra.

During the development of a female, similar processes occur to form the urethra. The problem usually

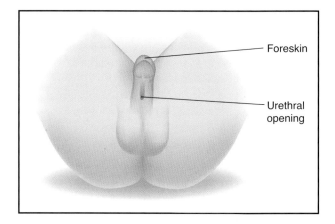

In hypospadias, the urethra opens along the penile shaft rather than at the penile tip. *(Illustration by Argosy Inc.)*

is insufficient length of the tube that becomes the urethra. As a result, the urethra opens in an abnormal location, resulting in a hypospadias. Occasionally, fissures form in the bladder. These may extend to the surface of the abdomen and fuse with the adjacent skin. This most often is identified as a defect in the bladder although it is technically an epispadias.

Hypospadias in males generally occur alone. Female hypospadias may be associated with abnormalities of the genital tract, since the urinary and genital tracts are formed in the same embryonic process.

Because it represents incomplete development of the penis, some experts think that insufficient male hormone may be responsible for hypospadias.

In males, the incidence of hypospadias is approximately one per 250 to 300 live births. Epispadias is much less common, having an incidence of about one per 100,000 live male births.

In females, hypospadias is much less common than in males. It appears about once in every 500,000 live female births. Epispadias is even rarer. Reliable estimates of the prevalence of epispadias in females are not available. Epispadias in females is often diagnosed and recorded as a bladder anomaly.

Causes and symptoms

Hypospadias and epispadias are congenital defects of the urinary tract. This means they occur during intrauterine development. There is no genetic basis for the defects. Specific causes for hypospadias are not known. This means that blood relatives do not have increased chances of developing them. Reports have shown some rise in prevalence of hypospadias among offspring of mothers who work in certain occupations where they may be exposed to chemicals that disrupt the endocrine system. However, a large trial ending in 2003 showed that aside from a slight increased risk among women who were hairdressers from 1992-1996, there is no evidence that maternal occupation or certain chemical exposure increases risk of hypospadias. The role of chemicals in the development of the defect remains uncertain.

Concern was once raised that use of the antihistamine loratadine (Claritin) early in **pregnancy** might cause hypospadias. However, a national clinical trial revealed in 2004 that there was no link between the drug and risk of second- or third-degree hypospadias.

Hypospadias usually is not associated with other defects of the penis or urethra. In males, it can occur at any site along the underside of the penis. In females, the urethra exits the body in an abnormal location. This usually is due to inadequate length of the urethra.

Epispadias is associated with bladder abnormalities. In females, the front wall of the bladder does not fuse or close. The bladder fissure may extend to the external abdominal wall. In such a rare case, the front of the pelvis also is widely separated. In males, the bladder fissure extends into the urethra and simply becomes an opening somewhere along the upper surface of the penis.

Hypospadias is associated with difficulty in assigning gender to babies. This occurs when gender is not obvious at birth because of deformities in the sex organs.

Diagnosis

Male external urinary tract defects are discovered at birth during the first detailed examination of the newborn. Female urethral defects may not be discovered for some time due to the difficulty in viewing the infant vagina.

Treatment

Surgery is the treatment of choice for both hypospadias and epispadias. All surgical repairs should be undertaken early and completed without delay. This minimizes psychological trauma.

In males with hypospadias, one surgery usually is sufficient to repair the defect. With more complicated hypospadias (more than one abnormally situated urethral opening), multiple surgeries may be required. In females with hypospadias, surgical repair technically is more complicated but can usually be completed in a brief interval of time.

Repairing an epispadias is more difficult. In males, this may involve other structures in the penis. Males should not be circumcised since the foreskin often is needed for the repair. Unfortunately, choices may be required that affect the ability to inseminate a female partner. Reproduction requires that the urethral meatus be close to the tip of the penis. Cosmetic appearance and ability to urinate (urinary continence) usually are the primary goals. Surgery for these defects is successful 70 to 80% of the time. Modern treatment of complete male epispadias allows for an excellent genital appearance and achievement of urinary continence.

In females, repair of epispadias may require multiple surgical procedures. Urinary continence and cosmetic appearance are the usual primary considerations. Urinary continence usually is achieved although cosmetic appearance may be somewhat compromised. Fertility is not usually affected. Repair rates that are similar or better than those for males usually can be achieved for females.

Hypospadias in both males and females is more of a nuisance and hindrance to reproduction than a threat to health. If surgery is not an option, the condition may be allowed to persist. This usually leads to an increased risk of infections in the lower urinary tract.

Prognosis

With adequate surgical repair, most males with simple hypospadias can lead normal lives with a penis that appears and functions in a normal manner. This includes fathering children. Females with simple hypospadias also have normal lives, including conceiving and bearing children.

The prognosis for epispadias depends on the extent of the defect. Most males with relatively minor epispadias lead normal lives, including fathering children. As the extent of the defect increases, surgical reconstruction generally is acceptable. However, many of these men are unable to conceive children. Most epispadias in females can be surgically repaired. The chances of residual disfigurement increase as the extent of the epispadias increases. Fertility in females is not generally affected by epispadias.

In hypospadias, the urethra opens along the penile shaft rather than at the penile tip.

Resources

BOOKS

Nelson, Waldo E., et al., editors. "Anomalies of the Bladder" In *Nelson Textbook of Pediatrics.* Philadelphia: W. B. Saunders, 2000, pp. 1639-1642.

Nelson, Waldo E., et al., editors. "Anomalies of the penis and urethra" In *Nelson Textbook of Pediatrics.* Philadelphia: W. B. Saunders, 2000, pp. 1645-1650.

PERIODICALS

Kubetin, Sally Koch. "Hypospadias, Loratidine Use in Pregnacy: No Link." *Pediatric News* July 2004.
"Molecular Epidemiology of Hypospadias: Genetic and Environmental Risk Factors." *Health & Medicine Week* December 15, 2003: 424.
Vrijheid, M., et al. "Risk of Hypospadias in Relation to Maternal Occupational Exposure to Potential Endocrine Disrupting Chemicals." *Occupational and Environmental Medicine* August 2003: 543–548.

ORGANIZATIONS

Association for the Bladder Exstrophy Community. PO Box 1472, Wake Forest, NC 27588-1472. (919) 624-9447. < http://www.bladderexstrophy.com/support.htm >.
Hypospadias Association of America. 4950 S. Yosemite Street, Box F2-156, Greenwood Village, CO 80111. hypospadiasassn@yahoo.com. < http:// www.hypospadias.net >.
Support for Parents with Hypospadias Boys. < http:// clubs.yahoo.com/clubs/mumswithhypospadiaskids >.
University of California - San Francisco. < http:// itsa.ucsf.edu/~uroweb/Uro/hypospadias/index.html >.

OTHER

Hatch, David A., MD. "Abnormal Development of the Penis and Male Urethra." *Genitourinary Development.* < http://www.meddean.luc.edu/lumen/MedEd/urology/abnpendv.htm >.
"Hypospadias." *Atlas of Congenital Deformities of the External Genitalia.* < http://www.atlasperovic.com/ contents/9.htm >.
"Hypospadias." Columbia Presbyterian Hospital. < http:// cpmcnet.cpmc.columbia.edu/dept/urology/pediatric/ hypospadias.html >.
"Hypospadias." University of Michigan. < http:// www.urology.med.umich.edu/clinic/pediatric/ hypospadias.html >.
Johns Hopkins University Pediatric Urology Center. "Epispadias." Johns Hopkins Exstrophy Database. < http://www.med.jhu.edu/pediurol/pediatric/ exstrophy/database/web4d.html >.
The Penis.com. < http://www.the-penis.com/ hypospadias.html >.
Society for Pediatric Urology. < http://www.spu.org/ >.

L. Fleming Fallon, Jr., MD, PhD, DrPH
Teresa G. Odle

Hypotension

Definition

Hypotension is the medical term for low blood pressure.

Description

The pressure of the blood in the arteries rises and falls as the heart and muscles handle demands of daily living, such as **exercise**, sleep and **stress**. Some healthy people have blood pressure well below the average for their age, even though they have a completely normal heart and blood vessels. This is often true of athletes who are in superior shape. The term "hypotension" is usually used only when blood pressure has fallen so far that enough blood can no longer reach the brain, causing **dizziness** and **fainting**.

Causes and symptoms

Postural hypotension is the most common type of low blood pressure. In this condition, symptoms appear after a person sits up or stands quickly. In normal people, the cardiovascular system must make a quick adjustment to raise blood pressure slightly to account for the change in position. For those with postural hypotension, the blood pressure adjustment is not adequate or it doesn't happen. Postural hypotension may occur if someone is taking certain drugs or medicine for high blood pressure. It also happens to diabetics when nerve damage has disrupted the reflexes that control blood pressure.

Many people have a chronic problem with low blood pressure that is not particularly serious. This may include people who require certain medications, who are pregnant, have bad veins, or have arteriosclerosis (hardening of the arteries).

The most serious problem with low blood pressure occurs when there is a sudden drop, which can be life-threatening due to widespread ischemia (insufficient supply of blood to an organ due to blockage in an artery). This type of low blood pressure may be due to a wide variety of causes, including:

- trauma with extensive blood loss
- serious burns
- shock from various causes (e.g. anaphylaxis)
- heart attack
- adrenal failure (Addisonian crisis)
- cancer
- severe fever
- serious infection (septicemia)

Diagnosis

Blood pressure is a measure of the pressure in the arteries created by the heart contracting. During the day, a normal person's blood pressure changes constantly, depending on activity. Low blood pressure can be diagnosed by taking the blood pressure with a sphygmomanometer. This is a device with a soft rubber cuff that is inflated around the upper arm until it's tight enough to stop blood flow. The cuff is then slowly deflated until the health care worker, listening to the artery in the arm with a stethoscope, can hear the blood first as a beat forcing its way along the artery. This is the systolic pressure. The cuff is then deflated more until the beat disappears and the blood flows steadily through the open artery; this gives the diastolic pressure.

Blood pressure is recorded as systolic (higher) and diastolic (lower) pressures. A healthy young adult has a blood pressure of about 110/75, which typically rises with age to about 140/90 by age 60 (a reading now considered mildly elevated).

Treatment

Treatment of low blood pressure depends on the underlying cause, which can usually be resolved. For

KEY TERMS

Arteriosclerosis—A group of disorders that causes thickening and loss of elasticity in artery walls.

those people with postural hypotension, a medication adjustment may help prevent the problem. These individuals may find that rising more slowly, or getting out of bed in slow stages, helps the problem. Low blood pressure with no other symptoms does not need to be treated.

Prognosis

Low blood pressure as a result of injury or other underlying condition can usually be successfully treated if the trauma is not too extensive or is treated in time. Less serious forms of chronic low blood pressure have a good prognosis and do not require treatment.

Resources

BOOKS

Smeltzer, Suzanne C., and Brenda G. Bare. *Brunner and Suddarth's Textbook of Medical and Surgical Nursing.* 8th ed. Philadelphia:Lippincott-Raven Publishers, 1996.

Carol A. Turkington

Hypothermia

Definition

Hypothermia, a potentially fatal condition, occurs when body temperature falls below 95 °F (35 °C).

Description

Although hypothermia is an obvious danger for people living in cold climates, many cases have occurred when the air temperature is well above the freezing mark. Elderly people, for instance, have succumbed to hypothermia after prolonged exposure to indoor air temperatures of 50–65 °F (10–18.3 °C). In the United States, hypothermia is primarily an urban phenomenon associated with **alcoholism**, drug **addiction**, mental illness, and cold—water immersion accidents. The victims are often homeless male alcoholics. Officially, 11,817 deaths were attributed to hypothermia in the United States from 1979 to 1994, but experts suspect that many fatal cases go unrecognized. Nearly half the victims were 65 or older, with males dominating every age group. Nonwhites were also overrepresented in the statistics. Among males 65 and older, nonwhites outnumbered whites by more than four to one.

Causes and symptoms

Measured orally, a healthy person's body temperature can fluctuate between 97 °F (36.1 °C) and 100 °F (37.8 °C). Survival depends on maintaining temperature stability within this range by balancing the heat produced by metabolism with the heat lost to the environment through (for the most part) the skin and lungs. When environmental or other changes cause heat loss to outpace heat production, the brain triggers physiological and behavioral responses to restore the balance. The involuntary muscular activity of shivering, for example, aids heat production by accelerating metabolism. But if the cold **stress** is too great and the body's defenses are overwhelmed, body temperature begins to fall. Hypothermia is considered to begin once body temperature reaches 95 °F (35 °C), though even smaller drops in temperature can have an adverse effect.

Hypothermia is divided into two types: primary and secondary. Primary hypothermia occurs when the body's heat-balancing mechanisms are working properly but are subjected to extreme cold, whereas secondary hypothermia affects people whose heat-balancing mechanisms are impaired in some way and cannot respond adequately to moderate or perhaps even mild cold. Primary hypothermia typically involves exposure to cold air or immersion in cold water. The cold air variety usually takes at least several hours to develop, but immersion hypothermia will occur within about an hour of entering the water, since water draws heat away from the body much faster than air does. In secondary hypothermia, the body's heat-balancing mechanisms can fail for any number of reasons, including strokes, diabetes, **malnutrition**, bacterial infection, thyroid disease, spinal cord injuries (which prevent the brain from receiving crucial temperature-related information from other parts of the body), and the use of medications and other substances that affect the brain or spinal cord. Alcohol is one such substance. In smaller amounts it can put people at risk by interfering with their ability to recognize and avoid cold-weather dangers. In larger amounts it shuts down the body's heat-balancing mechanisms.

Secondary hypothermia is often a threat to the elderly, who may be on medications or suffering from illnesses that affect their ability to conserve heat. Malnutrition and immobility can also put the elderly at risk. Some medical research suggests as well that shivering and blood vessel narrowing—two of the body's defenses against cold—may not be triggered as quickly in older people. For these and other reasons, the elderly can, over a period of days or even weeks, fall victim to hypothermia in poorly insulated homes or other surroundings that family, friends, and caregivers may not recognize as life threatening. Another risk for the elderly is the fact that hypothermia can easily be misdiagnosed as a **stroke** or some other common illness of old age.

The signs and symptoms of hypothermia follow a typical course, though the body temperatures at which they occur vary from person to person depending on age, health, and other factors. The impact of hypothermia on the nervous system often becomes apparent quite early. Coordination, for instance, may begin to suffer as soon as body temperature reaches 95 °F (35 °C). The early signs of hypothermia also include cold and pale skin and intense shivering; the latter stops between 90 °F (32.2 °C) and 86 °F (30 °C). As body temperature continues to fall, speech becomes slurred, the muscles go rigid, and the victim becomes disoriented and experiences eyesight problems. Other harmful consequences include **dehydration** as well as liver and kidney failure. Heart rate, respiratory rate, and blood pressure rise during the first stages of hypothermia, but fall once the 90 °F (32.2 °C) mark is passed. Below 86 °F (30 °C) most victims are comatose, and below 82 °F (27.8 °C) the heart's rhythm becomes dangerously disordered. Yet even at very low body temperatures, people can survive for several hours and be successfully revived, though they may appear to be dead.

Diagnosis

Information on the patient's prior health and activities often helps doctors establish a correct diagnosis and treatment plan. Pulse, blood pressure, temperature, and respiration require immediate monitoring. Because the temperature of the mouth is not an accurate guide to the body's core temperature, readings are taken at one or two other sites, usually the ear, rectum, or esophagus. Other diagnostic tools include **electrocardiography**, which is used to evaluate heart rhythm, and blood and urine tests, which provide several kinds of key information; a **chest x ray** is also required. A computed tomography scan (CT scan) or **magnetic resonance imaging** (MRI) may be needed to check for head and other injuries.

Treatment

Emergency medical help should be summoned whenever a person appears hypothermic. The danger signs include intense shivering; stiffness and **numbness** in the arms and legs; stumbling and clumsiness; sleepiness, confusion, disorientation, **amnesia**, and irrational behavior; and difficulty speaking. Until emergency help arrives, a victim of outdoor hypothermia should be brought to shelter and warmed by removing wet clothing and footwear, drying the skin, and wrapping him or her in warm blankets or a sleeping bag. Gentle handling is necessary when moving the victim to avoid disturbing the heart. Rubbing the skin or giving the victim alcohol can be harmful, though warm drinks such as clear soup and tea are recommended for those who can swallow. Anyone who aids a victim of hypothermia should also look for signs of **frostbite** and be aware that attempting to rewarm a frostbitten area of the body before emergency help arrives can be extremely dangerous. For this reason, frostbitten areas must be kept away from heat sources such as campfires and car heaters.

Rewarming is the essence of hospital treatment for hypothermia. How rewarming proceeds depends on the body temperature. Different approaches are used for patients who are mildly hypothermic (the patient's body temperature is 90–95 °F [32.2–35 °C]), moderately hypothermic (86–90 °F [30–32.2 °C]), or severely hypothermic (less than 86 °F [30 °C]). Other considerations, such as the patient's age or the condition of the heart, can also influence treatment choices.

Mild hypothermia is reversed with passive rewarming. This technique relies on the patient's own metabolism to rewarm the body. Once wet clothing is removed and the skin is dried, the patient is covered with blankets and placed in a warm room. The goal is to raise the patient's temperature by 0.5–2 °C an hour.

Moderate hypothermia is often treated first with active external rewarming and then with passive rewarming. Active external rewarming involves applying heat to the skin, for instance by placing the patient in a warm bath or wrapping the patient in electric heating blankets.

Severe hypothermia requires active internal rewarming, which is recommended for some cases of moderate hypothermia as well. There are several types of active internal rewarming. Cardiopulmonary bypass, in which the patient's blood is circulated through a rewarming device and then returned to the body, is considered the best, and can raise body temperature by 1–2 °C every 3–5 minutes. However, many hospitals are not equipped to offer this treatment. The alternative is to introduce warm oxygen or fluids into the body.

KEY TERMS

Antibiotics—Substances used against microorganisms that cause infection.

Computed tomography—A process that uses x rays to create three-dimensional images of structures inside the body.

Esophagus—A muscular tube through which food and liquids pass on their way to the stomach.

Insulin—A substance that regulates blood glucose levels. Glucose is a sugar.

Magnetic resonance imaging—The use of electromagnetic energy to create images of structures inside the body.

Metabolism—The chemical changes by which the body breaks down food and other substances and builds new substances necessary for life.

Nervous system—The system that transmits information, in the form of electrochemical impulses, throughout the body. It comprises the brain, spinal cord, and nerves.

Rectum—The lower section of the large intestine. The intestines are part of the digestive system.

Stroke—A condition involving loss of blood flow to the brain.

Thyroid—A gland (fluid-secreting structure) in the neck. It plays an important role in metabolism.

Hypothermia treatment can also include, among other things, insulin, **antibiotics**, and fluid replacement therapy. When the heart has stopped, both **cardiopulmonary resuscitation (CPR)** and rewarming are necessary. Once a patient's condition has stabilized, he or she may need treatment for an underlying problem such as alcoholism or thyroid disease.

Prognosis

Victims of mild or moderate hypothermia usually enjoy a complete recovery. In regard to severely hypothermic patients, the prognosis for survival varies due to differences in people's physiological responses to cold.

Prevention

People who spend time outdoors in cold weather can reduce heat loss by wearing their clothing loosely and in layers and by keeping their hands, feet, and head well covered (30–50% of body heat is lost through the head). Because water draws heat away from the body so easily, staying dry is important, and wet clothing and footwear should be replaced as quickly as possible. Wind- and water-resistant outer garments are also crucial. Alcohol should be avoided because it promotes heat loss by expanding the blood vessels that carry body heat to the skin.

Preventing hypothermia among the elderly requires vigilance on the part of family, friends, and caregivers. An elderly person's home should be properly insulated and heated, with living areas kept at a temperature of 70 °F (21.1 °C). Warm clothing and bedding are essential, as are adequate food, rest, and **exercise**; warming the bed and bedroom before going to sleep is also recommended. Older people who live alone should be visited regularly—at least once a day during very cold weather—to ensure that their health remains sound and that they are taking good care of themselves. For help and advice, family members and others can turn to government and social service agencies. Meals on wheels and visiting nurse programs, for instance, may be available, and it may be possible to obtain financial aid for winterizing and heating homes.

Resources

BOOKS

Petty, Kevin J. "Hypothermia." In *Harrison's Principles of Internal Medicine*, edited by Anthony S. Fauci, et al. New York: McGraw-Hill, 1997.

Howard Baker

Hypothyroidism

Definition

Hypothyroidism, or underactive thyroid, develops when the thyroid gland fails to produce or secrete as much thyroxine (T_4) as the body needs. Because T_4 regulates such essential functions as heart rate, digestion, physical growth, and mental development, an insufficient supply of this hormone can slow life-sustaining processes, damage organs and tissues in every part of the body, and lead to life-threatening complications.

Description

Hypothyroidism is one of the most common chronic diseases in the United States. Symptoms may not appear until years after the thyroid has stopped functioning and they are often mistaken for signs of other illnesses, **menopause**, or **aging**. Although this condition is believed to affect as many as 11 million adults and children, as many as two of every three people with hypothyroidism may not know they have the disease.

Nicknamed "Gland Central" because it influences almost every organ, tissue, and cell in the body, the thyroid is shaped like a butterfly and located just below the Adam's apple. The thyroid stores iodine the body gets from food and uses this mineral to create T_4. Low T_4 levels can alter weight, appetite, sleep patterns, body temperature, sex drive, and a variety of other physical, mental, and emotional characteristics.

There are three types of hypothyroidism. The most common is primary hypothyroidism, in which the thyroid doesn't produce an adequate amount of T_4. Secondary hypothyroidism develops when the pituitary gland does not release enough of the thyroid-stimulating hormone (TSH) that prompts the thyroid to manufacture T_4. Tertiary hypothyroidism results from a malfunction of the hypothalamus, the part of the brain that controls the endocrine system. Drug-induced hypothyroidism, an adverse reaction to medication, occurs in two of every 10,000 people, but rarely causes severe hypothyroidism.

Hypothyroidism is at least twice as common in women as it is in men. Although hypothyroidism is most common in women who are middle-aged or older, the disease can occur at any age. Newborn infants are tested for congenital thyroid deficiency (cretinism) using a test that measures the levels of thyroxine in the infant's blood. Treatment within the first few months of life can prevent **mental retardation** and physical abnormalities. Older children who develop hypothyroidism suddenly stop growing.

Factors that increase a person's risk of developing hypothyroidism include age, weight, and medical history. Women are more likely to develop the disease after age 50; men, after age 60. Obesity also increases risk. A family history of thyroid problems or a personal history of **high cholesterol** levels or such autoimmune diseases as lupus, **rheumatoid arthritis**, or diabetes can make an individual more susceptible to hypothyroidism.

Causes and symptoms

Hypothyroidism is most often the result of Hashimoto's disease, also known as chronic thyroiditis (inflammation of the thyroid gland). In this disease, the immune system fails to recognize that the thyroid gland is part of the body's own tissue and attacks it as if it were a foreign body. The attack by the immune system impairs thyroid function and sometimes destroys the gland. Other causes of hypothyroidism include:

- Radiation. Radioactive iodine used to treat hyperthyroidism (overactive thyroid) or radiation treatments for head or neck cancers can destroy the thyroid gland.

- Surgery. Removal of the thyroid gland because of **cancer** or other thyroid disorders can result in hypothyroidism.

- Viruses and bacteria. Infections that depress thyroid hormone production usually cause permanent hypothyroidism.

- Medication. Nitroprusside, lithium, or iodides can induce hypothyroidism. Because patients who use these medications are closely monitored by their doctors, this side effect is very rare.

- Pituitary gland malfunction. This is a rare condition in which the pituitary gland fails to produce enough TSH to activate the thyroid's production of T_4.

- Congenital defect. One of every 4,000 babies is born without a properly functioning thyroid gland.

- Diet. Because the thyroid makes T_4 from iodine drawn from food, an iodine-deficient diet can cause hypothyroidism. Adding iodine to table salt and other common foods has eliminated iodine deficiency in the United States. Certain foods (cabbage, rutabagas, peanuts, peaches, soybeans, spinach) can interfere with thyroid hormone production.

- Environmental contaminants. Certain man-made chemicals—such as PCBs—found in the local environment at high levels may also cause hypothyroidism.

Hypothyroidism is sometimes referred to as a "silent" disease because early symptoms may be so mild that no one realizes anything is wrong. Untreated symptoms become more noticeable and severe, and can lead to confusion and mental disorders, breathing difficulties, heart problems, fluctuations in body temperature, and **death**.

Someone who has hypothyroidism will probably have more than one of the following symptoms:

- fatigue
- decreased heart rate
- progressive **hearing loss**
- weight gain
- problems with memory and concentration
- depression
- goiter (enlarged thyroid gland)
- muscle **pain** or weakness
- loss of interest in sex
- numb, **tingling** hands
- dry skin
- swollen eyelids
- dryness, loss, or premature graying of hair
- extreme sensitivity to cold
- **constipation**
- irregular menstrual periods
- hoarse voice

Hypothyroidism usually develops gradually. When the disease results from surgery or other treatment for **hyperthyroidism**, symptoms may appear suddenly and include severe muscle cramps in the arms, legs, neck, shoulders, and back.

It's important to see a doctor if any of these symptoms appear unexpectedly. People whose hypothyroidism remains undiagnosed and untreated may eventually develop myxedema. Symptoms of this rare but potentially deadly complication include enlarged tongue, swollen facial features, hoarseness, and physical and mental sluggishness.

Myxedema **coma** can cause unresponsiveness; irregular, shallow breathing; and a drop in blood pressure and body temperature. The onset of this medical emergency can be sudden in people who are elderly or have been ill, injured, or exposed to very cold temperatures; who have recently had surgery; or who use sedatives or anti-depressants. Without immediate medical attention, myxedema coma can be fatal.

Diagnosis

Diagnosis of hypothyroidism is based on the patient's observations, medical history, physical examination, and thyroid function tests. Doctors who specialize in treating thyroid disorders (endocrinologists) are most apt to recognize subtle symptoms and physical indications of hypothyroidism. A blood test known as a thyroid-stimulating hormone (TSH) assay, thyroid nuclear medicine scan, and **thyroid ultrasound** are used to confirm the diagnosis. A woman being tested for hypothyroidism should let her doctor know if she is pregnant or breastfeeding and all patients should be sure their doctors are aware of any recent procedures involving radioactive materials or contrast media.

The TSH assay is extremely accurate, but some doctors doubt the test's ability to detect mild hypothyroidism. They advise patients to monitor their basal (resting) body temperature for below-normal readings that could indicate the presence of hypothyroidism.

Treatment

Natural or synthetic **thyroid hormones** are used to restore normal (euthyroid) thyroid hormone levels. Synthetic hormones are more effective than natural substances, but it may take several months to determine the correct dosage. Patients start to feel better within 48 hours, but symptoms will return if they stop taking the medication.

Most doctors prescribe levothyroxine sodium tablets, and most people with hypothyroidism will take the medication for the rest of their lives. Aging, other medications, and changes in weight and general health can affect how much replacement hormone a patient needs, and regular TSH tests are used to monitor hormone levels. Patients should not switch from one brand of thyroid hormone to another without a doctor's permission.

Regular **exercise** and a high-fiber diet can help maintain thyroid function and prevent constipation.

Alternative treatment

Alternative treatments are primarily aimed at strengthening the thyroid and will not eliminate the need for thyroid hormone medications. Herbal remedies to improve thyroid function and relieve symptoms of hypothyroidism include bladder wrack (*Fucus vesiculosus*), which can be taken in capsule form or as a tea. Some foods, including cabbage, peaches, radishes, soybeans, peanuts, and spinach, can interfere with the production of thyroid hormones. Anyone with hypothyroidism may want to avoid these foods. The Shoulder Stand **yoga** position (at least once daily for 20 minutes) is believed to improve thyroid function.

Prognosis

Thyroid **hormone replacement therapy** generally maintains normal thyroid hormone levels unless treatment is interrupted or discontinued.

KEY TERMS

Cretinism—Severe hypothyroidism that is present at birth.

Endocrine system—The network of glands that produce hormones and release them into the bloodstream. The thyroid gland is part of the endocrine system.

Hypothalamus—The part of the brain that controls the endocrine system.

Myxedema—A condition that can result from a thyroid gland that produces too little of its hormone. In addition to a decreased metabolic rate, symptoms may include anemia, slow speech, an enlarged tongue, puffiness of the face and hands, loss of hair, coarse and thickened skin, and sensitivity to cold.

Pituitary gland—Small, oval endocrine gland attached to the hypothalamus. The pituitary gland releases TSH, the hormone that activates the thyroid gland.

Thyroid-stimulating hormone (TSH)—A hormone secreted by the pituitary gland that controls the release of T_4 by the thyroid gland.

Thyroxine (T_4)—Thyroid hormone that regulates many essential body processes.

Prevention

Primary hypothyroidism can't be prevented, but routine screening of adults could detect the disease in its early stages and prevent complications.

Resources

ORGANIZATIONS

American Thyroid Association. Montefiore Medical Center, 111 E. 210th St., Bronx, NY 10467.

Endocrine Society. 4350 East West Highway, Suite 500, Bethesda, MD 20814-4410. (301) 941-0200.

Thyroid Foundation of America, Inc. Ruth Sleeper Hall, RSL 350, Boston, MA 02114-2968. (800) 832-8321 or (617) 726-8500.

Thyroid Society for Education and Research. 7515 S. Main St., Suite 545, Houston, TX 77030. (800) THYROID or (713) 799-9909.

Maureen Haggerty

Hypotonic duodenography

Definition

Hypotonic duodenography is an x-ray procedure that produces images of the duodenum. The duodenum is the first part of the small intestine.

Purpose

Hypotonic duodenography may be ordered to detect tumors of the head of the pancreas or the area where the pancreatic and bile ducts meet the small intestine. Lesions causing upper abdominal **pain** may be demonstrated by duodenography, and the procedure can aid in the diagnosis of chronic **pancreatitis**.

Precautions

Some patients with narrowing of the tubes in the upper gastrointestinal tract should not receive duodenography. Patients with certain heart disorders and **glaucoma** are cautioned against receiving an agent called anticholinergic, which is administered during the procedure to lessen intestinal **muscle spasms**. A hormone called glucagon may also be used to relax the intestines, but its use is not recommended in patients with most forms of diabetes.

Description

Hypotonic duodenography is also referred to as x ray of the duodenum or simply as duodenography. The patient is seated while the radiologist places a catheter in the nose and down into the stomach. Then the patient lies down and the tube is continued to the duodenum. The radiologist is guided in this placement by a fluoroscopic image. (Fluoroscopic equipment shows an immediate x ray. In this case, the x ray shows the location of the catheter as it is moved into the stomach and duodenum.) Next, either the glucagon is administered intravenously or anticholinergic is injected into the patient to relax the muscles of the intestine.

After several minutes, the physician will administer barium through the catheter. Barium is a contrast agent that will help highlight the area on the fluoroscopy screen and x rays. After a few films are taken, some of the barium is withdrawn and air is sent in through the catheter. Additional images are acquired and the catheter is then removed. The procedure takes from 30–60 minutes.

Preparation

Patients are required to fast from midnight before the test until after the test, or about 6–12 hours. Just prior to the exam, patients should remove dentures, glasses, and other objects that may interfere with the procedure. The patient may be instructed to empty his or her bladder just prior to duodenography.

Aftercare

The barium should be expelled within two to three days. Extra fluids and/or an agent given by the physician to help encourage bowel movement may aid in barium elimination. Physicians and patients should watch for possible reactions to the anticholinergic or glucagon. If an anticholinergic is used, patients are advised to empty their bladder within a few hours after the exam and to wait two hours for clearing of vision or have someone drive them home. Patients will notice that their stools are chalky white from the barium for one to three days following the procedure.

Risks

Abdominal cramping may occur when the physician instills air into the duodenum, but aside from the discomfort, there are few risks associated with this procedure. Side effects from the contrast, hormones or agents may occur. Those patients with diabetes, heart disease, or glaucoma run the highest risk of reaction and should not receive anticholinergic or glucagon, depending on their specific conditions. Elderly patients or those who are extremely ill, must be closely monitored during the procedure for possible return of fluid, or gastric reflux.

Normal results

The linings of the duodenum and surrounding tissues will look smooth and even. The shape of the head of the pancreas will appear normal and near the duodenal wall.

Abnormal results

Any masses or irregular nodules on the wall of the duodenum may indicate tumors or abnormality of tissue. Tumors of the head of the pancreas or of the opening into the intestine from the pancreatic and bile ducts may be seen. Chronic pancreatitis may be indicated on the x rays. In many instances, follow-up laboratory or imaging studies may be ordered to further study the abnormal findings and confirm a diagnosis.

KEY TERMS

Anticholinergic—A drug that lessens muscle spasms in the intestines, lungs, bladder, and eye muscles.

Fluoroscopic (fluoroscopy)—An x-ray procedure that produces immediate images and motion on a screen. The images look like those seen at airport baggage security stations.

Glucagon—A hormone that changes glycogen, a carbohydrate stored in muscles and the liver, into glucose. It can be used to relax muscles for a procedure such as duodenography.

Pancreas—A five-inch-long gland that lies behind the stomach and next to the duodenum. The pancreas releases glucagon, insulin and some of the enzymes which aid digestion. Pancreatitis is the swelling of the pancreas which can nausea, jaundice, and severe pain and may be fatal.

Resources

ORGANIZATIONS

American College of Radiology. 1891 Preston White Drive, Reston, VA 22091. (800) 227-5463. < http:// www.acr.org >.

National Cancer Institute. Building 31, Room 10A31, 31 Center Drive, MSC 2580, Bethesda, MD 20892-2580. (800) 422-6237. < http://www.nci.nih.gov >.

Teresa Odle

Hypovolemic shock *see* **Shock**

Hysterectomy

Definition

Hysterectomy is the surgical removal of the uterus. In a total hysterectomy, the uterus and cervix are removed. In some cases, the fallopian tubes and ovaries are removed along with the uterus (called hysterectomy with bilateral salpingo-oophorectomy). In a subtotal hysterectomy, only the uterus is removed. In a radical hysterectomy, the uterus, cervix, ovaries, oviducts, lymph nodes, and lymph channels are removed. The type of hysterectomy performed depends on the reason for the procedure. In all cases,

menstruation stops and a woman loses the ability to bear children.

Purpose

Hysterectomy is the second most common operation performed in the United States. About 556,000 of these surgeries are done annually. By age 60, approximately one out of every three American women will have had a hysterectomy. Yet it's estimated that 30 percent of hysterectomies are unnecessary.

About 10% of hysterectomies are performed to treat cancer of the cervix, ovaries, or uterus. Women with **cancer** in one or more of these organs almost always have the organ(s) removed as one part of their cancer treatment.

The most frequent reason for hysterectomy in the United States is to remove fibroid tumors, accounting for 30% of these surgeries. Fibroid tumors are noncancerous (benign) growths in the uterus, which can cause pelvic and **low back pain** and heavy or lengthy menstrual periods. They occur in 30–40% of women over age 40, and are three times more likely to be present in African-American women than in Caucasian women. Fibroids do not need to be removed unless they are causing symptoms that interfere with a woman's normal activities.

Treatment of **endometriosis** is the reason for 20% of hysterectomies. The endometrium is the lining of the uterus. Endometriosis is a condition that occurs when the cells from the endometrium begin growing outside the uterus. The outlying endometrial cells respond to the hormones that control the menstrual cycle, bleeding each month the way the lining of the uterus does. This causes irritation of the surrounding tissue, leading to pain and scarring.

Another 20% percent of hysterectomies are done because of heavy or abnormal vaginal bleeding that can not be linked to any specific cause and cannot be controlled by other means. The remaining 20% of hysterectomies are performed to treat prolapsed uterus, **pelvic inflammatory disease**, and endometrial hyperplasia, a potentially precancerous condition.

Alternatives

There are several alternatives to hysterectomy today. They include:

Embolization

Uterine artery embolization is not a surgical procedure. Instead, interventional radiologists put a catherter into the artery that leads to the uterus and inject polyvinyl alcohol particles right where the artery leads to the blood vessels that nourish the fibroids. By killing off those blood vessels, the fibroids have no more blood supply, and they die off. Severe cramping and **pain** after the procedure is common, but serious complications are less than 5 percent and it may protect fertility.

Myomectomy

A **myomectomy** is a surgery used to remove fibroids, thus avoiding a hysterectomy. Hysteroscopic myomectomy, in which a surgical "telescope," or laparascope, is inserted into the uterus through the vagina can be done on an outpatient basis. If there are large fibroids, however, an abdominal incision is required. Then women typically are hospitalized for two to three days, and require up to six weeks recovery. However, laparascopic myomectomies are also being done more often. They only require three small incisions in the abdomen, and have a much shorter hospitalization and recovery time.

Once the fibroids have been removed, the surgeon must repair the wall of the uterus to eliminate future bleeding or infection.

Endometrial ablation

In this surgical procedure, recommended for women with small fibroids, the entire lining of the uterus is removed. Women are no longer fertile, however. The uterine cavity is filled with fluid and a **hysteroscopy**, or telescope, inserted to provide a clear view of the uterus. Then the uterus is destroyed using a laser beam or electric voltage. The procedure is typically done under anesthesia, although women can go home the same day as the surgery. Another, newer procedure involves using a balloon, which is filled with superheated liquid and inflated until it fills the uterus. The liquid kills the lining, and after 8 minutes the balloon is removed.

Endometrial resection

Like endometrial ablation, the uterine lining is also destroyed during this procedure, only instead of a laser, an electrosurgical wire loop is used.

Total hysterectomy

A total hysterectomy, sometimes called a simple hysterectomy, removes the entire uterus and the cervix. The ovaries are not removed and continue to secrete hormones. Total hysterectomies are always performed in the case of uterine and cervical cancer. This is the most common kind of hysterectomy.

Sometimes, in addition to a total hysterectomy a procedure called a bilateral salpingo-oophorectomy is performed. This surgery removes the ovaries and the fallopian tubes. Removal of the ovaries eliminates the main source of the hormone estrogen, so **menopause** occurs immediately. Removal of the ovaries and fallopian tubes is performed in about one-third of hysterectomy operations, often to reduce the risk of **ovarian cancer**.

Subtotal hysterectomy

If the reason for the hysterectomy is to remove uterine fibroids, treat abnormal bleeding, or relieve pelvic pain, it may be possible to remove only the uterus and leave the cervix. This procedure, called a subtotal hysterectomy (or partial hysterectomy), removes the least amount of tissue. The opening to the cervix is left in place. Some women feel that leaving the cervix intact aids in their achieving sexual satisfaction. This procedure, which used to be rare, is now performed more frequently when requested.

Subtotal hysterectomy is easier to perform than a total hysterectomy, but leaves a woman at risk for **cervical cancer**. She will still need to get yearly pap smears.

Radical hysterectomy

Radical hysterectomies are performed on women with cervical cancer or **endometrial cancer** that has spread to the cervix. A radical hysterectomy removes the uterus, cervix, top part of the vagina, ovaries, fallopian tubes, lymph nodes, lymph channels, and tissue in the pelvic cavity that surrounds the cervix. This type of hysterectomy removes the most tissue and requires the longest hospital stay and longer recovery period.

Precautions

The frequency with which hysterectomies are performed in the United States has been questioned in recent years. It has been suggested that a large number of hysterectomies are performed unnecessarily. The United States has the highest rate of hysterectomies (number of hysterectomies per thousand women) of any country in the world. Also, the frequency of this surgery varies across different regions of the United States. Rates are highest in the South and Midwest, and are higher for African American women. In recent years, although the number of hysterectomies

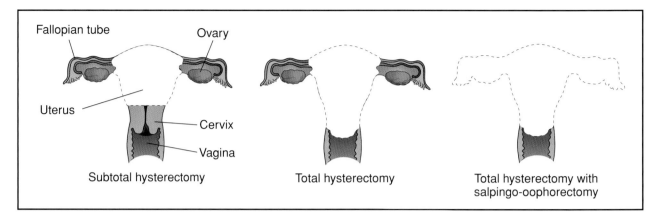

Three types of hysterectomies: subtotal, total, and total with salpingo-oophorectomy. *(Illustration by Electronic Illustrators Group.)*

performed has declined, the number of hysterectomies performed on younger women in their 30s and 40s is increasing, and 55 percent of all hysterectomies are performed on women 35 to 49.

Women for whom a hysterectomy is recommended should discuss possible alternatives with their doctor and consider getting a second opinion, since this is major surgery with life-changing implications. Alternative treatments exist for many conditions. Whether these alternatives are appropriate for any individual woman is a decision she and her doctor should make together.

As in all major surgery, the health of the patient affects the risk of the operation. Women who have chronic heart or lung diseases, diabetes, or iron-deficiency anemia may not be good candidates for this operation. Heavy **smoking, obesity**, use of steroid drugs, and use of illicit drugs add to the surgical risk.

Description

There are two ways that hysterectomies can be performed. The choice of method depends on the type of hysterectomy, the doctor's experience, and the reason for the hysterectomy.

Abdominal hysterectomy

About 75% of hysterectomies performed in the United States are abdominal hysterectomies. The surgeon makes a four to six inch incision either horizontally across the pubic hair line from hip bone to hip bone or vertically from navel to pubic bone. Horizontal incisions leave a less noticeable scar, but vertical incisions give the surgeon a better view of the abdominal cavity. The blood vessels, fallopian tubes, and ligaments are cut away from the uterus, which is lifted out.

Abdominal hysterectomies take from one to three hours. The hospital stay is three to five days, and it takes four to eight weeks to return to normal activities.

The advantages of an abdominal hysterectomy are that the uterus can be removed even if a woman has internal scarring (**adhesions**) from previous surgery or her fibroids are large. The surgeon has a good view of the abdominal cavity and more room to work. Also, surgeons have the most experience with this type of hysterectomy. The abdominal incision is more painful than with vaginal hysterectomy and the recovery period is longer.

Vaginal hysterectomy

With a vaginal hysterectomy, the surgeon makes an incision near the top of the vagina. The surgeon then reaches through this incision to cut and tie off the ligaments, blood vessels, and fallopian tubes. Once the uterus is cut free, it is removed through the vagina. The operation takes one to two hours. The hospital stay is usually one to three days, and return to normal activities takes about four weeks.

The advantages of this procedure are that it leaves no visible scar and is less painful. The disadvantage is that it is more difficult for the surgeon to see the uterus and surrounding tissue. This makes complications more common. Large fibroids cannot be removed using this technique. It is very difficult to remove the ovaries during a vaginal hysterectomy, so this approach may not be possible if the ovaries are involved.

Vaginal hysterectomy can also be performed using a laparoscopic technique. With this surgery, a tube containing a tiny camera is inserted through an incision in the navel. This allows the surgeon to see the uterus on a video monitor. The surgeon then inserts two slender instruments through small incisions in the abdomen and uses them to cut and tie off the blood vessels, fallopian tubes, and ligaments. When the uterus is detached, it is removed though a small incision at the top of the vagina.

This technique, called laparoscopic-assisted vaginal hysterectomy, allows surgeons to perform a vaginal hysterectomy that might be too difficult otherwise. The hospital stay is usually only one day. Recovery time is about two weeks. The disadvantage is that this operation is relatively new and requires great skill by the surgeon.

Any vaginal hysterectomy may have to be converted to an abdominal hysterectomy during surgery if complications develop.

Preparation

Before surgery the doctor will order blood and urine tests. The woman may also meet with the anesthesiologist to evaluate any special conditions that might affect the administration of anesthesia. On the evening before the operation, the woman should eat a light dinner and then avoid eating or drinking anything.

Aftercare

After surgery a woman will feel pain. The degree of discomfort varies, and is generally greatest in abdominal hysterectomies because of the incision. Hospital stays vary from about two days (laparoscopic-assisted vaginal hysterectomy) to five or six days (abdominal hysterectomy with bilateral **salpingo-oophorectomy**). During the hospital stay, the doctor will probably order more blood tests.

Return to normal activities such as driving and working takes anywhere from two to eight weeks, again depending on the type of surgery. Some women have emotional changes following a hysterectomy. Women who have had their ovaries removed will probably start taking **hormone replacement therapy**.

Risks

Hysterectomy is a relatively safe operation, although like all major surgery it carries risks. These include unanticipated reaction to anesthesia, internal bleeding, **blood clots**, damage to other organs such as the bladder, and post-surgery infection. The risk of **death** is about one in every 1,000 (1/1,000) women having the operation.

KEY TERMS

Cervix—The lower part of the uterus extending into the vagina.

Fallopian tubes—Slender tubes that carry eggs (ova) from the ovaries to the uterus.

Lymph nodes—Small, compact structures lying along the channels that carry lymph, a yellowish fluid. Lymph nodes produce white blood cells (lymphocytes), which are important in forming antibodies that fight disease.

Prolapsed uterus—A uterus that has slipped out of place, sometimes protruding down through the vagina.

Other complications sometimes reported after a hysterectomy include changes in sex drive, weight gain, **constipation**, and pelvic pain. Hot flashes and other symptoms of menopause can occur if the ovaries are removed. Women who have both ovaries removed and who do not take estrogen replacement therapy run an increased risk for heart disease and **osteoporosis** (a condition that causes bones to be brittle). Women with a history of psychological and emotional problems before the hysterectomy are more likely to experience psychological difficulties after the operation.

Normal results

Although there is some concern that hysterectomies may be performed unnecessarily, there are many conditions for which the operation improves a woman's quality of life. In the Maine Woman's Health Study, 71% of women who had hysterectomies to correct moderate or severe painful symptoms reported feeling better mentally, physically, and sexually after the operation.

Resources

ORGANIZATIONS

American Cancer Society. (800) 227-2345. < http://www.cancer.org >.

National Cancer Institute. (800) 4-CANCER. < http://www.nci.nih.gov >.

OTHER

Parker, William H. "A Gynecologist's Second Opinion." < http://www.gynsecondopinion.com >.

Debra Gordon

Hysteria

Definition

The term "hysteria" has been in use for over 2,000 years and its definition has become broader and more diffuse over time. In modern psychology and psychiatry, hysteria is a feature of hysterical disorders in which a patient experiences physical symptoms that have a psychological, rather than an organic, cause; and histrionic personality disorder characterized by excessive emotions, dramatics, and attention-seeking behavior.

Description

Hysterical disorders

Patients with hysterical disorders, such as conversion and somatization disorder experience physical symptoms that have no organic cause. Conversion disorder affects motor and sensory functions, while somatization affects the gastrointestinal, nervous, cardiopulmonary, or reproductive systems. These patients are not "faking" their ailments, as the symptoms are very real to them. Disorders with hysteric features typically begin in adolescence or early adulthood.

Histrionic personality disorder

Histrionic personality disorder has a prevalence of approximately 2–3% of the general population. It begins in early adulthood and has been diagnosed more frequently in women than in men. Histrionic personalities are typically self-centered and attention seeking. They operate on emotion, rather than fact or logic, and their conversation is full of generalizations and dramatic appeals. While the patient's enthusiasm, flirtatious behavior, and trusting nature may make them appear charming, their need for immediate gratification, mercurial displays of emotion, and constant demand for attention often alienates them from others.

Causes and symptoms

Hysterical disorders

Hysteria may be a defense mechanism to avoid painful emotions by unconsciously transferring this distress to the body. There may be a symbolic function for this, for example a **rape** victim may develop paralyzed legs. Symptoms may mimic a number of physical and neurological disorders which must be ruled out before a diagnosis of hysteria is made.

Histrionic personality disorder

According to the *Diagnostic and Statistical Manual of Mental Disorders,* Fourth Edition (*DSM-IV*), individuals with histrionic personality possess at least five of the following symptoms or personality features:

- a need to be the center of attention
- inappropriate, sexually seductive, or provocative behavior while interacting with others
- rapidly changing emotions and superficial expression of emotions
- vague and impressionistic speech (gives opinions without any supporting details)
- easily influenced by others
- believes relationships are more intimate than they are.

Diagnosis

Hysterical disorders frequently prove to be actual medical or neurological disorders, which makes it important to rule these disorders out before diagnosing a patient with hysterical disorders. In addition to a patient interview, several clinical inventories may be used to assess the patient for hysterical tendencies, such as the Minnesota Multiphasic Personality Inventory-2 (**MMPI-2**) or the Millon Clinical Multiaxial Inventory-III (MCMI-III). These tests may be administered in an outpatient or hospital setting by a psychiatrist or psychologist.

Treatment

Hysterical disorders

For people with hysterical disorders, a supportive healthcare environment is critical. Regular appointments with a physician who acknowledges the patient's physical discomfort are important. Psychotherapy may be attempted to help the patient gain insight into the cause of their distress. Use of behavioral therapy can help to avoid reinforcing symptoms.

Histrionic personality disorder

Psychotherapy is generally the treatment of choice for histrionic personality disorder. It focuses on supporting the patient and on helping develop the skills needed to create meaningful relationships with others.

JEAN MARTIN CHARCOT (1825–1893)

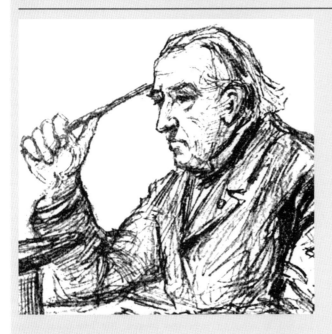

(Library of Congress.)

Jean Martin Charcot was born to a carriage maker on November 29, 1825, in Paris, France. Charcot attended the University of Paris, earning his medical degree in 1853. In 1860, he accepted a position at the university as a professor of pathological anatomy until 1862, when he was named senior physician at the Salpêtrière, a hospital for the treatment of mental illness.

Charcot's research and work on psychoneuroses and hysterical disorders untimately helped to dispell the belief that hysteria was a disorder found only in women. Charcot also explored the possibility that physiological abnormalities of the nervous system played a part when behavioral problems were exhibited. He became known for his ability to diagnose and locate these abnormalities of the central nervous system. Finally, Charcot's most notable contribution to the field of psychiatry was his successful use of hypnotism in the diagnosis and treatment of hysteria. He found that, while hypnotized, the patient recalled details, which were not readily available to the individual in a conscious state. In addition, Charcot found that the therapist could more easily influence the hypnotized patient during therapy. In 1882, Charcot presented his research findings to the French Academy of Sciences with favorable results.

Charcot was a prolific writer and a talented artist. Between 1888 and 1894, his complete works were compiled into nine volumes. His most noted work *Lectures on the Diseases of the Nervous System* was published in 1877. Charcot died on August 16, 1893.

KEY TERMS

Conversion disorder—A psychological disorder that alters motor or sensory functions. Paralysis, blindness, anesthesia (lack of feeling), coordination or balance problems, and seizures are all common symptoms of the disorder.

Somatization disorder—The appearance of physical symptoms in the gastrointestinal system, the nervous system, the cardiopulmonary system, or the reproductive system that have no organic cause.

Prognosis

Hysterical disorders

The outcome for hysterical disorders varies by type. Somatization is typically a lifelong disorder, while conversion disorder may last for months or years. Symptoms of hysterical disorders may suddenly disappear, only to reappear in another form later.

Histrionic personality disorder

Individuals with histrionic personality disorder may be at a higher risk for suicidal gestures, attempts, or threats in an effort to gain attention. Providing a supportive environment for patients with both hysterical disorders and histrionic personality disorder is key to helping these patients.

Resources

ORGANIZATIONS

American Psychiatric Association. 1400 K Street NW, Washington DC 20005. (888) 357-7924. <http://www.psych.org>.

American Psychological Association (APA). 750 First St. NE, Washington, DC 20002-4242. (202) 336-5700. <ttp://www.apa.org>.

National Alliance for the Mentally Ill (NAMI). Colonial Place Three, 2107 Wilson Blvd., Ste. 300, Arlington, VA 22201-3042. (800) 950-6264. <http://www.nami.org>.

Paula Anne Ford-Martin

Hysterosalpingography

Definition

Hysterosalpingography is a procedure where x rays are taken of a woman's reproductive tract after a dye is injected. *Hystero* means uterus and *salpingo* means tubes, so hysterosalpingography literally means to take pictures of the uterus and fallopian tubes. This procedure may also be called hysterography (or HSG).

Purpose

Hysterosalpingography is used to determine if the fallopian tubes are open, or if there are any apparent abnormalities or defects in the uterus. It can be used to detect tumors, scar tissue, or tears in the lining of the uterus. This procedure is often used to help diagnose **infertility** in women. The fallopian tubes are the location where an egg from the ovary joins with sperm to produce a fertilized ovum. If the fallopian tubes are blocked or deformed, the egg may not be able to descend or the sperm may be blocked from moving up to meet the egg. Up to 30% of all cases of infertility are due to damaged or blocked fallopian tubes.

Precautions

This procedure should not be done on women who suspect they might be pregnant or who may have a pelvic infection. Women who have had an allergic reaction to dye used in previous x-ray procedures should inform their doctor.

Description

As with other types of pelvic examinations, the woman will lie on her back on an examination table with her legs sometimes raised in stirrups. The x-ray equipment is placed above the abdomen.

A speculum is inserted into the vagina and a catheter (a thin tube) is inserted into the uterus through the cervix (the opening to the uterus). A small balloon in the catheter is inflated to hold it in place. A liquid water-based or oil-based dye is then injected through the catheter into the uterus. This process can cause cramping, **pain**, and uterine spasms.

As the dye spreads through the reproductive tract, the doctor may watch for blockages or abnormalities on an x-ray monitor. Several x rays will also be taken.

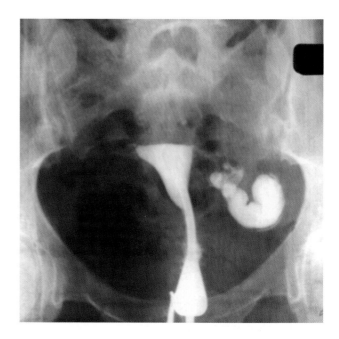

A hysterosalpingogram of the abdomen of a woman whose fallopian tubes are blocked. The fallopian tube (right on image) is blocked near the uterus, the triangular shape at center. The other fallopian tube is obstructed at a point further from the uterus where dilatation has occurred. *(Photo Researchers, Inc. Reproduced by permission.)*

The procedure takes approximately 15–30 minutes. The x rays will be developed while the patient waits, but the final reading and interpretation of the x rays by a radiologist (a doctor who specializes in x rays) may not be available for a few days.

Interestingly, sometimes the hysterosalpingography procedure itself can be considered a treatment. The dye used can sometimes open up small blockages in the fallopian tubes. The need for additional test procedures or surgical treatments to deal with infertility should be discussed with the doctor.

Preparation

This procedure is generally done in the x-ray department of a hospital or large clinic. **General anesthesia** is not needed. A pain reliever may be taken prior to the procedure to lessen the severity of cramping.

Aftercare

While no special aftercare is required after a hysterosalpingography, the woman may be observed for some period after the procedure to ensure that she does not have any allergic reactions to the dye. A sanitary napkin may be worn after

KEY TERMS

Catheter—A thin tube, usually made of plastic, that is inserted into the body to allow the passage of fluid into or out of a site.

Fallopian tubes—The narrow ducts leading from a woman's ovaries to the uterus. After an egg is released from the ovary during ovulation, fertilization (the union of sperm and egg) normally occurs in the fallopian tubes.

Hysterography—Another term for the x-ray procedure of the uterus and fallopian tubes.

Hysterosalpingogram—The term for the x ray taken during a hysterosalpingography procedure.

Speculum—A plastic or stainless steel instrument that is inserted into the opening of the vagina so the cervix (the opening of the uterus) and interior of the vagina can be examined.

the procedure to absorb dye that will flow out through the vaginal opening. If a blockage is seen in a tube, the patient may be given an antibiotic. A woman should notify her doctor if she experiences excessive bleeding, extensive pelvic pain, **fever**, or an unpleasant vaginal odor after the procedure. These symptoms may indicate a pelvic infection. Counseling may be necessary to interpret the results of the x rays, and to discuss any additional procedures to treat tubal blockages or uterine abnormalities found.

Risks

Cramps during the procedure are common. Complications associated with hysterosalpingography include abdominal pain, pelvic infection, and allergic reactions. It is also possible that abnormalities of the fallopian tubes and uterus will not be detected by this procedure.

Normal results

A normal hysterosalpingography will show a healthy, normally shaped uterus and unblocked fallopian tubes.

Abnormal results

Blockage of one or both of the fallopian tubes or abnormalities of the uterus may be detected.

Resources

ORGANIZATIONS

American Society for Reproductive Medicine. 1209 Montgomery Highway, Birmingham, AL 35216-2809. (205) 978-5000. < http://www.asrm.com >.

Altha Roberts Edgren

Hysteroscopy

Definition

Hysteroscopy is a procedure that allows a physician to look through the vagina and neck of the uterus (cervix) to inspect the cavity of the uterus. A telescope-like instrument called a hysteroscope is used. Hysteroscopy is used as both a diagnostic and a treatment tool.

Purpose

Diagnostic hysteroscopy may be used to evaluate the cause of **infertility**, to determine the cause of repeated miscarriages, or to help locate polyps and fibroids.

The procedure is also used to treat gynecological conditions, often instead of or in addition to **dilatation and curettage** (D&C). A D&C is a procedure for scraping the lining of the uterus. A D&C can be used to take a sample of the lining of the uterus for analysis. Hysteroscopy is an advance over D&C because the doctor can take tissue samples of specific areas or actually see fibroids, polyps, or structural abnormalities.

When used for treatment, the hysteroscope is used with other devices to remove polyps, fibroids, or IUDs that have become embedded in the wall of the uterus.

Precautions

The procedure is not performed on women with **cervical cancer**, **endometrial cancer**, or acute pelvic inflammation.

Description

Diagnostic hysteroscopy is performed in either a doctor's office or hospital. Before inserting the hysteroscope, the doctor injects a local anesthetic around the cervix. Once it has taken effect, the doctor dilates the cervix and then inserts a narrow lighted tube (the

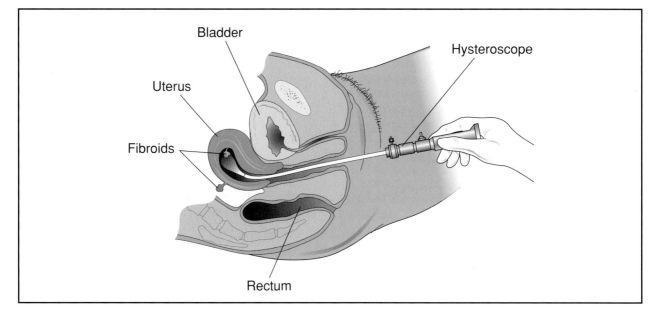

Bladder

Hysteroscope

Uterus

Fibroids

Rectum

Hysteroscopy is a procedure that allows inspection of the uterus by using a telescope-like instrument called a hysteroscope. *(Illustration by Electronic Illustrators Group.)*

hysteroscope) through the cervix to reveal the inside of the uterus. Ordinarily, the walls of the uterus are touching each other. In order to get a better view, the uterus is inflated with carbon dioxide gas or fluid. Hysteroscopy takes about 30 minutes, and can cost anywhere from $750 to $4,000 depending on the extent of the procedure.

Treatment involving the use of hysteroscopy is usually performed as a day surgical procedure with regional or **general anesthesia**. Tiny surgical instruments are inserted through the hysteroscope, and are used to remove polyps or fibroids. A small sample of tissue lining the uterus is often removed for examination, especially if there is any abnormal bleeding.

Preparation

If the procedure is done in the doctor's office, the patient will be given a mild **pain** reliever before the procedure to ease cramping. The doctor will wash the vagina and cervix with an antiseptic solution.

If the procedure is done in the hospital under general anesthesia, the patient should not eat or drink anything (not even water) after midnight the night before the procedure.

Aftercare

Many women experience light bleeding for several days after surgical hysteroscopy. Mild cramping or

pain is common after operative hysteroscopy, but usually fades away within eight hours. If carbon dioxide gas was used, there may also be some shoulder pain. Nonprescription pain relievers may help ease discomfort. Women may want to take the day off and relax after having hysteroscopy.

Risks

Diagnostic hysteroscopy is a fairly safe procedure that only rarely causes complications. The primary risk is prolonged bleeding or infection, usually following surgical hysteroscopy to remove a growth.

Very rare complications include perforation of the uterus, bowel, or bladder. Surgery under general anesthesia causes the additional risks typically associated with anesthesia.

Patients should alert their health care provider if they develop any of these symptoms:

- abnormal discharge
- heavy bleeding
- fever over 101 °F (38.3 °C)
- severe lower abdominal pain

Normal results

A normal, healthy uterus with no fibroids or other growths.

Fibroid—A benign tumor of the uterus

Polyp—A growth that projects from the lining of the cervix, the nose, or any other mucus membrane.

Septum—A condition present at birth in which there is an extra fold of tissue down the center of the uterus that can cause infertility. This tissue can be removed with a wire electrode and a hysteroscope.

Abnormal results

Using hysteroscopy, the doctor may find **uterine fibroids** or polyps (often the cause of abnormal bleeding) or a septum (extra fold of tissue down the center of the uterus) that can cause infertility. Sometimes, precancerous or malignant growths are discovered.

Resources

PERIODICALS

Anon. "Looking Inside the Uterus." *Harvard Women's Health Watch* 4, no. 5 (January 1997): 4-5.

Carol A. Turkington

Hysterosonography

Definition

Hysterosonography, which is also called sonohysterography, is a new noninvasive technique that involves the slow infusion of sterile saline solution into a woman's uterus during ultrasound imaging. Hysterosonography allows the doctor to evaluate abnormal growths inside the uterus; abnormalities of the tissue lining the uterus (the endometrium); or disorders affecting deeper tissue layers. Hysterosonography does not require either radiation or contrast media, or invasive surgical procedures

Purpose

Hysterosonography is used to evaluate patients in the following groups:

- peri- or postmenopausal women with unexplained vaginal bleeding

- women whose endometrium appears abnormal during baseline ultrasound imaging

- women with fertility problems. **Infertility** is sometimes related to polyps, leiomyomas (fibroids), or **adhesions** inside the uterus. Adhesions are areas of tissue that have grown together to form bands or membranes across the inside of the uterus.

- women receiving tamoxifen therapy for **breast cancer**

Hysterosonography is useful as a screening test to minimize the use of more invasive diagnostic procedures, such as tissue biopsies and dilation and curettage (D&C). Hysterosonography can also be used as a follow-up after uterine surgery to evaluate its success.

Precautions

Hysterosonography is difficult to perform in patients with certain abnormalities:

- Cervical stenosis. Cervical stenosis means that the lower end of the uterus is narrowed or tightened. It complicates the insertion of a tube (catheter).

- Adhesions or large fibroids. These growths sometimes block the flow of saline fluid into the uterus.

Patients with active **pelvic inflammatory disease** (PID) should not be tested with hysterosonography until the disease is brought under control. Women with chronic PID or heart problems are given **antibiotics** before the procedure.

Description

A hysterosonography is preceded by a baseline ultrasound examination performed through the vagina. This allows the doctor to detect an unsuspected **pregnancy** and to assess the thickness and possible abnormalities of the patient's endometrium. The doctor then inserts a catheter into the uterus and injects sterile saline fluid while ultrasound imaging is recorded on film or videotape. The procedure takes about 10 to 15 minutes.

Preparation

Patients do not require special preparation apart from the timing of the procedure. Patients with fertility problems are examined during the first 10 days of the menstrual cycle. Patients who may have polyps are usually examined at a later phase in the cycle. The best time for examining women with fibroids is still under discussion.

KEY TERMS

Adhesion—An abnormal union or attachment of two areas of tissue.

Contrast medium—A chemical substance used to make an organ or body part opaque on x ray.

Dilation and curettage (D&C)—A surgical procedure in which the patient's cervix is widened (dilated) and the endometrium is scraped with a scoop-shaped knife (curette).

Endometrium—The tissue that lines the uterus.

Fibroid—Another word for leiomyoma.

Leiomyoma—A benign tumor composed of muscle tissue. Leiomyomas in the uterus are sometimes called fibroids.

Pelvic inflammatory disease (PID)—An inflammation of the fallopian tubes, usually caused by bacterial infection.

Polyp—A growth projecting from the lining of the uterus. Polyps can cause fertility problems or abnormal vaginal bleeding.

Saline solution—A solution of sterile water and salt used in a variety of medical procedures. In hysterosonography, saline solution is used to fill the uterus for diagnostic imaging.

Transvaginal ultrasound (US)—The diagnostic imaging procedure that serves as the baseline for a hysterosonographic examination.

Aftercare

Aftercare consists of advising the patient to contact her doctor in case of abnormal bleeding, **fever**, or abdominal **pain**. Some spotting or cramping is common, however, and can usually be treated with **nonsteroidal anti-inflammatory drugs**, such as ibuprofen.

Risks

The chief risks are mild spotting and cramping after the procedure.

Normal results

Normal findings include a symmetrical uterus with a normal endometrium and no visible masses or tumors.

Abnormal results

Abnormal findings include adhesions; polyps; leiomyomas; abnormal thickening of the endometrium; or tissue changes related to tamoxifen (Nolvadex), which is a drug given for breast **cancer**.

Resources

PERIODICALS

Cullinan, Joanne, et al. "Sonohysterography: A Technique for Endometrial Evaluation." *RadioGraphics* 15 (May 1995): 501-514.

Rebecca J. Frey, PhD

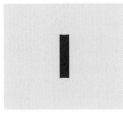

IBS *see* **Irritable bowel syndrome**

Ibuprophen *see* **Nonsteroidal anti-inflammatory drugs**

Ichthyosis

Definition

Derived from two Greek words meaning "fish" and "disease," ichthyosis is a congenital (meaning present at birth) dermatological (skin) disease that is represented by thick, scaly skin.

Description

The ichthyoses are a group of skin diseases caused by an abnormality in skin growth that results in drying and scaling. There are at least 20 types of ichthyosis. Ichthyosis can be more or less severe, sometimes accumulating thick scales and cracks that are painful and bleed. Ichthyosis is not contagious. Some forms of ichthyosis are inherited while others are acquired in later life as a symptom of systemic disorders.

The most common form of ichthyosis, accounting for 95% of all cases of ichthyosis, is called ichthyosis vulgaris (*vulgaris* is the Latin word for "common"), and occurs in approximately one person in every 250. It is inherited in an autosomal dominant manner. The most rare types of ichthyosis occur in fewer than one person in one million and are inherited in an autosomal recessive manner. Ichthyosis occurs regardless of the part of the world the child is from, or the ethnic background of the parents.

Acquired ichthyosis is extremely rare; neither its incidence in the United States nor its incidence in the rest of the world are known as of 2003.

Both inherited and acquired ichthyoses affect males and females equally.

Causes and symptoms

Inherited ichthyoses

Depending on the specific type of ichthyosis, the inheritance can be autosomal recessive, autosomal dominant, X-linked recessive, X-linked dominant, or sporadic. Autosomal recessive means that the altered gene for the disease or trait is located on one of the first 22 pairs of chromosomes, which are also called "autosomes." Males and females are equally likely to have an autosomal recessive disease or trait. Recessive means that two copies of the altered gene are necessary to express the condition. Therefore, a child inherits one copy of the altered gene from each parent, who are called carriers (because they have only one copy of the altered gene). Since carriers do not express the altered gene, parents usually do not know they carry the altered gene that causes ichthyosis until they have an affected child. Carrier parents have a 1-in-4 chance (or 25%) with each **pregnancy**, to have a child with ichthyosis.

Autosomal dominant inheritance also means that both males and females are equally likely to have the disease but only one copy of the altered gene is necessary to have the condition. An individual with ichthyosis has a 50/50 chance to pass the condition to his or her child.

The skin is made up of several layers, supported underneath by a layer of fat that is thicker or thinner depending on location. The lower layers contain blood vessels, the middle layers contain actively growing cells, and the upper layer consists of dead cells that serve as a barrier to the outside world. This barrier is nearly waterproof and highly resistant to infection. Scattered throughout the middle layers are hair follicles, oil and sweat glands, and nerve endings. The upper layer is constantly flaking off and being replaced from beneath by new tissue. In ichthyosis, the skin's natural shedding process is slowed or inhibited; and in some types, skin cells are produced too rapidly.

The abnormality in skin growth and hydration called ichthyosis may present with symptoms at birth or in early childhood. Ichthyosis can itch relentlessly, leading to such complications of scratching as lichen simplex (**dermatitis** characterized by raw patches of skin). Either the cracking or the scratching can introduce infection, bringing with it discomfort and complications.

Acquired ichthyoses

The mildest form of acquired ichthyosis is called xeroderma, or dry flaky skin. It is not associated with any systemic diseases. Xeroderma occurs most often on the lower legs of middle-aged and elderly adults during cold weather, or on the lower legs of people who bathe too often. It is characterized chiefly by mild or moderate **itching**.

Ichthyosis may also be an early symptom of such disorders as **AIDS**, lymphoma, **hypothyroidism**, or **leprosy**. In these cases the ichthyosis is most noticeable on the patient's trunk and legs.

A few rare cases of acquired ichthyosis have been attributed to the use of certain drugs, specifically cimetidine (Tagamet), triparanol (Metasqualene), dixyrazine (a phenothiazine derivative used as an antipsychotic), nicotinic acid (vitamin B_3, butyrophenone antipsychotics (Haldol, Inapsine, Orap), and clofazimine (Lamprene).

Diagnosis

A dermatologist will often make the diagnosis of ichthyosis based on findings from a clinical examination. However, a **skin biopsy**, or DNA study (from a small blood sample) is necessary to confirm the diagnosis. Evaluation for associated problems is done by a complete physical medical examination.

For some types of ichythyosis, the abnormal gene has been identified and prenatal testing is available. At present this is true for the autosomal recessive congenital ichythoses, which include: lamellar ichthyosis (LI), autosomal recessive lamellar ichthyosis (ARLI), congenital ichthyosiform erythroderma (CIE), and non-bullous congenital ichthyosiform erythroderma (NBCIE).

There are four different genes that have been located for the autosomal recessive congenital ichthyoses. Testing, however, is available for only one gene, known as transglutaminase-1 (TGM1). This gene is located on chromosome 14. Once a couple has had a child with ichthyosis, and they have had the genetic cause identified by DNA studies (performed from a small blood sample), prenatal testing for future pregnancies may be considered. (Note that prenatal testing may not be possible if both mutations cannot be identified.) Prenatal diagnosis is available via either **chorionic villus sampling** (CVS) or **amniocentesis**. CVS is a biopsy of the placenta performed in the first trimester of pregnancy under ultrasound guidance. Ultrasound is the use of sound waves to visualize the developing fetus. The genetic makeup of the placenta is identical to the fetus and therefore the TGM1 gene can be studied from this tissue. There is approximately a one in 100 chance for **miscarriage** with CVS. Amniocentesis is a procedure done under ultrasound guidance in which a long thin needle is inserted through the mother's abdomen into the uterus, to withdraw a couple of tablespoons of amniotic fluid (fluid surrounding the developing baby) to study. The TGM1 gene can be studied using cells from the amniotic fluid. Other genetic tests, such as a chromosome analysis, may also be performed through either CVS or amniocentesis.

Acquired ichthyosis is usually diagnosed in the course of identifying the underlying disorder. With the exception of acquired ichthyosis related to lymphoma, a doctor cannot tell the difference between inherited and acquired ichthyosis by examining skin samples through a microscope.

Treatment

Most treatments for ichthyosis are topical, which means that they are applied directly to the skin, not taken internally. Xeroderma is eaily treated by minimizing bathing and applying an emollient cream or mineral oil after bathing while the skin is still moist. Some forms of ichthyosis require two forms of treatment—a reduction in the amount of scale buildup and moisturizing of the underlying skin. Several agents are available for each purpose. Reduction in the amount of scale is achieved by keratolytics. Among this class of drugs are urea, lactic acid, and salicylic acid. Petrolatum, 60% propylene glycol, and glycerin are successful moisturizing agents, as are many commercially available products. Increased humidity of the ambient air is also helpful in preventing skin dryness.

KEY TERMS

Amniocentesis—A procedure performed at 16–18 weeks of pregnancy in which a needle is inserted through a woman's abdomen into her uterus to draw out a small sample of the amniotic fluid from around the baby. Either the fluid itself or cells from the fluid can be used for a variety of tests to obtain information about genetic disorders and other medical conditions in the fetus.

Amniotic fluid—The fluid that surrounds a developing baby during pregnancy.

Autosomal dominant—A pattern of genetic inheritance where only one abnormal gene is needed to display the trait or disease.

Autosomal recessive inheritance—A pattern of genetic inheritance where two abnormal genes are needed to display the trait or disease.

Dermatologist—A physician that specializes in diagnosing and treating disorders of the skin.

Emollients—Petroleum or lanolin-based skin lubricants.

Keratin—A tough, nonwater-soluble protein found in the nails, hair, and the outermost layer of skin. Human hair is made up largely of keratin.

Keratinocytes—Skin cells.

Keratolytic—An agent that dissolves or breaks down the outer layer of skin (keratins).

Retinoids—A derivative of synthetic Vitamin A.

Sporadic—Isolated or appearing occasionally with no apparent pattern.

X-linked dominant inheritance—The inheritance of a trait by the presence of a single gene on the X chromosome in a male or female, passed from an affected female who has the gene on one of her X chromosomes.

X-linked recessive inheritance—The inheritance of a trait by the presence of a single gene on the X chromosome in a male, passed from a female who has the gene on one of her X chromosomes, and who is referred to as an unaffected carrier.

Because the skin acts as a barrier to the outside environment, medicines have a hard time penetrating, especially through the thick skin of the palms of the hands and the soles of the feet. This resistance is diminished greatly by maceration (softening the skin). Soaking hands in water macerates skin so that it looks like prune skin. Occlusion (covering) with rubber gloves or plastic wrap will also macerate skin. Applying medicines and then covering the skin with an occlusive dressing will facilitate entrance of the medicine and greatly magnify its effect.

Secondary treatments are necessary to control pruritus (itching) and infection. Commercial products containing camphor, menthol, eucalyptus oil, aloe, and similar substances are very effective as antipruritics. If the skin cracks deeply enough, a pathway for infection is created. **Topical antibiotics** like bacitracin are effective in prevention and in the early stages of these skin infections. Cleansing with hydrogen peroxide inhibits infection as well.

Finally, there are topical and internal derivatives of vitamin A called retinoids that improve skin growth and are used for severe cases of **acne**, ichthyosis, and other skin conditions. Tazarotene (Tazorac), a retinoid that was originally developed to treat **psoriasis** and acne, appears to give good results in treating ichthyosis with fewer side effects than other retinoids.

Prognosis

This condition requires continuous care throughout a lifetime. Properly treated, in most cases it is a cosmetic problem. There are a small number of lethal forms, such as harlequin fetus.

Resources

BOOKS

Beers, Mark H., MD, and Robert Berkow, MD, editors. "Ichthyosis." Section 10, Chapter 121. In *The Merck Manual of Diagnosis and Therapy*. Whitehouse Station, NJ: Merck Research Laboratories, 2004.

PERIODICALS

Fleckman, P. "Management of the Ichthyoses." *Skin Therapy Letter* 8 (September 2003): 3–7.

Hatsell, S. J., H. Stevens, A. P. Jackson, et al. "An Autosomal Recessive Exfoliative Ichthyosis with Linkage to Chromosome 12q13." *British Journal of Dermatology* 149 (July 2003): 174–180.

Lefevre, C., S. Audebert, F. Jobard, et al. "Mutations in the Transporter ABCA12 Are Associated with Lamellar Ichthyosis Type 2." *Human Molecular Genetics* 12 (September 15, 2003): 2369–2378.

Marulli, G. C., E. Campione, M. S. Chimenti, et al. "Type I Lamellar Ichthyosis Improved by Tazarotene 0.1% Gel." *Clinical and Experimental Dermatology* 28 (July 2003): 391–393.

Okulicz, Jason F., MD, and Robert A. Schwartz, MD, MPH. "Ichthyosis Vulgaris, Hereditary and Acquired." *eMedicine* November 1, 2001. < http://www.emedicine.com/derm/topic678.htm >.

ORGANIZATIONS

Alliance of Genetic Support Groups. 4301 Connecticut Ave. NW, Suite 404, Washington, DC 20008. (202) 966-5557. Fax: (202) 966-8553. <http://www.geneticalliance.org>.

Foundation for Ichthyosis and Related Skin Types (FIRST). 650 N. Cannon Ave., Suite 17, Landsdale, PA 19446. (215) 631-1411 or (800) 545-3286. Fax: (215) 631-1413. <http://www.scalyskin.org>.

National Organization for Rare Disorders, Inc. (NORD). 55 Kenosia Avenue, P. O. Box 1968, Danbury, CT 06813. (800) 999-6673 or (203) 744-0100. <http://www.rarediseases.org>.

OTHER

Immune Deficiency Foundation Website. <www.primaryimmune.org>.

Catherine L. Tesla, MS, CGC
Rebecca J. Frey, PhD

Icterus *see* **Jaundice**

Idiopathic hypertrophic subaortic stenosis *see* **Hypertrophic cardiomyopathy**

▌ Idiopathic infiltrative lung diseases

Definition

The term *idiopathic* means "cause unknown." The idiopathic infiltrative lung diseases, also known as interstitial lung diseases, are a group of more than a hundred disorders seen in both adults and (less often) in children, whose cause is unknown but which tend to spread, or "infiltrate" through much or all of the lung tissue. They range from mild conditions that respond well to treatment, to progressive, nonresponsive disease states that severely limit lung function and may cause **death**.

Description

The body produces inflammatory cells in response to a variety of conditions, including a number of different diseases, pollutants, certain infections, exposure to organic dust or toxic fumes and vapors, and various drugs and poisons. When white blood cells and tissue fluid rich in protein collect in the small air sacs of the lungs, or alveoli, the sacs become inflamed (alveolitis). In time, the fluid may solidify and cause scar formation that replaces the normal lung tissue. This process is known as **pulmonary fibrosis**. In about half of all patients, no specific cause is ever found; they are said to have idiopathic pulmonary fibrosis.

Some patients have special types of interstitial lung disease that may occur in certain types of patients, or feature typical pathological changes when a sample of lung tissue is examined under a microscope. They include:

- Usual interstitial pneumonitis. Disease occurs in a patchy form throughout the lungs. Parts of the lungs can appear normal while others have dense scar tissue and lung cysts, often the end result of pulmonary fibrosis. This disease progresses quite slowly. Both children and adults may be affected.

- Desquamative interstitial pneumonitis. Similar-appearing lesions are present throughout the lungs. Both inflammatory cells and cells that have separated from the air sac linings ("desquamated") are present. Some researchers believe this is an early form of usual interstitial pneumonitis.

- Lymphocytic interstitial pneumonitis. Most of the cells infiltrating the lungs are the type of white blood cells called lymphocytes. Both the breathing tubes (bronchi) and blood vessels of the lungs become thickened. In children, this condition tends to occur when the immune system is not operating properly as occurs with Acquired Immune Deficiency Syndrome (AIDS).

Causes and symptoms

By definition, the causes of *idiopathic* infiltrative lung diseases are not known. Some forms of pulmonary fibrosis, however, do have specific causes and these may provide a clue as to what may cause idiopathic diseases. Known causes of pulmonary fibrosis include diseases that impair the body's immune function; infection by viruses and the bacterium causing **tuberculosis**; and exposure to such mineral dusts as silica or asbestos, or such organic materials as bird droppings. Other cases of pulmonary fibrosis result from exposure to fumes and vapors, radiation (in industry or medically), and certain drugs used to treat disease.

Patients with interstitial lung disease usually have labored breathing when exerting themselves. Often they **cough** and feel overly tired ("no stamina"). **Wheezing** is uncommon. When the physician listens to the patient's chest with a stethoscope, dry, crackling sounds may be heard. Some patients have vague chest **pain**. When disease progresses, the patient may breathe very rapidly, have mottled blue skin (because of getting too little oxygen), and lose weight. The fingertips may appear thick or club-shaped.

Diagnosis

Both **scars** in the lung and cysts (air-filled spaces) can be seen on a **chest x ray**. Up to 10% of patients, however, may have normal x rays even if their symptoms are severe. A special type of x ray, high-resolution computed tomography scan (CT scan), often is helpful in adult patients. Tests of lung function will show that the lungs cannot hold enough air with each breath, and there is too little oxygen in the blood, especially after exercising. In a procedure called bronchoalveolar lavage, a tube is placed through the nose and windpipe into the bronchi and a small amount of saline is released and then withdrawn. This fluid can then be analyzed for cells. A tiny piece of lung tissue can be sampled using the same instrument. If necessary, a larger sample (a biopsy) is taken through an incision in the chest wall and examined under a microscope.

Treatment

The first medication given, providing scarring is not too extensive, is usually a steroid drug such as prednisone. An occasional patient will improve dramatically if steroid therapy stops the inflammation. Most patients, however, improve to a limited extent. It may take 6–12 weeks for a patient to begin to respond. Patients must be watched closely for a gain in body weight, high blood pressure, and depression. Steroids can also result in diabetes, ulcer disease, and cataract. Patients treated with steroids are at risk of contracting serious infection. If steroids have not proved effective or have caused serious side effects, other anti-inflammatory drugs, such as cyclophosphamide (Cytoxan) or azathioprine (Imuran), can be tried. Cytoxan sometimes is combined with a steroid, but it carries its own risks, which include bladder inflammation and suppression of the bone marrow. Some patients will benefit from a bronchodilator drug that relaxes the airway and makes breathing easier.

Some patients with interstitial lung disease, especially children, will need **oxygen therapy**. Usually oxygen is given during sleep or **exercise**, but if the blood oxygen level is very low it may be given constantly. A program of conditioning, training in how to breathe efficiently, energy-saving tips, and a proper diet will help patients achieve the highest possible level of function given the state of their illness. All patients should be vaccinated each year against **influenza**. A last resort for those with very advanced disease who do not respond to medication is **lung transplantation**. This operation is being done more widely, and it is even possible to replace both lungs.

KEY TERMS

Bronchoalveolar lavage—A way of obtaining a sample of fluid from the airways by inserting a flexible tube through the windpipe. Used to diagnose the type of lung disease.

Desquamation—Shedding of the cells lining the insides of the air sacs. A feature of desquamative interstitial pneumonitis.

Idiopathic—A disease whose cause is unknown.

Immune system—A set of body chemicals and specialized cells that attack an invading agent (such as a virus) by forming antibodies that can engulf and destroy it.

Infiltrative—A process whereby inflammatory or other types of disease spread throughout an organ such as the lungs.

Interstitial—Refers to the connective tissue that supports the "working parts" of an organ, in the case of the lungs the air sacs.

Pulmonary fibrosis—A scarring process that is the end result of many forms of long-lasting lung disease.

Prognosis

A scoring system based on lung function and x ray appearances has been designed to help monitor a patient's course. In general, idiopathic forms of interstitial lung disease cause a good deal of illness, and a significant number of deaths. A majority of patients get worse over time, although survival for many years is certainly possible. An estimated one in five affected children fail to survive. In different series, survival times average between four and ten years. Early diagnosis gives the best chance of a patient recovering or at least stabilizing. Once the lungs are badly scarred, nothing short of lung transplantation offers hope of restoring lung function. Patients with desquamative interstitial pneumonitis tend to respond well to steroid treatment, and live longer than those with other types of infiltrative lung disease.

Prevention

Since we do not understand what causes idiopathic interstitial lung diseases, there is no way to prevent them. What can be done is to prevent extensive scarring of the lungs by making the diagnosis shortly after the first symptoms develop, and trying steroids or other drugs in hope of suppressing lung inflammation. Every effort should be made to avoid exposure to dusts, gases, chemicals, and even pets. Keeping fit and learning how to breathe efficiently will help maintain lung function as long as possible.

Resources

ORGANIZATIONS

American Lung Association. 1740 Broadway, New York, NY 10019. (800) 586-4872. < http://www.lungusa.org > .

David A. Cramer, MD

Idiopathic primary renal hematuric/proteinuric syndrome

Definition

This syndrome includes a group of disorders characterized by blood and protein in the urine and by damage to the kidney glomeruli (filtering structures) that may lead to kidney failure.

Description

This syndrome, also known as Berger's disease or IgA nephropathy, arises when internal kidney structures called glomeruli become inflamed and injured. It can occur at any age, but the great majority of patients are 16–35 when diagnosed. Males seem to be affected more often than females, and whites are more often affected than blacks. Blood in the urine (hematuria), either indicated by a visible change in the color of the urine or detected by laboratory testing, is a hallmark of this syndrome, and it may occur continuously or sporadically. The pattern of occurrence is not indicative of the severity of kidney damage.

Causes and symptoms

The glomeruli are the kidney structures that filter the blood and extract waste, which is then excreted as urine. The barrier between the blood and the urine side of the filter mechanism is a membrane only one cell layer thick. Anything that damages the membrane will result in hematuria. Symptoms of idiopathic primary renal hematruic/proteinuric syndrome are caused by inflammation of the glomeruli and deposit of IgA antibodies in kidney tissue. Although a genetic basis

for this syndrome is suspected, this has not been proven. Symptoms often appear 24–48 hours after an upper respiratory or gastrointestinal infection. Symptoms of the syndrome include:

- blood in the urine (hematuria)
- protein in the urine (proteinuria)
- pain in the lower back or kidney area
- elevated blood pressure (20–30% of cases)
- nephrotic syndrome (less than 10% of cases)
- swelling (occasionally)

This condition usually does not get worse with time, although renal failure occasionally results. In patients with large amounts of IgA deposits in their glomeruli, the long-term prognosis may not be favorable. The syndrome can go into remission spontaneously, although this is more common in children than in adults.

Diagnosis

One of the objectives of diagnosis is to distinguish glomerular from non-glomerular kidney diseases. Idiopathic primary hematuric/proteinuric syndrome involves the glomeruli. The presence of fragmented or distorted red blood cells in the urine is evidence of glomerular disease. A high concentration of protein in the urine is also evidence for glomerular disease. The hematuria associated with this syndrome must be distinguished from that caused by urinary tract diseases, which can also cause a loss of blood into the urine. Biopsy of the patient's kidney shows deposits of IgA antibodies. Detecting IgA-antibody deposits rules out thin membrane disease as the cause of the hematuria and proteinuria. Test values are normal for ASO, complement, rheumatoid factor, antinuclear antibodies, anti-DNase, and cryoglobulins, all of which are associated with different types of **kidney disease**. A diagnosis of idiopathic primary renal hematuric/proteinuric syndrome is largely made by ruling out other diseases and their causes, leaving this syndrome as the remaining possible diagnosis.

Treatment

Many patients do not need specific treatment, except for those who have symptoms indicating a poor prognosis. Oral doses of **corticosteroids** are effective in patients with mild proteinuria and good kidney function. Other treatments, such as medications to lower blood pressure, are aimed at slowing or

KEY TERMS

Glomeruli (singular, glomerulus)—Filtering structures in the kidneys.

Hematuria—The presence of hemoglobin or red blood cells in the urine.

Idiopathic—Refers to a disease that arises from an obscure or unknown cause.

Nephrotic syndrome—A kidney disorder characterized by fluid retention (edema) and proteinuria. It is caused by damage to the kidney glomeruli.

Proteinuria—The presence of protein in the urine exceeding normal levels.

preventing kidney damage. If kidney failure develops, dialysis or **kidney transplantation** is necessary.

Prognosis

Idiopathic primary renal hematuric/proteinuric syndrome progresses slowly and in many cases does not progress at all. Risk for progression of the disorder is considered higher if there is:

- high blood pressure
- large amounts of protein in the urine
- increased levels of urea and creatinine in the blood (indications of kidney function)

About 25–35% of patients may develop kidney failure within about 25 years.

Prevention

Since the underlying causes of this syndrome are so poorly understood, there is no known prevention.

Resources

BOOKS

Greenberg, A. *Primer on Kidney Diseases*. San Diego: Academic Press, 1998.

ORGANIZATIONS

IgA Nephropathy Support Network. 964 Brown Ave., Huntington Valley, PA 19006. (215) 663–0536.

National Kidney Foundation. 30 East 33rd St., New York, NY 10016. (800) 622-9010. < http://www.kidney.org >.

John T. Lohr, PhD

Idiopathic thrombocytopenic purpura

Definition

Idiopathic thrombocytopenic purpura, or ITP, is a bleeding disorder caused by an abnormally low level of platelets in the patient's blood. Platelets are small plate-shaped bodies in the blood that combine to form a plug when a blood vessel is injured. The platelet plug then binds certain proteins in the blood to form a clot that stops bleeding. ITP's name describes its cause and two symptoms. Idiopathic means that the disorder has no apparent cause. ITP is now often called immune thrombocytopenic purpura rather than idiopathic because of recent findings that ITP patients have autoimmune antibodies in their blood. **Thrombocytopenia** is another word for a decreased number of blood platelets. Purpura refers to a purplish or reddishbrown skin rash caused by the leakage of blood from broken capillaries into the skin. Other names for ITP include purpura hemorrhagica and essential thrombocytopenia.

Description

ITP may be either acute or chronic. The acute form is most common in children between the ages of two and six years; the chronic form is most common in adult females between 20 and 40. Between 10% and 20% of children with ITP have the chronic form. ITP does not appear to be related to race, lifestyle, climate, or environmental factors.

ITP is a disorder that affects the overall *number* of blood platelets rather than their function. The normal platelet level in adults is between 150,000 and 450,000/mm^3. Platelet counts below 50,000 mm^3 increase the risk of dangerous bleeding from trauma; counts below 20,000/mm^3 increase the risk of spontaneous bleeding.

Causes and Symptoms

In adults, ITP is considered an autoimmune disorder, which means that the body produces antibodies that damage some of its own products–in this case, blood platelets. Some adults with chronic ITP also have other immune system disorders, such as **systemic lupus erythematosus** (SLE). In children, ITP is usually triggered by a virus infection, most often **rubella**, **chickenpox**, **measles**, cytomegalovirus, or Epstein-Barr virus. It usually begins about two or three weeks after the infection.

Acute ITP

Acute ITP is characterized by bleeding into the skin or from the nose, mouth, digestive tract, or urinary tract. The onset is usually sudden. Bleeding into the skin takes the form of purpura or petechiae. Purpura is a purplish or reddish-brown rash or discoloration of the skin; petechiae are small round pinpoint hemorrhages. Both are caused by the leakage of blood from tiny capillaries under the skin surface. In addition to purpura and petechiae, the patient may notice that he or she **bruises** more easily than usual. In extreme cases, patients with ITP may bleed into the lungs, brain, or other vital organs.

Chronic ITP

Chronic ITP has a gradual onset and may have minimal or no external symptoms. The low **platelet count** may be discovered in the course of a routine blood test. Most patients with chronic ITP, however, will consult their primary care doctor because of the purpuric skin rash, nosebleeds, or bleeding from the digestive or urinary tract. Women sometimes go to their gynecologist for unusually heavy or lengthy menstrual periods.

The risk factors for the development of chronic ITP include:

• female sex

• age over 10 years at onset of symptoms

• slow onset of bruising

• presence of other autoantibodies in the blood

Diagnosis

ITP is usually considered a diagnosis of exclusion, which means that the doctor arrives at the diagnosis by a process of ruling out other possible causes. If the patient belongs to one or more of the risk groups for chronic ITP, the doctor may order a blood test for autoantibodies in the blood early in the diagnostic process.

Physical examination

If the doctor suspects ITP, he or she will examine the patient's skin for bruises, purpuric areas, or petechiae. If the patient has had nosebleeds or bleeding from the mouth or other parts of the body, the doctor will examine these areas for other possible causes of bleeding. Patients with ITP usually look and feel healthy except for the bleeding.

The most important features that the doctor will be looking for during the **physical examination** are the condition of the patient's spleen and the presence of **fever**. Patients with ITP do not have fever, whereas patients with lupus and some other types of thrombocytopenia are usually feverish. The doctor will have the patient lie flat on the examining table in order to feel the size of the spleen. If the spleen is noticeably enlarged, ITP is not absolutely ruled out but is a less likely diagnosis.

Laboratory testing

The doctor will order a complete **blood count** (CBC), a test of clotting time, a bone marrow test, and a test for antiplatelet antibodies if it is available in the hospital laboratory. Patients with ITP usually have platelet counts below $20,000/mm^3$ and prolonged **bleeding time**. The size and appearance of the platelets may be abnormal. The red blood cell count (RBC) and white blood cell count (WBC) are usually normal, although about 10% of patients with ITP are also anemic. The blood marrow test yields normal results. Detection of antiplatelet antibodies in the blood is considered to confirm the diagnosis of ITP.

Treatment

General care and monitoring

There is no specific treatment for ITP. In most cases, the disorder will resolve without medications or surgery within two to six weeks. Nosebleeds can be treated with ice packs when necessary.

General care includes explaining ITP to the patient and advising him or her to watch for bruising, petechiae, or other signs of recurrence. Children should be discouraged from rough contact sports or other activities that increase the risk of trauma. Patients are also advised to avoid using **aspirin** or ibuprofen (Advil, Motrin) as **pain** relievers because these drugs lengthen the clotting time of blood.

Emergency treatment

Patients with acute ITP who are losing large amounts of blood or bleeding into their central nervous system require emergency treatment. This includes transfusions of platelets, intravenous immunoglobulins, or prednisone. Prednisone is a steroid medication that decreases the effects of antibody on platelets and eventually lowers antibody production. If the patient has a history of ITP that has not responded to prednisone or immunoglobulins, the surgeon may remove the patient's spleen. This operation is called a **splenectomy**. The reason for removing the spleen when ITP does not respond to other forms of

KEY TERMS

Autoimmune disorder—A disorder in which the patient's immune system produces antibodies that destroy some of the body's own products. ITP in adults is thought to be an autoimmune disorder.

Idiopathic—Of unknown cause. Idiopathic refers to a disease that is not preceded or caused by any known dysfunction or disorder in the body.

Petechiae—Small pinpoint hemorrhages in skin or mucous membranes caused by the rupture of capillaries.

Platelet—A blood component that helps to prevent blood from leaking from broken blood vessels. ITP is a bleeding disorder caused by an abnormally low level of platelets in the blood.

Prednisone—A corticosteroid medication that is used to treat ITP. Prednisone works by decreasing the effects of antibody on blood platelets. Long-term treatment with prednisone is thought to decrease antibody production.

Purpura—A skin discoloration of purplish or brownish red spots caused by bleeding from broken capillaries.

Splenectomy—Surgical removal of the spleen.

Thrombocytopenia—An abnormal decline in the number of platelets in the blood.

treatment is that the spleen sometimes keeps platelets out of the general blood circulation.

Medications and transfusions

Patients with chronic ITP can be treated with prednisone, immune globulin, or large doses of intravenous gamma globulin. Although 90% of patients respond to immunoglobulin treatment, it is very expensive. About 80% of patients respond to prednisone therapy. Platelet transfusions are not recommended for routine treatment of ITP. If the patient's platelet level does not improve within one to four months, or requires high doses of prednisone, the doctor may recommend splenectomy. All medications for ITP are given either orally or intravenously; intramuscular injection is avoided because of the possibility of causing bleeding into the skin.

Surgery

Between 80% and 85% of adults with ITP have a remission of the disorder after the spleen is removed.

Splenectomy is usually avoided in children younger than five years because of the increased risk of a severe infection after the operation. In older children, however, splenectomy is recommended if the child has been treated for 12 months without improvement; if the ITP is very severe or the patient is getting worse; if the patient begins to bleed into the head or brain; and if the patient is an adolescent female with extremely heavy periods.

Prognosis

The prognosis for recovery from acute ITP is good; 80% of patients recover without special treatment. The prognosis for chronic ITP is also good; most patients experience long-term remissions. In rare instances, however, ITP can cause life-threatening hemorrhage or bleeding into the central nervous system.

Resources

BOOKS

Linker, Charles A. "Blood." In *Current Medical Diagnosis and Treatment, 1998,* edited by Stephen McPhee, et al., 37th ed. Stamford: Appleton & Lange, 1997.

Rebecca J. Frey, PhD

IHSS *see* **Hypertrophic cardiomyopathy**

Ileal conduit *see* **Urinary diversion surgery**

Ileocol *see* **Crohn's disease**

Ileostomy *see* **Enterostomy**

Ileus

Definition

Ileus is a partial or complete non-mechanical blockage of the small and/or large intestine. The term "ileus" comes from the Latin word for **colic**.

Description

There are two types of **intestinal obstructions**, mechanical and non-mechanical. Mechanical obstructions occur because the bowel is physically blocked and its contents can not pass the point of the obstruction. This happens when the bowel twists on itself (volvulus) or as the result of hernias, impacted feces, abnormal tissue growth, or the presence of foreign bodies in the intestines.

Unlike mechanical obstruction, non-mechanical obstruction, called ileus or paralytic ileus, occurs because peristalsis stops. Peristalsis is the rhythmic contraction that moves material through the bowel. Ileus is most often associated with an infection of the peritoneum (the membrane lining the abdomen). It is one of the major causes of bowel obstruction in infants and children.

Another common cause of ileus is a disruption or reduction of the blood supply to the abdomen. Handling the bowel during abdominal surgery can also cause peristalsis to stop, so people who have had abdominal surgery are more likely to experience ileus. When ileus results from abdominal surgery the condition is often temporary and usually lasts only 48–72 hours.

Ileus sometimes occurs as a complication of surgery on other parts of the body, including **joint replacement** or chest surgery.

Ileus can also be caused by kidney diseases, especially when potassium levels are decreased. Heart disease and certain **chemotherapy** drugs, such as vinblastine (Velban, Velsar) and vincristine (Oncovin, Vincasar PES, Vincrex), also can cause ileus. Infants with **cystic fibrosis** are more likely to experience meconium ileus (a dark green material in the intestine). Over all, the total rate of bowel obstruction due both to mechanical and non-mechanical causes is one in one thousand people (1/1,000).

Causes and symptoms

When the bowel stops functioning, the following symptoms occur:

- abdominal cramping
- abdominal distention
- nausea and vomiting
- failure to pass gas or stool

Diagnosis

When a doctor listens with a stethoscope to the abdomen there will be few or no bowel sounds, indicating that the intestine has stopped functioning. Ileus can be confirmed by x rays of the abdomen, **computed tomography scans** (CT scans), or ultrasound. It may be necessary to do more invasive tests, such as a **barium enema** or upper GI series, if the obstruction is mechanical. Blood tests also are useful in diagnosing paralytic ileus.

Barium studies are used in cases of mechanical obstruction, but may cause problems by increasing pressure or intestinal contents if used in ileus. Also, in cases of suspected mechanical obstruction involving the gastrointestinal tract (from the small intestine downward) use of barium x rays are contraindicated, since they may contribute to the obstruction. In such cases a barium enema should always be done first.

Treatment

Patients may be treated with supervised bed rest in a hospital and bowel rest. Bowel rest means that nothing is taken by mouth and patients are fed intravenously or through the use of a nasogastric tube. A nasogastric tube is a tube inserted through the nose, down the throat, and into the stomach. A similar tube can be inserted in the intestine. The contents are then suctioned out. In some cases, especially where there is a mechanical obstruction, surgery may be necessary.

Drug therapies that promote intestinal motility (ability of the intestine to move spontaneously), such as cisapride and vasopressin (Pitressin), are sometimes prescribed.

Alternative treatment

Alternative practitioners offer few treatment suggestions, but focus on prevention by keeping the bowels healthy through eating a good diet, high in fiber and low in fat. If the case is not a medical emergency, homeopathic treatment and **traditional Chinese medicine** can recommend therapies that may help to reinstate peristalsis.

Prognosis

The outcome of ileus varies depending on its cause.

Prevention

Most cases of ileus are not preventable. Surgery to remove a tumor or other mechanical obstruction will help prevent a recurrence.

Some measures that have been recommended to minimize the severity of postoperative ileus or shorten its duration include making sure that any electrolyte imbalances are corrected, and using nonopioid medications to relieve **pain**, as opioid drugs (including morphine, oxycodone, and codeine) tend to cause **constipation**. One group of drugs that shows promise for treating abdominal pain is a class of medications known as kappa-opioid agonists. As of 2004, however,

KEY TERMS

Computed tomography scan (or CT scan)—A computer enhanced x-ray study performed to detect abnormalities that do not show up on normal x rays.

Meconium—A greenish fecal material that forms the first bowel movement of an infant.

Peritoneum—The transparent membrane lining the abdominal cavity that holds internal organs in place.

these drugs are still under investigation for controlling visceral pain in humans.

Resources

BOOKS

Beers, Mark H., MD, and Robert Berkow, MD, editors. "Ileus." Section 3, Chapter 25. In *The Merck Manual of Diagnosis and Therapy*. Whitehouse Station, NJ: Merck Research Laboratories, 2004.

PERIODICALS

Baig, M. K., and and S. D. Wexner. "Postoperative Ileus: A Review." *Diseases of the Colon and Rectum* 47 (April 2004): 516–526.

Lassandro, F., N. Gagliardi, M. Scuderi, et al. "Gallstone Ileus Analysis of Radiological Findings in 27 Patients." *European Journal of Radiology* 50 (April 2004): 23–29.

Pavone, P., T. Johnson, P. S. Saulog, et al. "Perioperative Morbidity in Bilateral One-Stage Total Knee Replacements." *Clinical Orthopaedics and Related Research* 421 (April 2004): 155–161.

Riviere, P. J. "Peripheral Kappa-Opioid Agonists for Visceral Pain." *British Journal of Pharmacology* 141 (April 2004): 1331–1334.

OTHER

"Bowel Paralysis." *Trigan Oncology Associates Page.* < http://www.trigan.com/ileus.htm >.

"Intestinal Obstruction." *HealthAnswers.com.* < http://www.healthanswers.com/database/ami/converted/000260.html >.

Tish Davidson, A. M.
Rebecca J. Frey, PhD

Immobilization

Definition

Immobilization refers to the process of holding a joint or bone in place with a splint, cast, or brace. This is done to prevent an injured area from moving while it heals.

Purpose

Splints, casts, and braces support and protect broken bones, dislocated joints, and such injured soft tissue as tendons and ligaments. Immobilization restricts motion to allow the injured area to heal. It can help reduce **pain**, swelling, and muscle spasm. In some cases, splints and casts are applied after surgical procedures that repair bones, tendons, or ligaments. This allows for protection and proper alignment early in the healing phase.

Precautions

There are no special precautions for immobilization.

Description

When an arm, hand, leg, or foot requires immobilization, the cast, splint, or brace will generally extend from the joint above the injury to the joint below the injury. For example, an injury to the mid-calf requires immobilization from the knee to the ankle and foot. Injuries of the hip and upper thigh or shoulder and upper arm require a cast that encircles the body and extends down the injured leg or arm.

Casts and splints

Casts are generally used for immobilization of a broken bone. Once the doctor makes sure the two broken ends of the bone are aligned, a cast is put on to keep them in place until they are rejoined through natural healing. Casts are applied by a physician, a nurse, or an assistant. They are custom-made to fit each person, and are usually made of plaster or fiberglass. Fiberglass weighs less than plaster, is more durable, and allows the skin more adequate airflow than plaster. A layer of cotton or synthetic padding is first wrapped around the skin to cover the injured area and protect the skin. The plaster or fiberglass is then applied over this.

Most casts should not be gotten wet. However, some types of fiberglass casts use Gore-tex padding that is waterproof and allows the person to completely immerse the cast in water when taking a shower or bath. There are some circumstances when this type of cast material can not be used.

A splint is often used to immobilize a dislocated joint while it heals. Splints are also often used for finger injuries, such as **fractures** or baseball finger. Baseball finger is an injury in which the tendon at the

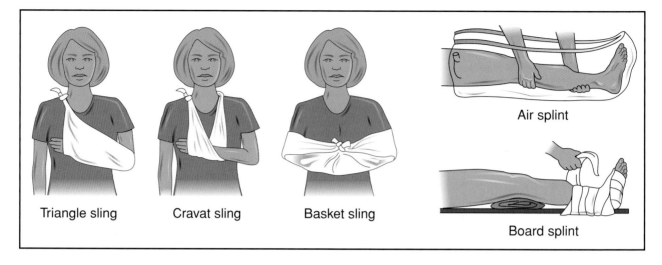

Immobilization refers to the process of immobilizing or fixating the position of a joint, bone, extremity, or torso with a splint, cast, or brace. Immobilization can help reduce pain, swelling, and muscle spasms. The illustrations above feature several types of immobilization techniques. *(Illustration by Electronic Illustrators Group.)*

end of the finger is separated from the bone as a result of trauma. Splinting also is used to immobilize an injured arm or leg immediately after an injury. Before moving a person who has injured an arm or leg some type of temporary splint should be applied to prevent further injury to the area. Splints may be made of acrylic, polyethylene foam, plaster of paris, or aluminum. In an emergency, a splint can be made from a piece of wood or rolled magazine.

Slings

Slings are often used to support the arm after a fracture or other injury. They are generally used along with a cast or splint, but sometimes are used alone as a means of immobilization. They can be used in an emergency to immobilize the arm until the person can be seen by a doctor. A triangular bandage is placed under the injured arm and then tied around the neck.

Braces

Braces are used to support, align, or hold a body part in the correct position. Braces are sometimes used after a surgical procedure is performed on an arm or leg. They can also be used for an injury. Since some braces can be easily taken off and put back on, they are often used when the person must have physical therapy or **exercise** the limb during the healing process. Many braces can also be adjusted to allow for a certain amount of movement.

Braces can be custom-made, or a ready-made brace can be used. The off-the-shelf braces are made in a variety of shapes and sizes. They generally have

Velcro straps that make the brace easy to adjust, and to put on and take off. Both braces and splints offer less support and protection than a cast and may not be a treatment option in all circumstances.

Collars

A collar is generally used for neck injuries. A soft collar can relieve pain by restricting movement of the head and neck. They also transfer some of the weight of the head from the neck to the chest. Stiff collars are generally used to support the neck when there has been a fracture in one of the bones of the neck. Cervical collars are widely used by emergency personnel at the scene of injuries when there is a potential neck or **head injury**.

Traction

Immobilization may also be secured by **traction**. Traction involves using a method for applying tension to correct the alignment of two structures (such as two bones) and hold them in the correct position. For example, if the bone in the thigh breaks, the broken ends may have a tendency to overlap. Use of traction will hold them in the correct position for healing to occur. The strongest form of traction involves inserting a stainless steel pin through a bony prominence attached by a horseshoe-shaped bow and rope to a pulley and weights suspended over the end of the patient's bed.

Traction must be balanced by countertraction. This is obtained by tilting the bed and allowing the patient's body to act as a counterweight. Another technique involves applying weights pulling in the opposite direction.

Traction for neck injuries may be in the form of a leather or cotton cloth halter placed around the chin and lower back of the head. For very severe neck injuries that require maximum traction, tongs that resemble ice tongs are inserted into small holes drilled in the outer skull.

All traction requires careful observation and adjustment by doctors and nurses to maintain proper balance and alignment of the traction with free suspension of the weights.

Immobilization can also be secured by a form of traction called skin traction. This is a combination of a splint and traction that is applied to the arms or legs by strips of adhesive tape placed over the skin of the arm or leg. Adhesive strips, moleskin, or foam rubber traction strips are applied on the skin. This method is effective only if a moderate amount of traction is required.

Preparation

There are many reasons for immobilization using splints, casts, and braces. Each person should understand his or her diagnosis clearly.

Aftercare

After a cast or splint has been put on, the injured arm or leg should be elevated for 24 to 72 hours. It is recommended that the person lie or sit with the injured arm or leg raised above the level of the heart. Rest combined with elevation will reduce pain and speed the healing process by minimizing swelling.

Fingers or toes can be exercised as much as can be tolerated after casting. This has been found to decrease swelling and prevent stiffness. If excessive swelling is noted, the application of ice to the splint or cast may be helpful.

After the cast, splint, or brace is removed, gradual exercise is usually performed to regain muscle strength and motion. The doctor may also recommend **hydrotherapy**, **heat treatments**, and other forms of physical therapy.

Risks

For some people, such as those in traction, immobilization will require long periods of bedrest. Lying in one position in bed for an extended period of time can result in sores on the skin (decubitus ulcers) and skin infection. Long periods of bedrest can also cause a buildup of fluid in the lungs or an infection in the lungs (**pneumonia**). Urinary infection can also be a result of extended bedrest.

KEY TERMS

Decubitus ulcers — A pressure sore resulting from ulceration of the skin occurring in persons confined to bed for long periods of time

Ligament—Ligaments are structures that hold bones together and prevent excessive movement of the joint. They are tough, fibrous bands of tissue.

Pneumonia — An acute or chronic disease characterized by inflammation of the lungs and caused by viruses, bacteria, or other microorganisms.

Tendon—Tendons are structures that attach bones to muscles and muscles to other muscles.

People who have casts, splints, or braces on their arms or legs will generally spend several weeks not using the injured arm or leg. This lack of use can result in decreased muscle tone and shrinkage of the muscle (atrophy). Much of this loss can usually be regained, however, through **rehabilitation** after the injury has healed.

Immobility can also cause psychological **stress**. An individual restricted to a bed with a traction device may become frustrated and bored, and perhaps even depressed, irritable, and withdrawn.

There is the possibility of decreased circulation if the cast, splint, or brace fits too tightly. Excessive pressure over a nerve can cause irritation or possible damage if not corrected. If the cast, splint, or brace breaks or malfunctions, the healing process of the bone or soft tissue can be disrupted and lead to deformity.

Normal results

Normally, the surgical or injured area heals appropriately with the help of immobilization. The form of immobilization can be discontinued, which is followed by an appropriate rehabilitation program under the supervision of a physical therapist to regain range of motion and strength.

Resources

OTHER

"Casts & Splints." *The Center for Orthopaedics and Sports Medicine.* < http://www.arthroscopy.com >.

Jeffrey P. Larson, RPT

Immune complex detection *see* **Immune complex test**

Immune complex test

Definition

These tests evaluate the immune system, whose function is to defend the body against such invaders as bacteria and viruses. The immune system also plays a role in the control of **cancer**, and is responsible for the phenomena of allergy, hypersensitivity, and rejection problems when organs or tissue are transplanted.

One of the ways the immune system protects the body is by producing proteins called antibodies. Antibodies are formed in response to another type of protein called an antigen (anything foreign or different from a natural body protein). Immune complex reactions occur when large numbers of antigen-antibody complexes accumulate in the body.

Purpose

The purpose of the immune complex test is to demonstrate circulating immune complexes in the blood, to estimate the severity of immune complex disease, and to monitor response to therapy.

Precautions

Because this test is requested when the physician suspects that a patient's immune system is not functioning properly, special care should be taken during and after blood is drawn. For example, the venipuncture site should be kept clean and dry to avoid any chance of infection.

Description

Immune complexes are normally not detected in the blood. However, when immune complexes are produced faster than they can be cleared by the system, immune complex disease may occur. Examples of such disorders are drug sensitivity, **rheumatoid arthritis**, and a disease called **systemic lupus erythematosus**, or SLE.

The method generally used for detecting immune complexes is examination of a tissue obtained by biopsy (removal and examination of tissue sample) and the subsequent use of different staining techniques with specific antibodies. However, since tissue biopsies do not provide information about the level of complexes still in the circulatory system, serum assays obtained from blood samples which indirectly detect circulating immune complexes are useful. However, due to the variability of these complexes, several test

methods may be used. Also, as most immune complex assays have not been standardized, more than one test may be required to achieve accurate results.

Preparation

This test requires a blood sample. It is not necessary for the patient to be in a **fasting** (nothing to eat or drink) state before the test.

Risks

Risks for this test are minimal, but may include slight bleeding from the blood-drawing site, **fainting** or feeling lightheaded after venipuncture, or hematoma (blood accumulating under the puncture site).

Normal results

Normally, immune complexes are not detected in the blood.

Abnormal results

The presence of detectable immune complexes in the blood is important in the diagnosis of autoimmune

> ### KEY TERMS
>
> **Antibody**—A (immunoglobulin) molecule that interacts with a specific antigen. Antibodies provide protection from microscopic invaders like bacteria.
>
> **Antigen**—Any substance that is capable under certain circumstances of producing an immune response either from antibodies or T-cells; bacteria are often antigens.
>
> **Autoimmune disorder**—A disorder caused by a reaction of an individual's immune system against the organs or tissues of the body. Autoimmune processes can have different results: slow destruction of a particular type of cell or tissue, stimulation of an organ into excessive growth, or interference in function.
>
> **Biopsy**—The removal and examination, usually under a microscope, of tissue from the living body. Used for diagnosis.
>
> **Systemic lupus erythematosus**—A chronic disease of the connective tissues in the body; characterized by involvement of the skin, joints, kidneys, and serosal membranes (membranes that form the outer covering of organs in the abdomen or chest).

diseases, such as SLE and rheumatoid arthritis. However, for definitive diagnosis, the results of other studies must be considered with the presence of any immune complex. For example, immune complexes are associated with high numbers of a component called antinuclear antibodies in the diagnosis of systemic lupus erythematosus. A different example are the kidneys. Because of their filtering functions, elements in the kidneys called renal glomeruli can be affected by immune complexes. In such cases, renal biopsy is used to provide conclusive evidence for immune complex.

Resources

BOOKS

Jacobs, David S., et al. *Laboratory Test Handbook.* 4th ed. New York: Lexi-Comp Inc., 1996.

Janis O. Flores

Immunodeficiency

Definition

Immunodeficiency disorders are a group of disorders in which part of the immune system is missing or defective. Therefore, the body's ability to fight infections is impaired. As a result, the person with an immunodeficiency disorder will have frequent infections that are generally more severe and last longer than usual.

Description

The immune system is the body's main method for fighting infections. Any defect in the immune system decreases a person's ability to fight infections. A person with an immunodeficiency disorder may get more frequent infections, heal more slowly, and have a higher incidence of some cancers.

The normal immune system involves a complex interaction of certain types of cells that can recognize and attack "foreign" invaders, such as bacteria, viruses, and fungi. It also plays a role in fighting **cancer**. The immune system has both innate and adaptive components. Innate immunity is made up of immune protections people are born with. Adaptive immunity develops throughout life. It adapts to fight off specific invading organisms. Adaptive immunity is divided into two components: humoral immunity and cellular immunity.

The innate immune system is made up of the skin (which acts as a barrier to prevent organisms from entering the body), white blood cells called phagocytes, a system of proteins called the complement system, and chemicals called interferons. When phagocytes encounter an invading organism, they surround and engulf it to destroy it. The complement system also attacks bacteria. The elements in the complement system create a hole in the outer layer of the target cell, which leads to the death of the cell.

The adaptive component of the immune system is extremely complex, and is still not entirely understood. Basically, it has the ability to recognize an organism or tumor cell as not being a normal part of the body, and to develop a response to attempt to eliminate it.

The humoral response of adaptive immunity involves a type of cell called B lymphocytes. B lymphocytes manufacture proteins called antibodies (which are also called immunoglobulins). Antibodies attach themselves to the invading foreign substance. This allows the phagocytes to begin engulfing and destroying the organism. The action of antibodies also activates the complement system. The humoral response is particularly useful for attacking bacteria.

The cellular response of adaptive immunity is useful for attacking viruses, some parasites, and possibly cancer cells. The main type of cell in the cellular response is T lymphocytes. There are helper T lymphocytes and killer T lymphocytes. The helper T lymphocytes play a role in recognizing invading organisms, and they also help killer T lymphocytes to multiply. As the name suggests, killer T lymphocytes act to destroy the target organism.

Defects can occur in any component of the immune system or in more than one component (combined immunodeficiency). Different immunodeficiency diseases involve different components of the immune system. The defects can be inherited and/or present at birth (congenital) or acquired.

Congenital immunodeficiency disorders

Congenital immunodeficiency is present at the time of birth, and is the result of genetic defects. These immunodeficiency disorders are also called primary immunodeficiencies. Even though more than 70 different types of congenital immunodeficiency disorders have been identified, they rarely occur. About 50,000 new cases are diagnosed in the United States each year. Congenital immunodeficiencies may occur as a result of defects in B lymphocytes, T lymphocytes, or both. They also can occur in the innate immune system.

HUMORAL IMMUNITY DISORDERS. Bruton's agammaglobulinemia, also known as **X-linked agammaglobulinemia**, a congenital immunodeficiency disorder. The defect results in a decrease or absence of B lymphocytes, and therefore a decreased ability to make antibodies. People with this disorder are particularly susceptible to infections of the throat, skin, middle ear, and lungs. It is seen only in males because it is caused by a genetic defect on the X chromosome. Since males have only one X chromosome, they always have the defect if the gene is present. Females can have the defective gene, but since they have two X chromosomes, there will be a normal gene on the other X chromosome to counter it. Women may pass the defective gene on to their male children.

B LYMPHOCYTE DEFICIENCIES. If there is an abnormality in either the development or function of B lymphocytes, the ability to make antibodies will be impaired. This allows the body to be susceptible to recurrent infections.

A type of B lymphocyte deficiency involves a group of disorders called selective immunoglobulin deficiency syndomes. Immunoglobulin is another name for antibody, and there are five different types of immunoglobulins (called IgA, IgG, IgM, IgD, and IgE). The most common type of immunoglobulin deficiency is selective IgA deficiency, occurring in about one in every 500 white persons. The amounts of the other antibody types are normal. Some patients with selective IgA deficiency experience no symptoms, while others have occasional lung infections and **diarrhea**. In another immunoglobulin disorder, IgG and IgA antibodies are deficient and there is increased IgM. People with this disorder tend to get severe bacterial infections.

Common variable immunodeficiency is another type of B lymphocyte deficiency. In this disorder, the production of one or more of the immunoglobulin types is decreased and the antibody response to infections is impaired. It generally develops around the age of 10-20. The symptoms vary among affected people. Most people with this disorder have frequent infections, and some also will experience anemia and **rheumatoid arthritis**. Many people with common variable immunodeficiency develop cancer.

T LYMPHOCYTE DEFICIENCIES. Severe defects in the ability of T lymphocytes to mature results in impaired immune responses to infections with viruses, fungi, and certain types of bacteria. These infections are usually severe and can be fatal.

DiGeorge syndrome is a T lymphocyte deficiency that starts during fetal development and is the result of a deletion in a particular chromosome. Children with DiGeorge syndrome either do not have a thymus or have an underdeveloped thymus. Since the thymus is a major organ that directs the production of T-lymphocytes, these patients have very low numbers of T-lymphocytes. They are susceptible to recurrent infections, and usually have physical abnormalities as well. For example, they may have low-set ears, a small receding jawbone, and wide-spaced eyes. People with DiGeorge syndrome are particularly susceptible to viral and fungal infections.

In some cases, no treatment is required for DiGeorge syndrome because T lymphocyte production improves. Either an underdeveloped thymus begins to produce more T lymphocytes or organ sites other than the thymus compensate by producing more T lymphocytes.

COMBINED IMMUNODEFICIENCIES. Some types of immunodeficiency disorders affect both B lymphocytes and T lymphocytes. For example, **severe combined immunodeficiency** disease (SCID) is caused by the defective development or function of these two types of lymphocytes. It results in impaired humoral and cellular immune responses. SCID usually is recognized during the first year of life. It tends to cause a fungal infection of the mouth (thrush), diarrhea, **failure to thrive**, and serious infections. If not treated with a bone marrow transplant, a person with SCID will generally die from infections before age two. In 2003, a report showed a new form of severe SCID with severe mutation of T receptor cells.

DISORDERS OF INNATE IMMUNITY. Disorders of innate immunity affect phagocytes or the complement system. These disorders also result in recurrent infections.

Acquired immunodeficiency disorders

Acquired immunodeficiency is more common than congenital immunodeficiency. It is the result of an infectious process or other disease. For example, the human immunodeficiency virus (HIV) is the virus that causes acquired immunodeficiency syndrome (AIDS). However, this is not the most common cause of acquired immunodeficiency.

Acquired immunodeficiency often occurs as a complication of other conditions and diseases. For example, the most common causes of acquired immunodeficiency are **malnutrition**, some types of cancer, and infections. People who weigh less than 70% of the average weight of persons of the same age and gender are considered to be malnourished. Examples of types of infections that can lead to immunodeficiency are **chickenpox**, cytomegalovirus, German **measles**, measles, **tuberculosis**, **infectious mononucleosis** (Epstein-Barr virus), chronic hepatitis, lupus, and bacterial and fungal infections.

In 2003, a new infection emerged that produces immunodeficiency. **Severe acute respiratory syndrome (SARS)** mysteriously appeared in a hospital in China. It eventually affected 8,000 people in Asia and Canada, killing 800 altogether. The virus is characterized by **fever**, lower respiratory tract symptoms, and abnormal chest x rays. However, it also produces immunodeficiency. No cases of the disease were reported from July 2003 through December 2003, but scientists feared it would reappear.

Sometimes, acquired immunodeficiency is brought on by drugs used to treat another condition. For example, patients who have an organ transplant are given drugs to suppress the immune system so the body will not reject the organ. Also, some **chemotherapy** drugs, which are given to treat cancer, have the side effect of killing cells of the immune system. During the period of time that these drugs are being taken, the risk of infection increases. It usually returns to normal after the person stops taking the drugs.

Causes and symptoms

Congenital immunodeficiency is caused by genetic defects, which generally occur while the fetus is developing in the womb. These defects affect the development and/or function of one or more of the components of the immune system. Acquired immunodeficiency is the result of a disease process, and it occurs later in life. The causes, as described above, can be diseases, infections, or the side effects of drugs given to treat other conditions.

People with an immunodeficiency disorder tend to become infected by organisms that do not usually cause disease in healthy persons. The major symptoms of most immunodeficiency disorders are repeated infections that heal slowly. These chronic infections cause symptoms that persist for long periods of time. People with chronic infection tend to be pale and thin. They may have skin **rashes**. Their lymph nodes tend to be larger than normal and their liver and spleen also may be enlarged. The lymph nodes are small organs that house antibodies and lymphocytes. Broken blood vessels, especially near the surface of the skin, may be seen. This can result in black-and-blue marks in the skin. The person may lose hair from their head.

Sometimes, a red inflammation of the lining of the eye (**conjunctivitis**) is present. They may have a crusty appearance in and on the nose from chronic nasal dripping.

Diagnosis

Usually, the first sign that a person might have an immunodeficiency disorder is that they do not improve rapidly when given **antibiotics** to treat an infection. Strong indicators that an immunodeficiency disorder may be present is when rare diseases occur or the patient gets ill from organisms that do not normally cause diseases, especially if the patient gets repeatedly infected. If this happens in very young children it is an indication that a genetic defect may be causing an immunodeficiency disorder. When this situation occurs in older children or young adults, their medical history will be reviewed to determine if childhood diseases may have caused an immunodeficiency disorder. Other possibilities will then be considered, such as recently acquired infections–for example, HIV, hepatitis, tuberculosis, etc.

Laboratory tests are used to determine the exact nature of the immunodeficiency. Most tests are performed on blood samples. Blood contains antibodies, lymphocytes, phagocytes, and complement components—all of the major immune components that might cause immunodeficiency. A blood cell count will determine if the number of phagocytic cells or lymphocytes is below normal. Lower than normal counts of either of these two cell types correlates with immunodeficiencies. The blood cells also are checked for their appearance. Sometimes a person may have normal cell counts, but the cells are structurally defective. If the lymphocyte cell count is low, further testing is usually done to determine whether any particular type of lymphocyte is lower than normal. A lymphocyte proliferation test is done to determine if the lymphocytes can respond to stimuli. The failure to respond to stimulants correlates with immunodeficiency. Antibody levels can be measured by a process called electrophoresis. Complement levels can be determined by immunodiagnostic tests.

Treatment

There is no cure for immunodeficiency disorders. Therapy is aimed at controlling infections and, for some disorders, replacing defective or absent components.

Patients with Bruton's agammaglobulinemia must be given periodic injections of a substance called gamma globulin throughout their lives to make up for their decreased ability to make antibodies. The gamma globulin preparation contains antibodies against common invading bacteria. If left untreated, the disease usually is fatal.

Common variable immunodeficiency also is treated with periodic injections of gamma globulin throughout life. Additionally, antibiotics are given when necessary to treat infections.

Patients with selective IgA deficiency usually do not require any treatment. Antibiotics can be given for frequent infections.

In some cases, no treatment is required for DiGeorge syndrome because T lymphocyte production improves on its own. Either an underdeveloped thymus begins to produce more T lymphocytes or organ sites other than the thymus compensate by producing more T lymphocytes. In some severe cases, a bone marrow transplant or thymus transplant can be done to correct the problem.

For patients with SCID, **bone marrow transplantation** is necessary. In this procedure, healthy bone marrow from a donor who has a similar type of tissue (usually a relative, like a brother or sister) is removed. The bone marrow is a substance that resides in the cavity of bones. It is the factory that produces blood, including some of the white blood cells that make up the immune system. The bone marrow of the person receiving the transplant is destroyed, and is then replaced with marrow from the donor.

Treatment of the HIV infection that causes AIDS consists of drugs called antiretrovirals. These drugs attempt to inhibit the process that the virus goes through to kill T lymphocytes. Several of these drugs used in various combinations with one another can prolong the period of time before the disease becomes apparent. However, this is not a cure. Other treatments for people with AIDS are aimed at the particular infections and conditions that arise as a result of the impaired immune system. SARS is a relatively new acquired disease. Treatment to date involves combination therapy with steroids and interferon and supplemental oxygen for breathing difficulties. In 2004, reports in the United States said that a drug called octagam 5%, an intravenous immunoglobulin, was used to treat primary immunodeficiency diseases. The drug has been used in Europe for the same purpose.

In most cases, immunodeficiency caused by malnutrition is reversible. The health of the immune system is directly linked to the nutritional status of the patient. Among the essential nutrients required by the immune system are proteins, **vitamins**, iron, and zinc.

For people being treated for cancer, periodic relief from chemotherapy drugs can restore the function of the immune system.

In general, people with immunodeficiency disorders should maintain a healthy diet. This is because malnutrition can aggravate immunodeficiencies. They also should avoid being near people who have colds or are sick because they can easily acquire new infections. For the same reason, they should practice good personal hygiene, especially dental care. People with immunodeficiency disorders also should avoid eating undercooked food because it might contain bacteria that could cause infection. This food would not cause infection in normal persons, but in someone with an immunodeficiency, food is a potential source of infectious organisms. People with immunodeficiency should be given antibiotics at the first indication of an infection.

Prognosis

The prognosis depends on the type of immunodeficiency disorder. People with Bruton's agammaglobulinemia who are given injections of gamma globulin generally live into their 30s or 40s. They often die from chronic infections, usually of the lung. People with selective IgA deficiency generally live normal lives. They may experience problems if given a blood **transfusion**, and therefore they should wear a Medic Alert bracelet or have some other way of alerting any physician who treats them that they have this disorder.

SCID is the most serious of the immunodeficiency disorders. If a bone marrow transplant is not successfully performed, the child usually will not live beyond two years old.

People with HIV/AIDS are living longer than in the past because of the **antiretroviral drugs** that became available in the mid 1990s. However, AIDS still is a fatal disease. People with AIDS usually die of opportunistic infections, which are infections that occur because the impaired immune system is unable to fight them.

Prevention

There is no way to prevent a congenital immunodeficiency disorder. However, someone with a congenital immunodeficiency disorder might want to consider getting **genetic counseling** before having children to find out if there is a chance they will pass the defect on to their children.

Some of the infections associated with acquired immunodeficiency can be prevented or treated before they cause problems. For example, there are effective treatments for tuberculosis and most bacterial and fungal infections. HIV infection can be prevented by practicing "safe sex" and not using illegal intravenous drugs. These are the primary routes of transmitting the virus. For people who do not know the HIV status of the person with whom they are having sex, safe sex involves using a **condom**.

Malnutrition can be prevented by getting adequate **nutrition**. Malnutrition tends to be more of a problem in developing countries.

Resources

PERIODICALS

"2003 Begins With SARS, Ends With Flu." *Medical Letter on the CDC & FDA* January 11, 2004: 24.

Cooper, Megan A., Thomas L. Pommering, and Katalin Koranyi. "Primary Immunodeficiencies." *American Family Physician* November 15, 2003: 2001.

Fischer, Alain. "Have We Seen the Last Variant of Severe Combined Immunodeficiency?" *The New England Journal of Medicine* November 6, 2003: 1789.

Low, Donald E., and Allison McGreer. "SARS— One Year Later." *The New England Journal of Medicine* December 18, 2003: 2381.

"Octagam is Efficacious for Treating Primary Immuno deficiency Diseases." *Medical Letter on the CDC & FDA* July 11, 2004: 52.

"Preliminary Report Suggests Combination Therapy May Help Treat SARS." *Drug Week* January 9, 2004: 557.

John T. Lohr, PhD
Teresa G. Odle

Immunoelectrophoresis

Definition

Immunoelectrophoresis, also called gamma globulin electrophoresis, or immunoglobulin electrophoresis, is a method of determining the blood levels of three major immunoglobulins: immunoglobulin M (IgM), immunoglobulin G (IgG), and immunoglobulin A (IgA).

Purpose

Immunoelectrophoresis is a powerful analytical technique with high resolving power as it combines separation of antigens by electrophoresis with immunodiffusion against an antiserum. The increased resolution is of benefit in the immunological examination of serum proteins. Immunoelectrophoresis aids in the diagnosis and evaluation of the therapeutic response in many disease states affecting the immune system. It is usually requested when a different type of electrophoresis, called a serum **protein electrophoresis**, has indicated a rise at the immunoglobulin level. Immunoelectrophoresis is also used frequently to diagnose **multiple myeloma**, a disease affecting the bone marrow.

Precautions

Drugs that may cause increased immunoglobulin levels include therapeutic gamma globulin, hydralazine, isoniazid, phenytoin (Dilantin), procainamide, **oral contraceptives**, **methadone**, steroids, and **tetanus** toxoid and antitoxin. The laboratory should be notified if the patient has received any vaccinations or immunizations in the six months before the test. This is mainly because prior immunizations lead to the increased immunoglobulin levels resulting in false positive results.

It should be noted that, because immunoelectrophoresis is not quantitative, it is being replaced by a procedure called immunofixation, which is more sensitive and easier to interpret.

Description

Serum proteins separate in agar gels under the influence of an electric field into albumin, alpha 1, alpha 2, and beta and gamma globulins. Immunoelectrophoresis is performed by placing serum on a slide containing a gel designed specifically for the test. An electric current is then passed through the gel, and immunoglobulins, which contain an electric charge, migrate through the gel according to the difference in their individual electric charges. Antiserum is placed alongside the slide to identify the specific type of immunoglobulin present. The results are used to identify different disease entities, and to aid in monitoring the course of the disease and the therapeutic response of the patient to such conditions as immune deficiencies, autoimmune disease, chronic infections, chronic viral infections, and intrauterine fetal infections.

There are five classes of antibodies: IgM, IgG, IgA, IgE, and IgD.

IgM is produced upon initial exposure to an antigen. For example, when a person receives the first tetanus **vaccination**, antitetanus antibodies of the IgM class are produced 10 to 14 days later. IgM is abundant in the blood but is not normally present in organs or tissues. IgM is primarily responsible for ABO blood grouping and rheumatoid factor, yet is involved in the immunologic reaction to other infections, such as hepatitis. Since IgM does not cross the placenta, an elevation of this immunoglobulin in the newborn indicates intrauterine infection such as **rubella**, cytomegalovirus (CMV) or a sexually transmitted disease (STD).

IgG is the most prevalent type of antibody, comprising approximately 75% of the serum immunoglobulins. IgG is produced upon subsequent exposure to an antigen. As an example, after receiving a second tetanus shot, or booster, a person produces IgG antibodies in five to seven days. IgG is present in both the blood and tissues, and is the only antibody to cross the placenta from the mother to the fetus. Maternal IgG protects the newborn for the first months of life, until the infant's immune system produces its own antibodies.

IgA constitutes approximately 15% of the immunoglobulins within the body. Although it is found to some degree in the blood, it is present primarily in the secretions of the respiratory and gastrointestinal tract, in saliva, colostrum (the yellowish fluid produced by the breasts during late **pregnancy** and the first few days after **childbirth**), and in tears. IgA plays an important role in defending the body against invasion of germs through the mucous membrane-lined organs.

IgE is the antibody that causes acute allergic reactions; it is measured to detect allergic conditions. IgD, which constitutes the smallest portion of the immunoglobulins, is rarely evaluated or detected, and its function is not well understood.

Preparation

This test requires a blood sample.

Aftercare

Because this test is ordered when either very low or very high levels of immunoglobulins are suspected, the patient should be alert for any signs of infection after the test, including **fever**, chills, rash, or skin ulcers. Any bone **pain** or tenderness should also be immediately reported to the physician.

Risks

Risks for this test are minimal, but may include slight bleeding from the blood-drawing site, **fainting** or feeling lightheaded after venipuncture, or bruising.

Normal results

Reference ranges vary from laboratory to laboratory and depend upon the method used. For adults, normal values are usually found within the following ranges (1 mg = approximately 0.000035 oz. and 1 dL = approximately 0.33 oz.):

- IgM: 60–290 mg/dL
- IgG: 700–1,800 mg/dL
- IgA: 70–440 mg/dL

Abnormal results

Increased IgM levels can indicate Waldenström's macroglobulinemia, a malignancy caused by secretion of IgM at high levels by malignant lymphoplasma cells. Increased IgM levels can also indicate chronic infections, such as hepatitis or mononucleosis and autoimmune diseases, like **rheumatoid arthritis**.

Decreased IgM levels can be indicative of **AIDS**, immunosuppression caused by certain drugs like steroids or dextran, or leukemia.

Increased levels of IgG can indicate chronic **liver disease**, autoimmune diseases, hyperimmunization reactions, or certain chronic infections, such as **tuberculosis** or **sarcoidosis**.

Decreased levels of IgG can indicate **Wiskott-Aldrich syndrome**, a genetic deficiency caused by inadequate synthesis of IgG and other immunoglobulins. Decreased IgG can also be seen with AIDS and leukemia.

Increased levels of IgA can indicate chronic liver disease, chronic infections, or inflammatory bowel disease.

Decreased levels of IgA can be found in ataxia, a condition affecting balance and gait, limb or eye movements, speech, and telangiectasia, an increase in the size and number of the small blood vessels in an area of skin, causing redness. Decreased

IgA levels are also seen in conditions of low blood protein (hypoproteinemia), and drug immunosuppression.

Resources

BOOKS

Fischbach, Frances T. *A Manual of Laboratory Diagnostic Tests*. Philadelphia: Lippincott Williams & Wilkins, 1999.

Pagana, Kathleen D., and Timothy J. Pagana. *Mosby's Manual of Diagnostic and Laboratory Tests*. St. Louis, MO: Mosby, Inc., 1999.

Janis O. Flores

Immunoglobulin *see* **Gammaglobulin**

Immunoglobulin deficiency syndromes

Definition

Immunoglobulin deficiency syndromes are a group of **immunodeficiency** disorders in which the patient has a reduced number of or lack of antibodies.

Description

Immunoglobulins (Ig) are antibodies. There are five major classes of antibodies: IgG, IgM, IgA, IgD, and IgE.

- IgG is the most abundant of the classes of immunoglobulins. It is the antibody for viruses, bacteria, and antitoxins. It is found in most tissues and plasma.

- IgM is the first antibody present in an immune response.

- IgA is an early antibody for bacteria and viruses. It is found in saliva, tears, and all other mucous secretions.

- IgD activity is not well understood.

- IgE is present in the respiratory secretions. It is an antibody for parasitic diseases, **Hodgkin's disease**, hay **fever**, **atopic dermatitis**, and allergic **asthma**.

All antibodies are made by B-lymphocytes (B-cells). Any disease that harms the development or function of B-cells will cause a decrease in the amount of antibodies produced. Since antibodies are essential in fighting infectious diseases, people with immunoglobulin deficiency syndromes become ill more often. However, the cellular immune system is still functional, so these patients are more prone to infection caused by organisms usually controlled by antibodies. Most of these invading germs (microbes) make capsules, a mechanism used to confuse the immune system. In a healthy body, antibodies can bind to the capsule and overcome the bacteria's defenses. The bacteria that make capsules include the streptococci, meningococci, and *Haemophilus influenzae*. These organisms cause such diseases as otitis, **sinusitis**, **pneumonia**, **meningitis**, **osteomyelitis**, septic arthritis, and **sepsis**. Patients with immunoglobulin deficiencies are also prone to some viral infections, including echovirus, enterovirus, and **hepatitis B**. They may also have a bad reaction to the attenuated version of the **polio** virus vaccine.

There are two types of immunodeficiency diseases: primary and secondary. Secondary disorders occur in normally healthy bodies that are suffering from an underlying disease. Once the disease is treated, the immunodeficiency is reversed. Immunoglobulin deficiency syndromes are primary immunodeficiency diseases, occurring because of defective B-cells or antibodies. They account for 50% of all primary immunodeficiencies, and they are, therefore, the most prevalent type of immunodeficiency disorders.

- **X-linked agammaglobulinemia** is an inherited disease. The defect is on the X chromosome and, consequently, this disease is seen more frequently in males than females. The defect results in a failure of B-cells to mature. Mature B-cells are capable of making antibodies and developing "memory," a feature in which the B-cell will rapidly recognize and respond to an infectious agent the next time it is encountered. All classes of antibodies are decreased in agammaglobulinemia.

- Selective IgA deficiency is an inherited disease, resulting from a failure of B-cells to switch from making IgM, the early antibody, to IgA. Although the B-cell numbers are normal, and the B-cells are otherwise normal (they can still make all other classes of antibodies), the amount of IgA produced is limited. This results in more infections of mucosal surfaces, such as the nose, throat, lungs, and intestines.

- Transient hypogammaglobulinemia of infancy is a temporary disease of unknown cause. It is believed to be caused by a defect in the development of T-helper cells (cells that recognize foreign antigens and activate T- and B-cells in an immune response). As the child ages, the number and condition of T-helper cells improves and this situation corrects itself. Hypogammaglobulinemia is characterized by low levels of **gammaglobulin** (antibodies) in the blood. During the disease period, patients have decreased levels of IgG and IgA antibodies. In lab tests, the antibodies that are present do not react well with infectious bacteria.

- Common variable immunodeficiency is a defect in both B cells and T-lymphocytes. It results in a near complete lack of antibodies in the blood.

- Ig heavy chain deletions is a genetic disease in which part of the antibody molecule is not produced. It results in the loss of several antibody classes and subclasses, including most IgG antibodies and all IgA and IgE antibodies. The disease occurs because part of the gene for the heavy chain has been lost.

- Selective IgG subclass deficiencies is a group of genetic diseases in which some of the subclasses of IgG are not made. There are four subclasses in the IgG class of antibodies. As the B-cell matures, it can switch from one subclass to another. In these diseases there is a defect in the maturation of the B-cells that results in a lack of switching.

- IgG deficiency with hyper-IgM is a disease that results when the B-cell fails to switch from making IgM to IgG. This produces an increase in the amount of IgM antibodies present and a decrease in the amount of IgG antibodies. This disease is the result of a genetic mutation.

Causes and symptoms

Immunoglobulin deficiencies are the result of congenital defects affecting the development and function

KEY TERMS

Antibody—Another term for immunoglobulin. A protein molecule that specifically recognizes and attaches to infectious agents.

T-helper cell—A type of cell that recognizes foreign antigens and activates T- and B-cells in an immune response.

of B lymphocytes (B-cells). There are two main points in the development of B-cells when defects can occur. First, B-cells can fail to develop into antibody-producing cells. X-linked agammaglobulinemia is an example of this disease. Secondly, B-cells can fail to make a particular type of antibody or fail to switch classes during maturation. Initially, when B-cells start making antibodies for the first time, they make IgM. As they mature and develop memory, they switch to one of the other four classes of antibodies. Failures in switching or failure to make a subclass of antibody leads to immunoglobulin deficiency diseases. Another mechanism that results in decreased antibody production is a defect in T-helper cells. Generally, defects in T-helper cells are listed as severe combined immunodeficiencies.

Symptoms are persistent and frequent infections, **diarrhea**, **failure to thrive**, and malabsorption (of nutrients).

Diagnosis

An immunodeficiency disease is suspected when children become ill frequently, especially from the same organisms. The profile of organisms that cause infection in patients with immunoglobulin deficiency syndrome is unique and is preliminary evidence for this disease. Laboratory tests are performed to verify the diagnosis. Antibodies can be found in the blood. Blood is collected and analyzed for the content and types of antibodies present. Depending on the type of immunoglobulin deficiency the laboratory tests will show a decrease or absence of antibodies or specific antibody subclasses.

Treatment

Immunodeficiency diseases cannot be cured. Patients are treated with **antibiotics** and immune serum. Immune serum is a source of antibodies. Antibiotics are useful for fighting bacteria infections. There are some drugs that are effective against fungi, but very few drugs that are effective against viral diseases.

Bone marrow transplantation can, in most cases, completely correct the immunodefiency.

Prognosis

Patients with immunoglobulin defiency syndromes must practice impeccable health maintenance and care, paying particular attention to optimal dental care, in order to stay in good health.

Resources

BOOKS

Berkow, Robert, editor. *Merck Manual of Medical Information*. Whitehouse Station, NJ: Merck Research Laboratories, 1997.

Jacqueline L. Longe

Immunoglobulin electrophoresis *see* **Immunoelectrophoresis**

Immunoglobulins G, A, and M test *see* **Immunoelectrophoresis**

Immunologic therapies

Definition

Immunologic therapy is the treatment of disease using medicines that boost the body's natural immune response.

Purpose

Immunologic therapy is used to improve the immune system's natural ability to fight diseases such as **cancer**, hepatitis and **AIDS**. These drugs may also be used to help the body recover from immunosuppression resulting from treatments such as **chemotherapy** or **radiation therapy**.

Description

Most drugs in this category are synthetic versions of substances produced naturally in the body. In their natural forms, these substances help defend the body against disease. For example, aldesleukin (Proleukin) is an artificially made form of interleukin-2, which helps white blood cells work. Aldesleukin is administered to patients with kidney cancers and skin cancers that have

spread to other parts of the body. Filgrastim (Neupogen) and sargramostim (Leukine) are versions of natural substances called colony stimulating factors, which drive the bone marrow to make new white blood cells. Another type of drug, epoetin (Epogen, Procrit), is a synthetic version of human erythropoietin that stimulates the bone marrow to make new red blood cells. Thrombopoietin stimulates the production of platelets, disk-shaped bodies in the blood that are important in clotting. Interferons are substances the body produces naturally using immune cells to fight infections and tumors. The synthetic interferons carry brand names such as Alferon, Roferon or Intron A. Some of the interferons that are currently in use as drugs are Recombinant Interferon Alfa-2a, Recombinant Interferon Alfa-2b, interferon alfa-n1 and Interferon Alfa-n3. Alfa interferons are used to treat **hairy cell leukemia**, **malignant melanoma** and AIDs-related **Kaposi's sarcoma**. In addition interferons are also used for other conditions such as laryngeal papillomatosis, **genital warts** and certain types of hepatitis.

Recommended dosage

The recommended dosage depends on the type of immunologic therapy. For some medicines, the physician will decide the dosage for each patient, taking into account a patient's weight and whether he/she is taking other medicines. Some drugs used in immunologic therapy are given only in a hospital, under a physician's supervision. For those that patients may give themselves, check with the physician who prescribed the medicine or the pharmacist who filled the prescription for the correct dosage.

Most of these drugs come in injectable form. These drugs are generally administered by the cancer care provider.

Precautions

Aldesleukin

This medicine may temporarily increase the chance of getting infections. It may also lower the number of platelets in the blood, and thus possibly interfering with the blood's ability to clot. Taking these precautions may reduce the chance of such problems:

- Avoid people with infections, if possible.

- Be alert to signs of infection, such as **fever**, chills, **sore throat**, **pain** in the lower back or side, **cough**, hoarseness, or painful or difficulty with urination. If any of these symptoms occur, get in touch with a physician immediately.

- Be alert to signs of bleeding problems, such as black, tarry stools, tiny red spots on the skin, blood in the urine or stools, or any other unusual bleeding or bruising.

- Take care to avoid cuts or other injuries. Be especially careful when using knives, razors, nail clippers and other sharp objects. Check with a dentist for the best ways to clean the teeth and mouth without injuring the gums. Do not have dental work done without checking with a physician.

- Wash hands frequently, and avoid touching the eyes or inside of the nose unless the hands have just been washed.

Aldesleukin may make some medical conditions worse, such as **chickenpox**, **shingles** (herpes zoster), **liver disease**, lung disease, heart disease, underactive thyroid, **psoriasis**, immune system problems and mental problems. The medicine may increase the chance of seizures (convulsions) in people who are prone to having them. Also, the drug's effects may be greater in people with **kidney disease**, because their kidneys are slow to clear the medicine from their bodies.

Colony stimulating factors

Certain drugs used in treating cancer reduce the body's ability to fight infections. Although colony stimulating factors help restore the body's natural defenses, the process takes time. Getting prompt treatment for infections is important, even while taking this medicine. Call the physician at the first sign of illness or infection, such as a sore throat, fever or chills.

People with certain medical conditions could have problems if they take colony stimulating factors. People who have kidney disease, liver disease or conditions caused by inflammation or immune system problems can worsen these problems with colony stimulating factors. Those who have heart disease may be more likely to experience side effects such as water retention and heart rhythm problems while taking these drugs. Finally, patients who have lung disease might increase their chances of suffering from **shortness of breath**. Those who have any of these medical conditions should check with their personal physicians before using colony stimulating factors.

Epoetin

Epoetin is a medicine that may cause seizures (convulsions), especially in people who are prone to having them. No one who takes these drugs should drive, use machines or do anything considered dangerous in case of a seizure.

Epoetin helps the body make new red blood cells, but it is not effective unless there is adequate iron in the body. The physician may recommend taking iron supplements or certain **vitamins** that help supply the body with iron. It is necessary to follow the physician's advice in this instance—recommendations for iron in this case, as with any supplements should only come from a physician.

In studies of laboratory animals, epoetin taken during **pregnancy** caused **birth defects**, including damage to the bones and spine. However, the drug has not been reported to cause problems in human babies whose mothers take it. Women who are pregnant or who may become pregnant should check with their physicians for the most up-to-date information on the safety of taking this medicine during pregnancy.

People with certain medical conditions may have problems if they take this medicine. For example, the chance of side effects may be greater in people with high blood pressure, heart or blood vessel disease or a history of **blood clots**. Epoetin may not work properly in people who have bone problems or sickle cell anemia.

Interferons

Interferons can add to the effects of alcohol and other drugs that slow down the central nervous system, such as **antihistamines**, cold medicine, allergy medicine, sleep aids, medicine for seizures, tranquilizers, some pain relievers, and **muscle relaxants**. They may also add to the effects of anesthetics, including those used for dental procedures. Those taking interferons should check with their physicians before taking any of the above.

Some people experience **dizziness**, unusual **fatigue**, or become less alert than usual while being treated with these drugs. Because of these possible problems, anyone who takes these drugs should not drive, use machines or do anything else considered dangerous until they have determined how the drugs affect them.

Interferons often cause flu-like symptoms, including fever and chills. The physician who prescribes this medicine may recommend taking **acetaminophen** (Tylenol) before—and sometimes after—each dose to keep the fever from getting too high. If the physician recommends this, follow instructions carefully.

Like aldesleukin, interferons may temporarily increase the chance of getting infections and lower the number of platelets in the blood, leading to clotting problems. To help prevent these problems, follow the precautions for reducing the risk of infection and bleeding listed for aldesleukin.

People who have certain medical conditions may have problems if they take interferons. For example, the drugs may worsen some medical conditions, including heart disease, kidney disease, liver disease, lung disease, diabetes, bleeding problems and mental problems. In people who have overactive immune systems, these drugs can even increase the activity of the immune system. People who have shingles or chickenpox, or who have recently been exposed to chickenpox may increase their risk of developing severe problems in other parts of the body if they take interferons. People with a history of seizures or mental problems could at risk if taking interferon.

In teenage women, interferons may cause changes in the menstrual cycle. Young women should discuss this possibility with their physicians. Older people may be more sensitive to the effects of interferons. This may increase the chance of side effects.

These drugs are not known to cause fetal **death**, birth defects or other problems in humans when taken during pregnancy. Women who are pregnant or who may become pregnant should ask their physicians for the latest information on the safety of taking these drugs during pregnancy.

Women who are breastfeeding their babies may need to stop while taking this medicine. Whether interferons pass into breast milk is not known. Because of the chance of serious side effects to the baby, breastfeeding while taking interferon is discouraged. Check with a physician for advice.

General precautions for all types of immunologic therapy

Regular physician visits are necessary during immunologic therapy treatment. This gives the physician a chance to make sure the medicine is working and to check for unwanted side effects.

Anyone who has had unusual reactions to drugs used in immunologic therapy should let the physician know before resuming the drugs. Any **allergies** to foods, dyes, preservatives, or other substances should also be reported.

Side effects

Aldesleukin

In addition to its helpful effects, this medicine may cause serious side effects. Generally, it is given only in a hospital, where medical professionals can watch for early signs of problems. Medical tests might be performed to check for unwanted effects.

Anyone who has breathing problems, fever or chills while being given aldesleukin should check with a physician immediately.

Other side effects should be brought to a physician's attention as soon as possible:

- dizziness
- drowsiness
- confusion
- agitation
- depression
- **nausea and vomiting**
- **diarrhea**
- sores in the mouth and on the lips
- **tingling** of hands or feet
- decrease in urination
- unexplained weight gain of five or more pounds

Some side effects are usually temporary and do not need medical attention unless they are bothersome. These include dry skin; itchy or burning skin rash or redness followed by peeling; loss of appetite; and a general feeling of illness or discomfort.

Colony stimulating factors

As this medicine starts to work, the patient might experience mild pain in the lower back or hips. This is nothing to cause undue concern, and will usually go away within a few days. If the pain is intense or causes discomfort, the physician may prescribe a painkiller.

Other possible side effects include **headache**, joint or muscle pain and skin rash or **itching**. These side effects tend to disappear as the body adjusts to the medicine, and do not need medical treatment. If they continue, or they interfere with normal activities, check with a physician.

Epoetin

This medicine may cause flu-like symptoms, such as muscle aches, bone pain, fever, chills, shivering, and sweating, within a few hours after it is taken. These symptoms usually go away within 12 hours. If they do not, or if they are troubling, check with a physician. Other possible side effects that do not need medical attention are diarrhea, **nausea** or **vomiting** and fatigue or weakness.

Certain side effects should be brought to a physician's attention as soon as possible. These include headache, vision problems, increased blood pressure, fast heartbeat, weight gain and swelling of the face, fingers, lower legs, ankles or feet.

Anyone who has chest pain or seizures after taking epoetin should seek professional emergency medical attention immediately.

Interferons

This medicine may cause temporary hair loss (**alopecia**). While upsetting, it is not a sign that something is seriously wrong. The hair should grow back normally after treatment ends.

As the body adjusts to the medicine many other side effects usually go away during treatment. These include flu-like symptoms, taste alteration, loss of appetite (anorexia), nausea and vomiting, skin rash, and unusual fatigue. If these problems persist, or if they interfere with normal life, check with a physician.

A few more serious side effects should be brought to a physician's attention as soon as possible:

- confusion
- difficulty thinking or concentrating
- nervousness
- depression
- sleep problems
- numbness or tingling in the fingers, toes and face

General caution regarding side effects for all types of immunologic therapy

Other side effects are possible with any type of immunologic therapy. Anyone who has unusual symptoms during or after treatment with these drugs should should contact the physician immediately.

Interactions

Anyone who has immunologic therapy should let the physician know all other medicines being taken. Some combinations of drugs may interact, that can increase or decrease the effects of one or both drugs or can increase the likelihood of side effects. Consultation with a physician is highly recommended to get the insight on whether the possible interactions can interfere with drug therapy or cause harmful effects.

Immunoprevention

Considering that most of the biological modifiers such as cytokines elicit immune response that inhibit incipient tumors before they are clinically evident, immunoprevention has been proposed as a recent strategy for combating cancer. Treatment involving immune molecules (such as cytokines) prepared synthetically or that are not produced by the patients themselves is called as passive immunotherapy. Conversely, a vaccine is a form of active immune therapy because it elicits an immune response in patients. A cancer vaccine may be made of whole tumor cell or of substances or fragments contained in the tumor called antigens.

Newer types of immunologic therapy that are still considered investigational as of 2003 include cell-based therapies. Instead of using synthetic chemicals that resemble substances produced by the body, cell-based therapies use modified stem cells or dendritic cells as vaccines against cancer. Stem cells are undifferentiated cells whose daughter cells can develop into various types of specialized cells, while dendritic cells are cells that are able to initiate and modify the immune system's responses to cancer by activating B cells and T cells. Dendritic cells appear to offer a promising new form of immunotherapy for cancer.

Another investigational form of treatment is the development of cell-free tumor-specific peptide vaccines. Peptides are subunits of protein molecules that contain two or more amino acids. Peptide vaccines are intended to induce responses in the patient's T cells that inhibit tumor growth. As of late 2003, however, peptide-based tumor vaccines have been shown to shrink cancerous tumors only in patients with limited disease.

Adoptive immunotherapy

Adoptive immunotherapy involves stimulating T lymphocytes by exposing them to tumor antigens. These modified cells are grown in the laboratory and then injected into patients. Since the cells taken from a different individual for this purpose often results in rejection, patients serve both as donor and recipient of their own T cells. Adoptive immunotherapy is particularly effective in patients who have received massive doses of radiation and chemotherapy. In such patients, therapy results in immunosuppression (weakened immune systems), making them vulnerable to viral infections. For example, CMV-specific T cells can reduce the risk of cytomegalovirus (CMV) infection in transplant patients.

Resources

PERIODICALS

Fishman, M. N., and S. J. Antonia. "Cell-Based Immune Therapy for Metastatic Renal Cancer." *Expert Review of Anticancer Therapy* 3 (December 2003): 837–849.

"Immunoprevention of Cancer: Is the time Ripe?" *Cancer Research* 60 (May 15, 2000): 2571–2575.

National Cancer Institute. *Treating Cancer with Vaccine Therapy.* June 29, 2001. < http://cancertrials.nci.nih.gov/news/features/vaccine/html/page05.htm 2000 >.

Nieda, M., M. Tomiyama, and K. Egawa. "Ex vivo Enhancement of Antigen-Presenting Function of Dendritic Cells and Its Application for DC-Based Immunotherapy." *Human Cell* 16 (December 2003): 199–204.

Paczesny, S., H. Ueno, J. Fay, et al. "Dendritic Cells as Vectors for Immunotherapy of Cancer." *Seminars in Cancer Biology* 13 (December 2003): 439–447.

Rosenberg, S. A. "Progress in Human Tumor Immunology and Immunotherapy." *Nature* 411, no. 6835 (2001): 380–385.

Scheibenbogen, C., A. Letsch, A. Schmittel, et al. "Rational Peptide-Based Tumour Vaccine Development and T Cell Monitoring." *Seminars in Cancer Biology* 13 (December 2003): 423–429.

Nancy Ross-Flanigan
Kausalya Santhanam, PhD
Teresa G. Odle
Rebecca J. Frey, PhD

Immunosuppressant drugs

Definition

Immunosuppressant drugs, also called **anti-rejection drugs**, are used to prevent the body from rejecting a transplanted organ.

Purpose

When an organ, such as a liver, a heart or a kidney, is transplanted from one person (the donor) into another (the recipient), the immune system of the recipient triggers the same response against the new organ it would have to any foreign material, setting off a chain of events that can damage the transplanted organ. This process is called rejection and it can occur rapidly (acute rejection), or over a long period of time (chronic rejection). Rejection can occur despite close matching of the donated organ and the transplant patient. Immunosuppressant drugs greatly decrease the risks of rejection, protecting the new organ and preserving its function. These drugs act by blocking the immune system so that it is less likely to react against the transplanted organ. A wide variety of drugs are available to achieve this aim but work in different ways to reduce the risk of rejection.

In addition to being used to prevent organ rejection, immunosuppressant drugs are also used to treat such severe skin disorders as **psoriasis** and such other diseases as **rheumatoid arthritis**, **Crohn's disease** (chronic inflammation of the digestive tract) and patchy hair loss (**alopecia** areata). Some of these conditions are termed "autoimmune" diseases, indicating that the immune system is acting against the body itself.

Description

Immunosuppressant drugs can be classified according to their specific molecular mode of action. The three main immunosuppressant drugs currently used in organ transplantations are the following:

- Cyclosporins (Neoral, Sandimmune, SangCya). These drugs act by inhibiting T-cell activation, thus preventing T-cells from attacking the transplanted organ.

- Azathioprines (Imuran). These drugs disrupt the synthesis of DNA and RNA and cell division.

- **Corticosteroids** such as prednisolone (Deltasone, Orasone). These drugs suppress the inflammation associated with transplant rejection.

Most patients are prescribed a combination of drugs after their transplant, one from each of the above main groups; for example cyclosporin, azathioprine and prednisolone. Over a period of time, the doses of each drug and the number of drugs taken may be reduced as the risks of rejection decrease. However, most patients need to take at least one immunosuppressive for the rest of their lives.

Immunosuppressants can also be classified depending on the specific transplant:

- basiliximab (Simulect) is also used in combination with such other drugs as cyclosporin and corticosteroids, in kidney transplants

- daclizumab (Zenapax) is also used in combination with such other drugs as cyclosporin and corticosteroids, in kidney transplants

- muromonab CD3 (Orthoclone OKT3) is used, along with cyclosporin, in kidney, liver and heart transplants

- tacrolimus (Prograf) is used in liver transplants and is under study for kidney, bone marrow, heart, pancreas, pancreatic island cell, and small bowel transplantation

Some immunosuppressants are also used to treat a variety of autoimmune diseases:

- Azathioprine (Imuran) is used not only to prevent organ rejection in kidney transplants, but also in treatment of rheumatoid arthritis. It has been used to treat chronic **ulcerative colitis**, but it has been of limited value for this use.

- Cyclosporin (Sandimmune, Neoral) is used in heart, liver, kidney, pancreas, bone marrow and heart/lung transplantation. The Neoral form has been used to treat psoriasis and rheumatoid arthritis. The drug has also been used for many other conditions including **multiple sclerosis**, diabetes and myesthenia gravis.

- Glatiramer acetate (Copaxone) is used in treatment of relapsing-remitting multiple sclerosis. In one study, glatiramer reduced the frequency of multiple sclerosis attacks by 75% over a two-year period.

- Mycopehnolate (CellCept) is used along with cyclosporin in kidney, liver and heart transplants. It has also been used to prevent the kidney problems associated with lupus erythematosus.

- Sirolimus (Rapamune) is used in combination with other drugs including cyclosporin and corticosteroids, in kidney transplants. The drug is also used for the treatment of psoriasis.

Recommended dosage

Immunosuppressant drugs are available only with a physician's prescription. They come in tablet, capsule, liquid and injectable forms.

The recommended dosage depends on the type and form of immunosuppressant drug and the purpose for which it is being used. Doses may be different for different patients. The prescribing physician or the pharmacist who filled the prescription will advise on correct dosage.

Taking immunosuppressant drugs exactly as directed is very important. Smaller, larger or more frequent doses should never be taken, and the drugs should never be taken for longer than directed. The physician will decide exactly how much of the medicine each patient needs. Blood tests often are necessary to monitor the action of the drug.

The prescribing physician should be consulted before stopping an immunosuppressant drug.

Precautions

Seeing a physician regularly while taking immuno-suppressant drugs is important. These regular check-ups will allow the physician to make sure the drug is working as it should and to watch for unwanted side effects. These drugs are very powerful and can cause serious side effects, such as high blood pressure, kidney problems and liver problems. Some side effects may not show up until years after the medicine is used. Anyone who has been advised to take immunosuppressant drugs should thoroughly discuss the risks and benefits with the prescribing physician

Immunosuppressant drugs lower a person's resistance to infection and can make infections harder to treat. The drugs can also increase the chance of uncontrolled bleeding. Anyone who has a serious infection or injury while taking immunosuppressant drugs should get prompt medical attention and should make sure that the treating physician knows about the immunosuppressant prescription. The prescribing physician should be immediately informed if signs of infection, such as **fever** or chills, **cough** or hoarseness, **pain** in the lower back or side, or painful or difficult urination, bruising or bleeding, blood in the urine, bloody or black, tarry stools occur. Other ways of preventing infection and injury include washing the hands frequently, avoiding sports in which injuries may occur, and being careful when using knives, razors, fingernail clippers or other sharp objects. Avoiding contact with people who have infections is also important. In addition, people who are taking or have been taking immunosuppressant drugs should not have immunizations, such as **smallpox** vaccinations, without checking with their physicians. Because of their low resistance to infection, people taking these drugs might get the disease that the vaccine is designed to prevent. People taking immunosuppressant drugs also should avoid contact with anyone who has taken the oral **polio** vaccine, as there is a chance the virus could be passed on to them. Other people living in their home should not take the oral polio vaccine.

Immunosuppressant drugs may cause the gums to become tender and swollen or to bleed. If this happens, a physician or dentist should be notified. Regular brushing, flossing, cleaning and gum massage may help prevent this problem. A dentist can provide advice on how to clean the teeth and mouth without causing injury.

Special conditions

People who have certain medical conditions or who are taking certain other medicines may have problems if they take immunosuppressant drugs. Before taking these drugs, the prescribing physician should be informed about any of these conditions:

ALLERGIES. Anyone who has had unusual reactions to immunosuppressant drugs in the past should let his or her physician know before taking the drugs again. The physician should also be told about any **allergies** to foods, dyes, preservatives, or other substances.

PREGNANCY. Azathioprine may cause **birth defects** if used during **pregnancy**, or if either the male or female is using it at time of conception. Anyone taking this medicine should use a barrier method of birth control, such as a **diaphragm** or condoms. Birth control pills should not be used without a physician's approval. Women who become pregnant while taking this medicine should check with their physicians immediately.

The medicine's effects have not been studied in humans during pregnancy. Women who are pregnant or who may become pregnant and who need to take this medicine should check with their physicians.

BREASTFEEDING. Immunosuppressant drugs pass into breast milk and may cause problems in nursing babies whose mothers take it. Breastfeeding is not recommended for women taking this medicine.

OTHER MEDICAL CONDITIONS. People who have certain medical conditions may have problems if they take immunosuppressant drugs. For example:

- People who have **shingles** (herpes zoster) or **chickenpox**, or who have recently been exposed to chickenpox, may develop severe disease in other parts of their bodies when they take these medicines.

- The medicine's effects may be greater in people with **kidney disease** or **liver disease**, because their bodies are slow to get rid of the medicine.

- The effects of oral forms of this medicine may be weakened in people with intestinal problems, because the medicine cannot be absorbed into the body.

Before using immunosuppressant drugs, people with these or other medical problems should make sure their physicians are aware of their conditions.

USE OF CERTAIN MEDICINES. Taking immunosuppressant drugs with certain other drugs may affect the way the drugs work or may increase the chance of side effects.

Side effects

Increased risk of infection is a common side effect of all the immunosuppressant drugs. The immune system protects the body from infections and when the immune system is suppressed, infections are more likely. Taking

KEY TERMS

Antibody—Protein produced by the immune system in response to the presence in the body of an antigen.

Antigen—Any substance or organism that is foreign to the body. Examples of antigens are: bacteria, bacterial toxins, viruses, or other cells or proteins.

Autoimmune disease—A disease in which the immune system is overactive and has lost the ability to distinguish between self and non-self.

Chronic—A word used to describe a long-lasting condition. Chronic conditions often develop gradually and involve slow changes.

Corticosteroids—A class of drugs that are synthetic versions of the cortisone produced by the body. They rank among the most powerful anti-inflammatory agents.

Cortisone—Glucocorticoid produced by the adrenal cortex in response to stress. Cortisone is a steroid with anti-inflammatory and immunosuppressive properties.

Inflammation—A process occurring in body tissues, characterized by increased circulation and the accumulation of white blood cells. Inflammation also occurs in such disorders as arthritis and causes harmful effects.

Inflammatory—Pertaining to inflammation.

Immune response—Physiological response of the body controlled by the immune system that involves the production of antibodies to fight off specific foreign substances or agents (antigens).

Immune system—The network of organs, cells, and molecules that work together to defend the body from foreign substances and organisms causing infection and disease such as: bacteria, viruses, fungi and parasites.

Immunosuppressant—Any chemical substance that suppresses the immune response.

Immunosuppressive—Any agent that suppresses the immune response of an individual.

Immunosuppresive cytotoxic drugs—A class of drugs that function by destroying cells and suppressing the immune response.

Lymphocyte—Lymphocytes are white blood cells that participate in the immune response. The two main groups are the B cells that have antibody molecules on their surface and T cells that destroy antigens.

Psoriasis—A skin disease characterized by itchy, scaly, red patches on the skin.

Rejection—Rejection occurs when the body recognizes a new transplanted organ as "foreign" and turns on the immune system of the body.

T cells—Any of several lymphocytes that have specific antigen receptors, and that are involved in cell-mediated immunity and destruction of antigen-bearing cells.

Transplantation—The removal of tissue from one part of the body for implantation to another part of the body; or the removal of tissue or an organ from one individual and its implantation in another individual by surgery.

such **antibiotics** as co-trimoxazole prevents some of these infections. Immunosuppressant drugs are also associated with a slightly increased risk of **cancer** because the immune system also plays a role in protecting the body against some forms of cancer. For example, long-term use of immunosuppressant drugs carries an increased risk of developing skin cancer as a result of the combination of the drugs and exposure to sunlight.

Other side effects of immunosuppressant drugs are minor and usually go away as the body adjusts to the medicine. These include loss of appetite, **nausea** or **vomiting**, increased hair growth, and trembling or shaking of the hands. Medical attention is not necessary unless these side effects continue or cause problems.

The treating physician should be notified immediately if any of the following side effects occur:

- unusual tiredness or weakness

- fever or chills

- frequent need to urinate

Interactions

Immunosuppressant drugs may interact with other medicines. When this happens, the effects of one or both drugs may change or the risk of side effects may be greater. Other drugs may also have an adverse effect on immunosuppressant therapy. This is particularly important for patients taking cyclosporin or tacrolimus. For example, some drugs can cause the blood levels to rise, while others can cause the blood levels to fall and it is important to avoid such contraindicated combinations. Other examples are:

- The effects of azathioprine may be greater in people who take allopurinol, a medicine used to treat gout.

- A number of drugs, including female hormones (estrogens), male hormones (androgens), the antifungal drug ketoconazole (Nizoral), the ulcer drug cimetidine (Tagamet) and the **erythromycins** (used to treat infections), may increase the effects of cyclosporine.

- When sirolimus is taken at the same time as cyclosporin, the blood levels of sirolimus may be increased to a level where there are severe side effects. Although these two drugs are usually used together, the sirolimus should be taken four hours after the dose of cyclosporin.

- Tacrolimus is eliminated through the kidneys. When the drug is used with other drugs that may harm the kidneys, such as cyclosporin, the antibiotics gentamicin and amikacin, or the antifungal drug amphotericin B, blood levels of tacrolimus may be increased. Careful kidney monitoring is essential when tacrolimus is given with any drug that might cause kidney damage.

- The risk of cancer or infection may be greater when immunosuppressant drugs are combined with certain other drugs which also lower the body's ability to fight disease and infection. These drugs include corticosteroids such as prednisone; the **anticancer drugs** chlorambucil (Leukeran), cyclophosphamide (Cytoxan) and mercaptopurine (Purinethol); and the monoclonal antibody muromonab-CD3 (Orthoclone), which also is used to prevent transplanted organ rejection.

Not every drug that may interact with immunosuppressant drugs is listed here. Anyone who takes immunosuppressant drugs should let the physician know all other medicines he or she is taking and should ask whether the possible interactions can interfere with treatment.

Resources

BOOKS

Abbas, A. K., and A. H. Lichtman. *Basic Immunology: Functions and Disorders of the Immune System.* Philadelphia: W. B. Saunders Co., 2001.

Sompayrac, L. M. *How the Immune System Works.* Boston: Blackwell Science, 1999.

Travers, P. *Immunobiology: The Immune System in Health and Disease.* 5th edition. New York: Garland Publishers, 2001.

Nancy Ross-Flanigan

Immunotherapy *see* **Immunologic therapies**

Impacted tooth

Definition

An impacted tooth is any tooth that is prevented from reaching its normal position in the mouth by tissue, bone, or another tooth.

Description

The teeth that most commonly become impacted are the third molars, also called wisdom teeth. These large teeth are the last to develop, beginning to form when a person is about nine years old, but not breaking through the gum tissue until the late teens or early twenties. By this time, the jaws have stopped growing and may be too small to accommodate these four additional teeth. As the wisdom teeth continue to move, one or more may become impacted, either by running into the teeth next to them or becoming blocked within the jawbone or gum tissue. An impacted tooth can cause further dental problems, including infection of the gums, displacement of other teeth, or decay. At least one wisdom tooth becomes impacted in nine of every ten people.

Causes and Symptoms

The movement of an erupting wisdom tooth and any subsequent impaction may produce **pain** at the back of the jaw. Pain may also be the result of infection, either from decay in any exposed portion of the tooth or from trapped food and plaque in the surrounding gum tissue. Infection typically produces an unpleasant taste when biting down and **bad breath**. Another source of pain may be pericoronitis, a gum condition in which the crown of the incompletely erupted tooth produces inflammation, redness, and tenderness of the gums. Less common symptoms of an impacted tooth are swollen lymph nodes in the neck, difficulty opening the mouth, and prolonged **headache**.

Diagnosis

Upon visual examination, the dentist may find signs of infection or swelling in the area where the tooth is present or only partially erupted. Dental x rays are necessary to confirm tooth impaction.

Treatment

Because impacted teeth may cause dental problems with few if any symptoms to indicate damage,

Resources

ORGANIZATIONS

American Association of Oral and Maxillofacial Surgeons. 9700 West Bryn Mawr Ave., Rosemont, IL 60018-5701. (847) 678-6200. < http://www.aaoms.org >.

Bethany Thivierge

KEY TERMS

Dry socket—A painful condition following tooth extraction in which a blood clot does not properly fill the empty socket, leaving the bone underneath exposed to air and food.

Eruption—The process of a tooth breaking through the gum tissue to grow into place in the mouth.

Extraction—The removal of a tooth from its socket in the bone.

Pericoronitis—A gum condition in which irritation and inflammation are produced by the crown of an incompletely erupted tooth.

Wisdom tooth—One of the four last teeth on the top and bottom rows of teeth. Also called a third molar.

dentists commonly recommend the removal of all wisdom teeth, preferably while the patient is still a young adult. A dentist may perform an extraction with forceps and local anesthetic if the tooth is exposed and appears to be easily removable in one piece. However, he or she may refer a difficult extraction to an oral surgeon, a specialist who administers either nitrous oxide-oxygen (commonly called "laughing gas"), an intravenous sedative, or a general anesthetic to alleviate any pain or discomfort during the surgical procedure. Extracting an impacted tooth typically requires cutting through gum tissue to expose the tooth, and may require removing portions of bone to free the tooth. The tooth may have to be removed in pieces to minimize destruction to the surrounding structures. The extraction site may or may not require one or more stitches to help the incision heal.

Prognosis

The prognosis is very good when impacted teeth are removed from young healthy adults without complications. Potential complications include postoperative infection, temporary **numbness** from nerve irritation, jaw fracture, and jaw joint pain. An additional condition which may develop is called dry socket: when a blood clot does not properly form in the empty tooth socket, or is disturbed by an oral vacuum (such as from drinking through a straw or **smoking**), the bone beneath the socket is painfully exposed to air and food, and the extraction site heals more slowly.

Impedance phlebography

Definition

Impedance phlebography is a noninvasive test that uses electrical monitoring to measure blood flow in veins of the leg. Information from this test helps a doctor to detect **deep vein thrombosis** (**blood clots** or **thrombophlebitis**).

Purpose

Impedance phlebography may be done in order to:

- detect blood clots lodged in the deep veins of the leg
- screen patients who are likely to have blood clots in the leg
- detect the source of blood clots in the lungs (pulmonary emboli)

Blood clots in the legs can lead to more serious problems. If a clot breaks loose from a leg vein, it may travel to the lungs and lodge in a blood vessel in the lungs. Blood clots are more likely to occur in people who have recently had leg injuries, surgery, **cancer**, or a long period of bed rest.

Precautions

Because this test is not invasive, it can be done on all patients. However, the accuracy of the results will be affected if the patient does not breathe normally or keep the leg muscles relaxed. Compression of the veins because of pelvic tumors or decreased blood flow, due to **shock** or any condition that reduces the amount of blood the heart pumps, may also change the test results.

Description

Impedance phlebography works by measuring the resistance to the transmission of electrical energy (impedance). This resistance changes depending on the volume of blood flowing through the veins. By graphing the impedance, a doctor or technician can tell whether a clot is obstructing blood flow.

Using conductive jelly, the examiner puts electrodes on the patient's calf. These electrodes are connected to an instrument called a plethysmograph, which records the changes in electrical resistance that occur during the test.

The patient lies down and raises one leg at a 30° angle, so that the calf is above the level of the heart. The examiner wraps a pressure cuff around the patient's thigh and inflates it to a pressure of 45–60 cm of water for 45 seconds. The plethysmograph records the electrical changes that correspond to changes in the volume of blood in the vein at the time the pressure is exerted and again three seconds after the cuff is deflated. This procedure is repeated several times in both legs.

This test takes 30 to 45 minutes. Impedance phlebography is also called an impedance test of blood flow or impedance plethysmography.

Preparation

Patients undergoing this test do not need to alter their diet, change their normal activities, or stop taking any medications. They will wear a surgical gown during the test, and be asked to urinate before the test starts. If keeping the legs elevated causes discomfort, mild **pain** medication will be given.

Aftercare

The patient may resume normal or postoperative activities after the test.

Risks

Impedance phlebography is painless and safe. It presents no risk to the patient.

Normal results

Normally, inflating the pressure cuff will cause a sharp rise in the pressure in the veins of the calf because blood flow is blocked. When the cuff is released, the pressure decreases rapidly as the blood flows away.

Abnormal results

If a clot is present, the pressure in the calf veins will already be high. It does not become sharply higher

---

KEY TERMS

Thrombophlebitis—Inflammation of a vein, associated with the formation of a blood clot.

---

when the pressure cuff is tightened. When the pressure cuff is deflated, the clot blocks the flow of blood out of the calf vein. The decrease in pressure is not as rapid as when no clot is present, and the shape of the resulting graph is different.

Resources

OTHER

Griffith, H. Winter. "Complete Guide to Medical Tests." *ThriveOnline.* < http://thriveonline.oxygen.com >.

Tish Davidson, A.M.

Impedance plethysmography *see* **Impedance phlebography**

Impedance test of blood flow *see* **Impedance phlebography**

Impetigo

Definition

Impetigo refers to a very localized bacterial infection of the skin. There are two types, bullous and epidemic.

Description

Impetigo is a skin infection that tends primarily to afflict children. Impetigo caused by the bacterium *Staphylococcus aureus* (also known as staph) affects children of all ages. Impetigo caused by the bacteria called group A streptococci (also know as strep) are most common in children ages two to five.

The bacteria that cause impetigo are very contagious. They can be spread by a child from one part of his or her body to another by scratching, or contact with a towel, clothing, or stuffed animal. These same methods can pass the bacteria on from one person to another.

Impetigo tends to develop in areas of the skin that have already been damaged through some other mechanism (a cut or scrape, burn, insect bite, or vesicle from **chickenpox**).

Causes and symptoms

The first sign of bullous impetigo is a large bump on the skin with a clear, fluid-filled top (called a vesicle). The bump develops a scab-like, honey-colored crust. There is usually no redness or **pain**, although the area may be quite itchy. Ultimately, the skin in this area will become dry and flake away. Bullous impetigo is usually caused by staph bacteria.

Epidemic impetigo can be caused by staph or strep bacteria, and (as the name implies) is very easily passed among children. Certain factors, such as heat and humidity, crowded conditions, and poor hygiene increase the chance that this type of impetigo will spread rapidly among large groups of children. This type of impetigo involves the formation of a small vesicle surrounded by a circle of reddened skin. The vesicles appear first on the face and legs. When a child has several of these vesicles close together, they may spread to one another. The skin surface may become eaten away (ulcerated), leaving irritated pits. When there are many of these deep, pitting ulcers, with pus in the center and brownish-black scabs, the condition is called ecthyma. If left untreated, the type of bacteria causing this type of impetigo has the potential to cause a serious **kidney disease** called **glomerulonephritis**. Even when impetigo is initially caused by strep bacteria, the vesicles are frequently secondarily infected with staph bacteria.

Impetigo is usually an uncomplicated skin condition. Left untreated, however, it may develop into a serious disease, including **osteomyelitis** (bone infection), septic arthritis (joint infection), or **pneumonia**. If large quantities of bacteria are present and begin circulating in the bloodstream, the child is in danger of developing an overwhelming systemic infection known as **sepsis**.

Diagnosis

Characteristic appearance of the skin is the usual method of diagnosis, although fluid from the vesicles can be cultured and then examined in an attempt to identify the causative bacteria.

Treatment

Uncomplicated impetigo is usually treated with a topical antibiotic cream called mupirocin. In more serious, widespread cases of impetigo, or when the child has a **fever** or swollen glands, **antibiotics** may be

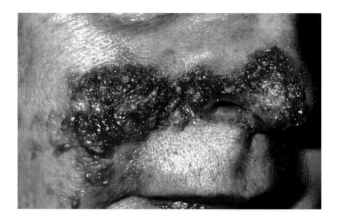

Impetigo is a contagious bacterial skin infection that mostly affects the area around the nose and mouth. Usually caused by staphylococci, this person's impetigo was triggered by herpes simplex. *(Photo Researchers, Inc. Reproduced by permission.)*

KEY TERMS

Systemic—Involving the whole body; the opposite of localized.

Ulcer—An irritated pit in the surface of a tissue.

Vesicle—A bump on the skin filled with fluid.

---

given by mouth or even through a needle placed in a vein (intravenously).

Prognosis

Prognosis for a child with impetigo is excellent. The vast majority of children recover quickly, completely, and uneventfully.

Prevention

Prevention involves good hygiene. Handwashing; never sharing towels, clothing, or stuffed animals; and keeping fingernails well-trimmed are easy precautions to take to avoid spreading the infection from one person to another.

Resources

PERIODICALS

"Bullous Impetigo." *Archives of Pediatrics and Adolescent Medicine* 151, no. 11 (November 1997): 1168 +.

Rosalyn Carson-DeWitt, MD

Implant therapy *see* **Radioactive implants**

Implantable cardioverter-defibrillator

Definition

The implantable cardioverter-defibrillator is an electronic device to treat life-threatening heartbeat irregularities. It is surgically implanted.

Purpose

The implantable cardioverter-defibrillator is used to detect and stop serious ventricular **arrhythmias** and restore a normal heartbeat in people who are at high risk of sudden **death**. The American Heart Association recommends that implantable cardioverter-defibrillators only be considered for patients who have a life-threatening arrhythmia. A recent study by the National Heart, Lung, and Blood Institute demonstrated that implantable cardioverter-defibrillators are the treatment of choice instead of drug therapy for patients who have had a cardiac arrest or **heart attack** and are at risk for developing **ventricular tachycardia**, which is a very rapid heartbeat, or **ventricular fibrillation**, which is an ineffective, irregular heart activity. Other studies suggest that 20% of these high risk patients would die within two years without an implantable cardioverter-defibrillator. With the device, the five-year risk of sudden death drops to five percent.

Precautions

The implantable cardioverter-defibrillator should not be used on patients who faint from causes other than a known life-threatening ventricular arrhythmia, to treat slow heart rates, or during an emergency.

Description

According to the American College of Cardiology, more than 80,000 Americans currently have an implantable cardioverter-defibrillator; 17,000 of these were implanted in 1995 alone. The battery-powered device rescues the patient from a life-threatening arrhythmia by rapid pacing and/or delivering electrical shock(s) to suspend heart activity and then allow it to initiate a normal rhythm. Before the development of the implantable cardioverter-defibrillator, most people who experienced ventricular fibrillation and were not near a hospital with a well equipped emergency team died within minutes.

The implantable cardioverter-defibrillator is like a mini computer connected to the patient's heart. Newer

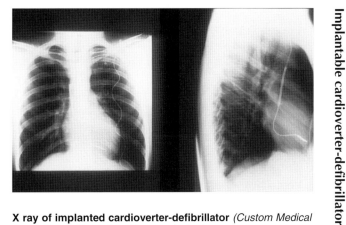

X ray of implanted cardioverter-defibrillator *(Custom Medical Stock Photo. Reproduced by permission.)*

models weigh less than 10 ounces and can be implanted beneath the skin of the chest in the pectoral region, without major surgery. A lead from the device is then inserted into the heart through a vein. The procedure is performed in an operating room under **general anesthesia**. Earlier versions of implantable cardioverter-defibrillators were implanted in the abdomen and required open-chest surgery to connect the electrodes to the left and right ventricles.

The implantable cardioverter-defibrillator is set above the patient's **exercise** heart rate. Once the device is in place, many tests will be conducted to ensure that the device is sensing and defibrillating properly. The newer implantable cardioverter-defibrillators last seven or eight years. Technology and procedures continue to evolve.

Preparation

Before the procedure, a complete medical history and physical exam will be done. **Electrocardiography**, special electrophysiologic testing, **chest x ray**, **urinalysis**, and a blood test are usually also required.

Aftercare

The patient is monitored for arrhythmias and to ensure that the implantable cardioverter-defibrillator is working properly. The physician also watches for signs of infection. Before the patient leaves the hospital, the device is tested again. Antiarrhythmia drug therapy is necessary in more than half of all patients with implantable cardioverter-defibrillators, but the number of drugs and the dosages are usually reduced. Any time a significant change in anti-arrhythmia medication is made, the device will be tested again.

KEY TERMS

Arrhythmia—A variation of the normal rhythm of the heartbeat.

Cardioverter—A device to apply electric shock to the chest to convert an abnormal heartbeat into a normal heartbeat.

Defibrillation—An electronic process which helps re-establish a normal heart rhythm.

Ventricles—The two large lower chambers of the heart which pump blood to the lungs and the rest of the human body.

Ventricular fibrillation—An arrhythmia in which the heart beats very fast but blood is not pumped out to the body. Ventricular fibrillation can quickly become fatal if not corrected.

Ventricular tachycardia—An arrhythmia in which the heart rate is more than 100 beats per minute.

The patient is taught how the device works, and that the shock it delivers will feel like a punch or kick in the chest. The patient is told to notify his/her physician when the implantable cardioverter-defibrillator delivers a shock, and to go to the emergency room if multiple shocks are sent within a short period of time.

Although most patients with implantable cardioverter-defibrillators are glad that they have the device and feel that it has extended their lives, they do experience fear and **anxiety**. This stems from the sensation of the shock(s), the unpredictable circumstances under which shock(s) occurs, and unknown outcomes.

Risks

There can be serious complications to the implantation of a cardioverter-defibrillator. These include inflammation of the pericardium, the sac that surrounds the heart; heart attack; congestive **heart failure**; and post-operative **stroke**. Serious infections can develop in the area around the device while the patient is initially hospitalized or up to several months later. Death due to the device's failure while being tested during surgery is an uncommon risk. The risk of death from the implantation procedure is about the same as that for a pacemaker, less than one percent. There are also potentially serious risks associated with the device's improper functioning once it is in place.

Resources

ORGANIZATIONS

American Heart Association. 7320 Greenville Ave. Dallas, TX 75231. (214) 373-6300. < http://www.americanheart.org >.

Texas Heart Institute. Heart Information Service. PO Box 20345, Houston, TX 77225-0345. < http://www.tmc.edu/thi >.

Lori De Milto

Impotence

Definition

Impotence, often called **erectile dysfunction**, is the inability to achieve or maintain an erection long enough to engage in sexual intercourse.

Description

Under normal circumstances, when a man is sexually stimulated, his brain sends a message down the spinal cord and into the nerves of the penis. The nerve endings in the penis release chemical messengers, called neurotransmitters, that signal the corpora cavernosa (the two spongy rods of tissue that span the length of the penis) to relax and fill with blood. As they expand, the corpora cavernosa close off other veins that would normally drain blood from the penis. As the penis becomes engorged with blood, it enlarges and stiffens, causing an erection. Problems with blood vessels, nerves, or tissues of the penis can interfere with an erection.

Causes and symptoms

It is estimated that up to 20 million American men frequently suffer from impotence and that it strikes up to half of all men between the ages of 40 and 70. Doctors used to think that most cases of impotence were psychological in origin, but they now recognize that, at least in older men, physical causes may play a primary role in 60% or more of all cases. In men over the age of 60, the leading cause is **atherosclerosis**, or narrowing of the arteries, which can restrict the flow of blood to the penis. Injury or disease of the connective tissue, such as **Peyronie's disease**, may prevent the corpora cavernosa from completely expanding. Damage to the nerves of the penis, from certain types of surgery or neurological conditions, such as

Parkinson's disease or **multiple sclerosis**, may also cause impotence. Men with diabetes are especially at risk for impotence because of their high risk of both atherosclerosis and a nerve disease called **diabetic neuropathy**.

Certain types of blood pressure medications, anti-ulcer drugs, **antihistamines**, tranquilizers (especially before intercourse), antifungals (hetoconazole), antipsychotics, **antianxiety drugs**, and antidepressants, known as **selective serotonin reuptake inhibitors** (SSRIs, including Prozac and Paxil), can interfere with erectile function. **Smoking**, excessive alcohol consumption, and illicit drug use may also contribute. In rare cases, low levels of the male hormone testosterone may contribute to erectile failure. Finally, psychological factors, such as **stress**, guilt, or **anxiety**, may also play a role, even when the impotence is primarily due to organic causes.

Diagnosis

The doctor also obtains a thorough medical history to find out about past pelvic surgery, diabetes, cardiovascular disease, **kidney disease**, and any medications the man may be taking. The **physical examination** should include a genital examination, a measurement of blood flow through the penis, hormone tests, and a glucose test for diabetes.

In some cases, nocturnal penile tumescence testing is performed to find out whether the man has erections while asleep. Healthy men usually have about four or five erections throughout the night. The man applies a device to the penis called a Rigiscan before going to bed at night, and the device can determine whether he has had erections. (If a man is able to have normal erections at night, this suggests a psychological cause for his impotence.)

Treatment

Years ago, the standard treatment for impotence was an implantable penile prosthesis or long-term psychotherapy. Although physical causes are now more readily diagnosed and treated, individual or marital counseling is still an effective treatment for impotence when emotional factors play a role. Fortunately, other approaches are now available to treat the physical causes of impotence.

Medications

The first line and by far the most common treatment today is with the prescription drug **sildenafil citrate**, sold under the brand name Viagra. An estimated 20 million prescriptions for the pill have been filled since it was approved by the FDA in March 1998. It is also the most effective treatment with a success rate of more than 60%. The drug boosts levels of a substance called cyclic GMP, which is responsible for widening the blood vessels of the penis. In clinical studies, Viagra produced headaches in 16% of men who took it, and other side effects included flushing, **indigestion**, and stuffy nose.

The primary drawback to Viagra, which works about an hour after it is taken, it that the FDA cautions men with heart disease or low blood pressure to be thoroughly examined by a physician before obtaining a prescription.

In the summer of 2002, two investigational drugs were announced to become available in the near future to also treat erectile dysfunction. Vardenafil and tadalafil both helped men who also had such conditions as diabetes, high blood pressure and benign prostatic hypertrophy. The drugs are awaiting final FDA approval.

Vardenafil and tadalafil belong to the same group of chemical compounds as sildenafil, namely phosphodiesterase type 5 (PDE-5) inhibitors. Some men cannot benefit from sildenafil or the two newer PDE-5 inhibitors because they have low levels of nitric oxide. British investigators reported in late 2002 that three different types of compounds are being studied as possible medications for men with low levels of nitric oxide. They are Rho-kinase inhibitors, soluble guanylate cyclase activators, and nitric oxide-releasing PDE-5 inhibitors.

Other medications under investigation as treatments for impotence are topical agents. Topical means that they are applied externally to the skin rather than being injected or taken by mouth. If approved, these drugs would provide a noninvasive alternative for men who cannot take sildenafil or other oral medications for impotence.

Injection therapy involves injecting a substance into the penis to enhance blood flow and cause an erection. The Food and Drug Administration (FDA) approved a drug called alprostadil (Caverject) for this purpose in July of 1995. Alprostadil relaxes smooth muscle tissue to enhance blood flow into the penis. It must be injected shortly before intercourse. Another, similar drug that is sometimes used is papaverine—not yet been approved by the FDA for this use. Either drug may sometimes cause painful erections or **priapism** (uncomfortable, prolonged erections) that must be treated with a shot of epinephrine.

Alprostadil may also be administered into the urethral opening of the penis. In MUSE (medical urethral system for erection), the man inserts a thin tube the width of a vermicelli noodle into his urethral opening and presses down on a plunger to deliver a tiny pellet containing alprostadil into his penis. The drug takes about 10 minutes to work and the erection lasts about an hour. The main side effect is a sensation of **pain** and burning in the urethra, which can last about five to 15 minutes.

Mechanical and surgical treatments

Another approach is vacuum therapy. The man inserts his penis into a clear plastic cylinder and uses a pump to force air out of the cylinder. This forms a partial vacuum around the penis, which helps to draw blood into the corpora cavernosa. The man then places a special ring over the base of the penis to trap the blood inside it. The only side effect with this type of treatment is occasional bruising if the vacuum is left on too long.

Implantable **penile prostheses** are usually considered a last resort for treating impotence. They are implanted in the corpora cavernosa to make the penis rigid without the need for blood flow. The semi-rigid type of prosthesis consists of a pair of flexible silicone rods that can be bent up or down. This type of device has a low failure rate but, unfortunately, it causes the penis to always be erect, which can be difficult to conceal under clothing.

The inflatable type of device consists of cylinders that are implanted in the corpora cavernosa, a fluid reservoir implanted in the abdomen, and a pump placed in the scrotum. The man squeezes the pump to move fluid into the cylinders and cause them to become rigid. (He reverses the process by squeezing the pump again.) While these devices allow for intermittent erections, they have a slightly higher malfunction rate than the silicon rods.

Men can return to sexual activity six to eight weeks after implantation surgery. Since implants affect the corpora cavernosa, they permanently take away a man's ability to have a natural erection.

In rare cases, if narrowed or diseased veins are responsible for impotence, surgeons may reroute the blood flow into the corpus cavernosa or remove leaking vessels. However, the success rate with these procedures has been very low, and they are still considered experimental.

Gene therapy

A newer investigational approach to the treatment of erectile dysfunction is **gene therapy**. As of late 2002, several preclinical studies have shown promise, but none of the gene-based strategies so far have yet been tested for safety.

Alternative treatment

A number of herbs have been promoted for treating impotence. The most widely touted herbs for this purpose are *Coryanthe yohimbe* (available by prescription as yohimbine, with the trade name Yocon) and gingko (*Gingko biloba*), although neither has been conclusively shown to help the condition in controlled studies. In addition, gingko carries some risk of abnormal blood clotting and should be avoided by men taking blood thinners such as coumadin. Other herbs promoted for treating impotence include true unicorn root (*Aletrius farinosa*), **saw palmetto** (*Serenoa repens*), ginseng (*Panax ginseng*), and Siberian ginseng (*Eleuthrococcus senticosus*). *Strychnos Nux vomica* has been recommended, especially when impotence is caused by excessive alcohol, cigarettes, or dietary indiscretions, but it can be very toxic if taken improperly, so it should be used only under the strict supervision of a physician trained in its use.

Prognosis

With proper diagnosis, impotence can nearly always be treated or managed successfully. Unfortunately, fewer than 10% of impotent men seek treatment.

Prevention

There is no specific treatment to prevent impotence. Perhaps the most important measure is to maintain general good health and avoid atherosclerosis by exercising regularly, controlling weight, controlling **hypertension** and **high cholesterol** levels, and avoiding smoking. Avoiding excessive alcohol intake may also help.

Resources

BOOKS

Beers, Mark H., MD, and Robert Berkow, MD, editors. "Erectile Dysfunction." Section 17, Chapter 220. In *The Merck Manual of Diagnosis and Therapy*. Whitehouse Station, NJ: Merck Research Laboratories, 2004.

Miller, Lucinda G., and Wallace J. Murray, editors. *Herbal Medicinals: A Clinician's Guide*. Binghamton, N.Y.: Haworth Press, 1999.

Pelletier, Kenneth R., MD. *The Best Alternative Medicine*, Part II. "CAM Therapies for Specific Conditions: Impotence." New York: Simon & Schuster, 2002.

KEY TERMS

Alprostadil—A smooth muscle relaxant sometimes injected into the penis or applied to the urethral opening to treat impotence.

Atherosclerosis—A disorder in which plaques of cholesterol, lipids, and other debris build up on the inner walls of arteries, narrowing them.

Corpus cavernosum (plural, corpora cavernosa)—One of two rods of spongy tissue in the penis that become engorged with blood in order to produce an erection.

Gene therapy—A menthod of treating a disorder by replacing damaged or abnormal genes with normal ones. Some researchers think that gene therapy may offer a new way to treat impotence.

Neurotransmitters—Chemicals that modify or help transmit impulses between nerve synapses.

Papaverine—A smooth muscle relaxant sometimes injected into the penis as a treatment for impotence.

Peyronie's disease—A disease resulting from scarring of the corpus cavernosa, causing painful erections.

Topical—A type of medication that is applied to a specific and limited area of skin, and affects only the area to which it is applied.

Urethra—The small tube that drains urine from the bladder, as well as serving as a conduit for semen during ejaculation in men.

Viagra—Trade name of an orally administered drug for erectile failure first cleared for marketing in the United States in March 1998. Its generic name is sildenafil citrate.

PERIODICALS

Campbell, Adam. "Soft Science: The Exclusive World on Which Sex Supplements may Help and Which Won't." *Men's Health* May 2002: 100.

Cellek, S., R. W. Rees, and J. Kalsi. "A Rho-Kinase Inhibitor, Soluble Guanylate Cyclase Activator and Nitric Oxide-Releasing PDE5 Inhibitor: Novel Approaches to Erectile Dysfunction." *Expert Opinion on Investigational Drugs* 11 (November 2002): 1563–1573.

Christ, G. J. "Gene Therapy for Erectile Dysfunction: Where Is It Going?" *Current Opinion in Urology* 12 (November 2002): 497–501.

Cowley, Geoffrey. "Looking Beyond Viagra." *Newsweek* April 24, 2000: 77.

Gresser, U., and C. H. Gleiter. "Erectile Dysfunction: Comparison of Efficacy and Side Effects of the PDE-5 Inhibitors Sildenafil, Vardenafil and Tadalafil— Review of the Literature." *European Journal of Medical Research* 7 (October 29, 2002): 435–446.

"Is Viagra Safe?" *Internal Medicine Alert* June 29, 2002: 90.

Norton, Patrice G.W. "Investigational Drugs in Erectile Dysfunction. (Vardenafil, Tadalafil)." *Internal Medicine News* June 1, 2002: 50.

Yap, R. L., and K. T. McVary. "Topical Agents and Erectile Dysfunction: Is There a Place?" *Current Urology Reports* 3 (December 2002): 471–476.

"Yohimbe Tree Bark: Herbal Viagra Better Gotten by Rx." *Environmental Nutrition* February 1999: 8.

ORGANIZATIONS

American Foundation for Urologic Disease. 1128 North Charles Street, Baltimore, MD 21201. (410) 468-1800.

American Urological Association (AUA). 1120 North Charles Street, Baltimore, MD 21201. (410) 727-1100. < www.auanet.org >.

Center for Biologics Evaluation and Research (CBER), U. S. Food and Drug Administration (FDA). 1401 Rockville Pike, Rockville, MD 20852-1448. (800) 835-4709 or (301) 827-1800. < www.fda.gov/cber >.

Impotence Institute of America, Impotents Anonymous. 10400 Little Patuxent Parkway, Suite 485, Columbia, MD 21044-3502. (800) 669-1603.

National Kidney and Urologic Diseases Information Clearinghouse. 3 Information Way, Bethesda, MD 20892-3580. (800) 891-5390.

Ken R. Wells
Rebecca J. Frey, PhD

Impulse control disorders

Definition

Impulse control disorders are characterized by an inability to resist the impulse to perform an action that is harmful to one's self or others. This is a relatively new class of **personality disorders**, and the most common of these are **intermittent explosive disorder**, kleptomania, pyromania, compulsive gambling disorder, and trichotillomania.

Description

All of these impulse control disorders involve the loss or lack of control in certain specific situations. The hallmark of these disorders is the individual's inability to stop impulses that may cause harm to themselves or others. Affected individuals often feel anxiety or tension in considering these behaviors. This anxiety or tension is relieved or diminished once the action is performed.

Intermittent explosive disorder is more common among men, and involves aggressive outbursts that lead to assaults on others or destruction of property. These outburst are unprovoked or seem to be out of proportion to the event that precedes them.

Kleptomania is more common among women, and involves the theft of objects that are seemingly worthless. The act of stealing relieves tension and is seen by the individual to be rewarding. The actual stealing is not preplanned, and the concept of punishment for the crime does not occur to these individuals, although they are aware that what they are doing is wrong.

Pyromania is more common among men, and involves setting fires in order to feel pleasure and relieve tension.

Pathological gambling occurs in roughly 1-3% of the population, and involves excessive gambling despite heavy monetary losses. These losses actually act as a motivating factor in continuing gambling in order to recoup some of what was lost.

Trichotillomania involves pulling hair from one's own scalp, face, or body, and is more common in women. It often begins in childhood, and is often associated with major depression or **attention-deficit/ hyperactivity disorder**.

Causes and symptoms

The exact causes of impulse control disorders are not fully understood as of 2004. Individuals who have had serious head injuries, however, can be at a higher risk for developing impulse control disorders, as are those with epilepsy.

Some cases of impulse control disorders appear to be side effects of general medical conditions. As of 2004, several groups of researchers have noted that some older adults with Parkinson's disease become compulsive gamblers as the disease progresses. It is thought that this gambling behavior is a side effect of dopaminergic drugs, as it does not respond to standard treatments for compulsive gambling but only to changes in the patient's medication.

Another medical condition that is associated with impulse control disorders is carcinoid syndrome. In one group of 20 consecutive patients with the syndrome, 75% met DSM-IV diagnostic criteria for one or another impulse control disorder. The researchers attribute the connection to the high levels of serotonin (a neurotransmitter) produced by carcinoid tumors.

Diagnosis

A diagnosis of any of these impulse control disorders can be made only after other medical and psychiatric disorders that may cause the same symptoms have been ruled out.

Some doctors may administer questionnaires or similar psychiatric screeners as part of the differential diagnosis. Two instruments that have been devised in the early 2000s to specifically target impulsive behavior are the Gambling Urge Scale (GUS) and the Lifetime History of Impulsive Behaviors (LHIB) Interview.

Intermittent explosive disorder involves severe acts of assault or destruction of property. The aggression seen during these acts is vastly out of proportion to events that may seem to have precipitated the acts.

Kleptomania involves stealing objects that are unnecessary and of little monetary value. The act of stealing is not an expression of anger or vengeance. Again, there is an increased tension before the act is committed, and this is resolved or relieved once the object is stolen.

Pyromania is classified by the deliberate setting of fires more than once. The individual will exhibit a fascination and attraction to fire and any objects associated with it. Before the fire is set, there is tension, with a resolving relief once the fire is set. Acts of true pyromania are not done for monetary gain, to express anger, to conceal criminal behavior, or in response to hallucination.

Pathological gambling is a disorder to gamble despite continuing losses and monetary insufficiency. This disorder typically begins in youth, and affected individuals are often competitive, easily bored, restless, and generous.

For a diagnosis of pathological gambling, five or more of the following symptoms must be present:

- a preoccupation with gambling

- a need to gamble with more money to achieve the thrill of winning

- repeated attempts to control or stop gambling

- irritability or restlessness due to repeated attempts of control

- gambling as an escape from stress

- lying to cover up gambling

KEY TERMS

Carcinoid syndrome—The pattern of symptoms (often including asthma and diarrhea) associated with carcinoid tumors of the digestive tract or lungs.

Compulsive gambling disorder—An impulse control disorder in which an individual cannot resist gambling despite repeated losses.

Intermittent explosive disorder—A personality disorder in which an individual is prone to intermittent explosive episodes of aggression during which he or she causes bodily harm or destroys property.

Kleptomania—An impulse control disorder in which one steals objects that are of little or no value.

Pyromania—An impulse control disorder in which one sets fires.

Trichotillomania—An impulse or compulsion to pull out one's own hair.

- conducting illegal activities, such as embezzling or fraud, to finance gambling

- losing a job or personal relationship due to gambling

- borrowing money to fund gambling

Trichotillomania is the continuous pulling out of one's own hair. Again, there is an increased sense of tension before pulling the hair, which is relieved once it is pulled out. Recurrent pulling out of one's hair resulting in noticeable hair loss. Affected individuals can undergo significant distress and impaired social, occupational, and functional behavior.

Treatment

A combination of psychological counseling and medication are the preferred treatments for the impulse control disorders. For kleptomania, pyromania, and trichotillomania, behavior modification is usually the treatment of choice. Children with trichotillomania are often helped by antidepressant medication. For pathological gambling, treatment usually involves an adaptation of the model set forth by Alcoholics Anonymous. Individuals are counseled with the goal of eventual response to appropriate social limits. In the case of intermittent explosive disorder, anger management and medication may be used in extreme cases of aggression.

Prognosis

These disorders can usually be controlled with medication, although it may need to be continued long-term to help prevent further aggressive outbursts. Long-term counseling is usually necessary as well. Support groups and meetings may also help these individuals.

The prognosis for intermittent explosive disorder, kleptomania, and pyromania is fair. Little is known about the prognosis for trichotillomania, and studies have shown that the condition can disappear for long periods (months to years) without any psychological counseling. For pathological gambling, the prognosis varies greatly from person to person. While total cure for this condition is unlikely, much like **alcoholism**, long periods of abstinence or continuous abstinence are possible.

Prevention

There are no known preventive treatments or measures for impulse control disorders.

Resources

BOOKS

American Psychiatric Association. *Diagnostic and Statistical Manual of Mental Disorders.* 4th ed., revised. Washington, D.C.: American Psychiatric Association, 2000.

PERIODICALS

Avanzi, M., E. Uber, and F. Bonfa. "Pathological Gambling in Two Patients on Dopamine Replacement Therapy for Parkinson's Disease." *Neurological Sciences* 25 (June 2004): 98–101.

Kurlan, R. "Disabling Repetitive Behaviors in Parkinson's Disease." *Movement Disorders* 19 (April 2004): 433–437.

Raylu, N., and T. P. Oei. "The Gambling Urge Scale: Development, Confirmatory Factor Validation, and Psychometric Properties." *Psychology of Addictive Behaviors* 18 (June 2004): 100–105.

Russo, S., J. C. Boon, I. P. Kema, et al. "Patients with Carcinoid Syndrome Exhibit Symptoms of Aggressive Impulse Dysregulation." *Psychosomatic Medicine* 66 (May-June 2004): 422–425.

Schmidt, C. A., A. E. Fallon, and E. F. Coccaro. "Assessment of Behavioral and Cognitive Impulsivity: Development and Validation of the Lifetime History of Impulsive Behaviors Interview." *Psychiatry Research* 126 (April 30, 2004): 107–121.

Tay, Y. K., M. L. Levy, and D. W. Metry. "Trichotillomania in Childhood: Case Series and Review." *Pediatrics* 113 (May 2004): 494–498.

ORGANIZATIONS

American Psychiatric Association. 1400 K Street, NW, Washington, DC 20005. < http://www.psych.org >.

Gamblers Anonymous International Service Office. PO Box 17173, Los Angeles, CA 90017. (213) 386-8789, Fax: (213) 386-0030. < http://www.gamblersanonymous. org/ >.

National Institute of Mental Health. 6001 Executive Boulevard, Room 8184, MSC 9663, Bethesda, MD 20892-9663. (301) 443-4513. < http:// www.nimh.nih.gov >.

Trichotillomania Learning Center, Inc. 1215 Mission Street, Suite 2, Santa Cruz, CA 95060. (831) 457-1004, Fax: (831) 426-4383. < http://www.trich.org >.

Liz Meszaros
Rebecca Frey, PhD

In vitro fertilization

Definition

In vitro fertilization (IVF) is a procedure in which eggs (ova) from a woman's ovary are removed. They are fertilized with sperm in a laboratory procedure, and then the fertilized egg (embryo) is returned to the woman's uterus.

Purpose

IVF is one of several assisted reproductive techniques (ART) used to help infertile couples to conceive a child. If after one year of having sexual intercourse without the use of birth control a woman is unable to get pregnant, **infertility** is suspected. Some of the reasons for infertility are damaged or blocked fallopian tubes, hormonal imbalance, or **endometriosis** in the woman. In the man, low sperm count or poor quality sperm can cause infertility.

IVF is one of several possible methods to increase the chance for an infertile couple to become pregnant. Its use depends on the reason for infertility. IVF may be an option if there is a blockage in the fallopian tube or endometriosis in the woman or low sperm count or poor quality sperm in the man. There are other possible treatments for these conditions, such as surgery for blocked tubes or endometriosis, which may be tried before IVF.

IVF will not work for a woman who is not capable of ovulating or a man who is not able to produce at least a few healthy sperm.

Precautions

The screening procedures and treatments for infertility can become a long, expensive, and sometimes, disappointing process. Each IVF attempt takes at least an entire menstrual cycle and can cost $5,000-$10,000, which may or may not be covered by health insurance. The **anxiety** of dealing with infertility can challenge both individuals and their relationship. The added **stress** and expense of multiple clinic visits, testing, treatments, and surgical procedures can become overwhelming. Couples may want to receive counseling and support throughout the process.

Description

In vitro fertilization is a procedure where the joining of egg and sperm takes place outside of the woman's body. A woman may be given fertility drugs before this procedure so that several eggs mature in the ovaries at the same time. Eggs (ova) are removed from a woman's ovaries using a long, thin needle. The physician gains access to the ovaries using one of two possible procedures. One procedure involves inserting the needle through the vagina (transvaginally). The physician guides the needle to the location of the ovaries with the help of an ultrasound machine. In the other procedure, called **laparoscopy**, a small thin tube with a viewing lens is inserted through an incision in the navel. This allows the physician to see inside the patient, and locate the ovaries, on a video monitor.

Once the eggs are removed, they are mixed with sperm in a laboratory dish or test tube. (This is where the term *test tube baby* comes from.) The eggs are monitored for several days. Once there is evidence that fertilization has occurred and the cells begin to divide, they are then returned to the woman's uterus.

In the procedure to remove eggs, enough may be gathered to be frozen and saved (either fertilized or unfertilized) for additional IVF attempts. A 2004 study from the Mayo Clinic found that frozen sperm was as effective as fresh sperm for IVF.

IVF has been used successfully since 1978, when the first child to be conceived by this method was born in England. Over the past 20 years, thousands of couples have used this method of ART or similar procedures to conceive.

Other types of assisted reproductive technologies might be used to achieve **pregnancy**. A procedure called intracytoplasmic sperm injection (ICSI) uses a manipulation technique that must be performed using a microscope to inject a single sperm into each egg. The

PATRICK CHRISTOPHER STEPTOE (1913–1988)

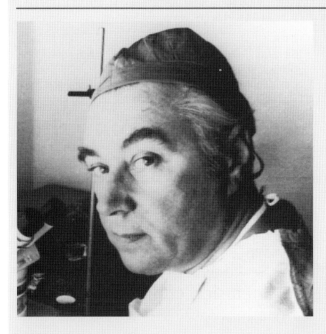

(Archive. Reproduced by permission.)

Patrick Christopher Steptoe was born in Oxfordshire, England, on June 9, 1913. His mother was a social worker and his father was a church organist. Steptoe entered the University of London's St. George Hospital Medical School, earning his physician's license in 1939 and becoming a member of the Royal College of Surgeons. When Steptoe volunteered as a naval surgeon during World War II, he was captured and held as a prisoner until his release in 1943. Following his release, Steptoe studied obstetrics and gynecology and moved to Manchester to start a private practice in 1948. In 1951, Steptoe accepted a position at Oldham General and District Hospital in England.

During his time at Oldham, Steoptoe continued his study of fertility problems. Using a laparoscope, he developed a method to remove eggs from a woman's ovaries. In 1966, Steptoe teamed with physiologist Robert G. Edwards who had successfully fertilized eggs outside of the body. In 1968, the pair had a breakthrough when Edwards successfully fertilized an egg that Steptoe had removed, but their attempts to implant the embryo failed repeatedly. However, Steptoe and Edwards experienced success when a fertilized egg was implanted into the uterus of Leslie Brown. Brown gave birth to a healthy baby girl on July 25, 1978.

Steptoe retired and built a clinic in Cambridge. He and Edwards were named Commanders of the British Empire, and Steptoe was honored with fellowship in the Royal Society. He and his wife had two children. Steptoe died on March 21, 1988.

fertilized eggs can then be returned to the uterus, as in IVF. In gamete intrafallopian tube transfer (GIFT) the eggs and sperm are mixed in a narrow tube and then deposited in the fallopian tube, where fertilization normally takes place. Another variation on IVF is zygote intrafallopian tube transfer (ZIFT). As in IVF, the fertilization of the eggs occurs in a laboratory dish. And, similar to GIFT, the embryos are placed in the fallopian tube (rather than the uterus as with IVF).

Preparation

Once a woman is determined to be a good candidate for in vitro fertilization, she will generally be given "fertility drugs" to stimulate ovulation and the development of multiple eggs. These drugs may include gonadotropin releasing hormone agonists (GnRHa), Pergonal, Clomid, or human chorionic gonadotropin (hcg). The maturation of the eggs is then monitored with ultrasound tests and frequent blood tests. If enough eggs mature, the physician will perform the procedure to remove them. The woman may be given a sedative prior to the procedure. A local anesthetic agent may also be used to reduce discomfort during the procedure.

Aftercare

After the IVF procedure is performed the woman can resume normal activities. A pregnancy test can be done approximately 12–14 days later to determine if the procedure was successful.

Risks

The risks associated with in vitro fertilization include the possibility of **multiple pregnancy** (since several embryos may be implanted) and **ectopic pregnancy** (an embryo that implants in the fallopian tube or in the abdominal cavity outside the uterus). There is a slight risk of ovarian rupture, bleeding, infections, and complications of anesthesia. If the procedure is successful and pregnancy is achieved, the pregnancy would carry the same risks as any pregnancy achieved without assisted technology.

Normal results

Success rates vary widely between clinics and between physicians performing the procedure and implantation does not guarantee pregnancy. Therefore, the procedure may have to be repeated more than once to achieve pregnancy. However, success rates have improved in recent years, up from 20% in 1995 to 27% in 2001.

Abnormal results

An ectopic or multiple pregnancy may abort spontaneously or may require termination if the health of the mother is at risk. The number of multiple pregnancies has decreased in recent years as technical advances and professional guidelines have led to implanting of fewer embryos per attempt.

Resources

PERIODICALS

"Frozen, Fresh Sperm Both Effective for In Vitro Fertilization." *Obesity, Fitness & Wellness Week* June 5, 2004: 1059.

"Multiple Births Via In Vitro Fertilization Are Declining." *Women's Health Weekly* May 6, 2004: 16.

ORGANIZATIONS

American Society for Reproductive Medicine. 1209 Montgomery Highway, Birmingham, AL 35216-2809. (205) 978-5000. < asrm@asrm.com > < http://www.asrm.com >.

Center for Fertility and In Vitro Fertilization Loma Linda University. 11370 Anderson St., Loma Linda, CA 92354. (909) 796-4851. < http://www.llu.edu/llumc/fertility >.

Resolve. 1310 Broadway, Somerville, MA 02144-1731. (617) 623-0744. < http://www.resolve.org >.

OTHER

"Infertility." *HealthWorld Online Page.* < http://www.healthy.net >.

"In vitro Fertilization: A Teacher's Guide from Newton's Apple." *PBS Page.* < http://www.pbs.org/ktca/newtons/11/invitro.html >.

Altha Roberts Edgren
Teresa G. Odle

Inclusion blennorrhea *see* **Inclusion conjunctivitis**

Inclusion conjunctivitis

Definition

Inclusion **conjunctivitis** is an inflammation of the conjunctiva (the membrane that lines the eyelids and covers the white part, or sclera, of the eyeball) by *Chlamydia trachomatis*. Chlamydia is a sexually transmitted organism.

Description

Inclusion conjunctivitis, known as neonatal inclusion conjunctivitis in the newborn and adult inclusion conjunctivitis in the adult, is also called inclusion blennorrhea, chlamydial conjunctivitis, or swimming pool conjunctivitis. This disease affects four of 1,000 (0.4%) live births. Approximately half of the infants born to untreated infected mothers will develop the disease.

Causes and symptoms

Inclusion conjunctivitis in the newborn results from passage through an infected birth canal and develops 5–14 days after birth. Both eyelids and conjunctivae are swollen. There may be a discharge of pus from the eyes.

Most instances of adult inclusion conjunctivitis result from exposure to infected genital secretions. It is transmitted to the eye by fingers and occasionally by the water in swimming pools, poorly chlorinated hot tubs, or by sharing makeup. In adult inclusion conjunctivitis, one eye is usually involved, with a stringy discharge of mucus and pus. There may be little bumps called follicles inside the lower eyelid and the eye is red. Occasionally, the condition damages the cornea, causing cloudy areas and a growth of new blood vessels (neovascularization).

Diagnosis

Inclusion conjunctivitis is usually considered when the patient has a follicular conjunctivitis that will not go away, even after using **topical antibiotics**. Diagnosis depends upon tests performed on the discharge from the eye. Gram stains determine the type of microorganism, while culture and sensitivity tests determine which antibiotic will kill the harmful microorganism. Conjuntival scraping determines whether chlamydia is present in cells taken from the conjunctiva.

Treatment

Treatment in the newborn consists of administration of tetracycline ointment to the conjunctiva and erythromycin orally or through intravenous therapy for fourteen days. The mother should be treated for **cervicitis** and the father for **urethritis**, even if they do not have symptoms of these diseases.

In adults, tetracycline ointment or drops should be applied to the conjunctiva and oral tetracycline, amoxacillin, or erythromycin should be taken for three weeks, or doxycycline for one week.

Patients should have weekly checkups so the doctor can monitor the healing.

Oral tetracycline should not be administered to children whose permanent teeth have not erupted. It should also not be given to nursing or pregnant women.

Prognosis

Untreated inclusion conjunctivitis in the newborn persists for 3–12 months and usually heals; however, there may be scarring or neovascularization. In the adult, if left untreated, the disease may continue for months and cause corneal neovascularization. Even if treated, **antibiotics** usually do not reverse damage that may have occurred, but they may help prevent it if given early enough.

Prevention

The neonatal infection may be prevented by instilling erythromycin ointment in the conjunctival cul-de-sac at birth. It is not prevented by silver nitrate.

Chlamydia is a contagious, sexually transmitted disease. Some systemic symptoms include a history of

> **KEY TERMS**
>
> **Cervicitis**—Cervicitis is an inflammation of the cervix or neck of the uterus.
>
> **Conjunctiva**—The conjunctiva is the membrane that lines the eyelids and covers the white part of the eyeball (sclera).
>
> **Cornea**—The clear dome-shaped structure that covers the colored part of the eye (iris).
>
> **Neovascularization**—Neovascularization is the growth of new blood vessels.
>
> **Urethritis**—Urethritis is an inflammation of the urethra, the canal for the discharge of urine that extends from the bladder to the outside of the body.

vaginitis, **pelvic inflammatory disease**, or urethritis. Patients with symptoms of these diseases should be treated by a physician.

Resources

BOOKS

Newell, Frank W. *Ophthalmology: Principles and Concepts.* 8th ed. St. Louis: Mosby, 1996.

ORGANIZATIONS

American Academy of Ophthalmology. 655 Beach Street, PO Box 7424, San Francisco, CA 94120-7424. < http://www.eyenet.org >.
American Optometric Association. 243 North Lindbergh Blvd., St. Louis, MO 63141. (314) 991-4100. < http://www.aoanet.org >.

Lorraine Steefel, RN

Incompetent cervix

Definition

A cervix (the structure at the bottom of the uterus) that is incompetent is abnormally weak, and therefore it can gradually widen during **pregnancy**. Left untreated, this can result in repeated pregnancy losses or premature delivery.

Description

Incompetent cervix is the result of an anatomical abnormality. Normally, the cervix remains closed throughout pregnancy until labor begins. An incompetent cervix gradually opens due to the pressure from the developing fetus after about the 13th week of pregnancy. The cervix begins to thin out and widen without any contractions or labor. The membranes surrounding the fetus bulge down into the opening of the cervix until they break, resulting in the loss of the baby or a very premature delivery.

Causes and symptoms

Some factors that can contribute to the chance of a woman having an incompetent cervix include trauma to the cervix, physical abnormality of the cervix, or having been exposed to the drug diethylstilbestrol (DES) in the mother's womb. Some women have cervical incompetence for no obvious reason.

Diagnosis

Incompetent cervix is suspected when a woman has three consecutive spontaneous pregnancy losses during the second trimester (the fourth, fifth and sixth months of the pregnancy). The likelihood of this happening by random chance is less than 1%. Spontaneous losses due to incompetent cervix account for 20–25% of all second trimester losses. A spontaneous second trimester pregnancy loss is different from a **miscarriage**, which usually happens during the first three months of pregnancy.

The physician can check for abnormalities in the cervix by performing a manual examination or by an ultrasound test. The physician can also check to see if the cervix is prematurely widened (dilated). Because incompetent cervix is only one of several potential causes for this, the patient's past history of pregnancy losses must also be considered when making the diagnosis.

Treatment

Treatment for incompetent cervix is a surgical procedure called cervical cerclage. A stitch (suture) is used to tie the cervix shut to give it more support. It is most effective if it is performed somewhere between 14–16 weeks into the pregnancy. The stitch is removed near the end of pregnancy to allow for a normal birth.

Cervical cerclage can be performed under spinal, epidural, or **general anesthesia**. The patient will need to stay in the hospital for one or more days. The procedure to remove the suture is done without the need for anesthesia. The vagina is held open with an instrument called a speculum and the stitch is cut and removed.

KEY TERMS

Diethylstilbestrol (DES)—DES is a drug given to women a generation ago to prevent miscarriage. At that time it was not known that female children born of women who had been given DES would show a higher rate for cervical and other reproductive abnormalities, as well as a rare form of vaginal cancer, when they reached reproductive age.

Effacement—The thinning out of the cervix that normally occurs along with dilation shortly before delivery.

Preterm labor—Labor before the thirty-seventh week of pregnancy.

This may be slightly uncomfortable, but should not be painful.

Some possible risks of cerclage are premature rupture of the amniotic membranes, infection of the amniotic sac, and preterm labor. The risk of infection of the amniotic sac increases as the pregnancy progresses. For a cervix that is dilated 3 centimeters (cm), the risk is 30%.

After cerclage, a woman will be monitored for any preterm labor. The woman needs to consult her obstetrician immediately if there are any signs of contractions.

Cervical cerclage can not be performed if a woman is more than 4 cm dilated, if the fetus has already died in her uterus, or if her amniotic membranes are torn and her water has broken.

Prognosis

The success rate for cerclage correction of incompetent cervix is good. About 80-90% of the time women deliver healthy infants. The success rate is higher for cerclage done early in pregnancy.

Resources

OTHER

Weiss, Robin. "Incompetent Cervix." *The Mining Co. Guide to Pregnancy/Childbirth Page*. March 1998. < http:// www.pregnancy.miningco.com/library/weekly/ aa011298.htm >.

Tish Davidson, A.M.

Incontinence *see* **Urinary incontinence**

Indigestion

Definition

Indigestion, which is sometimes called **dyspepsia**, is a general term covering a group of nonspecific symptoms in the digestive tract. It is often described as a feeling of fullness, bloating, **nausea**, **heartburn**, or gassy discomfort in the chest or abdomen. The symptoms develop during meals or shortly afterward. In most cases, indigestion is a minor problem that often clears up without professional treatment.

Description

Indigestion or dyspepsia is a widespread condition, estimated to occur in 25% of the adult population of the United States. Most people with indigestion do not feel sick enough to see a doctor; nonetheless, it is a common reason for office visits. About 3% of visits to primary care doctors are for indigestion.

Causes and symptoms

Physical causes

The symptoms associated with indigestion have a variety of possible physical causes, ranging from commonplace food items to serious systemic disorders:

- Diet. Milk, milk products, alcoholic beverages, tea, and coffee cause indigestion in some people because they stimulate the stomach's production of acid.

- Medications. Certain prescription drugs as well as over-the-counter medications can irritate the stomach lining. These medications include **aspirin**, NSAIDs, some **antibiotics**, digoxin, theophylline, **corticosteroids**, iron (ferrous sulfate), **oral contraceptives**, and tricyclic antidepressants.

- Disorders of the pancreas and gallbladder. These include inflammation of the gallbladder or pancreas, **cancer** of the pancreas, and **gallstones**.

- Intestinal parasites. Parasitic infections that cause indigestion include **amebiasis**, fluke and tapeworm infections, **giardiasis**, and strongyloidiasis.

- Systemic disorders, including diabetes, thyroid disease, collagen vascular disease.

- Cancers of the digestive tract.

- Conditions associated with women's reproductive organs. These conditions include menstrual cramps, **pregnancy**, and pelvic inflammatory disease.

Psychologic and emotional causes

Indigestion often accompanies an emotional upset, because the part of the nervous system involved in the so-called "fight-or-flight" response also affects the digestive tract. People diagnosed with **anxiety** or **somatoform disorders** frequently have problems with indigestion. Many people in the general population, however, will also experience heartburn, "butterflies in the stomach," or stomach cramps when they are in upsetting situations–such as school examinations, arguments with family members, crises in their workplace, and so on. Some people's digestive systems appear to react more intensely to emotional **stress** due to hypersensitive nerve endings in their intestinal tract.

Specific gastrointestinal disorders

In some cases, the patient's description of the symptoms suggests a specific digestive disorder as the cause of the indigestion. Some doctors classify these cases into three groups:

ESOPHAGITIS TYPE. Esophagitis is an inflammation of the tube that carries food from the throat to the stomach (the esophagus). The tissues of the esophagus can become irritated by the flow (reflux) of stomach acid backward into the lower part of the esophagus. If the patient describes the indigestion in terms of frequent or intense heartburn, the doctor will consider gastroesophageal reflux disease (GERD) as a possible cause. GERD is a common disorder in the general population, affecting about 30% of adults.

PEPTIC ULCER TYPE. Patients who smoke and are over 45 are more likely to have indigestion of the peptic ulcer type. This group also includes people who find that their indigestion is relieved by taking **antacids** or eating a small amount of food. Patients in this category are often found to have *Helicobacter pylori* infections. *H. pylori* is a rod-shaped bacterium that lives in the tissues of the stomach and causes irritation of the mucous lining of the stomach walls. Most people with *H. pylori* infections do not develop chronic indigestion, but the organism appears to cause peptic ulcer disease (PUD) in a vulnerable segment of the population.

NONULCER TYPE. Most cases of chronic indigestion–as many as 65%–fall into this third category. Nonulcer dyspepsia is sometimes called functional dyspepsia because it appears to be related to abnormalities in the way that the stomach empties its contents into the intestine. In some people, the stomach empties either too slowly or too rapidly. In others, the stomach's muscular contractions are irregular and uncoordinated. These disorders of stomach movement (motility) may be caused by hypersensitive nerve endings in the stomach tissues. Patients in this group are likely to be younger than 45 and have a history of taking medications for anxiety or depression.

Diagnosis

Patient history

Because indigestion is a nonspecific set of symptoms, patients who feel sick enough to seek medical attention are likely to go to their primary care doctor. The history does not always point to an obvious diagnosis. The doctor can, however, use the process of history-taking to evaluate the patient's mood or emotional state in order to assess the possibility of a psychiatric disturbance. In addition, asking about the location, intensity, timing, and recurrence of the indigestion can help the doctor weigh the different diagnostic possibilities.

An important part of the history-taking is asking about symptoms that may indicate a serious illness. These warning symptoms include:

- Weight loss
- Persistent vomiting
- Difficulty or **pain** in swallowing
- Vomiting blood or passing blood in the stools
- Anemia.

Imaging studies

If the doctor thinks that the indigestion should be investigated further, he or she will order an endoscopic examination of the stomach. An endoscope is a slender tube-shaped instrument that allows the doctor to look at the lining of the patient's stomach. If the patient has indigestion of the esophagitis type or nonulcer type, the stomach lining will appear normal. If the patient has PUD, the doctor will be able to see breaks or ulcerated areas in the tissue. He or she may also order ultrasound imaging of the abdomen, or a radionuclide scan to evaluate the motility of the stomach.

Laboratory tests

BLOOD TESTS. If the patient is over 45, the doctor will have the patient's blood analyzed for a complete blood cell count, measurements of liver enzyme levels, electrolyte and serum calcium levels, and thyroid function.

TESTS FOR *HELICOBACTER PYLORI.* Doctors can now test patients for the presence of *H. pylori* without having to take a tissue sample from the stomach. One of these noninvasive tests is a blood test and the other is a breath test.

Treatment

Since most cases of indigestion are not caused by serious disorders, many doctors prefer to try medications and other treatment measures before ordering an endoscopy.

Diet and stress management

Many patients benefit from the doctor's reassurance that they do not have a serious or fatal disorder. Cutting out alcoholic beverages and drinks containing **caffeine** often helps. The patient may also be asked to keep a record of food intake, daily schedule, and symptom severity. Food diaries sometimes reveal psychologic or dietary factors that influence indigestion.

Medications

Patients with the esophagitis type of indigestion are often treated with H_2 antagonists. H_2 antagonists are drugs that block the secretion of stomach acid. They include ranitidine (Zantac) and famotidine (Pepcid).

Patients with motility disorders may be given prokinetic drugs. Prokinetic medications speed up the emptying of the stomach and increase intestinal motility. They include metoclopramide (Reglan) and cisapride (Propulsid). These drugs relieve symptoms in 60–80% of patients.

Removal of H. pylori

It is not clear that patients with *H. pylori* infections who have *not* developed gastric ulcers need to have the bacterium removed. Some studies indicate, however, that these patients may benefit from antibiotic therapy.

Alternative treatment

Herbal medicine

Practitioners of Chinese traditional herbal medicine might recommend medicines derived from peony (*Paeonia lactiflora*), hibiscus (*Hibiscus sabdariffa*), or hare's ear (*Bupleurum chinense*) to treat indigestion. Western herbalists are likely to prescribe fennel (*Foeniculum vulgare*), lemon balm (*Melissa officinalis*), or peppermint (*Mentha piperita*) to relieve stomach cramps and heartburn.

KEY TERMS

Dyspepsia—Another name for indigestion.

Endoscope—A slender tubular instrument used to examine the inside of the stomach.

Gastroesophageal reflux disease (GERD)—A disorder of the lower end of the esophagus, caused by stomach acid flowing backward into the esophagus and irritating the tissues.

H₂ antagonist—A type of drug that relieves indigestion by reducing the production of stomach acid.

Heartburn—A popular term for an uncomfortable burning sensation in the stomach and lower esophagus, sometimes caused by the reflux of small amounts of stomach acid.

Helicobacter pylori—A gram-negative rod-shaped bacterium that lives in the tissues of the stomach and causes inflammation of the stomach lining.

Motility—The movement or capacity for movement of an organism or body organ. Indigestion is sometimes caused by abnormal patterns in the motility of the stomach.

Peptic ulcer disease (PUD)—A stomach disorder marked by corrosion of the stomach lining due to the acid in the digestive juices.

Prokinetic—A drug that works to speed up the emptying of the stomach and the motility of the intestines.

Reflux—The backward flow of a body fluid or secretion. Indigestion is sometimes caused by the reflux of stomach acid into the esophagus.

Prognosis

Most cases of mild indigestion do not need medical treatment. For patients who consult a doctor and are given an endoscopic examination, 5-15% are diagnosed with GERD and 15-25% with PUD. About 1% of patients who are endoscoped have **stomach cancer**. Most patients with functional dyspepsia do well on either H₂ antagonists or prokinetic drugs, depending on the cause of their indigestion.

Prevention

Indigestion can often be prevented by attention to one's diet, general stress level, and ways of managing stress. Specific preventive measures include:

• Stop **smoking**.

• Cutting down on or eliminating alcohol, tea, or coffee.

• Avoiding foods that are highly spiced or loaded with fat.

• Eating slowly and keeping mealtimes relaxed.

• Practicing yoga or meditation.

• Not taking aspirin or other medications on an empty stomach.

• Keeping one's weight within normal limits.

Resources

OTHER

"Indigestion." *ThriveOnline.* April 6, 1998. < http:// thriveonline.oxygen.com >.

Rebecca J. Frey, PhD

Homeopathy

Homeopaths tailor their remedies to the patient's overall personality profile as well as the specific symptoms. Depending on the patient's reaction to the indigestion and some of its likely causes, the homeopath might choose *Gelsemium* (*Gelsemium sempervirens*), *Carbo vegetalis*, *Nux vomica*, or *Pulsatilla* (*Pulsatilla nigricans*).

Other treatments

Some alternative treatments are aimed at lowering the patient's stress level or changing attitudes and beliefs that contribute to indigestion. These therapies and practices include **Reiki**, **reflexology**, **hydrotherapy**, therapeutic massage, **yoga**, and **meditation**.

Indinavir *see* **Protease inhibitors**

Indirect Coombs' test *see* **Coombs' tests**

Indium scan of the body

Definition

A scanning procedure in which a patient's white blood cells are first labeled with the radioactive substance indium, and then the patient's body is scanned as a way of tracking the white blood cells at the site of possible infection.

Purpose

The procedure is used to detect inflammatory processes in the body such as infections. By labelling the leukocytes (white blood cells), radiologists or nuclear medicine specialists can then watch their migration toward an **abscess** or other infection.

Description

A nuclear medicine technologist withdraws about 50 ml. of blood. White blood cells are collected, exposed to indium, and reinjected by IV back into the patient.

The scan is scheduled for between 18 and 24 hours after the white blood cells have been labelled with indium. (In some cases, more scanning may be scheduled 48 hours after labelling).

For the scan, the patient lies on a special scanning table, as either a single camera passing underneath the table or two cameras (one above the table and one underneath) are placed as close as possible to the body, slowly scanning the person's body.

The radiologist may need extra pictures, but these take only a few minutes each.

While the patient must remain perfectly still during the scan, there should be no discomfort.

Aftercare

After the scan, the patient should be able to continue with normal daily activities with no problems.

Risks

The only risk during this scanning procedure could be to a patient who is pregnant, as with any type of injectable radioactive substance. If the woman is pregnant, the radiologist must be notified; if the scan is cleared, the radiologist may use a lower dosage of indium.

Normal results

The scan should reveal no infection or pathology.

Abnormal results

The scan will reveal details, such as location, about an infection in the patient's body.

Carol A. Turkington

Induction of labor

Definition

Induction of labor involves using artificial means to assist the mother in delivering her baby.

Purpose

Labor is brought on, or induced, when the **pregnancy** has extended significantly beyond the expected delivery date and the mother shows no signs of going into labor. Generally, if the unborn baby is more than two weeks past due, labor will be induced. In most cases, a mother delivers her baby between 38–42 weeks of pregnancy. This usually means that labor is induced if the pregnancy has lasted more than 42 weeks. Labor is also induced if the mother is suffering from diseases (**preeclampsia**, chronic **hypertension**), if there is an Rh blood incompatibility between the baby and the mother, or if the mother or baby has a medical problem that requires delivery of the baby (like a premature rupture of the membranes).

Description

The uterus is the hollow female organ that supports the development and nourishment of the unborn baby during pregnancy. Sometimes labor is induced by the rupturing the amniotic membrane to release amniotic fluid. This is an attempt to mimic the normal process of "breaking water" that occurs early in the normal birth process. This method is sometimes enough stimulation to induce contractions in the mother's uterus. If labor fails to start, drugs are used.

Most labor is induced by using the drug Pitocin, a synthetic form of oxytocin. Oxytocin is a natural hormone produced in the body by the pituitary gland. During normal labor, oxytocin causes contractions. When labor does not occur naturally, the doctor may

KEY TERMS

Cesarean section—Delivery of a baby through an incision in the mother's abdomen instead of through the vagina; also called a C-section.

Preeclampsia—Hypertension (high blood pressure) experienced during pregnancy.

Rh blood incompatibility—A blood type problem between mother (who is Rh negative) and baby (who is Rh positive), making the immune system of the mother attack her unborn baby. During delivery of the first pregnancy, the mother's immune system becomes sensitive to the Rh positive blood of the baby. The mother's system may then attack later pregnancies and cause severe illness or death to those babies.

Vasoconstriction—Constriction of a blood vessel.

give the mother Pitocin to start the contractions. Pitocin makes the uterus contract with strength and force almost immediately. This drug is given through a vein in a steady flow that allows the doctor to control the amount the mother is given.

Sometimes vaginal gels are used to induce labor. Normally, the baby will pass through the opening of the uterus (the cervix) into the birth canal during delivery. Because of this, the cervix softens and begins to enlarge (dilate) during the early part of labor to make room for the baby to pass through. The cervix will continue to dilate, and the contractions will eventually push the baby out of the mother's body. When labor needs to be induced, the cervix is often small, hard, and not ready for the process. The doctor may need to prepare or "ripen" the cervix to induce labor. The hormone prostaglandin in a gel form may be applied high in the vagina to soften and dilate the cervix, making the area ready for labor. This may be enough to stimulate contractions on its own. More often, prostaglandin gel is used in conjunction with Pitocin.

If all attempts to induce labor fail, a **cesarean section** is performed.

Risks

Once labor has been induced, the unborn baby is monitored to guard against a reduction in its oxygen supply, or hypoxia. The drugs used to induce labor cause vasoconstriction, which can decrease blood supply to the unborn baby. Throughout the process, the baby's heart rate is monitored by an electronic device placed on top of the mother's abdomen. The heart rate is one sign that the unborn baby is getting enough oxygen and remains healthy. Once the membranes are broken, prolonged labor may result in infection to either the newborn or the mother.

Normal results

Once labor is induced and the cervix has dilated, labor usually proceeds normally. When performed properly, induced labor is a safe procedure for both mother and baby.

Resources

BOOKS

Berkow, Robert, et al., editors. *The Merck Manual of Medical Information.* Whitehouse Station, NJ: Merck Research Laboratories, 2004.

John T. Lohr, PhD

Infant massage

Definition

Infant massage refers to **massage therapy** as specifically applied to infants. In most cases, oil or lotion is used as it would be on an adult subject by a trained and licensed massage therapist. Medical professionals caring for infants might also use massage techniques on infants born prematurely, on those with motor or gastrointestinal problems, or on those who have been exposed to **cocaine** in utero.

Purpose

Research from experiments conducted at the Touch Research Institutes at the University of Miami School of Medicine and Nova Southeastern University has been cited for the clinical benefits massage has on infants and children. Tiffany Field, Ph. D., director, noted that the research "... suggests that touch is as important to infants and children as eating and sleeping. Touch therapy triggers many physiological changes that help infants and children grow and develop. For example, massage can stimulate nerves in the brain which facilitate food absorption, resulting in faster weight gain. It also lowers level of **stress** hormones, resulting in improved immune function."

The benefits of infant massage include:

- Relaxation
- relief from stress
- interaction with adults
- stimulation of the nervous system

The results of several studies showed that infant massage alleviates the stress that newborns experience as a result of the enormous change that birth brings about in their lives after the 6–9 months they have spent in the womb. Both premature infants and full-term babies need the relaxation that comes from massaging and moving their limbs and muscles. In infants with **colic**, massage provides the relief necessary to disperse gas, ease muscle spasm, tone the digestive system and help it work efficiently. Some techniques even help bring relief from teething and emotional stress. The stimulation an infant receives from massage can aid circulation, strengthen muscles, help digestion, and relieve **constipation**. The bonding that occurs with massage between a parent and child enhances the entire process of bonding that comes with contact through all of the senses, including touch, voice, and sight. It affords a physical experience of quality time between the parents and the child as well as with any significant others in a baby's life.

Description

Origins

The practice of massaging infants dates back to ancient times, particularly in Asian and Pacific Island cultures; that is, massage was a component of the baby's regular bath routine among the Maoris and Hawaiians. Touch in these cultures is considered healthful both physically and spiritually. In the West, however, infant massage has received more attention in recent years in conjunction with the popularity of natural **childbirth** and midwife-assisted births. Dr. Frédéric Leboyer, a French physician who was one of the leaders of the natural childbirth movement, helped to popularize infant massage through his photojournalistic book on the Indian art of baby massage.

Infant massage was introduced formally into the United States in 1978 when Vimala Schneider McClure, a **yoga** practitioner who served in an orphanage in Northern India, developed a training program for instructors at the request of childbirth educators. An early research study by R. Rice in 1976 had showed that premature babies who were massaged surged ahead in weight gain and neurological development over those who were not massaged. From McClure's training in India, her knowledge of Swedish massage and **reflexology**, along with her knowledge of yoga postures that she had already adapted for babies, she became the foremost authority on infant massage. In 1986 she founded the International Association of Infant Massage (IAIM), which has 27 chapters worldwide as of 2000.

Various techniques are used in infant massage, with the different strokes specific to a particular therapy. Special handling is used for treating a baby with gas and colic. Some of the strokes are known as "Indian milking," which is a gentle stroking of the child's legs; and the "twist and squeeze" stroke, a gentle squeeze of the muscles in the thigh and calf. The light "feather" strokes often employed in regular Swedish massage are applied at the end of a massage. The procedure is not unlike certain forms of adult massage, but with extra care taken for the fragility of the infant.

There are also specific Chinese techniques of pediatric massage, including massage of children with special needs. In China, these forms of massage can be given by medical professionals, but parents are often taught how to do the simpler forms for home treatment of their children.

Preparations

If lotions or oils are used, care is taken to ensure their safety on a baby's delicate skin. The most important consideration is to use vegetable oils rather than mineral oils, which can clog the pores in the skin. The oil that is used should be warmed in the caregiver's hands before applying it to the baby's skin. The environment in which the massage is given to an infant should be comfortably warm, and as calm and non-threatening as possible.

Precautions

Extreme caution is necessary when performing infant massage. Strokes are made with the greatest delicacy in order not to harm the infant in any way. Proper techniques are taught by licensed massage therapists ensuring that the infant is treated with appropriate physical touch. Anyone who is unfamiliar with handling a baby should receive appropriate instruction before beginning infant massage.

Side effects

No adverse side effects have been reported when infant massage is done properly after careful instruction, or by a licensed massage therapist who specializes in infant care.

Research and general acceptance

In addition to the study already noted regarding touch therapy, a website devoted to infant massage lists research published as early as 1969, and cites hundreds of individual projects that have been conducted throughout the world focusing on infant massage. Many of the studies are related to the benefits of massage and touch for premature infants and others born with such risk factors as drug dependence. Conclusions regarding the benefits are overwhelmingly positive. The proliferation of therapists licensed in infant massage across the United States and worldwide indicates that infant massage is increasingly recognized as a legitimate health care treatment.

Resources

BOOKS

Cline, Kyle. *Chinese Massage for Infants and Children: Traditional Techniques for Alleviating Colic, Teething Pain, Earache, and Other Common Childhood Conditions.* Inner Traditions International, Limited, 1999.

Fan, Ya-Li. *Chinese Pediatric Massage Therapy: Traditional Techniques for Alleviating Colic, Colds, Earaches, and Other Common Childhood Conditions,* edited by Bob Flaws. Blue Poppy Enterprises, 1999.

Gordon, Jay, and Brenda Adderly. *Brighter Baby: Boosting Your Child's Intelligence, Health and Happiness through Infant Therapeutic Massage.* New York: Regnery Publishing, Inc. 1999.

ORGANIZATIONS

International Association of Infant Massage. P.O. Box 1045. Oak View, CA 93022.

International Institute of Infant Massage. 605 Bledsoe Rd. NW. Albuquerque, NM 87107. (505) 341-9381. Fax: (505) 341-9386. < http://www.infantmassage.com >.

Jane Spehar

Infant respiratory distress syndrome *see* **Respiratory distress syndrome**

Infantile paralysis *see* **Polio**

Infarct avid imaging *see* **Technetium heart scan**

Infarction *see* **Stroke**

▌Infection control

Definition

Infection control refers to policies and procedures used to minimize the risk of spreading infections, especially in hospitals and human or animal health care facilities.

Purpose

The purpose of infection control is to reduce the occurrence of infectious diseases. These diseases are usually caused by bacteria or viruses and can be spread by human to human contact, animal to human contact, human contact with an infected surface, airborne transmission through tiny droplets of infectious agents suspended in the air, and, finally, by such common vehicles as food or water. Diseases that are spread from animals to humans are known as zoonoses; animals that carry disease agents from one host to another are known as vectors.

Infection control in hospitals and other health care settings

Infections contracted in hospitals are also called nosocomial infections. They occur in approximately 5% of all hospital patients. These infections result in increased time spent in the hospital and, in some cases, **death**. There are many reasons nosocomial infections are common, one of which is that many hospital patients have a weakened immune system which makes them more susceptible to infections. This weakened immune system can be caused either by the patient's diseases or by treatments given to the patient. Second, many medical procedures can increase the risk of infection by introducing infectious agents into the patient. Thirdly, many patients are admitted to hospitals because of infectious disease. These infectious agents can then be transferred from patient to patient by hospital workers or visitors.

Infection control has become a formal discipline in the United States since the 1950s, due to the spread of **staphylococcal infections** in hospitals. Because there is both the risk of health care providers acquiring infections themselves, and of them passing infections on to patients, the Centers for Disease Control and Prevention (CDC) established guidelines for infection control procedures. In addition to hospitals, infection control is important in nursing homes, clinics, child care centers, and restaurants, as well as in the home.

ELIZABETH LEE HAZEN
(1885–1975)

Elizabeth Lee Hazen was born on August 24, 1885, in Rich, Mississippi. Hazen, born the middle of three children to Maggie (Harper) and William Edgar Hazen, was orphaned before she turned four. She and her sister went to live with their aunt and uncle shorly after her younger brother died. Hazen attended the Mississippi Industrial Institute and College at Columbus, receiving her B.S. degree in 1910. During college, Hazen became interested in science and she studied biology at Columbia University, earning her M.S. in 1917. After working in the U.S. Army laboratories during World War I, she returned to Columbia where she received her Ph.D. in microbiology in 1927. Following her work as an instructor at Columbia, Hazen accepted a position with the New York Department of Health where she researched bacterial diseases.

In 1948, Hazen and Rachel Brown began researching fungal infections found in humans due to antibiotic treatments and diseases. Some of the antibiotics they discovered did indeed kill the fungus; however, they also killed the test mice. Finally, Hazen located a microorganism on a farm in Virginia, and Brown's tests indicated that the microorganism produced two antibiotics, one of which proved effective for treating fungus and candidiasis in humans. Brown purified the antibiotic which was patented under the name *nystatin*. In 1954, the antibiotic became available in pill form. Hazen and Brown continued their research and discovered two other antibiotics. Hazen received numerous awards individually and with her research partner, Rachel Brown. Elizabeth Hazen passed away on June 24, 1975.

Selected Infectious Diseases And Corresponding Treatment

Disease	Symptoms	Transmittal	Treatment
Chicken pox	Rash, low-grade **fever**	Person to person	None
Common cold/ Influenza	Runny nose, **sore throat**, **cough**, fever, **headache**, muscle aches	Person to person	None
Hepatitis	Jaundice, flu-like symptoms	Sexual contact with an infected person, contaminated blood, food, or water	None
Legionnaire's Disease	Flu symptoms, peneumonia, **diarrhea**, **vomiting**, kidney failure, respiratory failure	Air conditioning or water systems	Antibiotics
Measles	Skin rash, runny nose and eyes, fever, cough	Person to person	None
Meningitis	Neck **pain**, headache, pain caused by exposure to light, fever, **nausea**, drowsiness	Person to person	Antibiotics for bacterial meningitis, hospital care for viral meningitis
Mumps	Swelling of salivary glands	Person to person	Anti-inflammatory drugs
Ringworm	Skin rash	Contact with infected animal or person	Antifungal drugs applied topically
Tetanus	Lockjaw, other spasms	Soil infection of wounds	Antibiotics, antitoxins, muscle relaxers

To lower the risk of nosocomial infections, the CDC began a national program of hospital inspection in 1970 known as the National Nosocomial Infections Surveillance system, or NNIS. The CDC reported that over 300 hospitals participate in the NNIS system as of the early 2000s. Data collected from the participating hospitals show that infection control programs can siginificantly improve patient safety, lower infection rates, and lower patient mortality.

Dental health care settings are similar to hospitals in that both personnel and equipment can transmit infection if proper safeguards are not observed. The CDC issued new guidelines in 2003 for the proper maintenance and sterilization of dental equipment, hand hygiene for dentists and dental hygienists, dental radiology, medications, and oral surgery, environmental infection control, and standards for dental laboratories.

The newest addition to the infection control specialist's resources is molecular typing, which speeds up the identification of a disease agent. Rapid identification in turn allows for timely containment of a disease outbreak.

Threat of emerging infectious diseases

Due to constant changes in our lifestyles and environments, new diseases are constantly appearing that people are susceptible to, making protection from the threat of infectious disease urgent. Many new contagious diseases have been identified in the past 30 years, such as **AIDS**, Ebola, and hantavirus. Increased travel between continents makes the world-wide spread of disease a bigger concern than it once was. Additionally, many common infectious diseases have become resistant to known treatments.

The emergence of the **severe acute respiratory syndrome (SARS)** epidemic in Asia in February 2003 was a classic instance of an emerging disease that spread rapidly because of the increased frequency of international and intercontinental travel. In addition, the SARS outbreak demonstrated the vulnerability of hospitals and health care workers to emerging diseases. Clusters of cases within hospitals occurred in the early weeks of the epidemic when the disease had not yet been recognized and the first SARS patients were admitted without **isolation** precautions.

The SARS epidemic also raised a number of ethical and legal questions regarding current attitudes toward infection control.

Problems of antibiotic resistance

Because of the overuse of **antibiotics**, many bacteria have developed a resistance to common antibiotics. This means that newer antibiotics must continually be developed in order to treat an infection. However, further resistance seems to come about almost simultaneously. This indicates to many scientists that it might become more and more difficult to treat infectious diseases. The use of antibiotics outside of medicine also contributes to increased antibiotic resistance. One example of this is the use of antibiotics in animal husbandry. These negative trends can only be reversed by establishing a more rational use of antibiotics through treatment guidelines.

Bioterrorism

The events of September 11, 2001, and the **anthrax** scare that followed in October 2001 alerted public health officials as well as the general public to the possible use of infectious disease agents as weapons of terrorism. The Centers for Disease Control and Prevention (CDC) now has a list of topics and resources related to bioterrorism on its web site.

Description

The goals of infection control programs are: immunizing against preventable diseases, defining precautions that can prevent exposure to infectious agents, and restricting the exposure of health care workers to an infectious agent. An infection control practitioner is a specially trained professional, oftentimes a nurse, who oversees infection control programs.

Commonly recommended precautions to avoid and control the spread of infections include:

- Vaccinate people and pets against diseases for which a vaccine is available. As of 2003, the vaccines used against infectious diseases are very safe compared to most drugs.

- Wash hands often.

- Cook food thoroughly.

- Use antibiotics only as directed.

- See a doctor for infections that do not heal.

- Avoid areas with a lot of insects.

- Be cautious around wild or unfamiliar animals, or any animals that are unusually aggressive. Do not purchase exotic animals as pets.

- Do not engage in unprotected sex or in intravenous drug use.

- Find out about infectious diseases when you make travel plans. Travelers' advisories and adult **vaccination** recommendations are available on the CDC web site or by calling the CDC's telephone service at 404-332-4559.

Because of the higher risk of spreading infectious disease in a hospital setting, higher levels of precautions are taken there. Typically, health care workers wear gloves with all patients, since it is difficult to know whether a transmittable disease is present or not. Patients who have a known infectious disease are isolated to decrease the risk of transmitting the infectious agent to another person. Hospital workers who come in contact with infected patients must wear gloves and gowns to decrease the risk of carrying the infectious agent to other patients. All articles of equipment that are used in an isolation room are decontaminated before reuse. Patients who are immunocompromised may be put in protective isolation to decrease the risk of infectious agents being brought into their room. Any hospital worker with infections, including colds, are restricted from that room.

Hospital infections can also be transmitted through the air. Thus care must be taken when handling infected materials so as to decrease the numbers of infectious agents that become airborne. Special care should also taken with hospital ventilation systems to prevent recirculation of contaminated air.

Resources

BOOKS

Beers, Mark H., MD, and Robert Berkow, MD, editors. "Immunizations for Adults." Section 13, Chapter 152. In *The Merck Manual of Diagnosis and Therapy*. Whitehouse Station, NJ: Merck Research Laboratories, 2004.

KEY TERMS

Acquired immune deficiency syndrome (AIDS)— A disease that weakens the body's immune system. It is also known as HIV infection.

Antibiotic—A substance, such as a drug, that can stop a bacteria from growing or destroy the bacteria.

Antibiotic resistance—The ability of infectious agents to change their biochemistry in such a way as to make an antibiotic no longer effective.

Bioterrorism—The intentional use of disease-causing microbes or other biologic agents to intimidate or terrorize a civilian population for political or military reasons.

Ebola—The disease caused by the newly described and very deadly Ebola virus found in Africa.

Epidemiology—The branch of medicine that deals with the transmission of infectious diseases in large populations and with detection of the sources and causes of epidemics.

Hantavirus—A group of arboviruses that cause hemorrhagic fever (characterized by sudden onset, fever, aching and bleeding in the internal organs).

Immunization—Immunity refers to the body's ability to protect itself from a certain disease after it has been exposed to that disease. Through immunization, also known as vaccination, a small amount of an infectious agent is injected into the body to stimulate the body to develop immunity.

Immunocompromized—Refers to the condition of having a weakened immune system. This can happen due to genetic factors, drugs, or disease.

Nosocomial infection—An infection acquired in a hospital setting.

Staphylococcal infection—An infection caused by the organism *Staphlococcus*. Infection by this agent is common and is often resistant to antibiotics.

Vector—An animal carrier that transfers an infectious organism from one host to another.

Zoonosis (plural, zoonoses)—Any disease of animals that can be transmitted to humans under natural conditions. Lyme disease, rabies, psittacosis (parrot fever), cat-scratch fever, and monkeypox are examples of zoonoses.

PERIODICALS

Ashford, D. A., R. M. Kaiser, M. E. Bales, et al. "Planning Against Biological Terrorism: Lessons from Outbreak Investigations." *Emerging Infectious Diseases* 9 (May 2003): 515–519.

Gostin, L. O., R. Bayer, and A. L. Fairchild. "Ethical and Legal Challenges Posed by Severe Acute Respiratory Syndrome: Implications for the Control of Severe Infectious Disease Threats." *Journal of the American Medical Association* 290 (December 24, 2003): 3229–3237.

Ho, P. L., X. P. Tang, and W. H. Seto. "SARS: Hospital Infection Control and Admission Strategies." *Respirology* 8, Supplement (November 2003): S41–S45.

Jacobson, R. M., K. S. Zabel, and G. A. Poland. "The Overall Safety Profile of Currently Available Vaccines Directed Against Infectious Diseases." *Expert Opinion on Drug Safety* 2 (May 2003): 215–223.

Jarvis, W. R. "Benchmarking for Prevention: the Centers for Disease Control and Prevention's National Nosocomial Infections Surveillance (NNIS) System Experience." *Infection* 31, Supplement 2 (December 2003): 44–48.

Kohn, W. G., A. S. Collins, J. L. Cleveland, et al. "Guidelines for Infection Control in Dental Health-Care Settings—2003." *Morbidity and Mortality Weekly Reports: Reports and Recommendations* 52, RR-17 (December 19, 2003): 1–61.

Peng, P. W., D. T. Wong, D. Bevan, and M. Gardam. "Infection Control and Anesthesia: Lessons Learned from the Toronto SARS Outbreak." *Canadian Journal of Anaesthesiology* 50 (December 2003): 989–997.

Petrak, R. M., D. J. Sexton, M. L. Butera, et al. "The Value of an Infectious Diseases Specialist." *Clinical Infectious Diseases* 36 (April 15, 2003): 1013–1017.

Sehulster, L., and R. Y. Chinn. "Guidelines for Environmental Infection Control in Health-Care Facilities. Recommendations of CDC and the Healthcare Infection Control Practices Advisory Committee (HICPAC)." *Morbidity and Mortality Recommendations and Reports* 52, RR-10 (June 6, 2003): 1–42.

Subramanian, D., J. A. Sandoe, V. Keer, and M. H. Wilcox. "Rapid Spread of Penicillin-Resistant *Streptococcus pneumoniae* Among High-Risk Hospital Inpatients and the Role of Molecular Typing in Outbreak Confirmation." *Journal of Hospital Infection* 54 (June 2003): 99–103.

ORGANIZATIONS

American College of Epidemiology. 1500 Sunday Drive, Suite 102, Raleigh, NC 27607. (919) 861-5573. < http://www.acepidemiology.org >.

American Public Health Association (APHA). 800 I Street NW, Washington, DC 20001-3710. (202) 777-APHA. < http://www.apha.org >.

American Veterinary Medical Association (AVMA). 1931 North Meacham Road, Suite 100, Schaumburg, IL 60173-4360. < http://www.avma.org >.

Centers for Disease Control and Prevention. 1600 Clifton Rd., NE, Atlanta, GA 30333. (800) 311-3435, (404) 639-3311. < http://www.cdc.gov >.

National Institute of Allergy and Infectious Diseases (NIAID). 31 Center Drive, Room 7A50 MSC 2520, Bethesda, MD, 20892. (301) 496-5717. <http://www.niaid.nih.gov>.

Cindy L. A. Jones, PhD
Rebecca J. Frey, PhD

Infectious arthritis

Definition

Infectious arthritis, which is sometimes called septic arthritis or pyogenic arthritis, is a serious infection of the joints characterized by **pain**, **fever**, occasional chills, inflammation and swelling in one or more joints, and loss of function in the affected joints. It is considered a medical emergency.

Description

Infectious arthritis can occur in any age group, including newborns and children. In adults, it usually affects the wrists or one of the patient's weight-bearing joints–most often the knee–although about 20% of adult patients have symptoms in more than one joint. Multiple joint infection is common in children and typically involves the shoulders, knees, and hips.

Some groups of patients are at greater risk for developing infectious arthritis. These high-risk groups include:

- Patients with chronic **rheumatoid arthritis**.
- Patients with certain systemic infections, including **gonorrhea** and HIV infection. Women and male homosexuals are at greater risk for gonorrheal arthritis than are male heterosexuals.
- Patients with certain types of **cancer**.
- IV drug abusers and alcoholics.
- Patients with artificial (prosthetic) joints.
- Patients with diabetes, sickle cell anemia, or **systemic lupus erythematosus** (SLE).
- Patients with recent joint injuries or surgery, or patients receiving medications injected directly into a joint.

Causes and symptoms

In general, infectious arthritis is caused by the spread of a bacterial, viral, or fungal infection through the bloodstream to the joint. The disease agents may enter the joint directly from the outside as a result of an injury or a surgical procedure, or they may be carried to the joint by the blood from infections elsewhere in the body. The specific organisms vary somewhat according to age group. Newborns are most likely to acquire gonococcal infections of the joints from a mother with gonorrhea. Children may also acquire infectious arthritis from a hospital environment, often as a result of catheter placement. The organisms involved are usually either *Haemophilus influenzae* (in children under two years of age) or *Staphylococcus aureus*. In older children or adults, the infectious organisms include *Streptococcus pyogenes* and *Streptococcus viridans* as well as *Staphylococcus aureus*. *Staphylococcus epidermidis* is usually involved in joint infections related to surgery. Sexually active teenagers and adults frequently develop infectious arthritis from *Neisseria gonorrhoeae* infections. Older adults are often vulnerable to joint infections caused by gram-negative bacilli, including *Salmonella* and *Pseudomonas*.

Infectious arthritis often has a sudden onset, but symptoms sometimes develop over a period of three to 14 days. The symptoms include swelling in the infected joint and pain when the joint is moved. Infectious arthritis in the hip may be experienced as pain in the groin area that becomes much worse if the patient tries to walk. In 90% of cases, there is some leakage of tissue fluid into the affected joint. The joint is sore to the touch; it may or may not be warm to the touch, depending on how deep the infection lies within the joint. In most cases the patient will have fever and chills, although the fever may be only low-grade. Children sometimes develop **nausea and vomiting**.

Septic arthritis is considered a medical emergency because of the damage it causes to bone as well as cartilage, and its potential for creating **septic shock**, which is a potentially fatal condition. *Staphylococcus aureus* is capable of destroying cartilage in one or two days. Destruction of cartilage and bone in turn leads to **dislocations** of the joints and bones. If the infection is caused by bacteria, it can spread to the blood and surrounding tissues, causing abscesses or even blood **poisoning**. The most common complication of infectious arthritis is **osteoarthritis**.

Diagnosis

The diagnosis of infectious arthritis depends on a combination of laboratory testing with careful history-taking and **physical examination** of the affected joint. It is important to keep in mind that infectious arthritis can coexist with other forms of arthritis, **gout**, **rheumatic fever**, **Lyme disease**, or other disorders that can cause a combination of joint pain and fever. In some cases, the doctor may consult a specialist in orthopedics or rheumatology to avoid misdiagnosis.

Patient history

The patient's history will tell the doctor whether he or she belongs to a high-risk group for infectious arthritis. Sudden onset of joint pain is also important information.

Physical examination

The doctor will examine the affected joint for swelling, soreness, warmth, and other signs of infection. Location is sometimes a clue to diagnosis; infection of an unusual joint, such as the joints between the breastbone and collarbone, or the pelvic joints, often occurs in drug abusers.

Laboratory tests

Laboratory testing is necessary to confirm the diagnosis of infectious arthritis. The doctor will perform an arthrocentesis, which is a procedure that involves withdrawing a sample of synovial fluid (SF) from the joint with a needle and syringe. SF is a lubricating fluid secreted by tissues surrounding the joints. Patients should be warned that arthrocentesis is a painful procedure. The fluid sample is sent for culture in the sealed syringe. SF from infected joints is usually streaked with pus or looks cloudy and watery. Cell counts usually indicate a high level of white cells; a level higher than 100,000 cells/mm^3 or a neutrophil proportion greater than 90% suggests septic arthritis. A Gram's stain of the culture obtained from the SF is usually positive for the specific disease organism.

Doctors sometimes order a biopsy of the synovial tissue near the joint if the fluid sample is negative. Cultures of other body fluids, such as urine, blood, or cervical mucus, may be taken in addition to the SF culture.

Diagnostic imaging

Diagnostic imaging is not helpful in the early stages of infectious arthritis. Destruction of bone or cartilage does not appear on x rays until 10–14 days after the onset of symptoms. Imaging studies are sometimes useful if the infection is in a deep-seated joint.

Treatment

Infectious arthritis requires usually requires several days of treatment in a hospital, with follow-up medication and physical therapy lasting several weeks or months.

Medications

Because of the possibility of serious damage to the joint or other complications if treatment is delayed, the patient will be started on intravenous **antibiotics** before the specific organism is identified. After the disease organism has been identified, the doctor may give the patient a drug that targets the specific bacterium or virus. **Nonsteroidal anti-inflammatory drugs** are usually given for viral infections.

Intravenous antibiotics are given for about two weeks, or until the inflammation has disappeared. The patient may then be given a two- to four-week course of oral antibiotics.

Surgery

In some cases, surgery is necessary to drain fluid from the infected joint. Patients who need surgical drainage include those who have not responded to antibiotic treatment, those with infections of the hip or other joints that are difficult to reach with arthrocentesis, and those with joint infections related to gunshot or other penetrating **wounds**.

Patients with severe damage to bone or cartilage may need **reconstructive surgery**, but it cannot be performed until the infection is completely gone.

Monitoring and supportive treatment

Infectious arthritis requires careful monitoring while the patient is in the hospital. The doctor will drain the joint on a daily basis and remove a small sample of fluid for culture to check the patient's response to the antibiotic.

Infectious arthritis often causes intense pain. Patients are given medications to relieve pain, together with hot compresses or ice packs on the affected joint. In some cases the patient's arm or leg is put in a splint to protect the sore joint from accidental movement. Recovery can be speeded up, however, if the patient practices range-of-motion exercises to the extent that the pain allows.

Prognosis

The prognosis depends on prompt treatment with antibiotics and drainage of the infected

KEY TERMS

Arthrocentesis—A procedure in which the doctor inserts a needle into the patient's joint to withdraw fluid for diagnostic testing or to drain infected fluid from the joint.

Pyogenic arthritis—Another name for infectious arthritis. Pyogenic means that pus is formed during the disease process.

Sepsis—Invasion of the body by disease organisms or their toxins. Generalized sepsis can lead to shock and eventual death.

Septic arthritis—Another name for infectious arthritis.

Synovial fluid (SF)—A fluid secreted by tissues surrounding the joints that lubricates the joints.

joint. About 70% of patients will recover without permanent joint damage. However, many patients will develop osteoarthritis or deformed joints. Children with infected hip joints sometimes suffer damage to the growth plate. If treatment is delayed, infectious arthritis has a mortality rate between 5% and 30% due to septic **shock** and **respiratory failure**.

Prevention

Some cases of infectious arthritis are preventable by lifestyle choices. These include avoidance of self-injected drugs; sexual abstinence or monogamous relationships; and prompt testing and treatment for suspected cases of gonorrhea. Patients receiving corticosteroid injections into the joints for osteoarthritis may want to weigh this treatment method against the increased risk of infectious arthritis.

Resources

BOOKS

Hellman, David B., "Arthritis & Musculoskeletal Disorders." In *Current Medical Diagnosis and Treatment, 1998*, edited by Stephen McPhee, et al., 37th ed. Stamford: Appleton & Lange, 1997.

Rebecca J. Frey, PhD

Infectious hepatitis *see* **Hepatitis A**

▌Infectious mononucleosis

Definition

Infectious mononucleosis is a contagious illness caused by the Epstein-Barr virus that can affect the liver, lymph nodes, and oral cavity. While mononucleosis is not usually a serious disease, its primary symptoms of **fatigue** and lack of energy can linger for several months.

Description

Infectious mononucleosis, frequently called "mono" or the "kissing disease," is caused by the Epstein-Barr virus (EBV) found in saliva and mucus. The virus affects a type of white blood cell called the B lymphocyte producing characteristic atypical lymphocytes that may be useful in the diagnosis of the disease.

While anyone, even young children, can develop mononucleosis, it occurs most often in young adults between the ages of 15 and 35 and is especially common in teenagers. The mononucleosis infection rate among college students who have not previously been exposed to EBV has been estimated to be about 15%. In younger children, the illness may not be recognized.

The disease typically runs its course in four to six weeks in people with normally functioning immune systems. People with weakened or suppressed immune systems, such as **AIDS** patients or those who have had organ transplants, are particularly vulnerable to the potentially serious complications of infectious mononucleosis.

Causes and symptoms

The EBV that causes mononucleosis is related to a group of herpes viruses, including those that cause cold sores, chicken pox, and **shingles**. Most people are exposed to EBV at some point during their lives. Mononucleosis is most commonly spread by contact with virus-infected saliva through coughing, sneezing, kissing, or sharing drinking glasses or eating utensils.

In addition to general weakness and fatigue, symptoms of mononucleosis may include any or all of the following:

- **Sore throat** and/or swollen tonsils
- Fever and chills
- Nausea and **vomiting**, or decreased appetite
- Swollen lymph nodes in the neck and armpits
- Headaches or joint **pain**

- Enlarged spleen
- Jaundice
- Skin rash.

Complications that can occur with mononucleosis include a temporarily enlarged spleen or inflamed liver. In rare instances, the spleen may rupture, producing sharp pain on the left side of the abdomen, a symptom that warrants immediate medical attention. Additional symptoms of a ruptured spleen include light headedness, rapidly beating heart, and difficulty breathing. Other rare, but potentially life-threatening, complications may involve the heart or brain. The infection may also cause significant destruction of the body's red blood cells or platelets.

Symptoms do not usually appear until four to seven weeks after exposure to EBV. An infected person can be contagious during this incubation time period and for as many as five months after the disappearance of symptoms. Also, the virus will be excreted in the saliva intermittently for the rest of their lives, although the individual will experience no symptoms. Contrary to popular belief, the EBV is not highly contagious. As a result, individuals living in a household or college dormitory with someone who has mononucleosis have a very small risk of being infected unless they have direct contact with the person's saliva.

Diagnosis

If symptoms associated with a cold persist longer than two weeks, mononucleosis is a possibility; however, a variety of other conditions can produce similar symptoms. If mononucleosis is suspected, a physician will typically conduct a **physical examination**, including a "Monospot" antibody blood test that can indicate the presence of proteins or antibodies produced in response to infection with the EBV. These antibodies may not be detectable, however, until the second or third weeks of the illness. Occasionally, when this test is inconclusive, other blood tests may be conducted.

Treatment

The most effective treatment for infectious mononucleosis is rest and a gradual return to regular activities. Individuals with mild cases may not require bed rest but should limit their activities. Any strenuous activity, athletic endeavors, or heavy lifting should be avoided until the symptoms completely subside, since excessive activity may cause the spleen to rupture.

KEY TERMS

Antibody—A specific protein produced by the immune system in response to a specific foreign protein or particle called an antigen.

Herpes viruses—A group of viruses that can cause cold sores, shingles, chicken pox, and congenital abnormalities. The Epstein-Barr virus which causes mononucleosis belongs to this group of viruses.

Reye's syndrome—A very serious, rare disease, most common in children, which involves an upper respiratory tract infection followed by brain and liver damage.

The sore throat and **dehydration** that usually accompany mononucleosis may be relieved by drinking water and fruit juices. Gargling salt water or taking throat lozenges may also relieve discomfort. In addition, taking over-the-counter medications, such as **acetaminophen** or ibuprofen, may relieve symptoms, but **aspirin** should be avoided because mononucleosis has been associated with **Reye's syndrome**, a serious illness aggravated by aspirin.

While **antibiotics** do not affect EBV, the sore throat accompanying mononucleosis can be complicated by a streptococcal infection, which can be treated with antibiotics. Cortisone anti-inflammatory medications are also occasionally prescribed for the treatment of severely swollen tonsils or throat tissues.

Prognosis

While the severity and length of illness varies, most people diagnosed with mononucleosis will be able to return to their normal daily routines within two to three weeks, particularly if they rest during this time period. It may take two to three months before a person's usual energy levels return. One of the most common problems in treating mononuclcosis, particularly in teenagers, is that people return to their usual activities too quickly and then experience a relapse of symptoms. Once the disease has completely run its course, the person cannot be re-infected.

Prevention

Although there is no way to avoid becoming infected with EBV, paying general attention to good hygiene and avoiding sharing beverage glasses or having close contact with people who have mononucleosis or cold symptoms can help prevent infection.

Resources

ORGANIZATIONS

National Institute of Allergy and Infectious Disease. Building 31, Room 7A-50, 31 Center Drive MSC 2520, Bethesda, MD 20892-2520. (301) 496-5717. < http://www.niaid.nih.gov/default.htm >.

OTHER

"Communicable Disease Fact Sheet." New York State Department of Health.
"Mononucleosis: A Tiresome Disease." *Mayo Clinic Online.* < http://www.mayo.ivi.com/mayo/9701/htm/ mono.htm >.

Susan J. Montgomery

Infertility

Definition

Infertility is the failure of a couple to conceive a **pregnancy** after trying to do so for at least one full year. In primary infertility, pregnancy has never occurred. In secondary infertility, one or both members of the couple have previously conceived, but are unable to conceive again after a full year of trying.

Description

Currently, in the United States, about 20% of couples struggle with infertility at any given time. Infertility has increased as a problem over the last 30 years. Some studies pin the blame for this increase on social phenomena, including the tendency for marriage to occur at a later age, which means that couples are trying to start families at a later age. It is well known that fertility in women decreases with increasing age, as illustrated by the following statistics:

• Infertility in married women ages 16–20 = 4.5%

• Infertility in married women ages 35–40 = 31.8%

• Infertility in married women over the age of 40 = 70%.

Today, individuals often have multiple sexual partners before they marry and try to have children. This increase in numbers of sexual partners has led to an increase in **sexually transmitted diseases**. Scarring from these infections, especially from **pelvic inflammatory disease** (a serious infection of the female reproductive organs, most commonly caused by **gonorrhea**) seems to be in part responsible for the increase in infertility noted. Furthermore, use of some forms of a contraceptive called the intrauterine device (**IUD**) contributed to an increased rate of pelvic inflammatory disease, with subsequent scarring. However, newer IUDs do not lead to this increased rate of infection.

To understand issues of infertility, it is first necessary to understand the basics of human reproduction. Fertilization occurs when a sperm from the male merges with an egg (ovum) from the female, creating a zygote that contains genetic material (DNA) from both the father and the mother. If pregnancy is then established, the zygote will develop into an embryo, then a fetus, and ultimately a baby will be born.

The male contribution to fertilization and the establishment of pregnancy is the sperm. Sperm are small cells that carry the father's genetic material. This genetic material is contained within the oval head of the sperm. The sperm are mixed into a fluid called semen, which is discharged from the penis during sexual intercourse. The whip-like tail of the sperm allows the sperm to swim up the female reproductive tract, in search of the egg it will try to fertilize.

The female makes many contributions to fertilization and the establishment of pregnancy. The ovum is the cell that carries the mother's genetic material. These ova develop within the ovaries. Once a month, a single mature ovum is produced, and leaves the ovary in a process called ovulation. This ovum enters a tube leading to the uterus (the fallopian tube). The ovum needs to meet up with the sperm in the fallopian tube if fertilization is to occur.

When fertilization occurs, the resulting cell (which now contains genetic material from both the mother and the father) is called the zygote. This single cell will divide into multiple other cells within the fallopian tube, and the resulting cluster of cells (called a blastocyst) will then move into the womb (uterus). The uterine lining (endometrium) has been preparing itself to receive a pregnancy by growing thicker. If the blastocyst successfully reaches the inside of the uterus and attaches itself to the wall of the uterus, then implantation and pregnancy have been achieved.

Causes and symptoms

Unlike most medical problems, infertility is an issue requiring the careful evaluation of two separate individuals, as well as an evaluation of their interactions with each other. In about 3–4% of couples, no cause for their infertility will be discovered. About 40% of the time, the root of the couple's infertility is due to a problem with the male partner; about 40% of the time, the root of the infertility is due to the female partner; and about 20% of the time, there are fertility problems with both the man and the woman. Recently, a study in Great Britain reported that **smoking** adds to infertility problems for both men and women. In addition, men and women who smoke are less likely to respond to infertility treatment.

The main factors involved in causing infertility, listing from the most to the least common, include:

- Male problems: 35%
- Ovulation problems: 20%
- Tubal problems: 20%
- **Endometriosis**: 10%
- Cervical factors: 5%.

Male factors

Male infertility can be caused by a number of different characteristics of the sperm. To check for these characteristics, a sample of semen is obtained and examined under the microscope (**semen analysis**). Four basic characteristics are usually evaluated:

- Sperm count refers to the number of sperm present in a semen sample. The normal number of sperm present in just one milliliter (ml) of semen is more than 20 million. An individual with only 5–20 million sperm per ml of semen is considered subfertile, an individual with less than 5 million sperm per ml of semen is considered infertile.

- Sperm are also examined to see how well they swim (sperm motility) and to be sure that most have normal structure.

- Not all sperm within a specimen of semen will be perfectly normal. Some may be immature, and some may have abnormalities of the head or tail. A normal semen sample will contain no more than 25% abnormal forms of sperm.

- Volume of the semen sample is important. An abnormal amount of semen could affect the ability of the sperm to successfully fertilize an ovum.

Another test can be performed to evaluate the ability of the sperm to penetrate the outer coat of the ovum. This is done by observing whether sperm in a semen sample can penetrate the outer coat of a guinea pig ovum; fertilization cannot occur, of course, but this test is useful in predicting the ability of the individual's sperm to penetrate a human ovum.

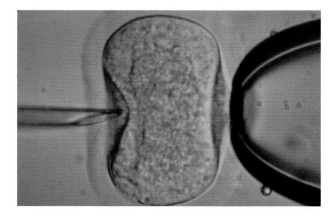

A microscopic image of a needle (left) injecting sperm cells directly into a human egg (center). The broad object at right is a pipette used to hold the ovum steady. *(Phototake NYC. Reproduced by permission.)*

Any number of conditions result in abnormal findings in the semen analysis. Men can be born with testicles that have not descended properly from the abdominal cavity (where testicles develop originally) into the scrotal sac, or may be born with only one instead of the normal two testicles. Testicle size can be smaller than normal. Past infection (including **mumps**) can affect testicular function, as can a past injury. The presence of abnormally large veins (varicocele) in the testicles can increase testicular temperature, which decreases sperm count. History of having been exposed to various toxins, drug use, excess alcohol use, use of anabolic steroids, certain medications, diabetes, thyroid problems, or other endocrine disturbances can have direct effects on the formation of sperm (spermatogenesis). Problems with the male anatomy can cause sperm to be ejaculated not out of the penis, but into the bladder, and scarring from past infections can interfere with ejaculation.

Treatment of male infertility includes addressing known reversible factors first; for example, discontinuing any medication known to have an effect on spermatogenesis or ejaculation, as well as decreasing alcohol intake, and treating thyroid or other endocrine disease. Varicoceles can be treated surgically. Testosterone in low doses can improve sperm motility.

Other treatments of male infertility include collecting semen samples from multiple ejaculations, after which the semen is put through a process that allows the most motile sperm to be sorted out. These motile sperm are pooled together to create a concentrate that can be deposited into the female partner's uterus at a time that coincides with ovulation. In cases where the male partner's sperm is proven to be absolutely unable to cause pregnancy in the female partner, and with the consent of both partners, donor sperm may be used for this process. Depositing the male partner's sperm or donor sperm by mechanical means into the female partner are both forms of artificial insemination.

Ovulatory problems

The first step in diagnosing ovulatory problems is to make sure that an ovum is being produced each month. A woman's morning body temperature is slightly higher around the time of ovulation. A woman can measure and record her temperatures daily and a chart can be drawn to show whether or not ovulation has occurred. Luteinizing hormone (LH) is released just before ovulation. A simple urine test can be done to check if LH has been released around the time that ovulation is expected.

Treatment of ovulatory problems depends on the cause. If a thyroid or pituitary problem is responsible, simply treating that problem can restore fertility. (The thyroid and pituitary glands release hormones that also are involved in regulating a woman's menstrual cycle.) Medication can also be used to stimulate fertility. The most commonly used of these are called Clomid and Pergonal. These drugs increase the risk of multiple births (twins, triplets, etc.). Other possible medications include gonadotropin medications, which are injected medications made up of hormones produced in the pituitary glands. They may directly stimulate the ovaries to produce eggs. Follicle stimulating hormone (FSH) has a 95% chance of simulating ovulation in women with an ovulatory problem. However, its use does not guarantee a successful pregnancy and may lead to multiple pregnancies.

Pelvic adhesions and endometriosis

Pelvic **adhesions** and endometriosis can cause infertility by preventing the sperm from reaching the egg or interfering with fertilization.

Pelvic adhesions are fibrous **scars**. These scars can be the result of past infections, such as pelvic inflammatory disease, or infections following abortions or prior births. Previous surgeries can also leave behind scarring.

Endometriosis may lead to pelvic adhesions. Endometriosis is the abnormal location of uterine tissue outside of the uterus. When uterine tissue is planted elsewhere in the pelvis, it still bleeds on a monthly basis with the start of the normal menstrual period. This leads to irritation within the pelvis around the site of this abnormal tissue and bleeding, and may cause scarring.

Pelvic adhesions cause infertility by blocking the fallopian tubes. The ovum may be prevented from traveling down the fallopian tube from the ovary or the sperm may be prevented from traveling up the fallopian tube from the uterus.

A hysterosalpingogram (HSG) can show if the fallopian tubes are blocked. This is an x-ray exam that tests whether dye material can travel through the patient's fallopian tubes. A few women become pregnant following this x-ray exam. It is thought that the dye material in some way helps flush out the tubes, decreasing any existing obstruction. Scarring also can be diagnosed by examining the pelvic area through the use of a scope that can be inserted into the abdomen through a tiny incision made near the naval. This scoping technique is called **laparoscopy**.

Pelvic adhesions can be treated during laparoscopy. The adhesions are cut using special instruments. Endometriosis can be treated with certain medications, but may also require surgery to repair any obstruction caused by adhesions.

Cervical factors

The cervix is the opening from the vagina into the uterus through which the sperm must pass. Mucus produced by the cervix helps to transport the sperm into the uterus. Injury to the cervix or scarring of the cervix after surgery or infection can result in a smaller than normal cervical opening, making it difficult for the sperm to enter. Injury or infection can also decrease the number of glands in the cervix, leading to a smaller amount of cervical mucus. In other situations, the mucus produced is the wrong consistency (perhaps too thick) to allow sperm to travel through. In addition, some women produce antibodies (immune cells) that are specifically directed to identify sperm as foreign invaders and to kill them.

Cervical mucus can be examined under a microscope to diagnose whether cervical factors are contributing to infertility. The interaction of a live sperm sample from the male partner and a sample of cervical mucus from the female partner can also be examined. This procedure is called a post-coital test.

Treatment of cervical factors includes **antibiotics** in the case of an infection, steroids to decrease production of anti-sperm antibodies, and artificial insemination techniques to completely bypass the cervical mucus.

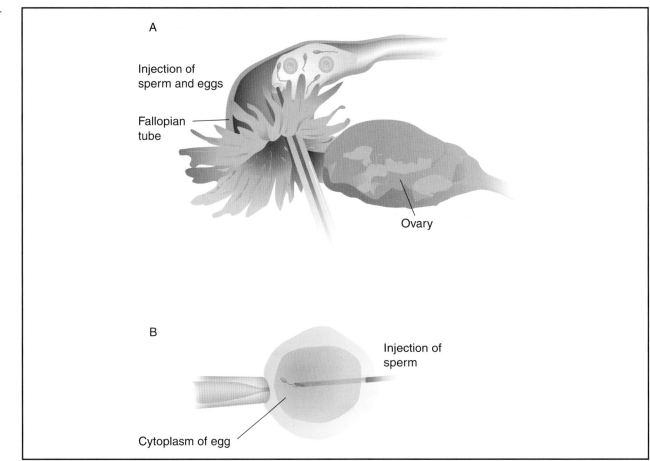

A. An egg and sperm are injected into the fallopian tube to encourage natural fertilization in a procedure called gamete intrafallopian transfer (GIFT). B. An alternative to GIFT is the injection of sperm directly into an egg using microscopic needles. *(Illustration by Argosy Inc.)*

Treatment

Assisted reproductive techniques include **in vitro fertilization** (IVF), gamete intrafallopian transfer (GIFT), and zygote intrafallopian tube transfer (ZIFT). These are usually used after other techniques to treat infertility have failed.

In vitro fertilization involves the use of a drug to induce the simultaneous release of many eggs from the female's ovaries, which are retrieved surgically. Meanwhile, several semen samples are obtained from the male partner, and a sperm concentrate is prepared. The ova and sperm are then combined in a laboratory, where several of the ova may be fertilized. Cell division is allowed to take place up to the embryo stage. While this takes place, the female may be given drugs to ensure that her uterus is ready to receive an embryo. Three or four of the embryos are transferred to the female's uterus, and the wait begins to see if any or all of them implant and result in an actual pregnancy.

Success rates of IVF are still rather low. Most centers report pregnancy rates between 10–20%. Since most IVF procedures put more than one embryo into the uterus, the chance for a multiple birth (twins or more) is greatly increased in couples undergoing IVF.

GIFT involves retrieval of both multiple ova and semen, and the mechanical placement of both within the female partner's fallopian tubes, where one hopes that fertilization will occur. ZIFT involves the same retrieval of ova and semen, and fertilization and growth in the laboratory up to the zygote stage, at which point the zygotes are placed in the fallopian tubes. Both GIFT and ZIFT seem to have higher success rates than IVF.

Prognosis

It is very hard to obtain statistics regarding the prognosis of infertility because many different problems may exist within and individual or couple trying to conceive. In general, it is believed that of all couples who undergo a complete evaluation of infertility followed by treatment, about half will ultimately have a successful pregnancy. Of those couples who do not choose to undergo evaluation or treatment, about 5% will go on to conceive after a year or more of infertility.

Resources

BOOKS

Martin, Mary C. "Infertility." In *Current Obstetric and Gynecologic Diagnosis and Treatment*, edited by Alan H. Cecherney and Martin L. Pernoll. Norwalk, CT: 1994.

PERIODICALS

"Infertility; Treatment." *NWHRC Health Center* March 10, 2004.
Kmietowicz, Zosia. "Smoking is Causing Impotence, Miscarriages, and Infertility." *British Medical Journal* February 14, 2004: 364.

ORGANIZATIONS

American Society for Reproductive Medicine. 1209 Montgomery Highway, Birmingham, AL 35216-2809. (205) 978-5000. < http://www.asrm.com >.
International Center for Infertility Information Dissemination. < http://www.inciid.org >.

Rosalyn Carson-DeWitt, MD
Teresa G. Odle

Infertility drugs

Definition

Infertility drugs are medicines that help bring about **pregnancy**.

Purpose

Infertility is the inability of a man and woman to achieve pregnancy after at least a year of having regular sexual intercourse without any type of birth control. There are many possible reasons for infertility, and finding the most effective treatment for a couple may involve many tests to find the problem. For pregnancy to occur, the woman's reproductive system must release eggs regularly—a process called ovulation. The man must produce healthy sperm that are able to reach and unite with an egg. And once an egg is fertilized, it must travel to the woman's uterus (womb), become implanted and remain there to be nourished.

If a couple is infertile because the woman is not ovulating, infertility drugs may be prescribed to stimulate ovulation. The first step usually is to try a drug such as clomiphene. If that does not work, human chorionic gonadotropin (HCG) may be tried, usually in combination with other infertility drugs.

Clomiphene and HCG may also be used to treat other conditions in both males and females.

Description

Clomiphene (Clomid, Serophene) comes in tablet form and is available only with a physician's prescription. Human chorionic gonadotropin is given as an injection, only under a physician's supervision.

Clomiphene citrate is used to increase the natural production of the hormones that stimulate ovulation in otherwise healthy women. When clomiphene is administered, the body produces higher levels of luteinizing hormone (LH), follicle stimulating hormone (FSH), and gonadotropins. These hormones induce ovulation.

Human chorionic gonadotropin (hCG) is sold under many brand names including Gonic, Pregnyl and Profasi. This hormone stimulates the gonads in both men and women. In men, hCG increases androgen production. In women, it increases the levels of progesterone. Human chorionic gonadotropin can help stimulate ovulation in women.

Although some people believe that hCG can help lose weight, there is no evidence that this hormone offers any benefit in weight loss programs. It should not be used for this purpose.

A number of other natural and synthetic hormones are used to induce ovulation. Urofollitropins (Fertinex) is a concentrated preparation of human hormones, while follitropin alfa (Gonal-F) and follitropin beta (Follistim) are human FSH preparations of recombinant DNA origin. Developments in this field are continuous. For example, in June 2004, the U.S. Food and Drug Administration (FDA) approved a follitropin beta injection in individualized doses for women to self-inject.

Menotropins (Pergonal, Humegon, Repronex) are given with human chorionic gonadotropin to stimulate ovulation in women and sperm production in men.

Recommended dosage

The dosage may be different for different patients. The physician who prescribed the drug or the pharmacist who filled the prescription will recommend the correct dosage.

Clomiphene must be taken at certain times during the menstrual cycle and patients should follow directions exactly.

Precautions

Seeing a physician regularly while taking infertility drugs is important.

Treatment with infertility drugs increases the chance of multiple births. Although this may seem like a good thing to couples who want children very badly,

multiple fetuses can cause problems during pregnancy and delivery and can even threaten the babies' survival.

Having intercourse at the proper time in the woman's menstrual cycle helps increase the chance of pregnancy. The physician may recommend using an ovulation prediction test kit to help determine the best times for intercourse.

Some people feel dizzy or lightheaded, or less alert when using clomiphene. The medicine may also cause blurred vision and other vision changes. Anyone who takes clomiphene should not drive, use machines or do anything else that might be dangerous until they have found out how the drugs affect them.

Questions remain about the safety of long-term treatment with clomiphene. Women should not have more than six courses of treatment with this drug and should ask their physicians for the most up-to-date information about its use.

Special conditions

People who have certain medical conditions or who are taking certain other medicines may have problems if they take infertility drugs. Before taking these drugs, patients should tell the physician about any of these conditions:

ALLERGIES. Anyone who has had unusual reactions to infertility drugs in the past should let his or her physician know before taking the drugs again. The physician should also be told about any allergies to foods, dyes, preservatives, or other substances.

PREGNANCY. Clomiphene may cause birth defects if taken during pregnancy. Women who think they have become pregnant while taking clomiphene should stop taking the medicine immediately and check with their physicians.

OTHER MEDICAL CONDITIONS. Infertility drugs may make some medical conditions worse. Before using infertility drugs, people with any of these medical problems should make sure their physicians are aware of their conditions:

- Endometriosis
- Fibroid tumors of the uterus
- Unusual vaginal bleeding
- Ovarian cyst
- Enlarged ovaries
- Inflamed veins caused by blood clots
- Liver disease, now or in the past
- Depression.

KEY TERMS

Endometriosis—A condition in which tissue like that normally found in the lining of the uterus is present outside the uterus. The condition often causes pain and bleeding.

Fetus—A developing baby inside the womb.

Fibroid tumor—A noncancerous tumor formed of fibrous tissue.

Ovary—A reproductive organ in females that produces eggs and hormones.

USE OF CERTAIN MEDICINES. Taking infertility drugs with certain other medicines may affect the way the drugs work or may increase the chance of side effects.

Side effects

When used in low doses for a short time, clomiphene and HCG rarely cause side effects. However, anyone who has stomach or pelvic **pain** or bloating while taking either medicine should check with a physician immediately. Infertility drugs may also cause less serious symptoms such as hot flashes, breast tenderness or swelling, heavy menstrual periods, bleeding between menstrual periods, **nausea** or **vomiting**, **dizziness**, lightheadedness, irritability, nervousness, restlessness, **headache**, tiredness, sleep problems, or depression. These problems usually go away as the body adjusts to the drug and do not require medical treatment unless they continue or they interfere with normal activities.

Other side effects are possible. Anyone who has unusual symptoms after taking infertility drugs should get in touch with a physician.

Interactions

Infertility drugs may interact with other medicines. When this happens, the effects of one or both of the drugs may change or the risk of side effects may be greater. Anyone who takes infertility drugs should let the physician know all other medicines she is taking.

Resources

PERIODICALS

Georgi, Kristen. "News from the FDA." *Patient Care* June 2004: 10.

Nancy Ross-Flanigan
Teresa G. Odle

Infertility therapies

Definition

Infertility is the inability of a man and a woman to conceive a child through sexual intercourse. There are many possible reasons for the problem, which can involve the man, the woman, or both partners. Various treatments are available that enable a woman to become pregnant; the correct one will depend on the specific cause of the infertility.

Purpose

Infertility treatment is aimed at enabling a woman to have a baby by treating the man, the woman, or both partners. During normal conception of a child, the man's sperm will travel to the woman's fallopian tubes, where, if conditions are right, it will encounter an egg that has been released from the ovary. The sperm will fertilize the egg, which will enter the uterus where it implants and begins to divide, forming an embryo. The embryo will develop during **pregnancy** into a baby.

Infertility treatment attempts to correct or compensate for any abnormalities in this process that prevent the fertilization of an egg or development of an embryo.

Precautions

It is important for a couple contemplating infertility treatment to examine their own ideas and feelings about the process and consider ethical objections before the woman becomes pregnant from such treatment.

Description

About 90% of women who are trying to get pregnant and use no birth control will do so within one year. If, after one year of having frequent sexual intercourse with no **contraception** a couple has not conceived, they should seek the advice of a physician. Tests can be performed to look for possible infertility problems.

Treating an underlying infection or illness is the first step in infertility treatment. The physician may also suggest improving general health, dietary changes, reducing **stress**, and counseling.

Treatment

Low sperm count treatments

The most common cause of male infertility is failure to produce enough healthy sperm. For fertilization to happen, the number of sperm cells in the man's semen (the fluid ejected during sexual intercourse) must be sufficient, and the sperm cells must have the right shape, appearance, and activity (motility).

Defects in the sperm can be caused by an infection resulting from a sexually transmitted disease, a blockage caused by a varicose vein in the scrotum (varicocele), an endocrine imbalance, or problems with other male reproductive organs (such as the testicles, prostate gland, or seminal vesicles).

If a low sperm count is the problem, it is possible to restore fertility by:

- Treating underlying infections.

- Timing sex to coincide with the time the woman is ovulating, which means that the egg is released from the ovary and is beginning to travel down the fallopian tube (the site of fertilization).

- Having sex less often to build up the number of sperm in the semen.

- Treating any endocrine imbalance with drugs.

- Having a surgical procedure to remove a varicocele (varicocelectomy).

Fertility drugs

If infertility is due to a woman's failure to release eggs from the ovary (ovulate), fertility drugs can help bring hormone levels into balance, stimulating the ovaries and triggering egg production.

Surgical repair

In some women, infertility is due to blocked fallopian tubes. The egg is released from the ovary, but the sperm is prevented from reaching it because of a physical obstruction in the fallopian tube. If this is the case, surgery may help repair the damage. Microsurgery can sometimes repair the damage to scarred fallopian tubes if it is not too severe. Not all tube damage can be repaired, however, and most tubal problems are more successfully treated with **in vitro fertilization**.

Fibroid tumors in the uterus also may cause infertility, and they can be surgically treated. **Endometriosis**, a condition in which parts of the lining of the uterus become imbedded on other internal organs (such as the ovaries or fallopian tubes) may contribute to infertility. It may be necessary to surgically remove the endometrial tissue to improve fertility.

Artificial insemination

Artificial insemination may be tried if sperm count is low, the man is impotent, or the woman's vagina creates a hostile environment for the sperm. The procedure is not always successful. In this procedure, the semen is collected and placed into the woman's cervix with a small syringe at the time of ovulation. From the cervix, it can travel to the fallopian tube where fertilization takes place. If the partner's sperm count is low, it can be mixed with donor sperm before being transferred into the uterus.

If there is no sperm in the male partner's semen, then artificial insemination can be performed using a donor's sperm obtained from a sperm bank.

Assisted reproductive technologies

Some fertility treatments require removal of the eggs and/or sperm and manipulation of them in certain ways in a laboratory to assist fertilization. These techniques are called assisted reproductive technologies.

IN VITRO FERTILIZATION (IVF). When infertility cannot be treated by other means or when the cause is not known, it is still possible to become pregnant through in vitro fertilization (IVF), a costly, complex procedure that achieves pregnancy 20% of the time.

In this procedure, a woman's eggs are removed by withdrawing them with a special needle. Attempts are then made to fertilize the eggs with sperm from her partner or a donor. This fertilization takes place in a petri dish in a laboratory. The fertilized egg (embryo) is then returned to the woman's uterus.

Often, three to six fertilized eggs are returned at the same time into the uterus. Usually one or two of the embryos survive and grow into fetuses, but sometimes three or more fetuses result.

A child born in this method is popularly known as a "test tube baby," but in fact the child actually develops inside the mother. Only the fertilization of the egg takes place in the laboratory.

INTRACYTOPLASMIC SPERM INJECTION (ICSI). In a variation of IVF called intracytoplasmic sperm injection (ICSI), single sperm cells are injected directly into each egg. This may be helpful for men with severe infertility.

GAMETE INTERFALLOPIAN TRANSFER (GIFT). In this technique, sperm and eggs are placed directly into the woman's fallopian tubes to encourage fertilization to occur naturally. This procedure is done with the help of **laparoscopy**. In laparoscopy, a small tube with a viewing lens at one end is inserted into the

KEY TERMS

Gamete—An egg (ovum) from the female or a mature sperm from the male.

Laparoscopy—A procedure in which a viewing tube is inserted through the abdominal wall to examine a woman's reproductive organs.

Ovulation—The release of an egg from the ovary. Fertilization can occur within a day or two of ovulation.

Zygote—A fertilized egg.

abdomen through a small incision. The lens allows the physician to see inside the patient on a video monitor.

ZYGOTE INTRAFALLOPIAN TRANSFER (ZIFT). If infertility is caused by a low sperm count, zygote intrafallopian transfer (ZIFT) can be tried. This technique combines GIFT and IVF. This procedure is also called a "tubal embryo transfer."

In this technique, in-vitro fertilization is first performed, so that the actual fertilization takes place and is confirmed in the laboratory. Two days later, instead of placing the embryo in the uterus, the physician performs laparoscopy to place the embryos in the fallopian tube, much like the GIFT procedure.

A woman must have at least one functioning fallopian tube in order to participate in ZIFT.

Preparation

Couples who are having fertility problems may want to limit or avoid:

• Tobacco

• Alcohol

• Caffeine

• Stress

• Tight-fitting undershorts (men)

• Hot tubs, saunas and steam rooms (high temperatures can kill sperm).

Risks

Women who take fertility drugs have a higher likelihood of getting pregnant with more than one child at once. There are also rare but serious side effects to fertility drugs.

Normal results

Typically, at least half of all couples who are infertile will respond to treatment with a successful pregnancy. For those who cannot become pregnant with treatment or insemination, surrogate parenting or adopting may be a workable option.

Resources

ORGANIZATIONS

American Society for Reproductive Medicine. 1209 Montgomery Highway, Birmingham, AL 35216. (205) 978-5000.

Resolve. 1310 Broadway, Somerville, MA 02144-1731. (617) 623-0744. < http://www.resolve.org >.

Carol A. Turkington

Influenza

Definition

Usually referred to as the flu or grippe, influenza is a highly infectious respiratory disease. The disease is caused by certain strains of the influenza virus. When the virus is inhaled, it attacks cells in the upper respiratory tract, causing typical flu symptoms such as **fatigue**, **fever** and chills, a hacking **cough**, and body aches. Influenza victims are also susceptible to potentially life-threatening secondary infections. Although the stomach or intestinal "flu" is commonly blamed for stomach upsets and **diarrhea**, the influenza virus rarely causes gastrointestinal symptoms. Such symptoms are most likely due to other organisms such as rotavirus, *Salmonella*, *Shigella*, or ***Escherichia coli***.

Description

The flu is considerably more debilitating than the **common cold**. Influenza outbreaks occur suddenly, and infection spreads rapidly. The annual **death** toll attributable to influenza and its complications averages 20,000 in the United States alone. In the 1918-1919 Spanish flu pandemic, the death toll reached a staggering 20–40 million worldwide. Approximately 500,000 of these fatalities occurred in America.

Influenza outbreaks occur on a regular basis. The most serious outbreaks are pandemics, which affect millions of people worldwide and last for several months. The 1918–1919 influenza outbreak serves as the primary example of an influenza pandemic. Pandemics also occurred in 1957 and 1968 with the Asian flu and Hong Kong flu, respectively. The Asian flu was responsible for 70,000 deaths in the United States, while the Hong Kong flu killed 34,000.

Epidemics are widespread regional outbreaks that occur every two to three years and affect 5–10% of the population. The Russian flu in the winter of 1977 is an example of an epidemic. A regional epidemic is shorter lived than a pandemic, lasting only several weeks. Finally, there are smaller outbreaks each winter that are confined to specific locales.

The earliest existing descriptions of influenza were written nearly 2500 years ago by the ancient Greek physician Hippocrates. Historically, influenza was ascribed to a number of different agents, including "bad air" and several different bacteria. In fact, its name comes from the Italian word for "influence," because people in eighteenth-century Europe thought that the disease was caused by the influence of bad weather. It was not until 1933 that the causative agent was identified as a virus.

There are three types of influenza viruses, identified as A, B, and C. Influenza A can infect a range of animal species, including humans, pigs, horses, and birds, but only humans are infected by types B and C. Influenza A is responsible for most flu cases, while infection with types B and C virus are less common and cause a milder illness.

In the United States, 90% of all deaths from influenza occur among persons older than 65. Flu-related deaths have increased substantially in the United States since the 1970s, largely because of the **aging** of the American population. In addition, elderly persons are vulnerable because they are often reluctant to be vaccinated against flu.

A new concern regarding influenza is the possibility that hostile groups or governments could use the virus as an agent of bioterrorism. A report published in early 2003 noted that Type A influenza virus has a high potential for use as such an agent because of the virulence of the Type A strain that broke out in Hong Kong in 1997 and the development of laboratory methods for generating large quantities of the virus. The report recommended the stockpiling of present **antiviral drugs** and speeding up the development of new ones.

Causes and symptoms

Approximately one to four days after infection with the influenza virus, the victim is hit with an array of symptoms. "Hit" is an appropriate term, because symptoms are sudden, harsh, and unmistakable. Typical influenza symptoms include the abrupt onset of a **headache**, dry cough, and chills, rapidly followed by overall achiness and a fever that may run as high as 104°F (40°C). As the fever subsides, nasal congestion and a **sore throat** become noticeable. Flu victims feel extremely tired and weak and may not return to their normal energy levels for several days or even a couple of weeks.

Influenza complications usually arise from bacterial infections of the lower respiratory tract. Signs of a secondary respiratory infection often appear just as the victim seems to be recovering. These signs include high fever, intense chills, chest pains associated with breathing, and a productive cough with thick yellowish green sputum. If these symptoms appear, medical treatment is necessary. Other secondary infections, such as sinus or ear infections, may also require medical intervention. Heart and lung problems, and other chronic diseases, can be aggravated by influenza, which is a particular concern with elderly patients.

With children and teenagers, it is advisable to be alert for symptoms of **Reye's syndrome**, a rare, but serious complication. Symptoms of Reye's syndrome are **nausea and vomiting**, and more seriously, neurological problems such as confusion or **delirium**. The syndrome has been associated with the use of **aspirin** to relieve flu symptoms.

Diagnosis

Although there are specific tests to identify the flu virus strain from respiratory samples, doctors typically rely on a set of symptoms and the presence of influenza in the community for diagnosis. Specific tests are useful to determine the type of flu in the community, but they do little for individual treatment. Doctors may administer tests, such as throat cultures, to identify secondary infections.

Since 1999, however, seven rapid diagnostic tests for flu have become commercially available. These tests appear to be especially useful in diagnosing flu in children, allowing doctors to make more accurate treatment decisions in less time.

Treatment

Essentially, a bout of influenza must be allowed to run its course. Symptoms can be relieved with bed rest and by keeping well hydrated. A steam vaporizer may make breathing easier, and **pain** relievers will take care of the aches and pain. Food may not seem very appetizing, but an effort should be made to consume

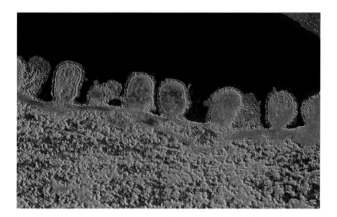

A transmission electron microscopy (TEM) image of influenza viruses budding from the surface of an infected cell. *(Photo Researchers, Inc. Reproduced by permission.)*

nourishing food. Recovery should not be pushed too rapidly. Returning to normal activities too quickly invites a possible relapse or complications.

Drugs

Since influenza is a viral infection, **antibiotics** are useless in treating it. However, antibiotics are frequently used to treat secondary infections.

Over-the-counter medications are used to treat flu symptoms, but it is not necessary to purchase a medication marketed specifically for flu symptoms. Any medication that is designed to relieve symptoms, such as pain and coughing, will provide some relief. Medications containing alcohol, however, should be avoided because of the dehydrating effects of alcohol. The best medicine for symptoms is simply an analgesic, such as aspirin, **acetaminophen**, or naproxen. Without a doctor's approval, aspirin is generally not recommended for people under 18 owing to its association with Reye's syndrome, a rare aspirin-associated complication seen in children recovering from the flu. To be on the safe side, children should receive acetaminophen or ibuprofen to treat their symptoms.

There are four antiviral drugs marketed for treating influenza as of 2003. To be effective, treatment should begin no later than two days after symptoms appear. Antivirals may be useful in treating patients who have weakened immune systems or who are at risk for developing serious complications. They include amantadine (Symmetrel, Symadine) and rimantadine (Flumandine), which work against Type A influenza, and zanamavir (Relenza) and oseltamivir phosphate (Tamiflu), which work against both Types A and B influenza. Amantadine and rimantadine can cause side effects

such as nervousness, **anxiety**, lightheadedness, and **nausea**. Severe side effects include seizures, delirium, and hallucination, but are rare and are nearly always limited to people who have kidney problems, seizure disorders, or psychiatric disorders. The new drugs zanamavir and oseltamivir phosphate have few side effects but can cause **dizziness**, jitters, and **insomnia**.

Alternative treatments

There are several alternative treatments that may help in fighting off the virus and recovering from the flu, in addition to easing flu symptoms.

- **Acupuncture** and **acupressure**. Both are said to stimulate natural resistance, relieve nasal congestion and headaches, fight fever, and calm coughs, depending on the acupuncture and acupressure points used.

- Aromatherapy. Aromatherapists recommend gargling daily with one drop each of the essential oils of tea tree (*Melaleuca* spp.) and lemon mixed in a glass of warm water. If already suffering from the flu, two drops of tea tree oil in a hot bath may help ease the symptoms. Essential oils of eucalyptus (*Eucalyptus globulus*) or peppermint (*Mentha piperita*) added to a steam vaporizer may help clear chest and nasal congestion.

- Herbal remedies. Herbal remedies can be used stimulate the immune system (**echinacea**), as antivirals (*Hydrastis canadensis*) goldenseal and garlic (*Allium sativum*), or directed at whatever symptoms arise as a result of the flu. For example, an infusion of boneset (*Eupatroium perfoliatum*) may counteract aches and fever, and yarrow (*Achillea millefolium*) or elderflower tinctures may combat chills.

- Homeopathy. To prevent flu, a homeopathic remedy called *Oscillococcinum* may be taken at the first sign of flu symptoms and repeated for a day or two. Although oscillococcinum is a popular flu remedy in Europe, however, a research study published in 2003 found it to be ineffective. Other homeopathic remedies recommended vary according to the specific flu symptoms present. *Gelsemium* (*Gelsemium sempervirens*) is recommended to combat weakness accompanied by chills, a headache, and nasal congestion. *Bryonia* (*Bryonia alba*) may be used to treat muscle aches, headaches, and a dry cough. For restlessness, chills, hoarseness, and achy joints, poison ivy (*Rhus toxicodendron*) is recommended. Finally, for achiness and a dry cough or chills, *Eupatorium perfoliatum* is suggested.

- Hydrotherapy. A bath to induce a fever will speed recovery from the flu by creating an environment in the body where the flu virus cannot survive. The patient should take a bath as hot as he/she can tolerate and remain in the bath for 20–30 minutes. While in the bath, the patient drinks a cup of yarrow or elderflower tea to induce sweating. During the bath, a cold cloth is held on the forehead or at the nape of the neck to keep the temperature down in the brain. The patient is assisted when getting out of the bath (he/she may feel weak or dizzy) and then gets into bed and covers up with layers of blankets to induce more sweating.

- Traditional Chinese medicine (TCM). Practitioners of TCM recommend mixtures of herbs to prevent flu as well as to relieve symptoms once a person has fallen ill. There are several different recipes for these remedies, but most contain ginger and Japanese honeysuckle in addition to other ingredients.

- Vitamins. For adults, 2–3 grams of vitamin C daily may help prevent the flu. Increasing the dose to 5–7 grams per day during the flu can felp fight the infection. (The dose should be reduced if diarrhea develops.)

Prognosis

Following proper treatment guidelines, healthy people under the age of 65 usually suffer no long-term consequences associated with flu infection. The elderly and the chronically ill are at greater risk for secondary infection and other complications, but they can also enjoy a complete recovery.

Most people recover fully from an influenza infection, but it should not be viewed complacently. Influenza is a serious disease, and approximately 1 in 1,000 cases proves fatal.

Prevention

The Centers for Disease Control and Prevention recommend that people get an influenza vaccine injection each year before flu season starts. In the United States, flu season typically runs from late December to early March. Vaccines should be received two to six weeks prior to the onset of flu season to allow the body enough time to establish immunity. Adults only need one dose of the yearly vaccine, but children under nine years of age who have not previously been immunized should receive two doses with a month between each dose.

Each season's flu vaccine contains three virus strains that are the most likely to be encountered in the coming flu season. When there is a good match between the anticipated flu strains and the strains used in the vaccine, the vaccine is 70–90% effective in people under 65. Because immune response diminishes somewhat with age, people over 65 may not receive the same level of protection from the vaccine, but even if they do contract the flu, the vaccine diminishes the severity and helps prevent complications.

The virus strains used to make the vaccine are inactivated and will not cause the flu. In the past, flu symptoms were associated with vaccine preparations that were not as highly purified as modern vaccines, not to the virus itself. In 1976, there was a slightly increased risk of developing **Guillain-Barré syndrome**, a very rare disorder, associated with the swine flu vaccine. This association occurred only with the 1976 swine flu vaccine preparation and has never recurred.

Serious side effects with modern vaccines are extremely unusual. Some people experience a slight soreness at the point of injection, which resolves within a day or two. People who have never been exposed to influenza, particularly children, may experience one to two days of a slight fever, tiredness, and muscle aches. These symptoms start within 6–12 hours after the **vaccination**.

It should be noted that certain people should not receive an influenza vaccine. Infants six months and younger have immature immune systems and will not benefit from the vaccine. Since the vaccines are prepared using hen eggs, people who have severe **allergies** to eggs or other vaccine components should not receive the influenza vaccine. As an alternative, they may receive a course of amantadine or rimantadine, which are also used as a protective measure against influenza. Other people who might receive these drugs are those that have been immunized after the flu season has started or who are immunocompromised, such as people with advanced HIV disease. Amantadine and rimantadine are 70–90% effective in preventing influenza.

Certain groups are strongly advised to be vaccinated because they are at increased risk for influenza-related complications:

- All people 65 years and older

- Residents of nursing homes and chronic-care facilities, regardless of age

- Adults and children who have chronic heart or lung problems, such as **asthma**

- Adults and children who have chronic metabolic diseases, such as diabetes and renal dysfunction, as well as severe anemia or inherited hemoglobin disorders

- Children and teenagers who are on long-term aspirin therapy

- Women who will be in their second or third trimester during flu season or women who are nursing

- Anyone who is immunocompromised, including HIV-infected persons, **cancer** patients, organ transplant recipients, and patients receiving steroids, **chemotherapy**, or **radiation therapy**

- Anyone in contact with the above groups, such as teachers, care givers, health-care personnel, and family members

- Travelers to foreign countries.

A person need not be in one of the at-risk categories listed above, however, to receive a flu vaccination. Anyone who wants to forego the discomfort and inconvenience of an influenza attack may receive the vaccine.

As of early 2003, researchers are working on developing an intranasal flu vaccine in aerosol form. An aerosol vaccine using a weakened form of Type A influenza virus has been tested in pilot studies and awaits further clinical trials.

Resources

BOOKS

Beers, Mark H., MD, and Robert Berkow, MD, editors. "Respiratory Viral Diseases: Influenza." Section 13, Chapter 162. In *The Merck Manual of Diagnosis and Therapy.* Whitehouse Station, NJ: Merck Research Laboratories, 2004.

Pelletier, Kenneth R., MD. *The Best Alternative Medicine,* Part II. "CAM Therapies for Specific Conditions: Colds/Flu." New York: Simon & Schuster, 2002.

PERIODICALS

Elkins, Rita. "Combat Colds and Flu." *Let's Live.* 68 (January 2000): 81 +.

Jonas, W. B., T. J. Kaptchuk, and K. Linde. "A Critical Overview of Homeopathy." *Annals of Internal Medicine* 138 (March 4, 2003): 393–399.

Krug, R. M. "The Potential Use of Influenza Virus as an Agent for Bioterrorism." *Antiviral Research* 57 (January 2003): 147–150.

Oxford, J. S., S. Bossuyt, S. Balasingam, et al. "Treatment of Epidemic and Pandemic Influenza with Neuraminidase and M2 Proton Channel Inhibitors." *Clinical Microbiology and Infection* 9 (January 2003): 1–14.

Roth, Y., J. S. Chapnik, and P. Cole. " Feasibility of Aerosol Vaccination in Humans." *Annals of Otology, Rhinology, and Laryngology* 112 (March 2003): 264–270.

Shortridge, K. F., J. S. Peiris, and Y. Guan. "The Next Influenza Pandemic: Lessons from Hong Kong." *Journal of Applied Microbiology* 94, Supplement (2003): 70S–79S.

Storch, G. A. "Rapid Diagnostic Tests for Influenza." *Current Opinion in Pediatrics* 15 (February 2003): 77–84.

Thompson, W. W., D. K. Shay, E. Weintraub, et al. "Mortality Associated with Influenza and Respiratory Syncytial Virus in the United States." *Journal of the American Medical Association* 289 (January 8, 2003): 179–186.

ORGANIZATIONS

Centers for Disease Control and Prevention. 1600 Clifton Rd., NE, Atlanta, GA 30333. (800) 311-3435, (404) 639-3311. <http://www.cdc.gov>.

National Institute of Allergy and Infectious Diseases (NIAID). 31 Center Drive, MSC 2520, Bethesda, MD 20892-2520. <http://www.niaid.nih.gov>.

OTHER

NIAID Fact Sheet: Flu. Bethesda, MD: NIAID, January 2003. <http://www.niaid.nih.gov/factsheets/flu.htm>.

Julia Barrett
Rebecca J. Frey, PhD

Infrequent menstruation *see* **Oligomenorrhea**

Inhalation therapies

Definition

Inhalation therapies are a group of respiratory, or breathing, treatments designed to help restore or improve breathing function in patients with a variety of diseases, conditions, or injuries. The treatments range from at-home **oxygen therapy** for patients with chronic obstructive pulmonary disease to mechanical ventilation for patients with acute **respiratory failure**. Inhalation therapies usually include the following categories:

- Oxygen therapy
- Incentive spirometry
- Continuous positive airway pressure (CPAP)
- Oxygen chamber therapy
- Mechanical ventilation
- Newborn **life support**.

Purpose

Inhalation therapies are ordered for various stages of diseases which are causing progressive or sudden respiratory failure. Although physicians generally follow guidelines to assign specific therapy according the type and stage of a disease, the ultimate decision is based on a number of tests indicating pulmonary function and the presence or absence of oxygen in body organs and tissues.

Oxygen therapy

Oxygen therapy is most commonly ordered to support patients with **emphysema** and other chronic obstructive pulmonary disease (COPD). The oxygen therapy is usually ordered once decreased oxygen saturation in the blood or tissues is demonstrated. Oxygen therapy may also be used in the hospital setting to help return a patient's breathing and oxygen levels to normal.

Incentive spirometry

Spirometry is a diagnostic method for measuring gases and respiratory function. Incentive spirometry may be ordered to help patients practice and improve controlled breathing. It may be ordered after surgery to the abdomen, lungs, neck, or head.

Continuous positive airway pressure (CPAP)

Common uses of continuous positive airway pressure include **sleep apnea**, **respiratory distress syndrome** in infants, and **adult respiratory distress syndrome**. Signs of **atelectasis** (absence of gas from the lungs) or abnormalities of the lower airways may also indicate CPAP.

Oxygen chamber therapy

Oxygen chamber therapy is ordered for various causes that indicate immediate need for oxygen saturation in the blood. Divers with decompression illness, climbers in high altitude, patients suffering from severe carbon dioxide **poisoning**, and children or adults in acute respiratory distress may require oxygen chamber therapy. In recent years, physicians have also used the forced pressure of oxygen chambers to help heal **burns** and other **wounds**, since the pressure under which the oxygen is delivered can reach areas that are blocked off or suffering from poor circulation.

Mechanical ventilation

Mechanical ventilation is ordered for patients in acute respiratory distress, and is often used in an intensive care situation. In some cases, mechanical ventilation is a final attempt to continue the breathing function in a patient and may be considered "life-sustaining."

Newborn life support

Newborn babies, particularly those who were premature, may require inhalation therapies immediately upon birth, since the lungs are among the last organs to fully develop. Some newborns suffer from serious respiratory problems or birth complications, such as respiratory distress syndrome, neonatal wet lung syndrome, apnea of **prematurity** or persistent fetal circulation, which may require inhalation therapies.

Precautions

There are numerous indications for not prescribing various inhalation therapies.

Oxygen therapy

Patients and family members who smoke should not have oxygen prescribed or should avoid **smoking** in the area to prevent combustion. Sedatives should be avoided for patients on oxygen therapy.

Incentive spirometry

Patients who are unable or unwilling to properly and consistently practice incentive spirometry as prescribed should not receive this form of treatment.

Continuous positive airway pressure (CPAP)

Patients unable or unwilling to comply with the physician's instructions for use of CPAP are not likely to have it prescribed. Extremely obese patients may have less success with this form of therapy for the treatment of sleep apnea.

Oxygen chamber therapy

Complications may arise from this form of treatment and during transport to or from the oxygen chamber. Therefore, some patients may not receive enough benefit to outweigh possible complications. All patients, particularly children, must be carefully monitored.

Mechanical ventilation

Use of mechanical ventilation will be carefully weighed against benefit and possible risks. Some patients will require **sedation** to prevent fighting of the ventilator, which can increase the risk of complications.

Newborn life support

Not all infants with breathing problems will require measures as severe as mechanical ventilation. The physician will make the determination based on weight and condition of the infant. Newborns with patent ductus arteriosis, a handicap affecting the pulmonary artery, are more likely to suffer pulmonary hemorrhage from mechanical ventilation.

Description

Oxygen therapy

Once a patient shows hypoxemia, or decreased oxygen in arterial blood, supplemental oxygen may be ordered. The main purpose of the oxygen is to prevent damage to vital organs resulting from inadequate oxygen supply. The lowest possible saturation will be given to keep the patient's measurements at a minimum acceptable level. The oxygen is administered through a mask or nasal tube, or sometimes directly into the trachea. The amount of oxygen prescribed is measured in liters of flow per minute. Patients with chronic hypoxemia, most likely in late stages of COPD, will often receive long-term oxygen therapy.

Most patients will receive their long-term oxygen therapy through home oxygen use. A physician must prescribe home oxygen and levels will be monitored to ensure that the correct amount of oxygen is administered. Some patients will receive oxygen therapy only at night or when exercising.

The choice of type of home oxygen systems will vary depending on availability, cost considerations, and the mobility of the patient. Those patients who are ambulatory, especially those who work, will need a system with a small portable tank. Depending on the system chosen, frequent deliveries of oxygen and filling of portable tanks will be necessary.

In the case of respiratory distress in newborns or adults, oxygen therapy may be attempted before mechanical ventilation since it is a noninvasive and less expensive choice. Oxygen has been found effective in treating patients with other diseases such as **cystic fibrosis**, chronic congestive **heart failure**, or other lung diseases.

Incentive spirometry

Incentive spirometry is also referred to as sustained maximal inspiration. It is designed to mimic natural sighs and yawns. A device provides positive feedback when a patient inhales at a predetermined rate and sustains the breath for a specific period of time. This helps teach the patient to take long, slow, and deep breaths. A spirometer, or equipment that measures pulmonary function, is provided to the patient and a respiratory therapist will work with the patient to demonstrate and explain the technique. Once patients show mastery of the technique, they are instructed to practice the exercises frequently on their own.

Continuous positive airway pressure (CPAP)

Patients with sleep apnea will receive continuous positive airway pressure to prevent upper airway collapse. It is usually administered through a tight-fitting mask as humidified oxygen. The pressure of flow is constant during both exhaling and inhaling and the level of pressure is determined based on each individual. Most patients undergoing CPAP in a hospital setting will receive continuous monitoring of some vital signs and periodic sampling of blood gas values.

Oxygen chamber therapy

Also known as hyperbaric oxygen chamber or hyperbaric oxygen therapy (HBO), this treatment delivers pure oxygen under pressure equal to that of 2–3 times normal atmospheric pressure. For years, this treatment has been especially effective on scuba divers who suffer from the "bends," or decompression illness. The patient enters the chamber, a plastic cylinder-shaped structure that is normally transparent. In most cases, just one patient will enter by being rolled into the chamber on a type of stretcher. Once inside, the oxygen will be delivered under forced pressure and the patient is free to read, nap, or listen to the radio. The therapy usually lasts one hour, although it can take up to five hours in serious decompression cases. Before exiting the chamber, the pressure will eventually be lowered to normal atmospheric level.

Mechanical ventilation

In general, mechanical ventilation replaces or supports the normal ventilatory lung function of a patient. Although normally delivered in a hospital, often to treat serious illness, mechanical ventilation may be performed at home under the order and supervision of a physician and home health agency. The patient will usually be intubated and the ventilator machine "takes over" the breathing function.

There are several modes and methods of mechanical ventilation, each offering different advantages and disadvantages. In assist/control ventilation, the oldest mode of ventilation, the physician predetermines settings and the ventilator delivers a breath each time the patient makes an effort to inhale. In synchronized intermittent mandatory ventilation, the machine senses a patient's effort to inhale and delivers the preset amount. The amount cannot be increased by the patient's effort. Pressure-control ventilation involves the physician's selection of a peak pressure and this method is most useful for patients suffering from obstructive airways disease. In cases of severe hypoventilation, an endotracheal tube must be inserted. If a patient will be on mechanical ventilation for more than two weeks, a tracheostomy, or surgical incision, will be performed for placement of the breathing tubes.

There are other modes of ventilation that may be used, including high-frequency ventilation, a newer technique that delivers 100 to 200 breaths per minute to the patient. The breaths are delivered through a humidified, high-pressure gas jet. High-frequency ventilation may be ordered when a patient does not respond to conventional mechanical ventilation or for certain conditions and circumstances.

Newborn life support

Premature infants, especially those born before the 28th week of gestation, have underdeveloped breathing muscles and immature structures within the lungs. These infants will require breathing support, often in the form of mechanical ventilation. The support delivers warm, humidified, oxygen-enriched gases either by oxygen hood or through mechanical ventilation. In serious cases, the infant may require mechanical ventilation with CPAP or positive-end expiratory pressure (PEEP) through a tightly fitting face mask or even by endotracheal intubation.

Need for continued resuscitation for newborns depends not only on gestational age, but on signs indicating ineffective breathing, including color, heart rate, and respiratory effort. CPAP will be delivered through nasal or endotracheal tubes with a continuous-flow ventilator specifically designed for infants. An alarm system alerts the neonatal staff to problems and monitoring of breathing and other vital functions will accompany the therapy. As respiratory distress syndrome begins to resolve, usually in four or five days, the type of support will be reduced accordingly and the infant may be weaned from the ventilator and moved to only CPAP or an oxygen hood.

Preparation

Preparation for any of these treatments is normally not necessary, and in fact, these therapies may be administered as a result of an emergency situation. Some of the methods, particularly incentive spirometry, or at-home oxygen or ventilation, will require education and cooperation with a home health agency or respiratory therapist. Pretreatment testing of various indicators of respiratory function and oxygen saturation will be performed to determine exact needs of individual patients.

Aftercare

Pulmonary function tests and other tests will be performed to verify that treatments have been successful or to monitor and adjust treatments. Mechanical ventilation will require weaning from the equipment and may also require care for the area surrounding the intubation.

Risks

Inhalation therapies may carry risks, complications or side effects including:

Oxygen therapy

At-home oxygen therapy carries risk if improper care is taken to follow instructions when handling the oxygen. Patients are cautioned not to smoke near the oxygen supply and to keep the supply away from other sources that may cause electrical spark, flames, or intense heat. Patients on home oxygen therapy should avoid use of sedatives.

Incentive spirometry

The major risk associated with incentive spirometry relates to improper use. Patients must be carefully instructed in the technique and monitored periodically for compliance and improvement. Barotrauma, injury to the middle ear or sinuses caused by imbalance between the affected cavity and the outside, or ambient pressure, can result form incentive spirometry. A patient may also suffer discomfort or **fatigue**.

Continuous positive airway pressure (CPAP)

The effectiveness of CPAP may be limited if patients do not cooperate. Possible side effects of CPAP include skin abrasions from the mask, leakage from the tube or mask, nasal congestion, nasal or oral dryness, or discomfort from the pressure of delivery.

Oxygen chamber therapy

Hyperbaric oxygen therapy is painless. The only risk would be associated with improper administration of the pressure levels, which should not occur, since respiratory staff and the supervising physician should be thoroughly trained in performance of this therapy. The drawback to hyperbaric oxygen treatment is the limited availability of chambers. Many cities do not have readily available chambers.

Mechanical ventilation

The biggest risk of mechanical ventilation is sometimes considered to be a patient's dependence on the machine and the difficulty of weaning the patient. The physician will carefully select and monitor the mode of ventilation, the machine's settings, and the patient's progress to prevent this complication. A patient may therefore be left on a ventilator after sufficient progress is made to gradually wean breathing dependence.

Intubation and mechanical ventilation are frightening and uncomfortable for many patients and they may fight the ventilator. If this occurs, the physician may order a sedative to ensure cooperation and effectiveness of the therapy. Intubation often results in irritation to the trachea and larynx. Tracheostomy is associated with risk of bleeding, **pneumothorax**, local infection, and increased incidence of aspiration.

Newborn life support

Infants are continuously monitored to determine even small changes in breathing function. Mechanical ventilation can result in increases in respiratory distress or other complications. It is possible for the ventilator to be accidentally disconnected and staff is trained to watch for signs or alarms indicating disconnection. Mechanical ventilation increases risk of infection in premature babies. Complications of PEEP or CPAP may include pneumothorax or decreased cardiac output.

Normal results

Oxygen therapy

In the case of COPD, oxygen therapy does not treat the disease but can prolong life, quality of life, and onset of more serious symptoms. Effective oxygen therapy for any patient should lead to improved or sustained levels of oxygen in arterial blood.

Incentive spirometry

With proper use of incentive spirometry, the physician should observe improved pulse rate, decreased respiratory rate, improved respiratory muscle performance, and other indicators of improved function. Lung function following lung resection should show marked improvement following incentive spirometry.

Continuous positive airway pressure

Successful CPAP will result in reduction in apnea for those suffering from sleep apnea. A study reported on in 1998 demonstrated that CPAP was effective in the majority of patients with sleep apnea, with the exception of significantly obese patients with blood gas values that were worse during waking hours at rest and at **exercise**. Hospitalized patients on CPAP therapy should show improvement in blood gas and other pulmonary measurements as expected by the treating physician.

Oxygen chamber therapy

Divers undergoing emergency treatment in a **hyperbaric chamber** should show immediate improvement in oxygen levels throughout the body, regardless of blood flow restrictions, after one or two treatments. Those patients receiving oxygen chamber therapy for difficult wounds may continue to receive treatments daily for several weeks before satisfactory results are reached. Patients with carbon dioxide poisoning should show improvement in or recovery of neurologic function. Results of hyperbaric chamber therapy depend largely on how quickly the patient was brought to the chamber, as well as the severity of the initial condition.

Mechanical ventilation

Successful mechanical ventilation will result in gradual decrease in dependence on the ventilator and weaning from the machine. Reduction of therapy to another form, such as CPAP or oxygen therapy, indicates that ventilation has worked as expected. In the case of COPD, exacerbation may be successfully treated with mechanical ventilation and the patient may return to home oxygen therapy. Pediatric patients will demonstrate normal growth and development as a normal result of long-term mechanical ventilation at home. Some patients, particularly those in a hospital intensive care unit, will not be able to breathe again without the ventilator and families and physicians will face tough choices about continued life support.

Newborn life support

Neonates will be constantly monitored to measure lung function. Those measurements will help caregivers determine if and when mechanical ventilation can be reduced and CPAP or oxygen mask begun. CPAP is considered successful when the infant's respiratory rate is reduced by 30–40%, a chest radiograph shows improved lung volume and appearance, stabilization of oxygen levels is documented and caregivers observe improvement in the infant's comfort. Evidence that there is no infection from ventilation is also considered normal. In some cases, inhalation therapy, including mechanical

ventilation, will not work and the infant's parents and physicians will face tough decisions about invasive procedures with associated high risks or cessation of life support.

Resources

ORGANIZATIONS

American Association for Respiratory Care. 11030 Ables Lane, Dallas, TX 75229. (972) 243-2272, Fax (972) 484-2720.
American Lung Association. 1740 Broadway, New York, NY 10019. (800) 586-4872. < http://www.lungusa.org >.
National Heart, Lung and Blood Institute. P.O. Box 30105, Bethesda, MD 20824-0105. (301) 251-1222. < http://www.nhlbi.nih.gov >.

OTHER

Hyperbaric Research and Treatment Center Page. < http://www.hyperbaricrx.com >.

Teresa Odle

Inner ear infection *see* **Labyrinthitis**

Insecticide poisoning

Definition

Insecticide **poisoning** is exposure to a group of chemicals designed to eradicate insects that cause affected persons to develop clinical signs that can progress to **death**.

Description

Insecticides belong to a group of chemicals called organophosphates used to protect against insects. Their use is popular since they are effective and do not remain in the environment, disintegrating within a few days. Organophosphates act to inhibit an enzyme in humans called acetyl cholinesterase. This enzyme functions to degrade a chemical called acetylcholine, which excites nerve cells. The resultant effect of organophosphates would be an increase in acetylcholine, thus causing initial excitation of nerve cells.

Poisoning can occur with a broad range of symptoms affecting the functioning of nerves and initial symptoms similar to the flu such as **vomiting**, abdominal **pain**, **dizziness**, and **headache**. Common names for insecticides include dichlorvos, chlorpyrifos, diazinon, fenthion, malathion, parathion, and carbamate. A special type of insecticide called paraquat is very lethal and responsible for approximately 1,000 deaths per year just in Japan. Paraquat poisoning releases oxygen free radicals that destroy lung and kidney tissues. When poisoning is suspected, a comprehensive management and assessment plan should be performed. This initial assessment should include:

• Description of toxins: names of chemical(s).

• Magnitude of exposure: determination of amount of exposure.

• Progression of symptoms: determining the progression of symptoms can provide information concerning **life support** and overall outcome.

• Time of exposure: knowing the time of exposure is vital since symptoms may be delayed, and it may assist to develop a management plan.

• Medical history: underlying diseases and therapeutic mediations may worsen toxic manifestations.

Causes and symptoms

Exposure to insecticides can occur by ingestion, inhalation, or exposure to skin or eyes. The chemicals are absorbed through the skin, lungs, and gastrointestinal tract and then widely distributed in tissues. Symptoms cover a broad spectrum and affect several organ systems:

• Gastrointestinal: **nausea**, vomiting, cramps, excess salivation, and loss of bowel movement control

• Lungs: increases in bronchial mucous secretions, coughing, **wheezing**, difficulty breathing, and water collection in the lungs (this can progress to breathing cessation)

• Skin: sweating

• Eyes: blurred vision, smaller sized pupil, and increased tearing

• Heart: slowed heart rate, block of the electrical conduction responsible of heartbeat, and lowered blood pressure

• Urinary system: urinary frequency and lack of control

• Central nervous system: convulsions, confusion, **paralysis**, and **coma**

Diagnosis

The confirmatory diagnosis for insecticide poisoning is the measurement of blood acetyl cholinesterase less than 50% of normal. The chemicals can also be detected by specific urine testing. Signs and

KEY TERMS

Acetylcholine—A chemical called a neurotransmitter that functions to excite nerve cells.

Acetylcholinesterase—An enzyme that breaks down acetylcholine.

Central nervous system—Consists of the brain and spinal cord and integrates and processes information.

Enzyme—A protein that speeds up a chemical reaction, but is not consumed during the process.

Oxygen free radicals—Reactive molecules containing oxygen and can cause cell damage.

symptoms in addition to a comprehensive poisoning assessment are essential for diagnosis. Carbamate insecticide poisoning exhibits symptoms similar to organophosphate poisoning but without central nervous system signs.

Treatment

Decontaminate exposed clothing and wash with soap and water immediately. Emergency measures may focus on ventilator support and heart monitoring. If inhalation is suspected, the patient should be removed from the site of exposure. If the eyes were the entry site, they should be flushed with large amounts of water. If the chemicals were ingested, the stomach may be washed out and **activated charcoal** may be administered. Atropine or glycopyrrolate (Robinul) is the drug of choice for carbamate insecticide poisoning. It reverses many symptoms, but is only partially effective for central nervous symptom effects such as coma and convulsions. A medication called Pralidoxime is also commonly indicated to reactivate acetylcholinesterase and to reverse typical symptoms due to organophosphate poisoning. Additionally, the patient is monitored for heart, lung, liver functioning, specific blood tests, and oxygen levels in blood.

Prognosis

Prognosis depends on the specific chemical of exposure, magnitude and time of exposure, progression of symptoms (severity), and onset for medical attention.

Prevention

Adherence to accepted guidelines for handling and management is the key to preventing insecticide poisoning. These may include masks, gowns, gloves, goggles, respiratory breathing machines, or hazardous material suits.

Resources

BOOKS

Behrman, Richard E., et al, editors. *Nelson Textbook*. 16th ed. W. B. Saunders Company, 2000.

Goldman, Lee, et al. *Cecil's Textbook of Medicine*. 21st ed. W. B. Saunders Company, 2000.

Rakel, Robert E., et al. *Conn's Current Therapy*. 53rd ed. W. B. Saunders Company, 2001.

PERIODICALS

Blain, P. G. "Effects of Insecticides." *Lancet* 357 (5 May 2001).

OTHER

Material Safety Data Sheets. < http://oshweb.me.tut.fi >.

National Toxicology Program. < http://ntp-server.niehs. nih.gov/main_Pages/NTP_ALL_STDY_PG.html >.

Laith Farid Gulli, M.D.

Insomnia

Definition

Insomnia is the inability to obtain an adequate amount or quality of sleep. The difficulty can be in falling asleep, remaining asleep, or both. People with insomnia do not feel refreshed when they wake up. Insomnia is a common symptom affecting millions of people that may be caused by many conditions, diseases, or circumstances.

Description

Sleep is essential for mental and physical restoration. It is a cycle with two separate states: rapid eye movement (REM), the stage in which most dreaming occurs; and non-REM (NREM). Four stages of sleep take place during NREM: stage I, when the person passes from relaxed wakefulness; stage II, an early stage of light sleep; stages III and IV, which are increasing degrees of deep sleep. Most stage IV sleep (also called delta sleep), occurs in the first several hours of sleep. A period of REM sleep normally follows a period of NREM sleep.

Insomnia is more common in women and older adults. People who are divorced, widowed, or separated are more likely to have the problem than those who are married, and it is more frequently reported by those with lower socioeconomic status. Short-term, or transient, insomnia is a common occurrence and usually lasts only a few days. Long-term, or chronic insomnia lasts more than three weeks and increases the risk for injuries in the home, at the workplace, and while driving because of daytime sleepiness and decreased concentration. Chronic insomnia can also lead to **mood disorders** like depression.

Causes and symptoms

Transient insomnia is often caused by a temporary situation in a person's life, such as an argument with a loved one, a brief medical illness, or **jet lag**. When the situation is resolved or the precipitating factor disappears, the condition goes away, usually without medical treatment.

Chronic insomnia usually has different causes, and there may be more than one. These include:

- A medical condition or its treatment, including **sleep apnea**
- Use of substances such as **caffeine**, alcohol, and nicotine
- Psychiatric conditions such as mood or **anxiety disorders**
- **Stress**, such as sadness caused by the loss of a loved one or a job
- Disturbed sleep cycles caused by a change in work shift
- Sleep-disordered breathing, such as **snoring**
- Periodic jerky leg movements (*nocturnal myoclonus*), which happen just as the individual is falling asleep
- Repeated nightmares or panic attacks during sleep.

Another cause is excessive worrying about whether or not a person will be able to go to sleep, which creates so much **anxiety** that the individual's bedtime rituals and behavior actually trigger insomnia. The more one worries about falling asleep, the harder it becomes. This is called psychophysiological insomnia.

Symptoms of insomnia

People who have insomnia do not start the day refreshed from a good night's sleep. They are tired. They may have difficulty falling asleep, and commonly lie in bed tossing and turning for hours. Or the individual may go to sleep without a problem but wakes in the early hours of the morning and is either unable to go back to sleep, or drifts into a restless unsatisfying sleep. This is a common symptom in the elderly and in those suffering from depression. Sometimes sleep patterns are reversed and the individual has difficulty staying awake during the day and takes frequent naps. The sleep at night is fitful and frequently interrupted.

Diagnosis

The diagnosis of insomnia is made by a physician based on the patient's reported signs and symptoms. It can be useful for the patient to keep a daily record for two weeks of sleep patterns, food intake, use of alcohol, medications, **exercise**, and any other information recommended by the physician. If the patient has a bed partner, information can be obtained about whether the patient snores or is restless during sleep. This, together with a medical history and **physical examination**, can help confirm the doctor's assessment.

A wide variety of healthcare professionals can recognize and treat insomnia, but when a patient with chronic insomnia does not respond to treatment, or the condition is not adequately explained by the patient's physical, emotional, or mental circumstances, then more extensive testing by a specialist in **sleep disorders** may be warranted.

Treatment

Treatment of insomnia includes alleviating any physical and emotional problems that are contributing to the condition and exploring changes in lifestyle that will improve the situation.

Changes in behavior

Patients can make changes in their daily routine that are simple and effective in treating their insomnia. They should go to bed only when sleepy and use the bedroom only for sleep. Other activities like reading, watching television, or snacking should take place somewhere else. If they are unable to go to sleep, they should go into another room and do something that is relaxing, like reading. Watching television should be avoided because it has an arousing effect. The person should return to bed only when they feel sleepy. Patients should set the alarm and get up every morning at the same time, no matter how much they have slept, to establish a regular sleep-wake pattern. Naps during the day should be avoided, but if absolutely necessary, than a 30 minute nap early in the afternoon may not interfere with sleep at night.

Another successful technique is called sleep-restriction therapy, which restricts the amount of time spent in bed to the actual time spent sleeping. This approach allows a slight sleep debt to build up, which increases the individual's ability to fall asleep and stay asleep. If a patient is sleeping five hours a night, the time in bed is limited to 5–5 1/2 hours. The time in bed is gradually increased in small segments, with the individual rising at the same time each morning; at least 85% of the time in bed must be spent sleeping.

Drug therapy

Medications given for insomnia include sedatives, tranquilizers, and **antianxiety drugs**. All require a doctor's prescription and may become habit-forming. They can lose effectiveness over time and can reduce alertness during the day. The medications should be taken two to four times daily for approximately three to four weeks, though this will vary with the physician and patient. If the insomnia is related to depression, then an antidepressant medication may be helpful. Over-the-counter drugs such as **antihistamines** are not very effective in bringing about sleep and can affect the quality of sleep.

Other measures

Relaxing before going to bed will help a person fall asleep faster. Learning to substitute pleasant thoughts for unpleasant ones (imagery training) is a technique that can be very helpful in reducing worry. Another effective measure is the use of audiotapes which combine the sounds of nature with soft relaxing music. These, alone or in combination with other relaxation techniques, can safely promote sleepiness.

Changes in diet and exercise routines can also have a have a beneficial effect. Dietary items to be avoided include drinks that contain caffeine such as coffee, tea and colas, chocolate (which contains a stimulant), and alcohol, which initially makes a person sleepy but a few hours later can have the opposite effect. Maintaining a comfortable bedroom temperature, reducing noise and eliminating light are also helpful. Regularly scheduled morning or afternoon exercise can relax the body. This should be done 3–4 times a week and be sufficient to produce a light sweat.

Alternative treatments

Many alternative treatments are effective in treating both the symptom of insomnia and its underlying causes. Incorporating relaxation techniques into bedtime rituals will help a person go to sleep faster, as well as improve the quality of sleep. These methods include **meditation**, massage, breathing exercises, and a warm bath, scented with rose, lavender (*Lavendula officinalis*), marjoram, or chamomile (*Matricaria recutita*). Eating a healthy diet rich in calcium, magnesium, and the B **vitamins** is also beneficial. A high protein snack like yogurt before going to bed is recommended, or a cup of herb tea made with chamomile, hops (*Humulus lupulus*), passionflower (*Passiflora incarnata*), or St John's Wort (*Hypericum perforatum*) to encourage relaxation. **Acupuncture** and **biofeedback** have also proven useful.

Prevention

Prevention of insomnia centers around promotion of a healthy lifestyle. A balance of rest, recreation and exercise in combination with stress management, regular physical examinations, and a healthy diet can do much to reduce the risk.

Resources

ORGANIZATIONS

American Sleep Disorders Association. 1610 14th St. NW, Ste. 300, Rochester, MN 55901. (507) 287-6006. < http://www.asda.org >.

OTHER

"What to Do When You Can't Sleep." *The Virtual Hospital Page.* University of Iowa. < http://www.vh.org >.

Donald G. Barstow, RN

Insulin *see* **Antidiabetic drugs**

Insulin resistance

Definition

Insulin resistance is not a disease as such but rather a state or condition in which a person's body tissues have a lowered level of response to insulin, a hormone secreted by the pancreas that helps to regulate the level of glucose (sugar) in the body. As a result, the person's body produces larger quantities of insulin to maintain normal levels of glucose in the blood. There is considerable individual variation in sensitivity to insulin within the general population, with the most insulin-sensitive persons being as much as six times as sensitive to the hormone as those identified as most resistant. Some doctors use an arbitrary number, defining insulin resistance as a need for 200 or more units of insulin per day to control blood sugar levels. Various researchers have estimated that 3–16 percent of the general population in the United States and Canada is insulin-resistant; another figure that is sometimes given is 70–80 million Americans.

Insulin resistance can be thought of as a set of metabolic dysfunctions associated with or contributing to a range of serious health problems. These disorders include type 2 diabetes (formerly called adult-onset or non-insulin-dependent diabetes), the metabolic syndrome (formerly known as syndrome X), **obesity**, and **polycystic ovary syndrome**. Some doctors prefer the term "insulin resistance syndrome" to "metabolic syndrome."

Description

To understand insulin resistance, it may be helpful for the reader to have a brief account of the way insulin works in the body. After a person eats a meal, digestive juices in the small intestine break down starch or complex sugars in the food into glucose, a simple sugar. The glucose then passes into the bloodstream. When the concentration of glucose in the blood reaches a certain point, the pancreas is stimulated to release insulin into the blood. As the insulin reaches cells in muscle and fatty (adipose) tissues, it attaches itself to molecules called insulin receptors on the surface of the cells. The activation of the insulin receptors sets in motion a series of complex biochemical signals within the cells that allow the cells to take in the glucose and convert it to energy. If the pancreas fails to produce enough insulin or the insulin receptors do not function properly, the cells cannot take in the glucose and the level of glucose in the blood remains high.

The insulin may fail to bind to the insulin receptors for any of several reasons. Some persons inherit a gene mutation that leads to the production of a defective form of insulin that cannot bind normally to the insulin receptor. Others may have one of two types of abnormalities in the insulin receptors themselves. In type A, the insulin receptor is missing from the cell surface or does not function properly. In type B, the person's immune system produces autoantibodies to the insulin receptor.

In the early stages of insulin resistance, the pancreas steps up its production of insulin in order to control the increased levels of glucose in the blood. As a result, it is not unusual for patients to have high blood sugar levels and high blood insulin levels (a condition known as hyperinsulinemia) at the same time. If insulin resistance is not detected and treated, however, the islets of Langerhans (the insulin-secreting groups of cells) in the pancreas may eventually shut down and decrease in number.

Causes & symptoms

Causes

The reasons for the development of insulin resistance are not completely understood as of the early 2000s, but several factors that contribute to it have been identified:

- Genetic factors. Insulin resistance is known to run in families. Genetic mutations may affect the insulin receptor, the signaling proteins within cells, or the mechanisms of glucose transport.

- Obesity. Being overweight keeps the muscles from using insulin properly, as it decreases the number of insulin receptors on cell surfaces.

- Low level of physical activity. Because muscle tissue takes up 95 percent of the glucose that insulin helps the body utilize (brain cells and blood cells do not depend on insulin to help them use glucose), inactivity further reduces the muscles ability to use insulin effectively.

- **Aging**. The aging process affects the efficiency of glucose transport.

- Other diseases and disorders. Some disorders—most notably Cushing syndrome and cirrhosis—and such stresses on the body as trauma, surgery, **malnutrition**, or severe infections speed up the breakdown of insulin or interfere with its effects.

- Certain medications. Some drugs, including cyclosporine, niacin, and the **protease inhibitors** used to treat HIV infection, may contribute to insulin resistance.

Symptoms

The symptoms of insulin resistance vary considerably from person to person. Some people may have no noticeable symptoms until they develop signs of heart disease or are diagnosed with high blood pressure during a routine checkup. Other patients may come to the doctor with extremely high levels of blood sugar (hyperglycemia) and such classical symptoms of diabetes as thirst, frequent urination, and weight loss. A small percentage of patients—most commonly women with polycystic ovary syndrome—develop a velvet-textured blackish or dark brown discoloration of the skin known as acanthosis nigricans. This symptom, which is most commonly found on the neck, groin, elbows, knees, knuckles, or armpits, is thought to appear when high levels of insulin in the blood spill over into the skin. This spillover activates insulin receptors in the skin and causes it to develop an abnormal texture and color. Acanthosis nigricans occurs more frequently in Hispanic and African American patients than in Caucasians.

Disorders associated with insulin resistance

Insulin resistance became an important field of research in the late 1980s, when doctors first began to understand it as a precondition of several common but serious threats to health. As of the early 2000s, insulin resistance is associated with the following disorders:

- Obesity. Obesity is not only the most common cause of insulin resistance but is a growing health concern in its own right. According to the National Institutes of Health (NIH), the percentage of American adults who meet the criteria for obesity rose from 25 percent to 33 percent between 1990 and 2000—an increase of a third within the space of a decade. Obesity is a risk factor for the development of type 2 diabetes, high blood pressure, and coronary artery disease.

- Pre-diabetes and type 2 diabetes. The NIH estimates that about 6.3 percent of the American population has diabetes. Of these 18.3 million people, 5.2 million are undiagnosed. Type 2 diabetes is much more common than type 1, accounting for 90–95 percent of patients with diabetes. Diabetes increases a person's risk of blindness, **kidney disease**, heart disease and **stroke**, disorders of the nervous system, complications during **pregnancy**, and dental problems; it also worsens the prognosis for such infectious diseases as **influenza** or **pneumonia**. About 41 million Americans are thought to have pre-diabetes, which is a condition marked by elevated levels of blood glucose after **fasting** or after a 2-hour test for glucose tolerance. According to the NIH, a majority of pre-diabetic people will develop type 2 diabetes within 10 years unless they lose between 5 and 7 percent of their body weight.

• Heart disease. Insulin resistance has been linked to a group of risk factors for heart disease and stroke known as the metabolic syndrome (formerly called syndrome X). The metabolic syndrome, like obesity, has become increasingly prevalent in the United States since the 1990s; as of the early 2000s, about a quarter of the general adult population is thought to have it, with the rate rising to 40 percent for adults over the age of 60. To be diagnosed with the metabolic syndrome, a person must have three or more of the following risk factors: a waist circumference greater than 40 in (102 cm) in men or 35 in (88 cm) in women; a level of blood triglycerides of 150 milligrams per deciliter (mg/dL) or higher; blood pressure of 130/85 Hg or higher; fasting blood sugar level of 110 mg/dL or higher; and a blood level of high-density lipoprotein (HDL) cholesterol (the so-called "good" cholesterol) lower than 50 mg/dL for men or 40 mg/dL for women.

• Polycystic ovary syndrome (PCOS). PCOS is an endocrine disorder that develops in 3–10 percent of premenopausal women as a result of the formation of cysts (small fluid-filled sacs) in the ovaries. Women with PCOS do not have normal menstrual periods; they are often infertile and may develop **hirsutism** (excess body hair) or other indications of high levels of androgens (male sex hormones) in the blood. This condition is called hyperandrogenism, and has been linked to insulin resistance in women with PCOS. Weight loss in these patients usually corrects hyperandrogenism and often restores normal ovulation patterns and fertility.

Diagnosis

Patient history and physical examination

Because insulin resistance is a silent condition in many people, the National Institute of Diabetes and Digestive and Kidney Diseases (NIDDK) recommends that all adults over the age of 45 be tested for type 2 diabetes. People younger than 45 who are overweight and have one or more of the following risk factors should also visit their doctor to be tested:

• One or more family members with diabetes.

• High levels of triglycerides and low levels of HDL cholesterol as defined by the criteria for metabolic syndrome.

• Hypertension (high blood pressure).

• A history of **smoking**.

• A history of diabetes during pregnancy (**gestational diabetes**).

• Giving birth to a baby weighing more than 9 pounds. In addition to increasing the mother's risk of developing type 2 diabetes, children who are large for their gestational age (LGA) at birth have an increased risk of developing insulin resistance and metabolic syndrome in later life.

• Having African American, Hispanic, Native American, or Asian American/Pacific Islander heritage.

Some signs and symptoms associated with insulin resistance can be detected by a primary care physician during a routine office visit. Blood pressure, weight, body shape, and the condition of the skin can be checked, as well as determining whether the patient meets the criteria for obesity or is less severely overweight. Obesity is determined by the patient's body mass index, or BMI. The BMI, which is an indirect measurement of the amount of body fat, is calculated in English units by multiplying a person's weight in pounds by 703.1, and dividing that number by the person's height in inches squared. A BMI between 19 and 24 is considered normal; 25–29 is overweight; 30–34 is moderately obese; 35–39 is severely obese; and 40 or higher is defined as morbidly obese. The doctor may also evaluate the patient for obesity in the office by measuring the thickness of the skinfold at the back of the upper arm.

The distribution of the patient's weight is also significant, as insulin resistance is associated with a so-called "apple-shaped" figure, in which much of the excess weight is carried around the abdomen. People whose excess weight is carried on the hips (the "pear-shaped" figure) or distributed more evenly on the body are less likely to develop insulin resistance. One way of measuring weight distribution is the patient's waist-to-hip ratio; a ratio greater than 1.0 in men or 0.8 in women is strongly correlated with insulin resistance.

Laboratory tests

There is no single laboratory test that can be used to diagnose insulin resistance by itself as of 2005. Doctors usually evaluate individual patients on the basis of specific symptoms or risk factors. The tests most commonly used include the following:

- Blood glucose tests. A high level of blood glucose may indicate either that the body is not producing enough insulin or is not using it effectively. Two common tests used to screen for insulin resistance are the fasting glucose test and the glucose tolerance test. In the fasting glucose test, the person takes no food after midnight and has their blood glucose level measured early in the morning. Normal blood glucose levels after several hours without food should be below 100 milligrams per deciliter (mg/dL). If the level is between 100 and 125 mg/dL, the person has impaired fasting glucose (IFG) or pre-diabetes. If the level is over 126 and is confirmed by a second test, the person has diabetes. In the glucose tolerance test, the person is given a sugar solution to drink and their blood glucose level is measured 2 hours later. A normal level is 140 mg/dL; 140–199 mg/dL indicates impaired glucose tolerance (IGT) or pre-diabetes, while a level of 200 mg/dL or higher indicates diabetes.

- Tests of blood insulin levels. These help to determine whether high blood glucose levels are the result of insufficient production of insulin or inefficient use of insulin.

- Lipid profile test. This test measures the amount of total cholesterol, high-density lipoprotein (HDL) cholesterol, low-density lipoprotein (LDL) cholesterol, and triglycerides. Patients with insulin resistance will have high levels of LDL cholesterol and triglycerides with low levels of HDL cholesterol.

- Measurement of blood electrolytes and uric acid. Many patients with the metabolic syndrome have high blood levels of uric acid.

A highly accurate technique for measuring insulin resistance is called the euglycemic clamp technique. The patient's blood insulin level is kept ("clamped") at a high but steady level by continual insulin infusion while the blood glucose level is monitored at frequent intervals. Glucose concentrations in the blood are maintained at a normal level by an adjustable-rate glucose drip. The amount of glucose needed to maintain a normal blood glucose level over a given unit of time indicates the degree of insulin resistance. This test, however, requires complex equipment and careful monitoring; it is considered too cumbersome to use in routine screening and is used mostly by researchers.

Treatment

Lifestyle modifications

Lifestyle modifications are the first line of treatment in dealing with insulin resistance:

- Weight reduction. Losing weight increases the body's sensitivity to insulin. It is not necessary, however, for patients to reduce their weight to the ideal levels listed on life insurance charts. In recent years, researchers have found that even a modest weight loss—usually defined as 10 percent of the patient's pretreatment weight—is enough to control or at least improve insulin resistance and other health complications of obesity. Weight reduction is usually accomplished by a combination of reduced calorie intake and increased physical activity. Insulin sensitivity is reported to improve within a few days of lowered calorie intake, even before the patient loses a measurable amount of weight.

- **Exercise**. Regular exercise improves the body's sensitivity to insulin by increasing the muscles' uptake of glucose from the bloodstream, by increasing the efficiency of the circulatory system and glucose transport, and by reducing the amount of fat around the patient's abdomen. The American Academy of Family Practice (AAFP) recommends 30 minutes of moderately intense physical activity on most or all days of the week for people diagnosed with insulin resistance. Walking is a very good form of exercise because it does not require any special equipment other than comfortable walking shoes, can be combined with doing errands, and can be done either alone or with a group of friends. Riding a bicycle is another form of exercise recommended for weight control.

- Adding foods high in fiber to the diet. A diet high in natural fiber, found in whole grains and vegetables, lowers the levels of blood insulin as well as lowering the patient's risk of developing high blood pressure.

- Quitting smoking. Giving up smoking lowers the risk of heart disease, stroke, or lung **cancer** as well as increasing the body's sensitivity to insulin.

- Limiting alcohol consumption. Alcohol is a source of "empty" calories with little nutritional value of its own.

Medications

There are several different types of medications that can be used to treat patients with abnormal blood sugar or insulin levels:

- Biguanides. Biguanides are drugs that improve the body's sensitivity to insulin by lowering the absorption of glucose in the small intestine, decreasing the liver's production of glucose, and increasing the uptake of glucose in muscle and fatty tissues. Metformin (Glucophage), a drug used in the treatment of type 2 diabetes, is the most commonly used biguanide in treating insulin resistance. It has also been studied as a possible treatment in preventing or delaying the onset of type 2 diabetes.

- Thiazolidinediones. These drugs stimulate glucose uptake in the muscles and fatty tissues by activating specific receptors in the cell nucleus. They also lower blood insulin levels in patients with hyperinsulinemia. The thiazolidinediones include pioglitazone (Actos) and rosiglitazone (Avandia).

- Glucocorticoids. These drugs may be given to patients with insulin resistance caused by anti-insulin antibodies produced by their immune system. Prednisone (Deltasone) is the most commonly used glucocorticoid.

- Insulin itself. Some patients with insulin resistance benefit from injectable insulin to reduce their blood sugar levels.

As of early 2005, however, the Food and Drug Administration (FDA) has not approved any drugs for the treatment of insulin resistance by itself. For this reason, the American Diabetes Association does not recommend treating insulin resistance with medications unless the patient has already been diagnosed with diabetes.

The patient's doctor may also prescribe medications to treat specific health problems associated with insulin resistance. These drugs may include **diuretics** and other medications to lower blood pressure; **aspirin** to reduce the risk of **heart attack**; medications to lower the levels of triglycerides and LDL cholesterol in the blood; and weight-control drugs. The drugs most frequently prescribed in the early 2000s to help patients lose weight are orlistat (Xenical) and sibutramine (Meridia).

Acanthosis nigricans may be treated with topical preparations containing Retin-A, 20% urea, or salicylic acid; however, many patients find that the skin disorder improves by itself following weight loss.

Surgery

Insulin resistance by itself does not require surgical treatment; however, patients who have already developed heart disease may require coronary artery bypass surgery. In addition, very obese patients—those with a BMI of 40 or higher—may benefit from **bariatric surgery**. Bariatric surgery includes such procedures as vertical banded gastroplasty and gastric bypass, which limit the amount of food that the stomach can contain.

Alternative treatment

Some alternative treatments for insulin resistance and type 2 diabetes have been studied by the Agency for Healthcare Research and Quality (AHRQ). One study reported in 2004 that **omega-3 fatty acids**, a dietary supplement commonly derived from fish, canola, or soybean oil, did not appear to have any significant effect on blood sugar levels or blood insulin levels in patients diagnosed with type 2 diabetes or the metabolic syndrome. An earlier study of **Ayurvedic medicine**, the traditional medical system of India, reported in 2001 that certain herbs used to make Ayurvedic medicines, such as fenugreek, holy basil, *Coccinia indica*, and *Gymnema sylvestre* appear to be effective in lowering blood sugar levels and merit further study. The AHRQ report also noted that the Ayurvedic practice of combining herbal medicines with **yoga** and other forms of physical activity should be investigated further.

Other alternative treatments for insulin resistance and type 2 diabetes include chromium supplements, ginseng, **biofeedback**, and **acupuncture**. The connection between chromium supplementation and insulin resistance is that the body needs chromium to produce a substance called glucose tolerance factor, which increases the effectiveness of insulin. Further studies need to be done, however, before recommendations about dietary chromium as a treatment for insulin resistance can be made.

Prognosis

Since insulin resistance is a condition that precedes the appearance of symptoms of a number of different disorders, its prognosis depends in part on the patient's age, ethnicity, family history, and severity of any current health problems. Some patients diagnosed with insulin resistance eventually develop type 2 diabetes, but it is not yet known why the others do not; for example, some patients do not develop diabetes in spite of a high degree of insulin resistance. What is known at present is that weight reduction and exercise can control or even reverse insulin resistance in many people.

KEY TERMS

Acanthosis nigricans—A dark brownish or blackish discoloration of the skin related to overweight and high levels of insulin in the blood. Acanthosis nigricans is most likely to develop in the groin or armpits, or around the back of the neck.

Bariatrics—The branch of medicine that deals with the prevention and treatment of obesity and related disorders.

Body mass index (BMI)—A measurement that has replaced weight as the preferred determinant of obesity. The BMI can be calculated (in English units) as 703.1 times a person's weight in pounds divided by the square of the person's height in inches.

Glucose—A simple sugar produced when carbohydrates are broken down in the small intestine. It is the primary source of energy for the body. Various tests that measure blood glucose levels are used in diagnosing insulin resistance.

Hyperandrogenism—Excessive secretion of androgens (male sex hormones).

Hyperinsulinemia—The medical term for high levels of insulin in the blood.

Insulin—A protein hormone secreted by the islets of Langerhans in the pancreas in response to eating. Insulin carries glucose and amino acids to muscle and adipose cells and promotes their efficient use and storage.

Islets of Langerhans—Special structures in the pancreas responsible for insulin secretion among other functions. They are named for Paul Langerhans, the German researcher who first identified them in 1869.

Lipids—A group of fats and fat-like substances that are not soluble in water, are stored in the body, and serve as a source of fuel for the body.

Metabolic syndrome—A group of risk factors for heart disease, diabetes, and stroke. It includes abdominal obesity, high blood pressure, high blood glucose levels, and low levels of high-density lipoprotein (HDL) cholesterol. The metabolic syndrome is sometimes called the insulin resistance syndrome.

Metabolism—The sum of an organism's physical and chemical processes that produce and maintain living tissue, and make energy available to the organism. Insulin resistance is a disorder of metabolism.

Obesity—Excessive weight gain due to accumulation of fat in the body, sometimes defined as a BMI of 30 or higher, or body weight greater than 30 percent above one s desirable weight on standard height-weight tables.

Pancreas—A large gland located behind the stomach near the spleen that secretes digestive enzymes into the small intestine and insulin into the bloodstream.

Syndrome—In general, a set of symptoms that occur together as signs of a disease or disorder.

Syndrome X—A term that was sometimes used for metabolic syndrome when the syndrome was first identified in the 1960s.

Triglycerides—Fatty compounds synthesized from carbohydrates during the process of digestion and stored in the body's adipose (fat) tissues. High levels of triglycerides in the blood are associated with insulin resistance.

Type 2 diabetes mellitus—One of the two major types of diabetes mellitus, characterized by late age of onset (30 years or older), insulin resistance, high levels of blood sugar, and little or no need for supplemental insulin. It was formerly known as adult-onset or non-insulin-dependent diabetes.

Prevention

Genetic factors contributing to insulin resistance cannot be changed as of the early 2000s.

With regard to lifestyle factors, the National Institute of Diabetes and Digestive and Kidney Diseases (NIDDK) reported the findings of a study of the effects of lifestyle changes or metformin on the incidence of diabetes in a group of over 3200 overweight people with impaired glucose tolerance, which is a risk factor for developing type 2 diabetes. The researchers found that the subjects in the lifestyle modification group, who lowered their food intake and took 30-minute walks five days a week, had a 58-percent lower incidence of diabetes. The subjects who received metformin had a 31-percent lower incidence of diabetes. Lifestyle changes were most effective in volunteers over the age of 60, while metformin was most effective in younger subjects. In short, the 2002 study confirmed the beneficial effects of lowered food intake and increased activity as preventive measures against type 2 diabetes.

Another important part of preventing insulin resistance is patient education. A number of resources on weight control and exercise written for the general public are available from the Weight-Control Information Network (WIN) on the NIDDK website at http://win.niddk.nih.gov/publications/physical.htm. Some pamphlets are available in Spanish as well as English. Patient education materials on insulin resistance in relation to heart disease and diabetes can be downloaded free of charge from the American Heart Association and American Diabetes Associan websites.

Resources

BOOKS

"Diabetes Mellitus." Section 2, Chapter 13 in *The Merck Manual of Diagnosis and Therapy*, edited by Mark H. Beers, MD, and Robert Berkow, MD. Whitehouse Station, NJ: Merck Research Laboratories, 2004.

Flancbaum, Louis, MD, with Erica Manfred and Deborah Biskin. *The Doctor's Guide to Weight Loss Surgery*. West Hurley, NY: Fredonia Communications, 2001.

"Nutritional Disorders: Obesity." Section 1, Chapter 5 in *The Merck Manual of Diagnosis and Therapy*, edited by Mark H. Beers, MD, and Robert Berkow, MD. Whitehouse Station, NJ: Merck Research Laboratories, 2004.

Pelletier, Kenneth R., MD. *The Best Alternative Medicine*. New York: Simon & Schuster, 2002.

PERIODICALS

Boney, C. M., A. Verma, R. Tucker, and B. R. Vohr. "Metabolic Syndrome in Childhood: Association with Birth Weight, Maternal Obesity, and Gestational Diabetes Mellitus." *Pediatrics* 115 (March 2005): 290–296.

Diabetes Prevention Program Research Group. "Reduction in the Incidence of Type 2 Diabetes with Lifestyle Intervention or Metformin." *New England Journal of Medicine* 346 (February 7, 2002): 393–403.

Ford, Earl S., MD, MPH, Wayne H. Giles, MD, MSc, and William H. Dietz, MD, PhD. "Prevalence of the Metabolic Syndrome Among US Adults." *Journal of the American Medical Association* 287 (January 16, 2002): 356–359.

Litonjua, P., A. Pinero-Pilona, L. Aviles-Santa, and P. Raskin. "Prevalence of Acanthosis Nigricans in Newly-Diagnosed Type 2 Diabetes." *Endocrine Practice* 10 (March–April 2004): 101–106.

Olatunbosun, Samuel, MD, and Samuel Dagogo-Jack, MD. "Insulin Resistance." *eMedicine*, 3 June 2004. < http:// www.emedicine.com/med/topic1173.htm >.

Rao, Goutham, MD. "Insulin Resistance Syndrome." *American Family Physician* 63 (March 15, 2001): 1159–1166.

Scheinfeld, N. S. "Obesity and Dermatology." *Clinical Dermatology* 22 (July-August 2004): 303–309.

Sivitz, William I., MD. "Understanding Insulin Resistance: What Are the Clinical Implications?" *Postgraduate Medicine* 116 (July 2004): 41–48.

ORGANIZATIONS

American Academy of Dermatology (AAD). P. O. Box 4014, Schaumburg, IL 60168-4014. (847) 330-0230. Fax: (847) 330-0050. < http://www.aad.org >.

American Diabetes Association. 1701 North Beauregard Street, Alexandria, VA 22311. (800) 342-2383. < http:// www.diabetes.org >.

American Heart Association National Center. 7272 Greenville Avenue, Dallas, TX 75231. (800) 242-8721. < http://www.americanheart.org >.

American Obesity Association (AOA). 1250 24th Street NW, Suite 300, Washington, DC 20037. (202) 776-7711 or (800) 98-OBESE. < www.obesity.org >.

National Diabetes Information Clearinghouse (NDIC). 1 Information Way, Bethesda, MD 20892-3560. (800) 860-8747. Fax: (703) 738-4929.

OTHER

Agency for Healthcare Research and Quality (AHRQ). Evidence Report/Technology Assessment: Number 41. *Ayurvedic Interventions for Diabetes Mellitus*. Rockville, MD: AHRQ, 2001. < http://www.ahrq.gov/ clinic/epcsums/ayurvsum.htm >.

Agency for Healthcare Research and Quality (AHRQ). Evidence Report/Technology Assessment: Number 89. *Effects of Omega-3 Fatty Acids and Glycemic Control in Type II Diabetes and the Metabolic Syndrome and on Inflammatory Bowel Disease, Rheumatoid Arthritis, Renal Disease, Systemic Lupus Erythematosus, and Osteoporosis*. Rockville, MD: AHRQ, 2004. < http:// www.ahrq.gov/clinic/epcsums/o3lipidsum.htm >.

Mayo Clinic Staff. *Metabolic Syndrome*. < http:// www.mayoclinic.com/invoke.cfm?id=DS00522 >.

National Diabetes Information Clearinghouse (NDIC). *Insulin Resistance and Pre-Diabetes*. NIH Publication No. 04-4893. Bethesda, MD: National Institute of Diabetes and Digestive and Kidney Diseases (NIDDK), 2004. < http://diabetes.niddk.nih.gov/dm/ pubs/insulinresistance >.

National Institute of Diabetes and Digestive and Kidney Diseases (NIDDK) News Brief, 6 February 2002. "Diet and Exercise Delay Diabetes and Normalize Blood Glucose." < http://www.niddk.nih.gov/welcome/ releases/02-06-02.htm >.

Rebecca Frey, PhD

Intelligence tests *see* **Stanford-Binet intelligence scales; Wechsler intelligence test**

Intention tremor *see* **Tremors**

Interferon *see* **Antiviral drugs; Immunologic therapies**

Interleukin-2 *see* **Immunologic therapies**

Intermittent claudication

Definition

Intermittent claudicationis a **pain** in the leg that a person experiences when walking or exercising. The pain is intermittent and goes away when the person rests.

Description

Claudication comes from the Latin word that means "to limp," and the condition is characterized by intermittent pain in the leg muscles. Poor circulation produces the pain. The legs do not receive the oxygen-rich blood supply needed for activities like walking and exercising. The decreased blood flow is caused by the narrowing of arteries that bring blood to the leg and foot.

The leg pain produced by claudication is usually experienced as cramping in the thighs, calves, hips, and feet. The pain stops several minutes after the person rests, but returns when the person performs activities that use the leg muscles. If untreated, claudication is no longer intermittent and occurs when a person is resting.

People age 50 or older are at risk of intermittent claudication. The risk increases with age. Statistically, 5% of men and 2.5% of women experience symptoms of this condition, according to the Vascular Disease Foundation (VDF). Many people with this condition have cholesterol plaque build-up in the leg's arteries. **Smoking** raises the risk, as do high blood pressure, **obesity**, lack of **exercise**, and diabetes.

Intermittent claudication is the main symptom of peripheral arterial disease (PAD), which is also known as **peripheral vascular disease**, and or occlusive arterial disease. Intermittent claudication is an early symptom of the condition that affects peripheral arteries, those blood vessels located outside the heart. PAD is caused by arteriosclerosis, the narrowing and hardening of the arteries.

Women with diabetes are 7.6 times as likely to experience PAD as those without diabetes, according to the American Diabetes Association (ADA). Furthermore, intermittent claudication is related to a two to three times increased risk of coronary heart disease, **stroke**, or cardiac failure in men with diabetes, according to the association.

Causes & symptoms

Intermittent claudication is caused by poor circulation and is experienced in a person's muscle groups. It affects the peripheral arteries that convey oxygen-rich blood from the heart to the legs. A person with this condition feels pain shortly after beginning to exercise. Walking may trigger the pain in an inactive person. Activities such as climbing stairs, walking rapidly or dancing can cause the pain to increase.

The person feels the pain as tightness in the calf, thigh, or buttocks. The pain stops after the person rests for several minutes. However, it returns when the person reaches the exertion level that previously produced the pain.

Intermittent claudication is the primary symptom of PAD, the condition causing reduced flow of blood and oxygen to tissues. If the intermittent condition is not treated, the person will find that resting does not relieve pain. As arteries become more clogged, the person could feel pain even when not exercising. Symptoms include cold or numb feet and toes, poor balance when standing, a drop in leg strength, sores that heal slowly, and **erectile dysfunction** (**impotence**).

In the advanced stages of PAD, the person experiences pain when resting. This condition, ischemic rest pain, is characterized by symptoms visible on the feet and toes. These include ulcers, loss of hair, and the change to red color when feet are suspended. Other symptoms include blue or purple markings on the legs, feet and toes. The coloring is a sign that less oxygen is reaching these areas. Furthermore, black skin on the legs and feet is a sign of **gangrene** infection.

Diagnosis

People experiencing symptoms of intermittent claudication should contact their doctor immediately. The doctor will review the patient's medical history and examine the person for signs of the condition. This examination includes checking for a lower pulse or the absence of a pulse behind the knee, on the ankle, foot, and groin.

The doctor may order an ankle-brachial index (ABI) test to determine whether arteries are blocked. This procedure will verify if the person has PAD and provides information on the severity of the condition. The ABI measures blood pressure in the arms and ankle. Readings are taken when the person is at rest and after exercising lightly by walking on a treadmill. The ABI index is found by dividing the ankle blood pressure by the pressure for the arm. An ABI below 0.90 in a person at rest is a sign of PAD.

The physician may also order a Doppler ultrasound exam to measure the flow of blood through the arteries. Cuffs are placed on four places on each leg. The doctor then moves an ultrasound probe over arteries in the foot. The probe detects signals from the artery.

Testing can last from 20 minutes to an hour. Costs vary by location and facility. In March of 2005, the ABI test was priced from $45 to $150. Some facilities offered a package of tests for around $200. The procedures are usually covered by medical insurance.

Treatment

Lifestyle changes are the primary form of treating intermittent claudication. Physicians advise people to quit smoking, exercise, and to follow the American Heart Association's healthy diet guidelines. Diabetics need to control blood sugar levels. The patient may need to lower blood pressure and cholesterol levels. Those measurements should drop when a person makes lifestyle changes.

The goal of treatment is stop development of PAD. By exercising, eating a diet that includes fiber and low-fat foods, and not smoking, a person could also reverse the build-up that clogs arteries. After several months of this regimen, many people experience a lessening of leg pain. If pain continues, the doctor may prescribe medication. Furthermore, surgery may be needed in some cases.

Walking

Walking is frequently an important treatment for intermittent claudication. A person experiencing the pain of intermittent claudication may not feel like walking. However, walking can increase the capacity to exercise. Before starting an exercise program, the person should consult with consult with a doctor.

The physician reviews the patient's medical history, does a physical and may order an exercise **stress test** on a treadmill. The test shows how long a person walks before claudication starts. Information such as blood pressure is used to evaluate the person's ability to walk. The findings are also used to develop a medically supervised exercise program.

At the beginning, the treadmill is set to cause claudication symptoms in three to five minutes,

according to the Vascular Disease Foundation. The person walks until pain is moderately severe. A rest period is scheduled after the person walks eight to 10 minutes.

The person walks and rests, with the goal of walking for a total of 35 minutes. The person walks at least three times weekly. If a treadmill is not available, VDF recommends that people walk on a track. Generally, a person walking three times weekly will be able to walk longer after three to 12 months.

Medications

People diagnosed with PAD are at a high risk for a stroke and **heart attack**. They should take **aspirin** to reduce this risk. Clopidogrel, a drug marketed as Plavix, worked even better than aspirin in a study. However, it was more costly, with 30 tablets selling for about $119 in 2005. The dosage is one tablet daily.

A doctor may also prescribe cilostazol—sold under the name Pletal—which extends the distance people can walk without pain. One tablet is taken twice daily. The medication cost around $112 for 60 tablets.

Surgical procedures

Surgical procedures may be necessary in cases where intermittent claudication is disabling. The person experiences pain when resting, has open sores that do not heal, or symptoms of gangrene like dying skin in the leg or foot.

Bypass surgery directs blood through a grafted blood vessel, bypassing the damaged artery. The grafted vessel is either a healthy artery or vein or an artificial vessel.

Angioplasty is a procedure to open blocked blood vessels. A catheter (tube) is inserted in the groin and moved to the artery. Then a tiny balloon is inflated to open the artery. Another angioplasty procedure involves the insertion of a stent, a metal device that keeps the vessel open.

Angioplasty is a minimally invasive procedure. **Local anesthesia** is used, and a person is able to resume normal activities within one to two days. The cost averaged $6,502, according to a 2001 Dartmouth Medical School study. Bypass surgery cost $12,422 on average, according to the study. A non-invasive procedure is not as risky as surgery. However, a bypass may be needed when multiple sections of blood vessels are blocked.

Once a person is diagnosed with intermittent claudication, health plans usually cover part of treatment costs. A study on the overall costs of this condition from diagnosis through treatment should be completed by the end of 2005, according to a Sheryl Benjamin, VDF executive director.

Alternative treatment

Ginkgo biloba extract, an herbal remedy, has been used by people with intermittent claudication. The extract made from the dried leaves of the Gingko tree is thought to improve blood flow, allowing people to walk longer without pain.

However, herbal remedies are not regulated the U.S. Food and Drug Administration, and people should consult with their doctors before taking Ginkgo. Furthermore, use of this remedy could interact adversely when taken with Vitamin E and some medications.

Prognosis

If untreated, intermittent claudication will advance and eventually restrict a person's mobility. In later stages, people feel pain when resting. The leg or foot may feel cold. In the extreme stage, the person might need a cane, walker, or wheelchair. There is more risk of gangrene developing, and **amputation** might be necessary. Diabetics face an increased risk of amputation.

PAD also increases the risk of heart attacks and strokes.

Prevention

A healthy lifestyle is the best method for preventing intermittent claudication. Cigarette smokers should quit smoking. Regular exercise and a healthy diet help reduce the risk of this condition. If necessary, people should work to lower cholesterol and blood pressure. Diabetics should strive to manage that condition, obese people should lose weight.

The methods of preventing intermittent claudication are also the means for managing the risks associated with a diagnosis of PAD.

People can learn more about peripheral vascular disease through public education programs like the free Legs for Life screenings held at sites across the nation. The program started the Society of Interventional Radiology features a free ABI testing.

Resources

PERIODICALS

"New Treatment for Leg Pain–Conference News Update."*Clinician Reviews*, April 2002 [cited March 25, 2005]. < http://www.findarticles.com/p/articles/mi_m0BUY/is_4_12/ai_86050499 >.

Warkentin, Donald L. "Intermittent Claudication." *Clinical Reference Systems*. January 1, 2004, 1813.

ORGANIZATIONS

American Diabetes Association. 1701 North Beauregard Street, Alexandria, VA 22311. 800-342-2383. < http://www.diabetes.org >.

Society of Interventional Radiology. 10201 Lee Highway, Suite 500, Fairfax, VA 22030. 703-691-1805. < http://www.sirweb.org/index.shtml >.

Vascular Disease Foundation. 1075 S. Yukon Street, Suite 320, Lakewood, CO 80226. 866-723-4636. < http://www.vdf.org/Contact_Frame.htm >.

OTHER

"Intermittent Claudication: 8 Ways to Ease the Pain." The Doctors Book of Home Remedies, Rodale. [cited March 25, 2005]. < http://www.mothernature.com/Library/Bookshelf/Books/47/85.cfm >.

"Peripheral Arterial Disease of the Legs." Kaiser Permanente. Updated November 3, 2003 [cited March 25, 2005]. < http://prospectivemembers.kaiserpermanente.org >.

Liz Swain

Intermittent explosive disorder

Definition

Intermittent explosive disorder (IED) is a mental disturbance that is characterized by specific episodes of violent and aggressive behavior that may involve harm to others or destruction of property. IED is discussed in the *Diagnostic and Statistical Manual of Mental Disorders* fourth edition (DSM-IV) under the heading of "Impulse-Control Disorders Not Elsewhere Classified." As such, it is grouped together with kleptomania, pyromania, and pathological gambling.

A person must meet certain specific criteria to be diagnosed with IED:

- There must be several separate episodes of failure to restrain aggressive impulses that result in serious assaults against others or property destruction.

- The degree of aggression expressed must be out of proportion to any provocation or other stressor prior to the incidents.

- The behavior cannot be accounted for by another mental disorder, **substance abuse**, medication side effects, or such general medical conditions as epilepsy or head injuries.

The reader should note that DSM-IV's classification of IED is not universally accepted. Many psychiatrists do not place intermittent explosive disorder into a separate clinical category but consider it a symptom of other psychiatric and mental disorders. In many cases individuals diagnosed with IED do in fact have a dual psychiatric diagnosis. IED is frequently associated with mood and **anxiety disorders**, substance **abuse** and eating disorders, and narcissistic, paranoid, and antisocial **personality disorders**.

Description

People diagnosed with IED sometimes describe strong impulses to act aggressively prior to the specific incidents reported to the doctor and/or the police. They may experience racing thoughts or a heightened energy level during the aggressive episode, with **fatigue** and depression developing shortly afterward. Some report various physical sensations, including tightness in the chest, **tingling** sensations, tremor, hearing echoes, or a feeling of pressure inside the head.

Many people diagnosed with IED appear to have general problems with anger or other impulsive behaviors between explosive episodes. Some are able to control aggressive impulses without acting on them while others act out in less destructive ways, such as screaming at someone rather than attacking them physically.

Although the editors of DSM-IV stated in 2000 that IED "is apparently rare," a group of researchers in Chicago reported in 2004 that it is more common than previously thought. They estimate that 1.4 million persons in the United States currently meet the criteria for IED, with a total of 10 million meeting the lifetime criteria for the disorder.

With regard to sex and age group, 80% of individuals diagnosed with IED in the United States are adolescent and adult males. Women do experience IED, however, and have reported it as part of **premenstrual syndrome** (PMS).

Causes and symptoms

Causes

As with other impulse-control disorders, the cause of IED has not been determined. As of 2004, researchers disagree as to whether it is learned behavior, the result of biochemical or neurological abnormalities, or a combination of factors. Some scientists have reported abnormally low levels of serotonin, a neurotransmitter that affects mood, in the cerebrospinal fluid of some anger-prone persons, but the relationship of this finding to IED is not clear. Similarly, some individuals diagnosed with IED have a medical history that includes migraine headaches, seizures, attention-deficit hyperactivity disorder, or developmental problems of various types, but it is not clear that these cause IED, as most persons with migraines, learning problems, or other neurological disorders do not develop IED.

Some psychiatrists who take a cognitive approach to mental disorders believe that IED results from rigid beliefs and a tendency to misinterpret other people's behavior in accordance with these beliefs. According to Dr. Aaron Beck, a pioneer in the application of cognitive therapy to violence-prone individuals, most people diagnosed with IED believe that other people are basically hostile and untrustworthy, that physical force is the only way to obtain respect from others, and that life in general is a battlefield. Beck also identifies certain characteristic errors in thinking that go along with these beliefs:

- Personalizing. The person interprets others' behavior as directed specifically against him.

- Selective perception. The person notices only those features of situations or interactions that fit his negative view of the world rather than taking in all available information.

- Misinterpreting the motives of others. The person tends to see neutral or even friendly behavior as either malicious or manipulative.

- Denial. The person blames others for provoking his violence while denying or minimizing his own role in the fight or other outburst.

Symptoms

The symptoms of IED are described by the DSM-IV criteria for diagnosing the disorder.

Diagnosis

The diagnosis of IED is basically a diagnosis of exclusion, which means that the doctor will eliminate such other possibilities as neurological disorders, mood or substance abuse disorders, **anxiety** syndromes, and personality disorders before deciding that the patient meets the DSM-IV criteria for IED. In addition to taking a history and performing a **physical examination** to rule out general medical conditions, the doctor may administer one or more psychiatric inventories or screeners to determine whether the person meets the criteria for other mental disorders.

In some cases the doctor may order imaging studies or refer the person to a neurologist to rule out brain tumors, traumatic injuries of the nervous system, epilepsy, or similar physical conditions.

Treatment

Emergency room treatment

A person brought to a hospital emergency room by family members, police, or other emergency personnel after an explosive episode will be evaluated by a psychiatrist to see whether he can safely be released after any necessary medical treatment. If the patient appears to be a danger to himself or others, he may be committed against his will for further treatment. In terms of legal issues, a doctor is required by law to notify the specific individuals as well as the police if the patient threatens to harm particular persons. In most states, the doctor is also required by law to report suspected abuse of children, the elderly, or other vulnerable family members.

The doctor will perform a thorough medical examination to determine whether the explosive outburst was related to substance abuse, withdrawal from drugs, head trauma, **delirium**, or other physical conditions. If the patient becomes assaultive inside the hospital, he may be placed in restraints or given a tranquilizer (usually either lorazepam [Ativan] or diazepam [Valium]), most often by injection. In addition to the physical examination, the doctor will obtain as detailed a history as possible from the family members or others who accompanied the patient.

Medications

Medications that have been shown to be beneficial in treating IED in nonemergency situations include lithium, carbamazepine (Tegretol), propranolol (Inderal), and such **selective serotonin reuptake inhibitors** as fluoxetine (Prozac) and sertraline (Zoloft).

Adolescents diagnosed with IED have been reported to respond well to clozapine (Clozaril), a drug normally used to treat **schizophrenia** and other psychotic disorders.

Psychotherapy

Some persons with IED benefit from cognitive therapy in addition to medications, particularly if they are concerned about the impact of their disorder on their education, employment, or interpersonal relationships. Psychoanalytic approaches are not useful in treating IED.

Prognosis

The prognosis of IED depends on several factors that include the individual's socioeconomic status, the stability of his or her family, the values of the surrounding neighborhood, and his or her motivation to change. One reason why the Chicago researchers think that IED is more common than previously thought is that most people who meet the criteria for the disorder do not seek help for the problems in their lives that result from it. The researchers found that although 88% of the 253 individuals with IED that they studied were upset by the results of their explosive outbursts, only 13% had ever asked for treatment in dealing with it.

Prevention

Since the cause(s) of IED are not fully understood as of the early 2000s, preventive strategies should focus on treatment of young children (particularly boys) who may be at risk for IED before they enter adolescence.

Resources

BOOKS

American Psychiatric Association. *Diagnostic and Statistical Manual of Mental Disorders,* 4th ed., revised. Washington, D.C.: American Psychiatric Association, 2000.

Beck, Aaron T., MD. *Prisoners of Hate: The Cognitive Basis of Anger, Hostility, and Violence.* New York: HarperCollins Publishers, 1999.

Beers, Mark H., MD., and Robert Berkow, MD, editors. "Psychiatric Emergencies." Section 15, Chapter 194. In *The Merck Manual of Diagnosis and Therapy.* Whitehouse Station, NJ: Merck Research Laboratories, 2004.

PERIODICALS

Citrome, Leslie L., MD, MPH, and Jan Volavka, MD. "Aggression." *eMedicine.* February 8, 2002. < http://www.emedicine.com/Med/topic3005.htm >.

KEY TERMS

Cognitive therapy—A form of short-term psychotherapy that focuses on changing people's patterns of emotional reaction by correcting distorted patterns of thinking and perception.

Delirium—An acute but temporary disturbance of consciousness marked by confusion, difficulty paying attention, delusions, hallucinations, or restlessness. Delirium may be caused by drug intoxication, high fever related to infection, head trauma, brain tumors, kidney or liver failure, or various metabolic disturbances.

Kleptomania—A mental disorder characterized by impulsive stealing.

Neurotransmitter—Any of a group of chemicals that transmit nerve impulses across the gap (synapse) between two nerve cells.

Pyromania—A mental disorder characterized by setting fires.

Serotonin—A neurotransmitter or brain chemical that is responsible for transporting nerve impulses.

Coccaro, E. F., C. A. Schmidt, J. F. Samuels, and G. Nestadt. "Lifetime and 1-Month Prevalence Rates of Intermittent Explosive Disorder in a Community Sample." *Journal of Clinical Psychiatry* 65 (June 2004): 820–824.

Grant, J. E., and M. N. Potenza. "Impulse Control Disorders: Clinical Characteristics and Pharmacological Management." *Annals of Clinical Psychiatry* 16 (January–March 2004): 27–34.

Kant, R., R. Chalansani, K. N. Chengappa, and M. F. Dieringer. "The Off-Label Use of Clozapine in Adolescents with Bipolar Disorder, Intermittent Explosive Disorder, or Posttraumatic Stress Disorder." *Journal of Child and Adolescent Psychopharmacology* 14 (Spring 2004): 57–63.

McElroy, Susan L. "Recognition and Treatment of DSM-IV Intermittent Explosive Disorder." *Journal of Clinical Psychiatry* (1999): 12–16.

ORGANIZATIONS

American Academy of Child and Adolescent Psychiatry. 3615 Wisconsin Avenue, NW, Washington, DC 20016-3007. (202) 966-7300. Fax: (202) 966-2891. < http://www.aacap.org >.

American Psychiatric Association. 1400 K Street, NW, Washington, DC 20005. < http://www.psych.org >.

National Institute of Mental Health. 6001 Executive Boulevard, Room 8184, MSC 9663, Bethesda, MD 20892-9663. (301) 443-4513. < http://www.nimh.nih.gov >.

OTHER

Padgitt, Steven T. "Treating Intermittent Explosive Disorder with Neurofeedback" Behavenet.com. May 7, 2001. < http://www.behavenet.com/capsules/disorders/explosivedis.htm >.

Janie F. Franz
Rebecca Frey, PhD

Internal fetal monitoring *see* **Electronic fetal monitoring**

Internuclear ophthalmoplegia *see* **Ophthalmoplegia**

Interpositional reconstruction *see* **Arthroplasty**

Intersex states

Definition

Intersex states are conditions where a newborn's sex organs (genitals) look unusual, making it impossible to identify the sex of the baby from its outward appearance.

Description

All developing babies start out with external sex organs that look female. If the baby is male, the internal sex organs mature and begin to produce the male hormone testosterone. If the hormones reach the tissues correctly, the external genitals that looked female change into the scrotum and penis. Sometimes, the genetic sex (as indicated by chromosomes) may not match the appearance of the external sex organs. About 1 in every 2,000 births results in a baby whose sex organs look unusual.

Patients with intersex states can be classified as a true hermaphrodite, a female pseudohermaphrodite, or a male pseudohermaphrodite. This is determined by examining the internal and external structures of the child.

A true hermaphrodite is born with both ovaries and testicles. They also have mixed male and female external genitals. This condition is extremely rare.

A female pseudohermaphrodite is a genetic female. However, the external sex organs have been masculinized and look like a penis. This may occur if the mother takes the hormone progesterone to prevent

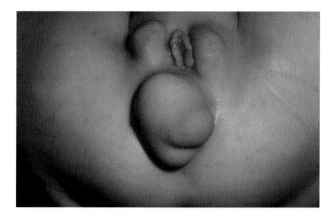

This infant was born with female and male genitalia. *(Photography by Mike Peres, Custom Medical Stock Photo. Reproduced by permission.)*

a **miscarriage**, but more often it is caused by an over-production of certain hormones.

A male pseudohermaphrodite is a genetic male. However, the external sex organs fail to develop normally. Intersex males may have testes and a female-like vulva, or a very small penis.

Causes and symptoms

Any abnormality in chromosomes or sex hormones, or in the unborn baby's response to the hormones, can lead to an intersex state in a newborn.

Intersex states may also be caused by a condition called **congenital adrenal hyperplasia**, which occurs in about 1 out of every 5,000 newborns. This disease blocks the baby's metabolism and can cause a range of symptoms, including abnormal genitals.

Diagnosis

When doctors are uncertain about a newborn's sex, a specialist in infant hormonal problems is consulted as soon as possible. Ultrasound can locate a uterus behind the bladder and can determine if there is a cervix or uterine canal. Blood tests can check the levels of sex hormones in the baby's blood, and chromosome analysis (called karyotyping) can determine sex. Explorative surgery or a biopsy of reproductive tissue may be necessary. Only after thorough testing can a correct diagnosis and determination of sex be made.

Treatment

Treatment of intersex states is controversial. Traditional treatment assigns sex according to test

results, the potential for the child to identify with a sex, and the ease of genital surgery to make the organs look more normal. Treatment may then include **reconstructive surgery** followed by hormone therapy. Babies born with congenital adrenal hyperplasia can be treated with cortisone-type drugs and sometimes surgery.

Counseling should be given to the entire family of an intersex newborn. Families should explore all available medical and surgical options. Counseling should also be provided to the child when he or she is old enough.

Prognosis

Since the mid-1950s, doctors have typically assigned a sex to an intersex infant based on how easy reconstructive surgery would be. The American Academy of Pediatrics states that children with these types of genitals can be raised successfully as members of either sex, and recommends surgery within the first 15 months of life.

Some people are critical of this approach, including intersex adults who were operated on as children. The remolded genitals do not function sexually and can be the source of lifelong **pain**. They suggest that surgery be delayed until the patient can make informed choices about surgery and intervention.

Resources

ORGANIZATIONS

Ambiguous Genitalia Support Network. P.O. Box 313, Clements, CA 95227. (209) 727-0313.

Intersex Society. P.O. Box 31791, San Francisco, CA 94131.

Carol A. Turkington

Interstitial microwave thermal therapy

Definition

Interstitial microwave thermal therapy is a type of hyperthermia treatment for **cancer**, in which heat produced by microwaves (which are a non-ionizing form of radiation) is used in conjunction with other cancer treatments, such as radiation or **chemotherapy**, to kill cancer cells associated with tumors located deep with the body.

Purpose

The purpose of interstitial microwave thermal therapy is to damage and kill cancer cells associated with tumors that are deep within the body. Interstitial microwave therapy is a type of hyperthermia cancer treatment procedure (also called thermal therapy or thermotherapy) in which body tissue and the cancerous tumor are exposed to high temperatures (up to 113°F). Hyperthermia kills cancer cells with usually only minimal injury to normal tissues by damaging proteins and structures within the cells. Thermal therapy is usually used with other forms of cancer therapy, such as radiation and chemotherapy. The increased temperatures may make some cancer cells more sensitive to radiation or may harm some cancer cells that radiation cannot damage.

Precautions

If a patient has become insensitive to **pain** due to disease, radiation, surgery, anesthetics, or other conditions, hyperthermia treatment cannot be used to treat tumors. Also the excessive heating of normal surrounding tissue is prevented by normal blood perfusion, so hyperthermia should not be used in patients with known circulatory problems in the heated areas or in patients who are taking vasoconstrictive drugs.

Description

Interstitial microwave thermal therapy is used to treat tumors that are deep within the body, such as brain, cervical, breast, prostate, and neck tumors. This technique allows the tumor to be heated to higher temperatures than external thermal therapy techniques allow. Probes or needles are inserted into the tumor, guided by the use of imaging techniques, such as ultrasound, to make sure that the probe is properly located within the tumor. A new type of microwave generator includes electronic phase control that allows the operator to electronically direct and shape the pattern of hyperthermia treatments based on the positioning the microwave antennae array that is used in treating the tumor. The treatment pattern can be electronically targeted on the tumor position, shape, and size.

Tissues are heated as the electromagnetic energy produced by the microwave treatment results in heating through molecular excitation. This energy is dissipated in normal living tissue by the blood that perfuses through the tissue. However, since large solid malignant tumors have less blood perfusion than the surrounding normal tissue, for a given absorbed thermal dose, the tumor reaches a higher temperature than the normal tissue. Tumors present within normal tissue will therefore be preferentially heated and will reach higher temperatures than the surrounding tissue.

As cancerous tumors grow rapidly, their need for blood quickly begins to exceed the available blood supply, and major portions of the tumors become blood-starved. These blood-starved tumors are resistant to both radiation and chemotherapy. Chemotherapy drugs carried through the blood cannot effectively penetrate tumors that have poor blood flow. Poor blood flow also means that the tumors are oxygen-starved (hypoxic), making it difficult for **radiation therapy** to make the oxygen radicals that are needed to destroy the DNA of cancer cells. Hypoxic cancer cells, which are an especially dangerous type of cancer, for they have a tendency to metastasize and spread the cancer to other parts of the body, are three times more resistant to ionizing radiation than are normal cells.

When the tumor is heated to **fever** levels through the use of microwave thermal therapy, its blood vessels expand so that more blood can flow into the tumor in order to carry away the excess heat. With the increased blood flow, more blood-borne chemotherapy drugs can be carried into the tumor. Blood is also the source of oxygen for tumors, so with increased blood flow due to the thermal therapy, radiation therapy can form the necessary oxygen radicals to kill the cancer cells. The increased temperature also acts as a drug activator, accelerating chemical reactions and pulling increased oxygen molecules into the tumor tissue for chemical reactions with the chemotherapy drug. **Hypothermia** also enhances the effectiveness of chemotherapy drugs encapsulated in liposomes, increasing the penetration of the drug into the tumor.

When tumors are heated to higher temperatures for at least an hour, the tumors in some cases have been shown to decrease in size and to exhibit necrosis (death of the tumor cells). Therefore, hyperthermia by itself also tends to shrink tumors, often dramatically, due to the collapse of dead cancer cells, making it easier to remove the tumor by surgical techniques. For tumors of the head and neck, a smaller tumor due to hyperthermia treatment may reduce the disfiguration associated with surgical removal of the tumor.

Hyperthermia is being studied as a means of enhancing **gene therapy** by acting as an activator to turn on new biological therapies, by speeding up gene production by thousands of times. In addition, hyperthermia is used as an essential tool to turn on anti-tumor vaccines that are based on heat shock proteins. Hyperthermia has been shown to prevent a cancererous tumor from growing new blood vessels to expand its blood supply. With regards to quality of life, hyperthermia lessens pain and stimulates the immune system, thus helping patients recover from toxic cancer therapies such as ionizing radiation and chemotherapy. Even in patients with terminal cancer, hyperthermia can provide benefits through the alleviation of bleeding, pain, and infection.

As of 2005, the use of hyperthermia alone and in conjunction with radiation therapy has been approved by the United States Food and Drug Administration for the treatment of advanced, recurrent, and persistent tumors, upon authorization of a licensed practitioner. When used with radiation, the treatment regimen usually consists of 10 hyperthermia treatments delivered twice a week, at 72 hour intervals. The prescribed radiation is administered within 30 minutes of the hyperthermia treatment. During each heat treatment, the temperature within the tumor is usually maintained at 42.5 degrees centigrade for 60 minutes. The use of hyperthermia in conjunction with chemotherapy is presently investigational in the United States as of 2005.

The effectiveness of treatment is related to the temperature achieved during the treatment process, the length of the treatment, and cell and tissue characteristics. The temperature within the tumor must be monitored to ensure that the appropriate temperature is achieved, but not exceeded, in the treatment area. Monitoring is accomplished by inserting small needles or tubes with small thermometers into the treatment area. Imaging techniques such as computed tomography (CT) are used to make sure that the temperature probes are positioned appropriately.

Preparation

The safety and effectiveness of hyperthermia treatment is dependent on careful placement of the temperature probes and careful monitoring of tissue temperatures during treatment.

Aftercare

During the treatment period, which may last for weeks, the patient must be instructed in proper care of implanted catheters and temperature probe sites to avoid the risk of infection.

Risks

Excessive heating of normal tissues may result in areas of thermal aseptic necrosis that will require medical care. The electromagnetic radiation from the microwave equipment can interfere with electronic devices such as cardiac **pacemakers** or other implanted electronic devices. Thermal treatment of tumors in the neck or head may result in inadvertent heating of thermoregulatory centers in the brain stem, thus resulting in overheating of the body, beyond levels that the patient can tolerate. Metallic implants, such as joint protheses or dental braces may become excessively and preferentially overheated and adversely affect the patient.

Normal results

The effectiveness of interstitial microwave thermal therapy varies among cancer patients. For example, studies have shown in Phase III clinical trials, when hyperthermia was used with ionizing radiation treatment, that the following treatment improvements were seen, as compared to the use of ionizing radiation therapy alone:

- complete response for recurrent **breast cancer** increased from 38% to 60%

- 2-year survival for globlastoma (brain cancer) increased from 15% to 31%

- complete response for advanced **cervical cancer** increased from 57% to 83%

Known side effects of hypothermia are associated with direct effects of heat on tissues and indirect effects of tumor necrosis. These side effects, as determined in various medical studies, include:

- surface **burns** and blistering in the area of application of heat by the microwave applicators; experienced in about 10% of the tumor sites studied.

- localized and temporary pain in the area of and during the delivery of the heat by the microwave applicators; experienced in about 8% of the tumor sites studied.

- ulceration from rapid tumor necrosis following successful hyperthermia treatment, resulting in fever from toxemia and patient discomfort through drainage and bleeding; experienced in about 4% of the tumor sites studied.

- local and systematic (rarely) infections from placement of the temperature probes and from ulceration related to tumor necrosis; experienced in about 2% of the tumor sites studied.

Abnormal results

Hyperthermia has the potential for producing the following adverse reactions as a result of exposure to electromagnetic radiation:

- cataracts

- permanent or temporary male sterility

- exacerbation of existing diseases due to additional systemic stress

- enhanced drug activity

- thermal stress

Resources

BOOKS

Rosenbaum, Ernest, Dollinger, Malin, Tempero, Margaret, and Mulvihill, Sean. *Everyone's Guide to Cancer Therapy. 4th Edition.* Kansas City, KS: Andrews McMeel Publishing, 2002

PERIODICALS

Falk, M.H., and Issels, R.D. "Hyperthermia in Oncology." *International Journal of Hyperthermia.* 2001, (17) 1–18.

van der Zee, J. "Heating the Patient: A Promising Approach?" *Annals of Oncology* 2002, (13) 1173–1184.
Wust, P., Hildebrandt, B., Sreenivasa, G. et al. "Hyperthermia in Combined Treatment of Cancer." *The Lancet Oncology* 2002, (3) 487–497.

ORGANIZATION

Hyperthermia in Cancer Treatment. National Cancer Institute. < www.cis.nci.gov/fact/7_3.htm >
Society for Thermal Medicine. < www.thermaltherapy.org >.

Judith L. Sims

Intestinal culture *see* **Stool culture**

Intestinal lymphangiectasia *see* **Malabsorption syndrome**

Intestinal obstructions

Definition

Intestinal obstruction refers to the partial or complete mechanical or nonmechanical blockage of the small or large intestine.

Description

There are two types of intestinal obstructions, mechanical and nonmechanical. Mechanical obstructions occur because the bowel is physically blocked and its contents cannot get past the obstruction. Mechanical obstructions can occur for several reasons. Sometimes the bowel twists on itself (volvulus) or telescopes into itself (**intussusception**). Mechanical obstruction can also result from hernias, impacted feces, abnormal tissue growth, the presence of foreign bodies in the intestines (including **gallstones**), or inflammatory bowel disease (**Crohn's disease**). Nonmechanical obstruction, called **ileus**, occurs because the wavelike muscular contractions of the intestine (peristalsis) that ordinarily move food through the digestive tract stop.

Mechanical obstruction in infants

Infants under one year of age are most likely to have intestinal obstruction caused by meconium ileus, volvulus, and intussusception. Meconium ileus, which is the inability to pass the first fecal excretion after birth (meconium), is a disorder of newborns. It is an early clue that the infant has **cystic fibrosis**, but may also occur in very low birth weight (VLBW) infants. In meconium ileus, the material that is blocking the intestine is thick and stringy, rather than the collection of mucus and bile that is passed by normal infants. The abnormal meconium must be removed with an enema or through surgery.

Volvulus is the medical term for twisting of either the small or large bowel. The twisting may cut off the blood supply to the bowel, leading to tissue **death** (**gangrene**). This development is called a strangulating obstruction.

In intussusception, the bowel telescopes into itself like a radio antenna folding up. Intussusception is most common in children between the ages of three and nine months, although it also occurs in older children. Almost twice as many boys suffer intussusception as girls. It is, however, difficult for doctors to predict which infants will suffer from intestinal obstruction.

Mechanical obstruction in adults

Obstructions in adults are usually caused by tumors, trauma, volvulus, the presence of foreign bodies such as gallstones, or hernias, although they have also been reported in adults with cystic fibrosis. Volvulus occurs most often in elderly adults and psychiatrically disturbed patients. Intussusception in adults is usually associated with tumors in the bowel, whether benign or malignant.

More recently, gastroenterologists have described a postsurgical complication known as early postoperative small bowel obstruction, or EPSBO. Although this condition was at one time confused with postoperative ileus, it is now known to be caused by mechanical obstructions resulting from **radiation therapy** for **cancer** or laparoscopic surgery. Most casses can be succesfully treated within 10–14 days of surgery.

Causes and symptoms

One of the earliest signs of mechanical intestinal obstruction is abdominal **pain** or cramps that come and go in waves. Infants typically pull up their legs and cry in pain, then stop crying suddenly. They will then behave normally for as long as 15–30 minutes, only to start crying again when the next cramp begins. The cramping results from the inability of the muscular contractions of the bowel to push the digested food past the obstruction.

Vomiting is another symptom of intestinal obstruction. The speed of its onset is a clue to the location of the obstruction. Vomiting follows shortly after the pain if the obstruction is in the small intestine but is delayed if it is in the large intestine. The vomited

material may be fecal in character. When the patient has a mechanical obstruction, the doctor will first hear active, high-pitched gurgling and splashing bowel sounds while listening with a stethoscope. Later these sounds decrease, then stop. If the blockage is complete, the patient will not pass any gas or feces. If the blockage is only partial, however, the patient may have **diarrhea**. Initially there is little or no **fever**.

When the material in the bowel cannot move past the obstruction, the body reabsorbs large amounts of fluid and the abdomen becomes sore to the touch and swollen. The balance of certain important chemicals (electrolytes) in the blood is upset. Persistent vomiting can cause the patient to become dehydrated. Without treatment, the patient can suffer **shock** and kidney failure.

Strangulation occurs when a loop of the intestine is cut off from its blood supply. Strangulation occurs in about 25% of cases of small bowel obstruction. It is a serious condition that can progress to gangrene within six hours.

Diagnosis

Imaging studies

If the doctor suspects intestinal obstruction based on the **physical examination** and patient history, he or she will order x rays, a computed tomography scan (CT scan), or an ultrasound evaluation of the abdomen. In many cases the patient is given a **barium enema**. Barium sulfate, which is a white powder, is inserted through the rectum and the intestinal area is photographed. Barium acts as a contrast material and allows the location of the obstruction to be pinpointed on film.

Laboratory tests

The first blood test of a patient with an intestinal obstruction usually gives normal results, but later tests indicate electrolyte imbalances. There is no way to determine if an obstruction is simple or strangulated except surgery.

Treatment

Initial assessment

All patients with suspected intestinal obstruction are hospitalized. Treatment must be rapid, because strangulating obstructions can be fatal. The first step in treatment is inserting a nasogastric tube to suction out the contents of the stomach and intestines. The patient is then given intravenous fluids to prevent **dehydration** and correct electrolyte imbalances.

KEY TERMS

Electrolytes—Salts and minerals that ionize in body fluids. Electrolytes control the body's fluid balance as well as performing other important functions.

Gangrene—The death of soft tissue in any part of the body when the blood supply is obstructed.

Ileus—Obstruction of the intestines caused by the absence of peristalsis.

Intussusception—The slipping or telescoping of one part of the intestine into the section next to it.

Meconium—A greenish fecal material that forms the first bowel movement of an infant.

Peristalsis—The waves of muscular contraction in the intestines that push the food along during the process of digestion.

Strangulated obstruction—An obstruction in which a loop of the intestine has its blood supply cut off.

Volvulus—A twisting of the intestine that causes an obstruction.

Nonsurgical approaches

Surgery can be avoided for some patients. In some cases of volvulus, guiding a rectal tube into the intestines will straighten the twisted bowels. In infants, a barium enema may reverse intussusception in 50–90%. An air enema is sometimes used instead of a barium enema. This treatment successfully relieves the obstruction in many infants. The children are usually hospitalized for observation for two to three days after these procedures. In patients with only partial obstruction, a barium enema may dissolve the blockage.

Surgical treatment

If these efforts fail, surgery is necessary. Strangulated obstructions require emergency surgery. The obstructed area is removed and part of the bowel is cut away. If the obstruction is caused by tumors, polyps, or scar tissue, they are removed. Hernias, if present, are repaired. **Antibiotics** are given to reduce the possibility of infection.

Alternative treatment

Alternative practitioners offer few suggestions for treatment. They focus on preventive strategies,

particularly the use of high-fiber **diets** to keep the bowels healthy through regular elimination.

Prognosis

Mortality

Untreated intestinal obstructions can be fatal. Delayed diagnosis of volvulus in infants has a mortality rate of 23–33% with prompt diagnosis and treatment the mortality rate is 3–9%. The bowel either strangulates or perforates, causing massive infection. With prompt treatment, however, most patients recover without complications.

Recurrence

As many as 80% of patients whose volvulus is treated without surgery have recurrences. Recurrences in infants with intussusception are most likely to happen during the first 36 hours after the blockage has been cleared. The mortality rate for unsuccessfully treated infants is 1–2%.

Prevention

Most cases of intestinal obstruction are not preventable. Surgery to remove tumors, polyps, or gallstones helps prevent recurrences.

Resources

BOOKS

Beers, Mark H., MD, and Robert Berkow, MD, editors. "Mechanical Intestinal Obstruction." Section 3, Chapter 25. In *The Merck Manual of Diagnosis and Therapy*. Whitehouse Station, NJ: Merck Research Laboratories, 2004.

PERIODICALS

Chahine, A. Alfred, MD. "Intussusception." *eMedicine* June 10, 2004. < http://www.emedicine.com/ped/topic1208.htm >.

Dray, X., T. Bienvenu, N. Desmazes-Dufeu, et al. "Distal Intestinal Obstruction Syndrome in Adults with Cystic Fibrosis." *Clinical Gastroenterology and Hepatology* 2 (June 2004): 498–503.

Emil, S., T. Nguyen, J. Sills, and G. Padilla. "Meconium Obstruction in Extremely Low-Birth-Weight Neonates: Guidelines for Diagnosis and Management." *Journal of Pediatric Surgery* 39 (May 2004): 731–737.

Hebra, Andre, MD, and Melissa Miller, MD. "Intestinal Volvulus." *eMedicine* February 25, 2004. < http://www.emedicine.com/ped/topic1205.htm >.

Sajja, S. B., and M. Schein. "Early Postoperative Small Bowel Obstruction." *British Journal of Surgery* 91 (June 2004): 683–691.

OTHER

HealthAnswers.com. "Intestinal Obstruction." < http://www.healthanswers.com/database/ami/converted/000260.html >.

"Intussusception: A Case Study for Nurses." *University of New Brunswick Nursing Faculty Page.* < http://www.unb.ca/courses/nur4284/intu.htm >.

Tish Davidson, A.M.
Rebecca Frey, PhD

Intestinal polyps

Definition

The word polyp refers to any overgrowth of tissue from the surface of mucous membranes. Intestinal polyps grow out of the lining of the small and large bowels. Polyps come in a variety of shapes–round, droplet, and irregular being the most common.

Description

Polyps are one of many forms of tissue over-production that can occur in the body. Cells in many body tissues sometimes keep growing beyond their usual limits. Medical scientists call this process *neoplasia*, which means simply "new growth." An individual overgrowth is called a neoplasm. In most cases these growths are limited, and the result is a benign swelling or mass of cells called a tumor. If the new growth occurs on the surface of the tissue instead of inside an organ it is often called a polyp. **Cancer** is another type of neoplasm marked by unlimited tissue growth. The essential feature that distinguishes cancer from nonmalignant neoplasms is that it does not stop growing.

Intestinal polyps are a common form of neoplasm. All intestinal polyps arise from the inner lining of the intestinal wall. This layer of mucosal tissue does the work of digestion. About 30% of the general population will develop intestinal polyps at some point in life, with the likelihood increasing with age. Most of these polyps are never noticed during a person's lifetime because they cause no problems. They are often discovered accidentally at **autopsy**. The primary importance of intestinal polyps is that 1% of them become cancerous. Because the polyps that eventually turn malignant cannot be identified in advance, they are all suspect.

Location of intestinal polyps

The chances of a polyp's becoming cancerous depend to some extent on its location within the digestive tract.

COLON. Ninety-five percent of all intestinal polyps develop inside the large bowel. There are several hereditary diseases that produce large numbers of intestinal polyps. These disorders include:

- Familial polyposis of the colon.
- Gardner's syndrome.
- Lynch's syndrome.
- Turcot's syndrome.
- Peutz-Jeghers syndrome.
- Juvenile polyposis.

All of these disorders are inherited in what is called an autosomal dominant pattern. This pattern means that the disorders are not sex-linked and that a child can inherit the disorder from either parent. In all of these hereditary disorders, the intestinal polyps appear during or after **puberty**. The first four diseases on the list have such a high rate of cancer of the large bowel (colon)–virtually 100% by the age of 40–that persons diagnosed with any of them should have the colon removed surgically in early adulthood.

STOMACH. The stomach's lining is host to polyps of a similar appearance, but there is no agreement as to their potential for becoming **stomach cancer**.

SMALL INTESTINE. Polyps in the small bowel do not seem to have malignant potential. Instead they can produce obstruction in either of two ways. A large polyp can obstruct the bowel by its sheer size. Smaller polyps can be picked up by the rhythmic contractions (peristalsis) of the intestines and pull the part of the bowel to which they are attached into the adjoining section. The result is a telescoping of one section of bowel into another, called **intussusception**.

Causes and symptoms

Population studies of **colon cancer** suggest that diet plays an important role in the disease, and by implication in the formation of colon polyps. The most consistent interpretation of these data is that animal fats—though not vegetable fats—are the single most important dietary factor. Lack of fiber in the diet may also contribute to polyp formation. Other types of polyps are too rare to produce enough data for evaluation.

Most polyps cause no symptoms. Large ones eventually cause intestinal obstruction, which produces cramping abdominal **pain** with **nausea and vomiting**. As colon polyps evolve into cancers, they begin to produce symptoms that include bleeding and altered bowel habits.

Diagnosis

Routine screening for bowel cancer is recommended for everyone over the age of 40. Screening may be as simple as testing the stool for blood or as elaborate as **colonoscopy**. Colonoscopy is a procedure in which the doctor threads an instrument called a colonoscope up through the entire large bowel. Most polyps are in the lower segment of the colon, called the sigmoid colon. These polyps can be seen with a shorter scope called a sigmoidoscope. X ray imaging can also used to look for polyps. For x rays, the colon is first filled with barium, which is a white substance that shows up as a shadowed area on the film. The colon can also be filled with barium and air, which is called a double contrast study.

Because polyps take about five years to turn into cancers, routine examinations are recommended every three years.

Treatment

All polyps should be removed as preventive care. Most of them can be taken out through a colonoscope. Complications like obstruction and intussusception are surgical emergencies.

Prevention

Patients with hereditary disorders associated with polyps must undergo total colectomy early in adult life. All children of parents with these disorders should be screened early in adulthood, because half of them will have the same disease. For the bulk of the population, increased dietary fiber and decreased animal fat are the best preventives known at present. For the occasional intestinal polyp that arises in spite of good dietary habits, routine screening should prevent it from becoming cancerous.

Resources

BOOKS

Silverstein, Fred E. "Gastrointestinal Endoscopy." In *Harrison's Principles of Internal Medicine*, edited Anthony S. Fauci, et al. New York: McGraw-Hill, 1997.

J. Ricker Polsdorfer, MD

Intestinal strangulation *see* **Intestinal obstructions**

Intoxication confusional state *see* **Delirium**

Intracavity therapy *see* **Radioactive implants**

Intracranial abscess *see* **Brain abscess**

Intrapartum monitoring *see* **Electronic fetal monitoring**

Intrauterine device *see* **IUD**

Intrauterine growth retardation

Definition

Intrauterine growth retardation (IUGR) occurs when the unborn baby is at or below the 10th weight percentile for his or her age (in weeks).

Description

There are standards or averages in weight for unborn babies according their age in weeks. When the baby's weight is at or below the 10th percentile for his or her age, it is called intrauterine growth retardation or fetal growth restriction. These babies are smaller than they should be for their age. How much a baby weighs at birth depends not only on how many weeks old it is, but the rate at which it has grown. This growth process is complex and delicate. There are three phases associated with the development of the baby. During the first phase, cells multiply in the baby's organs. This occurs from the beginning of development through the early part of the fourth month. During the second phase, cells continue to multiply and the organs grow. In the third phase (after 32 weeks of development), growth occurs quickly and the baby may gain as much as 7 ounces per week. If the delicate process of development and weight gain is disturbed or interrupted, the baby can suffer from restricted growth.

IUGR is usually classified as symmetrical or asymmetrical. In symmetrical IUGR, the baby's head and body are proportionately small. In asymmetrical IUGR, the baby's brain is abnormally large when compared to the liver. In a normal infant, the brain weighs about three times more than the liver. In asymmetrical IUGR, the brain can weigh five or six times more than the liver.

Causes and symptoms

Doctors think that the two types of IUGR may be linked to the time during development that the problem occurs. Symmetrical IUGR may occur when the unborn baby experiences a problem during early development. Asymmetrical IUGR may occur when the unborn baby experiences a problem during later development. While not true for all asymmetrical cases, doctors think that sometimes the placenta may allow the brain to get more oxygen and **nutrition** while the liver gets less.

There are many IUGR risk factors involving the mother and the baby. A mother is at risk for having a growth restricted infant if she:

- Has had a previous baby who suffered from IUGR

- Is small in size

- Has poor weight gain and nutrition during **pregnancy**

- Is socially deprived

- Uses substances (like tobacco, **narcotics**, alcohol) that can cause abnormal development or **birth defects**

- Has a vascular disease (like **preeclampsia**)

- Has chronic **kidney disease**

- Has a low total blood volume during early pregnancy

- Is pregnant with more than one baby

- Has an antibody problem that can make successful pregnancy difficult (antiphospholipid antibody syndrome).

KEY TERMS

Preeclampsia—Hypertension (high blood pressure) during pregnancy.

Additionally, an unborn baby may suffer from IUGR if it has:

- Exposure to an infection, including German **measles** (**rubella**), cytomegalovirus, **tuberculosis**, **syphilis**, or **toxoplasmosis**

- A birth defect (like a severe cardiovascular defect)

- A chromosome defect, especially trisomy 18 (**Edwards' syndrome**)

- A primary disorder of bone or cartilage

- A chronic lack of oxygen during development (hypoxia)

- Placenta or umbilical cord defects

- Developed outside of the uterus.

Diagnosis

IUGR can be difficult to diagnose and in many cases doctors are not able to make an exact diagnosis until the baby is born. A mother who has had a growth restricted baby is at risk of having another during a later pregnancy. Such mothers are closely monitored during pregnancy. The length in weeks of the pregnancy must be carefully determined so that the doctor will know if development and weight gain are appropriate. Checking the mother's weight and abdomen measurements can help diagnose cases when there are no other risk factors present. Measuring the girth of the abdomen is often used as a tool for diagnosing IUGR. During pregnancy, the healthcare provider will use a tape measure to record the height of the upper portion of the uterus (the uterine fundal height). As the pregnancy continues and the baby grows, the uterus stretches upward in the direction of the mother's head. Between 18 and 30 weeks of gestation, the uterine fundal height (in cm.) equals the weeks of gestation. If the uterine fundal height is more than 2–3 cm below normal, then IUGR is suspected. Ultrasound is used to evaluate the growth of the baby. Usually, IUGR is diagnosed after week 32 of pregnancy. This is during the phase of rapid growth when the baby should be gaining more weight. IUGR caused by genetic factors or infection may sometimes be detected earlier.

Treatment

There is no treatment that improves fetal growth, but IUGR babies who are at or near term have the best outcome if delivered promptly. If IUGR is caused by a problem with the placenta and the baby is otherwise healthy, early diagnosis and treatment of the problem may reduce the chance of a serious outcome.

Prognosis

Babies who suffer from IUGR are at an increased risk for **death**, low blood sugar (**hypoglycemia**), low body temperature (**hypothermia**), and abnormal development of the nervous system. These risks increase with the severity of the growth restriction. The growth that occurs after birth cannot be predicted with certainty based on the size of the baby when it is born. Infants with asymmetrical IUGR are more likely to catch up in growth after birth than are infants who suffer from prolonged symmetrical IUGR. However, as of 1998, doctors cannot reliably predict an infant's future progress. Each case is unique. Some infants who have IUGR will develop normally, while others will have complications of the nervous system or intellectual problems like **learning disorders**. If IUGR is related to a disease or a genetic defect, the future of the infant is related to the severity and the nature of that disorder.

Resources

BOOKS

Cunningham, F. Gary, et al. *Williams Obstetrics.* 20th ed. Stamford: Appleton & Lange, 1997.

Linda Jones

Intravenous nutrition *see* **Nutrition through an intravenous line**

Intravenous pyelography *see* **Intravenous urography**

Intravenous rehydration

Definition

Sterile water solutions containing small amounts of salt or sugar, are injected into the body through a tube attached to a needle which is inserted into a vein.

Purpose

Fever, **vomiting**, and **diarrhea** can cause a person to become dehydrated fairly quickly. Infants and children are especially vulnerable to **dehydration**. Patients can become dehydrated due to an illness, surgery, or accident. Athletes who have overexerted themselves may also require rehydration with IV fluids. An IV for rehydration can be used for several hours to several days, and is generally used if a patient cannot drink fluids.

Precautions

Patients receiving IV therapy need to be monitored to ensure that the IV solutions are providing the correct amounts of fluids and **minerals** needed. People with kidney and heart disease are at increased risk for **overhydration**, so they must be carefully monitored when receiving IV therapy.

Description

Basic IV solutions are sterile water with small amounts of sodium (salt) or dextrose (sugar) supplied in bottles or thick plastic bags that can hang on a stand mounted next to the patient's bed. Additional minerals like potassium and calcium, **vitamins**, or drugs can be added to the IV solution by injecting them into the bottle or bag with a needle.

Preparation

A doctor orders the IV solution and any additional nutrients or drugs to be added to it. The doctor also specifies the rate at which the IV will be infused. The IV solutions are prepared under the supervision of a doctor, pharmacist, or nurse, using sanitary techniques that prevent bacterial contamination. Just like a prescription, the IV is clearly labeled to show its contents and the amounts of any additives. The skin around the area where the needle is inserted is cleaned and disinfected. Once the needle is in place, it will be taped to the skin to prevent it from dislodging.

Aftercare

Patients need to take fluids by mouth before an IV solution is discontinued. After the IV needle is removed, the site should be inspected for any signs of bleeding or infection.

Risks

There is a small risk of infection at the injection site. It is possible that the IV solution may not provide all of the nutrients needed, leading to a deficiency or an imbalance. If the needle becomes dislodged, it is possible that the solution may flow into tissues around the injection site rather than into the vein.

Resources

OTHER

Martinez-Bianchi, Viviana, Michelle Rejman-Peterson, and Mark A. Graber. "Pediatrics: Vomiting, Diarrhea, and Dehydration." *Family Practice Handbook*. University of Iowa. < http://www.vh.org/Providers/ClinRef/ FPHandbook/Chapter10/17-10.html >.

Toth, Peter P. "Gastroenterology: Acute Diarrhea." *Family Practice Handbook*. University of Iowa. < http://www.vh.org/Providers/ClinRef/ FPHandbook/Chapter04/01-4.html >.

Altha Roberts Edgren

Intravenous urography

Definition

Intravenous urography is a test which x rays the urinary system using intravenous dye for diagnostic purposes.

Of the many ways to obtain images of the urinary system, the intravenous injection of a contrast agent has been traditionally considered the best. The kidneys excrete the dye into the urine. X rays can then create pictures of every structure through which the urine passes.

The procedure has several variations and many names.

- Intravenous pyelography (IVP).

- Urography.

- Pyelography.

- Antegrade pyelography differentiates this procedure from "retrograde pyelography," which injects dye into the lower end of the system, therefore flowing backward or "retrograde." Retrograde pyelography is better able to define problems in the lower parts of the system and is the only way to get x rays if the kidneys are not working well.

- Nephrotomography is somewhat different in that the x rays are taken by a moving x ray source onto a film moving in the opposite direction. By accurately coordinating the movement, all but a single plane of tissue is blurred, and that plane is seen without overlying shadows.

Every method available gives good pictures of this system, and the question becomes one of choosing among many excellent alternatives. Each condition has special requirements, while each technique has distinctive benefits and drawbacks.

- Nuclear scans rely on the radiation given off by certain atoms. Chemicals containing such atoms are injected into the bloodstream. They reach the kidneys, where images are constructed by measuring the radiation emitted. The radiation is no more dangerous than standard x rays. The images require considerable training to interpret, but unique information is often available using this technology. Different chemicals can concentrate the radiation in different types of tissue. This technique may require several days for the chemical to concentrate at its destination. It also requires a special detector to create the image.

- Ultrasound is a quick, safe, simple, and inexpensive way to obtain views of internal organs. Although less detailed than other methods, it may be sufficient.

- Retrograde pyelography is better able to define problems in the lower parts of the system and is the only way to get x rays if the kidneys are not working well. Dye is usually injected through an instrument (cystoscope) passed into the bladder through the urethra.

- Computed tomography scans (CT or CAT scanning) uses the same kind of radiation used in x rays, but it collects information by computer in such a way that three dimensional images can be constructed, eliminating interference from nearby structures. CT scanning requires a special apparatus.

- Magnetic resonance imaging (MRI) uses magnetic fields and radio frequency signals, instead of ionizing radiation, to create computerized images. This form of energy is entirely safe as long as the patient has no metal on board. The technique is far more versatile than CT scanning. MRI requires special apparatus and, because of the powerful magnets needed, even a special building all by itself. It is quite expensive.

Purpose

Most diseases of the kidneys, ureters, and bladder will yield information to this procedure, which actually has two phases. First, it requires a functioning kidney to filter the dye out of the blood into the urine. The time required for the dye to appear on x rays correlates accurately with kidney function. The second phase gives detailed anatomical images of the urinary tract. Within the first few minutes the dye "lights up" the kidneys, a phase called the nephrogram. Subsequent pictures follow the dye down the ureters and into the bladder. A final film taken after urinating reveals how well the bladder empties.

IVPs are most often done to assess structural abnormalities or obstruction to urine flow. If kidney function is at issue, more films are taken sooner to catch the earliest phase of the process.

- Stones, tumors and congenital malformations account for many of the findings.

- Kidney cysts and cancers can be seen.

- Displacement of a kidney or ureter suggests a space-occupying lesion like a **cancer** pushing it out of the way.

- Bad valves where the ureters enter the bladder will often show up.

- Bladder cancers and other abnormalities are often outlined by the dye in the bladder.

- An **enlarged prostate** gland will show up as incomplete bladder emptying and a bump at the bottom of the bladder.

Precautions

The only serious complication of an IVP is allergy to the iodine-containing dye that is used. Such an allergy is rare, but it can be dramatic and even lethal. Emergency measures taken immediately are usually effective.

Description

IVPs are usually done in the morning. In the x ray suite, the patient will undress and lie down. There are two methods of injecting the dye. An intravenous line can be established, through which the dye will be consistently fed through the body during the procedure. The other method is to give the dye all at once through a needle that is immediately withdrawn. X rays are taken until the dye has reached the bladder, an interval of half an hour or less. The patient will be asked to empty the bladder before one last x ray.

Preparation

Emptying the bowel with **laxatives** or **enemas** prevents bowel shadows from obscuring the details of the urinary system. An empty stomach prevents the complications of **vomiting**, a rare effect of the contrast agent. Therefore, the night before the IVP the patient will be asked to evacuate the bowels and to drink sparingly.

Risks

Allergy to the contrast agent is the only risk. Anyone with a possible iodine allergy or a previous reaction to x ray dye must be particularly careful to inform the x ray personnel.

Resources

BOOKS

Merrill, Vinta. *Atlas of Roentgenographic Positions and Standard Radiologic Procedures.* Saint Louis: The C.V. Mosby Co., 1975.

J. Ricker Polsdorfer, MD

Intussusception

Definition

Intussusception is the enfolding of one segment of the intestine within another. It is characterized and initially presents with recurring attacks of cramping abdominal **pain** that gradually become more painful.

Description

Intussusception occurs when part of the bowel or intestine is wrapped around itself producing a mass-like object on the right side of the abdomen during palpation (a procedure used during a **physical examination**, when the examiner touches the abdomen with his/her hand, usually feeling for mass, pain, or discomfort). The number of new cases of intussuscetion is approximately 1.5 to four cases per 1,000 live births. The onset of abdominal pain is usually abrupt and severe. Just as fast as the onset of pain appears, it disappears and the child resumes activity normally. This process of sudden severe abdominal pain appearing out of the blue then disappearing is repeated with duration of painful attacks. The pain usually increases after approximately five hours of recurrent cycles of severe abdominal pain followed by relaxation. **Vomiting** and **diarrhea** occur in about 90% of cases with six to 12 hours after initial onset of symptoms.

Physical examination and palpation usually reveal a sausage shaped mass of enfolded bowel in the right upper mid portion of the abdomen. Within a few hours approximately 50% of cases have bloody, mucus filled bowel movements. At about this time the child is visibly very ill with **fever**, tenderness, and distended abdomen. Intussusception is the most frequent cause of intestinal obstruction during the first two years of life and commonly affects children between three to 12 months of age. The disease is three times more common in males than in females. In about 85% of cases the cause is idiopathic (meaning unknown). The remaining 15% of cases can be caused by a variety of other diseases such as tumors of the lymph nodes (lymphoma), fat tumors (lipomas), foreign bodies/objects, or from infections that mobilize immune cells to the area causing and an inflammatory reaction and intestinal blockage. Most cases of intussusception do not strangulate the affected bowel within the first 24 hours. If the disease is not treated after this time, the possibility of intestinal **gangrene**, **shock**, and **death** increases.

Causes and symptoms

The major symptom of intussusception is when a healthy child suddenly and without warning experiences severe abdominal pain that subsides and usually results in continuation of normal activities such as playing. The duration of the painful attacks increases as the hours go by. Usually, the child develops **nausea**, vomiting, and diarrhea soon afterwards in about 90% of all cases. The child becomes weak, exhausted, and develops a fever. The affected child may also expel bloody, mucus-like bowel movements. These blood filled bowel movements are usually due to impaired blood flow to the obstructed area. During palpation there may be a sausage-shaped mass located on the upper right mid portion of the abdomen. If the disease progresses and

is undetected, the child may develop necrosis death of cells within the affected area. Additionally, there may be perforation or hole in the intussusception bowel that can cause a life threatening infection in the peritoneum (a layer of tissue that protects the organs and intestines within the abdominal cavity). This infection of the peritoneum is called **peritonitis**. Some patients may exhibit altered states of consciousness or seizures.

Diagnosis

A presumed diagnosis can be made by history alone. If the clinician suspect's intussusception x-ray films should be performed, which may reveal a mass in the right upper mid abdominal region. Two classical clinical signs are mucus-blood filled stools and a "coiled string" appearance in the affected bowel as visualized during an x ray with a **barium enema**. Blood chemistry analysis is not specific for intussusception. Depending on vomiting and blood loss through the stools, blood chemistry may reflect signs of **dehydration** and anemia.

Treatment

Treating intussusception by reduction (alleviating the source of blockage) is an emergency procedure. The barium examination is not only the diagnostic tool of choice, but also frequently curative. Infusion by gravity from a catheter placed in the rectum will tend to relieve pressure buildup. If this does not relieve the area, then air can be pumped into the colon to clear blockage. If these procedures are unsuccessful then surgery is required. Approximately 25% of affected children require surgical intervention. Surgery in the affected bowel is advantageous since the actual cause can be removed, and the procedure decreases the possibility of recurrences. In general without surgical correction of the affected bowel, there is a 5–10% chance of recurrence. Recurrence usually appears within the first 24 to 48 hours after barium procedure.

Prognosis

The outcome of intussusception depends on the duration of symptoms before treatment initiation. Most infants will recover if treatment is initiated within the first 24 hours. Untreated intussusception is almost always fatal. Overall even with treatment, approximately 1–2% of affected children will die.

Prevention

Prevention of death can be accomplished with immediate medical care, within the first 24 hours. Once intussusception is suspected, emergency measures should be initiated. Untreated intussusception is almost always fatal. There is an increased chance for death if the disorder is not treated within 48 hours.

Resources

BOOKS

Behrman, Richard E., et al, editors. *Nelson Textbook of Pediatrics*. 16th ed. W. B. Saunders Company, 2000.

Townsend, Courtney M., et al. *Sabiston Textbook of Surgery*. 16th ed. W. B. Saunders Company, 2001.

OTHER

University of Maryland. 2001. < http://www.umm.edu >.

Laith Farid Gulli, M.D.

Intussusception *see* **Intestinal obstructions**

Iodine *see* **Antiseptics**

Iodine uptake test *see* **Thyroid nuclear medicine scan**

Ipecac

Definition

Ipecac is a medicine commonly used to induce **vomiting** in cases of accidental **poisoning**. It is also a homeopathic remedy.

Purpose

Treatment of poisoning

At one time, standard medical practice recommended syrup of ipecac to cause vomiting in cases of poisoning in order to remove the toxic substance from the stomach before absorption occurs. More recently, however, doctors are discouraging the use of ipecac in emergency treatment of poisoning. The reason for this change in practice is that ipecac has not been shown to be more effective than **activated charcoal** or gastric lavage; in addition, its use may delay the administration of these other methods of treatment. In 2004 the American College of Toxicology updated a 1997 position paper on the use of syrup of ipecac to treat poisoning with the following statement: "There is no evidence from clinical studies that ipecac improves the outcome of poisoned patients and its routine administration in the emergency department should be abandoned."

Ipecac should *never* be used to induce vomiting if the poison is one of the following:

- strychnine
- alkalis (lye)
- strong acids
- kerosene
- fuel oil
- gasoline
- coal oil
- paint thinner
- cleaning fluid

In cases of poisoning, it is always best to contact a local poison control center, local hospital emergency room, or the family doctor for instructions before using syrup of ipecac.

Ipecac's reputation for inducing vomiting has encouraged some bulimics to take it on a regular basis in order to purge the contents of the stomach after an eating binge. This misuse of ipecac is extremely dangerous; it can cause heart problems, tears in the esophagus or stomach lining, vomiting blood, seizures, or even **death**.

Homeopathy

The homeopathic remedy made from ipecac is called *Ipecacuanha*. Homeopathic preparations are given for a reason completely opposite from that of standard allopathic treatment. In homeopathy, ipecac is given to stop vomiting rather than to induce it. According to Hahnemann's law of similars, a substance that would cause vomiting in large doses when given to a healthy person will stimulate a sick person's natural defenses when given in extremely dilute and carefully prepared doses. *Ipecacuanha* is a favorite homeopathic remedy for morning sickness associated with **pregnancy**. It is also given to stop **nausea** that is not relieved by vomiting; when the vomitus is

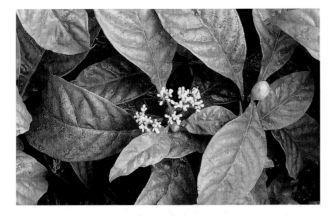

Ipecac plant (*Cephaelis ipecacuanha*). *(PlantaPhile Germany. Reproduced by permission.)*

slimy and white; when there is gagging and heavy salivation; when the tongue is clean despite the patient's feelings of nausea; and when the patient is not thirsty. The nausea may be accompanied by a **headache**, **cough**, or heavy menstrual bleeding. The modalities (circumstances) that suggest *Ipecacuanha* as the appropriate homeopathic remedy is that the patient feels worse lying down; in dry weather; in winter; and when exercising or moving about.

A homeopathic practitioner would not necessarily prescribe ipecac for all cases of nausea. *Arsenicum* would be given when the nausea is caused by **food poisoning** and accompanied by strong thirst, *Nux vomica* when the nausea is the result of overindulgence in food or alcohol and accompanied by gas or **heartburn**. A sick child might be given *Pulsatilla*, particularly if rich foods have been eaten.

On the other hand, a homeopathic practitioner may prescribe ipecac for any of the following conditions that are not related to **nausea and vomiting**.

- Nosebleeds producing bright red blood.
- Dental bleeding.
- Diarrhea with cramping abdominal **pain**. The stools are green with froth or foam.
- Asthma of sudden onset. The patient has to sit up in order to breathe, but cannot bring up any mucus in spite of violent coughing.
- Hoarseness or loss of voice following a cold.
- Physical or mental exhaustion.

Description

The medicinal effects of ipecac were recognized centuries ago by the Portuguese who settled in South America. They found a plant that can make people vomit and appropriately named it *Caephalis ipecacuanha*, meaning sick-making plant. Syrup of ipecac is now considered the safest drug to treat poisoning and is often the most effective. There are different types of ipecac preparations that vary greatly in strength. Syrup of ipecac is best for use at home to treat accidental poisoning. Ipecac fluid extract and ipecac tincture should be avoided as they are much stronger compounds and can be toxic.

Ipecacuanha is a homeopathic remedy made from ipecac by a process of dilution and succussion (shaking). In contrast to syrup of ipecac, it is given to relieve vomiting.

Recommended dosage

Syrup of ipecac

Syrup of ipecac is made from the dried roots and rhizomes (underground stems) of *Cephaelis ipecacuanha*. It is available over the counter in 0.5–1 oz bottles. Larger bottles require a doctor's prescription. The dosage for infants under 6 months old should be prescribed by the family doctor or poison control center. For children six months to one year, the usual dose is 5–10 ml or 1–2 tsp. One-half or one full glass (4–8 oz) of water should be taken immediately before or after the dose. The dose may be repeated once after 20–30 minutes if vomiting does not occur. For children one to 12 years of age, the usual dose is 15 ml (1 tbsp) to be taken with one full glass (8 oz) of water. Adults and teenagers should take 15–30 ml of ipecac with at least 1 full glass of water. Syrup of ipecac should not be taken with milk or soda drinks as these foods may prevent it from working properly. If vomiting does not occur within 20–30 minutes after the first dose, a second dose may be needed. If the second dose fails to induce vomiting, the patient should be taken to a hospital emergency room.

If both activated charcoal and syrup of ipecac are recommended to treat poison, ipecac must be used first. Activated charcoal should not be taken until 30 minutes after taking syrup of ipecac, or until the vomiting caused by ipecac stops.

Homeopathic preparations

Ipecacuanha is available as an over-the-counter remedy in 30x potency. This is a decimal potency, which means that one part of ipecac has been mixed with nine parts of alcohol or water; 30x means that this decimal dilution has been repeated 30 times. The dilute solution of ipecac is then added to sugar tablets so that the remedy can be taken in tablet form.

Precautions

Syrup of ipecac

For inducing vomiting in cases of accidental poisoning, only the syrup form of ipecac should be used. Syrup of ipecac should not be mixed with milk or carbonated drinks as they may prevent vomiting.

Syrup of ipecac should not be used in the following situations (contact poison control center or family doctor for alternative treatments).

- Poisoning caused by strychnine; sustained-release theophylline; such corrosive substances as strong alkalis (lye); strong acids (such as toilet bowl cleaner); and such petroleum products as kerosene, gasoline, coal oil, fuel oil, paint thinner, or cleaning fluids.
- Overdoses of medications given for depression.
- Excessive vomiting.
- A serious heart condition.
- Timing. Do not give ipecac more than 4–6 hours after the poison was ingested.
- Pregnancy.
- Very young children (less than six months old). Infants and very young children may choke on their own vomit or get vomit into their lungs.
- Drowsy or unconscious patients.
- Seizures.

Homeopathic preparations

Ipecacuanha should not be given after *Arsenicum* or *Tabac* because these remedies will counteract it.

Side effects

The following side effects have been associated with the use of syrup of ipecac:

- Loose bowel movements.
- Diarrhea.
- Fast irregular heartbeat.
- Inhaling or **choking** on vomit.
- Stomach cramps or pains.
- Coughing.
- Weakness.
- Aching.

KEY TERMS

Bulimia nervosa—An eating disorder characterized by episodic binge eating followed by self-induced vomiting or laxative abuse.

Cephaeline—A chemical compound found in ipecac that irritates the stomach lining and triggers the vomiting reflex.

Fluid extract—A concentrated preparation of a drug.

Law of similars—A principle of homeopathic treatment according to which substances that cause specific symptoms in healthy people are given to sick people with similar symptoms.

Modality—A factor or circumstance that makes a patient's symptoms better or worse. Modalities include such factors as time of day, room temperature, the patient's level of activity, sleep patterns, etc.

Tincture—An alcoholic solution of a chemical or drug.

- Muscle stiffness.
- Severe heart problems often occur in cases of ipecac **abuse**. Because ipecac stays in the body for a long time, damage to the heart frequently occurs in persons who repeatedly take ipecac to induce vomiting.
- Seizures. These are most likely to occur in patients who accidentally swallow ipecac or in ipecac abusers.
- Death. Deaths have been reported due to ipecac abuse in bulimic persons.

Homeopathic *Ipecacuanha* has been highly diluted and is relatively nontoxic.

Interactions

If used to induce vomiting, ipecac should not be given together with other drugs because it can decrease their effectiveness and increase their toxicity. If both syrup of ipecac and activated charcoal are needed to treat suspected poisons, ipecac should be given first. Activated charcoal should not be given until vomiting induced by ipecac has stopped. Carbonated beverages should also be avoided because they can cause the stomach to swell. The person should lie on the stomach or side in case vomiting occurs.

Homeopathic *Ipecacuanha* is considered complementary to *Arnica* and *Cuprum*. It is counteracted by *Arsenicum* and *Tabac*.

Resources

BOOKS

Beers, Mark H., MD, and Robert Berkow, MD, editors. "Bulimia Nervosa." Section 15, Chapter 196. In *The Merck Manual of Diagnosis and Therapy*. Whitehouse Station, NJ: Merck Research Laboratories, 2004.

Beers, Mark H., MD, and Robert Berkow, MD, editors. "Poisoning." Section 23, Chapter 307. In *The Merck Manual of Diagnosis and Therapy*. Whitehouse Station, NJ: Merck Research Laboratories, 2004.

PDR Nurse's Drug Handbook. Montvale, NJ: Delmar Publishers, 2000.

PERIODICALS

"Position Paper: Ipecac Syrup." *Journal of Toxicology: Clinical Toxicology* 42 (February 2004): 133–143.

ORGANIZATIONS

American College of Toxicology (ACT). 9650 Rockville Pike, Bethesda, MD 20814. (301) 634-7840. Fax: (301) 634-7852. <http://www.actox.org>.

American Foundation for Homeopathy. 1508 S. Garfield, Alhambra, CA 91801.

Homeopathic Educational Services. 2124B Kittredge St. Berkeley, CA 94704. (510) 649-0294. Fax: (510) 649-1955.

Rebecca J. Frey, PhD

Ipratropium *see* **Bronchodilators**

I.Q. tests *see* **Stanford-Binet intelligence scales; Wechsler intelligence test**

Iridocyclitis *see* **Uveitis**

Iritis *see* **Uveitis**

Iron-binding capacity test *see* **Iron tests**

Iron-utilization anemias *see* **Sideroblastic anemia**

Iron deficiency anemia

Definition

Anemia can be caused by iron deficiency, folate deficiency, vitamin B_{12} deficiency, and other causes. The term iron deficiency anemia means anemia that is due to iron deficiency. Iron deficiency anemia is characterized by the production of small red blood cells. When examined under a microscope, the red blood cells also appear pale or light colored. For this reason, the anemia that occurs with iron deficiency is also called hypochronic microcytic anemia.

Description

Iron deficiency anemia is the most common type of anemia throughout the world. In the United States, iron deficiency anemia occurs to a lesser extent than in developing countries because of the higher consumption of red meat and the practice of food fortification (addition of iron to foods by the manufacturer). Anemia in the United States is caused by a variety of sources, including excessive losses of iron in menstrual fluids and excessive bleeding in the gastrointestinal tract. In developing countries located in tropical climates, the most common cause of iron deficiency anemia is infestation with hookworm.

Causes and symptoms

Infancy is a period of increased risk for iron deficiency. The human infant is born with a built-in supply of iron, which can be tapped during periods of drinking low-iron milk or formula. Both human milk and cow milk contain rather low levels of iron (0.5–1.0 mg iron/liter). However, the iron in human milk is about 50% absorbed by the infant, while the iron of cow milk is only 10% absorbed. During the first six months of life, growth of the infant is made possible by the milk in the diet and by the infant's built-in supply. However, premature infants have a lower supply of iron and, for this reason, it is recommended that pre-term infants (beginning at 2 months of age) be given oral supplements of 7 mg iron/day, as ferrous sulfate. Iron deficiency can be provoked where infants are fed formulas that are based on unfortified cow milk. For example, unfortified cow milk is given free of charge to mothers in Chile. This practice has the fortunate result of preventing general **malnutrition**, but the unfortunate result of allowing the development of mild iron deficiency.

The normal rate of blood loss in the feces is 0.5–1.0 ml per day. These losses can increase with colorectal **cancer**. About 60% of colorectal cancers result in further blood losses, where the extent of blood loss is 2-10 ml/day. Cancer of the colon and rectum can provoke losses of blood, resulting in iron deficiency anemia. The fecal blood test is widely used to screen for the presence of cancer of the colon or rectum. In the absence of testing, colorectal cancer may be first detected because of the resulting iron deficiency anemia.

Infection with hookworm can provoke iron deficiency and iron deficiency anemia. The hookworm is a parasitic worm. It thrives in warm climates, including in the southern United States. The hookworm enters the body through the skin, as through bare feet. The hookworm then migrates to the small intestines where it attaches itself to the villi (small sausage-shaped structures in the intestines that are used for the absorption of all nutrients). The hookworm provokes damage to the villi, resulting in blood loss, and they produce anti-coagulants which promote continued bleeding. Each worm can provoke the loss of up to 0.25 ml of blood per day.

Bleeding and blood losses through gastrointestinal tract can be provoked by colorectal cancer and hookworms, as mentioned above, but also by **hemorrhoids**, anal fissures, **irritable bowel syndrome**, aspirin-induced bleeding, blood clotting disorders, and **diverticulosis** (a condition caused by an abnormal opening from the intestine or bladder). Several genetic diseases exist which lead to bleeding diorders, and these include **hemophilia** A, hemophilia B, and von Willebrand's disease. Of these, only von Willebrand's disease leads to gastrointestinal bleeding.

The symptoms of iron deficiency anemia include weakness and **fatigue**. These symptoms result because of the lack of function of the red blood cells, and the reduced ability of the red blood cells to carry iron to exercising muscles. Iron deficiency can also affect other tissues, including the tongue and fingernails. Prolonged iron deficiency can result in changes of the tongue, and it may become smooth, shiny, and reddened. This condition is called glossitis. The fingernails may grow abnormally, and acquire a spoon-shaped appearance.

Decreased iron intake is a contributing factor in iron deficiency and iron deficiency anemia. The iron content of cabbage, for example, is about 1.6 mg/kg food, while that of spinach (33 mg/kg), lima beans (15 mg/kg), potato (14 mg/kg), tomato (3 mg/kg), apples (1.5 mg/kg), raisins (20 mg/kg), whole wheat bread (43 mg/kg), eggs (20 mg/kg), canned tuna (13 mg/kg), chicken (11 mg/kg), beef (28 mg/kg), corn oil (0.6 mg/kg), and peanut butter (6.0 mg/kg), are indicated. One can see that apples, tomatoes, and vegetable oil are relatively low in iron, while whole wheat bread and beef are relatively high in iron. The assessment of whether a food is low or high in iron can also be made by comparing the amount of that food eaten per day with the recommended dietary allowance (RDA) for iron. The RDA for iron for the adult male is 10 mg/day, while that for the adult woman is 15 mg/day. The RDA during **pregnancy** is 30 mg/day. The RDA for infants of 0–0.5 years of age is 6 mg/day, while that for infants of 0.5–1.0 years of age is 10 mg/day. The RDA values are based on the assumption that the consumer eats a mixture of plant and animal foods.

The above list of iron values alone may be deceptive, since the availability of iron in fruits, vegetables, and grains is very low, while that the availability from meat is much higher. The availability of iron in plants ranges from only 1–10%, while that in meat, fish, chicken, and liver is 20–30%. The term availability means the percent of dietary iron that is absorbed via the gastrointestinal tract to the bloodstream. Non-absorbed iron is lost in the feces.

Interactions between various foods can influence the absorption of dietary iron. Vitamin C can increase the absorption of dietary iron. Orange juice is a rich source of vitamin C. Thus, if a plant food, such as rice, is consumed with orange juice, then the orange juice can enhance the absorption of the iron of the rice. Vitamin C is also added to infant formulas, and the increased use of formulas fortified with both iron and vitamin C have led to a marked decline in anemia in infants and young children in the United States (Dallman, 1989). In contrast, if rice is consumed with tea, certain chemicals in the tea (tannins) can reduce the absorption of the iron. Phytic acid is a chemical that naturally occurs in legumes, cereals, and nuts. Phytic acid, which can account for 1–5% of the weight of these foods, is a potent inhibitor of iron absorption. The increased availability of the iron in meat products is partly due to the fact that heme-iron is absorbed to a greater extent than free iron salts, and to a greater extent than iron in the phytic acid/iron complex. Nearly all of the iron in plants is nonheme-iron. Much of the iron in meat is nonheme-iron as well. The nonheme-iron in meat, fish, chicken and liver may be about 20% available. The heme-iron of meat may be close to 30% available. The most available source of iron is human milk (50% availability).

Diagnosis

Iron deficiency anemia in infants is defined as a hemoglobin level below 109 mg/ml of whole blood, and a **hematocrit** of under 33%. Anemia in adult males is defined as a hemoglobin under 130 mg/ml and a hematocrit of under 38%. Anemia in adult females is defined as hemoglobin under 120 mg/ml and a hematocrit of under 32%. Anemia in pregnant women is defined as hemoglobin of under 110 mg/ml and hematocrit of under 31%.

When an abnormally high presence of blood is found in the feces during a **fecal occult blood test**, the physician needs to examine the gastrointestinal tract to determine the cause of bleeding. Here, the diagnosis for iron deficiency anemia includes the examination using a sigmoidoscope. The sigmoidoscope is an instrument that consists of a flexible tube that permits examination of the colon to a distance of 60 cm. A **barium enema**, with an x ray, may also be used to detect abnormalities that can cause bleeding.

The diagnosis of iron deficiency anemia should include a test for oral iron absorption, where evidence suggests that oral iron supplements fail in treating anemia. The oral iron absorption test is conducted by eating 64 mg iron (325 mg ferrous sulfate) in a single dose. Blood samples are then taken after 2 hours and 4 hours. The iron content of the blood serum is then measured. The concentration of iron should rise by an increment of about 22 micromolar, where iron absorption is normal. Lesser increases in concentration mean that iron absorption is abnormal, and that therapy should involve injections or infusions of iron.

Treatment

Oral iron supplements (pills) may contain various iron salts. These iron salts include ferrous sulfate, ferrous gluconate, or ferrous fumarate. Injections and infusions of iron can be carried out with a preparation called iron dextran. In patients with poor iron absorption (by the gut), therapy with injection or infusion is preferable over oral supplements. Treatment of iron deficiency anemia sometimes requires more than therapy with iron. Where iron deficiency was provoked by hemorrhoids, surgery may prove essential to prevent recurrent iron deficiency anemia. Where iron deficiency is provoked by bleeding due to **aspirin** treatment, aspirin should be discontinued. Where iron deficiency is provoked by hookworm infections, therapy for this parasite should be used, along with protection of the feet by wearing shoes whenever walking in hookworm-infested soil.

Prognosis

The prognosis for treating and curing iron deficiency anemia is excellent. Perhaps the main problem is failure to take iron supplements. In cases of pregnant women, the health care worker may recommend taking 100–200 mg iron/day. This dose is rather

high, and can lead to **nausea**, **diarrhea**, or abdominal **pain** in 10–20% of women taking this dose. The reason for using this high dose is to effect a rapid cure for anemia, where the anemia is detected at a mid-point during the pregnancy. The above problems of side-effects and noncompliance can be avoided by taking iron doses (100–200 mg) only once a week, where supplements are initiated some time prior to conception, or continuously throughout the fertile period of life. The problem of compliance is not an issue where infusions are used, however a fraction of patients treated with iron infusions experience side effects, such as flushing, **headache**, nausea, **anaphylaxis**, or seizures. A number of studies have shown that iron deficiency anemia in infancy can result in reduced intelligence, where intelligence was measured in early childhood. It is not certain if iron supplementation of children with reduced intelligence, due to iron-deficiency anemia in infancy, has any influence in allowing a "catch-up" in intellectual development.

Prevention

In the healthy population, all of the mineral deficiencies can be prevented by the consumption of inorganic nutrients at levels defined by the RDA. Iron deficiency anemia in infants and young children can be prevented by the use of fortified foods. Liquid cow milk-based infant formulas are generally supplemented with iron (12 mg/L). The iron in liquid formulas is added as ferrous sulfate or ferrous gluconate. Commercial infant cereals are also fortified with iron, and here small particles of elemental iron are added. The levels used are about 0.5 gram iron/kg dry cereal. This amount of iron is about 10-fold greater than that of the iron naturally present in the cereal.

Resources

PERIODICALS

Walter, T., P. Pino, F. Pizarro, and B. Lozoff. "Prevention of Iron-deficiency Anemia: Comparison of High- and Low-iron Formulas in Term Healthy Infants after Six Months of Life." *Journal of Pediatrics* 132 (1998): 635-640.

Tom Brody, PhD

Iron overload *see* **Hemochromatosis**

Iron tests

Definition

Iron tests are a group of blood tests that are done to evaluate the iron level in blood serum, the body's capacity to absorb iron, and the amount of iron actually stored in the body. Iron is an essential trace element; it is necessary for the formation of red blood cells and certain enzymes. At the other extreme, high levels of iron can be poisonous.

Purpose

There are four different types of tests that measure the body's iron levels and storage. They are called iron level tests, total iron-binding capacity (TIBC) tests, ferritin tests, and transferrin tests. These tests are given for several reasons:

- To help in the differential diagnosis of different types of anemia.

- To assess the severity of anemia and monitor the treatment of patients with chronic anemia.

- To evaluate protein depletion and other forms of **malnutrition**.

- To check for certain liver disorders.

- To evaluate the possibility of chronic gastrointestinal bleeding. Blood loss from the digestive tract is a common cause of **iron deficiency anemia**.

- To help diagnose certain unusual disorders, including iron **poisoning**, **thalassemia**, hemosiderosis, and **hemochromatosis**.

A serum iron test can be used without the others to evaluate cases of iron poisoning.

Precautions

Patients should not have their blood tested for iron within four days of a blood **transfusion** or tests and treatments that use radioactive materials. Recent high **stress** levels or sleep deprivation are additional reasons for postponing iron tests.

Blood samples for iron tests should be taken early in the morning because serum iron levels vary during the day. This precaution is especially important in evaluating the results of iron replacement therapy.

Description

Iron tests are performed on samples of the patient's blood, withdrawn from a vein into a vacuum tube. The amount of blood taken is between 6 mL and 10 mL (1/3 of a fluid ounce). The procedure, which is called a venipuncture, takes about five minutes.

Iron level test

The iron level test measures the amount of iron in the blood serum that is being carried by a protein (transferrin) in the blood plasma.

Medications and substances that can cause *increased* iron levels include chloramphenicol, estrogen preparations, dietary iron supplements, alcoholic beverages, methyldopa, and birth control pills.

Medications that can cause *decreased* iron levels include ACTH, colchicine, deferoxamine, methicillin, and testosterone.

Total iron-binding capacity (TIBC) test

The TIBC test measures the amount of iron that the blood would carry if the transferrin were fully saturated. Since transferrin is produced by the liver, the TIBC can be used to monitor liver function and **nutrition**.

Medications that can cause *increased* TIBC levels include fluorides and birth control pills.

Medications that can cause *decreased* TIBC levels include chloramphenicol and ACTH.

Transferrin test

The transferrin test is a direct measurement of transferrin–which is also called siderophilin–levels in the blood. Some laboratories prefer this measurement to the TIBC. The saturation level of the transferrin can be calculated by dividing the serum iron level by the TIBC.

Ferritin test

The ferritin test measures the level of a protein in the blood that stores iron for later use by the body.

Medications that can cause *increased* ferritin levels include dietary iron supplements. In addition, some diseases that do not directly affect the body's iron storage can cause artificially high ferritin levels. These disorders include infections, late-stage cancers, lymphomas, and severe inflammations. Alcoholics often have high ferritin levels.

Preparation

Patient history

Before patients are tested for iron, they should be checked for any of the following factors:

- Prescription medications that affect iron levels, absorption, or storage
- Blood transfusion or radioactive medications within the last four days
- Recent extreme stress or sleep deprivation
- Recent eating habits. Test results can be affected by eating large amounts of iron-rich foods shortly before the blood test.

Fasting

Patients scheduled for an iron level, TIBC, or transferrin test should fast for 12 hours before the blood is drawn. They are allowed to drink water. Patients scheduled for a ferritin test do not need to fast but they should not have any alcoholic beverages before the test.

Aftercare

Aftercare consists of routine care of the area around the venipuncture.

Risks

The primary risk is the possibility of a bruise or swelling in the area of the venipuncture. The patient can apply moist warm compresses if there is any discomfort.

Normal results

Iron level test

Normal serum iron values are as follows:

- Adult males: 75–175 micrograms/dL
- Adult females: 65–165 micrograms/dL
- Children: 50–120 micrograms/dL
- Newborns: 100–250 micrograms/dL.

TIBC test

Normal TIBC values are as follows:

- Adult males: 300–400 micrograms/dL
- Adult females: 300–450 micrograms/dL.

Transferrin test

Normal transferrin values are as follows:

- Adult males: 200–400 mg/dL
- Adult females: 200–400 mg/dL
- Children: 203–360 mg/dL
- Newborns: 130–275 mg/dL.

Normal transferrin saturation values are between 30–40%.

Ferritin test

Normal ferritin values are as follows:

- Adult males: 20–300 ng/mL
- Adult females: 20–120 ng/mL
- Children (one month): 200–600 ng/mL
- Children (two to five months): 50–200 ng/mL
- Children (six months to 15 years): 7–140 ng/mL
- Newborns: 25–200 ng/mL.

Abnormal results

Iron level test

Serum iron level is *increased* in thalassemia, hemochromatosis, severe hepatitis, **liver disease**, **lead poisoning**, acute leukemia, and **kidney disease**. It is also increased by multiple blood transfusions and intramuscular iron injections.

Anemia—A disorder marked by low hemoglobin levels in red blood cells, which leads to a deficiency of oxygen in the blood.

Ferritin—A protein found in the liver, spleen, and bone marrow that stores iron.

Hemochromatosis—A disorder of iron absorption characterized by bronze-colored skin. It can cause painful joints, diabetes, and liver damage if the iron concentration is not lowered.

Hemosiderosis—An overload of iron in the body resulting from repeated blood transfusions. Hemosiderosis occurs most often in patients with thalassemia.

Iron poisoning—A potentially fatal condition caused by swallowing large amounts of iron dietary supplements. Most cases occur in children who have taken adult- strength iron formulas. The symptoms of iron poisoning include vomiting, bloody diarrhea, convulsions, low blood pressure, and turning blue.

Plasma—The liquid part of blood.

Siderophilin—Another name for transferrin.

Thalassemia—A hereditary form of anemia that occurs most frequently in people of Mediterranean origin.

Transferrin—A protein in blood plasma that carries iron derived from food intake to the liver, spleen, and bone marrow.

Iron levels above 350–500 micrograms/dL are considered toxic; levels over 1000 micrograms/dL indicate severe iron poisoning.

Serum iron level is *decreased* in iron deficiency anemia, chronic blood loss, chronic diseases (lupus, **rheumatoid arthritis**), late **pregnancy**, chronically heavy menstrual periods, and thyroid deficiency.

TIBC test

The TIBC is *increased* in iron deficiency anemia, **polycythemia vera**, pregnancy, blood loss, severe hepatitis, and the use of birth control pills.

The TIBC is *decreased* in malnutrition, severe **burns**, hemochromatosis, anemia caused by infections and chronic diseases, **cirrhosis** of the liver, and kidney disease.

Transferrin test

Transferrin is *increased* in iron deficiency anemia, pregnancy, **hormone replacement therapy** (HRT), and the use of birth control pills.

Transferrin is *decreased* in protein deficiency, liver damage, malnutrition, severe burns, kidney disease, chronic infections, and certain genetic disorders.

Ferritin test

Ferritin is *increased* in liver disease, iron overload from hemochromatosis, certain types of anemia, acute leukemia, **Hodgkin's disease**, **breast cancer**, thalassemia, infections, inflammatory diseases, and hemosiderosis. Ferritin levels may be normal or slightly above normal in patients with kidney disease.

Ferritin is *decreased* in chronic iron deficiency and severe protein depletion.

Resources

BOOKS

Pagana, Kathleen Deska. *Mosby's Manual of Diagnostic and Laboratory Tests.* St. Louis: Mosby, Inc., 1998.

Rebecca J. Frey, PhD

Irregular bite *see* **Malocclusion**

Irritable bowel syndrome

Definition

Irritable bowel syndrome (IBS) is a common intestinal condition characterized by abdominal **pain** and cramps; changes in bowel movements (**diarrhea**, **constipation**, or both); gassiness; bloating; **nausea**; and other symptoms. There is no cure for IBS. Much about the condition remains unknown or poorly understood; however, dietary changes, drugs, and psychological treatment are often able to eliminate or substantially reduce its symptoms.

Description

IBS is the name people use today for a condition that was once called–among other things–colitis, mucous colitis, spastic colon, nervous colon, spastic bowel, and functional bowel disorder. Some of these names reflected the now outdated belief that IBS is a purely psychological disorder, a product of the patient's imagination. Although modern medicine

GALE ENCYCLOPEDIA OF MEDICINE

recognizes that **stress** can trigger IBS attacks, medical specialists agree that IBS is a genuine physical disorder–or group of disorders–with specific identifiable characteristics.

No one knows for sure how many Americans suffer from IBS. Surveys indicate a range of 10–20%, with perhaps as many as 30% of Americans experiencing IBS at some point in their lives. IBS normally makes its first appearance during young adulthood, and in half of all cases symptoms begin before age 35. Women with IBS outnumber men by two to one, for reasons that are not yet understood. IBS is responsible for more time lost from work and school than any medical problem other than the **common cold**. It accounts for a substantial proportion of the patients seen by specialists in diseases of the digestive system (gastroenterologists). Yet only half–possibly as few as 15%–of IBS sufferers ever consult a doctor.

Causes and symptoms

Symptoms

The symptoms of IBS tend to rise and fall in intensity rather than growing steadily worse over time. They always include abdominal pain, which may be relieved by defecation; diarrhea or constipation; or diarrhea alternating with constipation. Other symptoms–which vary from person to person–include cramps; gassiness; bloating; nausea; a powerful and uncontrollable urge to defecate (urgency); passage of a sticky fluid (mucus) during bowel movements; or the feeling after finishing a bowel movement that the bowels are still not completely empty. The accepted diagnostic criteria–known as the Rome criteria–require at least three months of continuous or recurrent symptoms before IBS can be confirmed. According to Christine B. Dalton and Douglas A. Drossman in the *American Family Physician,* an estimated 70% of IBS cases can be described as "mild;" 25% as "moderate;" and 5% as "severe." In mild cases the symptoms are slight. As a general rule, they are not present all the time and do not interfere with work and other normal activities. Moderate IBS occasionally disrupts normal activities and may cause some psychological problems. People with severe IBS often find living a normal life impossible and experience crippling psychological problems as a result. For some the physical pain is constant and intense.

Causes

Researchers remain unsure about the cause or causes of IBS. It is called a functional disorder because it is thought to result from changes in the activity of the major part of the large intestine (the colon). After food is digested by the stomach and small intestine, the undigested material passes in liquid form into the colon, which absorbs water and salts. This process may take several days. In a healthy person the colon is quiet during most of that period except after meals, when its muscles contract in a series of wavelike movements called peristalsis. Peristalsis helps absorption by bringing the undigested material into contact with the colon wall. It also pushes undigested material that has been converted into solid or semisolid feces toward the rectum, where it remains until defecation. In IBS, however, the normal rhythm and intensity of peristalsis is disrupted. Sometimes there is too little peristalsis, which can slow the passage of undigested material through the colon and cause constipation. Sometimes there is too much, which has the opposite effect and causes diarrhea. A Johns Hopkins University study found that healthy volunteers experienced 6–8 contractions of the colon each day, compared with up to 25 contractions a day for volunteers suffering from IBS with diarrhea, and an almost complete absence of contractions among constipated IBS volunteers. In addition to differences in the number of contractions, many of the IBS volunteers experienced powerful spasmodic contractions affecting a larger-than-normal area of the colon–"like having a Charlie horse in the gut," according to one of the investigators.

DIET. Some kinds of food and drink appear to play a key role in triggering IBS attacks. Food and drink that healthy people can ingest without any trouble may disrupt peristalsis in IBS patients, which probably explains why IBS attacks often occur shortly after meals. Chocolate, milk products, **caffeine** (in coffee, tea, colas, and other drinks), and large quantities of alcohol are some of the chief culprits. Other kinds of food have also been identified as problems, however, and the pattern of what can and cannot be tolerated is different for each person. Characteristically, IBS symptoms rarely occur at night and disrupt the patient's sleep.

STRESS. Stress is an important factor in IBS because of the close nervous system connections between the brain and the intestines. Although researchers do not yet understand all of the links between changes in the nervous system and IBS, they point out the similarities between mild digestive upsets and IBS. Just as healthy people can feel nauseated or have an upset stomach when under stress, people with IBS react the same way, but to a greater degree. Finally, IBS symptoms sometimes intensify during menstruation, which suggests that female reproductive hormones are another trigger.

Diagnosis

Diagnosing IBS is a fairly complex task because the disorder does not produce changes that can be identified during a **physical examination** or by laboratory tests. When IBS is suspected, the doctor (who can be either a family doctor or a specialist) needs to determine whether the patient's symptoms satisfy the Rome criteria. The doctor must rule out other conditions that resemble IBS, such as **Crohn's disease** and **ulcerative colitis**. These disorders are ruled out by questioning the patient about his or her physical and mental health (the medical history), performing a physical examination, and ordering laboratory tests. Normally the patient is asked to provide a stool sample that can be tested for blood and intestinal parasites. In some cases x rays or an internal examination of the colon using a flexible instrument inserted through the anus (a sigmoidoscope or colonoscope) is necessary. The doctor also may ask the patient to try a lactose-free diet for two or three weeks to see whether **lactose intolerance** is causing the symptoms.

Treatment

Dietary changes, sometimes supplemented by drugs or psychotherapy, are considered the key to successful treatment. The following approach, offered by Dalton and Drossman, is typical of the advice found in the medical literature on IBS. The authors tie their approach to the severity of the patient's symptoms:

Mild symptoms

Dalton and Drossman recommend a low-fat, high-fiber diet. Problem-causing substances such as lactose, caffeine, beans, cabbage, cucumbers, broccoli, fatty foods, alcohol, and medications should be identified and avoided. Bran or 15-25 grams a day of an over-the-counter psyllium laxative (Metamucil or Fiberall) may also help both constipation and diarrhea. The patient can still have milk or milk products if lactose intolerance is not a problem. People with irregular bowel habits–particularly constipated patients–may be helped by establishing set times for meals and bathroom visits.

Moderate symptoms

The advice given by Dalton and Drossman in mild cases applies here as well. They also suggest that

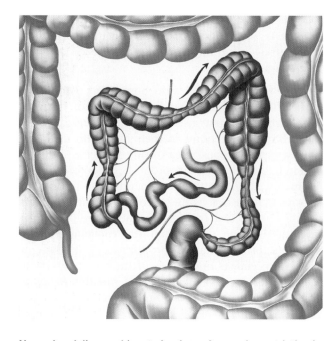

Normal and diseased (center) colons. Areas of constriction in the colon cause constipation, while areas of distention cause diarrhea. *(John Bavosi/Science Photo Library. Custom Medical Stock Photo. Reproduced by permission.)*

patients keep a diary of symptoms for two or three weeks, covering daily activities including meals, and emotional responses to events. The doctor can then review the diary with the patient to identify possible problem areas.

Although a high-fiber diet remains the standard treatment for constipated patients, such **laxatives** as lactulose (Chronulac) or sorbitol may be prescribed. Loperamide (Imodium) and cholestyramine (Questran) are suggested for diarrhea. Abdominal pain after meals can be reduced by taking **antispasmodic drugs** such as hyoscyamine (Anaspaz, Cystospaz, or Levsin) or dicyclomine (Bemote, Bentyl, or Di-Spaz) before eating.

Dalton and Drossman also suggest psychological counseling or behavioral therapy for some patients to reduce **anxiety** and to learn to cope with the pain and other symptoms of IBS. Relaxation therapy, hypnosis, **biofeedback**, and **cognitive-behavioral therapy** are examples of behavioral therapy.

Severe symptoms

When IBS produces constant pain that interferes with everyday life, **antidepressant drugs** can help by blocking pain transmission from the nervous system. Dalton and Drossman also underscore the importance

KEY TERMS

Anus—The opening at the lower end of the rectum.

Crohn's disease—A disease characterized by inflammation of the intestines. Its early symptoms may resemble those of IBS.

Defecation—Passage of feces through the anus.

Feces—Undigested food and other waste that is eliminated through the anus. Feces are also called fecal matter or stools.

Lactose—A sugar found in milk and milk products. Some people are lactose intolerant, meaning they have trouble digesting lactose. Lactose intolerance can produce symptoms resembling those of IBS.

Peristalsis—The periodic waves of muscular contractions that move food through the intestines during the process of digestion.

Ulcerative colitis—A disease that inflames and causes breaks (ulcers) in the colon and rectum, which are parts of the large intestine.

of an ongoing and supportive doctor-patient relationship.

Alternative treatment

Alternative and mainstream approaches to IBS treatment overlap to a certain extent. Like mainstream doctors, alternative practitioners advise a high-fiber diet to reduce digestive system irritation. They also suggest avoiding alcohol, caffeine, and fatty, gassy, or spicy foods. Recommended stress management techniques include **yoga**, **meditation**, hypnosis, biofeedback, and **reflexology**. Reflexology is a technique of foot massage that is thought to relieve diarrhea, constipation, and other IBS symptoms.

Alternative medicine also emphasizes such herbal remedies as ginger (*Zingiber officinale*), buckthorn (*Rhamnus purshiana*), and enteric-coated peppermint oil. Enteric coating prevents digestion until the peppermint oil reaches the small intestine, thus avoiding irritation of the upper part of the digestive tract. Chamomile (*Matricaria recutita*), valerian (*Valeriana officinalis*), rosemary (*Rosemarinus officinalis*), lemon balm (*Melissa officinalis*), and other herbs are recommended for their antispasmodic properties. The list of alternative treatments for IBS is in fact quite long. It includes **aromatherapy**, homeopathy, **hydrotherapy**,

juice therapy, **acupuncture**, **chiropractic**, **osteopathy**, **naturopathic medicine**, and Chinese traditional herbal medicine.

Prognosis

IBS is not a life-threatening condition. It does not cause intestinal bleeding or inflammation, nor does it cause other bowel diseases or **cancer**. Although IBS can last a lifetime, in up to 30% of cases the symptoms eventually disappear. Even if the symptoms cannot be eliminated, with appropriate treatment they can usually be brought under control to the point where IBS becomes merely an occasional inconvenience. Treatment requires a long-term commitment, however; six months or more may be needed before the patient notices substantial improvement.

Resources

ORGANIZATIONS

International Foundation for Functional Gastrointestinal Disorders. P.O. Box 17864, Milwaukee, WI 53217. (888) 964-2001. < http://www.iffgd.org >.

National Digestive Diseases Information Clearinghouse. 2 Information Way, Bethesda, MD 20892-3570. (800) 891-5389. < http://www.niddk.nih.gov/health/digest/nddic.htm >.

Howard Baker

Ischemia

Definition

Ischemia is an insufficient supply of blood to an organ, usually due to a blocked artery.

Description

Myocardial ischemia is an intermediate condition in **coronary artery disease** during which the heart tissue is slowly or suddenly starved of oxygen and other nutrients. Eventually, the affected heart tissue will die. When blood flow is completely blocked to the heart, ischemia can lead to a **heart attack**. Ischemia can be silent or symptomatic. According to the American Heart Association, up to four million Americans may have silent ischemia and be at high risk of having a heart attack with no warning.

Symptomatic ischemia is characterized by chest **pain** called **angina** pectoris. The American Heart Association estimates that nearly seven million Americans have angina pectoris, usually called angina. Angina occurs more frequently in women than in men, and in blacks and Hispanics more than in whites. It also occurs more frequently as people age–25% of women over the age of 85 and 27% of men who are 80–84 years old have angina.

People with angina are at risk of having a heart attack. Stable angina occurs during exertion, can be quickly relieved by resting or taking nitroglycerine, and lasts from three to twenty minutes. Unstable angina, which increases the risk of a heart attack, occurs more frequently, lasts longer, is more severe, and may cause discomfort during rest or light exertion.

Ischemia can also occur in the arteries of the brain, where blockages can lead to a **stroke**. About 80–85% of all strokes are ischemic. Most blockages in the cerebral arteries are due to a blood clot, often in an artery narrowed by plaque. Sometimes, a blood clot in the heart or aorta travels to a cerebral artery. A **transient ischemic attack** (TIA) is a "mini-stroke" caused by a temporary deficiency of blood supply to the brain. It occurs suddenly, lasts a few minutes to a few hours, and is a strong warning sign of an impending stroke. Ischemia can also effect intestines, legs, feet and kidneys. Pain, malfunctions, and damage in those areas may result.

Causes and symptoms

Ischemia is almost always caused by blockage of an artery, usually due to atherosclerotic plaque. Myocardial ischemia is also caused by **blood clots** (which tend to form on plaque), artery spasms or contractions, or any of these factors combined. Silent ischemia is usually caused by emotional or mental **stress** or by exertion, but there are no symptoms. Angina is usually caused by increased oxygen demand when the heart is working harder than usual, for example, during **exercise**, or during mental or physical stress. According to researchers at Harvard University, physical stress is harder on the heart than mental stress. A TIA is caused by a blood clot briefly blocking a cerebral artery.

Risk factors

The risk factors for myocardial ischemia are the same as those for coronary artery disease. For TIA, coronary artery disease is also a risk factor.

- Heredity. People whose parents have coronary artery disease are more likely to develop it. African Americans are also at higher risk.

- Sex. Men are more likely to have heart attacks than women, and to have them at a younger age.

- Age. Men who are 45 years of age and older and women who are 55 years of age and older are considered to be at risk.

- **Smoking**. Smoking increases both the chance of developing coronary artery disease and the chance of dying from it. Second hand smoke may also increase risk.

- **High cholesterol**. Risk of developing coronary artery disease increases as blood cholesterol levels increase. When combined with other factors, the risk is even greater.

- High blood pressure. High blood pressure makes the heart work harder, and with time, weakens it. When combined with **obesity**, smoking, high cholesterol, or diabetes, the risk of heart attack or stroke increases several times.

- Lack of physical activity. Lack of exercise increases the risk of coronary artery disease.

- Diabetes mellitus. The risk of developing coronary artery disease is seriously increased for diabetics.

- Obesity. Excess weight increases the strain on the heart and increases the risk of developing coronary artery disease, even if no other risk factors are present. Obesity increases blood pressure and blood cholesterol, and can lead to diabetes.

- Stress and anger. Some scientists believe that stress and anger can contribute to the development of coronary artery disease. Stress increases the heart rate and blood pressure and can injure the lining of the arteries. Angina attacks often occur after anger, as do many heart attacks and strokes.

Angina symptoms include:

- A tight, squeezing, heavy, burning, or **choking** pain that is usually beneath the breastbone—the pain may spread to the throat, jaw, or one arm

- A feeling of heaviness or tightness that is not painful

- A feeling similar to gas or indigestion

- Attacks brought on by exertion and relieved by rest.

If the pain or discomfort continues or intensifies, immediate medical help should be sought, ideally within 30 minutes.

TIA symptoms include:

- Sudden weakness, **tingling**, or **numbness**, usually in one arm or leg or both the arm and leg on the same side of the body, as well as sometimes in the face

- Sudden loss of coordination

- Loss of vision or double vision

- Difficulty speaking

- Vertigo and loss of balance.

Diagnosis

Diagnostic tests for myocardial ischemia include: resting, exercise, or ambulatory electrocardiograms; scintigraphic studies (radioactive heart scans); **echocardiography**; coronary **angiography**; and, rarely, **positron emission tomography**. Diagnostic tests for TIA include physician review of symptoms, **computed tomography scans** (CT scans), carotid artery ultrasound (**Doppler ultrasonography**), and **magnetic resonance imaging**. Angiography is the best test for ischemia of any organ.

An electrocardiogram (ECG) shows the heart's activity and may reveal a lack of oxygen. Electrodes covered with conducting jelly are placed on the patient's chest, arms, and legs. Impulses of the heart's activity are recorded on paper. The test takes about 10 minutes and is performed in a physician's office. About 25% of patients with angina have normal electrocardiograms. Another type of electrocardiogram, the exercise **stress test**, measures response to exertion when the patient is exercising on a treadmill or a stationary bike. It is performed in a physician's office or an exercise laboratory and takes 15 to 30 minutes. This test is more accurate than a resting ECG in diagnosing ischemia. Sometimes an ambulatory ECG is ordered. For this test, the patient wears a portable ECG machine called a Holter monitor for 12, 24, or 48 hours.

Myocardial perfusion scintigraphy and radionuclide angiography are nuclear studies involving the injection of a radioactive material (e.g., thallium) which is absorbed by healthy tissue. A gamma scintillation camera displays and records a series of images of the radioactive material's movement through the heart. Both tests are usually performed in a hospital's nuclear medicine department and take about 30 minutes to an hour. A perfusion scan is sometimes performed at the end of a stress test.

An echocardiogram uses sound waves to create an image of the heart's chambers and valves. The technician applies gel to a handheld transducer then presses it against the patient's chest. The heart's sound waves are converted into an image on a monitor. Performed in a cardiology outpatient diagnostic laboratory, the test takes 30 minutes to an hour. It can reveal abnormalities in the heart wall that indicate ischemia, but it doesn't evaluate the coronary arteries directly.

Coronary angiography is the most accurate diagnostic technique, but it is also the most invasive. It shows the heart's chambers, great vessels, and coronary arteries by using a contrast solution and x-ray technology. A moving picture is recorded of the blood flow through the coronary arteries. The patient is awake, but sedated, and connected to ECG electrodes and an intravenous line. A local anesthetic is injected. The cardiologist then inserts a catheter into a blood vessel and guides it into the heart. Coronary angiography is performed in a **cardiac catheterization** laboratory and takes from half an hour to two hours.

Positron emission tomography (PET) is a noninvasive nuclear test used to evaluate the heart tissue. A **PET** scanner traces high-energy gamma rays released from radioactive particles to provide three-dimensional images of the heart tissue. Performed at a hospital, it usually takes from one hour to one hour and 45 minutes. PET is very expensive and not widely available.

Computed tomography scans (CT scans) and magnetic resonance imaging (MRI) are computerized scanning methods. CT scanning uses a thin x-ray beam to show three-dimensional views of soft tissues. It is performed at a hospital or clinic and takes less than a minute. MRI uses a magnetic field to produce clear, cross-sectional images of soft tissues. The patient lies on a table which slides into a tunnel-like scanner. It is usually performed at a hospital and takes about 30 minutes.

Treatment

Angina is treated with drug therapy and surgery. Drugs such as nitrates, beta-blockers, and **calcium channel blockers** relieve chest pain, but they cannot clear blocked arteries. **Aspirin** helps prevent blood clots. Surgical procedures include percutaneous transluminal coronary **angioplasty** and **coronary artery bypass graft surgery**.

Nitroglycerin is the classic treatment for angina. It quickly relieves pain and discomfort by opening the coronary arteries and allowing more blood to flow to the heart. **Beta blockers** reduce the amount of oxygen required by the heart during stress. Calcium channel blockers help keep the arteries open and reduce blood

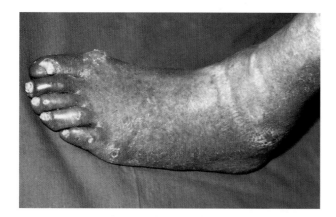

This patient's foot is affected with ischemia. Ischemia occurs when there is an insufficient supply of blood to a specific organ or tissue. *(Photograph by Dr. P. Marazzi, Photo Researchers, Inc. Reproduced by permission.)*

pressure. Aspirin helps prevent blood clots from forming on plaques.

Percutaneous transluminal coronary angioplasty and coronary artery bypass graft surgery are invasive procedures which improve blood flow in the coronary arteries. Percutaneous transluminal coronary angioplasty is a non-surgical procedure in which a catheter tipped with a balloon is threaded from a blood vessel in the thigh into the blocked artery. The balloon is inflated, compressing the plaque to enlarge the blood vessel and open the blocked artery. The balloon is deflated and the catheter is removed. The procedure is performed by a cardiologist in a hospital and generally requires a two-day stay. Sometimes a metal stent is placed in the artery to prevent closing of the artery.

In coronary artery bypass graft, called bypass surgery, a detour is built around the coronary artery blockage with a healthy leg vein or chest wall artery. The healthy vein or artery then supplies oxygen-rich blood to the heart. Bypass surgery is major surgery appropriate for patients with blockages in two or three major coronary arteries or severely narrowed left main coronary arteries, as well as those who have not responded to other treatments. It is performed in a hospital under **general anesthesia** using a heart-lung machine to support the patient while the healthy vein or artery is attached to the coronary artery.

There are several experimental surgical procedures: **atherectomy**, where the surgeon shaves off and removes strips of plaque from the blocked artery; laser angioplasty, where a catheter with a laser tip is inserted to burn or break down the plaque; and insertion of a metal coil, called a stent, that can be implanted permanently to keep a blocked artery

open. This stenting procedure is becoming more common. Another experimental procedure uses a laser to drill channels in the heart muscle to increase blood supply.

TIAs are treated by drugs that control high blood pressure and reduce the likelihood of blood clots and surgery. Aspirin is commonly used and anticoagulants are sometimes used to prevent blood clots. In some cases, carotid **endarterectomy** surgery is performed to help prevent further TIAs. The procedure involves removing arterial plaque from inside blood vessels.

The use of **chelation therapy**, a long-term injection by a physician of a cocktail of synthetic amino acid, ethylenediaminetetracetric acid, and **anticoagulant drugs** and nutrients, is controversial.

Alternative treatment

Ischemia can be life-threatening. Although there are alternative treatments for angina, traditional medical care may be necessary. Prevention of the cause of ischemia, primarily **atherosclerosis**, is primary. This becomes even more important for people with a family history of heart disease. Dietary modifications, especially the reduction or elimination of saturated fats (primarily found in meat), are essential. Increased fiber (found in fresh fruits and vegetables, grains, and beans) can help the body eliminate excessive cholesterol through the stools. Exercise, particularly aerobic exercise, is essential for circulation health. Not smoking will prevent damage from smoke and the harmful substances it contains.

Abana, a mixture of herbs and **minerals** used in **Ayurvedic medicine**, can reduce the frequency and severity of angina attacks. Western herbal medicine recommends hawthorn (*Crataegus laevigata* or *C. oxyacantha*) to relieve long-term angina, since it strengthens the contractility of the heart muscles. **Nutritional supplements** and botanical medicines that act as antioxidants, for example, **vitamins** C and E, selenium, gingko (*Gingko biloba*), bilberry (*Vaccinium myrtillus*), and hawthorn, can help prevent initial arterial injury that can lead to the formation of plaque deposits. Cactus (*Cactus grandiflorus*) is a homeopathic remedy used for pain relief during an attack. Mind/body relaxation techniques such as **yoga** and **biofeedback** can help control strong emotions and stress.

Prognosis

In many cases, ischemia can be successfully treated, but the underlying disease process of atherosclerosis is usually not "cured." New diagnostic techniques enable doctors to identify ischemia earlier. New technologies and surgical procedures can prevent angina from leading to a heart attack or TIA from resulting in a stroke. The outcome for patients with silent ischemia has not been well established.

Prevention

A healthy lifestyle, including eating right, getting regular exercise, maintaining a healthy weight, not smoking, drinking in moderation, not using illegal drugs, controlling **hypertension**, and managing stress are practices that can reduce the risk of ischemia progressing to a heart attack or stroke.

A healthy diet includes a variety of foods that are low in fat, especially saturated fat; low in cholesterol; and high in fiber. Plenty of fruits and vegetables should be eaten and sodium should be limited. Fat should comprise no more than 30% of total daily calories. Cholesterol should be limited to about 300 mg and sodium to about 2,400 mg per day.

Moderate aerobic exercise lasting about 30 minutes four or more times per week is recommended for maximum heart health, according to the Centers for Disease Control and Prevention and the American College of Sports Medicine. Three 10-minute exercise periods are also beneficial. If any risk factors are present, a physician's clearance should be obtained before starting exercise.

Maintaining a desirable body weight is also important. People who are 20% or more over their ideal body weight have an increased risk of developing coronary artery disease or stroke.

Smoking has many adverse effects on the heart and arteries, so should be avoided. Heart damage caused by smoking can be improved by quitting. Several studies have shown that ex-smokers face the same risk of heart disease as non-smokers within five to ten years of quitting.

Excessive drinking can increase risk factors for heart disease. Modest consumption of alcohol, however, can actually protect against coronary artery disease. The American Heart Association defines moderate consumption as one ounce of alcohol per day–roughly one cocktail, one 8-ounce glass of wine, or two 12-ounce glasses of beer.

Commonly used illegal drugs can seriously harm the heart and should never be used. Even stimulants like ephedra and **decongestants** like pseudoephedrine can be harmful to patients with hypertension or heart disease.

KEY TERMS

Atherosclerosis—A process in which the walls of the arteries thicken due to the accumulation of plaque in the blood vessels. Atherosclerosis is the cause of most coronary artery disease.

Coronary artery disease—A narrowing or blockage, due to atherosclerosis, of the arteries that provide oxygen and nutrients to the heart. When blood flow is cut-off, the result is a heart attack.

Plaque—A deposit of fatty and other substances that accumulate in the lining of the artery wall.

Stroke—A sudden decrease or loss of consciousness caused by rupture or blockage of a blood vessel by a blood clot or hemorrhage in the brain. Ischemic strokes are caused by blood clots in a cerebral artery.

Treatment should be sought for hypertension. High blood pressure can be completely controlled through lifestyle changes and medication. Stress, which can increase the risk of a heart attack or stroke, should also be managed. While it cannot always be avoided, it can be controlled.

Resources

ORGANIZATIONS

American Heart Association. 7320 Greenville Ave. Dallas, TX 75231. (214) 373-6300. < http:// www.americanheart.org >.

National Heart, Lung and Blood Institute. P.O. Box 30105, Bethesda, MD 20824-0105. (301) 251-1222. < http:// www.nhlbi.nih.gov >.

Texas Heart Institute. Heart Information Service. P.O. Box 20345, Houston, TX 77225-0345. < http:// www.tmc.edu/thi >.

Lori De Milto

Isocarboxazid *see* **Monoamine oxidase inhibitors**

Isolation

Definition

Isolation refers to the precautions that are taken in the hospital to prevent the spread of an infectious agent from an infected or colonized patient to susceptible persons.

Purpose

Isolation practices are designed to minimize the transmission of infection in the hospital, using current understanding of the way infections can transmit. Isolation should be done in a user friendly, well-accepted, inexpensive way that interferes as little as possible with patient care, minimizes patient discomfort, and avoids unnecessary use.

Precautions

The type of precautions used should be viewed as a flexible scale that may range from the least to the most demanding methods of prevention. These methods should always take into account that differences exist in the way that diseases are spread. Recognition and understanding of these differences will avoid use of insufficient or unnecessary interventions.

Description

Isolation practices can include placement in a private room or with a select roommate, the use of protective barriers such as masks, gowns and gloves, a special emphasis on handwashing (which is always very important), and special handling of contaminated articles. Because of the differences among infectious diseases, more than one of these precautions may be necessary to prevent spread of some diseases but may not be necessary for others.

The Centers for Disease Control and Prevention (CDC) and the Hospital Infection Control Practice Advisory Committee (HICPAC) have led the way in defining the guidelines for hospital-based infection precautions. The most current system recommended for use in hospitals consists of two levels of precautions. The first level is Standard Precautions which apply to all patients at all times because signs and symptoms of infection are not always obvious and therefore may unknowingly pose a risk for a susceptible person. The second level is known as Transmission-Based Precautions which are intended for individuals who have a known or suspected infection with certain organisms.

Frequently, patients are admitted to the hospital without a definite diagnosis, but with clues to suggest an infection. These patients should be isolated with the appropriate precautions until a definite diagnosis is made.

Standard Precautions

Standard Precautions define all the steps that should be taken to prevent spread of infection from person to person when there is an anticipated contact with:

- Blood
- Body fluids
- Secretions, such as phlegm
- Excretions, such as urine and feces (not including sweat) whether or not they contain visible blood
- Nonintact skin, such as an open wound
- Mucous membranes, such as the mouth cavity.

Standard Precautions includes the use of one or combinations of the following practices. The level of use will always depend on the anticipated contact with the patient:

- Handwashing, the most important **infection control** method
- Use of latex or other protective gloves
- Masks, eye protection and/or face shield
- Gowns
- Proper handling of soiled patient care equipment
- Proper environmental cleaning
- Minimal handling of soiled linen
- Proper disposal of needles and other sharp equipment such as scalpels
- Placement in a private room for patients who cannot maintain appropriate cleanliness or contain body fluids.

Transmission Based Precautions

Transmission Based Precautions may be needed in addition to Standard Precautions for selected patients who are known or suspected to harbor certain infections. These precautions are divided into three categories that reflect the differences in the way infections are transmitted. Some diseases may require more than one isolation category.

AIRBORNE PRECAUTIONS. Airborne Precautions prevent diseases that are transmitted by minute particles called droplet nuclei or contaminated dust particles. These particles, because of their size, can remain suspended in the air for long periods of time; even after the infected person has left the room. Some examples of diseases requiring these precautions are **tuberculosis**, **measles**, and **chickenpox**.

KEY TERMS

Colonized—This occurs when a microorganism is found on or in a person without causing a disease.

Disinfected—Decreased the number of microorganisms on or in an object.

Latex—A rubber material which gloves and condoms are made from.

Phlegm—Another word for sputum; material coughed up from a person's airways.

Stethoscope—A medical instrument for listening to a patient's heart and lungs.

A patient needing Airborne Precautions should be assigned to a private room with special ventilation requirements. The door to this room must be closed at all possible times. If a patient must move from the isolation room to another area of the hospital, the patient should be wearing a mask during the transport. Anyone entering the isolation room to provide care to the patient must wear a special mask called a respirator.

DROPLET PRECAUTIONS. Droplet Precautions prevent the spread of organisms that travel on particles much larger than the droplet nuclei. These particles do not spend much time suspended in the air, and usually do not travel beyond a several foot range from the patient. These particles are produced when a patient coughs, talks, or sneezes. Examples of disease requiring droplet precautions are meningococcal **meningitis** (a serious bacterial infection of the lining of the brain), **influenza**, **mumps**, and German measles (**rubella**).

Patients who require Droplet Precautions should be placed in a private room or with a roommate who is infected with the same organism. The door to the room may remain open. Health care workers will need to wear masks within 3 ft of the patient. Patients moving about the hospital away from the isolation room should wear a mask.

CONTACT PRECAUTIONS. Contact Precautions prevent spread of organisms from an infected patient through direct (touching the patient) or indirect (touching surfaces or objects that that been in contact with the patient) contact. Examples of patients who might be placed in Contact Precautions are those infected with:

- Antibiotic-resistant bacteria
- Hepatitis A
- Scabies
- Impetigo
- Lice.

This type of precaution requires the patient to be placed in a private room or with a roommate who has the same infection. Health care workers should wear gloves when entering the room. They should change their gloves if they touch material that contains large volumes of organisms such as soiled dressings. Prior to leaving the room, health care workers should remove the gloves and wash their hands with medicated soap. In addition, they may need to wear protective gowns if there is a chance of contact with potentially infective materials such as **diarrhea** or wound drainage that cannot be contained or if there is likely to be extensive contact with the patient or environment.

Patient care items, such as a stethoscope, that are used for a patient in Contact Precautions should not be shared with other patients unless they are properly cleaned and disinfected before reuse. Patients should leave the isolation room infrequently.

Resources

BOOKS

Edmond, M. "Isolation." In *A Practical Handbook for Hospital Epidemiologists*, edited by L. A. Herwaldt and M. D. Decker. Thorofare, NJ: Slack Inc., 1998.

Suzanne M. Lutwick, MPH

Isoniazid *see* **Antituberculosis drugs**

Isosorbide dinitrate *see* **Antiangina drugs**

Isotretinoin *see* **Antiacne drugs**

Isradipine *see* **Calcium channel blockers**

Itching

Definition

Itching is an intense, distracting irritation or tickling sensation that may be felt all over the skin's surface, or confined to just one area. The medical term for itching is pruritus.

Description

Itching instinctively leads most people to scratch the affected area. Different people can tolerate different amounts of itching, and anyone's threshold of tolerance can be changed due to **stress**, emotions, and other factors. In general, itching is more severe if the skin is warm, and if there are few distractions. This is why people tend to notice itching more at night.

Causes and symptoms

The biology underlying itching is not fully understood. It is believed that itching results from the interactions of several different chemical messengers. Although itching and **pain** sensations were at one time thought to be sent along the same nerve pathways, researchers reported the discovery in 2003 of itch-specific nerve pathways. Nerve endings that are specifically sensitive to itching have been named pruriceptors.

Research into itching has been helped by the recent invention of a mechanical device called the Matcher, which electrically stimulates the patient's left hand. When the intensity of the stimulation equals the intensity of itching that the patient is experiencing elsewhere in the body, the patient stops the stimulation and the device automatically records the measurement. The Matcher was found to be sensitive to immediate changes in the patient's perception of itching as well as reliable in its measurements.

Stress and emotional upset can make itching worse, no matter what the underlying cause. If emotional problems are the primary reason for the itch, the condition is known as psychogenic itching. Some people become convinced that their itch is caused by a parasite; this conviction is often linked to burning sensations in the tongue, and may be caused by a major psychiatric disorder.

Generalized itching

Itching that occurs all over the body may indicate a medical condition such as **diabetes mellitus**, **liver disease**, kidney failure, **jaundice**, thyroid disorders (and rarely, **cancer**). Blood disorders such as leukemia, and lymphatic conditions such as **Hodgkin's disease** may sometimes cause itching as well.

Some people may develop an itch without a rash when they take certain drugs (such as **aspirin**, codeine, **cocaine**); others may develop an itchy red "drug rash" or **hives** because of an allergy to a specific drug. Some medications given to cancer patients may also cause itching.

Itching also may be caused when any of the family of hookworm larvae penetrate the skin. This includes swimmer's itch and creeping eruption caused by cat or dog hookworm, and ground itch caused by the "true" hookworm.

Many skin conditions cause an itchy rash. These include:

- **Atopic dermatitis**
- Chickenpox
- **Contact dermatitis**
- **Dermatitis** herpetiformis (occasionally)
- Eczema
- Fungus infections (such as **athlete's foot**)
- Hives (urticaria)
- Insect bites
- Lice
- Lichen planus
- Neurodermatitis (**lichen simplex chronicus**)
- **Psoriasis** (occasionally)
- Scabies.

On the other hand, itching all over the body can be caused by something as simple as bathing too often, which removes the skin's natural oils and may make the skin too dry and scaly.

Localized itching

Specific itchy areas may occur if a person comes in contact with soap, detergents, and wool or other rough-textured, scratchy material. Adults who have **hemorrhoids**, anal fissure, or persistent **diarrhea** may notice itching around the anus (called "pruritus ani"). In children, itching in this area is most likely due to worms.

Intense itching in the external genitalia in women ("pruritus vulvae") may be due to **candidiasis**, hormonal changes, or the use of certain spermicides or vaginal suppositories, ointments, or deodorants.

It is also common for older people to suffer from dry, itchy skin (especially on the back) for no obvious reason. Younger people also may notice dry, itchy skin in cold weather. Itching is also a common complaint during **pregnancy**.

Diagnosis

Itching is a symptom that is quite obvious to its victim. Someone who itches all over should seek medical care. Because itching can be caused by such a wide variety of triggers, a complete physical exam and medical history will help diagnose the underlying problem. A variety of blood and stool tests may help determine the underlying cause.

Treatment

Antihistamines such as diphenhydramine (Benadryl) can help relieve itching caused by hives, but will not affect itching from other causes. Most antihistamines also make people sleepy, which can help patients sleep who would otherwise be awake from the itch.

Specific treatment of itching depends on the underlying condition that causes it. In general, itchy skin should be treated very gently. While scratching may temporarily ease the itch, in the long run scratching just makes it worse. In addition, scratching can lead to an endless cycle of itch–scratch–more itching.

To avoid the urge to scratch, a person can apply a cooling or soothing lotion or cold compress when the urge to scratch occurs. Soaps are often irritating to the skin, and can make an itch worse; they should be avoided, or used only when necessary.

Creams or ointments containing cortisone may help control the itch from insect bites, contact dermatitis or eczema. Cortisone cream should not be applied to the face unless a doctor prescribes it.

Probably the most common cause of itching is dry skin. There are a number of simple things a person can do to ease the annoying itch:

- Do not wear tight clothes
- Avoid synthetic fabrics
- Do not take long baths
- Wash the area in lukewarm water with a little baking soda
- For generalized itching, take a lukewarm shower
- Try a lukewarm oatmeal (or Aveeno) bath for generalized itching
- Apply bath oil or lotion (without added colors or scents) right after bathing.

Itching may also be treated with whole-body medications. In addition to antihistamines, some of these systemic treatments include:

- tricyclic antidepressants
- sedatives or tranquilizers
- such selective serotonin reputake inhibitors as paroxetine (Paxil) and sertraline (Zoloft)
- binding agents (such as cholestyramine which relieves itching associated with kidney or liver disease).
- aspirin
- cimetidine

People who itch as a result of mental problems or stress should seek help from a mental health expert.

Alternative and complementary therapies

A well-balanced diet that includes carbohydrates, fats, **minerals**, proteins, **vitamins**, and liquids will help to maintain skin health. Capsules that contain eicosapentaenoic acid, which is obtained from herring, mackerel, or salmon, may help to reduce itching. Vitamin A plays an important role in skin health. Vitamin E (capsules or ointment) may reduce itching. Patients should check with their treating physician before using supplements.

Homeopathy has been reported to be effective in treating systemic itching associated with hemodialysis.

Baths containing oil with milk or oatmeal are effective at relieving localized itching. Evening primrose oil may soothe itching and may be as effective as **corticosteroids**. Calendula cream may relieve short-term itching. Other herbal treatments that have been recently reported to relieve itching include sangre de drago, a preparation made with sap from a South American tree; and a mixture of honey, olive oil, and beeswax.

Distraction, **music therapy**, relaxation techniques, and visualization may be useful in relieving itching. Ultraviolet light therapy may relieve itching associated with conditions of the skin, kidneys, blood, and gallbladder. There are some reports of the use of **acupuncture** and transcutaneous electrical nerve stimulators (TENS) to relieve itching.

Prognosis

Most cases of itching go away when the underlying cause is treated successfully.

Prevention

There are certain things people can do to avoid itchy skin. Patients who tend toward itchy skin should:

- Avoid a daily bath
- Use only lukewarm water when bathing
- Use only gentle soap
- Pat dry, not rub dry, after bathing, leaving a bit of water on the skin
- Apply a moisture-holding ointment or cream after the bath
- Use a humidifier in the home.

Patients who are allergic to certain substances, medications, and so on can avoid the resulting itch if they

KEY TERMS

Atopic dermatitis—An intensely itchy inflammation often found on the face of people prone to allergies. In infants and early childhood, it is called infantile eczema.

Creeping eruption—Itchy irregular, wandering red lines on the foot made by burrowing larvae of the hookworm family and some roundworms.

Dermatitis herpetiformis—A chronic very itchy skin disease with groups of red lesions that leave spots behind when they heal. It is sometimes associated with cancer of an internal organ.

Eczema—A superficial type of inflammation of the skin that may be very itchy and weeping in the early stages; later, the affected skin becomes crusted, scaly, and thick. There is no known cause.

Hodgkin's disease—A type of cancer characterized by a slowly-enlarging lymph tissue; symptoms include generalized itching.

Lichen planus—A noncancerous, chronic itchy skin disease that causes small, flat purple plaques on wrists, forearm, ankles.

Neurodermatitis—An itchy skin disease (also called lichen simplex chronicus) found in nervous, anxious people.

Pruriceptors—Nerve endings specialized to perceive itching sensations.

Pruritus—The medical term for itching.

Psoriasis—A common, chronic skin disorder that causes red patches anywhere on the body. Occasionally, the lesions may itch.

Scabies—A contagious parasitic skin disease characterized by intense itching.

Swimmer's itch—An allergic skin inflammation caused by a sensitivity to flatworms that die under the skin, causing an itchy rash.

avoid contact with the allergen. Avoiding insect bites, bee stings, poison ivy and so on can prevent the resulting itch. Treating sensitive skin carefully, avoiding overdrying of the skin, and protecting against diseases that cause itchy **rashes** are all good ways to avoid itching.

Resources

BOOKS

Beers, Mark H., MD, and Robert Berkow, MD, editors. "Pruritus." Section 10, Chapter 109. In *The Merck Manual of Diagnosis and Therapy*. Whitehouse Station, NJ: Merck Research Laboratories, 2004.

PERIODICALS

Al-Waili, N. S. "Topical Application of Natural Honey, Beeswax and Olive Oil Mixture for Atopic Dermatitis or Psoriasis: Partially Controlled, Single-Blinded Study." *Complementary Therapies in Medicine* 11 (December 2003): 226–234.

Browning, J., B. Combes, and M. J. Mayo. "Long-Term Efficacy of Sertraline as a Treatment for Cholestatic Pruritus in Patients with Primary Biliary Cirrhosis." *American Journal of Gastroenterology* 98 (December 2003): 2736–2741.

Cavalcanti, A. M., L. M. Rocha, R. Carillo Jr., et al. "Effects of Homeopathic Treatment on Pruritus of Haemodialysis Patients: A Randomised Placebo-Controlled Double-Blind Trial." *Homeopathy* 92 (October 2003): 177–181.

Ikoma, A., R. Rukwied, S. Stander, et al. "Neurophysiology of Pruritus: Interaction of Itch and Pain." *Archives of Dermatology* 139 (November 2003): 1475–1478.

Jones, K. "Review of Sangre de Drago (*Croton lechleri*)—A South American Tree Sap in the Treatment of Diarrhea, Inflammation, Insect Bites, Viral Infections, and Wounds: Traditional Uses to Clinical Research." *Journal of Alternative and Complementary Medicine* 9 (December 2003): 877–896.

Ochoa, J. G. "Pruritus, a Rare but Troublesome Adverse Reaction of Topiramate." *Seizure* 12 (October 2003): 516–518.

Stener-Victorin, E., T. Lundeberg, J. Kowalski, et al. "Perceptual Matching for Assessment of Itch; Reliability and Responsiveness Analyzed by a Rank-Invariant Statistical Method." *Journal of Investigative Dermatology* 121 (December 2003): 1301–1305.

Zylicz, Z., M. Krajnik, A. A. Sorge, and M. Costantini. "Paroxetine in the Treatment of Severe Non-Dermatological Pruritus: A Randomized, Controlled Trial." *Journal of Pain and Symptom Management* 26 (December 2003): 1105–1112.

Carol A. Turkington
Rebecca J. Frey, PhD

IUD

Definition

An IUD is an intrauterine device made of plastic and/or copper that is inserted into the womb (uterus) by way of the vaginal canal. One type releases a hormone (progesterone), and is replaced each year. The second type is made of copper and can be left in place for five years. The most common shape in current use is a plastic "T" which is wrapped with copper wire.

Purpose

IUDs are used to prevent **pregnancy** and are considered to be 95-98% effective. It should be noted that IUDs offer no protection against the acquired immune deficiency syndrome (**AIDS**) virus or other **sexually transmitted diseases** (STDs).

Precautions

IUDs are placed in the uterus by physicians. Prior to placement the doctor will take a medical history, do a **physical examination**, and take a **Pap test**. Women who have had tubal pregnancies, an abnormal Pap smear, or abnormal vaginal bleeding are generally disqualified from using this form of **contraception**. Also, women who have STDs, an allergy to copper, severe **pain** with periods (menstruation), sex with multiple partners, or who are currently pregnant are not eligible for an IUD. There are no age restrictions.

Description

There is continuing controversy over exactly how IUDs prevent pregnancy. Some researchers think pregnancy is controlled by preventing conception (fertilization), while others believe that the devices prevent embryo attachment to the uterine wall (implantation).

IUDs which release a hormone may prevent pregnancy in several ways. Since one hormonal response is a thickening of the mucous at the entrance to the uterus, it is more difficult for the sperm to gain entry. This prevents the sperm from reaching an ovum. At the same time, the lining of the uterus becomes thinner, making it more difficult for a fertilized egg to implant itself in the uterus. The copper device slowly releases copper which is believed to weaken and perhaps kill sperm. An alternate explanation is that these objects "sweep" the uterus, dislodging any fertilized egg that attempts to implant itself. In addition, both devices tend to cause a mild inflammatory reaction in the lining of the uterus which also has an adverse impact on implantation.

Preparation

After the physician approves the use of an IUD, the woman's genital area is washed thoroughly with soap and water in preparation of IUD insertion. The opening into the uterus (cervix) will also be cleaned with an antiseptic such as an iodine solution. Actual IUD insertion takes about five minutes, during which

---

KEY TERMS

Antiseptic—An antiseptic is a chemical that prevents the growth of germs.

Hormone—Hormones are chemicals that are produced in an organ or gland and then are carried by the blood to another part of the body where they produce a special effect for which they were designed.

Pap test—This is a procedure by which cells are collected from the cervix and vagina by inserting a swab into the vaginal canal. These cells are then examined under a microscope in order to detect signs of early cancer.

---

a **local anesthesia** is used to reduce any discomfort associated with the procedure. A plastic string connected to the IUD will hang out of the uterus into the vagina. The string is used to periodically check the position of the IUD.

Aftercare

The woman will be taught to watch for the signs and symptoms of potential complications and how to check the string, which should be done at least once a week. To check the string, the woman should first wash her hands with soap and water. From a squatting position, or with one foot elevated (such as on a chair), she should gently insert her finger into the vagina until she nears the cervix. If she cannot feel the string, if the string feels longer than it should, or if she can feel part of the IUD, she should notify her physician immediately. Additional information that needs to be reported includes painful intercourse and unusual discharge from the vagina.

Risks

Serious risks are rare, but include heavy bleeding, pain, infection, cramps, **pelvic inflammatory disease**, perforation of the uterus, and **ectopic pregnancy**.

Resources

ORGANIZATIONS

Planned Parenthood Federation of America, Inc. 810 Seventh Ave., New York, NY,10019. (800) 669-0156. < http://www.plannedparenthood.org >.

Donald G. Barstow, RN

Ivory bones *see* **Osteopetroses**

Ivy method *see* **Bleeding time**

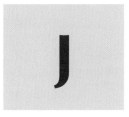

Japanese encephalitis

Definition

Japanese **encephalitis** is an infection of the brain caused by a virus. The virus is transmitted to humans by mosquitoes.

Description

The virus that causes Japanese encephalitis is called an arbovirus, which is an arthropod-borne virus. Mosquitoes are a type of arthropod. Mosquitoes in a number of regions carry this virus and are responsible for passing it along to humans. Many of these areas are in Asia, including Japan, Korea, China, India, Thailand, Indonesia, Malaysia, Vietnam, Taiwan, and the Philippines. Areas where the disease-causing arbovirus is always present are referred to as being endemic for the disease. In such areas, blood tests will reveal that more than 70% of all adults have been infected at some point with the arbovirus.

Because the virus that causes Japanese encephalitis is carried by mosquitoes, the number of people infected increases during those seasons when mosquitoes are abundant. This tends to be in the warmest, rainiest months. In addition to humans, other animals like wild birds, pigs, and horses are susceptible to infection with this arbovirus. Because the specific type of mosquito carrying the Japanese encephalitis arbovirus frequently breeds in rice paddies, the disease is considered to be primarily a rural problem.

Causes and symptoms

The virus is transferred to a human when an infected mosquito sucks that person's blood. Once in the body, the virus travels to various glands where it multiplies. The virus can then enter the bloodstream.

Ultimately, the virus settles in the brain, where it causes serious problems.

Japanese encephalitis begins with **fever**, severe **headache**, **nausea**, and **vomiting**. As the tissue covering the brain and spinal cord (the meninges) becomes infected and swollen, the patient will develop a stiff and painful neck. By day two or three, the patient begins to suffer the effects of swelling in the brain. These effects include:

- Problems with balance and coordination
- Paralysis of some muscle groups
- Tremors
- Seizures
- Lapses in consciousness
- A stiff, mask-like appearance of the face.

The patient becomes dehydrated and loses weight. If the patient survives the illness, the fever will decrease by about day seven and the symptoms will begin to improve by about day 14. Other patients will continue to have extremely high fevers and their symptoms will get worse. In these cases, **coma** and then **death** occur in 7-14 days. Many patients who recover have permanent disabilities due to brain damage.

Diagnosis

Most diagnostic techniques for Japanese encephalitis do not yield results very quickly. The diagnosis is made primarily on the basis of the patient's symptoms and the knowledge of the kinds of illnesses endemic to a particular geographic region.

Immunofluorescence tests, where special viral markers react with human antibodies that have been tagged with a fluorescent chemical, are used to verify the disease. However, these results tend to be unavailable until week two of the infection. Other tests involve comparing the presence and quantity of particular

KEY TERMS

Antibody—A type of cell made by the immune system that has the ability to recognize markers (antigens) on the surface of invading organisms, like bacteria and viruses.

Encephalitis—A swelling of the brain, potentially causing serious brain damage.

Endemic—Naturally and consistently present in a certain geographical region.

antibodies in the blood or spinal fluid during week one with those present during week two of the illness.

Treatment

There are no treatments available to stop or slow the progression of Japanese encephalitis. Only the symptoms of each patient can be treated. Fluids are given to decrease **dehydration** and medications are given to decrease fever and **pain**. Medications are available to attempt to decrease brain swelling. Patients in a coma may require mechanical assistance with breathing.

Prognosis

While the majority of people infected with arbovirus never become sick, those who develop Japanese encephalitis become very ill. Some outbreaks have a 50% death rate. A variety of long-term problems may haunt those who recover from the illness. These problems include:

- Movement difficulties where the arms, legs, or body jerks or writhes involuntarily
- Shaking
- Paralysis
- Inability to control emotions
- Loss of mental abilities
- Mental disturbances, including **schizophrenia** (which may affect as many as 75% of Japanese encephalitis survivors).

Young children are most likely to have serious, long-term problems after an infection.

Prevention

A three-dose vaccine is available for Japanese encephalitis and is commonly given to young children in areas where the disease is endemic. Travelers to these regions can also receive the vaccine.

Controlling the mosquito population with insecticides is another preventive measure. Visitors to regions with high rates of Japanese encephalitis should take precautions (like using mosquito repellents and sleeping under a bed net) to avoid contact with mosquitoes.

Resources

ORGANIZATIONS

Centers for Disease Control and Prevention. 1600 Clifton Rd., NE, Atlanta, GA 30333. (800) 311-3435, (404) 639-3311. < http://www.cdc.gov >.

Rosalyn Carson-DeWitt, MD

Jaundice

Definition

Jaundice is a condition in which a person's skin and the whites of the eyes are discolored yellow due to an increased level of bile pigments in the blood resulting from **liver disease**. Jaundice is sometimes called icterus, from a Greek word for the condition.

Description

In order to understand jaundice, it is useful to know about the role of the liver in producing bile. The most important function of the liver is the processing of chemical waste products like cholesterol and excreting them into the intestines as bile. The liver is the premier chemical factory in the body—most incoming and outgoing chemicals pass through it. It is the first stop for all nutrients, toxins, and drugs absorbed by the digestive tract. The liver also collects chemicals from the blood for processing. Many of these outward-bound chemicals are excreted into the bile. One particular substance, bilirubin, is yellow. Bilirubin is a product of the breakdown of hemoglobin, which is the protein inside red blood cells. If bilirubin cannot leave the body, it accumulates and discolors other tissues. The normal total level of bilirubin in blood serum is between 0.2 mg/dL and 1.2 mg/dL. When it rises to 3 mg/dL or higher, the person's skin and the whites of the eyes become noticeably yellow.

Bile is formed in the liver. It then passes into the network of hepatic bile ducts, which join to form a single tube. A branch of this tube carries bile to the gallbladder, where it is stored, concentrated, and released on a signal from the stomach. Food entering the stomach is the signal that stimulates the gallbladder to release the bile. The tube, which is called the common bile duct, continues to the intestines. Before the common bile duct reaches the intestines, it is joined by another duct from the pancreas. The bile and the pancreatic juice enter the intestine through a valve called the ampulla of Vater. After entering the intestine, the bile and pancreatic secretions together help in the process of digestion.

Causes and symptoms

There are many different causes for jaundice, but they can be divided into three categories based on where they start–before, in, or after the liver (prehepatic, hepatic and post-hepatic). When bilirubin begins its life cycle, it cannot be dissolved in water. The liver changes it so that it is soluble in water. These two types of bilirubin are called unconjugated (insoluble) and conjugated (soluble). Blood tests can easily distinguish between these two types of bilirubin.

Hemoglobin and bilirubin formation

Bilirubin begins as hemoglobin in the blood-forming organs, primarily the bone marrow. If the production of red blood cells (RBCs) falls below normal, the extra hemoglobin finds its way into the bilirubin cycle and adds to the pool.

Once hemoglobin is in the red cells of the blood, it circulates for the life span of those cells. The hemoglobin that is released when the cells die is turned into bilirubin. If for any reason the RBCs die at a faster rate than usual, bilirubin can accumulate in the blood and cause jaundice.

Hemolytic disorders

Many disorders speed up the death of red blood cells. The process of red blood cell destruction is called hemolysis, and the diseases that cause it are called hemolytic disorders. If red blood cells are destroyed faster than they can be produced, the patient develops anemia. Hemolysis can occur in a number of diseases, disorders, conditions, and medical procedures:

- **Malaria**. The malaria parasite develops inside red blood cells. When it is mature it breaks the cell apart and swims off in the blood. This process happens to most of the parasites simultaneously, causing the intermittent symptoms of the disease. When enough cells burst at once, jaundice may result from the large amount of bilirubin formed from the hemoglobin in the dead cells. The pigment may reach the urine in sufficient quantities to cause "blackwater fever," an often lethal form of malaria.

- Side effects of certain drugs. Some common drugs can cause hemolysis as a rare but sudden side effect. These medications include some antibiotic and antituberculosis medicines; drugs that regulate the heartbeat; and levodopa, a drug used to treat Parkinson's disease.

- Certain drugs in combination with a hereditary enzyme deficiency known as glucose-6-phosphate dehydrogenase (G6PD). G6PD is a deficiency that affects more than 200 million people in the world. Some of the drugs listed above are more likely to cause hemolysis in people with G6PD. Other drugs cause hemolysis only in people with this disorder. Most important among these drugs are anti-malarial medications such as quinine, and **vitamins** C and K.

- Poisons. Snake and spider venom, certain bacterial toxins, copper, and some organic industrial chemicals directly attack the membranes of red blood cells.

- Artificial heart valves. The inflexible moving parts of heart valves damage RBCs as they flutter back and forth. This damage is one reason to recommend pig valves and valves made of other organic materials.

- Hereditary RBC disorders. There are a number of hereditary defects that affect the blood cells. There are many genetic mutations that affect the hemoglobin itself, the best-known of which is **sickle cell disease**. Such hereditary disorders as spherocytosis weaken the outer membrane of the red cell. There are also inherited defects that involve the internal chemistry of RBCs.

- Enlargement of the spleen. The spleen is an organ that is located near the upper end of the stomach and filters the blood. It is supposed to filter out and destroy only worn-out RBCs. If it has become enlarged, it filters out normal cells as well. Malaria, other infections, cancers and leukemias, some of the hereditary **anemias** mentioned above, obstruction of blood flow from the spleen–all these and many more diseases can enlarge the spleen to the point where it removes too many red blood cells.

- Diseases of the small blood vessels. Hemolysis that occurs in diseased small blood vessels is called microangiopathic hemolysis. It results from damage caused by rough surfaces on the inside of the capillaries. The RBCs squeeze through capillaries one at a time and can easily be damaged by scraping against the vessel walls.

- Immune reactions to RBCs. Several types of **cancer** and immune system diseases produce antibodies that react with RBCs and destroy them. In 75% of cases, this reaction occurs all by itself, with no underlying disease to account for it.

- Transfusions. If a patient is given an incompatible blood type, hemolysis results.

- Kidney failure and other serious diseases. Several diseases are characterized by defective blood coagulation that can destroy red blood cells.

- **Erythroblastosis fetalis.** Erythroblastosis fetalis is a disease of newborns marked by the presence of too many immature red blood cells (erythroblasts) in the baby's blood. When a baby's mother has a different blood type, antibodies from the mother may leak into the baby's circulation and destroy blood cells. This reaction can produce severe hemolysis and jaundice in the newborn. Rh factor incompatibility is the most common cause.

- High bilirubin levels in newborns. Even in the absence of blood type incompatibility, the newborn's bilirubin level may reach threatening levels.

Normal jaundice in newborns

Normal newborn jaundice is the result of two conditions occurring at the same time–a pre-hepatic and a hepatic source of excess bilirubin. First of all, the baby at birth immediately begins converting hemoglobin from a fetal type to an adult type. The fetal type of hemoglobin was able to extract oxygen from the lower levels of oxygen in the mother's blood. At birth the infant can extract oxygen directly from his or her own lungs and does not need the fetal hemoglobin any more. So fetal hemoglobin is removed from the system and replaced with adult hemoglobin. The resulting bilirubin loads the system and places demands on the liver to clear it. But the liver is not quite ready for the task, so there is a period of a week or so when the liver has to catch up. During that time the baby is jaundiced.

Hepatic jaundice

Liver diseases of all kinds threaten the organ's ability to keep up with bilirubin processing. **Starvation**, circulating infections, certain medications, hepatitis, and **cirrhosis** can all cause hepatic jaundice, as can certain hereditary defects of liver chemistry, including Gilbert's syndrome and Crigler-Najjar syndrome.

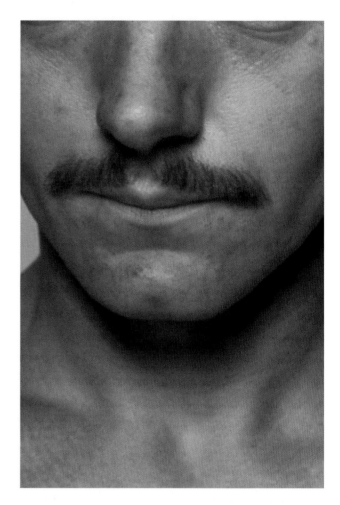

This patient suffers from obstructive jaundice, which is often caused by gallstones. *(Custom Medical Stock Photo. Reproduced by permission.)*

Post-hepatic jaundice

Post-hepatic forms of jaundice include the jaundices caused by failure of soluble bilirubin to reach the intestines after it has left the liver. These disorders are called obstructive jaundices. The most common cause of obstructive jaundice is the presence of **gallstones** in the ducts of the biliary system. Other causes have to do with **birth defects** and infections that damage the bile ducts; drugs; infections; cancers; and physical injury. Some drugs–and **pregnancy** on rare occasions–simply cause the bile in the ducts to stop flowing.

Symptoms and complications associated with jaundice

Certain chemicals in bile may cause **itching** when too much of them end up in the skin. In newborns, insoluble bilirubin may get into the brain and do permanent damage. Long-standing jaundice may upset the balance of chemicals in the bile and cause stones to form. Apart from these potential complications and the discoloration of skin and eyes, jaundice by itself is inoffensive. Other symptoms are determined by the disease producing the jaundice.

Diagnosis

Physical examination

In many cases the diagnosis of jaundice is suggested by the appearance of the patient's eyes and complexion. The doctor will ask the patient to lie flat on the examining table in order to feel (palpate) the liver and spleen for enlargement and to evaluate any abdominal **pain**. The location and severity of abdominal pain and the presence or absence of **fever** help the doctor to distinguish between hepatic and obstructive jaundice.

Laboratory tests

Disorders of blood formation can be diagnosed by more thorough examination of the blood or the bone marrow, where blood is made. Occasionally a **bone marrow biopsy** is required, but usually the blood itself will reveal the diagnosis. The spleen can be evaluated by an ultrasound examination or a nuclear scan if the **physical examination** has not yielded enough information.

Liver disease is usually assessed from blood studies alone, but again a biopsy may be necessary to clarify less obvious conditions. A **liver biopsy** is performed at the bedside. The doctor uses a thin needle to take a tiny core of tissue from the liver. The tissue sample is sent to the laboratory for examination under a microscope.

Assessment of jaundice in newborns

Newborns are more likely to have problems with jaundice if:

- They are premature.
- They are Asian or Native Americans.
- They have been bruised during the birth process.
- They have lost too much weight during the first few days.
- They are born at high altitude.
- The mother has diabetes.
- Labor had to be induced.

In 2003, research was continuing to find noninvasive methods to determine bilirubin levels in newborns

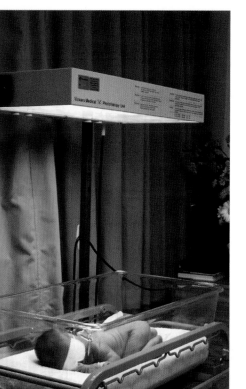

A newborn baby undergoes phototherapy with visible blue light to treat his jaundice. *(Photograph by Ron Sutherland, Photo Researchers, Inc. Reproduced by permission.)*

so that physicians did not have to rely on visual examination alone to determine which infants should receive blood tests. Once these measurements of skin pigment can be shown effective and cost-effective in clinical practice, they may become more available. Another study used this measurement method incorporated into home health visits to monitor babies within 24 hours of discharge from the hospital following birth.

Imaging studies

Disease in the biliary system can be identified by imaging techniques, of which there are many. X rays are taken a day after swallowing a contrast agent that is secreted into the bile. This study gives functional as well as anatomical information. There are several ways of injecting contrast dye directly into the bile ducts. It can be done through a thin needle pushed straight into the liver or through a scope passed through the stomach that can inject dye into the Ampulla of Vater. CT and MRI scans are very useful for imaging certain conditions like cancers in and around the liver or gallstones in the common bile duct.

Treatment

Jaundice in newborns

Newborns are the only major category of patients in whom the jaundice itself requires attention. Because the insoluble bilirubin can get into the brain, the amount in the blood must not go over certain levels. If there is reason to suspect increased hemolysis in the newborn, the bilirubin level must be measured repeatedly during the first few days of life. If the level of bilirubin shortly after birth threatens to go too high, treatment must begin immediately. Exchanging most of the baby's blood was the only way to reduce the amount of bilirubin until a few decades ago. Then it was discovered that bright blue light rendered the bilirubin harmless. Now jaundiced babies are fitted with eye protection and placed under bright fluorescent lights. The light chemically alters the bilirubin in the blood as it passes through the baby's skin. In 2003, researchers were testing a new drug called Stanate that showed promise in blocking bilirubin production. However, debate concerning the use of the drug for treatment of only those infants with jaundice or as a preventive measure was delaying its FDA approval and widespread use.

Hemolytic disorders

Hemolytic diseases are treated, if at all, with medications and blood transfusions, except in the case of a large spleen. Surgical removal of the spleen (**splenectomy**) can sometimes cure **hemolytic anemia**. Drugs that cause hemolysis or arrest the flow of bile must be stopped immediately.

Hepatic jaundice

Most liver diseases have no specific cure, but the liver is so robust that it can heal from severe damage and regenerate itself from a small remnant of its original tissue.

Post-hepatic jaundice

Obstructive jaundice frequently requires a surgical cure. If the original passageways cannot be restored, surgeons have several ways to create alternate routes. A popular technique is to sew an open piece of intestine over a bare patch of liver. Tiny bile ducts in that part of the liver will begin to discharge

KEY TERMS

Ampulla of Vater—The widened portion of the duct through which the bile and pancreatic juices enter the intestine. Ampulla is a Latin word for a bottle with a narrow neck that opens into a wide body.

Anemia—A condition in which the blood does not contain enough hemoglobin.

Biliary system/Bile ducts—The gall bladder and the system of tubes that carries bile from the liver into the intestines.

Bilirubin—A reddish pigment excreted by the liver into the bile as a breakdown product of hemoglobin.

Crigler-Najjar syndrome—A moderate to severe form of hereditary jaundice.

Erythroblastosis fetalis—A disorder of newborn infants marked by a high level of immature red blood cells (erythroblasts) in the infant's blood.

Gilbert's syndrome—A mild hereditary form of jaundice.

Glucose-6-phosphate dehydrogenase (G6PD) deficiency—A hereditary disorder that can lead to episodes of hemolytic anemia in combination with certain medications.

Hemoglobin—The red chemical in blood cells that carries oxygen.

Hemolysis—The destruction or breakdown of red blood cells.

Hepatic—Refers to the liver.

Icterus—Another name for jaundice.

Microangiopathic—Pertaining to disorders of the small blood vessels.

Pancreas—The organ beneath the stomach that produces digestive juices, insulin, and other hormones.

Sickle cell disease—A hereditary defect in hemoglobin synthesis that changes the shape of red cells and makes them more fragile.

Splenectomy—Surgical removal of the spleen.

their bile into the intestine, and pressure from the obstructed ducts elsewhere will find release in that direction. As the flow increases, the ducts grow to accommodate it. Soon all the bile is redirected through the open pathways.

Prevention

Erythroblastosis fetalis can be prevented by giving an Rh negative mother a gamma globulin solution called RhoGAM whenever there is a possibility that she is developing antibodies to her baby's blood. G6PD hemolysis can be prevented by testing patients before giving them drugs that can cause it. Medication side effects can be minimized by early detection and immediate cessation of the drug. Malaria can often be prevented by certain precautions when traveling in tropical or subtropical countries. These precautions include staying in after dark; using prophylactic drugs such as mefloquine; and protecting sleeping quarters with mosquito nets treated with insecticides and mosquito repellents. In 2003, new studies showed promise for a possible vaccine against malaria. Early trials showed that **vaccination** combination might stimulate T-cell activity against malaria, the best type of protection that researchers can hope to find. However, further studies will have to be done.

Resources

PERIODICALS

Grimm, David. "Baby Pigment Peril." *U.S. News & World Report* July 28, 2003: 39.

Lawrence, David. "Combination Malaria Vaccine Shows Early Promise in Human Trials." *The Lancet* May 31, 2003: 1875.

Morantz, Carrie, and Brian Torrey. "AHRQ Report on Neonatal Jaundice." *American Family Physician* June 1, 2003: 2417.

Richmond, Glenn, Melissa Brown, and Patricia Wagstaff. "Using a Home Care Model to Monitor Bilirubin Levels in Early Discharged Infants." *Topics in Health Information Management* January–March 2003: 39–43.

ORGANIZATIONS

American Liver Foundation. 1425 Pompton Ave., Cedar Grove, NJ 07009. (800) 223-0179. < http://www.liverfoundation.org >.

J. Ricker Polsdorfer, MD
Teresa G. Odle

Jaw wiring

Definition

Jaw wiring, also known as maxillomandibular fixation, is a surgical procedure where metal pins and wires are anchored into the jaw bones and surrounding tissues to keep the jaw from moving.

Purpose

Sports injuries, automobile accidents, falls, or fistfights are a few of the situations where the jaw might be fractured or broken. In these cases, jaw wiring may be necessary to keep the bones aligned and stable while the jaw heals. The presence of **cancer** or other diseased tissues may make removal and reconstruction of the jaw necessary. Wiring the jaws shut has been used in the past as a weight loss aid in cases of extreme **obesity** where other treatments had failed, although this procedure is rarely used for that purpose today.

Precautions

Traumatic injuries to the face can cause damage to facial nerves and salivary glands and ducts. These injuries can also leave **scars** that may require additional surgery to correct.

Description

Jaw wiring surgery can be performed by an oral or maxillofacial surgeon (a specially trained dentist), or by an otolaryngologist (a doctor specializing in surgeries of the head and neck). The procedure may be done in a medical or dental office if the office is staffed and equipped to handle this type of surgery. More often, this surgery is performed in a hospital or medical center surgical area. If jaw wiring is required due to an injury, the surgeon may set the fracture immediately before swelling sets in. It is also possible to wait (up to several weeks) until the swelling goes down and some of the soft tissue injuries have healed, prior to wiring the jaw fracture.

The surgeon realigns the fractured bones. Every effort is made to restore the shape and appearance of the original jaw line. If any teeth were damaged, repair or replacement may be done at the same time. Small incisions may be made through the skin and surrounding tissue so the pins and wires can be set into the jawbone to hold the fracture together. To prevent the lower jaw from moving during healing, pins and wires may be inserted into the top jaw, as well. The upper and lower jaws are then wired together in order to stabilize the fracture.

As with other types of bone **fractures**, the jaw may take several weeks to heal. Another type of jaw **immobilization** that has been developed more recently, rigid fixation uses small metal plates and screws rather than pins and wires to secure the jaw bones. The main benefit of this technique is that the jaws do not have to be wired shut, allowing the patient to return to a more normal lifestyle sooner.

KEY TERMS

Oral and maxillofacial surgeon—A dentist who is trained to perform surgery to correct injuries, defects, or conditions of the mouth, teeth, jaws, and face.

Otolaryngologist—A doctor who is trained to treat injuries, defects, or conditions of the head and neck.

Preparation

X rays of the fractured area may be taken prior to surgery. Depending on the extent of the facial injury or condition to be corrected, the patient may receive a sedative for relaxation, a local anesthetic drug to numb the area, and/or an anesthetic agent to induce unconsciousness prior to the surgery.

Aftercare

A patient whose jaw has been wired will not be able to eat solid foods for several weeks. In order for the bone and surrounding tissues to heal, it is important to maintain adequate **nutrition**. A liquid diet that can be consumed through a straw, will be required. Soft, precooked foods can be liquefied in a blender, however, it may be difficult for the patient to consume adequate calories, protein, **vitamins**, and **minerals** with this type of diet. Liquid diet formulas may be a good alternative. The patient will also have to be taught how to care for the mouth, teeth, and injured area while the wires are in place.

Risks

It is possible that scarring may occur due to the need to make small incisions in the skin in order to insert the wires. With any surgical procedure, there are risks associated with the anesthetic drugs used and the possibility of infection. If there is a risk that the patient may vomit, the jaw wiring may pose a **choking** hazard. It may be recommended that wire cutters be kept available in case the wires need to be cut in an emergency situation.

Resources

ORGANIZATIONS

American Association of Oral & Maxillofacial Surgeons. 9700 West Bryn Mawr Avenue; Rosemont, IL 60018-5701; (847) 678-6200.

American Dental Association. 211 E. Chicago Ave., Chicago, IL 60611. (312) 440-2500. < http://www.ada.org >.

OTHER

"Know the Score on Facial Sports Injuries" *The Virtual Hospital Page.* University of Iowa. < http://www.vh.org >.
"Topic: Maxillofacial Trauma." *Connecticut Maxillofacial Surgeons Page.* < http://www.cmsllc.com/toptrm.html >.

Altha Roberts Edgren

JC virus infection *see* **Progressive multifocal leukoencephalopathy**

Jejunostomy *see* **Enterostomy**

Jet lag

Definition

Jet lag is a condition marked by **fatigue, insomnia**, and irritability that is caused by air travel through changing time zones. It is commonplace: a 2002 study of international business travelers (IBTs) found that jet lag was one of the most common health problems reported, affecting as many as 74% of IBTs.

Description

Living organisms are accustomed to periods of night and day alternating at set intervals. Most of the human body's regulating hormones follow this cycle, known as circadian rhythm. The word circadian comes from the Latin, *circa*, meaning about, and *dies*, meaning day. These cycles are not exactly 24 hours long, hence the "circa." Each chemical has its own cycle of highs and lows, interacting with and influencing the other cycles. Body temperature, sleepiness, thyroid function, growth hormone, metabolic processes, adrenal hormones, and the sleep hormone melatonin all cycle with daylight. There is a direct connection between the retina (where light hits the back of the eye) and the part of the brain that controls all these hormones. Artificial light has some effect, but sunlight has much more.

When people are without clocks in a compartment that is completely closed to sunlight, most of them fall into a circadian cycle of about 25 hours. Normally, all the regulating chemicals follow one another in order like threads in a weaving pattern. Every morning the sunlight resets the cycle, stimulating the leading chemicals and thus compensating for the difference between the 24-hour day and the 25-hour innate rhythm.

When traveling through a number of time zones, most people reset their rhythms within a few days, demonstrating the adaptability of the human species. Some people, however, have upset rhythms that last indefinitely.

Causes and symptoms

Traveling through a few time zones at a time is not as disruptive to circadian rhythms as traveling around the world can be. The foremost symptom of jet lag is altered sleep pattern—sleepiness during the day, and insomnia during the night. Jet lag may also include **indigestion** and trouble concentrating. Individuals afflicted by jet lag will alternate in and out of a normal day-night cycle.

Treatment

Current treatments

In cases of short-term insomnia triggered by jet lag, a physician may recommend sleeping pills or prescription medication. Such medication should only be taken under the guidance of a health care professional.

Investigational treatments

In 2002, a team from Flanders University invented new jet lag sunglasses equipped with a vision device that used light to stimulate travelers brains. They believed that wearing the glasses before and during flights could help the human clock adjust more easily to changing time zones. The researchers were looking for a commercial partner to help them further study the glasses and make them widely available. The effectiveness of glasses or other head-mounted light devices is still uncertain, however. A team of researchers at Columbia University reported in the fall of 2002 that the use of a head-mounted light visor yielded only modest improvement in the test subjects' symptoms of jet lag.

A newer medication that is considered investigational is a melatonin agonist presently known as LY 156735. An agonist is a drug that stimulates activity at cell receptors that are normally stimulated by such naturally occurring substances as melatonin. LY 156735 was found to speed up the readaptation time of volunteer subjects following a simulated 9-hour time shift.

Another new area of research involves the genes that encode the proteins governing circadian rhythms. It is known as of late 2002 that differences among individuals in adaptability to time zone changes are to some extent genetically determined. Targeting the genes that affect this adaptability may yield new treatments for jet lag and other disorders of circadian rhythm.

Alternative treatment

Exposure to bright morning sunlight cures jet lag after a few days in most people. A few will have prolonged sleep phase difficulties. For these, there is a curious treatment that has achieved success. By forcing one's self into a 27 hour day, complete with the appropriate stimulation from bright light, all the errant chemical cycles will be able to catch up during one week.

When selecting an international flight, individuals should try to arrange an early evening arrival in their destination city. When an individual is traveling to a destination in the east, he or she can try going to bed and waking up a few hours earlier several days before their flight. If travel is to the west, going to bed and waking up later than usual can help the body start to adjust to the upcoming time change. More specific recommendations are available as of 2002, tailored to whether the person is traveling through six time zones, 7–9 zones, or 10 or more.

The following precautions taken during an international flight can help to limit or prevent jet lag:

- Stay hydrated. Drink plenty of water and juices to prevent **dehydration**. Beverages and foods with **caffeine** should be avoided because of their stimulant properties. Alcohol should also be avoided.

- Stretch and walk. As much movement as possible during a flight helps circulation, which moves nutrients and waste through the body and aids in elimination.

- Stay on time. Set watches and clocks ahead to the time in the destination city to start adjusting to the change.

- Sleep smart. Draw the shade and sleep during the evening hours in the destination city, even if it is still daylight outside of the airplane. Earplugs and sleep masks may be helpful in blocking noise and light. Many airlines provide these items on international flights.

- Dress comfortably. Wear or bring comfortable clothes and slippers that will make sleeping during the flight easier.

Once arriving in their destination city, individuals should spend as much time outdoors in the sunlight as possible during the day to reset their internal clock and lessen the symptoms of jet lag. Bedtime should be postponed until at least 10 P.M., with no daytime naps. If a daytime nap is absolutely necessary, it should be limited to no more than two hours.

To promote a restful sleeping environment in a hotel setting, individuals should request that the hotel desk hold all phone calls. Because sleeping in too late can also prolong jet lag, an early wake up call should be requested if an alarm clock is not available. If the hotel room is noisy, a portable white noise machine can help to block outside traffic and hallway noises. A room air conditioner or fan can serve the same purpose. The temperature in the room should also be adjusted for sleeping comfort.

All antioxidants help to decrease the effects of jet lag. Extra doses of **vitamins** A, C, and E, as well as zinc and selenium, two days before and two days after a flight help to alleviate jet lag. Melatonin, a hormone which helps to regulate circadian rhythms, can also help to combat jet lag. Melatonin is available as an over-the-counter supplement in most health food stores and pharmacies, but no more than 3 mg should be used in a 24-hour period.

If weather prevents an individual from spending time in the sunlight, light therapy may be beneficial in decreasing jet lag symptoms. Light therapy, or **phototherapy**, uses a device called a light box, which contains a set of fluorescent or incandescent lights in front of a reflector. Typically, the patient sits for 30 minutes next to a 10,000-lux box (which is about 50 times as bright as an ordinary indoor light). Light therapy is safe for most people, but those with eye diseases should consult a healthcare professional before undergoing the treatment.

Prognosis

Jet lag usually lasts 24–48 hours after travel has taken place. In that short time period, the body adjusts to the time change, and with enough rest and daytime exposure to sunlight, it returns to normal circadian rhythm.

Prevention

Eating a high protein diet that is low in calories before intended travel may help reduce the effects of jet lag.

Resources

PERIODICALS

Boulos, Z., M. M. Macchi, M. P. Sturchler, et al. "Light Visor Treatment for Jet Lag After Westward Travel Across Six Time Zones." *Aviation, Space, and Environmental Medicine* 73 (October 2002): 953–963.

"Jet Lag Sunglasses Help Body Clock Tick." *Optician* August 2, 2002: 1.

Monson, Nancy. "What Really Works for Jet Lag." *Shape* August 2002: 78.

Nickelsen, T., A. Samel, M. Vejvoda, et al. "Chronobiotic Effects of the Melatonin Agonist LY 156735 Following a Simulated 9h Time Shift: Results of a Placebo-Controlled Trial." *Chronobiology International* 19 (September 2002): 915–936.

Parry, B. L. "Jet Lag: Minimizing Its Effects with Critically Timed Bright Light and Melatonin Administration." *Journal of Molecular Microbiology and Biotechnology* 4 (September 2002): 463–466.

Rogers, H. L., and S. M. Reilly. "A Survey of the Health Experiences of International Business Travelers. Part One—Physiological Aspects." *Journal of the American Association of Occupational Health Nurses* 50 (October 2002): 449–459.

Wisor, J. P. "Disorders of the Circadian Clock: Etiology and Possible Therapeutic Targets." *Current Drug Targets: Cns and Neurological Disorders* 1 (December 2002): 555–566.

ORGANIZATIONS

American Sleep Disorders Association. 1610 14th Street NW, Suite 300. Rochester, MN 55901. (507) 287–6006.

National Sleep Foundation. 1367 Connecticut Avenue NW, Suite 200. Washington, DC 20036. (202) 785–2300.

Paula Anne Ford-Martin
Rebecca J. Frey, PhD

Jock itch

Definition

Also known as *Tinea cruris*, jock itch is a growth of fungus in the warm, moist area of the groin.

Description

Although there are many causes of jock itch, this term has become synonymous with *tinea cruris*, a common fungal infection that affects the groin and inner thighs of men and woman. *Tinea* is the name of the fungus; *cruris* comes from the Latin word for leg. Jock itch can develop when tight garments trap moisture and heat. This creates an environment in which fungi multiply and flourish. Athletes often get jock itch but non-athletic men who sweat a lot can also get it. Jock itch occurs more commonly in men, but can affect women as well. The jock itch fungus may cause a rash on the upper and inner thighs, the armpits, and the area just underneath the breasts. Many people with *tinea cruris* also have **athlete's foot**. Athlete's foot is called *tinea pedis*.

Causes & symptoms

The rash of jock itch starts in the groin fold usually on both sides. If the rash advances, it usually advances down the inner thigh. The advancing edge is redder and more raised than areas that have been infected longer. The advancing edge is usually scaly and very easily distinguished or well demarcated. The skin within the border turns a reddish-brown and loses much of its scale. Jock itch can spread to the pubic and genital regions and sometimes to the buttocks.

Jock itch caused by *T. rubrum* does not involve the scrotum or penis. If those areas are involved, the most likely agent is *Candida albicans*, the same type of yeast that causes vaginal yeast infections.

Diagnosis

Often a case of jock itch can be identified based on the characteristic description previously described. If assessed by a conventional doctor, the area of affected skin may be scraped onto a glass slide for definitive diagnosis under the microscope. In order to determine the exact type of fungus present, a small piece of affected skin maybe sent off to the lab for further study.

KEY TERMS

Fungus—A single-celled or multi-celled organism without chlorophyll that reproduces by spores and lives by absorbing nutrients from organic matter.

Scrotum—The external pouch of skin and muscle containing the testes (testicles).

Vaginal yeast infection—An overgrowth of fungus in the vaginal area.

Treatment

Typical conventional treatment for jock itch involves the use of an anti-fungal cream, spray, or powder twice a day for about two weeks. Three commonly used, over-the-counter anti-fungals are *miconazole* (Micatin), *clotrimazole* (Lotrimin) and *tolnaftate* (Tinactin). While the tendency to discontinue treatment once **itching** disappears is common, it is important to use the anti-fungal for a full two-week course in order to prevent recurrence of the infection.

Alternative treatment

Topical treatments include poultices of peppermint, oregano, or lavender. Tea tree oil, diluted with a carrier oil of almond oil, can be applied to the rash several times per day. Cedarwood and jasmine oils can relieve itching when applied in the same manner. Grapefruit seed extract can be taken as a strong solution of 15 drops in 1 oz of water.

Another alternative remedy for jock itch is to wash the groin area with the diluted juice of a freshly squeezed lemon, which can help dry up the rash. A hair dryer on the cool setting can also be used on the area after showering to dry it thoroughly. A warm bath relieves itching in many patients. The affected area should kept clean and dry, and loose-fitting, cotton underwear is recommended.

Prognosis

Treatment for jock itch is quick and usually effective, but the condition often comes back. With treatment, jock itch improves in two or three days and is completely gone in three or four weeks. The following people should be especially vigilant to prevent the problem from returning:

- Athletes
- People with fungal infections that affect other parts of the body (such as athlete's foot)

- People who wear tight clothing
- People with damaged or altered immune systems, including people with HIV or AIDS

Prevention

The best prevention of jock itch is cleanliness and sanitation. This includes keeping the groin area dry, wearing loose-fitting rather than tight clothing, wear boxer shorts rather than briefs, change sweat-covered clothes as soon as possible, showering immediately after working out or playing a sport and then applying talc, and washing workout clothes or sports uniforms after each use.

Resources

BOOKS

Icon Health Publications. *Jock Itch—A Medical Dictionary, Bibliography, and Annotated Research Guide to Internet References* San Diego: Icon Health Publications, 2003.

PERIODICALS

Grin, Caron. "Tinea: Diagnostic Clues, Treatment Keys." *Consultant* (February 2004): 214-216.
"Jock Itch." *Clinical Reference Systems* (January 1, 2004): 1859.
Schmitt, B. D. "Jock Itch for Teenagers." *Clinical Reference Systems* (January 1, 2004): 1858.

ORGANIZATIONS

American Academy of Dermatology. 1350 I St. NW, Suite 870, Washington, DC 20005. (202) 842-3555. < http://www.aad.org >.

OTHER

August 5, 2003. National Institutes of Health Medical Encyclopedia *Jock Itch* < http://www.nlm.nih.gov/medlineplus/print/ency/article/ooo876.htm >. (Accessed March 30, 2005).

Ken R. Wells,

Jock itch *see* **Ringworm**

Joint aspiration *see* **Joint fluid analysis**

▌Joint biopsy

Definition

A joint or synovial membrane biopsy refers to a procedure where a sample of the joint lining or synovial membrane is taken.

KEY TERMS

Joint—The point where two bones meet.
Pathology—The branch of medicine that looks at abnormal changes in cells and tissues which signal disease.
Synovial membrane—Membrane lining a joint.
Trocar—A sharp pointed tube through which a needle can be inserted.

Purpose

A joint biopsy is performed to determine why a joint is painful or swollen. It is usually reserved for more difficult cases where the diagnosis is not clear. The test can be used to diagnose bacterial or fungal infections, an abnormal buildup of iron, **cancer**, or other diseases.

Precautions

The procedure must be done under very sterile conditions to reduce the risk of infection.

Description

The test is performed either in the doctor's office, clinic, or hospital by a surgeon. There are many different ways to perform this biopsy: through an incision in the joint; with a scope inserted in the joint; or, more typically, by the insertion of a sharp instrument through the skin. The procedure can be taken from any joint, but the most common joint requiring biopsy is the knee. A sharp instrument (trocar) is pushed into the joint space. A needle with an attached syringe is inserted into the joint to withdraw fluid for laboratory analysis. The surgeon may instill numbing medicine into the joint and along the needle track before the needle is withdrawn. The trocar and then the biopsy needle is inserted and specimens taken. After the specimen is taken, both the trocar and the biopsy needle are removed, a bandage is placed over the joint, and the samples are sent to pathology for analysis.

Preparation

Blood tests will be done to check that blood clots properly. A mild sedative may be given before the procedure. With the patient lying down, the skin over the joint is disinfected and a local anesthetic is injected into the skin and tissue just below the skin.

Aftercare

The joint will need rest for at least one day. Normal activity can resume if there is no increased **pain** or swelling.

Risks

There is a chance of joint swelling or tenderness. Rarely, bleeding and infection can occur in the joint, or the biopsy needle could break off or strike a nerve or blood vessel. The risk of infection is higher if the patient has an immune deficiency.

Resources

BOOKS

Schumacher, H. Ralph, Jr. "Synovial Fluid Analysis and Synovial Biopsy." In *Textbook of Rheumatology*, edited by William N. Kelley, et al. Philadelphia: W. B. Saunders Co., 1997.

Jeanine Barone, Physiologist

Joint endoscopy *see* **Arthroscopy**

Joint fluid analysis

Definition

Joint fluid analysis, also called synovial fluid analysis, or arthrocentesis, is a procedure used to assess joint-related abnormalities, such as in the knee or elbow.

Purpose

The purpose of a joint fluid analysis is to identify the cause of swelling in the joints, to relieve **pain** and distention from fluid accumulation in the joint, and to diagnose certain types of arthritis and inflammatory joint diseases. The test is also a method to determine whether an infection, either bacterial or fungal, exists within the joint.

Precautions

Joint fluid analysis should not be performed on any patient who is uncooperative, especially if the patient cannot or will not keep the joint immobile throughout the procedure. Patients with certain infections should be excluded from the procedure, particularly those who have a local infection along the proposed needle track. The joint space should be accessible. Therefore, a poorly accessible joint space, such as in hip aspiration in an obese patient, should not be subject to this procedure.

Description

The test is also called arthrocentesis, joint tap, and closed joint aspiration. Normal synovial fluid is a clear or pale-yellow fluid found in small amounts in joints, bursae (fluid-filled sac found on points of friction, like joints), and tendon sheaths. The procedure is done by passing a needle into a joint space and sucking out (aspirating) synovial fluid for diagnostic analysis. When the sample is sent to the laboratory, the fluid is analyzed for color, clarity, quantity, and chemical composition. It is also examined microscopically to check for the presence of bacteria and other cells.

The procedure takes about 10 minutes. Prior to the procedure, any risks that are involved should be explained to the patient. No intravenous pain medications or sedatives are required, although the patient will be given a local anesthetic.

The patient is asked to lie on their back and remain relaxed. The local anesthetic, typically an injection of lidocaine, is then administered. The clinician is usually seated next to the patient. Then the clinician marks exactly where the needle is to enter. As the needle enters the joint, a "pop" may be felt or heard. This is normal. Correct placement of the needle in the joint space is normally painless. At this point, the clinician slowly drains some of the fluid into the syringe. The needle is then withdrawn and adhesive tape is placed over the needle site.

Preparation

Glucose, or sugar, in the joint can be a signal of arthritis. If the clinician will be doing a glucose test, the patient will be asked to fast for 6-12 hours preceding the procedure. If not, there is no special preparation required for a joint fluid analysis.

Aftercare

Some post-procedural pain may be experienced. For this reason, the patient should arrange to be driven home by someone else. Aftercare of the joints will depend on the results of the analysis.

Risks

While joint fluid analysis is generally a safe procedure, especially when performed on a large, easily accessible joint, such as the knee, some risks are

KEY TERMS

Aspirate—The removal by suction of a fluid from a body cavity using a needle.

Bursae—A closed sac lined with a synovial membrane and filled with fluid, usually found in areas subject to friction, such as where a tendon passes over a bone.

Hematoma—A localized mass of blood that is confined within an organ or tissue.

Synovial fluid—A transparent lubricating fluid secreted in a sac to protect an area where a tendon passes over a bone.

possible. Some of the complications to the procedure, although rare, include infection at the site of the needle stick, an accumulation of blood (hematoma) formation, local pain, injury to cartilage, tendon rupture, and nerve damage.

Normal results

The results of a normal joint fluid analysis include fluid of a clear or pale-yellow color and the absence of bacteria, fungus, and other cells, such as white blood cells.

Abnormal results

The results of an abnormal joint fluid analysis include fluid that is turbid, or cloudy. Also, white blood cells and other blood cells may be found, from which the clinician can make a diagnosis and arrive at a treatment for the joint problem. An abnormal result can indicate an infection caused by a bacteria, or **tuberculosis**. Or, there might be inflammation that is caused by **gout**, **rheumatoid arthritis**, or **osteoarthritis**.

Resources

BOOKS

Arnold, William J., and Robert W. Ike. "Specialized Procedures in the Management of Patients with Rheumatic Diseases." In *Cecil Textbook of Medicine*, edited by James B. Wyngaarden, et al. Philadelphia: W. B. Saunders Co., 1996.

Ron Gasbarro, PharmD

Joint infection *see* **Infectious arthritis**
Joint radiography *see* **Arthrography**

Joint replacement

Definition

Joint replacement is the surgical replacement of a joint with an artificial prosthesis.

Purpose

Great advances have been made in joint replacement since the first hip replacement was performed in the United States in 1969. Improvements have been made in the endurance and compatibility of materials used and the surgical techniques to install artificial joints. Custom joints can be made using a mold of the original joint that duplicate the original with a very high degree of accuracy.

The most common joints to be replaced are hips and knees. There is ongoing work on elbow and shoulder replacement, but some joint problems are still treated with joint resection (the surgical removal of the joint in question) or interpositional reconstruction (the reassembly of the joint from constituent parts).

Seventy percent of joint replacements are performed because arthritis has caused the joint to stiffen and become painful to the point where normal daily activities are no longer possible. If the joint does not respond to conservative treatment such medication, weight loss, activity restriction, and use of walking aids such as a cane, joint replacement is considered appropriate.

Patients with **rheumatoid arthritis** or other connective tissue diseases may also be candidates for joint replacement, but the results are usually less satisfactory in those patients. Elderly people who fall and break their hip often undergo hip replacement when the probability of successful bone healing is low.

More than 170,000 hip replacements are performed in the United States each year. Since the lifetime of the artificial joint is limited, the best candidates for joint replacement are over age 60.

Precautions

Joint replacements are performed successfully on an older-than-average group of patients. People with diseases that interfere with blood clotting are not good candidates for joint replacement. Joint replacement surgery should not be done on patients with infection, or any heart, kidney or lung problems that would make it risky to undergo **general anesthesia**.

Description

Joint replacements are performed under general or regional anesthesia in a hospital by an orthopedic surgeon. Some medical centers specialize in joint replacement, and these centers generally have a higher success rate than less specialized facilities. The specific techniques of joint replacement vary depending on the joint involved.

Hip Replacement

The surgeon makes an incision along the top of the thigh bone (femur) and pulls the thigh bone away from the socket of the hip bone (the acetabulum). An artificial socket made of metal coated with polyethylene (plastic) to reduce friction is inserted in the hip. The top of the thigh bone is cut, and a piece of artificial thigh made of metal is fitted into the lower thigh bone on one end and the new socket on the other.

The artificial hip can either be held in place by a synthetic cement or by natural bone in-growth. The cement is an acrylic polymer. It assures good locking of the prosthesis to the remaining bone. However, bubbles left in the cement after it cures may act as weak spots, causing the development of cracks. This promotes loosening of the prosthesis later in life. If additional surgery is needed, all the cement must be removed before surgery can be performed.

An artificial hip fixed by natural bone in-growth requires more precise surgical techniques to assure maximum contact between the remaining natural bone and the prosthesis. The prosthesis is made so that it contains small pores that encourage the natural bone to grow into it. Growth begins 6 to 12 weeks after surgery. The short term outcome with non-cemented hips is less satisfactory, with patients reporting more thigh **pain**, but the long term outlook is better, with fewer cases of hip loosening in non-cemented hips. The trend is to use the non-cemented technique. Hospital stays last from four to eight days.

Knee Replacement

The doctor puts a tourniquet above the knee, then makes a cut to expose the knee joint. The ligaments surrounding the knee are loosened, then the shin bone and thigh bone are cut and the knee removed. The artificial knee is then cemented into place on the remaining stubs of those bones. The excess cement is removed, and the knee is closed. Hospital stays range from three to six days.

In both types of surgery, preventing infection is very important. **Antibiotics** are given intravenously

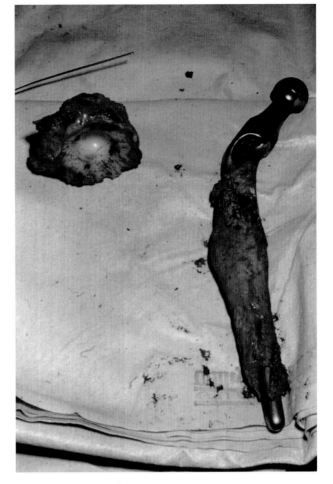

The components of a prosthetic hip joint, removed due to loosening. On the right is the metal shaft encased in the cement which fixed it to the inside of the femur. On the left is the plastic socket. *(Custom Medical Stock Photo. Reproduced by permission.)*

and continued in pill form after the surgery. Fluid and blood loss can be great, and sometimes blood transfusions are needed.

Preparation

Many patients choose to donate their own blood for **transfusion** during the surgery. This prevents any blood incompatibility problems or the transmission of bloodbourne diseases.

Prior to surgery, all the standard preoperative blood and urine tests are performed, and the patient meets with the anesthesiologist to discuss any special conditions that affect the administration of anesthesia. Patients receiving general anesthesia should not eat or drink for ten hours prior to the operation.

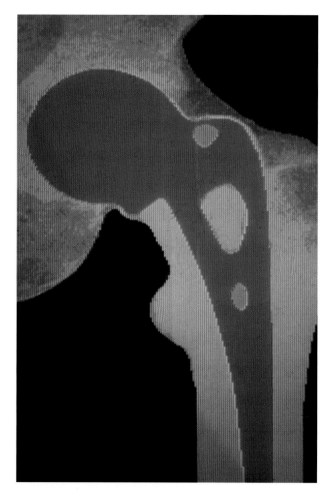

A false color x-ray image of the human pelvis showing a prosthetic hip joint. *(Custom Medical Stock Photo. Reproduced by permission.)*

Aftercare

Immediately after the operation the patient will be catheterized so that he or she will not have to get out of bed to urinate. The patient will be monitored for infection. Antibiotics are continued and pain medication is prescribed. Physical therapy begins (first passive exercises, then active ones) as soon as possible using a walker, cane, or crutches for additional support. Long term care of the artificial joint involves refraining from heavy activity and heavy lifting, and learning how to sit, walk, how to get out of beds, chairs, and cars so as not to dislocate the joint.

Risks

The immediate risks during and after surgery include the development of **blood clots** that may come loose and block the arteries, excessive loss of blood, and infection. Blood thinning medication is usually given to reduce the risk of clots forming. Some elderly people experience short term confusion and disorientation from the anesthesia.

Although joint replacement surgery is highly successful, there is an increased risk of nerve injury. Dislocation or fracture of the hip joint is also a possibility. Infection caused by the operation can occur as long as a year later and can be difficult to treat. Some doctors add antibiotics directly to the cement used to fix the replacement joint in place. Loosening of the joint is the most common cause of failure in hip joints that are not infected. This may require another joint replacement surgery in about 12% of patients within a 15-year period following the first procedure.

Normal results

More than 90% of patients receiving hip replacements achieve complete relief from pain and significant improvement in joint function. The success rate is slightly lower in knee replacements, and drops still more for other joint replacement operations.

Resources

PERIODICALS

Siopack, Jorge, and Harry Jergensen. "Total Hip Arthroplasty." In *Western Journal of Medicine* March 1995: 43–50.

Tish Davidson, A.M.

Joint resection *see* **Arthroplasty**

Joint x rays *see* **Arthrography**

Juvenile arthritis

Definition

Juvenile arthritis (JA), also called juvenile **rheumatoid arthritis** (JRA), refers to a number of different conditions, all of which strike children, and all of which have immune-mediated joint inflammation as their major manifestation. JRA is also known as juvenile idiopathic arthritis or JIA. The European League Against Rheumatism, or EULAR, refers to the disorder as juvenile chronic arthritis, or JCA.

Description

The skeletal system of the body is made up of different types of the strong, fibrous tissue known as connective tissue. Bone, cartilage, ligaments, and tendons are all forms of connective tissue which have different compositions, and thus different characteristics.

The joints are structures which hold two or more bones together. Some joints (synovial joints) allow for movement between the bones being joined (called articulating bones). The simplest model of a synovial joint involves two bones, separated by a slight gap called the joint cavity. The ends of each articular bone are covered by a layer of cartilage. Both articular bones and the joint cavity are surrounded by a tough tissue called the articular capsule. The articular capsule has two components: the fibrous membrane on the outside, and the synovial membrane (or synovium) on the inside. The fibrous membrane may include tough bands of fibrous tissue called ligaments, which are responsible for providing support to the joints. The synovial membrane has special cells and many capillaries (tiny blood vessels). This membrane produces a supply of synovial fluid which fills the joint cavity, lubricates it, and helps the articular bones move smoothly about the joint.

In JA, the synovial membrane becomes intensely inflamed. Usually thin and delicate, the synovium becomes thick and stiff, with numerous infoldings on its surface. The membrane becomes invaded by white blood cells, which produce a variety of destructive chemicals. The cartilage along the articular surfaces of the bones may be attacked and destroyed, and the bone, articular capsule, and ligaments may begin to be worn away (eroded). These processes severely interfere with movement in the joint.

JA specifically refers to chronic arthritic conditions which affect a child under the age of 16 years, and which last for a minimum of three to six months. JA is often characterized by a waxing and waning course, with flares separated by periods of time during which no symptoms are noted (remission). Some literature refers to JA as juvenile rheumatoid arthritis, although most types of JA differ significantly from the adult disease called rheumatoid arthritis, in terms of symptoms, progression, and prognosis.

Causes and symptoms

A number of different causes have been sought to explain the onset of JA. There seems to be some genetic link, based on the fact that the tendency to develop JA sometimes runs in a particular family, and based on the fact that certain genetic markers are more frequently found in patients with JA and other related diseases. Many researchers have looked for some infectious cause for JA, but no clear connection to a particular organism has ever been made. JA is considered by some to be an autoimmune disorder. **Autoimmune disorders** occur when the body's immune system mistakenly identifies the body's own tissue as foreign, and goes about attacking those tissues, as if trying to rid the body of an invader (such as a bacteria, virus, or fungi). While an autoimmune mechanism is strongly suspected, certain markers of such a mechanism (such as rheumatoid factor, often present in adults with such disorders) are rarely present in children with JA.

Joint symptoms of arthritis may include stiffness, **pain**, redness and warmth of the joint, and swelling. Bone in the area of an affected joint may grow too quickly, or too slowly, resulting in limbs which are of different lengths. When the child tries to avoid moving a painful joint, the muscle may begin to shorten from disuse. This is called a contracture.

Symptoms of JA depend on the particular subtype. According to criteria published by the American College of Rheumatology (ACR) in 1973 and modified in 1977, JRA is classified by the symptoms that appear within the first six months of the disorder:

- Pauciarticular JA: This is the most common and the least severe type of JA, affecting about 40–60% of all JA patients. This type of JA affects fewer than four joints, usually the knee, ankle, wrist, and/or elbow. Other more general (systemic) symptoms are usually absent, and the child's growth usually remains normal. Very few children (less than 15%) with pauciarticular JA end up with deformed joints. Some children with this form of JA experience painless swelling of the joint. Some children with JA have a serious inflammation of structures within the eye, which if left undiagnosed and untreated could even lead to blindness. This condition is known as **uveitis**, and affects about 20% of children diagnosed with JRA. While many children have cycles of flares and remissions, in some children the disease completely and permanently resolves within a few years of diagnosis.

- Polyarticular JA: About 40% of all cases of JA are of this type. More girls than boys are diagnosed with this form of JA. This type of JA is most common in children up to age three, or after the age of 10. Polyarticular JA affects five or more joints simultaneously. This type of JA usually affects the small joints of both hands and both feet, although other large joints may be affected as well. Some patients with arthritis in their knees will experience a different rate of growth in each leg. Ultimately, one leg will grow longer than the other. About half of all patients with polyarticular JA have arthritis of the spine and/or hip. Some patients with polyarticular JA will have other symptoms of a systemic illness, including anemia (low red blood cell count), decreased growth rate, low appetite, low-grade **fever**, and a slight rash. The disease is most severe in those children who are diagnosed in early adolescence. Some of these children will test positive for a marker present in other autoimmune disorders, called rheumatoid factor (RF). RF is found in adults who have rheumatoid arthritis. Children who are positive for RF tend to have a more severe course, with a disabling form of arthritis which destroys and deforms the joints. This type of arthritis is thought to be the adult form of rheumatoid arthritis occurring at a very early age.

- Systemic onset JA: Sometimes called Still disease (after a physician who originally described it), this type of JA occurs in about 10–20% of all patients with JA. Boys and girls are equally affected, and diagnosis is usually made between the ages of 5–10 years. The initial symptoms are not usually related to the joints. Instead, these children have high fevers; a rash; decreased appetite and weight loss; severe joint and muscle pain; swollen lymph nodes, spleen, and liver; and serious anemia. Some children experience other complications, including inflammation of the sac containing the heart (**pericarditis**); inflammation of the tissue lining the chest cavity and lungs (pleuritis); and inflammation of the heart muscle (**myocarditis**). The eye inflammation often seen in pauciarticular JA is uncommon in systemic onset JA. Symptoms of actual arthritis begin later in the course of systemic onset JA, and they often involve the wrists and ankles. Many of these children

continue to have periodic flares of fever and systemic symptoms throughout childhood. Some children will go on to develop a polyarticular type of JA.

- Spondyloarthropathy: This type of JA most commonly affects boys older than eight years of age. The arthritis occurs in the knees and ankles, moving over time to include the hips and lower spine. Inflammation of the eye may occur occasionally, but usually resolves without permanent damage.

- Psoriatic JA: This type of arthritis usually shows up in fewer than four joints, but goes on to include multiple joints (appearing similar to polyarticular JA). Hips, back, fingers, and toes are frequently affected. A skin condition called **psoriasis** accompanies this type of arthritis. Children with this type of JA often have pits or ridges in their fingernails. The arthritis usually progresses to become a serious, disabling problem.

As of 2003, there is some disagreement among specialists about the classification of JRA. Some prefer the EULAR classification, also introduced in 1977, to the ACR system. In 1997, the World Health Organization (WHO) met in Durban and issued a new classification system for JRA known as the Durban criteria, in an attempt to standardize definitions of the various subtypes of JRA. None of the various classification systems, however, are considered fully satisfactory as of early 2004.

Diagnosis

Diagnosis of JA is often made on the basis of the child's collection of symptoms. Laboratory tests often show normal results. Some nonspecific indicators of inflammation may be elevated, including white blood cell count, **erythrocyte sedimentation rate**, and a marker called **C-reactive protein**. As with any chronic disease, anemia may be noted. Children with an extraordinarily early onset of the adult type of rheumatoid arthritis will have a positive test for rheumatoid factor.

Treatment

Treating JA involves efforts to decrease the amount of inflammation, in order to preserve movement. Medications which can be used for this include nonsteroidal anti-inflammatory agents (such as ibuprofen and naproxen). Oral (by mouth) steroid medications are effective, but have many serious side effects with long-term use. Injections of steroids into an affected joint can be helpful. Steroid eye drops are used to treat eye inflammation. Other drugs which have been used to treat JA include methotrexate, sulfasalazine, penicillamine, and hydroxychloroquine. Physical therapy and exercises are often recommended in order to improve joint mobility and to strengthen supporting muscles. Occasionally, splints are used to rest painful joints and to try to prevent or improve deformities.

The Food and Drug Administration (FDA) approved a new drug, etanercept, marketed under the brand name Enbrel, in 1999. It is the most dramatic advancement in treating JRA in recent years. A study by Children's Hospital Medical Center in Cincinnati, Ohio, released in 1999, showed the drug was effective in 75% of children with severe JRA. The drug eases joint pain, reduces swelling, and improves mobility.

In 2003, a group of Japanese researchers noted that the blood serum of patients with JRA contains elevated levels of interleukin-6, a cytokine (nonantibody protein) that is critical to regulation of the immune system and blood cell formation. Because interleukin-6 is also associated with inflammation, the researchers think that compounds inhibiting the formation of interleukin-6 might provide new treatment options for JRA.

Alternative treatment

Alternative treatments that have been suggested for arthritis include juice therapy, which can work to detoxify the body, helping to reduce JA symptoms. Some recommended fruits and vegetables to include in the juice are carrots, celery, cabbage, potatoes, cherries, lemons, beets, cucumbers, radishes, and garlic. Tomatoes and other vegetables in the nightshade (potatoes, eggplant, red and green peppers) are discouraged. As an adjunct therapy, **aromatherapy** preparations utilize cypress, fennel, and lemon. Massage oils include rosemary, benzoin, chamomile, camphor, juniper, and lavender. Other types of therapy which have been used include **acupuncture**, **acupressure**, and body work. **Nutritional supplements** that may be beneficial include large amounts of antioxidants (**vitamins** C, A, E, zinc, selenium, and flavenoids), as well as B vitamins and a full complement of **minerals** (including boron, copper, manganese). Other nutrients that assist in detoxifying the body, including methionine, cysteine, and other amino acids, may also be helpful. A number of autoimmune disorders, including JA, seem to have a relationship to **food allergies**. Identification and elimination of reactive foods may result in a decrease in JA symptoms. Constitutional homeopathy can also work to

quiet the symptoms of JA and bring about balance to the whole person.

Prognosis

The prognosis for pauciarticular JA is quite good, as is the prognosis for spondyloarthropathy. Polyarticular JA carries a slightly worse prognosis. RF-positive polyarticular JA carries a difficult prognosis, often with progressive, destructive arthritis and joint deformities. Systemic onset JA has a variable prognosis, depending on the organ systems affected, and the progression to polyarticular JA. About 1-5% of all JA patients die of such complications as infection, inflammation of the heart, or **kidney disease**.

Prevention

Because so little is known about what causes JA, there are no recommendations available for how to avoid developing it.

KEY TERMS

Articular bones—Two or more bones which are connected with each other via a joint.

Cytokine—A general term for nonantibody proteins released by a specific type of cell as part of the body's immune response.

Idiopathic—Of unknown cause or spontaneous origin. JRA is sometimes called juvenile idiopathic arthritis or JIA because its causes are still not fully known.

Joint—A structure that holds two or more bones together.

Rheumatology—The branch of medicine that specializes in the diagnosis and treatment of disorders affecting the muscles and joints.

Synovial joint—A particular type of joint that allows for movement in the articular bones.

Synovial membrane—The membrane that lines the inside of the articular capsule of a joint and produces a lubricating fluid called synovial fluid.

Uveitis—Inflammation of the pigmented vascular covering of the eye, which includes the choroid, iris, and ciliary body. Uveitis is a common complication of JRA.

Resources

BOOKS

Beers, Mark H., MD, and Robert Berkow, MD., editors. "Juvenile Rheumatoid Arthritis." Section 19, Chapter 270 In *The Merck Manual of Diagnosis and Therapy*. Whitehouse Station, NJ: Merck Research Laboratories, 2002.

Behrman, Richard, et al., editors. *Nelson Textbook of Pediatrics*. 16th ed. Philadelphia: W. B. Saunders Co., 2000.

Kredich, Deborah Welt. "Juvenile Rheumatoid Arthritis." In *Rudolph's Pediatrics,* edited by Abraham M. Rudolph. Stamford:McGraw-Hill, 2002.

Peacock, Judith. *Juvenile Arthritis*. Mankato, MN: LifeMatters Books, 2000.

PERIODICALS

de Boer, J., N. Wulffraat, and A. Rothova. "Visual Loss in Uveitis of Childhood." *British Journal of Ophthalmology* 87 (July 2003): 879–884.

Henderson, Charles W. "Etancercept a Dramatic Advancement in Treatment, Say Researchers." *Immunotherapy Weekly* April 2, 2000.

Kotaniemi, K., A. Savolainen, A. Karma, and K. Aho. "Recent Advances in Uveitis of Juvenile Idiopathic Arthritis." *Survey of Ophthalmology* 48 (September-October 2003): 489–502.

Larkin, Marilynn. "Juvenile Arthritis Helped by Resistance Exercise." *Lancet* November 20, 1999: 1797.

Manners, P., J. Lesslie, D. Speldewinde, and D. Tunbridge. "Classification of Juvenile Idiopathic Arthritis: Should Family History Be Included in the Criteria?" *Journal of Rheumatology* 30 (August 2003): 1857–1863.

Moran, M. "Autoimmune Diseases Could Share Common Genetic Etiology." *American Medical News* 44, no. 38 (October 8, 2001): 38.

Yokota, S. "Interleukin 6 as a Therapeutic Target in Systemic-Onset Juvenile Idiopathic Arthritis." *Current Opinion in Rheumatology* 15 (September 2003): 581–586.

ORGANIZATIONS

American College of Rheumatology. 1800 Century Place, Suite 250, Atlanta, GA 30345. (404) 633-3777. < http://www.rheumatology.org >.

Arthritis Foundation. 1330 West Peachtree St., Atlanta, GA 30309. (404) 872-7100. < http://www.arthritis.org >.

National Arthritis and Musculoskeletal and Skin Diseases Information Clearinghouse. National Institutes of Health, 1 AMS Circle, Bethesda, MD 20892. (301) 495-4484. < http://www.nih.gov/niams >.

OTHER

National Institute of Arthritis and Musculoskeletal and Skin Diseases (NIAMS). *Questions and Answers About Juvenile Rheumatoid Arthritis*. NIH Publication No. 01-4942. Bethesda, MD: NIAMS, 2001. < http://www.niams.nih.gov/hi/topics/juvenile_arthritis/juvarthr.htm >.

Rosalyn Carson-DeWitt, MD
Rebecca J. Frey, PhD

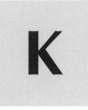

K

Kala-azar *see* **Leishmaniasis**

Kaposi's sarcoma

Definition

Kaposi's sarcoma is a form of skin **cancer** that can involve internal organs. It most often is found in patients with acquired **immunodeficiency** syndrome (**AIDS**), and can be fatal.

Description

Kaposi's sarcoma (KS) was once a very rare form of cancer, primarily affecting elderly men of Mediterranean and eastern European background, until the 1980s, when it began to appear among AIDS patients. It manifests in four distinct forms. The first form, called classic KS, was described by the Austrian dermatologist Moricz Kaposi more than a century ago. Classic KS usually affects older men of Mediterranean or eastern European backgrounds by producing tumors on the lower legs. Though at times painful and disfiguring, they generally are not life-threatening. The second form of the disease, African endemic KS, primarily affects boys and men. It can appear as classic KS, or in a more deadly form that quickly spreads to tissues below the skin, the bones and lymph system, leading to **death** within a few years of diagnosis. Another form of KS, iatrogenic KS, is observed in kidney and liver transplant patients who take immunosuppressive drugs to prevent rejection of their organ transplant. Iatrogenic KS usually reverses after the immunosuppressive drug is stopped. The fourth form of KS, AIDS-related KS, emerged as one of the first illnesses observed among those with AIDS. Unlike classic KS, AIDS-related KS

tumors generally appear on the upper body, including the head, neck, and back. The tumors also can appear on the soft palate and gum areas of the mouth. In more advanced cases, they can be found in the stomach and intestines, the lymph nodes, and the lungs.

Incidence of Kaposi's sarcoma has been reported as high as 20% in homosexual men who have HIV, 3% in heterosexual intravenous drug users, 3% in women and children, 3% in **transfusion** recipients, and 1% in hemophiliacs. Once regarded as only a defining illness for AIDS, KS has proven to be a progressive, fatal disease on its own, especially when the disease becomes systemic. Yet involvement throughout the body is not the only factor in patient mortality. Research in 2000 found that patients with KS in oral mucosa had a higher risk of death than those with KS appearing only on the skin.

Causes and symptoms

A variety of factors appear to contribute to the development of KS. One of the first avenues offered as causal agents was genetic predisposition. People with classic KS, and those who develop the tumors after transplantation, are more likely than others to possess a genetically determined immune factor called HLA-DR. Cases of KS that run in families, however, are rare.

The fact that the disease is more likely to afflict men than women suggests sex hormones, such as testosterone in men, may stimulate the growth of KS tumors, and that estrogen in women may retard their growth.

Immune suppression was the next likely cause since liver, kidney, and bone marrow patients who take immunosuppressive drugs to prevent transplant rejection frequently develop KS lesions. Similarly,

MORIZ KAPOSI, (1837–1902)

Moriz Kohn Kaposi was born in 1837 to very poor Hungarian parents. He studied dermatology under Ferdinand von Hebra at the University of Vienna, earning his medical degree in 1861. Kaposi took a position in Hebra's clinic and ultimately became a lecturer where he was responsible for educating numerous dermatologists. Kaposi and Hebra coauthored *The Handbook of Diseases of the Skin* which had great success. Kaposi married Hebra's daughter and the couple had one son, Hermann (1872). When Hebra died, Kaposi filled the vacant spot as director of the skin clinic and as Vienna's most renowned dermatologist.

Between 1872 and 1887, Kaposi discovered nine skin diseases that had not been previously documented. His discovery of a malignant disease that strikes the lymph nodes and skin (Kaposi's sarcoma 1872) has been documented as the most noteworthy. This disease was seen relatively rarely in the United States until the 1980s when it was tied to AIDS. This sarcoma has been the most common tumor found in AIDS patients. In 1872, Kaposi also studied cases of lupus erythematosus, which had no previous documentation. Kaposi was a prolific writer who published *Pathology and Treatment of Diseases of the Skin* in addition to numerous other publications, which he completed individually and with other authors. Kaposi died in 1902.

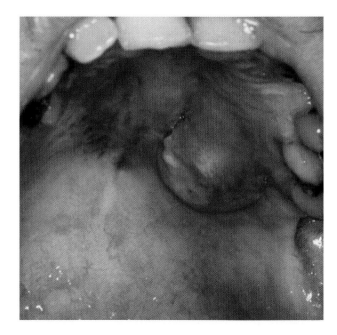

This HIV-positive patient is afflicted with Kaposi's sarcoma inside the mouth. (Custom Medical Stock Photo. Reproduced by permission.)

KS has been observed in patients receiving systemic treatment with high-dose **corticosteroids**, which also suppresses the immune system. Immune suppression is the hallmark of AIDS.

The current theory is the discovery of an infectious agent. A number of viruses have been proposed as possible causes, including cytomegalovirus and human papilloma virus, fragments of which have been found in KS tumor specimens. A more likely candidate, however, is a new herpes virus that has been called human herpes virus 8 (HHV-8) or KS-associated herpes virus (KSHV). Since fragments of the virus were first disclosed in KS samples in 1994, they have since been found in KS samples taken from patients with classic KS, African endemic KS, and KS in transplant patients. Fragments of HHV-8, however, also have been found in patients who have other skin diseases but who do not have KS.

Studies in 2000 showed that HHV-8 was indeed the culprit behind KS. Nevertheless, it does not work alone. In combination with a patient's altered response to cytokines (regulatory proteins produced

by the immune system) and the HIV-1 transactivating protein Tat which promotes the growth of endothelial cells, HHV-8 can then encode interleukin 6 viral proteins. These specific cytokines stimulate cell growth in the skin, becoming KS.

HHV-8 destroys the immune system further by directing a cell to remove the major histocompatibility complex (MHC-1) proteins that protect it from invasion. These proteins then are transferred to the interior of the cell and are destroyed. This leaves the cell unguarded and vulnerable to invaders which normally would be targeted for attack by the immune system.

Research in early 2001 showed that transmission of HHV-8 virus can be more casual than once was thought, giving rise to incidence among women and children. Women who are intravenous drug users and who also have had a sexually transmitted disease have been found to harbor HHV-8. This evidence shows that women can contract HHV-8 through blood. In addition, researchers in 2000 found that HHV-8 could be transmitted orally though kissing. This study found more HHV-8 virus in oral samples than in genital secretions. In fact, HHV-8 was difficult to find in genital samples. This may indicate why children and women who were not intravenous drug users have had KS.

Kaposi's sarcoma produces pink, purple, or brown tumors on the skin, mucous membranes, or internal organs.

Diagnosis

Many physicians will diagnose KS based on the appearance of the skin tumors and the patient's medical history. Unexplained **cough** or chest **pain**, as well as unexplained stomach or intestinal pain or bleeding, could suggest that the disease has moved beyond the skin. The most certain diagnosis can be achieved by taking a biopsy sample of a suspected KS lesion and examining it under high-power magnification. For suspected involvement of internal organs, physicians will use a bronchoscope to examine the lungs or an endoscope to view the stomach and intestinal tract.

Treatment

Treatment goals for KS are simple: to reduce the severity of symptoms, shrink tumors, and prevent disease progression. Unfortunately, there is no single best treatment plan that can achieve all of these goals. Treatments range from topical agents for mild disease with few tumors to more aggressive systemic **chemotherapy** for more serious KS that has spread to large areas of skin or the internal organs. Physicians will frequently combine topical, radiation, and various systemic chemotherapy drugs, depending on the sites of the body affected, the speed at which it is progressing, and the patient's overall health, among other considerations.

Local therapy

When the number of KS tumors is small and the disease appears to be progressing slowly, physicians have had great success with the application, by the patient, of a topical gel containing alitretinoin. This product is a naturally occurring retinoid (a derivative of vitamin A) that can inhibit cell growth and activate apoptosis (cell death). Patients tolerate the product well with only mild to moderate skin irritation at the site of application in some individuals. Duration of treatment is long term, with the patient seeing results after four to eight weeks of therapy. Treatment slows the progress of the disease and reduces the size of the lesions.

Other local treatments include **cryotherapy** (using a liquid nitrogen spray or probe to freeze the tumor), injections of vinblastine (a drug also used for systemic chemotherapy) directly into the tumor, laser therapy, or **radiation therapy** targeted at the tumor sites. These methods have some success, but they also have unpleasant side effects. Vinblastine injections are about 70% effective, but they do not resolve the lesions completely.

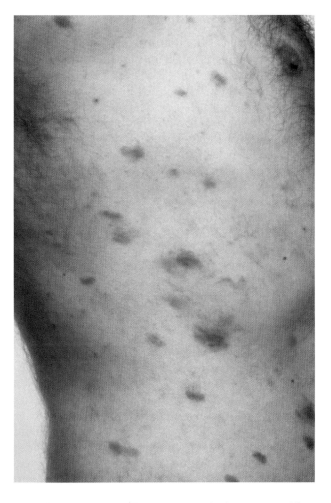

Kaposi's sarcoma usually appears on the lower extremities, as evidenced on this patient's hip. *(Custom Medical Stock Photo. Reproduced by permission.)*

Systemic chemotherapy

With widespread KS lesions over the body surface, or evidence of spread to other parts of the body, physicians will consider systemic chemotherapy drugs. A new class of chemotherapy drugs, called liposomal anthracyclines, appears to produce good results with fewer toxic side effects than do more conventional chemotherapy drugs. Two of these drugs, liposomal doxorubicin (Doxil) and liposomal daunorubicin (DaunoXone) have become the treatment of choice. These drugs last longer in the human body, demonstrate higher concentrations of the drug in tumors, and have fewer toxic side effects.

Paclitaxel (Taxol) is the newest drug in the KS arsenal. It has a 75% effective rate and is very effective in patients who are resistant to anthracycline drugs. The 3-hour infusion time and the incidence of bone marrow suppression, hair loss, and joint and muscle pain make it less attractive to patients.

Antiretroviral therapy

Evidence suggests that for some individuals, the class of AIDS drugs called **protease inhibitors**, in combination with other anti-HIV drugs, can reduce the levels of detectable HIV in the blood to nearly zero, and in some patients stabilize or reverse KS tumors. A study late in 2003 showed that highly active antiretroviral therapy (HAART) containing a protease inhibitor helped block KS tumor growth, invasion and distant spread. HAART is a treatment used to treat HIV patients. Since the discovery of HHV-8, interest in an antiviral approach to KS has increased. There is no evidence, however, that two **antiviral drugs** commonly prescribed for herpes, acyclovir and ganciclovir, have any effect on the disease. One study of 20,000 patients with HIV and AIDS found that those who took foscarnet, another antretroiviral medication that works in a different way than acyclovir and ganciclovir, were less likely to develop KS tumors.

Another treatment source is interferon-alpha, which is made by the body and has powerful effects on the immune system. Investigators have tried injecting it directly into lesions, and also in combination with other anti-HIV drugs such as zidovudine, with some success. It has been used with patients who have KS limited only to the skin and who have little immunosuppression. Interferon-alpha has had poor tumor response and significant toxic effects in patients, especially those with seriously-depressed immune systems.

Still other avenues of therapy being researched are sex hormones, thalidomide, SU5516 (an endothelial growth factor inhibitor), and angiogenesis inhibitors, which prevent the growth of blood vessels within a cell that supplies oxygen and nutrients. There also is some research involving the oral administration of alitretinoin.

Alternative treatment

The Bastyr University AIDS Research Study has been investigating and collecting data on treatment for KS and other opportunistic conditions that are AIDS-related. Among the treatments under investigation are nutritional and herbal therapies (both internal and external). Bastyr University is located in Seattle, Washington.

Prognosis

The prognosis for patients with classic KS is good. Tumors can frequently be controlled and patients frequently die of other causes before any serious spread. African endemic KS can progress rapidly and lead to

premature death, despite treatment. In AIDS-related KS, milder cases can frequently be controlled; the prognosis for more advanced and rapidly progressing cases is less certain and dependent on the patient's overall medical condition. There are indications that KS can be stabilized or reversed in patients whose level of HIV in the blood is reduced to undetectable levels via combined antiretroviral therapy.

Prevention

Safer sex practices may help to prevent AIDS-related KS by decreasing the risk of transmission of HHV-8 through sexual means. However, the addition of avoidance of deep kissing to those precautions may be necessary. Intravenous drug users should still be urged not to share needles. Treatment with antiretrovirals may help to preserve the function of the immune system in HIV patients and delay the appearance and progression of KS lesions. In fact, since the introduction of HAART in those infected with HIV, KS has decreased substantially. However, it still remains the most common cancer among those infected with HIV.

Large clinical trials underway in 2003 were showing some promise for preventing infection with HHV-8 through **prophylaxis** (preventive medication) with antiherpes drugs.

Resources

PERIODICALS

"Alitretinoin Gel Effective for Treating Lesions." *AIDS Weekly* February 12, 2001.

Cannon, Michael J., A. Scott Laney, and Philip E. Pellett. "Human Herpesvirus 8: Current Issues." *Clinical Infectious Diseases* July 1, 2003: 82–86.

Dezube, Bruce J. "AIDS-Related Kaposi Sarcoma." *Archives of Dermatology* 136, no. 2 (December 2000): 1554.

Henderson, Charles W. "Kissing May Spread Cause of Kaposi's Sarcoma." *Cancer Weekly* November 21, 2000: NA.

Mann, Arnold. "Kaposi's Lesions Benefit from Long-Term Alitretinoin Gel Use." *Family Practice News* 30, no. 19 (October 1, 2000): 12.

"Protease Inhibitors Used for Treating HIV also Block Kaposi Sarcoma." *Cancer Weekly* 30, no. 19 (November 4, 2003): 125.

Rohrmus, Bettina, Eva M. Thoma-Greber, Hohannes R. Bogner, and Martin Rocken. "Outlook in Oral and Cutaneous Kaposi's Sarcoma." *The Lancet* 356, no. 9248 (December 23, 2000): 2160.

Janie F. Franz
Teresa G. Odle

Kawasaki syndrome

Definition

Kawasaki syndrome is a potentially fatal inflammatory disease that affects several organ systems in the body, including the heart, circulatory system, mucous membranes, skin, and immune system. It occurs primarily in infants and children but has also been identified in adults as old as 34 years. Its cause is unknown.

Description

Kawasaki syndrome, also called mucocutaneous lymph node syndrome (MLNS), is an inflammatory disorder with potentially fatal complications affecting the heart and its larger arteries. Nearly twice as many males are affected as females. Although persons of Asian descent are affected more frequently than either black or white individuals, there does not appear to be a distinctive geographic pattern of occurrence. Eighty percent of cases involve children under the age of four. Although the disease usually appears in individuals, it sometimes affects several members of the same family and occasionally occurs in small epidemics.

Causes and symptoms

The specific cause of Kawasaki syndrome is unknown, although the disease resembles infectious illnesses in many ways. It has been suggested that Kawasaki syndrome represents an allergic reaction or other unusual response to certain types of infections. Some researchers think that the syndrome may be caused by the interaction of an immune cell, called the T cell, with certain poisons (toxins) secreted by bacteria.

Kawasaki syndrome has an abrupt onset, with **fever** as high as 104°F (40°C) and a rash that spreads over the patient's chest and genital area. The fever is followed by a characteristic peeling of the skin beginning at the fingertips and toenails. In addition to the body rash, the patient's lips become very red, with the tongue developing a "strawberry" appearance. The palms, soles, and mucous membranes that line the eyelids and cover the exposed portion of the eyeball (conjuntivae) become purplish-red and swollen. The lymph nodes in the patient's neck may also become swollen. These symptoms may last from two weeks to three months, with relapses in some patients.

In addition to the major symptoms, about 30% of patients develop joint pains or arthritis, usually in the large joints of the body. Others develop **pneumonia, diarrhea**, dry or cracked lips, **jaundice**, or an inflammation of the membranes covering the brain and spinal cord (**meningitis**). A few patients develop symptoms of inflammation in the liver (hepatitis), gallbladder, lungs, or tonsils.

About 20% of patients with Kawasaki syndrome develop complications of the cardiovascular system. These complications include inflammation of the heart tissue (**myocarditis**), disturbances in heartbeat rhythm (**arrhythmias**), and areas of blood vessel dilation (aneurysms) in the coronary arteries. Other patients may develop inflammation of an artery (arteritis) in their arms or legs. Complications of the heart or arteries begin to develop around the tenth day after the illness begins, when the fever and rash begin to subside. A few patients may develop **gangrene**, or the death of soft tissue, in their hands and feet. The specific causes of these complications are not yet known.

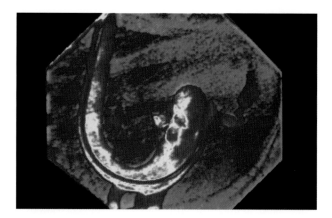

An angiogram showing abnormal coronary arteries in a child suffering from Kawasaki's disease. The coronary arteries are abnormal and weakened in that they bulge into balloon shapes, or aneurysms, along their lengths. This illness afflicts children between the ages of 1–2 years. *(Photograph by Mehau Kulyk, Photo Researchers, Inc. Reproduced by permission.)*

Diagnosis

Because Kawasaki syndrome is primarily a disease of infants and young children, the disease is most likely to be diagnosed by a pediatrician. The physician will first consider the possible involvement of other diseases that cause fever and skin **rashes**, including **scarlet fever**, **measles**, **Rocky Mountain spotted fever**, **toxoplasmosis** (a disease carried by cats), juvenile **rheumatoid arthritis**, and a blistering and inflammation of the skin caused by reactions to certain medications (Stevens-Johnson syndrome).

Once other diseases have been ruled out, the patient's symptoms will be compared with a set of diagnostic criteria. The patient must have a fever lasting five days or longer that does not respond to **antibiotics**, together with four of the following five symptoms:

- Inflammation of the conjunctivae of both eyes with no discharge

- At least one of the following changes in the mucous membranes of the mouth and throat: "strawberry" tongue; cracked lips; or swollen throat tissues

- At least one of the following changes in the hands or feet: swelling caused by excess fluid in the tissues; peeling of the skin; or abnormal redness of the skin

- A skin eruption or rash associated with fever (exanthem) on the patient's trunk

- Swelling of the lymph nodes in the neck to a size greater than 1.5 cm.

Since the cause of Kawasaki syndrome is unknown, there are no laboratory tests that can confirm the diagnosis. The following test results, however, are associated with the disease:

- Blood tests show a high white blood cell count, high **platelet count**, a high level of protein in the blood serum, and mild anemia

- Chest x ray may show enlargement of the heart (cardiomegaly)

- Urine may show the presence of pus or an abnormally high level of protein

- An electrocardiogram may show changes in the heartbeat rhythm

In addition to these tests, it is important to take a series of echocardiograms during the course of the illness because 20% of Kawasaki patients will develop coronary aneurysms or arteritis that will not appear during the first examination.

Treatment

Kawasaki syndrome is usually treated with a combination of **aspirin**, to control the patient's fever and skin inflammation, and high doses of intravenous immune globulin to reduce the possibility of coronary artery complications. Some patients with heart complications may be treated with drugs that reduce blood clotting or may receive corrective surgery.

Follow-up care includes two to three months of monitoring with chest x rays, **electrocardiography**, and **echocardiography**. Treatment with aspirin is often continued for several months.

Prognosis

Most patients with Kawasaki syndrome will recover completely, but about 1–2% will die as a result of **blood clots** forming in the coronary arteries or as a result of a **heart attack**. Deaths are sudden and unpredictable. Almost 95% of fatalities occur within six months of infection, but some have been reported as long as 10 years afterward. Long-term follow-up of patients with aneurysms indicates that about half show some healing of the aneurysm. The remaining half has a high risk of heart complications in later life.

Resources

BOOKS

Shandera, Wayne X., and Maria E. Carlini. "Infectious Diseases: Viral & Rickettsial." In *Current Medical*

KEY TERMS

Aneurysm—Dilation of an artery caused by thinning and weakening of the vessel wall.

Arrythmia—Abnormal heart rhythm.

Arteritis—Inflammation of an artery.

Cardiomegaly—An enlarged heart.

Conjunctivae—The mucous membranes that cover the exposed area of the eyeball and line the inner surface of the eyelids.

Exanthem—A skin eruption associated with a disease, usually one accompanied by fever as in Kawasaki syndrome.

Gangrene—The death of soft tissue in a part of the body, usually caused by obstructed circulation.

Hepatitis—Inflammation of the liver.

Meningitis—Inflammation of the membranes, called the meninges, covering the brain and spinal cord.

Mucocutaneous lymph node syndrome (MLNS)—Mucocutaneous lymph node syndrome, another name for Kawasaki syndrome. The name comes from the key symptoms of the disease, which involve the mucous membranes of the mouth and throat, the skin, and the lymph nodes.

Myocarditis—Inflammation of the heart muscle.

Stevens-Johnson syndrome—A severe inflammatory skin eruption that occurs as a result of an allergic reaction or respiratory infection.

T cell—A type of white blood cell that develops in the thymus gland and helps to regulate the immune system's response to infections or malignancy.

Diagnosis and Treatment, 1998, edited by Stephen McPhee, et al., 37th ed. Stamford: Appleton & Lange, 1997.

Rebecca J. Frey, PhD

Keloids

Definition

Keloids are overgrowths of fibrous tissue or **scars** that can occur after an injury to the skin. These heavy scars are also called cheloid or hypertrophic scars. In individuals prone to keloids, even minor traumas to the skin, such as ear **piercing**, can cause keloids. The word "keloid" itself comes from the Greek word for a crab's claw; it was first used by a French physician to describe the way that keloids grow sideways into normal skin.

Description

Keloids can occur anywhere on the body, but they are most common on the earlobes, upper back, shoulders, and chest. The pattern of distribution of keloids differs according to race, with facial keloids more common in Caucasians and relatively uncommon in Asians. African Americans are more likely to develop keloids on the legs or feet than either Asians or Caucasians. In general, keloids consist of hard, raised scars that may be slightly pink or whitish. These may itch and be painful, and some keloids can grow to be quite large.

Causes and symptoms

Although the cause of keloids is unknown, it is thought that they are due to the body's failure to turn off the healing process needed to repair skin. When this occurs, extra collagen forms at the site of the scar, and keeps forming because it is not shut off. This results in keloid formation.

Keloids occur most frequently in individuals of African-American descent and in those with darker skin. They are more common in Polynesians and Chinese than in people from India or Malaysia. Caucasians are the least frequently affected by keloids. Other risk factors include a family history of keloids, surgery, **acne**, **burns**, ear piercing, vaccinations, or even insect bites. Spontaneous keloids have been reported occasionally in siblings. In addition, women and young people under the age of 30 are more prone to develop them. Keloids are infrequent among the elderly.

Although the association of keloids with darker skin pigmentation suggests a genetic linkage of some sort, no specific genes have been identified in connection with keloids as of the early 2000s.

Initially, keloids will begin as a small lump where the skin has been injured. This lump grows and can eventually become very large and cosmetically unacceptable.

Diagnosis

A dermatologist can usually make the diagnosis of a keloid based on looking at the scar. In some cases, however, a biopsy may be necessary to rule out other types of **skin lesions**, such as tumors.

Treatment

The treatment of choice for keloids is usually an injection of corticosteroid drugs such as cortisone directly into the lesion. These injections cause the keloid to become atrophic, or thinner, and are repeated every three to four weeks until the keloid has been resolved to the individual's satisfaction. Other therapies include laser treatment or **radiation therapy**, and topical treatments are undergoing study.

Surgery is often used in combination with corticosteroid injections. The injections are given for several weeks, and then the keloid is surgically removed. The injections are then continued for several weeks. Surgical removal of the keloid may also be used in conjunction with radiation therapy, which delivers small amounts of radiation to the affected area.

Another surgical option is cryosurgery, in which liquid nitrogen is used to freeze the tissues in the keloid. The treatment may need to be repeated to remove as much of the keloid as possible; however, cryosurgery prevents keloids from recurring in about 70% of patients.

Newer approaches include silastic gel sheeting, which makes use of pressure to flatten the keloid. The gel is applied and kept securely in place with tape, cloth, or an Ace bandage. The dressing is to be changed every seven to 10 days for as long as 12 months.

Finally, researchers are now studying a type of tape that has been soaked with steroids, which are released slowly into the keloid, causing it to thin over time.

Newer treatments include injections of interferon directly into the keloids, and local application of 5% imiquimod cream, which induces the skin where it is applied to produce interferon. The imiquimod cream is reported to significantly lower the risk of keloid recurrence.

Prognosis

Although keloids are unsightly, they are not life-threatening. Keloids do not have a tendency to develop into malignancies, but they can become cosmetically unacceptable. Keloids can gradually lessen after treatment, but many recur. And just as they can occur spontaneously, they can also resolve spontaneously.

Prevention

Preventive measures include avoiding any trauma to the skin, and compression pressure dressing for high-risk patients who have suffered burns to their skin. Patients with a tendency to form keloids should avoid any sort of elective surgery. Individuals who are prone to develop keloids or who have a history of keloids should immediately care for any cuts or abrasions they may sustain.

To lower the risk of keloids, surgeons are advised to close incisions with as little tension on the sutures as possible, and to use buried sutures whenever possible.

Resources

BOOKS

Beers, Mark H., MD, and Robert Berkow, MD., editors. "Benign Tumors." Section 10, Chapter 125 In *The Merck Manual of Diagnosis and Therapy*. Whitehouse Station, NJ: Merck Research Laboratories, 2004.

PERIODICALS

Berman, Brian, MD, PhD, and Sonia Kapoor, MBBS. "Keloid and Hypertrophic Scar." *eMedicine* November 30, 2001. < http://www.emedicine.com/derm/topic205.htm >.

Dinh, Q., M. Veness, and S. Richards. "Role of Adjuvant Radiotherapy in Recurrent Earlobe Keloids." *Australasian Journal of Dermatology* 45 (August 2004): 162–166.

Food and Drug Administration (FDA). "General and Plastic Surgery Devices; Classification of Silicone Sheeting. Final Rule." *Federal Register* 69 (August 9, 2004): 48146–48148.

Mandal, A., D. Imran, and G. S. Rao. "Spontaneous Keloids in Siblings." *Irish Medical Journal* 97 (September 2004): 250–251.

ORGANIZATIONS

American Academy of Dermatology. 930 N. Meacham Road, PO Box 4014, Schaumburg, IL 60168-4014. (847) 330-0230. Fax: (847) 330-0050. < http://www.aad.org >.

United States Food and Drug Administration (FDA). 5600 Fishers Lane, Rockville, MD 20857-0001. (888) INFO-FDA. < http://www.fda.gov >.

OTHER

< http://www.skinsite.com >.

"Keloids." Black Women's Health. < http://www.black-womenshealth.com/Keloids.htm >.

Liz Meszaros
Rebecca J. Frey, PhD

Keratitis

Definition

Keratitis is an inflammation of the cornea, the transparent membrane that covers the colored part of the eye (iris) and pupil of the eye.

Description

There are many types and causes of keratitis. Keratitis occurs in both children and adults. Organisms cannot generally invade an intact, healthy cornea. However, certain conditions can allow an infection to occur. For example, a scratch can leave the cornea open to infection. A very dry eye can also decrease the cornea's protective mechanisms.

Risk factors that increase the likelihood of developing this condition include:

- poor contact lens care; overuse of contact lenses
- illnesses or other factors that reduce the body's ability to overcome infection
- cold sores, **genital herpes**, and other viral infections
- crowded, dirty living conditions; poor hygiene
- poor **nutrition** (especially a deficiency of Vitamin A, which is essential for normal vision)

Some common types of keratitis are listed below, however there are many other forms

Herpes simplex keratitis

A major cause of adult eye disease, herpes simplex keratitis may lead to:

- chronic inflammation of the cornea
- development of tiny blood vessels in the eye
- scarring

- loss of vision
- glaucoma

This infection generally begins with inflammation of the membrane lining the eyelid (conjunctiva) and the portion of the eyeball that comes into contact with it. It usually occurs in one eye. Subsequent infections are characterized by a pattern of lesions that resemble the veins of a leaf. These infections are called dendritic keratitis and aid in the diagnosis.

Recurrences may be brought on by **stress**, **fatigue**, or ultraviolet light (UV) exposure (e.g., skiing or boating increase the exposure of the eye to sunlight; the sunlight reflects off of the surfaces). Repeated episodes of dendritic keratitis can cause sores, permanent scarring, and **numbness** of the cornea.

Recurrent dendritic keratitis is often followed by disciform keratitis. This condition is characterized by clouding and deep, disc-shaped swelling of the cornea and by inflammation of the iris.

It is very important not to use topical **corticosteroids** with herpes simplex keratitis as it can make it much worse, possibly leading to blindness.

Bacterial keratitis

People who have bacterial keratitis wake up with their eyelids stuck together. There can be **pain**, sensitivity to light, redness, tearing, and a decrease in vision. This condition, which is usually aggressive, can be caused by wearing soft contact lenses overnight. One study found that overnight wear can increase risk by 10-15 times more than if wearing daily wear contact lenses. Improper lens care is also a factor. Contaminated makeup can also contain bacteria.

Bacterial keratitis makes the cornea cloudy. It may also cause abscesses to develop in the stroma, which is located beneath the outer layer of the cornea.

Fungal keratitis

Usually a consequence of injuring the cornea in a farm-like setting or in a place where plant material is present, fungal keratitis often develops slowly. This condition:

- usually affects people with weakened immune systems
- often results in infection within the eyeball
- may cause stromal abscesses

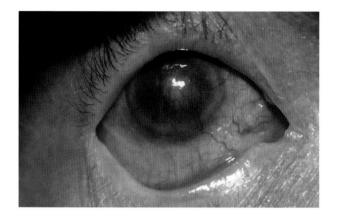

Close-up of a damaged cornea due to complications following cataract surgery. *(Custom Medical Stock Photo. Reproduced by permission.)*

Peripheral ulcerative keratitis

Peripheral ulcerative keratitis is also called marginal keratolysis or peripheral rheumatoid ulceration. This condition is often associated with active or chronic:

- rheumatoid arthritis

- relapsing polychondritis (connective-tissue inflammation)

- Wegener's granulomatosis, a rare condition characterized by **kidney disease** and development of nodules in the respiratory tract

Superficial punctate keratitis

Often associated with the type of viruses that cause upper respiratory infection (adenoviruses), superficial punctate keratitis is characterized by destruction of pinpoint areas in the outer layer of the cornea (epithelium). One or both eyes may be affected.

Acanthamoeba keratitis

This pus-producing condition is very painful. It is a common source of infection in people who wear soft or rigid contact lenses. It can be found in tap water, soil, and swimming pools.

Photokeratitis

Photokeratitis or snowblindness is caused by excess exposure to UV light. This can occur with sunlight, suntanning lamps, or a welding arc. It is called snowblindness because the sunlight is reflected off of the snow. It therefore can occur in water sports as well, because of the reflection of light off of the water. It is

very painful and may occur several hours after exposure. It may last one to two days.

Interstitial keratitis

Also called parenchymatous keratitis, interstitial keratitis is a chronic inflammation of tissue deep within the cornea. Interstitial keratitis is rare in the United States. Interstitial keratitis affects both eyes and usually occurs as a complication of congenital or acquired **syphilis**. In congenital syphilis it can occur between age two and **puberty**. It may also occur in people with **tuberculosis**, **leprosy**, or other diseases.

Causes and symptoms

In summary, keratitis can be caused by:

- bacterial, viral, or fungal infections

- dry eyes resulting from disorders of the eyelid or diminished ability to form tears

- exposure to very bright light

- **foreign objects** that injure or become lodged in the eye

- sensitivity or allergic reactions to eye makeup, dust, pollen, pollution, or other irritants

- vitamin A deficiency, which people with normal **diets** rarely develop

Symptoms of keratitis include, but are not limited to:

- tearing

- pain

- sensitivity to light

- inflammation of the eyelid

- decrease in vision

- redness

Diagnosis

A case history will be taken and the vision will be tested. Examination with a slit lamp, an instrument that's a microscope and focuses a beam of light on the eye is important for diagnosis. The cornea can be examined with fluorescein, a yellow dye which will highlight defects in the cornea. Deeper layers of the cornea can also be examined with the slit lamp. Infiltrates, hazy looking areas in the cornea, can be seen by the doctor and will aid in the diagnosis. Samples of infectious matter removed from the eye will be sent for laboratory analysis.

Abscess—A collection of pus.

Glaucoma—An eye disease characterized by an increase of pressure in the eye. Left untreated, blindness may result.

Infiltrate—A collection of cells not usually present in that area. In the cornea, infiltrates may be a collection of white blood cells.

Inflammation—A localized response to an injury. May include swelling, redness, and pain.

Treatment

Antibiotics, antifungals, and antiviral medication will be used to treat the appropriate organism. Broad spectrum antibiotics will be used immediately, but once the lab analysis determines the offending organism, the medication may be changed. Sometimes more than one medication is necessary. It depends upon the infection, but the patient should be clear on how often and how to use the medications.

A sterile, cotton-tipped applicator may be used to gently remove infected tissue and allow the eye to heal more rapidly. **Laser surgery** is sometimes performed to destroy unhealthy cells, and some severe infections require corneal transplants.

Antifungal, antibiotic, or antiviral eyedrops or ointments are usually prescribed to cure keratitis, but they should be used only by patients under a doctor's care. Inappropriate prescriptions or over-the-counter preparations can make symptoms more severe and cause tissue deterioration. Topical corticosteroids can cause great harm to the cornea in patient's with herpes simplex keratitis.

A patient with keratitis may wear a patch to protect the healing eye from bright light, foreign objects, the lid rubbing against the cornea, and other irritants. Sometimes a patch can make it worse, so again, the patient must discuss with the doctor whether or not a patch is necessary. The patient will probably return every day to the eye doctor to check on the progress.

Although early detection and treatment can cure most forms of keratitis, the infection can cause:

- glaucoma
- permanent scarring
- ulceration of the cornea
- blindness

Prevention

Children and adults who wear contact lenses should always use sterile lens-cleaning and disinfecting solutions. Tap water is not sterile and should not be used to clean contact lenses. It is important to go for follow-up checkups because small defects in the cornea can occur without the patient being aware of it. Do not overwear contact lenses. Remove them if the eyes become red or irritated. Replace contact lenses when scheduled to do so. Proteins and other things can deposit on the contacts, leading to an increased risk of infection. Rinse contact lens cases in hot water every night, if possible, and let them air dry. Replace contact lens cases every three months. Organisms have been cultured from contact lens cases.

Eating a well-balanced diet and wearing protective glasses when working or playing in potentially dangerous situations can reduce anyone's risk of developing keratitis. Protective goggles can even be worn mowing the lawn so that if twigs are tossed up they can't hurt the eye. Goggles or sunglasses with UV coatings can help protect against damage from UV light.

Resources

ORGANIZATIONS

American Academy of Ophthalmology. 655 Beach Street, P.O. Box 7424, San Francisco, CA 94120-7424. <http://www.eyenet.org>.

American Optometric Association. 243 North Lindbergh Blvd., St. Louis, MO 63141. (314) 991-4100. <http://www.aoanet.org>.

National Eye Institute. 2020 Vision Place, Bethesda, MD 20892-3655. (301) 496-5248. <http://www.nei.nih.gov>.

Prevent Blindness America. 500 East Remington Road, Schaumburg, IL 60173. (800) 331-2020. <http://www.preventblindness.org>.

Maureen Haggerty

Keratosis pilaris

Definition

Keratosis pilaris is a common skin condition that looks like small goose bumps, which are actually dead skin cells that build up around the hair follicle.

Description

Keratosis pilaris is a disorder that occurs around the hair follicles of the upper arms, thighs, and sometimes the buttocks. It presents as small, benign bumps or papules that are actually waxy build-ups of keratin. Normally skin sloughs off. However, around the hair follicle where the papules form, the keratinized skin cells slough off at a slower rate, clogging the follicles.

This is generally thought to be genetic disorder, although the symptoms of keratosis pilaris are often seen with **ichthyosis** and allergic **dermatitis**. It can also be observed in people of all ages who have either inherited it or have a **vitamin A deficiency** or have dry skin. Keratosis pilaris is a self-limiting disorder that disappears as the person ages. It can become more severe when conditions are dry such as during the winter months or in dry climates.

Causes and symptoms

The specific causes of this disorder are unknown. Since this disorder runs in families, it is thought to be hereditary. Keratosis pilaris is not a serious disorder and is not contagious.

The symptoms of keratosis pilaris are based on the development of small white papules the size of a grain of sand on the upper arms, thighs, and occasionally the buttocks and face. The papules occur around a hair follicle and are firm and white. They feel a little like coarse sandpaper, but they are not painful and there usually is no **itching** associated with them. They are easily removed and the material inside the papule usually contains a small, coiled hair.

Diagnosis

A dermatologist or a general practicioner can easily diagnose this disorder. A **physical examination** is all that is necessary to diagnose keratosis pilaris. Special tests are not needed.

Treatment

To treat keratosis pilaris patients can try several strategies to lessen the bumps. First, the patient can supplement the natural removal of dry skin and papules by using a loofah or another type of scrub showering or bathing. A variety of different over-the-counter (OTC) lotions, ointments, and creams can also be applied after showering while the skin is still moist and then several times a day to keep the area moist. Medicated lotions with urea, 15% alpha-hydroxy acids, or Retin A can also be prescribed by

---

KEY TERMS

Benign—Not cancerous.

Dermatologist—A physician that specializes in diseases and disorders of the skin.

Ichthyosis—A group of congenital disorders of keratinization characterized by dryness and scaling of the skin.

Keratin—The hard, waxy material that is made by the outer layer of skin cells.

---

the dermatologist and applied one to two times daily. Systemic (oral) medications are not prescribed for keratosis pilaris. However if papules are opened and become infected, **antibiotics** may be necessary to treat the infection.

Prognosis

Unfortunately, the treatment for keratosis pilaris is often disappointing. Although extreme cases of keratosis pilaris can occasionally be unsightly, the disorder is not life threatening and usually begins to disappear as the patient ages.

Prevention

Since keratosis pilaris is thought to be a genetic disorder and is observed in several members of the same family, there is nothing that can be done to prevent this disorder. Following the treatment advice above can alleviate the outward characteristics of keratosis pilaris.

Sally C. McFarlane-Parrott

Kidney biopsy

Definition

Kidney biopsy is a medical procedure in which a small piece of tissue is removed from the kidney for microscopic examination.

Purpose

The test is usually done to diagnose **kidney disease** and to evaluate the extent of damage to the kidney.

A biopsy is also frequently ordered to detect the reason for acute renal failure when normal office procedures and tests fail to establish the cause. In addition, information regarding the progression of the disease and how it is responding to medical treatment can be obtained from a biopsy. Occasionally a biopsy may be done to confirm a diagnosis of **kidney cancer**, to determine its aggressiveness, and decide on the mode of treatment.

Precautions

The biopsy is not recommended for patients who have any uncontrollable bleeding disorders. Platelets are blood cells that play an important role in the blood clotting process. If the bleeding disorder is caused by a low **platelet count** (less than 50,000 per cubic millimeter of blood), then a platelet **transfusion** can be done just before performing the biopsy.

Description

The kidneys, a pair of organs that are shaped like beans, lie on either side of the backbone, just above the waist. The periphery (parenchyma) of the kidney is made up of tiny tubes. These tubes filter and clean the blood by taking out the waste products and making urine. The urine is collected in the central portion of the kidney. Tubes called ureters drain the urine from the kidney into the bladder, where it is held until it is voided from the body.

A kidney specialist (nephrologist) performs the biopsy. It can be done either in the doctor's office or in a local hospital. The patient may be given a calming drug before the procedure to help him relax. The skin and muscles on the back overlying the site that is to be biopsied may be numbed with **local anesthesia**.

The patient will be asked to lie face down and a pad or a rolled towel may be placed under the stomach. Either the left or the right kidney may be biopsied depending on the results of the imaging tests: x rays, **computed tomography scans** (CT scans), **magnetic resonance imaging** (MRI), and ultrasound. The area that will be biopsied is cleaned with an antiseptic solution and sterile drapes are placed on it. The skin is numbed with local anesthesia. A small incision is made on the skin with a scalpel blade. Using a long needle, the physician injects local anesthesia into the incision so that it infiltrates down to the kidney. The biopsy needle is then advanced slowly through the incision. The patient is asked to hold his or her breath each time the needle is pushed forward. Once the wall (capsule) of the kidney has been penetrated, the patient can breathe normally. The tissue is collected for examination and the needle is withdrawn. The needle may be re-inserted into another part of the kidney so that tissue is collected from at least three different areas. The tissue samples are sent to the laboratory for examination. The entire procedure may last about an hour.

Preparation

Before performing the biopsy, the doctor should be made aware of all the medications that the patient is taking. The doctor should also be told whether the patient is allergic to any medications. The procedure and the risks of the procedure are explained to the patient and the necessary consent forms are obtained. The patient should be told that a kidney biopsy requires a 24-hour stay in the hospital after the biopsy.

Some doctors order blood tests to check for clotting problems before performing the biopsy. The patient's blood type may also be determined in case a transfusion becomes necessary.

Aftercare

Immediately after the biopsy, pulse, respiration, and temperature (vital signs) are measured. If they are stable, the patient is instructed to lie flat in bed for at least 12 hours. The pulse and blood pressure are checked at regular intervals by the nursing staff. All urine voided by the patient in the first 12–24 hours is examined in the laboratory for blood cells.

If bleeding is severe, iron levels in the blood drop significantly, or the patient complains of severe **pain** at the biopsy site, the physician should be contacted immediately. After the patient goes home, he should avoid heavy lifting, vigorous **exercise**, and contact sports for at least one or two weeks.

Risks

The risks of a kidney biopsy are very small. Severe bleeding may occur after the procedure. There is also a slight chance that an infection or a lump of blood under the skin that looks black and blue (hematoma) may develop. In most cases, the hematoma disappears by itself and does not cause any pain. However, severe pain or a drop in blood pressure and iron levels in the blood indicates that the hematoma is expanding. This condition could lead to complications and should be reported immediately to the doctor.

Very rarely, the patient may develop high blood pressure (**hypertension**), and the bleeding may be severe enough to require a transfusion. In extremely

KEY TERMS

Biopsy—The surgical removal and microscopic examination of living tissue for diagnostic purposes.

Computed tomography (CT) scan—A medical procedure in which a series of x rays are taken and put together by a computer in order to form detailed pictures of areas inside the body.

Magnetic resonance imaging (MRI)—A medical procedure used for diagnostic purposes in which pictures of areas inside the body can be created using a magnet linked to a computer.

Nephrologist—A doctor who specializes in the diseases and disorders of the kidneys.

Renal ultrasound—A painless and non-invasive procedure in which sound waves are bounced off the kidneys. These sound waves produce a pattern of echoes that are then used by the computer to create pictures of areas inside the kidney (sonograms).

rare circumstances, the kidney may rupture, or the surrounding organs (pancreas, bowel, spleen, and liver) may be punctured. **Death** occurs in about one in 3000 cases.

Normal results

The results are normal if no abnormalities can be seen in the tissue samples with the naked eye, with an electron microscope or through staining with a fluorescent dye (immunofluorescence).

Abnormal results

Any abnormalities in the size, color, and consistency of the sample will be reported as an abnormal result. In addition, any change in the structure of the renal tubules, the presence of red blood cells, or abnormalities in the cells are considered an abnormal result. If cancerous changes are detected in the kidney cells, they are further characterized in order to determine the stage of the tumor and decide on the appropriate mode of treatment.

Resources

ORGANIZATIONS

National Kidney Cancer Association. 1234 Sherman Ave., Suite 203, Evanston, IL 60202-1375. (800) 850-9132.

National Kidney Foundation. 30 East 33rd St., New York, NY 10016. (800) 622-9010. < http://www.kidney.org >.

Lata Cherath, PhD

Kidney cancer

Definition

Kidney **cancer** is a disease in which the cells in certain tissues of the kidney start to grow uncontrollably and form tumors. Renal cell carcinoma, which occurs in the cells lining the kidneys (epithelial cells), is the most common type of kidney cancer. Eighty-five percent of all kidney tumors are renal cell carcinomas. **Wilms' tumor** is a rapidly developing cancer of the kidney most often found in children under four years of age.

Description

The kidneys are a pair of organs shaped like kidney beans that lie on either side of the spine just above the waist. Inside each kidney are tiny tubes (tubules) that filter and clean the blood, taking out the waste products and making urine. The urine that is made by the kidney passes through a tube called the ureter into the bladder. Urine is held in the bladder until it is discharged from the body. Renal cell carcinoma generally develops in the lining of the tubules that filter and clean the blood. Cancer that develops in the central portion of the kidney (where the urine is collected and drained into the ureters) is known as transitional cell cancer of the renal pelvis. Transitional cell cancer is similar to **bladder cancer**.

Kidney cancer accounts for approximately 2–3% of all cancers. In the United States, kidney cancer is the tenth most common cancer and the incidence has increased by 43% since 1973; the **death** rate has increased by 16%. According to the American Cancer Society, 35,710 Americans were diagnosed with kidney cancer in 2004, and 12,480 died from the disease. RCC accounts for 90–95% of malignant neoplasms that originate from the kidney.

Causes and symptoms

The causes of kidney cancer are unknown, but men seem to have a greater risk than women of contracting the disease; the male:female ratio in the United States and Canada is 3:2 as of the early

2000s. There is a strong association between cigarette **smoking** and kidney cancer. Cigarette smokers are twice as likely as non-smokers are to develop kidney cancer. Working around coke ovens has been shown to increase people's risk of developing this cancer. Certain types of painkillers that contain the chemical phenacetin are associated with kidney cancer. The United States government discontinued use of **analgesics** containing phenacetin about 20 years ago. **Obesity** may be yet another risk factor for kidney cancer. Some studies show a loose association between kidney cancer and occupational exposure to cadmium, petroleum products, lead, dry-cleaning solvents, trichloroethylene (TCE), and asbestos. Other risk factors for the development of kidney cancer include Hispanic heritage and preexisting von Hippel-Lindau disease.

The most common symptom of kidney cancer is blood in the urine (hematuria). Other symptoms include painful urination, **pain** in the lower back or on the sides, abdominal pain, a lump or hard mass that can be felt in the kidney area, unexplained weight loss, **fever**, weakness, **fatigue**, and high blood pressure.

Other symptoms may occur if the cancer has spread beyond its original location. Spread of kidney cancer most commonly occurs to the lung (55%), liver (33%), bone (33%), adrenal (20%), and opposite kidney (10%). Lymph node spread is also common, occurring in about 25% of patients).

Diagnosis

A diagnostic examination for kidney cancer includes taking a thorough medical history and making a complete **physical examination** in which the doctor will probe (palpate) the abdomen for lumps. Blood tests will be ordered to check for changes in blood chemistry caused by substances released by the tumor. Laboratory tests may show abnormal levels of iron in the blood. Either a low red blood cell count (anemia) or a high red blood cell count (erythrocytosis) may accompany kidney cancer. Occasionally, patients will have high calcium levels.

If the doctor suspects kidney cancer, an intravenous pyelogram (IVP) may be ordered. An IVP is an x-ray test in which a dye in injected into a vein in the arm. The dye travels through the body, and when it is concentrated in the urine to be discharged, it outlines the kidneys, ureters, and the urinary bladder. On an x-ray image, the dye will reveal any abnormalities of the urinary tract. The IVP may miss small kidney cancers.

Renal ultrasound is a diagnostic test in which sound waves are used to form an image of the kidneys.

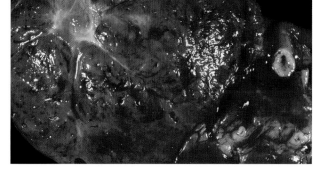

An extracted cancerous kidney. *(Custom Medical Stock Photo. Reproduced by permission.)*

Ultrasound is a painless and non-invasive procedure that can be used to detect even very small kidney tumors. Imaging tests such as **computed tomography scans** (CT scans) and **magnetic resonance imaging** (MRI) can be used to evaluate the kidneys and the surrounding organs. These tests are used to check whether the tumor has spread outside the kidney to other organs in the abdomen. If the patient complains of bone pain, a special x ray called a bone scan may be ordered to rule out spread to the bones. A **chest x ray** may be taken to rule out spread to the lungs.

A **kidney biopsy** is used to positively confirm the diagnosis of kidney cancer. During this procedure, a small piece of tissue is removed from the tumor and examined under a microscope. The biopsy will give information about the type of tumor, the cells that are involved, and the aggressiveness of the tumor (tumor stage).

Treatment

Each person's treatment is different and depends on several factors. The location, size, and extent of the tumor have to be considered in addition to the patient's age, general health, and medical history. In addition, much has changed in the treatment and management of kidney cancer since the 1980s, including new surgical techniques, new **anticancer drugs**, and the development of effective treatments for advanced disease.

The primary treatment for kidney cancer that has not spread to other parts of the body, which is a Stage I, II, or III tumor, is surgical removal of the diseased kidney (**nephrectomy**). Because most cancers affect only one kidney, the patient can function well with the remaining one. Two types of surgical procedure are used. Radical nephrectomy removes the entire kidney and the surrounding tissue. Sometimes, the lymph nodes surrounding the kidney are also removed. Partial nephrectomy removes only part of the kidney along with the tumor. This procedure is used either when the tumor is very small or when it is not practical to remove the entire kidney. It is not practical to remove a kidney when the patient has only one kidney or when both kidneys have tumors. There is a small (5%) chance of missing some of the cancer. Nephrectomy can also be useful for Stage IV cancers, but alternative surgical procedures such as transarterial angioinfarction may be used.

The rapid development and widespread use of laparoscopic techniques has made it possible for surgeons to remove small tumors while sparing the rest of the kidney. Most tumors removed by **laparoscopy** are 4 cm (1.6 in) in size or smaller. Laparoscopy also allows the surgeon to remove small tumors with cryoablation (destroying the tumor by freezing it) rather than cutting.

Radiation therapy, which consists of exposing the cancer cells to high-energy gamma rays from an external source, generally destroys cancer cells with minimal damage to the normal tissue. Side effects are **nausea**, fatigue, and stomach upsets. These symptoms disappear when the treatment is over. In kidney cancer, radiation therapy has been shown to alleviate pain and bleeding, especially when the cancer is inoperable. However, it has not proven to be of much use in destroying the kidney cancer cells. Therefore radiation therapy is not used very often as a treatment for cancer or as a routine adjuvant to nephrectomy. Radiotherapy, however, is used to manage metastatic kidney cancer.

Treatment of kidney cancer with anticancer drugs (**chemotherapy**) has not produced good results. However, new drugs and new combinations of drugs continue to be tested in clinical trials. One new drug, semaxanib (SU5416), is reported to have good results in treating patients with kidney cancer. As of 2004, however, semaxanib is still undergoing clinical trials in the United States.

Immunologic therapy (or immunotherapy), a form of treatment in which the body's immune system is harnessed to help fight the cancer, is a new mode of therapy that is being tested for kidney cancer. Clinical trials with substances produced by the immune cells (aldesleukin and interferon) have shown some promise in destroying kidney cancer cells. These substances have been approved for use but they can be very toxic and produce severe side effects. The benefits

derived from the treatment have to be weighed very carefully against the side effects in each case. Immunotherapy is the most promising systemic therapy for metastatic kidney cancer.

KEY TERMS

Biopsy—The surgical removal and microscopic examination of living tissue for diagnostic purposes.

Bone scan—An x-ray study in which patients are given an intravenous injection of a small amount of a radioactive material that travels in the blood. When it reaches the bones, it can be detected by x ray to make a picture of their internal structure.

Chemotherapy—Treatment with anticancer drugs.

Computed tomography (CT) scan—A medical procedure in which a series of x-ray images are made and put together by a computer to form detailed pictures of areas inside the body.

Cryoablation—A technique for removing tissue by destroying it with extreme cold.

Hematuria—Blood in the urine.

Immunotherapy—Treatment of cancer by stimulating the body's immune defense system.

Intravenous pyelogram (IVP)—A procedure in which a dye is injected into a vein in the arm. The dye travels through the body and concentrates in the urine to be discharged. It outlines the kidneys, ureters, and the urinary bladder. An x-ray image is then made and any abnormalities of the urinary tract are revealed.

Magnetic resonance imaging (MRI)—A medical procedure used for diagnostic purposes in which pictures of areas inside the body can be created using a magnet linked to a computer.

Nephrectomy—A medical procedure in which the kidney is surgically removed.

Radiation therapy—Treatment with high-energy radiation from x-ray machines, cobalt, radium, or other sources.

Renal ultrasound—A painless and non-invasive procedure in which sound waves are bounced off the kidneys. These sound waves produce a pattern of echoes that are then used by the computer to create pictures of areas inside the kidney (sonograms).

Prognosis

Because kidney cancer is often caught early and sometimes progresses slowly, the chances of a surgical cure are good. Length of survival depends on the size of the original tumor, the aggressiveness of the specific cells making up the tumor, and whether the cancer cells spread from the kidney to surrounding or distant tissues.

Kidney cancer is also one of the few cancers for which there are well-documented cases of spontaneous remission without therapy. Unfortunately, recurrences can occur even as long as ten years after the original diagnosis and treatment, and cancer can also crop up in the other, previously unaffected kidney.

Prevention

The exact cause of kidney cancer is not known, so it is not possible to prevent all cases. However, because a strong association between kidney cancer and tobacco has been shown, avoiding tobacco is the best way to lower one's risk of developing this cancer. Using care when working with cancer-causing agents such as asbestos and cadmium and eating a well-balanced diet may also help prevent kidney cancer.

Resources

BOOKS

Beers, Mark H., MD, and Robert Berkow, MD., editors. "Renal Cell Carcinoma (Hypernephroma; Adenocarcinoma of the Kidney)." Section 17, Chapter 233 In *The Merck Manual of Diagnosis and Therapy.* Whitehouse Station, NJ: Merck Research Laboratories, 2004.

Quek, Marcus L., and John P. Stein. "Malignant Tumors of the Urogenital Tract." In *Conn's Current Therapy 2001.* 53th ed. Philadlphia: W.B. Saunders Company, 2001.

PERIODICALS

Brauch, H., G. Weirich, B. Klein, et al. "VHL Mutations in Renal Cell Cancer: Does Occupational Exposure to Trichloroethylene Make a Difference?" *Toxicology Letters* 151 (June 15, 2004): 301–310.

Dutcher, J.P. "Immunotherapy: Are We Making a Difference?" *Current Opinion in Urology* September 2000: 435–9.

Godley, P.A., and K.I. Ataga. "Renal Cell Carcinoma." *Current Opinion in Oncology* May 2000: 260–4.

Griffiths, T. R., and J. K. Mellon. "Evolving Immunotherapeutic Strategies in Bladder and Renal Cancer." *Postgraduate Medical Journal* 80 (June 2004): 320–327.

Jennens, R. R., M. A. Rosenthal, G. J. Lindeman, and M. Michael. "Complete Radiological and Metabolic Response of Metastatic Renal Cell Carcinoma to SU5416 (Semaxanib) in a Patient with Probable von Hippel-Lindau Syndrome." *Urologic Oncology* 22 (May–June 2004): 193–196.

Lam, J. S., O. Svarts, and A. J. Pantuck. "Changing Concepts in the Surgical Management of Renal Cell Carcinoma." *European Urology* 45 (June 2004): 692–705.

Lotan, Y., D. A. Duchene, J. A. Cadeddu, et al. "Changing Management of Organ-Confined Renal Masses." *Journal of Endourology* 18 (April 2004): 263–268.

Moon, T. D., F. T. Lee, Jr., S. P. Hedican, et al. "Laparoscopic Cryoablation under Sonographic Guidance for the Treatment of Small Renal Tumors." *Journal of Endourology* 18 (June 2004): 436–440.

ORGANIZATIONS

American Cancer Society. 1599 Clifton Road, N.E., Atlanta, GA 30329. (800) 227-2345. <http://www.cancer.org>.

Cancer Research Institute (National Headquarters). 681 Fifth Avenue, New York, NY 10022. (800) 992-2623. <http://www.cancerresearch.org>.

National Cancer Institute (NCI). 9000 Rockville Pike, Building 31, Room 10A16, Bethesda, MD 20892. (800) 422-6237. <http://www.nci.nih.gov>.

National Kidney Cancer Association. 1234 Sherman Avenue, Suite 203, Evanston, IL 60202-1375. (800) 850-9132.

National Kidney Foundation. 30 East 33rd Street, New York, NY 10016. (800) 622-9010. <http://www.kidney.org>.

Rosalyn Carson-DeWitt, MD
Rebecca Frey, PhD

Kidney dialysis *see* **Dialysis, kidney**

Kidney disease

Definition

Kidney disease is a general term for any damage that reduces the functioning of the kidney. Kidney disease is also called renal disease.

Description

The kidneys are a pair bean-shaped, fist-sized organs that are located below the rib cage near the middle of the back. In adults they filter about 200 quarts (190 L) of blood every day to remove waste products that result from the normal activities of tissues in the body. These wastes circulate in the blood. and if not removed they would damage the body. The kidneys also play a crucial role in regulating the amount of water and chemicals (electrolytes) in the body such as sodium, potassium and phosphorous.

Inside the kidneys are about one million tiny units called nephrons. Inside each nephron is a very thin blood vessel called a capillary that twists around a very thin tube called a tubule. This combination of capillary and tubule inside the nephron is called a glomerulous and it is here that the blood is filtered. Water, electrolytes, and waste products (but not red blood cells) can pass across the capillary wall and into the tubule. The kidney then regulates how much water and which other substances can pass back into the blood in the capillary to keep the body in balance. Waste products, excess water, and excess electrolytes remain in the tubule and eventually leave the body as urine.

The kidneys also release three regulatory chemicals—erythropoietin, renin, and calcitriol—that affect other functions in the body. Erythropoietin stimulates the bone marrow to produce new red blood cells. Renin helps regulate blood pressure, and calcitriol is a form of vitamin D and is important in maintaining bones and the level of calcium in the body.

Because the kidney has many functions, there are many types of kidney disease. Congenital kidney diseases are disorders that are present at birth. **Polycystic kidney disease** (PKD) is a rare disorder in which children inherit defective genes from both parents that cause cysts full of fluid to develop in the kidneys and replace the blood filtering units. As a result, the kidneys cannot adequately remove wastes from the body. There are two other types of PDK. One is inherited, but does not appear until adulthood, and the other develops as a result of long-term kidney damage. In total, about half a million people in the United States have some form of PKD. Hereditary disease and **birth defects** are the most common causes of kidney disease in children up to age 14.

Acute kidney diseases are problems that develop suddenly. Many acute kidney diseases can be cured, but some may cause permanent damage. Common acute kidney diseases include kidney infection, hemolytic uremic syndrome, **nephrotic syndrome** in children, and damage caused by injury to the kidney or **poisoning**. Hemolytic uremic syndrome is a rare disease that usually affects children under age ten and is caused by eating food contaminated with bacteria. The bacteria release a poison that damages the kidney and causes **acute kidney failure**. Most children who develop this disease recover and their kidney function returns to normal.

Chronic kidney disease is disease that is slow to develop and usually does not show any symptoms until kidney damage is permanent. The National Kidney and Urologic Disease Information Clearinghouse, a federal agency, estimates that about 4.5% of people over age 20 have chronic kidney disease as indicated by tests that measure kidney function. The most common cause of chronic kidney disease in the United States is diabetes. It accounts for between 33% and 40% of all new cases of chronic kidney disease in the United States. In diabetes, the body cannot break down glucose (sugar). This extra glucose in the blood damages the nephrons so that they no longer filter blood effectively.

High or uncontrolled blood pressure (**hypertension**) is the second leading cause of chronic kidney disease. It accounts for between 27% and 30% of all new cases of chronic kidney disease. High blood pressure damages the capillaries in the nephron, so that they can no longer work with the tubules to filter the blood. Glomerulonephtitis is a term for several different chronic kidney diseases where damage to the nephrons causes protein or red blood cells pass into the urine. **Kidney cancer** is uncommon, accounting for only 2% of **cancer** cases.

Over-the-counter **analgesics** (**pain** medications) such as **aspirin**, **acetaminophen** (Tylenol), ibuprofen (Advil), naxopren sodium (Aleve), and similar medications that can be bought without a prescription may make kidney disease worse in individuals who already have kidney damage or cause kidney damage in healthy individuals who take these medications daily for several years. The chance of damage is increased when these pain medications are taken in combination with each other or with **caffeine** or codeine (Some painkilling tablets are a combination of pain medications and caffeine or codeine). Individuals who take these painkillers regularly or who have been told they have kidney damage should discuss the risk of these medications with their physician.

Chronic kidney disease can lead to end-stage renal disease (ESRD), in which there is almost total failure of the kidneys. If renal function is reduced to only 25% of normal, serious illness results. When this drops to 10–15% of normal, **death** occurs unless the individual receives dialysis or a kidney transplant. In 2002, there were over 100,300 new cases of ESRD, 44% of which were caused by diabetes. Treatment of ESRD in the United States cost about $25.2 billion in 2002.

Causes & symptoms

Causes of kidney disease are many and varied. Leading causes are diabetes, high blood pressure, inherited disease, and infection. Acute kidney disease is often marked by a lack of urination and increased fluid build up in the body. Chronic kidney disease is often called a "silent" killer, because no obvious symptoms develop until the kidneys are permanently damaged. The National Kidney Foundation estimated in 2005 that 20 million Americans had undetected moderate chronic kidney disease. Chronic kidney disease most often results from other diseases such as diabetes or hypertension.

Diagnosis

Simple blood and urine tests can indicated kidney disease, but more extensive testing may be needed to determine the exact nature of the disease. A blood test that measures serum creatinine, a waste product, can indicate how well the kidneys are working. Although normal levels of creatinine vary (an average range is 0.6–1.2 mg/dL), a higher than expected level in the blood may indicate kidney damage. A blood urea nitrogen (BUN) blood test measures waste products circulating in the blood. Normal levels range from 7%–20 mg/dL. The less well the kidney is working, the higher the BUN.

A 24-hour urine collection test will accurately measure how much urine the kidneys are producing in a day. A **urinalysis** can determine if protein or red blood cells are leaking into the urine indicating abnormal kidney function. A creatinine clearance test compares the amount of creatinine in a 24-hour urine sample with the amount of creatinine in the blood to determine how much blood the kidneys are filtering each minute.

Based on the results of blood and urine tests, other tests such as a CT scan, MRI, or **kidney biopsy** may be ordered.

Treatment

Most treatment for kidney disease involves treating the underlying cause of the disease, such as controlling high blood pressure or diabetes. Diuretic medication ("water pills") may be given to help relieve fluid accumulation. **Antibiotics** are used to treat kidney infections. Other drugs may be given to treat specific kidney diseases.

Diet and lifestyle changes are an important part of controlling kidney disease. **Obesity** increases blood pressure, so losing weight can help limit kidney damage, as can stopping **smoking**. Reducing sodium (salt) in the diet also helps control blood pressure. In certain kinds of kidney disease, potassium is removed in abnormally large quantities by the kidneys and

excreted in urine. Eating more foods such as bananas, dried beans and peas, nuts, and potatoes that are high in potassium or taking a potassium supplement pill help reverse this effect. When protein is found in the urine, some physicians recommend reducing the amount of protein (mainly found in meat) in the diet.

When kidneys fail completely in ESRD, there are only two alternatives: dialysis or kidney transplant. There are two types of dialysis. Peritoneal dialysis uses a membrane in the individual's abdomen to filter waste products. The most common kind of peritoneal dialysis is continuous ambulatory peritoneal dialysis (CAPD), in which the individual is hooked up to a bag of dialysis fluid that he carries with him, allowing continuous dialysis. The fluid is changed four times a day. In another form of peritoneal dialysis, the abdomen is filled with dialysis fluid. Wastes filter into the fluid for several hours often while the individual is asleep, the then the fluid is drained from the body. Peritoneal dialysis can be done at home without the need for a health care professional.

In hemodialysis, the individual must go to a dialysis center about three times a week. His blood is sent through a machine that filters out the waste and then returns the cleansed blood to his body. The process takes three to four hours and is done by a health care professional.

Kidney transplants can come from either a living donor or a deceased donor. Donors are matched with recipients based on blood type and must take drugs to prevent their immune system from rejecting the kidney after transplantation. The United Network for Organ Sharing (UNOS) coordinates matching donor kidneys with appropriate recipients. As of 2005, over 100 clinical trials were enrolling patients with various types of kidney disease. Information on current clinical trials can be found at < http://www.clinicaltrials.gov > .

Alternative treatment

Alternative treatments tend to focus on removing excess water from the body, but have limited effect on serious disease. Asparagus (*Asparagus officinalis*) birch tea(*Betula* species), goldenrod infusion(*Solidago* species), horsetail *Equisetum arvense*), and stinging nettle (*Urtica dioica*) all are used to stimulate urine production.

Prognosis

Many individuals recover normal kidney function after developing acute kidney disease, although in some cases, such as poisoning and injury, kidney

KEY TERMS

Congenital—Present at birth.

Diuretic—A substance that stimulates the kidney to excrete water.

Glomerulous—A twisted mass of blood capillaries and urine tubules in the kidney where filtering of waste products occurs.

Hormone—A chemical produced by living cells that travels through the circulatory system and affects tissue at some distance from where it was released.

Hypertension—High blood pressure.

Nephron—The smallest functional unit of the kidney involved in the removal of waste products and excess water from the blood.

damage may be permanent. Chronic kidney disease tends to get progressively worse as the individual ages. More than 15,000 kidney transplants are done each year, and there is a often long waiting list for donated kidneys. As of 2001 (last year for which statistics were available), 80.6% of individuals receiving a transplant from a deceased donor survived for at least 5 years, and 90.4% of individuals receiving a kidney donated from a living donor survived for at least 5 years.

Prevention

Maintaining a healthy body weight, getting regular **exercise**, and not smoking all promote kidney health. Controlling underlying diseases such as diabetes and high blood pressure are important in preventing chronic kidney diseases.

Resources

ORGANIZATIONS

American Association of Kidney Patients. 3505 East Frontage Road, Suite 315, Tampa, FL 33607. Telephone: 800-749-2257. < http://www.aakp.org >.

American Foundation for Urologic Disease. 1128 North Charles Street, Baltimore, MD 21201 Telephone: 800-242-2383. < http://www.afud.org >.

National Kidney Foundation. 30 East 33rd Street, New York, NY 10016 Telephone: 800-622-9010. < http://www.kidney.org >.

National Kidney and Urologic Disease Clearinghouse. 3 Information Way, Bethesda, MD 20892-3580. Telephone: 800-891-5390. < http://www.niddk.nih.gov >.

United Network for Organ Sharing (UNOS). P. O. Box 13770, Richmond, VA 23225. Telephone: 804-330-8500. < http://www.unos.org >.

OTHER

"Your Kidneys and How They Work." National Kidney and Urologic Disease Clearinghouse. July 2003 [cited 23 March 2005]. < http://www.kidney.niddke.nih.gov/kudiseases/pubs/yourkidneys/index.htm#rate >.

"Kidney Disease Overview." National Kidney Disease Education Program. 9 March 2005 [cited 23 March 2005]. < http://www.nkdep.nih.gov/patientspublic/kindeydiseaseoverview.htm#4 >.

Tish Davidson, A.M.

Kidney failure *see* **Acute kidney failure; Chronic kidney failure**

Kidney function tests

Definition

Kidney function tests is a collective term for a variety of individual tests and procedures that can be done to evaluate how well the kidneys are functioning.

Purpose

The kidneys, the body's natural filtration system, perform many vital functions, including removing metabolic waste products from the bloodstream, regulating the body's water balance, and maintaining the pH (acidity/alkalinity) of the body's fluids. Approximately one and a half quarts of blood per minute are circulated through the kidneys, where waste chemicals are filtered out and eliminated from the body (along with excess water) in the form of urine. Kidney function tests help to determine if the kidneys are performing their tasks adequately.

Precautions

A complete history should be taken prior to kidney function tests to assess the patient's food and drug intake. A wide variety of prescription and over-the-counter medications can affect blood and urine kidney function test results, as can some food and beverages.

Description

Many conditions can affect the ability of the kidneys to carry-out their vital functions. Some lead to a rapid (acute) decline in kidney function; others lead to a gradual (chronic) decline in function. Both result in a build-up of toxic waste substances in the blood. A number of clinical laboratory tests that measure the levels of substances normally regulated by the kidneys can help determine the cause and extent of kidney dysfunction. These tests are done on urine samples, as well as on blood samples.

Urine tests

There are a variety of urine tests that assess kidney function. A simple, inexpensive screening test, called a routine **urinalysis**, is often the first test administered if kidney problems are suspected. A small, randomly collected urine sample is examined physically for things like color, odor, appearance, and concentration (specific gravity); chemically for substances such as protein, glucose, and pH (acidity/ alkalinity); and microscopically for the presence of cellular elements (red blood cells, white blood cells, and epithelial cells), bacteria, crystals, and casts (structures formed by the deposit of protein, cells, and other substances in the kidneys' tubules). If results indicate a possibility of disease or impaired kidney function, one or more of the following additional tests is usually performed to more specifically diagnose the cause and the level of decline in kidney function.

- Creatinine clearance test. This test evaluates how efficiently the kidneys clear a substance called creatinine from the blood. Creatinine, a waste product of muscle energy metabolism, is produced at a constant rate that is proportional to the muscle mass of the individual. Because the body does not recycle it, all of the creatinine filtered by the kidneys in a given amount of time is excreted in the urine, making creatinine clearance a very specific measurement of kidney function. The test is performed on a timed urine specimen—a cumulative sample collected over a two to twenty-four hour period. Determination of the blood creatinine level is also required to calculate the urine clearance.

- Urea clearance test. Urea is a waste product that is created by protein metabolism and excreted in the urine. The urea clearance test requires a blood sample to measure the amount of urea in the bloodstream and two urine specimens, collected one hour apart, to determine the amount of urea that is filtered, or cleared, by the kidneys into the urine.

- Urine osmolality test. Urine osmolality is a measurement of the number of dissolved particles in urine. It is a more precise measurement than specific gravity for evaluating the ability of the kidneys to concentrate or dilute the urine. Kidneys that are functioning normally will excrete more water into the urine as fluid intake is increased, diluting the urine. If fluid intake is decreased, the kidneys excrete less water and the urine becomes more concentrated. The test may be done on a urine sample collected first thing in the morning, on multiple timed samples, or on a cumulative sample collected over a twenty-four hour period. The patient will typically be prescribed a high-protein diet for several days before the test and asked to drink no fluids the night before the test.

- Urine protein test. Healthy kidneys filter all proteins from the bloodstream and then reabsorb them, allowing no protein, or only slight amounts of protein, into the urine. The persistent presence of significant amounts of protein in the urine, then, is an important indicator of **kidney disease**. A positive screening test for protein (included in a routine urinalysis) on a random urine sample is usually followed-up with a test on a 24-hour urine sample that more precisely measures the quantity of protein.

Blood tests

There are also several blood tests that can aid in evaluating kidney function. These include:

- **Blood urea nitrogen test** (BUN). Urea is a by-product of protein metabolism. This waste product is formed in the liver, then filtered from the blood and excreted in the urine by the kidneys. The BUN test measures the amount of nitrogen contained in the urea. High BUN levels can indicate kidney dysfunction, but because blood urea nitrogen is also affected by protein intake and liver function, the test is usually done in conjunction with a blood creatinine, a more specific indicator of kidney function.

- Creatinine test. This test measures blood levels of creatinine, a by-product of muscle energy metabolism that, like urea, is filtered from the blood by the kidneys and excreted into the urine. Production of creatinine depends on an individual's muscle mass, which usually fluctuates very little. With normal kidney function, then, the amount of creatinine in the blood remains relatively constant and normal. For this reason, and because creatinine is affected very little by liver function, an elevated blood creatinine is a more sensitive indication of impaired kidney function than the BUN.

- Other blood tests. Measurement of the blood levels of other elements regulated in part by the kidneys can also be useful in evaluating kidney function. These include sodium, potassium, chloride, bicarbonate,

KEY TERMS

Blood urea nitrogen (BUN)—The nitrogen portion of urea in the bloodstream. Urea is a waste product of protein metabolism in the body.

Creatinine—The metabolized by-product of creatine, an organic acid that assists the body in producing muscle contractions. Creatinine is found in the bloodstream and in muscle tissue. It is removed from the blood by the kidneys and excreted in the urine.

Osmolality—A measurement of urine concentration that depends on the number of particles dissolved in it. Values are expressed as milliosmols per kilogram (mOsm/kg) of water.

Urea—A by-product of protein metabolism that is formed in the liver. Because urea contains ammonia, which is toxic to the body, it must be quickly filtered from the blood by the kidneys and excreted in the urine.

calcium, magnesium, phosphorus, protein, uric acid, and glucose.

Preparation

Patients will be given specific instructions for collection of urine samples, depending on the test to be performed. Some timed urine tests require an extended collection period of up to 24 hours, during which time the patient collects all urine voided and transfers it to a specimen container. Refrigeration and/or preservatives are typically required to maintain the integrity of such urine specimens. Certain dietary and/or medication restrictions may be imposed for some of the blood and urine tests. The patient may also be instructed to avoid **exercise** for a period of time before a test.

Aftercare

If medication was discontinued prior to a urine kidney function test, it may be resumed once the test is completed.

Risks

Risks for these tests are minimal, but may include slight bleeding from a blood-drawing site, hematoma (accumulation of blood under a puncture site), or **fainting** or feeling light-headed after venipuncture. In addition, suspension of medication or dietary changes imposed in preparation for some blood or urine tests may trigger side-effects in some individuals.

Normal results

Normal values for many tests are determined by the patient's age and sex. Reference values can also vary by laboratory, but are generally within the ranges that follow.

Urine tests

- Creatinine clearance. For a 24-hour urine collection, normal results are 90-139 ml/min for adult males less than 40 years old, and 80-125 ml/min for adult females less than 40 years old. For people over 40, values decrease by 6.5 ml/min for each decade of life.

- Urea clearance. With maximum clearance, normal is 64–99 ml/min.

- Urine osmolality. With restricted fluid intake (concentration testing), osmolality should be greater than 800 mOsm/kg of water. With increased fluid intake (dilution testing), osmolality should be less than 100 mOSm/kg in at least one of the specimens collected.

- Urine protein. A 24-hour urine collection should contain no more than 150 mg of protein.

Blood tests

- Blood urea nitrogen (BUN). 8–20 mg/dl.

- Creatinine. 0.8–1.2 mg/dl for males, and 0.6–0.9 mg/dl for females.

Abnormal results

Low clearance values for creatinine and urea indicate diminished ability of the kidneys to filter these waste products from the blood and excrete them in the urine. As clearance levels decrease, blood levels of creatinine and urea nitrogen increase. Since it can be affected by other factors, an elevated BUN, by itself, is suggestive, but not diagnostic, for kidney dysfunction. An abnormally elevated blood creatinine, a more specific and sensitive indicator of kidney disease than the BUN, is diagnostic of impaired kidney function.

Inability of the kidneys to concentrate the urine in response to restricted fluid intake, or to dilute the urine in response to increased fluid intake during osmolality testing may indicate decreased kidney function. Because the kidneys normally excrete almost no protein in the urine, its persistent presence, in amounts that exceed the normal 24-hour urine value, usually indicates some type of kidney disease as well.

Resources

ORGANIZATIONS

National Kidney Foundation. 30 East 33rd St., New York, NY 10016. (800) 622-9010. < http://www.kidney.org >.

Paula Anne Ford-Martin

Kidney nuclear medicine scan

Definition

A kidney nuclear medicine scan, or study, is a simple outpatient test that involves administering small amounts of radioactive substances, called tracers, into the body and then imaging the kidneys and bladder with a special camera. The images obtained can help in the diagnosis and treatment of certain kidney diseases.

Purpose

While many tests, such as x rays, ultrasound exams, or **computed tomography scans** (CT scans), can reveal the structure of the kidneys (its anatomy), the kidney nuclear medicine scan is unique in that it reveals how the kidneys are functioning. This is valuable information in helping a doctor make a diagnosis. Therefore, the kidney nuclear medicine scan is performed primarily to see how well the kidneys are working and, at the same time, they can identify some of the various structures that make up the kidney.

Precautions

If a patient is pregnant, it is generally recommended that she not have a kidney nuclear medicine scan. The unborn baby is more sensitive to radiation than an adult. If a woman thinks she might be pregnant, she should inform her doctor of this too.

Women who are breastfeeding should also inform their doctor. The doctor may recommend the woman stop breastfeeding for a day or two after a kidney nuclear medicine scan, depending on the particular tracer that was used since the tracer can accumulate in breast milk.

Description

Nuclear medicine is a branch of radiology that uses radioactive materials to diagnose or treat various diseases. These radioactive materials (tracers) may also be called radiopharmaceuticals, and they accumulate (collect) in specific organs in the body. Radiopharmaceuticals are able to yield valuable information about the particular organ being studied.

Whether outside the body or inside the body, tracers emit radioactive signals, called gamma rays, which can be collected and counted by a special device, called a gamma camera. The images of the kidney that the camera produces are called renal scans.

The kidney nuclear medicine scan can be performed on an outpatient basis, usually by a nuclear medicine technologist. The technologist helps prepare the patient for the exam by positioning him or her on an exam table or cart in the imaging area. The patient's position is usually flat on the back. The patient must lie still during imaging to prevent blurring of the images that will be taken. The technologist positions the camera as close to the kidney (or kidneys) as possible to obtain the best images.

In the next step of the procedure, the technologist injects the radiopharmaceutical into the patient. This may be done with one single injection or through an intravenous (IV) line. Immediately after the tracer is injected, imaging begins. It is important to obtain images right away because the tracer's radioactivity begins to diminish (decay). The time required for one-half of the tracer's activity to decay is called the tracer's half-life (T 1/2). The half-life is unique to each radiopharmaceutical. Also, it is important to see the kidney in its immediate state.

Serial pictures are taken with the gamma camera and may be seen on a computer or TV-like screen. The camera doesn't emit radiation, it only records it. The images then are stored on film.

A kidney nuclear medicine scan ranges from 45 minutes to three hours in length, depending on the goals of the test. But the test typically takes about an hour to an hour-and-a-half.

Once the images and curves are obtained, the nuclear medicine physician or radiologist analyzes, or reads, them. Various information can be provided to the doctor through these, depending on the test that was performed. A variety of kidney nuclear medicine studies are available for a doctor to help in making diagnoses. It is important to understand that kidney nuclear medicine scans are good at identifying when there is an abnormality, but they do not always identify the specific problem. They are very useful in providing information about how the various parts of the kidneys function, which, in turn, can assist in making a diagnosis.

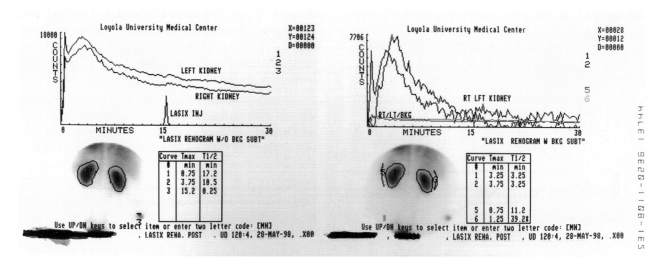

A computer-generated time activity curve generated from a renal scan. This time activity curve looks at the radiation count over a period of time. *(Photograph by Collette Placek. Reproduced by permission.)*

Studies may be performed to determine the rate at which the kidney's are filtering a patient's blood. These studies use a radiopharmaceutical, called Technetium DTPA (Tc 99m DTPA). This radiopharmaceutical also can identify obstruction (blockage) in the collecting system. To study how well the tubules and ducts of the kidney are functioning, the radiopharmaceutical Technetium MAG3 is used. Studying tubular function is a good indicator of overall renal function. In many renal diseases, one of the first things that disappears or diminishes is the tubular function.

Candidates for a kidney nuclear medicine scan are patients who have:

• Renal failure or chronic renal failure

• Obstruction in their urine collection systems

• **Renal artery stenosis**

• A kidney transplant.

Preparation

No preparation is necessary for a kidney nuclear medicine scan. The doctor may ask the patient to refrain from certain medications, however, before the scan if the medications might interfere with the test. For example, if a scan is being performed to study renal artery stenosis, the patient may have to refrain from taking medications for **hypertension**.

Aftercare

Patients can resume their normal daily activities immediately after the test. Most tracers are passed

---

KEY TERMS

Intravenous pyelogram (IVP)—X ray technique using dye to image the kidneys, ureters, and bladder.

Renal—Having to do with the kidneys.

Renal artery stenosis—Narrowing or constriction of the artery that supplies the kidney with blood.

---

naturally from the body, though drinking fluids after a kidney nuclear medicine scan can help flush the tracer into the urine and out of the body more quickly.

Risks

Nuclear medicine procedures are very safe. Unlike some of the dyes that may be used in x-ray studies, radioactive tracers rarely cause side effects. There are no long-lasting effects of the tracers themselves, because they have no functional effects on the body's tissues.

Normal results

The test reveals normal kidney function for age and medical situation.

Abnormal results

The test reveals a change in function that may be attributable to a disease process, such as obstruction or a malfunctioning kidney. If the test is abnormal, the patient may be recalled another day for a repeat study, performed differently, to narrow the list of causes.

Resources

ORGANIZATIONS

Society of Nuclear Medicine. 1850 Samuel Morse Dr., Reston, VA 10016. (703) 708-9000. <http://www.snm.org>.

Collette L. Placek

Kidney removal *see* **Nephrectomy**

Kidney stones

Definition

Kidney stones are solid accumulations of material that form in the tubal system of the kidney. Kidney stones cause problems when they block the flow of urine through or out of the kidney. When the stones move along the ureter, they cause severe **pain**.

Description

Urine is formed by the kidneys. Blood flows into the kidneys, and specialized tubes (nephrons) within the kidneys allow a certain amount of fluid from the blood, and certain substances dissolved in that fluid, to flow out of the body as urine. Sometimes, a problem causes the dissolved substances to become solid again. Tiny crystals may form in the urine, meet, and cling together to create a larger solid mass called a kidney stone.

Many people do not ever find out that they have stones in their kidneys. These stones are small enough to allow the kidney to continue functioning normally, never causing any pain. These are called "silent stones." Kidney stones cause problems when they interfere with the normal flow of urine. They can block (obstruct) the flow down the tube (the ureter) that carries urine from the kidney to the bladder. The kidney is not accustomed to experiencing any pressure. When pressure builds from backed-up urine, the kidney may swell (**hydronephrosis**). If the kidney is subjected to this pressure for some time, it may cause damage to the delicate kidney structures. When the kidney stone is lodged further down the ureter, the backed-up urine may also cause the ureter to swell (hydroureter). Because the ureters are muscular

tubes, the presence of a stone will make these muscular tubes spasm, causing severe pain.

About 10% of all people will have a kidney stone in his or her lifetime. Kidney stones are most common among:

- Caucasians
- Males
- People over the age of 30
- People who have had kidney stones previously
- Relatives of kidney stone patients

Causes and symptoms

Kidney stones can be composed of a variety of substances. The most common types of kidney stones include:

- Calcium stones. About 80% of all kidney stones fall into this category. These stones are composed of either calcium and phosphate, or calcium and oxalate. People with calcium stones may have other diseases that cause them to have increased blood levels of calcium. These diseases include primary parathyroidism, **sarcoidosis**, **hyperthyroidism**, **renal tubular acidosis**, **multiple myeloma**, hyperoxaluria, and some types of **cancer**. A diet heavy in meat, fish, and poultry can cause calcium oxalate stones.

- Struvite stones. About 10% of all kidney stones fall into this category. This type of stone is composed of magnesium ammonium phosphate. These stones occur most often when patients have had repeated urinary tract infections with certain types of bacteria. These bacteria produce a substance called urease, which increases the urine pH and makes the urine more alkaline and less acidic. This chemical environment allows struvite to settle out of the urine, forming stones.

- Uric acid stones. About 5% of all kidney stones fall into this category. Uric acid stones occur when increased amounts of uric acid circulate in the bloodstream. When the uric acid content becomes very high, it can no longer remain dissolved and solid bits of uric acid settle out of the urine. A kidney stone is formed when these bits of uric acid begin to cling to each other within the kidney, slowly growing into a solid mass. About half of all patients with this type of stone also have deposits of uric acid elsewhere in their body, commonly in the joint of the big toe. This painful disorder is called **gout**. Other causes of uric acid stones include **chemotherapy** for cancer, certain bone marrow disorders where blood cells

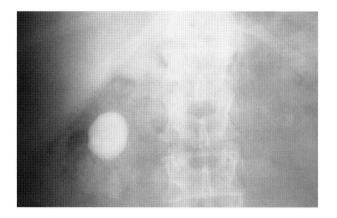

X ray of kidney stone. *(Custom Medical Stock Photo. Reproduced by permission.)*

are over-produced, and an inherited disorder called **Lesch-Nyhan syndrome**.

• Cystine stones. About 2% of all kidney stones fall into this category. Cystine is a type of amino acid, and people with this type of kidney stone have an abnormality in the way their bodies process amino acids in the diet.

Patients who have kidney stones usually do not have symptoms until the stones pass into the ureter. Prior to this, some people may notice blood in their urine. Once the stone is in the ureter, however, most people will experience bouts of very severe pain. The pain is crampy and spasmodic, and is referred to as "colic." The pain usually begins in the flank region, the area between the lower ribs and the hip bone. As the stone moves closer to the bladder, a patient will often feel the pain radiating along the inner thigh. In women, the pain may be felt in the vulva. In men, the pain may be felt in the testicles. **Nausea**, **vomiting**, extremely frequent and painful urination, and obvious blood in the urine are common. **Fever** and chills usually means that the ureter has become obstructed, allowing bacteria to become trapped in the kidney causing a kidney infection (**pyelonephritis**).

Diagnosis

Diagnosing kidney stones is based on the patient's history of the very severe, distinctive pain associated with the stones. Diagnosis includes laboratory examination of a urine sample and an x-ray examination. During the passage of a stone, examination of the urine almost always reveals blood. A number of x-ray tests are used to diagnose kidney stones. A plain x ray of the kidneys, ureters, and bladder may or may not reveal the stone. A series of x rays taken after injecting iodine dye into a vein is usually a more reliable way of seeing a stone. This procedure is called an intravenous pyelogram (IVP). The dye "lights up" the urinary system as it travels. In the case of an obstruction, the dye will be stopped by the stone or will only be able to get past the stone at a slow trickle.

When a patient is passing a kidney stone, it is important that all of his or her urine is strained through a special sieve. This is to make sure that the stone is caught. The stone can then be sent to a special laboratory for analysis so that the chemical composition of the stone can be determined. After the kidney stone has been passed, other tests will be required in order to understand the underlying condition that may have caused the stone to form. Collecting urine for 24 hours, followed by careful analysis of its chemical makeup, can often determine a number of reasons for stone formation.

Treatment

A patient with a kidney stone will say that the most important aspect of treatment is adequate pain relief. Because the pain of passing a kidney stone is so severe, narcotic pain medications (like morphine) are usually required. It is believed that stones may pass more quickly if the patient is encouraged to drink large amounts of water (2–3 quarts per day). If the patient is vomiting or unable to drink because of the pain, it may be necessary to provide fluids through a vein. If symptoms and urine tests indicate the presence of infection, **antibiotics** will be required.

Although most kidney stones will pass on their own, some will not. Surgical removal of a stone may become necessary when a stone appears too large to pass. Surgery may also be required if the stone is causing serious obstructions, pain that cannot be treated, heavy bleeding, or infection. Several alternatives exist for removing stones. One method involves inserting a tube into the bladder and up into the ureter. A tiny basket is then passed through the tube, and an attempt is made to snare the stone and pull it out. Open surgery to remove an obstructing kidney stone was relatively common in the past, but current methods allow the stone to be crushed with shock waves (called **lithotripsy**). These shock waves may be aimed at the stone from outside of the body by passing the necessary equipment through the bladder and into the ureter. The shock waves may be aimed at the stone from inside the body by placing the instrument through a tiny incision located near the stone. The stone fragments may then pass on their own or may be removed through the incision. All of these methods

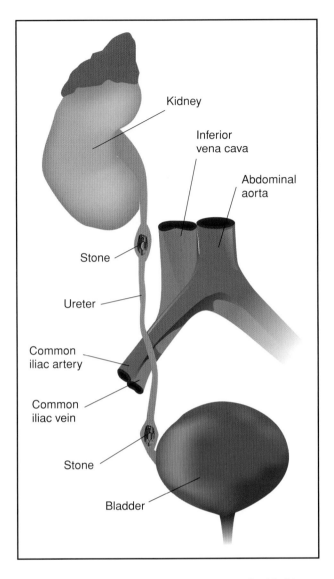

Kidney stones can occur in the ureter near the bladder or
kidney. *(Illustration by Argosy Inc.)*

reduce the patient's recovery time considerably when
compared to the traditional open operation.

Alternative treatment

Alternative treatments for kidney stones include the
use of herbal medicine, homeopathy, **acupuncture, acupressure**, hypnosis, or **guided imagery** to relieve pain.
Starfruit (*Averrhoa carambola*) is recommended to
increase the amount of urine a patient passes and to
relieve pain. Dietary changes can be made to reduce the
risk of future stone formation and to facilitate the resorp-
tion of existing stones. Supplementation with magnesium, a smooth muscle relaxant, can help reduce pain
and facilitate stone passing. Homeopathy and herbal

medicine, both western and Chinese, recommend a number of remedies that may help prevent kidney stones.

Prognosis

A patient's prognosis depends on the underlying
disorder causing the development of kidney stones. In
most cases, patients with uncomplicated calcium stones
will recover very well. About 60% of these patients,
however, will have other kidney stones. Struvite stones
are particularly dangerous because they may grow
extremely large, filling the tubes within the kidney.
These are called staghorn stones and will not pass out
in the urine. They will require surgical removal. Uric
acid stones may also become staghorn stones.

Prevention

Prevention of kidney stones depends on the type of
stone and the presence of an underlying disease. In almost
all cases, increasing fluid intake so that a person consistently drinks several quarts of water a day is an important
preventative measure. Patients with calcium stones may
benefit from taking a medication called a diuretic, which
has the effect of decreasing the amount of calcium passed
in the urine. Eating less meat, fish, and chicken may be
helpful for patients with calcium oxalate stones. Other
items in the diet that may encourage calcium oxalate
stone formation include beer, black pepper, berries, broccoli, chocolate, spinach, and tea. Uric acid stones may
require treatment with a medication called allopurinol.
Struvite stones will require removal and the patient
should receive an antibiotic. When a disease is identified
as the cause of stone formation, treatment specific to that
disease may lessen the likelihood of repeated stones.

Resources

ORGANIZATIONS

American Foundation for Urologic Disease. 300 West Pratt
St., Baltimore, MD 21201-2463. (800) 242-2383.
National Kidney Foundation. 30 East 33rd St., New York,
NY 10016. (800) 622-9010. < http://www.kidney.org >.

Rosalyn Carson-DeWitt, MD

Kidney transplantation

Definition

Kidney transplantation is a surgical procedure to
remove a healthy, functioning kidney from a living or

National Transplant Waiting List By Organ Type (June 2000)

Organ Needed	Number Waiting
Kidney	48,349
Liver	15,987
Heart	4,139
Lung	3,695
Kidney-Pancreas	2,437
Pancreas	942
Heart-Lung	212
Intestine	137

brain-dead donor and implant it into a patient with non-functioning kidneys.

Purpose

Kidney transplantation is performed on patients with **chronic kidney failure**, or end-stage renal disease (ESRD). ESRD occurs when a disease or disorder damages the kidneys so that they are no longer capable of adequately removing fluids and wastes from the body or of maintaining the proper level of certain kidney-regulated chemicals in the bloodstream. Without long-term dialysis or a kidney transplant, ESRD is fatal.

Precautions

Patients with a history of heart disease, lung disease, **cancer**, or hepatitis may not be suitable candidates for receiving a kidney transplant.

Description

Kidney transplantation involves surgically attaching a functioning kidney, or graft, from a brain-dead organ donor (a cadaver transplant) or from a living donor, to a patient with ESRD. Living donors may be related or unrelated to the patient, but a related donor has a better chance of having a kidney that is a stronger biological "match" for the patient.

The surgical procedure to remove a kidney from a living donor is called a *nephrectomy*. The kidney donor is administered **general anesthesia** and an incision is made on the side or front of the abdomen. The blood vessels connecting the kidney to the donor are cut and clamped, and the ureter is also cut between the bladder and kidney and clamped. The kidney and an attached section of ureter is removed from the donor. The vessels and ureter in the donor are then tied off and the incision is sutured together again. A similar procedure is used to harvest cadaver kidneys, although both kidneys are typically removed at once, and blood and cell samples for **tissue typing** are also taken.

Laparoscopic **nephrectomy** is a form of minimally-invasive surgery using instruments on long, narrow rods to view, cut, and remove the donor kidney. The surgeon views the kidney and surrounding tissue with a flexible videoscope. The videoscope and surgical instruments are maneuvered through four small incisions in the abdomen. Once the kidney is freed, it is secured in a bag and pulled through a fifth incision, approximately 3 in (7.6 cm) wide, in the front of the abdominal wall below the navel. Although this surgical technique takes slightly longer than a traditional nephrectomy, preliminary studies have shown that it promotes a faster recovery time, shorter hospital stays, and less post-operative **pain** for kidney donors.

Once removed, kidneys from live donors and cadavers are placed on ice and flushed with a cold preservative solution. The kidney can be preserved in this solution for 24–48 hours until the transplant takes place. The sooner the transplant takes place after harvesting the kidney, the better the chances are for proper functioning.

During the transplant operation, the kidney recipient patient is typically under general anesthesia and administered **antibiotics** to prevent possible infection. A catheter is placed in the bladder before surgery begins. An incision is made in the flank of the patient and the surgeon implants the kidney above the pelvic bone and below the existing, non-functioning kidney by suturing the kidney artery and vein to the patient's iliac artery and vein. The ureter of the new kidney is attached directly to the bladder of the kidney recipient. Once the new kidney is attached, the patient's existing, diseased kidneys may or may not be removed, depending on the circumstances surrounding the kidney failure.

Since 1973, Medicare has picked up 80% of ESRD treatment costs, including the costs of transplantation for both the kidney donor and recipient. Medicare also covers 80% of immunosuppressive medication costs for up to three years, although federal legislation was under consideration in early 1998 that may remove the time limit on these benefits. To qualify for Medicare ESRD benefits, a patient must be insured or eligible for benefits under Social Security, or be a spouse or child of an eligible American. Private insurance and state Medicaid programs often cover the remaining 20% of treatment costs.

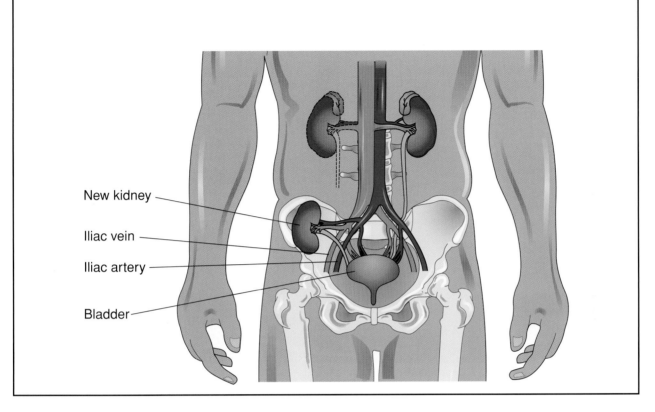

New kidney

Iliac vein

Iliac artery

Bladder

Kidney transplantation involves the surgical attachment of a functioning kidney, or graft, from a donor to a patient with end-stage renal disease (ESRD). During the procedure, the surgeon makes an incision in the patient's flank and implants the new kidney above the pelvic bone and below the non-functioning kidney by suturing the kidney artery and vein to the patient's iliac artery and vein. The ureter of the new kidney is then attached directly to the bladder of the patient. *(Illustration by Electronic Illustrators Group.)*

Preparation

Patients with chronic renal disease who need a transplant and do not have a living donor register with United Network for Organ Sharing (UNOS) will be placed on a waiting list for a cadaver kidney transplant. UNOS is a non-profit organization that is under contract with the federal government to administer the Organ Procurement and Transplant Network (OPTN) and the national Scientific Registry of Transplant Recipients (SR). Kidney availability is based on the patient's health status. The most important factor is that the kidney be compatible to the patient's body. A human kidney has a set of six antigens, substances that stimulate the production of antibodies. (Antibodies then attach to cells they recognize as foreign and attack them.) Donors are tissue-matched for 0 to 6 of the antigens, and compatibility is determined by the number and

strength of those matched pairs. Patients with a living donor who is a close relative have the best chance of a close match.

Potential kidney donors undergo a complete medical history and **physical examination** to evaluate their suitability for donation. Extensive blood tests are performed on both donor and recipient. The blood samples are used to tissue type for antigen matches, and confirm that blood types are compatible. A panel of reactive antibody (PRA) is performed by mixing white blood cells from the donor and serum from the recipient to ensure that the recipient antibodies will not have a negative reaction to the donor antigens. A urine test is performed on the donor to evaluate his kidney function. In some cases, a special dye that shows up on x rays is injected into an artery, and x rays are taken to show the blood supply of the donor kidney (a procedure called an arteriogram).

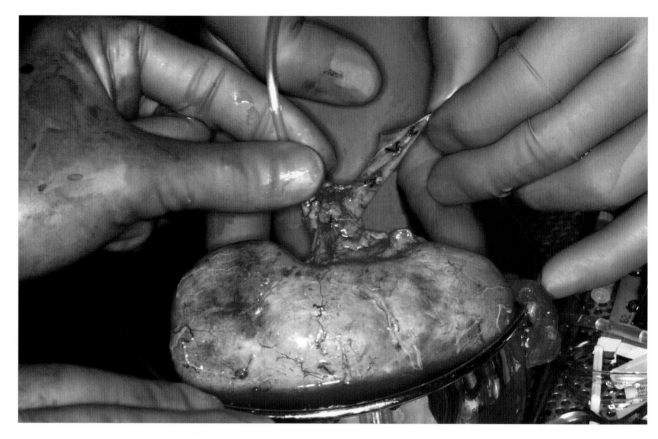

A human kidney is being prepped by medical personnel prior to transplantation. *(Photograph by Brad Nelson, Custom Medical Stock Photo. Reproduced by permission.)*

Once compatibility is confirmed and the physical preparations for kidney transplantation are complete, both donor and recipient may undergo a psychological or psychiatric evaluation to ensure that they are emotionally prepared for the transplant procedure and aftercare regimen.

Aftercare

Kidney donors and recipients will experience some discomfort in the area of the incision. Pain relievers are administered following the transplant operation. Patients may also experience **numbness**, caused by severed nerves, near or on the incision.

A regimen of immunosuppressive, or anti-rejection, medication is prescribed to prevent the body's immune system from rejecting the new kidney. Common immunosuppressants include cyclosporine, prednisone, and azathioprine. The kidney recipient will be required to take immunosuppressants for the life span of the new kidney. Intravenous antibodies may also be administered after transplant surgery. Daclizumab, a monoclonal antibody, is a promising new therapy that can be used in conjunction with standard immunosuppressive medications to reduce the incidence of organ rejection.

Transplant recipients may need to adjust their dietary habits. Certain immunosuppressive medications cause increased appetite or sodium and protein retention, and the patient may have to adjust his or her intake of calories, salt, and protein to compensate.

Risks

As with any surgical procedure, the kidney transplantation procedure carries some risk for both a living donor and a graft recipient. Possible complications include infection and bleeding (hemorrhage). The most common complication for kidney recipients is a urine leak. In approximately 5% of kidney transplants, the ureter suffers some damage, which results in the leak. This problem is usually correctable with follow-up surgery.

The biggest risk to the recovering transplant recipient is not from the operation or the kidney itself, but from the immunosuppressive medication he or she

KEY TERMS

Arteriogram—A diagnostic test that involves viewing the arteries and/or attached organs by injecting a contrast medium, or dye, into the artery and taking an x ray.

Dialysis—A blood filtration therapy that replaces the function of the kidneys, filtering fluids and waste products out of the bloodstream. There are two types of dialysis treatment—hemodialysis, which uses an artificial kidney, or dialyzer, as a blood filter; and peritoneal dialysis, which uses the patient's abdominal cavity (peritoneum) as a blood filter.

Iliac artery—Large blood vessel in the pelvis that leads into the leg.

Immunosuppressive medication—Drugs given to a transplant recipient to prevent his or her immune system from attacking the transplanted organ.

Rejection—The process in which the immune system attacks tissue it sees as foreign to the body.

Videoscope—A surgical camera.

must take. Because these drugs suppress the immune system, the patient is susceptible to infections such as cytomegalovirus (CMV) and varicella (**chickenpox**). The immunosuppressants can also cause a host of possible side effects, from high blood pressure to **osteoporosis**. Prescription and dosage adjustments can lessen side effects for some patients.

Normal results

The new kidney may start functioning immediately, or may take several weeks to begin producing urine. Living donor kidneys are more likely to begin functioning earlier than cadaver kidneys, which frequently suffer some reversible damage during the kidney transplant and storage procedure. Patients may have to undergo dialysis for several weeks while their new kidney establishes an acceptable level of functioning.

The success of a kidney transplant graft depends on the strength of the match between donor and recipient and the source of the kidney. Cadaver kidneys have a four-year survival rate of 66%, compared to an 80.9% survival rate for living donor kidneys. However, there have been cases of cadaver and living, related donor kidneys functioning well for over 25 years.

Studies have shown that after they recover from surgery, kidney donors typically have no long-term complications from the loss of one kidney, and their remaining kidney will increase its functioning to compensate for the loss of the other.

Abnormal results

A transplanted kidney may be rejected by the patient. Rejection occurs when the patient's immune system recognizes the new kidney as a foreign body and attacks the kidney. It may occur soon after transplantation, or several months or years after the procedure has taken place. Rejection episodes are not uncommon in the first weeks after transplantation surgery, and are treated with high-dose injections of **immunosuppressant drugs**. If a rejection episode cannot be reversed and kidney failure continues, the patient will typically go back on dialysis. Another transplant procedure can be attempted at a later date if another kidney becomes available.

Resources

ORGANIZATIONS

American Association of Kidney Patients. 100 S. Ashley Drive, #280, Tampa, FL 33602. (800) 749-2257. < http://www.aakp.org >.

American Kidney Fund (AKF). Suite 1010, 6110 Executive Boulevard, Rockville, MD 20852. (800) 638-8299. < http://www.arbon.com/kidney >.

National Kidney Foundation. 30 East 33rd St., New York, NY 10016. (800) 622-9010. < http://www.kidney.org >.

United Network for Organ Sharing (UNOS). 1100 Boulders Parkway, Suite 500, P.O. Box 13770, Richmond, VA 23225-8770. (804) 330-8500. < http://www.unos.org >.

United States Renal Data System (USRDS). The University of Michigan, 315 W. Huron, Suite 240, Ann Arbor, MI 48103. (734) 998-6611. < http://www.med.umich.edu/usrds >.

OTHER

Transweb. < http://www.transweb.org >.

Paula Anne Ford-Martin

Kidney ultrasound *see* **Abdominal ultrasound**

Kidney, ureter, and bladder x-ray study

Definition

A kidney, ureter, and bladder (KUB) x-ray study is an abdominal x ray. Despite its name, KUB does not show the ureters and only sometimes shows the kidneys and bladder and, even then, with uncertainty.

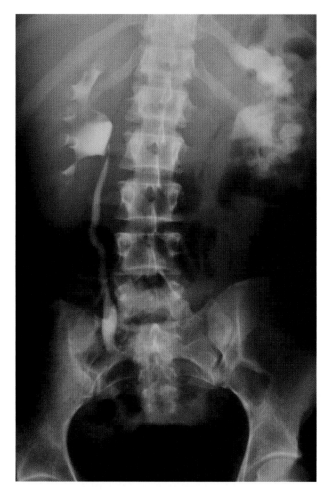

An x-ray image of a human torso and abdomen showing a blocked ureter. *(Custom Medical Stock Photo. Reproduced by permission.)*

Purpose

The KUB study is a diagnostic test used to detect **kidney stones** and to diagnose some gastrointestinal disorders. The KUB is also used as a follow-up procedure after the placement of devices such as ureteral stents and nasogastric or nasointestinal tubes (feeding tubes) to verify proper positioning.

Precautions

Because of the risks of radiation exposure to the fetus, pregnant women are advised to avoid this x-ray procedure.

A KUB study is a preliminary screening test for kidney stones, and should be followed by a more sophisticated series of diagnostic tests [such as an **abdominal ultrasound**, **intravenous urography**, or computed tomography scan (CT scan)] if kidney stones are suspected.

Description

A KUB is typically a single x-ray procedure. The patient lies flat on his back on an x-ray table. An x-ray plate is placed underneath him near the small of the back, and the x-ray camera is aimed at his abdomen. The patient is asked to hold his breath and lie still while the x ray is taken. Sometimes a second KUB will be ordered, with the patient standing, or if unable to do so, lying on his side.

Preparation

A KUB study requires no special diet, fluid restrictions, medications, or other preparation. The patient is typically required to wear a hospital gown or similar attire and to remove all jewelry so the x-ray camera has an unobstructed view of the abdomen. A lead apron may be placed over the abdominal areas of the body not being x rayed to shield the patient from unnecessary radiation.

Aftercare

No special aftercare treatment or regimen is required for a KUB study.

Risks

Because the KUB study is an x-ray procedure, it does involve minor exposure to radiation.

Normal results

Normal KUB x-ray films show two kidneys of a similar size and shape. A normal amount of intestinal gas is seen.

Abnormal results

Abnormal KUB films may show calculi (kidney stones). If both kidneys are visible, it may be possible to diagnose renal size discrepancies. The films may also show too much bowel gas indicating possible obstruction or soft tissue masses.

Resources

BOOKS

Pagana, Kathleen Deska. *Mosby's Manual of Diagnostic and Laboratory Tests.* St. Louis: Mosby, Inc., 1998.

Paula Anne Ford-Martin

Kinesiology, applied

Definition

Kinesiology is a series of tests that locate weaknesses in specific muscles reflecting imbalances throughout the body. Then specific massages or **acupressure** techniques are used in an attempt to rebalance what has been revealed by the kinesiology tests. Thus, kinesiology is used as both an assessment tool and as a limited therapeutic modality.

Purpose

Kinesiology claims to be a healing system that detects and corrects imbalances in the body before they develop into a disease, and which restores overall system balance and harmony. It is used to alleviate muscle, bone, and joint problems, treat all manner of aches and pains, and correct many areas of imbalance and discomfort.

Precautions

Since interpretation of the muscle tests is both complex and subjective, it should only be performed by a licensed health professional trained to look for "subclinical" symptoms (those which have not yet become a major problem). Kinesiology, itself, is more of a diagnostic technique and should not be thought of as a cure for any particular problem.

Description

Traditionally, the word "kinesiology" refers simply to the study of muscles and body movement. In 1964, however, American chiropractor George J. Goodheart founded what has become known as applied kinesiology when he linked oriental ideas about energy flow in the body with western techniques of muscle testing. First, Goodheart noted that all muscles are related to other muscles. He observed that for each movement a muscle makes, there is another muscle or group of muscles involved with that movement; one muscle contracts while another one relaxes. So when he was presented with a painful, overly-tight muscle, he would observe and treat the opposite, and necessarily weak, muscle to restore balance. This was then a very new technique.

Further, Goodheart argued that there is a definite and real connection between muscles, glands, and organs, and that by testing the strength of certain muscles he could learn about the health or condition of the gland or organ to which it was related.

Applied kinesiology is based on the idea that the body is an interacting unit made of different parts that interconnect and affect each other. Everything we do affects the body as a whole; therefore, a problem in one area can cause trouble in another area. According to kinesiology, the muscles eventually register and reflect anything that is wrong with any part of the body, whether physical or mental. Thus, a particular digestive problem might show up in the related and corresponding muscles of the legs. By testing the strength of certain muscles, the kinesiologist claims to be able to gain access to the body's communication system, and, thus, to read the health status of each of the body's major components.

The manual testing of muscles or muscle strength is not new, and was used in the late 1940s to evaluate muscle function and strength and to assess the extent of an injury. Applied kinesiology measures whether a muscle is stuck in the "on" position, acting like a tense muscle spasm, or is stuck "off," appearing weak or flaccid. It is called manual testing because it is done without instruments, using only the kinesiologist's fingertip pressure. During the first and longest appointment, which lasts about an hour, the kinesiologist conducts a complete consultation, asking about the patient's history and background. During the **physical examination**, patients sit or lie down, then the kinesiologist holds the patient's leg or arm to isolate a particular muscle. The practitioner then touches a point on the body which he believes is related to that muscle, and, with quick, gentle, and painless pressure, pushes down on the limb. Patients are asked to resist this pressure, and, if they cannot, an imbalance is suspected in the related organ, gland, or body part. This diagnostic technique uses muscles to find the cause of a problem, and is based on **traditional Chinese medicine** and its idea that the body has common energy meridians, or channels, for both organs and muscles. Kinesiologists also claim that they are able to locate muscle weaknesses that stem from a variety of causes such as **allergies**, mineral and vitamin deficiencies, as well as from problems with the lymph system. Once the exact cause is determined, the kinesiologist uses his fingertips to work the appropriate corresponding acupressure points in order to rebalance the flow of energy and restore health. Often he will recommend a complementary program of **nutrition** therapy.

Risks

There are no major risks associated with this gentle, noninvasive therapy. It is generally safe for people of all ages and has no side effects.

Normal results

If applied kinesiology does what it claims, patients should expect muscle testing to discover the cause of their physical complaint and to be told how to correct it.

Resources

ORGANIZATIONS

International College of Applied Kinesiology. 6405 Metcalf Ave., Suite 503, Shawnee Mission, KS 66202. (913) 384-5336. < http://www.icakusa.com > and < http://www.icak.com >.

Leonard C. Bruno, PhD

Kleine-Levin syndrome *see* **Sleep disorders**

Klinefelter syndrome

Definition

Klinefelter syndrome is a chromosomal disorder that affects only males. People with this condition are born with at least one extra X chromosome. The syndrome was first identified and described in 1942 by Harry Fitch Klinefelter, Jr., an American physician.

Description

Klinefelter syndrome is a condition in which one or more extra X chromosomes are present in a male. Boys with this condition appear normal at birth. They enter **puberty** normally, but by mid puberty have low levels of testosterone causing small testicles and the inability to make sperm. Affected males may also have learning disabilities and behavior problems such as **shyness** and immaturity, and an increased risk for certain other health problems.

Klinefelter syndrome is one of the most common chromosomal abnormalities. About 1 in every 500 to 800 males is born with this disorder; approximately 3000 affected boys are born each year in the United States. About 3% of the infertile male population have Klinefelter syndrome. The condition appears to affect all racial and ethnic groups equally.

Causes and symptoms

Chromosomes are found in the cells in the body. Chromosomes contain genes, structures that tell the body how to grow and develop. Chromosomes are responsible for passing on hereditary traits from parents to child. Chromosomes also determine whether the child will be male or female. Normally, a person has a total of 46 chromosomes in each cell, two of which are responsible for determining that individual's sex. These two sex chromosomes are called X and Y. The combination of these two types of chromosomes determines the sex of a child. Females have two X chromosomes (the XX combination); males have one X and one Y chromosome (the XY combination).

In Klinefelter syndrome, a problem very early in development results in an abnormal number of chromosomes. About 60% of embryos with Klinefelter syndrome do not survive the fetal period. Most commonly, a male with Klinefelter syndrome will be born with 47 chromosomes in each cell, rather than the normal number of 46. The extra chromosome is an X chromosome. This means that rather than having the normal XY combination, the male has an XXY combination. Because people with Klinefelter syndrome have a Y chromosome, they are all male.

Approximately 1/3 of all males with Klinefelter syndrome have other chromosomal abnormalities involving an extra X chromosome. Mosaic Klinefelter syndrome occurs when some of the cells in the body have an extra X chromosome and the others have normal male chromosomes. These males can have the same or milder symptoms than non-mosaic Klinefelter syndrome. Males with more than one additional extra X chromosome, such as 48,XXXY, are usually more severely affected than males with 47,XXY.

Klinefelter syndrome is not considered an inherited condition. The risk of Klinefelter syndrome reoccurring in another **pregnancy** is not increased above the general population risk.

The symptoms of Klinefelter syndrome are variable and not every affected person will have all of the features of the condition. Males with Klinefelter syndrome appear normal at birth and have normal male genitalia. From childhood, males with Klinefelter syndrome are taller than average with long limbs. Approximately 20–50% have a mild intention tremor, an uncontrolled shaking. Many males with Klinefelter syndrome have poor upper body strength and can be clumsy. Klinefelter syndrome does not cause homosexuality. Approximately 1/3 of males with Klinefelter syndrome have **gynecomastia** or breast growth, some requiring **breast reduction** surgery.

Most boys enter puberty normally, though some can be delayed. The Leydig cells in the testicles usually produce testosterone. With Klinefelter syndrome, the Leydig cells fail to work properly causing the testosterone production to slow. By mid-puberty, testosterone production is decreased to approximately half of normal. This can lead to decreased facial and pubic hair growth. The decreased testosterone also causes an increase in two other hormones, follicle stimulating hormone (FSH) and luteinizing hormone (LH). Normally, FSH and LH help the immature sperm cells grow and develop. In Klinefelter syndrome, there are few or no sperm cells. The increased amount of FSH and LH causes hyalinization and fibrosis, the growth of excess fibrous tissue, in the seminiferous tubules, where the sperm are normally located. As a result, the testicles appear smaller and firmer than normal. With rare exception, men with Klinefelter syndrome are infertile because they can not make sperm.

While it was once believed that all boys with Klinefelter syndrome are mentally retarded, doctors now know that the disorder can exist without retardation. However, children with Klinefelter syndrome frequently have difficulty with language, including learning to speak, read, and write. Approximately 50% of males with Klinefelter syndrome are dyslexic.

Some people with Klinefelter syndrome have difficulty with social skills and tend to be more shy, anxious, or immature than their peers. They can also have poor judgment and do not handle stressful situations well. As a result, they often do not feel comfortable in large social gatherings. Some people with Klinefelter syndrome can also have **anxiety**, nervousness and/or depression.

The greater the number of X chromosomes present, the greater the disability; each extra X chromosome lowers the child's IQ by about 15 points. Boys with several extra X-chromosomes have distinctive facial features, more severe retardation, deformities of bony structures, and even more disordered development of male features.

Diagnosis

Diagnosis of Klinefelter syndrome is made by examining chromosomes for evidence of more than one X chromosome present in a male. This can be done in pregnancy with prenatal testing such as a **chorionic villus sampling** or **amniocentesis**. Chorionic villus sampling is a procedure done early in pregnancy (approximately 10–12 weeks) to obtain a small sample of the placenta for testing. An amniocentesis is done further along in pregnancy (from approximately 16–18 weeks) to obtain a sample of fluid surrounding the baby for testing. Both procedures have a risk of **miscarriage**. Usually these procedures are done for a reason other than diagnosing Klinefelter syndrome. For example, a prenatal diagnostic procedure may be done on an older woman to determine if her baby has **Down syndrome**. If the diagnosis of Klinefelter syndrome is suspected in a young boy or adult male, chromosome testing can also be on a small blood or skin sample after birth.

Many men with Klinefelter syndrome go through life without being diagnosed. The two most common complaints leading to diagnosis of the condition are gynecomastia and **infertility**.

Treatment

There is no treatment available as of the early 2000s to change a person's chromosomal makeup. Children with Klinefelter syndrome may benefit from speech therapy for speech problems or other educational interventions for learning disabilities. Testosterone injections started around the time of puberty may help to produce more normal development including more muscle mass, hair growth and increased sex drive. Testosterone supplementation will not increase testicular size, decrease breast growth or correct infertility. Psychiatric consultation may be helpful when the boy reaches adolescence.

Some doctors recommend **mastectomy** as a surgical treatment for gynecomastia, on the grounds that the enlarged breasts are often socially stressful for affected males and significantly increase their risk of **breast cancer**.

Prognosis

While many men with Klinefelter syndrome go on to live normal lives, nearly 100% of these men will be sterile (unable to produce a child). However, a few men with Klinefelter syndrome have been reported who have fathered a child through the use of assisted fertility services.

Males with Klinefelter syndrome have an increased risk of several systemic conditions, including epilepsy, **osteoporosis**, such **autoimmune disorders** as lupus and arthritis, diabetes, and breast and germ cell tumors. One Danish study reported in 2004 that men with Klinefelter's syndrome have a slightly shortened life span, dying about 2.1 years earlier than men without the syndrome.

Resources

BOOKS

Beers, Mark H., MD, and Robert Berkow, MD., editors. "Chromosomal Abnormalities." Section 19, Chapter 261 In *The Merck Manual of Diagnosis and Therapy*. Whitehouse Station, NJ: Merck Research Laboratories, 2004.

Beers, Mark H., MD, and Robert Berkow, MD., editors. "Infertility." Section 18, Chapter 245 In *The Merck Manual of Diagnosis and Therapy*. Whitehouse Station, NJ: Merck Research Laboratories, 2004.

Probasco, Teri, and Gretchen A. Gibbs. *Klinefelter Syndrome*. Richmond, IN: Prinit Press, 1999.

PERIODICALS

Bojesen, A., S. Juul, N. Birkebaek, and C. H. Gravholt. "Increased Mortality in Klinefelter Syndrome." *Journal of Clinical Endocrinology and Metabolism* 89 (August 2004): 3830–3834.

Chen, Harold, MD. "Klinefelter Syndrome." *eMedicine* December 17, 2004. < http://emedicine.com/ped/topic1252.htm >.

Diamond, M., and L. A. Watson. "Androgen Insensitivity Syndrome and Klinefelter's Syndrome: Sex and Gender Considerations." *Child and Adolescent Psychiatric Clinics of North America* 13 (July 2004): 623–640.

Grosso, S., M. A. Farnetani, R. M. Di Bartolo, et al. "Electroencephalographic and Epileptic Patterns in X Chromosome Anomalies." *Journal of Clinical Neurophysiology* 21 (July-August 2004): 249–253.

Lanfranco, F., A. Kamischke, M. Zitzmann, and E. Nieschlag. "Klinefelter's Syndrome." *Lancet* 364 (July 17, 2004): 273–283.

Tyler, C., and J. C. Edman. "Down Syndrome, Turner Syndrome, and Klinefelter Syndrome: Primary Care throughout the Life Span." *Primary Care* 31 (September 2004): 627–648.

ORGANIZATIONS

Klinefelter's Organization. PO Box 60, Orpington, BR68ZQ. UK. < http://hometown.aol.com/KSCUK/index.htm >.

Klinefelter Syndrome and Associates, Inc. PO Box 119, Roseville, CA 95678-0119. (916) 773-2999 or (888) 999-9428. Fax: (916) 773-1449. ksinfo@genetic.org. < http://www.genetic.org/ks >.

National Organization for Rare Disorders (NORD). 55 Kenosia Avenue, P. O. Box 1968, Danbury, CT 06813-1968. (203) 744-0100. Fax: (203) 798-2291. < http://www.rarediseases.org >.

Carin Lea Beltz, MS
Rebecca J. Frey, PhD

Knee injuries

Definition

The five most common knee problems are arthritis, tendonitis, **bruises**, cartilage tears, and damaged ligaments. Knee injuries can be caused by accidents, impact, sudden or awkward movements, and gradual wear and tear of the knee joint.

Description

Because the knee joint is both vulnerable and used extensively in many activities, it is prone to injuries. The American Academy of Orthopaedic Surgeons estimates that 19.5 million visits to doctors' offices in 2002 were for knee problems. In some sports including football, skiing, and gymnastics, and racket sports, injury rates to avid practitioners can near 50 percent, and knee injuries are the most common reason patients visit orthopedic doctors. An estimated one in five runners gets a knee injury. The majority of knee injuries, however, are minor and do not require intensive treatment.

The knee, the largest joint in the body, connects the thighbone (femur) to the lower leg (tibia). It is a complex and efficient joint consisting of ligaments, cartilage, and the bone of the kneecap (patella). All of these parts can be injured. Inside the knee joint is synovial fluid that protects and lubricates the parts, which during injuries may increase and cause swelling. The bursa are sacs in the knee that contain synovial fluid and provide cushioning and lubrication.

Four ligaments comprise the knee joint. The medial collateral ligament (MCL) runs along the inside of the knee, while the lateral collateral ligament (LCL) is on the outside of the knee. The cruciate ligaments cross inside the knee. The anterior cruciate ligament (ACL) is deep inside the knee and limits rotation of the joint. The posterior cruciate ligament (PCL) is also inside the knee and limits the backward movement of the joint. Ligaments in the knee can be partially or completely torn, depending on the extent of the injury.

The minisci cartilage are two thin, oval-shaped tissues that act as cushions between the ends of the leg bones. The medial miniscus is the cartilage closest to the other leg while the lateral miniscus is nearer the outside of the knee. Injuries to the minisci include tears from injuries and impact and degenerative wearing away of the structure. The minisci can be partially or completely torn during injury.

The bones around the knee, including the kneecap, can be broken, fractured, or chipped. The patellar tendon connects the kneecap to the shinbone, while the quadriceps tendon connects the quadriceps muscle to the patella. The patellar tendon can be torn or can develop injury and **pain** from degeneration. It can also be fully dislocated or partially dislocated (called subluxation). The tendons in the knee may develop pain and inflammation known as tendonitis.

The bones of the knee joint are covered with tissue known as articular cartilage. This cartilage can be injured or fractured, and can also develop a degenerative condition called chondromalacia. **Osteoarthritis** is the pain associated with the wearing down of this cartilage.

Causes & symptoms

Arthritis may develop from an auto-immune disorder, known as **rheumatoid arthritis**, or may be caused by the gradual wear and tear of the joint, known as osteoarthritis. Symptoms of arthritis in the knee include pain ranging from dull aches to severe pain, and may be accompanied by swelling and range of movement loss. Arthritic symptoms may tend to be worst in the morning and decrease throughout the day as the knee is used. Arthritis can be caused by lupus, **Lyme disease**, and other infections. Knee swelling also may be caused by **bursitis**, the inflammation of the bursa.

Cartilage injuries may include chondromalacia, with symptoms including dull pain and pain while climbing stairs. Damage to the minisci cartilage often occurs from sudden twists, forceful plants, and awkward movements. A torn cartilage may make a popping sound, and may be accompanied by mild to severe pain, particularly while straightening the leg. Swelling, stiffening, and loss of movement are also symptoms of cartilage tears, as are clicking sounds and friction in the knee during movement.

Ligament injuries may cause dull or severe pain, swelling, loss of the range of movement of the joint, and loss of the stability and strength of the knee. Ligament injuries typically occur from strong blows and forces applied to the knee. Injuries to the MCL are the most common, often caused by impact to the side of the knee joint. Of the cruciate ligaments, the PCL is less commonly injured than the ACL. Typically, the PCL is injured by forceful blows to the knee, such as during car accidents, while the ACL can be injured by impacts and by sudden twists. Torn ligaments may be accompanied by a popping sound indicating the rupture, and may not always cause pain, so that some of them go unnoticed. Torn ligaments may weaken the knee and cause buckling or folding under weight.

Tendon injuries range from tendonitis to torn tendons. Symptoms of tendonitis include pain and swelling, while ruptured tendons can cause more intense pain, swelling, and loss of movement.

Osgood-Shlatter disease is a condition common in young boys who play running and jumping sports. Symptoms include inflammation of the patellar tendon and pain in the front of the knee during and after strenuous activity.

Iliotibial band syndrome is common in running and other repetitive sports, characterized by pain at the side of the knee caused by **stress** on the band of tendons there. Sometimes this condition causes a snapping sensation when the knee is straightened.

Diagnosis

Depending on the severity of the condition, family physicians or orthopedic physicians who specialize in the knee joint may be consulted. If arthritis is suspected, a rheumatologist may be consulted. The diagnosis process includes taking a complete patient history with details of the pain and the circumstances of the injury. The physician will give the patient a thorough **physical examination**, including utilizing several manual techniques of moving the knee joint and legs in various positions to help determine the type of injury. An experienced practitioner can often make an accurate diagnosis of injuries by performing a sequence of manual diagnostic tests.

Laboratory tests may be ordered to further or clarify the diagnosis. X rays can show damage to the bones as well as the narrowing of the knee space that may imply cartilage problems. For more in-depth diagnosis, a computerized axial tomographic (CAT) scan is an x-ray technique that can provide three-dimensional views of the bones in the knee. A **magnetic resonance imaging** (MRI) scan gives a computerized portrait of the interior of the knee, and may show damage to the ligaments and cartilage. **Arthroscopy** is a form of minor surgery that inserts a

tiny camera into the knee and gives a very accurate view of the joint. Radionuclide scanning (bone scans) use radioactive material injected into the bloodstream to monitor the blood flow in particular areas. If infection or rheumatoid arthritis is suspected, a physician may order blood tests for diagnosis. Biopsies, in which pieces of tissue are laboratory tested, may also be used for diagnosis.

Treatment

When a person suspects a knee injury, the first treatment recommended is R.I.C.E., which stands for rest, ice, compression, and elevation. First, the person should cease the activity which caused the injury and immediately rest and immobilize the joint. Ice may be applied to reduce pain and swelling, and compression, such as wraps and braces, may be used to immobilize the knee. Elevating the leg is also helpful in reducing swelling and aiding circulation. Immediate care will prevent the worsening of the injury.

Treatment options for knee injuries can range from rest and light activity, to physical therapy, to surgery. Most knee injuries are treated with proper rest, **exercise**, and strengthening programs recommended by physicians. For injuries that require surgery or deeper diagnosis, arthroscopy is the least invasive technique and has a quick recovery time associated with the procedure. Arthroscopy is commonly used to repair cartilage and partially torn ligaments. For severe knee injuries, **reconstructive surgery** or open knee surgery may be required. Full knee replacements may also be performed for severely damaged knees. After surgery, physical therapy programs for **rehabilitation** are recommended. Treatment for osteoarthritis includes over-the-counter painkillers, exercise, and weight reduction. For rheumatoid arthritis, more powerful prescription medications, such as steroids and stronger painkillers, and intensive physical therapy may be ordered. Knee injuries associated with infection may require **antibiotics**.

Alternative treatment

Alternative therapies for knee injuries focus on supporting the body's ability to heal itself. Various therapies may include bodywork and postural adjustments such as **chiropractic** and **Rolfing** work, in addition to physical therapy and gentle exercise routines. Herbal remedies and **nutritional supplements** may be used to aid the healing process and reduce symptoms. **Acupuncture** may be used for pain relief, and **yoga** is a low-impact exercise routine that increases flexibility, good alignment, and strength.

Prevention

The best prevention for knee injuries is being aware of activities that carry high risks for knee injuries and acting carefully. The knees can be strengthened by evenly building the muscles in the quadriceps and hamstrings. Increasing flexibility in the body through stretching can also help reduce injuries. Properly fitting shoes and other sports equipment are essential for preventing injury as well. Finally, before engaging in activities that stress the knee, a thorough and gradual warm-up routine, including aerobic activity and stretching, will lessen the chances of knee injury.

Resources

BOOKS

Grelsamer, Ronald, M.D. *What Your Doctor May Not Tell You about Knee Pain and Surgery.* Warner Books, 2002.

Halpern, Brian. *The Knee Crisis Handbook.* Rodale Books, 2003.

Scott, W. Norman. *Dr. Scott's Knee Book.* Fireside Books, 1996.

ORGANIZATIONS

American Academy of Orthopaedic Surgeons. P.O. Box 2058, Des Plaines, IL 60017. 800-824-BONE. < ttp://www.aaos.org >.

National Athletic Trainers' Association. 2952 Stemmons Freeway, Dallas, TX 75247-6196. (214) 637-6282. < http://www.nata.org >.

American Physical Therapy Association. 1111 North Fairfax St., Alexandria, VA 22314-1488. (703) 684-2782. < http://www.apta.org >.

Douglas Dupler

Knee replacement *see* **Joint replacement**

Kneecap removal

Definition

Kneecap removal, or patellectomy, is the surgical removal of the patella, commonly called the kneecap.

Purpose

Kneecap removal is done under three circumstances:

- When the kneecap is fractured or shattered
- When the kneecap dislocates easily and repeatedly
- When degenerative arthritis of the kneecap causes extreme **pain**

A person of any age can break a kneecap in an accident. When the bone is shattered beyond repair, the kneecap is removed. No prosthesis or artificial replacement part is put in its place.

Dislocation of the kneecap is most common in young girls between the ages of 10-14. Initially, the kneecap will pop back into place of its own accord, but pain may continue. If dislocation occurs too often, or the kneecap doesn't go back into place correctly, the patella may rub the other bones in the knee, causing an arthritis-like condition. Some people are born with **birth defects** that cause the kneecap to dislocate frequently.

Degenerative arthritis of the kneecap, also called patellar arthritis or *chondromalacia patellae*, can cause enough pain that it is necessary to remove the kneecap. As techniques of **joint replacement** have improved, arthritis in the knee is more frequently treated with total knee replacement.

Precautions

People who have had their kneecap removed for degenerative arthritis and then later have to have a total knee replacement are more likely to have problems with the stability of their artificial knee than those who only have total knee replacement. This is because the realigned muscles and tendons provide less support once the kneecap is removed.

Description

Kneecap removal is performed under either general or **local anesthesia** at a hospital or freestanding surgical center, by an orthopedic surgeon. The surgeon makes an incision around the kneecap. Then, the muscles and tendons attached to the kneecap are cut and the kneecap is removed. Next, the muscles are sewed back together, and the skin is closed with sutures or clips that stay in place about one week. Any hospital stay is generally brief.

Preparation

Prior to surgery, x rays and other diagnostic tests are done on the knee to determine if removing the kneecap is the appropriate treatment. Pre-operative blood and urine tests are also done.

Aftercare

Pain relievers may be prescribed for a few days. The patient will initially need to use a cane, or crutches, to walk. Physical therapy exercises to strengthen the knee should be begun immediately. Driving should be avoided for several weeks. Full recovery can take months.

Risks

Risks involved with kneecap removal are similar to those that occur in any surgical procedure, mainly allergic reaction to anesthesia, excessive bleeding, and infection.

Normal results

People who have kneecap removal because of a broken bone or repeated **dislocations** have the best chance for complete recovery. Those who have this operation because of arthritis may have less successful results, and later need a total knee replacement.

Resources

BOOKS

"Kneecap Removal." In *The Complete Guide to Symptoms, Illness and Surgery*, edited by H. Winter Griffith, et al, 3rd ed. New York: Berkeley Publishing, 1995.

Tish Davidson, A.M.

KOH test

Definition

The KOH test takes its name from the chemical formula for potassium hydroxide (KOH), which is the substance used in the test. The test, which is also called a potassium hydroxide preparation, is done to rapidly diagnose fungal infections of the hair, skin, or nails. A sample of the infected area is analyzed under a microscope following the addition of a few drops of potassium hydroxide.

Purpose

The primary purpose of the KOH test is the differential diagnosis of infections produced by dermatophytes and *Candida albicans* from other skin disorders. Dermatophytes are a type of fungus that invade the top layer of the skin, hair, or nails, and produce an infection commonly known as **ringworm**, technically known as tinea. It can appear as "jock itch" in the groin or inner thighs (tinea cruris); on the feet (tinea pedis); on the scalp and hair (tinea capitis); and on the nails (tinea unguium). Tinea versicolor appears anywhere on the skin and produces characteristic unpigmented patches. Tinea unguium affects the nails.

Similar symptoms of redness, scaling, and **itching** can be caused by other conditions, such as eczema and **psoriasis**. The KOH test is a quick, inexpensive test—often done in a physician's office—to see if these symptoms are caused by a dermatophyte. If a dermatophyte is found, treatment is started immediately; further tests are seldom necessary.

A yeast (candidal) infection of the skin or a mucous membrane, such as the mouth, often produces a white cheesy material at the infection site. This type of infection, known as thrush, is also identified with the KOH test.

Description

The KOH test involves the preparation of a slide for viewing under the laboratory microscope. KOH mixed with a blue-black dye is added to a sample from the infected tissues. This mixture makes it easier to see the dermatophytes or yeast under the microscope. The KOH dissolves skin cells, hair, and debris; the dye adds color. The slide is gently heated to speed up the action of the KOH. Finally the slide is examined under a microscope.

Dermatophytes are easily recognized under the microscope by their long branch-like structures.

KEY TERMS

Dermatophyte—A type of fungus that causes diseases of the skin, including tinea or ringworm.

KOH—The chemical formula for potassium hydroxide, which is used to perform the KOH test. The tests is also called a potassium hydroxide preparation.

Thrush—A disease of the mouth, caused by *Candida albicans* and characterized by a whitish growth and ulcers. It can be diagnosed with the KOH test.

Tinea—A superficial infection of the skin, hair, or nails, caused by a fungus and commonly known as ringworm.

Yeast cells look round or oval. The dermatophyte that causes tinea versicolor has a characteristic spaghetti-and-meatballs appearance.

If the KOH test is done in the doctor's office, the results are usually available while the person waits. If the test is sent to a laboratory, the results will be ready the same or following day. The KOH test is covered by insurance when medically necessary.

Preparation

The physician selects an infected area from which to collect the sample. Scales and cells from the area are scraped using a scalpel. If the test is to be analyzed immediately, the scrapings are placed directly onto a microscope slide. If the test will be sent to a laboratory, the scrapings are placed in a sterile covered container.

Normal results

A normal, or negative, KOH test shows no fungi (no dermatophytes or yeast).

Abnormal results

Dermatophytes or yeast seen on a KOH test indicate the person has a fungal infection. Follow-up tests are usually unnecessary.

Resources

PERIODICALS

Crissey, John Thorne. "Common Dermatophyte Infections. A Simple Diagnostic Test and Current Management."

Postgraduate Medicine February 1998: 191–192, 197–198, 200, 205.

Nancy J. Nordenson

Korsakoff's psychosis *see* **Korsakoff's syndrome**

Korsakoff's syndrome

Definition

Korsakoff's syndrome is a memory disorder which is caused by a deficiency of vitamin B_1, also called thiamine.

Description

In the United States, the most common cause of thiamine deficiency is **alcoholism**. Other conditions which cause thiamine deficiency occur quite rarely, but can be seen in patients undergoing dialysis (a procedure used primarily for patients suffering from kidney failure, during which the patient's blood circulates outside of the body, is mechanically cleansed, and then is circulated back into the body), pregnant women with a condition called **hyperemesis gravidarum** (a condition of extreme morning sickness, during which the woman vomits up nearly all fluid and food intake), and patients after surgery who are given vitamin-free fluids for a prolonged period of time. Thiamine deficiency is an important cause of disability in developing countries where the main source of food is polished rice (rice with the more nutritious outer husk removed).

An associated disorder, Wernicke's syndrome, often precedes Korsakoff's syndrome. In fact, they so often occur together that the spectrum of symptoms produced during the course of the two diseases is frequently referred to as Wernicke-Korsakoff syndrome. The main symptoms of Wernicke's syndrome include ataxia (difficulty in walking and maintaining balance), **paralysis** of some of the muscles responsible for movement of the eyes, and confusion. Untreated Wernicke's will lead to **coma** and then **death**.

Causes and symptoms

One of the main reasons that alcoholism leads to thiamine deficiency has to do with the high-calorie nature of alcohol. A person with a large alcohol intake often, in essence, substitutes alcohol for other, more nutritive calorie sources. Food intake drops off considerably, and multiple vitamin deficiencies develop. Furthermore, it is believed that alcohol increases the body's requirements for **B** **vitamins**, at the same time interfering with the absorption of thiamine from the intestine and impairing the body's ability to store and use thiamine. Direct neurotoxic (poisonous damage to the nerves) effects of alcohol may also play some role.

Thiamine is involved in a variety of reactions which provide energy to the neurons (nerve cells) of the brain. When thiamine is unavailable, these reactions cannot be carried out, and the important end-products of the reactions are not produced. Furthermore, certain other substances begin to accumulate, and are thought to cause damage to the vulnerable neurons. The area of the brain believed to be responsible for the symptoms of Korsakoff's syndrome is called the diencephalon, specifically the structures called the mamillary bodies and the thalamus.

An individual with Korsakoff's syndrome displays much difficulty with memory. The main area of memory affected is the ability to learn new information. Usually, intelligence and memory for past events is relatively unaffected, so that an individual may remember what occurred 20 years previously, but is unable to remember what occurred 20 minutes ago. This memory defect is referred to as anterograde **amnesia**, and leads to a peculiar symptom called "confabulation," in which a person suffering from Korsakoff's fills in the gaps in his or her memory with fabricated or imagined information. For instance, a person may insist that a doctor to whom he or she has just been introduced is actually an old high school classmate, and may have a lengthy story to back this up. When asked, as part of a memory test, to remember the name of three objects which the examiner listed ten minutes earlier, a person with Korsakoff's may list three entirely different objects and be completely convincing in his or her certainty. In fact, one of the hallmarks of Korsakoff's is the person's complete unawareness of the memory defect, and complete lack of worry or concern when it is pointed out.

Diagnosis

Whenever someone has a possible diagnosis of alcoholism, and then has the sudden onset of memory difficulties, it is important to seriously consider the diagnosis of Korsakoff's syndrome. While there is no specific laboratory test to diagnose Korsakoff's syndrome in a patient, a careful exam of the individual's mental state should be rather revealing. Although the patient's ability to confabulate answers may be convincing, checking the patient's retention of factual

information (asking, for example, for the name of the current president of the United States), along with the patient's ability to learn new information (repeating a series of numbers, or recalling the names of three objects ten minutes after having been asked to memorize them) should point to the diagnosis. Certainly a patient known to have just begun recovery from Wernicke's syndrome, who then begins displaying memory difficulties, would be very likely to have developed Korsakoff's syndrome. A **physical examination** may also show signs of Wernicke's syndrome, such as **peripheral neuropathy**.

Treatment

Treatment of both Korsakoff's and Wernicke's syndromes involves the immediate administration of thiamine. In fact, any individual who is hospitalized for any reason and who is suspected of being an alcoholic, should receive thiamine. The combined Wernicke-Korsakoff syndrome has actually been precipitated in alcoholic patients hospitalized for other medical illnesses, due to the administration of thiamine-free intravenous fluids (intravenous fluids are those fluids containing vital sugars and salts which are given to the patient through a needle inserted in a vein). Also, the vitamin therapy may be impaired by the feeding of carbohydrates prior to the giving of thiamine; since carbohydrates cannot be metabolized with thiamine.

Prognosis

Fifteen to twenty percent of all patients hospitalized for Wernicke's syndrome will die of the disorder.

Although the degree of ataxia nearly always improves with treatment, half of those who survive will continue to have some permanent difficulty walking. The paralysis of the eye muscles almost always resolves completely with thiamine treatment. Recovery from Wernicke's begins to occur rapidly after thiamine is given. Improvement in the symptoms of Korsakoff's syndrome, however, can take months and months of thiamine replacement. Furthermore, patients who develop Korsakoff's syndrome are almost universally memory-impaired for the rest of their lives. Even with thiamine treatment, the memory deficits tend to be irreversible, with less than 20% of patients even approaching recovery. The development of Korsakoff's syndrome often results in an individual requiring a supervised living situation.

Prevention

Prevention depends on either maintaining a diet with a sufficient intake of thiamine, or supplementing an inadequate diet with vitamin preparations. Certainly, one of the most important forms of prevention involves treating the underlying alcohol **addiction**.

Resources

ORGANIZATIONS

National Institute on Alcoholism Abuse and Alcoholism. 6000 Executive Boulevard, Willco Building, Bethesda, Maryland 20892-7003. < http://www.niaaa.nih.gov >.

Rosalyn Carson-DeWitt, MD

KUB *see* **Kidney, ureter, and bladder x-ray study**

Kuru *see* **Creutzfeldt-Jakob disease**

Kwashiorkor *see* **Protein-energy malnutrition**

Kyphosis

Definition

Kyphosis is the extreme curvature of the upper back also known as a hunchback.

Description

The upper back bone (thoracic region), is normally curved forward. If the curve exceeds 50° it is considered abnormal (kyphotic).

Causes and symptoms

Kyphosis can be divided into three ages of acquisition—birth, old age, and the time in between.

- Spinal **birth defects** can result in a fixed, exaggerated curve. Vertebrae can be fused together, shaped wrong, extraneous, or partially missing. Congenital and hereditary defects in bone growth weaken bone and result in exaggerated curves wherever gravity or muscles pull on them. Dwarfism is such a defect.

- During life, several events can distort the spine. Because the natural tendency of the thoracic spine is to curve forward, any weakness of the supporting structures will tend in that direction. A diseased thoracic vertebra (a spine bone) will ordinarily crumble its forward edge first, increasing the kyphotic curve. Conditions that can do this include **cancer**, **tuberculosis**, Scheuermann's disease, and certain kinds of arthritis. Healthy vertebra will fracture forward with rapid deceleration injuries, such as in car crashes when the victim is not wearing a seat belt.

- Later in life, kyphosis is caused from **osteoporosis**, bone weakness, and crumbling forward.

The **stress** caused by kyphosis produces such symptoms as an increase in musculoskeletal pains, tension headaches, back aches, and joint pains.

Diagnosis

A quick look at the back will usually identify kyphosis. X rays of the spine will confirm the diagnosis and identify its cause.

Treatment

Congenital defects have to be repaired surgically. The procedures are delicate, complicated, and lengthy. Often orthopedic hardware must be placed to stabilize the back bone. At other times, a device called a Milwaukee brace can hold the back in place from the outside. Fitting Milwaukee braces comfortably is difficult because they tend to rub and cause sores.

Kyphosis acquired during the younger years requires treatment directed at the cause, such as medications for tuberculosis. Surgical reconstruction or bracing may also be necessary.

Kyphosis induced by osteoporosis is generally not treated except to prevent further bone softening.

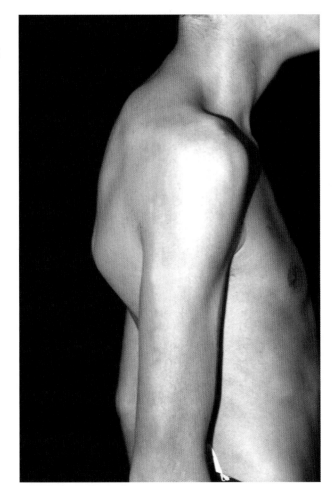

This patient's spine shows excessive backward curvature at the level of the upper chest. *(Custom Medical Stock Photo. Reproduced by permission.)*

Prognosis

Congenital kyphosis may be alleviated to some extent by surgery and bracing. Kyphosis occurring later in life may worsen over time.

Prevention

Preventing osteoporosis is within the grasp of modern medicine. Menopausal women must start early with estrogen replacement, calcium supplementation, and appropriate **exercise**. The treatment must continue through the remainder of life. Evidence suggests that a high calcium intake even during younger years delays the onset of symptomatic osteoporosis. Dairy products are the major dietary sources of calcium.

Resources

ORGANIZATIONS

Arthritis Foundation.1300 W. Peachtree St., Atlanta, GA 30309. (800) 283-7800. < http://www.arthritis.org >.

National Osteoporosis Foundation. 1150 17th St., Suite 500 NW, Washington, DC 20036-4603. (800) 223-9994. < http://www.nof.org >.

Osteoporosis and Related Bone Diseases-National Resource Center. 1150 17th S. NW, Ste. 500, Washington, DC 20036. (800) 624-2663.

J. Ricker Polsdorfer, MD

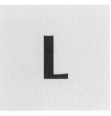

Labor and delivery *see* **Childbirth**

Labor induction *see* **Induction of labor**

Labyrinthitis

Definition

Labyrinthitis is an inflammation of the inner ear that is often a complication of **otitis media**. It is caused by the spread of bacterial or viral infections from the head or respiratory tract into the inner ear.

Description

Labyrinthitis is characterized by **dizziness** or feelings of **motion sickness** caused by disturbance of the sense of balance.

Causes and symptoms

Causes

The disease agents that cause labyrinthitis may reach the inner ear by one of three routes:

- Bacteria may be carried from the middle ear or the membranes that cover the brain.
- The viruses that cause **mumps**, **measles**, **influenza**, and colds may reach the inner ear following an upper respiratory infection.
- The **rubella** virus can cause labyrinthitis in infants prior to birth.

   Labyrinthitis can also be caused by toxic drugs.

Symptoms

The primary symptoms of labyrinthitis are vertigo (dizziness), accompanied by **hearing loss** and a sensation of ringing in the ears called **tinnitus**. Vertigo occurs because the inner ear controls the sense of balance as well as hearing. Some patients also experience **nausea and vomiting** and spontaneous eye movements in the direction of the unaffected ear. Bacterial labyrinthitis may produce a discharge from the infected ear.

Diagnosis

The diagnosis of labyrinthitis is based on a combination of the patient's symptoms and history–especially a history of a recent upper respiratory infection. The doctor will test the patient's hearing, and order a laboratory culture to identify the organism if the patient has a discharge.

If there is no history of a recent infection, the doctor will order extra tests in order to exclude injuries to the brain or Meniere's disease.

Treatment

Medication

Patients with labyrinthitis are given **antibiotics**, either by mouth or intravenously to clear up the infection. They may also be given meclizine (Antivert, Bonine) for vertigo and **nausea**.

Surgery

Some patients require surgery to drain the inner and middle ear.

Supportive care

Patients with labyrinthitis should rest in bed for three to five days until the acute dizziness subsides. Patients who are dehydrated by repeated **vomiting** may need intravenous fluid replacement. In addition, patients are advised to avoid driving or similar

KEY TERMS

Labyrinth—The bony cavity of the inner ear.

Meniere's syndrome—A disease of the inner ear marked by recurrent episodes of vertigo and roaring in the ears lasting several hours. Its cause is unknown.

Otitis media—Inflammation of the middle ear. It can lead to labyrinthitis.

Vertigo—A sensation of dizziness marked by the feeling that one's self or surroundings are spinning or whirling.

activities for four to six weeks after the acute symptoms subside, because they may have occasional dizzy spells during that period.

Prognosis

Most patients with labyrinthitis recover completely, although it often takes five to six weeks for the vertigo to disappear completely and the patient's hearing to return to normal. In a few cases the hearing loss is permanent.

Prevention

The most effective preventive strategy includes prompt treatment of middle ear infections, as well as monitoring of patients with mumps, measles, influenza, or colds for signs of dizziness or hearing problems.

Resources

BOOKS

Jackler, Robert K., and Michael J. Kaplan. "Ear, Nose, & Throat." In *Current Medical Diagnosis and Treatment, 1998* edited by Stephen McPhee, et al., 37th ed. Stamford: Appleton & Lange, 1997.

Rebecca J. Frey, PhD

Laceration repair

Definition

A laceration is a wound caused by a sharp object producing edges that may be jagged, dirty, or bleeding. Lacerations most often affect the skin, but any

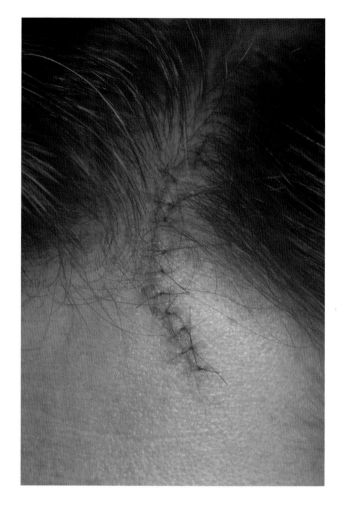

Eleven sutures are necessary to close up the laceration on this person's forehead. *(Custom Medical Stock Photo. Reproduced by permission.)*

tissue may be lacerated, including subcutaneous fat, tendon, muscle, or bone.

Purpose

A laceration should be repaired if it:

- Continues to bleed after application of pressure for ten to fifteen minutes
- Is more than one-eighth to one-fourth inch deep
- Exposes fat, muscle, tendon, or bone
- Causes a change in function surrounding the area of the laceration
- Is dirty or has visible debris in it
- Is located in an area where an unsightly scar is undesirable.

Precautions

Lacerations are less likely to become infected if they are repaired soon after they occur. Many physicians will not repair a laceration that is more than eight hours old because the risk of infection is too great.

Description

Laceration repair mends a tear in the skin or other tissue. The procedure is similar to repairing a tear in clothing. Primary care physicians, emergency room physicians, and surgeons usually repair lacerations. The four goals of laceration repair are to stop bleeding, prevent infection, preserve function, and restore appearance. Insurance companies do pay for the procedure. Cost depends upon the severity and size of the laceration.

Before repairing the laceration, the physician thoroughly examines the wound and the underlying tendons or nerves. If nerves or tendons have been injured, a surgeon may be needed to complete the repair. The laceration is cleaned by removing any foreign material or debris. Removing **foreign objects** from penetrating **wounds** can sometimes cause bleeding, so this type of wound must be cleaned very carefully. The wound is then irrigated with saline solution and a disinfectant. The disinfecting agent may be mild soap or a commercial preparation. An antibacterial agent may be applied.

Once the wound has been cleansed, the physician anesthetizes the area of the repair by injecting a local anesthetic. The physician may trim edges that are jagged or extremely uneven. Tissue that is too damaged to heal must be removed (**debridement**) to prevent infection. If the laceration is deep, several absorbable stitches (sutures) are placed in the tissue under the skin to help bring the tissue layers together. Suturing also helps eliminate any pockets where tissue fluid or blood can accumulate. The skin wound is closed with sutures. Suture material used on the surface of a wound is usually non-absorbable and will have to be removed later. A light dressing or an adhesive bandage is applied for 24-48 hours. In areas where a dressing is not feasible, an antibiotic ointment can be applied. If the laceration is the result of a human or

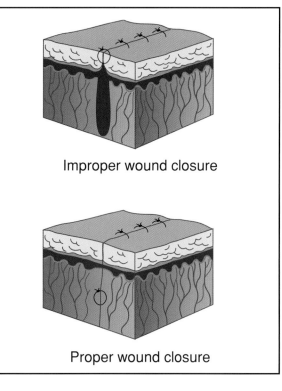

Improper wound closure

Proper wound closure

A laceration is a traumatic break in the skin caused by a sharp object producing edges that may be jagged, dirty, or bleeding. The underlying tissue may also be severed. In such instances, the physician may place absorbable sutures in the tissue to help bring the edges together before the skin is sutured close. *(Illustration by Electronic Illustrators Group.)*

animal bite, if it is very dirty, or if the patient has a medical condition that alters wound healing, oral **antibiotics** may be prescribed.

Aftercare

The laceration is kept clean and dry for at least 24 hours after the repair. Light bathing is generally permitted after 24 hours if the wound is not soaked. The physician will provide directions for any special wound care. Sutures are removed 3-14 days after the repair is completed. Timing of suture removal depends on the location of the laceration and physician preference.

The repair should be observed frequently for signs of infection, which include redness, swelling, tenderness, drainage from the wound, red streaks in the skin surrounding the repair, chills, or **fever**. If any of these occur, the physician should be contacted immediately.

Risks

The most common complication of any laceration repair is infection. Risk of infection can be minimized by cleansing the wound thoroughly. Wounds from bites or dirty objects or wounds that have a large amount of dirt in them are most likely to become infected.

All lacerations will heal with a scar. Wounds that are repaired with sutures are less likely to develop **scars** that are unsightly, but no one can predict how wounds will heal and who will develop unsightly scars. **Plastic surgery** can improve the appearance of many scars.

Resources

OTHER

"Caring for Cuts and Scrapes at Home." *Mayo Clinic Online.* < http://www.mayohealth.org/mayo/9611/htm/cuts_sb.htm >.
"Laceration Repair." *ThriveOnline.* < http://thriveonline.oxygen.com >.

Mary Jeanne Krob, MD, FACS

Lacerations *see* **Wounds**

Lacrimal duct obstruction

Definition

A lacrimal duct obstruction is blockage of the tear duct, the thin channel that normally drains tears from the surface of the eye.

Description

The lacrimal glands, located above each eyeball, produce tears. The tears flow over the eye, then drain through the nasolacrimal ducts. A tiny hole at the inner edge of each eyelid marks the opening of the ducts, which lead to the lacrimal sacs located on the side of the nose. The tears pass from the sacs into the nasolacrimal ducts and then into the nose.

When a tear duct becomes obstructed, tears may spill over the eyelids and run down the face. Stagnant tears within the system can become infected, leading to recurrent red eyes and infections. Excessive tearing can also produce secondary skin changes on the lower eyelids.

Causes and symptoms

An obstructed lacrimal tear duct can result in inflammation and infection of the lacrimal sac. The area beneath the eyes next to the nose can become red, inflamed, and sensitive to the touch. The area usually is swollen, and there may be a mucous discharge from the opening of the nasal corner of the eye. Common complaints include **itching**, irritation, burning, redness, foreign body sensation, and tearing.

Children frequently have a congenital lacrimal duct obstruction. Six to ten percent of all children are born before their tear ducts are open.

In adults, a common cause of lacrimal duct obstruction is involution, which is progressive degeneration occurring naturally with advancing age, resulting in shrivelling of organs or tissues. Other causes include **eyelid disorders**, infections by bacteria, viruses, fungi, and parasites, inflammations, the use of eye drops or excessive nasal spray, systemic **chemotherapy**, trauma from previous surgeries, injury to the bone at the side of the nose, foreign bodies, sinus disease, **nasal polyps**, and malignant or benign tumors.

Diagnosis

If the primary symptom is excessive tearing, the first step is for the health care professional to determine if the overflow of tears is due to an increase in tear production or a decrease in tear drainage. Causes of increased tear production may include trichiasis, a disease in which the eyelashes produce constant irritation, and eyelid malpositions and diseases. If abnormal tear production is ruled out, then obstructions in tear drainage is the most likely cause of the excessive tearing. Additional observations of swollen lacrimal sac area and purulent eye discharge indicate that there may be a lacrimal duct infection present. To further define the diagnosis, the lacrimal discharge may be cultured to determine possible infective agents, while various imaging techniques may be used to detect the type of obstruction. Dye tracer tests are also used to test for blockages.

Treatment

Lacrimal duct obstructions in children often resolve spontaneously, with 95% showing resolution before the child is one year old. Daily massaging of the lacrimal sac may help open the blockage. A topical antibiotic ointment may be applied if infection is present. If the blockage is not resolved after several weeks to months of this therapy, a physician may attempt forceful irrigation. Surgical probing to open up the duct under **general anesthesia** is a last resort, after a year or so of less invasive treatments.

In adults, conservative treatments are usually recommended. The infected or inflamed area may be massaged, with warm compresses applied to provide relief and speed the healing process. The health care

KEY TERMS

Lacrimal duct—A short canal leading from a small orifice at the medial angle of each eyelid to the lacrimal sac.

Lacrimal gland—An almond-shaped gland that secretes tears.

Lacrimal sac—The dilated upper end of the nasolacrimal duct in which the lacrimal ducts empty.

Nasolacrimal duct—A channel that transmits tears from the lacrimal sac to the nose.

Purulent—Consisting of or containing pus

Tear—A drop of the clear, salty fluid secreted by the lachrimal gland.

Trichiasis—A disease of the eye, in which the eyelashes, being turned in upon the eyeball, produce constant irritation by the motion of the lids.

provider may also massage or irrigate the infected area. Topical antibiotic ointments and oral **antibiotics** may also be used reduce infection. The use of **analgesics** such as **aspirin** may be recommended to control discomfort and reduce swelling. Severe cases may require surgical intervention to prevent future recurrences. Surgical approaches include insertion of a probe or catheter to remove an obstruction or creation of an artificial duct to bypass the obstruction.

Prognosis

If more conservative approaches fail to clear the obstruction, surgical procedures are available, with success rates greater than 90%.

Prevention

In many cases, the cause of a lacrimal duct obstruction is not known. However, in some cases, lacrimal duct obstruction may be caused by **smoking** and **abuse** of nasal sprays.

Resources

PERIODICALS

Camara, Jorge G., and Alfonso U. Bengzon. "Nasolacrimal Duct Obstruction." *eMedicine Journal* August 24, 2000. < http://www.emedicine.com/OPH/topic465.htm >.

Judith Sims

Lacrimal sac infection *see* **Dacryocystitis**

Lactate dehydrogenase isoenzymes test

Definition

The enzyme lactate dehydrogenase (also known as lactic dehydrogenase, or LDH) is found in the cells of almost all body tissues. The enzyme is especially concentrated in the heart, liver, red blood cells, kidneys, muscles, brain, and lungs. The total LDH can be further separated into five components or fractions labeled by number: LDH-1, LDH-2, LDH-3, LDH-4, and LDH-5. Each of these fractions, called isoenzymes, is used mainly by a different set of cells or tissues in the body. For this reason, the relative amounts of a particular isoenzyme of LDH in the blood can provide valuable diagnostic information.

Purpose

The LDH isoenzymes test assists in differentiating **heart attack**, anemia, lung injury, or **liver disease** from other conditions that may cause the same symptoms (differential diagnosis).

Precautions

Strenuous **exercise** may raise levels of total LDH, specifically the isoenzymes LDH-1, LDH-2, and LDH-5. Alcohol, anesthetics, **aspirin**, **narcotics**, procainamide, fluorides, and mithramycin may also raise levels of LDH. Ascorbic acid (vitamin C) can lower levels of LDH.

Description

LDH is found in the cells of almost all body tissues. When certain conditions injure cells in tissues containing LDH, it is released into the bloodstream. Because LDH is so widely distributed throughout the body, analysis of total LDH will not help make a diagnosis of a particular disease. Because this enzyme is actually composed of five different isoenzymes, however, analysis of the different LDH isoenzyme levels in the blood can help in the diagnosis of some diseases.

The five LDH isoenzymes are: LDH-1, LDH-2, LDH-3, LDH-4, and LDH-5. In general, each isoenzyme is used mostly by the cells in a specific tissue. LDH-1 is found mainly in the heart. LDH-2 is primarily associated with the system in the body that defends against infection (reticuloendothelial system). LDH-3 is found in the lungs and other tissues, LDH-4 in the kidney, placenta, and pancreas, and LDH-5 in liver and striated (skeletal) muscle. Normally, levels of LDH-2 are higher than those of the other isoenzymes.

Certain diseases have classic patterns of elevated LDH isoenzyme levels. For example, an LDH-1 level higher than that of LDH-2 is indicative of a heart attack or injury; elevations of LDH-2 and LDH-3 indicate lung injury or disease; elevations of LDH-4 and LDH-5 indicate liver or muscle disease or both. A rise of all LDH isoenzymes at the same time is diagnostic of injury to multiple organs. For example, a heart attack with congestive **heart failure** may cause symptoms of lung and liver congestion. Advanced **cancer** and autoimmune diseases such as lupus can also cause this pattern.

One of the most important diagnostic uses for the LDH isoenzymes test is in the differential diagnosis of myocardial infarction or heart attack. The total LDH level rises within 24–48 hours after a heart attack, peaks in two to three days, and returns to normal in approximately five to ten days. This pattern is a useful tool for a delayed diagnosis of heart attack. The LDH-1 isoenzyme level, however, is more sensitive and specific than the total LDH. Normally, the level of LDH-2 is higher than the level of LDH-1. An LDH-1 level higher than that of LDH-2, a phenomenon known as "flipped LDH," is strongly indicative of a heart attack. The flipped LDH usually appears within 12–24 hours after a heart attack. In about 80% of cases, flipped LDH is present within 48 hours of the incident. A normal LDH-1/LDH-2 ratio is considered reliable evidence that a heart attack has not occurred.

It should be noted that two conditions might cause elevated LDH isoenzymes at the same time and that one may confuse the other. For example, a patient with **pneumonia** may also be having an acute heart attack. In this instance, the LDH-1 level would rise with the LDH-2 and LDH-3. Because of this complication, some laboratories measure only the LDH-1 and consider an elevated LDH level with LDH-1 higher than 40% to be diagnostic of heart damage. LDH isoenzymes test is not used much anymore for diagnosis of heart attack. Tests for the protein troponin, which is found in myocardial cells, have been found to be more accurate.

Preparation

This test requires a blood sample. The patient need not fast (nothing to eat or drink) before the test unless requested to do so by the physician.

Risks

Risks for this test are minimal. The patient may experience slight bleeding from the blood-drawing site, **fainting** or feeling lightheaded after the vein is punctured (venipuncture), or an accumulation of blood under the puncture site (hematoma).

Normal results

Reference values for normal levels of LDH isoenzymes vary from laboratory to laboratory but can generally be found within the following ranges:

- LDH-1: 17-27%
- LDH-2: 27-37%
- LDH-3: 18-25%
- LDH-4: 8-16%
- LDH-5: 6-16%.

Abnormal results

Increased levels of LDH-1 are seen in myocardial infarction, red blood cell diseases like **hemolytic anemia**, **kidney disease** including **kidney transplantation** rejection, and testicular tumors. Increased levels of LDH-2 are found in lung diseases such as pneumonia and congestive heart failure, as well as in lymphomas and other tumors. Elevations of LDH-3 are significant in lung disease and certain tumors. Elevations of LDH-4 are greatly increased in **pancreatitis**. High levels of LDH-5 are found in liver disease, intestinal problems, and skeletal muscle disease and injury, such as **muscular dystrophy** and recent muscular trauma.

Diffuse disease or injury (for example, collagen disease, **shock**, low blood pressure) and advanced solid-tumor cancers cause significant elevations of all LDH isoenzymes at the same time.

Resources

BOOKS

Pagana, Kathleen Deska. *Mosby's Manual of Diagnostic and Laboratory Tests.* St. Louis: Mosby, Inc., 1998.

Janis O. Flores

Lactate dehydrogenase test

Definition

Lactate dehydrogenase, also called lactic dehydrogenase, or LDH, is an enzyme found in the cells of many body tissues, including the heart, liver, kidneys, skeletal muscle, brain, red blood cells, and lungs. It is responsible for converting muscle lactic acid into pyruvic acid, an essential step in producing cellular energy.

Purpose

Lactic dehydrogenase is present in almost all body tissues, so the LDH test is used to detect tissue alterations and as an aid in the diagnosis of **heart attack**, anemia, and **liver disease**. Newer injury markers are becoming more useful than LDH for heart attack diagnosis.

Precautions

Because the LDH enzyme is so widely distributed throughout the body, cellular damage causes an elevation of the total serum LDH. As a result, the diagnostic usefulness of this enzyme by itself is not as valuable as determination of the five fractions that comprise the LDH. These fractions are called isoenzymes and are better indicators of disease than is the total LDH. The fractions are LDH-1, LDH-2, LDH-3, LDH-4, and LDH-5. A normal total LDH level does not mean that individual isoenzyme levels should not be measured. Individual isoenzyme ranges can help differentiate a diagnosis.

Description

When disease or injury affects tissues containing LDH, the cells release LDH into the bloodstream, where it is identified in higher than normal levels.

KEY TERMS

Enzyme—A protein that regulates the rate of a chemical reaction in the body, increasing the speed at which the change occurs.

Isoenzyme—One of a group of enzymes that catalyze the same reaction but are differentiated by variations in physical properties.

For example, when a person has a heart attack, the LDH level begins to rise about 12 hours after the attack and usually returns to normal within 5-10 days. The LDH is also elevated in diseases of the liver, in certain types of anemia, and in cases of excessive destruction of cells, as in **fractures**, trauma, muscle damage, and **shock**.

Cancers can also elevate LDH level. Additionally, some patients have chronically elevated LDH with no identifiable cause and no apparent consequence.

Preparation

This test requires a blood sample. It is not necessary for the patient to fast (nothing to eat or drink) before the test unless the physician requests it.

Risks

Risks for this test are minimal, but may include slight bleeding from the blood-drawing site, **fainting** or feeling lightheaded after venipuncture, or hematoma (blood accumulating under the puncture site).

Normal results

Reference ranges for total LDH vary from laboratory to laboratory. Normal values are also higher in childhood. For adults, in most laboratories, the range can be up to approximately 200 units/L, but is usually found within 45-90 U/L.

Abnormal results

Due to the fact that many common disease processes cause elevations in the total LDH level, a breakdown of the five different isoenzymes that make up the total LDH is often helpful for diagnosis. In certain disorders, the total LDH may be within normal limits, but individual isoenzyme elevations can indicate specific organ or tissue damage. For example, the LDH-2 fraction is normally greater than LDH-1 in the blood.

After an acute heart attack, however, the LDH-1 rises over the LDH-2 in what is known as a "flipped LDH."

Certain diagnoses can be assisted by determination of the total LDH. One example is **infectious mononucleosis**, in which the LDH is usually more elevated than a liver enzyme called AST. Conversely, in cases of viral hepatitis, the liver enzymes AST and ALT are greatly increased over the LDH.

Resources

BOOKS

Pagana, Kathleen Deska. *Mosby's Manual of Diagnostic and Laboratory Tests.* St. Louis: Mosby, Inc., 1998.

Janis O. Flores

Lactation

Definition

Lactation is the medical term for yielding of milk by the mammary glands which leads to breastfeeding. Human milk contains the ideal amount of nutrients for the infant, and provides important protection from diseases through the mother's natural defenses.

Description

Early in a woman's **pregnancy** her milk-producing glands begin to prepare for her baby's arrival, and by the sixth month of pregnancy the breasts are ready to produce milk. Immediately after the baby is born, the placenta is delivered. This causes a hormone in the woman's body (prolactin) to activate the milk-producing glands. By the third to fifth day, the woman's breasts fill with milk.

Then, as the baby continues to suck each day, nursing triggers the continuing production of milk. The baby's sucking stimulates nerve endings in the nipple, which signal the mother's pituitary gland to release oxytocin, a hormone that causes the mammary glands to release milk to the nursing baby. This is called the "let-down reflex." While the baby's sucking is the primary stimulus for this reflex, a baby's cry, thoughts of the baby, or the sound of running water also may trigger the response. Frequent nursing will lead to increased milk production.

Breast milk cannot be duplicated by commercial baby food formulas, although both contain protein, fat, and carbohydrates. In particular, breast milk

changes to meet the specific needs of a baby. The composition of breast milk changes as the baby grows to meet the baby's changing needs. Most important, breast milk contains substances called antibodies from the mother that can protect the child against illness and **allergies**. Antibodies are part of the body's natural defense system against infections and other agents that can cause disease. Breast milk also helps a baby's own immune system mature faster. As a result, breast-fed babies have less **diarrhea** and fewer ear infections, **rashes**, allergies, and other medical problems than bottle-fed babies.

There are many other benefits to breast milk. Because it is easily digested, babies do not get constipated. Breast-fed babies may have fewer speech impediments, and breastfeeding can improve cheekbone development and jaw alignment.

Breastfeeding is also good for the mother. The act of breastfeeding releases hormones that stimulate the uterus to contract, helping it to return to normal size after delivery and reducing the risk of bleeding. The act of producing milk is thought to burn more calories, helping the mother to lose excess weight gained during pregnancy. However, research in 2004 disputed this belief when body composition changes of lactation and non-lactating women were compared at intervals for six months postpartum. Breastfeeding may be related to a lower risk of **breast cancer**, **ovarian cancer**, or **cervical cancer**. This benefit is stronger the younger a woman is when she breastfeeds; women who breastfeed before age 20 and nurse for at least six months have a 50% drop in the risk for breast **cancer**.

In addition, breastfeeding does not involve any formulas, bottles and nipples, or sterilizing equipment. Breast milk is free, and saves money by eliminating the need to buy formula, bottles, and nipples. Because breast-fed babies are healthier, health care costs for breast-fed infants are lower.

Procedure

Breastfeeding should begin as soon as possible after birth, and should continue every two to three hours. However, all babies are different; some need to nurse almost constantly at first, while others can go much longer between feedings. A baby should be fed at least 8-12 times in 24 hours. Because breast milk is easily digested, a baby may be hungry again as soon as one and one-half hours after the last meal.

Mothers should wear comfortable, loose, front-opening clothes and a good nursing bra. Mothers should find a comfortable chair with lots of pillows, supporting the arm and back. Feet should rest on a low footstool, with knees raised slightly. The baby should be level with the breast. The new mother may have to experiment with different ways of holding the baby before finding one that is comfortable for both the mother and baby.

Some babies have no trouble breastfeeding, while others may need some assistance. Once the baby begins to suck, the mother should make sure that the entire dark area around the nipple is in the baby's mouth. This will help stimulate milk flow, allowing the baby to get enough milk. It will also prevent nipple soreness.

Breastfeeding mothers will usually offer the baby both breasts at each feeding. Breastfeeding takes about 15-20 minutes on each side. After stopping the feeding on one side, the mother should burp the baby before beginning the feeding on the other breast. If the baby falls asleep at the breast, the next feeding should begin with the breast that was not nursed.

Mothers can tell if the baby is getting enough milk by checking diapers; a baby who is wetting between four to six disposable diapers (six to eight cloth) and who has three or four bowel movements in 24 hours is getting enough milk.

Nursing problems

New mothers may experience nursing problems, including:

- Engorged breasts. Breasts that are too full can prevent the baby from sucking. Expressing milk manually or with a breast pump can help.

- Sore nipples. In the early weeks nipples may become sore; a nipple shield can ease discomfort.

- Infection. Soreness and inflammation on the breast surface or a **fever** in the mother, may be an indication of breast infection. **Antibiotics** and continued nursing on the affected side may solve the problem.

Prognosis

There are no rules about when to stop breastfeeding. A baby needs breast milk for at least the first year of life; as long as a baby eats age-appropriate solid food, the mother may nurse for several years.

Prevention

Most common illnesses can not be transmitted via breast milk. However, some viruses, including HIV (the virus that causes **AIDS**) can be passed in breast milk; for this reason, women who are HIV-positive should not breastfeed.

KEY TERMS

Bromocriptine —A drug used to treat Parkinson's disease that can decrease a woman's milk supply.

Ergotamine—A drug used to prevent or treat migraine headaches. This can cause vomiting, diarrhea, and convulsions in infants.

Lithium—A drug used to treat manic depression (bipolar disorder) that can be transmitted in breast milk.

Methotrexate—An anticancer drug also used to treat arthritis that can suppress an infant's immune system when taken by a nursing mother.

Many medications have not been tested in nursing women, so it is not known if these drugs can affect a breast-fed child. A nursing woman should always check with her doctor before taking any medications, including over-the-counter drugs.

These drugs are not safe to take while nursing:

- Radioactive drugs for some diagnostic tests

- Chemotherapy drugs for cancer

- Bromocriptine

- Ergotamine

- Lithium

- Methotrexate

- Street drugs (including **marijuana**, heroin, amphetamines)

- Tobacco.

Resources

PERIODICALS

Wosje, Karen S., and Heidi J. Kalkwarf. "Lactation, Weaning, and Calcium Supplementation: Effects on Body Composition in Postpartum Women." *American Journal of Clinical Nutrition* August 2004: 676.

ORGANIZATIONS

International Lactation Consultants Assoc. 201 Brown Ave., Evanston, IL 60202. (708) 260-8874.

La Leche League International. 1400 North Meacham Rd., Schaumburg, IL 60173. (800) LA-LECHE.

National Alliance for Breastfeeding Advocacy. 254 Conant Rd., Weston, MA 02193. (617) 893-3553.

Carol A. Turkington
Teresa G. Odle

Lactic acid test

Definition

Lactic acid is an acid produced by cells during chemical processes in the body that do not require oxygen (anaerobic metabolism). Anaerobic metabolism occurs only when too little oxygen is present for the more usual aerobic metabolism (oxygen requiring). Lactic acid is a contributing factor in **muscle cramps**. It is also produced in tissues when conditions such as **heart attack** or **shock** reduce the blood supply responsible for carrying oxygen. Normally, lactic acid is removed from the blood by the liver. When an excess of lactic acid accumulates for any reason, the result is a condition called lactic acidosis.

Purpose

The lactic acid test is used as an indirect assessment of the oxygen level in tissues and to determine the cause and course of lactic acidosis.

Precautions

During blood collection, the patient should be instructed to relax the hand. Clenching and unclenching the fist will cause a build-up of potassium and lactic acid from the hand muscles that will falsely elevate the levels.

Description

The degree of acidity is an important chemical property of blood and other body fluids. Acidity is expressed on a pH scale where 7.0 is neutral, above 7.0 is basic (alkaline), and below 7.0 is acidic. A strong acid has a very low pH (near 1.0). A strong base has a very high pH (near 14.0). Blood is normally slightly alkaline or basic. It has a pH range of 7.35-7.45. The balance of acid to base in blood is precisely controlled. Even a minor deviation from the normal range can severely affect many organs.

Lactic acid (present in the blood as lactate ion) is a product of the breakdown of glucose to generate energy. It is found primarily in muscle cells and red blood cells. The lactate ion concentration in the blood depends on the rates of energy production and metabolism. Levels may increase significantly during **exercise**.

Together, lactic acid and another chemical (pyruvate) form a reversible reaction regulated by the oxygen supply to the blood and tissues. When oxygen levels are low, pyruvate converts to lactic acid; when oxygen levels are adequate, lactic acid converts to pyruvate. When the liver fails to metabolize lactose sufficiently or when too much pyruvate converts to lactate, lactic acidosis occurs. Measurement of blood lactate levels is recommended for all patients with symptoms of lactic acidosis. Testing is generally indicated if the blood pH level falls below 7.25-7.35.

Because of the close relationship between pyruvate and lactic acid, comparison of blood levels of the two substances can provide reliable information about tissue oxidation. However, pyruvate measurement is technically difficult and seldom performed. Lactic acid is measured more often, in either venous or arterial blood samples.

Preparation

This test requires a blood sample. The patient should have nothing to eat or drink (**fasting**) from midnight the night before the test. Because lactic acid is produced by exertion, the patient should rest for at least one hour before the test.

Risks

Risks for this test are minimal. The patient may experience slight bleeding from the blood-drawing site, **fainting** or feeling lightheaded after puncture of the vein (venipuncture), or an accumulation of blood under the puncture site (hematoma).

Normal results

Reference values vary from laboratory to laboratory but can be found within the following ranges:

- Venous blood: 4.5-19.8 mg/dL
- Arterial blood: 4.5-14.4 mg/dL

Abnormal results

High blood lactate levels, together with decreased oxygen in tissues, may be caused by strenuous muscle exercise, shock, hemorrhage, severe infection in the blood stream, heart attack, or cardiac arrest. When tissue oxygenation is low for no apparent reason, increased lactate levels may be caused by systemic disorders like diabetes, leukemia, **liver disease**, or kidney failure. Defects in enzymes may also be responsible, as in glycogen storage disease (von Gierke's disease). Lactate is also increased in certain instances of intestinal obstruction.

Lactic acidosis can be caused by taking large doses of **acetaminophen** and alcohol and by intravenous infusion of epinephrine, glucagon, fructose, or sorbitol. Antifreeze **poisoning** can also cause lactic acidosis. In rare instances, a diabetic medication, metformin (Glucophage), causes lactic acidosis. People with weak kidneys should not take metformin.

Resources

BOOKS

Pagana, Kathleen Deska, and Timothy James Pagana. *Mosby's Manual of Diagnostic and Laboratory Tests.* St. Louis: Mosby, Inc., 1998.

Paul A. Johnson, Ed.M.

Lactic acidosis *see* **Metabolic acidosis**

Lactogen test *see* **Prolactin test**

Lactogenic hormone test *see* **Prolactin test**

Lactose intolerance

Definition

Lactose intolerance refers to the inability of the body to digest lactose.

Description

Lactose is the form of sugar present in milk. The enzyme lactase, which is normally produced by cells lining the small intestine, breaks down lactose into substances that can be absorbed into the bloodstream. When dairy products are ingested, the lactose reaches the digestive system and is broken down by lactase into the simpler sugars glucose and galactose. The liver changes the galactose into glucose, which then enters the bloodstream and raises the blood glucose level. Lactose intolerance occurs when, due to a deficiency of lactase, lactose is not completely broken down and the glucose level does not rise. While not usually dangerous, lactose intolerance can cause severe discomfort.

From 30 to 50 million Americans suffer from the symptoms of lactose intolerance, but not everyone who is deficient in lactase experiences symptoms. Experts believe that 75% of the adult population worldwide does not produce enough lactase and is at risk for some or all of the symptoms of lactose intolerance.

Causes and symptoms

Lactose intolerance can be caused by some diseases of the digestive system and by injuries to the small intestine that result in a decreased production of lactase. While rare, some children are also born unable to produce the enzyme. For many, however, lactase deficiency develops naturally because, after about two years of age, the body produces less lactase.

Symptoms include **nausea**, cramps, **diarrhea**, bloating and gas. The symptoms usually occur between 30 minutes to two hours after eating or drinking lactose-containing foods.

Diagnosis

Usually, health care professionals measure the absorption of lactose in the digestive system by using the lactose tolerance test, hydrogen breath test or stool acidity test. Each of these can be performed outpatient, through a hospital, clinic or doctor's office.

People taking the lactose tolerance test must fast before being tested. They then drink a lactose-containing liquid for the test and medical personnel take blood samples during the next two hours to measure the patient's blood glucose level. The blood glucose level, or blood sugar level, indicates how well the body is digesting the lactose. A diagnosis of lactose intolerance is confirmed when blood glucose level does not rise. This test is not administered to infants and very young children because they are more prone to **dehydration**, which can result from diarrhea from the liquid.

Health care professionals measure the amount of hydrogen in the breath using the hydrogen breath test. Hydrogen is usually detected only in small amounts in the breath. However when undigested lactose found in the colon is fermented by bacteria, hydrogen in the breath is produced in greater quantities. The hydrogen is exhaled after being absorbed from the intestines and carried through the bloodstream to the lungs. The hydrogen breath test involves having the patient drink a lactose-containing beverage. Health care professionals monitor the breath at regular intervals to see if the hydrogen levels rise, which indicates improper lactose digestion. People taking the test who have had certain foods, medications or cigarettes before the test may get inaccurate results. While the test is available to children and adults, newborns and young children should not have it because of the risk of dehydration from drinking the beverage that can cause diarrhea in those who are lactose intolerant.

A stool acidity test measures the amount of acid in the stool. This is a safe test for newborns and young children. The test detects lactic acid and other short-chain fatty acids from undigested lactose fermented by bacteria in the colon. Glucose might also be in the stool sample, resulting form unabsorbed lactose in the colon.

Treatment

Pediatricians might recommend that parents of newborns and very young children who are suspected of having lactose intolerance simply change from cow's milk to a soya formula. Since there is no treatment that can improve the body's ability to produce lactase, lactose deficiency treatments instead, are focused on controlling the diet.

Most people affected by lactose intolerance do well if they limit their intake of lactose foods and drinks. People differ in the amounts they can handle before experiencing symptoms. Some have to stop lactose completely. People who are sensitive after ingesting small amounts of lactose can take lactase enzymes, which are available without a prescription. Using the liquid form, people can add a few drops in their milk, put the milk in the refrigerator and drink it after 24 hours, when the lactase enzymes have worked to reduce the lactose content by 70%. If the milk is heated first and double the amount of lactase liquid is added, the milk will be 90 percent lactose free. Recently, researchers have developed a chewable lactase enzyme tablet. By taking three to six tablets just before eating, the tablets help people digest lactose-containing solid foods. Supermarkets also carry lactose-reduced mild and other products, which contain the needed nutrients found in the regular products but without the lactose.

Foods that contain lactose are milk, low-fat milk, skim milk, chocolate milk, buttermilk, sweetened condensed milk, dried whole milk, instant nonfat dry milk, low-fat yogurts, frozen yogurts ice cream, ice

---

milk, sherbet, cheese, cottage cheese, low-fat cottage cheese, cream and butter. Other foods that may contain hidden lactose are: nondairy creamers, powdered artificial sweeteners, foods containing milk power or nonfat milk solids, bread, cake, margarine, creamed soups, pancakes, waffles, processed breakfast cereals, salad dressings, lunch meats, puddings, custards, confections and some meat products.

Prognosis

Lactose intolerance is easy to manage. People of all ages however, especially children, have to replace the calcium lost by cutting back on milk products by taking supplements and eating calcium-rich foods, such as broccoli, kale, canned salmon with bones, calcium-fortified foods and tofu. Many people who suffer with lactose intolerance will be able to continue eating some milk products. The condition is not considered dangerous.

Prevention

Often, lactose intolerance is a natural occurrence that cannot be avoided. However, people can prevent symptoms by managing the condition with diet and lactase supplements.

Resources

ORGANIZATIONS

American Dietetic Association. (800) 366-1655. < http://www.eatright.org/nfs/nfs43.html >.

OTHER

"Lactose Intolerance." Onebody.com. < http://www.onebody.com >.

Lisette Hilton

Lambliasis *see* **Giardiasis**

Laminectomy *see* **Disk removal**

Language disturbance *see* **Aphasia**

Laparoscopic cholecystectomy *see* **Cholecystectomy**

Laparoscopy

Definition

Laparoscopy is a type of surgical procedure in which a small incision is made, usually in the navel, through which a viewing tube (laparoscope) is inserted. The viewing tube has a small camera on the eyepiece. This allows the doctor to examine the abdominal and pelvic organs on a video monitor connected to the tube. Other small incisions can be made to insert instruments to perform procedures. Laparoscopy can be done to diagnose conditions or to perform certain types of operations. It is less invasive than regular open abdominal surgery (laparotomy).

Purpose

Since the late 1980s, laparoscopy has been a popular diagnostic and treatment tool. The technique dates back to 1901, when it was reportedly first used in a gynecologic procedure performed in Russia. In fact, gynecologists were the first to use laparoscopy to diagnose and treat conditions relating to the female reproductive organs: uterus, fallopian tubes, and ovaries.

Laparoscopy was first used with **cancer** patients in 1973. In these first cases, the procedure was used to observe and biopsy the liver. Laparoscopy plays a role in the diagnosis, staging, and treatment for a variety of cancers.

As of 2001, the use of laparoscopy to completely remove cancerous growths and surrounding tissues (in place of open surgery) is controversial. The procedure is being studied to determine if it is as effective as open surgery in complex operations. Laparoscopy is also being investigated as a screening tool for **ovarian cancer**.

Laparoscopy is widely used in procedures for noncancerous conditions that in the past required open surgery, such as removal of the appendix (**appendectomy**) and gallbladder removal (**cholecystectomy**).

Diagnostic procedure

As a diagnostic procedure, laparoscopy is useful in taking biopsies of abdominal or pelvic growths, as well as lymph nodes. It allows the doctor to examine the abdominal area, including the female organs, appendix, gallbladder, stomach, and the liver.

Laparoscopy is used to determine the cause of pelvic **pain** or gynecological symptoms that cannot be confirmed by a physical exam or ultrasound. For example, **ovarian cysts**, **endometriosis**, **ectopic pregnancy**, or blocked fallopian tubes can be diagnosed using this procedure. It is an important tool when trying to determine the cause of **infertility**.

Operative procedure

While laparoscopic surgery to completely remove cancerous tumors, surrounding tissues, and lymph nodes is used on a limited basis, this type of operation is widely used in noncancerous conditions that once required open surgery. These conditions include:

- Tubal ligation. In this procedure, the fallopian tubes are sealed or cut to prevent subsequent pregnancies.

- Ectopic **pregnancy**. If a fertilized egg becomes embedded outside the uterus, usually in the fallopian tube, an operation must be performed to remove the developing embryo. This often can be done with laparoscopy.

- Endometriosis. This is a condition in which tissue from inside the uterus is found outside the uterus in other parts of (or on organs within) the pelvic cavity. This can cause cysts to form. Endometriosis is diagnosed with laparoscopy, and in some cases the cysts and other tissue can be removed during laparoscopy.

- Hysterectomy. This procedure to remove the uterus can, in some cases, be performed using laparoscopy. The uterus is cut away with the aid of the laparoscopic instruments and then the uterus is removed through the vagina.

- Ovarian masses. Tumors or cysts in the ovaries can be removed using laparoscopy.

- Appendectomy. This surgery to remove an inflamed appendix required open surgery in the past. It is now routinely performed with laparoscopy.

- Cholecystectomy. Like appendectomy, this procedure to remove the gall bladder used to require open surgery. Now it can be performed with laparoscopy, in some cases.

In contrast to open abdominal surgery, laparoscopy usually involves less pain, less risk, less scarring, and faster recovery. Because laparoscopy is so much less invasive than traditional abdominal surgery, patients can leave the hospital sooner.

Cancer staging

Laparoscopy can be used in determining the spread of certain cancers. Sometimes it is combined with ultrasound. Although laparoscopy is a useful staging tool, its use depends on a variety of factors, which are considered for each patient. Types of cancers where laparoscopy may be used to determine the spread of the disease include:

- Liver cancer. Laparoscopy is an important tool for determining if cancer is present in the liver. When a patient has non-liver cancer, the liver is often checked to see if the cancer has spread there. Laparoscopy can identify up to 90% of malignant lesions that have spread to that organ from a cancer located elsewhere in the body. While computerized tomography (CT) can find cancerous lesions that are 0.4 in (10 mil) in size, laparoscopy is capable of locating lesions that are as small as 0.04 in (1 millimeter).

- Pancreatic cancer. Laparoscopy has been used to evaluate pancreatic cancer for years. In fact, the first reported use of laparoscopy in the United States was in a case involving pancreatic cancer.

- Esophageal and stomach cancers. Laparoscopy has been found to be more effective than **magnetic resonance imaging** (MRI) or computerized tomography (CT) in diagnosing the spread of cancer from these organs.

- **Hodgkin's disease**. Some patients with Hodgkin's disease have surgical procedures to evaluate lymph nodes for cancer. Laparoscopy is sometimes selected over laparotomy for this procedure. In addition, the spleen may be removed in patients with Hodgkin's disease. Laparoscopy is the standard surgical technique for this procedure, which is called a splenectomy.

- **Prostate cancer**. Patients with prostate cancer may have the nearby lymph nodes examined. Laparoscopy is an important tool in this procedure.

Cancer treatment

Laparoscopy is sometimes used as part of a palliative cancer treatment. This type of treatment is not a cure, but can often lessen the symptoms. An example is the feeding tube, which cancer patients may have if they are unable to take in food by mouth. The feeding tube provides **nutrition** directly into the stomach. Inserting the tube with a laparoscopy saves the patient the ordeal of open surgery.

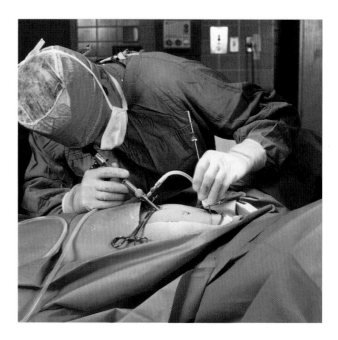

This surgeon is performing a laparoscopic procedure on a patient. *(Photo Researchers, Inc. Reproduced by permission.)*

Precautions

As with any surgury, patients should notify their physician of any medications they are taking (prescription, over-the-counter, or herbal) and of any **allergies**. Precautions vary due to the several different purposes for laparoscopy. Patients should expect to rest for several days after the procedure, and should set up a comfortable environment in their home (with items such as pain medication, heating pads, feminine products, comfortable clothing, and food readily accessible) prior to surgery.

Description

Laparoscopy is a surgical procedure that is done in the hospital under anesthesia. For diagnosis and biopsy, **local anesthesia** is sometimes used. In operative procedures, such as abdominal surgery, **general anesthesia** is required. Before starting the procedure, a catheter is inserted through the urethra to empty the bladder, and the skin of the abdomen is cleaned.

After the patient is anesthetized, a hollow needle is inserted into the abdomen in or near the navel, and carbon dioxide gas is pumped through the needle to expand the abdomen. This allows the surgeon a better view of the internal organs. The laparoscope is then inserted through this incision to look at the internal organs. The image from the camera attached to the end of the laparoscope is seen on a video monitor.

Sometimes, additional small incisions are made to insert other instruments that are used to lift the tubes and ovaries for examination or to perform surgical procedures.

Preparation

Patients should not eat or drink after midnight on the night before the procedure.

Aftercare

After the operation, nurses will check the vital signs of patients who had general anesthesia. If there are no complications, the patient may leave the hospital within four to eight hours. (Traditional abdominal surgery requires a hospital stay of several days).

There may be some slight pain or throbbing at the incision sites in the first day or so after the procedure. The gas that is used to expand the abdomen may cause discomfort under the ribs or in the shoulder for a few days. Depending on the reason for the laparoscopy in gynecological procedures, some women may experience some vaginal bleeding. Many patients can return to work within a week of surgery and most are back to work within two weeks.

Risks

Laparoscopy is a relatively safe procedure, especially if the physician is experienced in the technique. The risk of complication is approximately 1%.

The procedure carries a slight risk of puncturing a blood vessel or organ, which could cause blood to seep into the abdominal cavity. Puncturing the intestines could allow intestinal contents to seep into the cavity. These are serious complications and major surgery may be required to correct the problem. For operative procedures, there is the possibility that it may become apparent that open surgery is required. Serious complications occur at a rate of only 0.2%.

Rare complications include:

• hemorrhage

• inflammation of the abdominal cavity lining

• abscess

• problems related to general anesthesia

Laparoscopy is generally not used in patients with certain heart or lung conditions, or in those who have some intestinal disorders, such as bowel obstruction.

KEY TERMS

Biopsy—Microscopic evaluation of a tissue sample. The tissue is closely examined for the presence of abnormal cells.

Cancer staging—Determining the course and spread of cancer.

Cyst—An abnormal lump or swelling that is filled with fluid or other material.

Palliative treatment—A type treatment that does not provide a cure, but eases the symptoms.

Tumor—A growth of tissue, benign or malignant, often referred to as a mass.

Normal results

In diagnostic procedures, normal results would indicate no abnormalities or disease of the organs or lymph nodes that were examined.

Abnormal results

A diagnostic laparoscopy may reveal cancerous or benign masses or lesions. Abnormal findings include tumors or cysts, infections (such as **pelvic inflammatory disease**), **cirrhosis**, endometriosis, fibroid tumors, or an accumulation of fluid in the cavity. If a doctor is checking for the spread of cancer, the presence of malignant lesions in areas other than the original site of malignancy is an abnormal finding.

Resources

BOOKS

Kurtz, Robert C., and Robert J. Ginsberg. "Cancer Diagnosis: Endoscopy." In *Cancer: Principles & Practice of Oncology*, edited by Vincent T. DeVita, Jr. Philadelphia: Lippincott, Williams & Wilkins, 2001, pp. 725-27.

Lefor, Alan T. "Specialized Techniques in Cancer Management." In *Cancer: Principles & Practice of Oncology*, edited by Vincent T. DeVita Jr., et al., 6th ed. Philadelphia: Lippincott, Williams & Wilkins, 2001, pp. 739-57.

OTHER

Iannitti, David A. "The Role of Laparoscopy in the Management of Pancreatic Cancer." *Home Journal Library Index*. March 23, 2001. [cited June 27, 2001]. < http://bioscience.org/1998/v3/e/iannitti/e181-185.htm >.

Carol A. Turkington
Rhonda Cloos, R.N.

Laryngeal cancer

Laryngeal cancer

Definition

Laryngeal **cancer** is cancer of the larynx or voice box.

Description

The larynx is located where the throat divides into the esophagus and the trachea. The esophagus is the tube that takes food to the stomach. The trachea, or windpipe, takes air to the lungs. The area where the larynx is located is sometimes called the Adam's apple.

The larynx has two main functions. It contains the vocal cords, cartilage, and small muscles that make up the voice box. When a person speaks, small muscles tighten the vocal cords, narrowing the distance between them. As air is exhaled past the tightened vocal cords, it creates sounds that are formed into speech by the mouth, lips, and tongue.

The second function of the larynx is to allow air to enter the trachea and to keep food, saliva, and foreign material from entering the lungs. A flap of tissue called the epiglottis covers the trachea each time a person swallows. This blocks foreign material from entering the lungs. When not swallowing, the epiglottis retracts, and air flows into the trachea. During treatment for cancer of the larynx, both of these functions may be lost.

Cancers of the larynx develop slowly. About 95% of these cancers develop from thin, flat cells similar to skin cells called squamous epithelial cells. These cells line the larynx. Gradually, the squamous epithelial cells begin to change and are replaced with abnormal cells. These abnormal cells are not cancerous but are pre-malignant cells that have the potential to develop into cancer. This condition is called dysplasia. Most people with dysplasia never develop cancer. The condition simply goes away without any treatment, especially if the person with dysplasia stops **smoking** or drinking alcohol.

The larynx is made up of three parts, the glottis, the supraglottis, and the subglottis. Cancer can start in any of these regions. Treatment and survival rates depend on which parts of the larynx are affected and whether the cancer has spread to neighboring areas of the neck or distant parts of the body.

The glottis is the middle part of the larynx. It contains the vocal cords. Cancers that develop on the vocal cords are often diagnosed very early because even small vocal cord tumors cause hoarseness. In addition, the vocal cords have no connection to the lymphatic system. This means that cancers on the vocal cord do not spread easily. When confined to the vocal cords without any involvement of other parts of the larynx, the cure rate for this cancer is 75% to 95%.

The supraglottis is the area above the vocal cords. It contains the epiglottis, which protects the trachea from foreign materials. Cancers that develop in this region are usually not found as early as cancers of the glottis because the symptoms are less distinct. The supraglottis region has many connections to the lymphatic system, so cancers in this region tend to spread easily to the lymph nodes and may spread to other parts of the body (lymph nodes are small bean-shaped structures that are found throughout the body; they produce and store infection-fighting cells). In 25% to 50% of people with cancer in the supraglottal region, the cancer has already spread to the lymph nodes by the time they are diagnosed. Because of this, survival rates are lower than for cancers that involve only the glottis.

The subglottis is the region below the vocal cords. Cancer starting in the subglottis region is rare. When it does, it is usually detected only after it has spread to the vocal cords, where it causes obvious symptoms such as hoarseness. Because the cancer has already begun to spread by the time it is detected, survival rates are generally lower than for cancers in other parts of the larynx.

About 12,000 new cases of cancer of the larynx develop in the United States each year. Each year, about 3,900 die of the disease. Laryngeal cancer is between four and five times more common in men than in women. Almost all men who develop laryngeal cancer are over age 55. Laryngeal cancer is about 50% more common among African-American men than among other Americans.

It is thought that older men are more likely to develop laryngeal cancer than women because the two main risk factors for acquiring the disease are lifetime habits of smoking and alcohol **abuse**. More men are heavy smokers and drinkers than women, and more African-American men are heavy smokers than other men in the United States. However, as smoking becomes more prevalent among women, it seems likely that more cases of laryngeal cancer in females will be seen.

Causes and symptoms

Laryngeal cancer develops when the normal cells lining the larynx are replaced with abnormal cells

2162

(dysplasia) that become malignant and reproduce to form tumors. The development of dysplasia is strongly linked to life-long habits of smoking and heavy use of alcohol. The more a person smokes, the greater the risk of developing laryngeal cancer. It is unusual for someone who does not smoke or drink to develop cancer of the larynx. Occasionally, however, people who inhale asbestos particles, wood dust, paint or industrial chemical fumes over a long period of time develop the disease.

The symptoms of laryngeal cancer depend on the location of the tumor. Tumors on the vocal cords are rarely painful, but cause hoarseness. Anyone who is continually hoarse for more than two weeks or who has a **cough** that does not go away should be checked by a doctor.

Tumors in the supraglottal region above the vocal cords often cause more, but less distinct symptoms. These include:

- persistent **sore throat**

- **pain** when swallowing

- difficulty swallowing or frequent **choking** on food

- bad breath

- lumps in the neck

- persistent ear pain (called referred pain; the source of the pain is not the ear)

- change in voice quality

Tumors that begin below the vocal cords are rare, but may cause noisy or difficult breathing. All the symptoms above can also be caused other cancers as well as by less seriousness illnesses. However, if these symptoms persist, it is important to see a doctor and find their cause, because the earlier cancer treatment begins, the more successful it is.

Diagnosis

On the first visit to a doctor for symptoms that suggest laryngeal cancer, the doctor first takes a complete medical history, including family history of cancer and lifestyle information about smoking and alcohol use. The doctor also does a **physical examination**, paying special attention to the neck region for lumps, tenderness, or swelling.

The next step is examination by an otolaryngologist, or ear, nose, and throat (ENT) specialist. This doctor also performs a physical examination, but in addition will also want to look inside the throat at the larynx. Initially, the doctor may spray a local anesthetic on the back of the throat to prevent gagging,

then use a long-handled mirror to look at the larynx and vocal cords. This examination is done in the doctor's office. It may cause gagging but is usually painless.

A more extensive examination involves a **laryngoscopy**. In a laryngoscopy, a lighted fiberoptic tube called a laryngoscope that contains a tiny camera is inserted through the patient's nose and mouth and snaked down the throat so that the doctor can see the larynx and surrounding area. This procedure can be done with a sedative and local anesthetic in a doctor's office. More often, the procedure is done in an outpatient surgery clinic or hospital under **general anesthesia**. This allows the doctor to use tiny clips on the end of the laryngoscope to take biopsies (tissue samples) of any abnormal-looking areas.

Laryngoscopies are normally painless and take about one hour. Some people find their throat feels scratchy after the procedure. Since laryngoscopies are done under **sedation**, patients should not drive immediately after the procedure, and should have someone available to take them home. Laryngoscopy is a standard procedure that is covered by insurance.

The locations of the samples taken during the laryngoscopy are recorded, and the samples are then sent to the laboratory where they are examined under the microscope by a pathologist who specializes in diagnosing diseases through cell samples and laboratory tests. It may take several days to get the results. Based on the findings of the pathologist, cancer can be diagnosed and staged.

Once cancer is diagnosed, other tests will probably be done to help determine the exact size and location of the tumors. This information is helpful in determining which treatments are most appropriate. These tests may include:

- Endoscopy. Similar to a laryngoscopy, this test is done when it appears that cancer may have spread to other areas, such as the esophagus or trachea.

- Computed tomography (CT or CAT) scan. Using x-ray images taken from several angles and computer modeling, CT scans allow parts of the body to be seen as a cross section. This helps locate and size the tumors, and provides information on whether they can be surgically removed.

- Magnetic resonance imaging (MRI). MRI uses magnets and radio waves to create more detailed cross-sectional scans than computed tomography. This detailed information is needed if surgery on the larynx area is planned.

- Barium swallow. Barium is a substance that, unlike soft tissue, shows up on x rays. Swallowed barium coats the throat and allows x-ray pictures to be made of the tissues lining the throat.

- Chest x ray. Done to determine if cancer has spread to the lungs. Since most people with laryngeal cancer are smokers, the risk of also having lung cancer or **emphysema** is high.

- Fine needle aspiration (FNA) biopsy. If any lumps on the neck are found, a thin needle is inserted into the lump, and some cells are removed for analysis by the pathologist.

- Additional blood and urine tests. These tests do not diagnose cancer, but help to determine the patient's general health and provide information to determine which cancer treatments are most appropriate.

Treatment

Staging

Once cancer of the larynx is found, more tests will be done to find out if cancer cells have spread to other parts of the body. This is called staging. A doctor needs to know the stage of the disease to plan treatment. In cancer of the larynx, the definitions of the early stages depend on where the cancer started.

STAGE I. The cancer is only in the area where it started and has not spread to lymph nodes in the area or to other parts of the body. The exact definition of stage I depends on where the cancer started, as follows:

- Supraglottis: The cancer is only in one area of the supraglottis and the vocal cords can move normally.

- Glottis: The cancer is only in the vocal cords and the vocal cords can move normally.

- Subglottis: The cancer has not spread outside of the subglottis.

STAGE II. The cancer is only in the larynx and has not spread to lymph nodes in the area or to other parts of the body. The exact definition of stage II depends on where the cancer started, as follows:

- Supraglottis: The cancer is in more than one area of the supraglottis, but the vocal cords can move normally.

- Glottis: The cancer has spread to the supraglottis or the subglottis or both. The vocal cords may or may not be able to move normally.

- Subglottis: The cancer has spread to the vocal cords, which may or may not be able to move normally.

STAGE III. Either of the following may be true:

- The cancer has not spread outside of the larynx, but the vocal cords cannot move normally, or the cancer has spread to tissues next to the larynx.

- The cancer has spread to one lymph node on the same side of the neck as the cancer, and the lymph node measures no more than 3 centimeters (just over 1 inch).

STAGE IV. Any of the following may be true:

- The cancer has spread to tissues around the larynx, such as the pharynx or the tissues in the neck. The lymph nodes in the area may or may not contain cancer.

- The cancer has spread to more than one lymph node on the same side of the neck as the cancer, to lymph nodes on one or both sides of the neck, or to any lymph node that measures more than 6 centimeters (over 2 inches).

- The cancer has spread to other parts of the body.

RECURRENT. Recurrent disease means that the cancer has come back (recurred) after it has been treated. It may come back in the larynx or in another part of the body.

Treatment

Treatment is based on the stage of the cancer as well as its location and the health of the individual. Generally, there are three types of treatments for cancer of the larynx. These are surgery, radiation, and **chemotherapy**. They can be used alone or in combination based in the stage of the caner. Getting a second opinion after the cancer has been staged can be very helpful in sorting out treatment options and should always be considered.

SURGERY. The goal of surgery is to cut out the tissue that contains malignant cells. There are several common surgeries to treat laryngeal cancer.

Stage III and stage IV cancers are usually treated with total **laryngectomy**. This is an operation to remove the entire larynx. Sometimes other tissues around the larynx are also removed. Total laryngectomy removes the vocal cords. Alternate methods of voice communication must be learned with the help of a speech pathologist. Laryngectomy is treated in depth as a separate entry in this volume.

Smaller tumors are sometimes treated by partial laryngectomy. The goal is to remove the cancer but save as much of the larynx (and corresponding speech capability) as possible. Very small tumors or cancer in situ are sometimes successfully treated with laser excision surgery. In this type of surgery, a narrowly-targeted beam of light from a laser is used to remove the cancer.

Advanced cancer (Stages III and IV) that has spread to the lymph nodes often requires an operation called a neck dissection. The goal of a neck dissection is to remove the lymph nodes and prevent the cancer from spreading. There are several forms of neck dissection. A **radical neck dissection** is the operation that removes the most tissue.

Several other operations are sometimes performed because of laryngeal cancer. A **tracheotomy** is a surgical procedure in which an artificial opening is made in the trachea (windpipe) to allow air into the lungs. This operation is necessary if the larynx is totally removed. A **gastrectomy** tube is a feeding tube placed through skin and directly into the stomach. It is used to give **nutrition** to people who cannot swallow or whose esophagus is blocked by a tumor. People who have a total laryngectomy usually do not need a gastrectomy tube if their esophagus remains intact.

RADIATION. Radiation therapy uses high-energy rays, such as x rays or gamma rays, to kill cancer cells. The advantage of radiation therapy is that it preserves the larynx and the ability to speak. The disadvantage is that it may not kill all the cancer cells. Radiation therapy can be used alone in early stage cancers or in combination with surgery. Sometimes it is tried first with the plan that if it fails to cure the cancer, surgery still remains an option. Often, radiation therapy is used after surgery for advanced cancers to kill any cells the surgeon might not have removed.

There are two types of radiation therapy. External beam radiation therapy focuses rays from outside the body on the cancerous tissue. This is the most common type of radiation therapy used to treat laryngeal cancer. With internal radiation therapy, also called brachytherapy, radioactive materials are placed directly on the cancerous tissue. This type of radiation therapy is a much less common treatment for laryngeal cancer.

External radiation therapy is given in doses called fractions. A common treatment involves giving fractions five days a week for seven weeks. Clinical trials are underway to determine the benefits of accelerating the delivery of fractions (accelerated fractionation) or dividing fractions into smaller doses given more than once a day (hyperfractionation). Side effects of radiation therapy include **dry mouth**, sore throat, hoarseness, skin problems, trouble swallowing, and diminished ability to taste.

CHEMOTHERAPY. Chemotherapy is the use of drugs to kill cancer cells. Unlike radiation therapy, which is targeted to a specific tissue, chemotherapy drugs are either taken by mouth or intravenously (through a vein) and circulate throughout the whole body. They are used mainly to treat advanced laryngeal cancer that is inoperable or that has metastasized to a distant site. Chemotherapy is often used after surgery or in combination with radiation therapy. Clinical trials are underway to determine the best combination of treatments for advanced cancer.

The two most common chemotherapy drugs used to treat laryngeal cancer are cisplatin and 5-fluorouracil (5-FU). There are many side effects associated with chemotherapy drugs, including **nausea and vomiting**, loss of appetite, hair loss, **diarrhea**, and mouth sores. Chemotherapy can also damage the blood-producing cells of the bone marrow, which can result in low blood cell counts, increased chance of infection, and abnormal bleeding or bruising.

Alternative treatment

Alternative and complementary therapies range from herbal remedies, vitamin supplements, and special **diets** to spiritual practices, **acupuncture**, massage, and similar treatments. When these therapies are used in addition to conventional medicine, they are called complementary therapies. When they are used instead of conventional medicine, they are called alternative therapies.

Complementary or alternative therapies are widely used by people with cancer. One large study published in the *Journal of Clinical Oncology* in July, 2000 found that 83% of all cancer patients studied used some form of complementary or alternative medicine as part of their cancer treatment. No specific alternative therapies have been directed toward laryngeal cancer. However, good nutrition and activities that reduce **stress** and promote a positive view of life have no unwanted side-effects and appear to be beneficial in boosting the immune system in fighting cancer.

Unlike traditional pharmaceuticals, complementary and alternative therapies are not evaluated by the United States Food and Drug Administration (FDA) for either safety or effectiveness. These therapies may have interactions with traditional pharmaceuticals. Patients should be wary of "miracle cures" and notify their doctors if they are using herbal remedies, vitamin supplements or other unprescribed treatments. Alternative and experimental treatments normally are not covered by insurance.

Prognosis

Cure rates and survival rates can predict group outcomes, but can never precisely predict the outcome for a single individual. However, the earlier laryngeal cancer is discovered and treated, the more likely it will be cured.

Cancers found in stage 0 and stage 1 have a 75% to 95% cure rate depending on the site. Late stage cancers that have metastasized have a very poor survival rate, with intermediate stages falling somewhere in between. People who have had laryngeal cancer are at greatest risk for recurrence (having cancer come back), especially in the head and neck, during the first two to three years after treatment. Check-ups during the first year are needed every other month, and four times a year during the second year. It is rare for laryngeal cancer to recur after five years of being cancer-free.

Prevention

By far, the most effective way to prevent laryngeal cancer is not to smoke. Smokers who quit smoking also significantly decrease their risk of developing the disease. Other ways to prevent laryngeal cancer include limiting the use of alcohol, eating a well-balanced diet, seeking treatment for prolonged **heartburn**, and avoiding inhaling asbestos and chemical fumes.

Resources

PERIODICALS

Ahmad, I., B. N. Kumar, K. Radford, J. O'Connell, and A. J. Batch. "Surgical Voice Restoration Following Ablative Surgery for Laryngeal and Hypopharyngeal Carcinoma." *Journal or Laryngology and Otolaryngology* 114 (July 2000): 522–5.

ORGANIZATIONS

American Cancer Society. 1599 Clifton Rd. NE, Atlanta, GA 30329. 800 (ACS)-2345. < http://www.cancer.org >.

National Cancer Institute. Cancer Information Service. Bldg. 31, Room 10A19, 9000 Rockville Pike, Bethesda, MD 20892. (800) 4-CANCER. < http://www.nci.nih.gov/cancerinfo/index.html >.

National Cancer Institute Office of Cancer Complementary and Alternative Medicine. < http://occam.nci.nih.gov >.

National Center for Complementary and Alternative Medicine. P. O. Box 8218, Silver Spring, MD 20907-8281. (888) 644-6226. < http://nccam.nih.gov >.

OTHER

"Laryngeal Cancer." *CancerNet.* July 19, 2001. < http://www.graylab.ac.uk/cancernet/201519.html#3_STAGEEXPLANATION >.

"What you Need to Know About Cancer of the Larynx." *CancerNet* November 2000. [cited July 19, 2001]. < http://www.cancernet.nci.nih.gov >.

Tish Davidson, A.M.

Laryngeal cancer *see* **Head and neck cancer**

Laryngectomy

Definition

Laryngectomy is the partial or complete surgical removal of the larynx, usually as a treatment for **cancer** of the larynx.

Purpose

Normally a laryngectomy is performed to remove tumors or cancerous tissue. In rare cases, it may be done when the larynx is badly damaged by gunshot, automobile injuries, or similar violent accidents. Laryngectomies can be total or partial. Total laryngectomies are done when cancer is advanced. The entire larynx is removed. Often if the cancer has spread, other surrounding structures in the neck, such as lymph nodes, are removed at the same time. Partial laryngectomies are done when cancer is limited to one spot. Only the area with the tumor is removed. Laryngectomies may also be performed when other cancer treatment options, such as radiation or **chemotherapy**, fail.

Precautions

Laryngectomy is done only after cancer of the larynx has been diagnosed by a series of tests that allow the otolaryngologist (a specialist often called an ear, nose, and throat doctor) to look into the throat and take tissue samples (biopsies) to confirm and stage the cancer. People need to be in good general health to undergo a laryngectomy, and will have standard pre-operative blood work and tests to make sure they are able to safely withstand the operation.

Description

The larynx is located slightly below the point where the throat divides into the esophagus, which takes food to the stomach, and the trachea (windpipe), which takes air to the lungs. Because of its location, the larynx plays a critical role in normal breathing, swallowing, and speaking. Within the larynx, vocal folds (often called vocal cords) vibrate as air is exhaled past, thus creating speech. The epiglottis protects the trachea, making sure that only air gets into the lungs. When the larynx is removed, these functions are lost.

Once the larynx is removed, air can no longer flow into the lungs. During this operation, the surgeon removes the larynx through an incision in the neck. The surgeon also performs a **tracheotomy**. He makes an artificial opening called a stoma in the front of the neck. The upper portion of the trachea is brought to the stoma and secured, making a permanent alternate way for air to get to the lungs. The connection between the throat and the esophagus is not normally affected, so after healing, the person whose larynx has been removed (called a laryngectomee) can eat normally. However, normal speech is no longer possible. Several alternate means of vocal communication can be learned with the help of a speech pathologist.

Preparation

As with any surgical procedure, the patient will be required to sign a consent form after the procedure is thoroughly explained. Many patients prefer a second opinion, and some insurers require it.

Blood and urine studies, along with **chest x ray** and EKG may be ordered as the doctor deems necessary. The patient also has a pre-operative meeting with an anesthesiologist. If a complete laryngectomy is planned, it may be helpful to meet with a speech pathologist and/or an established laryngectomee for discussion of post-operative expectations and support.

Aftercare

A person undergoing a laryngectomy spends several days in intensive care (ICU) and receives intravenous (IV) fluids and medication. As with any major surgery, the blood pressure, pulse, and respirations are monitored regularly. The patient is encouraged to turn, **cough**, and deep breathe to help mobilize secretions in the lungs. One or more drains are usually inserted in the neck to remove any fluids that collect. These drains are removed after several days.

It takes two to three weeks for the tissues of the throat to heal. During this time, the laryngectomee cannot swallow food and must receive **nutrition** through a tube inserted through the nose and down the throat into the stomach. During this time, even people with partial laryngectomies are unable to speak.

When air is drawn in normally through the nose, it is warmed and moistened before it reaches the lungs. When air is drawn in through the stoma, it does not have the opportunity to be warmed and humidified. In order to keep the stoma from drying out and becoming crusty, laryngectomees are encouraged to breathe artificially humidified air. The stoma is usually covered with a light cloth to keep it clean and to keep unwanted particles from accidentally entering the lungs. Care of the stoma is extremely important, since it is the person's only way to get air to the lungs. After a laryngectomy, a healthcare professional will teach the laryngectomee and his or her caregivers how to care for the stoma.

Immediately after a laryngectomy, an alternate method of communication such as writing notes, gesturing, or pointing must be used. A partial laryngectomy patient will gradually regain some speech several weeks after the operation, but the voice may be hoarse, weak, and strained. A speech pathologist will work with a complete laryngectomee to establish new ways of communicating.

There are three main methods of vocalizing after a total laryngectomy. In esophageal speech the

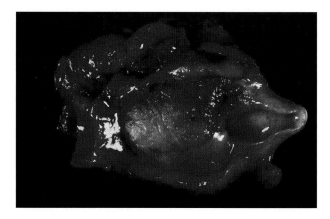

A pathology photograph of an extracted tumor found on the larynx. *(Custom Medical Stock Photo. Reproduced by permission.)*

laryngectomee learns how to "swallow" air down into the esophagus and creates sounds by releasing the air. This method requires quite a bit of coordination and learning, and produces short bursts (7 or 8 syllables) of low-volume sound.

Tracheoesophageal speech diverts air through a hole in the trachea made by the surgeon. The air then passes through an implanted artificial voice prosthesis (a small tube that makes a sound when air goes through it). Recent advances have been made in implanting voice prostheses that produce good voice quality.

The third method of artificial sound communication involves using a hand-held electronic device that translates vibrations into sounds. There are several different styles of these devices, but all require the use of at least one hand to hold the device to the throat. The choice of which method to use depends on many things including the age and health of the laryngectomee, and whether other parts of the mouth, such as the tongue, have also been removed.

Many patients resume daily activities after surgery. Special precautions must be taken during showering or shaving. Special instruction and equipment is also required for those who wish to swim or water ski, as it is dangerous for water to enter the windpipe and lungs through the stoma.

Regular follow-up visits are important following treatment for cancer of the larynx because there is a higher-than-average risk of developing a new cancer in the mouth, throat, or other regions of the head or neck. Many self-help and support groups are available to help patients meet others who face similar problems.

KEY TERMS

Larynx—Also known as the voice box, the larynx is composed of cartilage that contains the apparatus for voice production. This includes the vocal cords and the muscles and ligaments that move the cords.

Lymph nodes—Accumulations of tissue along a lymph channel, which produce cells called lymphocytes that fight infection.

Tracheostomy—A surgical procedure in which an artificial opening is made in the trachea (windpipe) to allow air into the lungs.

Risks

Laryngectomy is often successful in curing early stage cancers. However it does cause lifestyle changes. Laryngectomees must learn new ways of speaking. They must be continually concerned about the care of their stoma. Serious infections can occur if water or other foreign material enters the lungs through an unprotected stoma. Also, women who undergo partial laryngectomy or who learn some types of artificial speech will have a deep voice similar to that of a man. For some women this presents psychological challenges.

Normal results

Ideally, removal of the larynx will remove all cancerous material. The person will recover from the operation, make lifestyle adjustments, and return to an active life.

Abnormal results

Sometimes cancer has spread to surrounding tissues and it is necessary to remove lymph nodes, parts of the tongue, or other cancerous tissues. As with any major operation, post- surgical infection is possible. Infection is of particular concern to laryngectomees who have chosen to have a voice prosthesis implanted, and is one of the major reasons for having to remove the device.

Resources

ORGANIZATIONS

American Cancer Society. 1599 Clifton Road NE, Atlanta, GA 30329. (800) ACS -2345. < http://www.cancer.org >.

Cancer Information Service. National Cancer Institute, Building 31, Room 10A19, 9000 Rockville Pike, Bethesda, MD 20892. (800) 4-CANCER. < http://www.nci.nih.gov/cancerinfo/index.html >.

International Association of Laryngectomees(IAL). 7440 North Shadeland Ave., Suite 100, Indianapolis, IN 46250. < http://www.larynxlink.com/ >.

National Institute on Deafness and Other Communication Disorders. National Institutes of Health, 31 Center Drive, MSC 2320, Bethesda, MD 20892-2320. < http://www.nidcd.nih.gov >.

The Voice Center at Eastern Virginia Medical School. Norfolk, VA 23507. < http://www.voice-center.com >.

Kathleen D. Wright, RN
Tish Davidson, AM

Laryngitis

Definition

Laryngitis is caused by inflammation of the larynx, resulting in hoarseness of the voice.

Description

When air is breathed in (inspired), it passes through the nose and the nasopharynx or through the mouth and the oropharynx. These are both connected to the larynx, a tube made of cartilage. The vocal cords, responsible for setting up the vibrations necessary for speech, are located within the larynx. The air continues down the larynx to the trachea. The trachea then splits into two branches, the left and right bronchi (bronchial tubes). These bronchi branch into smaller air tubes which run within the lungs, leading to the small air sacs of the lungs (alveoli).

Either food, liquid, or air may be taken in through the mouth. While air goes into the larynx and the respiratory system, food and liquid are directed into the tube leading to the stomach, the esophagus. Because food or liquid in the bronchial tubes or lungs could cause a blockage or lead to an infection, the airway must be protected. The epiglottis is a leaf-like piece of cartilage extending upwards from the larynx. The epiglottis can close down over the larynx when someone is eating or drinking, preventing these substances from entering the airway.

In laryngitis, the tissues below the level of the epiglottis are swollen and inflamed. This causes swelling around the area of the vocal cords, so that they cannot vibrate normally. A hoarse sound to the voice is very characteristic of laryngitis. Laryngitis is a very common problem, and often occurs during the course of an upper respiratory tract infection (cold).

Causes and symptoms

Laryngitis is caused almost 100% of the time by a virus. The same viruses which cause the majority of simple upper respiratory infections (colds, etc.) are responsible for laryngitis. These include parainfluenzae virus, **influenza** virus, respiratory syncytial virus, rhinovirus, coronavirus, and echovirus. Extremely rarely, bacteria such as Group A streptococcus, M. catarrhalis, or that which causes **tuberculosis** may cause laryngitis. In people with faulty immune systems (particular due to acquired **immunodeficiency** syndrome, or **AIDS**), infections with fungi may be responsible for laryngitis.

Symptoms usually begin along with, or following, symptoms of a cold. A sore, scratchy throat, **fever**, runny nose, achiness, and **fatigue** may all occur. Difficulty swallowing sometimes occurs with **streptococcal infections**. The patient may **cough** and wheeze. Most characteristically, the patient's voice will sound strained, hoarse, and raspy.

In extremely rare cases, the swelling of the larynx may cause symptoms of airway obstruction. This is more common in infants, because the diameter of their airways is so small. In that case, the baby may have a greatly increased respiratory rate, and exhibit loud high-pitched sounds with breathing (called **stridor**).

Diagnosis

Diagnosis is usually made by learning the history of a cold followed by hoarseness. The throat usually appears red and somewhat swollen. Listening to the chest and back with a stethoscope may reveal some harsh **wheezing** sounds with inspiration (breathing in).

In long-standing (chronic laryngitis), tuberculosis may be suspected. Using a scope called a laryngoscope, examination of the airway will show redness, swelling, small bumps of tissue called nodules, and irritated pits in the tissue called ulcerations. Special skin testing (TB testing) will reveal that the individual has been exposed to the bacteria causing TB.

Treatment

Treatment of a simple, viral laryngitis simply addresses the symptoms. Gargling with warm salt water, **pain** relievers such as **acetaminophen**, the use of vaporizers to create moist air, and rest will help the illness resolve within a week.

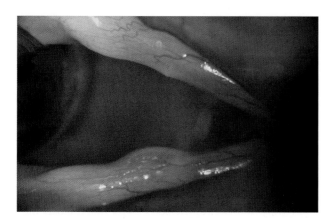

An endoscopic view of a patient's vocal cords with laryngitis.
(Custom Medical Stock Photo. Reproduced by permission.)

KEY TERMS

Epiglottis—A leaf-like piece of cartilage extending upwards from the larynx, which can close like a lid over the trachea to prevent the airway from receiving any food or liquid being swallowed.

Larynx—The part of the airway lying between the pharynx and the trachea.

Nasopharynx—The part of the airway into which the nose leads.

Oropharynx—The part of the airway into which the mouth leads.

Trachea—The part of the airway which leads into the bronchial tubes.

In an infant who is clearly struggling for air, it may be necessary to put in an artificial airway for a short period of time. This is very rarely needed.

An individual with tubercular laryngitis is treated with a combination of medications used to treat classic TB. In people with fungal laryngitis, a variety of antifungal medications are available.

Alternative treatment

Alternative treatments include **aromatherapy** inhalations made with benzoin, lavender, frankincense, thyme, and sandalwood. Decoctions (extracts made by boiling an herb in water) or infusions (extracts made by steeping an herb in boiling water) can be made with red sage (*Salvia officinalis* var. *rubra*) and yarrow (*Achillea millefolium*) or with licorice

(*Glycyrrhiza glabra*). These are used for gargling, and are said to reduce pain. **Echinacea** (*Echinacea* spp.) tincture taken in water every hour for 48 hours is recommended to boost the immune system. Antiviral herbs, including usnea (*Usnea* spp.), lomatium (*Lomatium dissectum*), and ligusticum (*Ligusticum porteri*), may help hasten recovery from laryngitis. Homeopathic remedies are recommended based on the patient's symptoms. Some people may get relief from placing cold compresses on the throat.

Prognosis

Prognosis for laryngitis is excellent. Recovery is complete, and usually occurs within a week's time.

Prevention

Prevention of laryngitis is the same as for any upper respiratory infections. The only way to even attempt to prevent such illnesses is by good handwashing, and by avoiding situations where one might come in contact with people who might be sick. However, even with relatively good hygiene practices, most people will get about five to six colds per year. It is unpredictable which of these may lead to laryngitis.

Resources

ORGANIZATIONS

American Academy of Otolaryngology-Head and Neck Surgery, Inc. One Prince St., Alexandria VA 22314-3357. (703) 836-4444. < http://www.entnet.org >.

Rosalyn Carson-DeWitt, MD

Laryngoscopy

Definition

Laryngoscopy refers to a procedure used to view the inside of the larynx (the voice box).

Description

The purpose and advantage of seeing inside the larynx is to detect tumors, foreign bodies, nerve or structural injury, or other abnormalities. Two methods allow the larynx to be seen directly during the examination. In one, a flexible tube with a fiber-optic device is threaded through the nasal passage and down into the throat. The other method uses a rigid viewing tube passed directly from the mouth, through the throat, into the larynx. A light and lens affixed to the endoscope are used in both methods. The endoscopic tube may also be equipped to suction debris or remove material for biopsy. **Bronchoscopy** is a similar, but more extensive procedure in which the tube is continued through the larynx, down into the trachea and bronchi.

Preparation

Laryngoscopy is done in the hospital with a local anesthetic spray to minimize discomfort and suppress the gag reflex. Patients are requested not to eat for several hours before the examination.

Aftercare

If the throat is sore, soothing liquids or lozenges will probably relieve any temporary discomfort.

Risks

This procedure carries no serious risks, although the patient may experience soreness of the throat or **cough** up small amounts of blood until the irritation subsides.

Normal results

A normal result would be the absence of signs of disease or damage.

Abnormal results

An abnormal finding, such as a tumor or an object lodged in the tissue, would either be removed or described for further medical attention.

Jill S. Lasker

Larynx removal *see* **Laryngectomy**

Laser-assisted in-situ keratomileusis *see* **Photorefractive keratectomy and laser-assisted in-**

Laser surgery

Definition

Laser (light amplification by stimulated emission of radiation) surgery uses an intensely hot, precisely focused beam of light to remove or vaporize tissue and control bleeding in a wide variety of non-invasive and minimally invasive procedures.

Purpose

Laser surgery is used to:

- Cut or destroy tissue that is abnormal or diseased without harming healthy, normal tissue
- Shrink or destroy tumors and lesions
- Cauterize (seal) blood vessels to prevent excessive bleeding.

Precautions

Anyone who is thinking about having laser surgery should ask his doctor to:

- Explain why laser surgery is likely to be more beneficial than traditional surgery
- Describe his experience in performing the laser procedure the patient is considering.

Because some lasers can temporarily or permanently discolor the skin of Blacks, Asians, and Hispanics, a dark-skinned patient should make sure that his surgeon has successfully performed laser procedures on people of color.

Some types of laser surgery should not be performed on pregnant women or on patients with severe cardiopulmonary disease or other serious health problems.

Description

The first working laser was introduced in 1960. The device was initially used to treat diseases and disorders of the eye, whose transparent tissues gave ophthalmic surgeons a clear view of how the narrow, concentrated beam was being directed. Dermatologic surgeons also helped pioneer laser surgery, and developed and improved upon many early techniques and more refined surgical procedures.

Types of lasers

The three types of lasers most often used in medical treatment are the:

- Carbon dioxide (CO_2) laser. Primarily a surgical tool, this device converts light energy to heat strong enough to minimize bleeding while it cuts through or vaporizes tissue.

- Neodymium:yttrium-aluminum-garnet (Nd:YAG) laser. Capable of penetrating tissue more deeply than other lasers, the Nd:YAG makes blood clot quickly and can enable surgeons to see and work on parts of the body that could otherwise be reached only through open (invasive) surgery.

- Argon laser. This laser provides the limited penetration needed for eye surgery and superficial skin disorders. In a special procedure known as photodynamic therapy (PDT), this laser uses light-sensitive dyes to shrink or dissolve tumors.

Laser applications

Sometimes described as "scalpels of light," lasers are used alone or with conventional surgical instruments in a diverse array of procedures that:

- improve appearance

- relieve **pain**

- restore function

- save lives

Laser surgery is often standard operating procedure for specialists in:

- cardiology

- dentistry

- dermatology

- gastroenterology (treatment of disorders of the stomach and intestines)

- gynecology

- neurosurgery

- oncology (**cancer** treatment)

- ophthalmology (treatment of disorders of the eye)

- orthopedics (treatment of disorders of bones, joints, muscles, ligaments, and tendons)

- otolaryngology (treatment of disorders of the ears, nose, and throat)

- pulmonary care (treatment of disorders of the respiratory system

- urology (treatment of disorders of the urinary tract and of the male reproductive system)

Routine uses of lasers include erasing **birthmarks**, skin discoloration, and skin changes due to **aging**, and removing benign, precancerous, or cancerous tissues or tumors. Lasers are used to stop **snoring**, remove tonsils, remove or transplant hair, and relieve pain and restore function in patients who are too weak to undergo major surgery. Lasers are also used to treat:

- angina (chest pain)

- cancerous or non-cancerous tumors that cannot be removed or destroyed

- cold and **canker sores**, gum disease, and tooth sensitivity or decay

- ectopic **pregnancy** (development of a fertilized egg outside the uterus)

- endometriosis

- fibroid tumors

- gallstones

- glaucoma, mild-to-moderate nearsightedness and **astigmatism**, and other conditions that impair sight

- migraine headaches

- non-cancerous enlargement of the prostate gland

- nosebleeds

- ovarian cysts

- ulcers

- varicose veins

- warts

- numerous other conditions, diseases, and disorders

Advantages of laser surgery

Often referred to as "bloodless surgery," laser procedures usually involve less bleeding than conventional surgery. The heat generated by the laser keeps the surgical site free of germs and reduces the risk of infection. Because a smaller incision is required, laser procedures often take less time (and cost less money) than traditional surgery. Sealing off blood vessels and nerves reduces bleeding, swelling, scarring, pain, and the length of the recovery period.

Disadvantages of laser surgery

Although many laser surgeries can be performed in a doctor's office rather than in a hospital, the person guiding the laser must be at least as thoroughly trained and highly skilled as someone performing the same procedure in a hospital setting. The American Society for Laser Medicine and Surgery, Inc. urges that:

- All operative areas be equipped with oxygen and other drugs and equipment required for **cardiopulmonary resuscitation (CPR)**

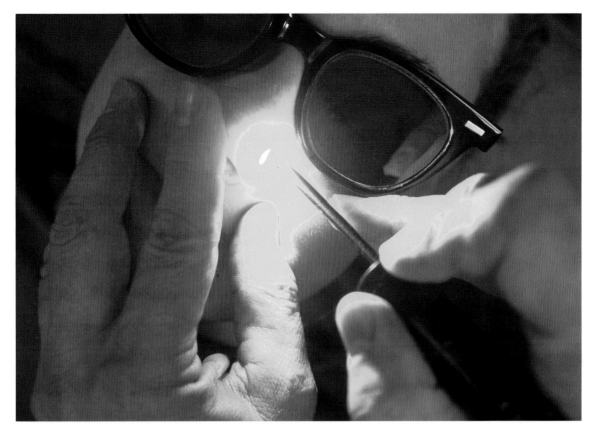

Cosmetic laser surgery in progress. The wavelengths of the laser's light can be matched to a specific target, enabling the physician to destroy the capillaries near the skin's surface without damaging the surrounding tissue. *(Photograph by Will & Deni McIntyre, Photo Researchers, Inc. Reproduced by permission.)*

- Non-physicians performing laser procedures be properly trained, licensed, and insured

- A qualified and experienced supervising physician be able to respond to and manage unanticipated events or other emergencies within five minutes of the time they occur

- Emergency transportation to a hospital or other acute-care facility be available whenever laser surgery is performed in a non-hospital setting.

Imprecisely aimed lasers can burn or destroy healthy tissue.

Preparation

Because laser surgery is used to treat so many dissimilar conditions, the patient should ask his physician for detailed instructions about how to prepare for a specific procedure. Diet, activities, and medications may not have to be limited prior to surgery, but some procedures require a **physical examination** and a medical history that:

- Determines the patient's general health and current medical status

- Describes how the patient has responded to other illnesses, hospital stays, and diagnostic or therapeutic procedures

- Clarifies what the patient expects the outcome of the procedure to be.

Aftercare

Most laser surgeries can be performed on an outpatient basis, and patients are usually permitted to leave the hospital or medical office when their vital signs have stabilized. A patient who has been sedated should not be discharged:

- Until he has recovered from the anesthesia and knows who and where he is

- Unless he is accompanied by a responsible adult.

The doctor may prescribe analgesic (pain-relieving) medication, and should provide easy-to-understand written instructions that describe how the patient's recovery should progress and what to do in case complications or emergency arise.

Risks

Like traditional surgery, laser surgery can be complicated by:

- hemorrhage
- infection
- perforation (piercing) of an organ or tissue

Laser surgery can also involve risks that are not associated with traditional surgical procedures. Being careless or not practicing safe surgical techniques can severely burn the patient's lungs or even cause them to explode. Patients must wear protective eye shields while undergoing laser surgery on any part of the face near the eyes or eyelids, and the United States Food and Drug Administration (FDA) has said that both doctors and patients must use special protective eyewear whenever a CO_2 laser is used.

Laser beams can burn or destroy healthy tissue, cause injuries that are painful and sometimes permanent, and actually compound problems they are supposed to solve. Errors or inaccuracies in laser surgery can worsen a patient's vision, for example, and lasers can scar and even change the skin color of some patients.

Normal results

The nature and severity of the problem, the skill of the surgeon performing the procedure, and the patient's general health and realistic expectations are among the factors that influence the outcome of laser surgery. Successful procedures can enable patients to:

- feel better
- look younger
- enjoy longer, fuller, more active lives

A patient who is considering any kind of laser surgery should ask his doctor to provide detailed information about what the outcome of the surgery is expected to be, what the recovery process will involve, and how long it will probably be before he regains a normal appearance and can resume his normal activities.

Abnormal results

A person who is considering any type of laser surgery should ask his doctor to provide specific and detailed information about what could go wrong during the procedure and what the negative impact on the patient's health or appearance might be.

KEY TERMS

Argon—A colorless, odorless gas.

Astigmatism—A condition in which one or both eyes cannot filter light properly and images appear blurred and indistinct.

Canker sore—A blister-like sore on the inside of the mouth that can be painful but is not serious.

Carbon dioxide—A heavy, colorless gas that dissolves in water.

Cardiopulmonary resuscitation—An emergency procedure used to restore circulation and prevent brain death to a person who has collapsed, is unconscious, is not breathing, and has no pulse.

Cauterize—To use heat or chemicals to stop bleeding, prevent the spread of infection, or destroy tissue.

Cornea—The outer, transparent lens that covers the pupil of the eye and admits light.

Endometriosis—An often painful gynecologic condition in which endometrial tissue migrates from the inside of the uterus to other organs inside and beyond the abdominal cavity.

Glaucoma—A disease of the eye in which increased pressure within the eyeball can cause gradual loss of vision.

Invasive surgery—A form of surgery that involves making an incision in the patient's body and inserting instruments or other medical devices into it.

Nearsightedness—A condition in which one or both eyes cannot focus normally, causing objects at a distance to appear blurred and indistinct. Also called myopia.

Ovarian cyst—A benign or malignant growth on an ovary. An ovarian cyst can disappear without treatment or become extremely painful and have to be surgically removed.

Vaporize—To dissolve solid material or convert it into smoke or gas.

Varicose veins—Swollen, twisted veins, usually occurring in the legs, that occur more often in women than in men.

Lighter or darker skin may appear, for example, when a laser is used to remove sun damage or age spots from an olive-skinned or dark-skinned individual. This abnormal pigmentation may or may not disappear in time.

Scarring or rupturing of the cornea is uncommon, but laser surgery on one or both eyes can:

- increase sensitivity to light or glare
- reduce night vision
- permanently cloud vision, or cause sharpness of vision to decline throughout the day

Signs of infection following laser surgery include:

- burning
- crusting of the skin
- itching
- pain
- scarring
- severe redness
- swelling

Resources

ORGANIZATIONS

American Society for Dermatologic Surgery. 930 N. Meacham Road, P.O. Box 4014, Schaumburg, IL 60168-4014. (847) 330-9830. < http://www.asds-net.org >.

American Society for Laser Medicine and Surgery. 2404 Stewart Square, Wausau, WI 54401. (715) 845-9283. < http://www.aslms.org >.

Cancer Information Service. 9000 Rockville Pike, Building 31, Suite 10A18, Bethesda, MD 20892. 1-800-4-CANCER. < http://wwwicic.nci.nih.gov >. 7.

National Cancer Institute. Building 31, Room 10A31, 31 Center Drive, MSC 2580, Bethesda, MD 20892-2580. (800) 422-6237. < http://www.nci.nih.gov >.

Maureen Haggerty

LASIK *see* **Photorefractive keratectomy and laser-assisted in-**

Lassa fever *see* **Hemorrhagic fevers**

Laxatives

Definition

Laxatives are products that promote bowel movements.

Purpose

Laxatives are used to treat constipation—the passage of small amounts of hard, dry stools, usually fewer than three times a week. Before recommending use of laxatives, differential diagnosis should be performed. Prolonged **constipation** may be evidence of a significant problem, such as localized **peritonitis** or **diverticulitis**. Complaints of constipation may be associated with **obsessive-compulsive disorder**. Use of laxatives should be avoided in these cases. Patients should be aware that patterns of defecation are highly variable, and may vary from two to three times daily to two to three times weekly.

Laxatives may also be used prophylacticly for patients, such as those recovering from a myocardial infarction or those who have had recent surgery, who should not strain during defecation.

Laxatives are also used to cleanse the lower bowel before a **colonoscopy** or similar diagnostic procedure.

Description

Laxatives may be grouped by mechanism of action.

Saline cathartics include dibasic sodium phosphate (Phospo-Soda), magnesium citrate, magnesium hydroxide (milk of magnesia), magnesium sulfate (Epsom salts), sodium biphosphate, and others. They act by attracting and holding water in the intestinal lumen, and may produce a watery stool. Magnesium sulfate is the most potent of the laxatives in this group.

Stimulant and irritant laxatives increase the peristaltic movement of the intestine. Examples include cascara and bisadocyl (Dulcolax.) Castor oil works in a similar fashion.

Bulk-producing laxatives increase the volume of the stool, and will both soften the stool and stimulate intestinal motility. Psyllium (Metamucil, Konsil) and methylcellulose (Citrucel) are examples of this type. The overall effect is similar to that of eating high-fiber foods, and this class of laxative is most suitable for regular use. Many primary care physicians suggest that patients try laxatives in this category before using saline or stimulant laxatives.

Docusate (Colace) is the only representative example of the stool softener class. It holds water within the fecal mass, providing a larger, softer stool. Docusate has no effect on acute constipation, since it must be present before the fecal mass forms to have any effect, but may be useful for prevention of constipation in patients with recurrent problems, or those who are about to take a constipating drug, such as narcotic **analgesics**.

Mineral oil is an emollient laxative. It acts by retarding intestinal absorption of fecal water, thereby softening the stool.

The hyperosmotic laxatives are glycerin and lactulose (Chronulac, Duphalac), both of which act by holding water within the intestine. Lactulose may also increase peristaltic action of the intestine.

Some newer options for the treatment of chronic constipation are being developed by various groups of researchers. These include such alternative therapies as **biofeedback**; newer drugs like tegaserod (Zelnorm) and prucalopride, which stimulate peristalsis; a nerve growth factor known as neurotrophin-3; and electrical stimulation of the colon.

Recommended dosage

See specific products.

Precautions

Short-term use of laxatives is generally safe except in **appendicitis**, fecal impaction, or intestinal obstruction. Lactulose is composed of two sugar molecules; galactose and fructose, and should not be administered to patients who require a low galactose diet.

Chronic use of laxatives may result in fluid and electrolyte imbalances, steatorrhea, osteomalacia, **diarrhea**, cathartic colon, and **liver disease**. Excessive intake of mineral oil may cause impaired absorption of oil soluble **vitamins**, particularly A and D. Excessive use of magnesium salts may cause hypermanesemia.

Lactulose and magnesium sulfate are **pregnancy** category B. Casanthranol, cascara sagrada, danthron, docusate sodium, docusate calcium, docusate potassium, mineral oil and senna are category C. Casanthranol, cascara sagrada and danthron are excreted in breast milk, resulting in a potential increased incidence of diarrhea in the nursing infant.

The American College of Toxicology states that cathartics should *not* be used as a means of clearing poisons from the digestive tract of a **poisoning** victim. Although some physicians have administered these laxatives along with **activated charcoal** in order to reduce the body's absorption of the poison, this treatment is no longer recommended.

Interactions

Mineral oil and docusate should not be used in combination. Docusate is an emulsifying agent which will increase the absorption of mineral oil.

KEY TERMS

Carbohydrates—Compounds, such as cellulose, sugar, and starch, that contain only carbon, hydrogen, and oxygen, and are a major part of the diets of people and other animals.

Cathartic colon—A poorly functioning colon, resulting from the chronic abuse of stimulant cathartics.

Colon—The large intestine.

Diverticulitis—Inflammation of the part of the intestine known as the diverticulum.

Fiber—Carbohydrate material in food that cannot be digested.

Hyperosmotic—Hypertonic, containing a higher concentration of salts or other dissolved materials than normal tissues.

Osteomalacia—A disease of adults, characterized by softening of the bone. Similar to rickets which is seen in children.

Pregnancy category—A system of classifying drugs according to their established risks for use during pregnancy. Category A: Controlled human studies have demonstrated no fetal risk. Category B: Animal studies indicate no fetal risk, but no human studies, or adverse effects in animals, but not in well-controlled human studies. Category C: No adequate human or animal studies, or adverse fetal effects in animal studies, but no available human data. Category D: Evidence of fetal risk, but benefits outweigh risks. Category X: Evidence of fetal risk. Risks outweigh any benefits.

Steatorrhea—An excess of fat in the stool.

Stool—The solid waste that is left after food is digested. Stool forms in the intestines and passes out of the body through the anus.

Bisacodyl tablets are enteric coated, and so should not be used in combination with **antacids**. The antacids will cause premature rupture of the enteric coating.

Resources

BOOKS

Beers, Mark H., MD, and Robert Berkow, MD., editors. "Diarrhea and Constipation." In *The Merck Manual of Diagnosis and Therapy*. Whitehouse Station, NJ: Merck Research Laboratories, 2004.

Karch, A. M. *Lippincott's Nursing Drug Guide*. Springhouse, PA: Lippincott Williams & Wilkins, 2003.

ORGANIZATIONS

American Society of Health-System Pharmacists (ASHP). 7272 Wisconsin Avenue, Bethesda, MD 20814. (301) 657-3000. < http://www.ashp.org >.

National Digestive Diseases Information Clearinghouse. 2 Information Way, Bethesda, MD 20892-3570. nddic@aerie.com. < http://www.niddk.nih.gov/Brochures/NDDIC.htm >.

United States Food and Drug Administration (FDA). 5600 Fishers Lane, Rockville, MD 20857-0001. (888) INFO-FDA. < http:/www.fda.gov >.

Samuel D. Uretsky, PharmD
Rebecca J. Frey, PhD

Lazy eye *see* **Amblyopia**

LCM *see* **Lymphocytic choriomeningitis**

LDH isoenzymes test *see* **Lactate dehydrogenase isoenzymes test**

LDH test *see* **Lactate dehydrogenase test**

Lead poisoning

Definition

Lead **poisoning** occurs when a person swallows, absorbs, or inhales lead in any form. The result can be damaging to the brain, nerves, and many other parts of the body. Acute lead poisoning, which is somewhat rare, occurs when a relatively large amount of lead is taken into the body over a short period of time. Chronic lead poisoning—a common problem in children—occurs when small amounts of lead are taken in over a longer period. The Centers for Disease Control and Prevention (CDC) defines childhood lead poisoning as a whole-blood lead concentration equal to or greater than 10 micrograms/dL.

Description

Lead can damage almost every system in the human body, and it can also cause high blood pressure (**hypertension**). It is particularly harmful to the developing brain of fetuses and young children. The higher the level of lead in a child's blood, and the longer this elevated level lasts, the greater the chance of ill effects. Over the long term, lead poisoning in a child can lead to learning disabilities, behavioral problems, and even

mental retardation. At very high levels, lead poisoning can cause seizures, **coma**, and even **death**. According to the National Center for Environmental Health, there were about 200 deaths from lead poisoning in the United States between 1979 and 1998. Most of the deaths were among males (74%), African Americans (67%), adults over the age of 45 (76%), and Southerners (70%).

About one out of every six children in the United States has a high level of lead in the blood, according to the Agency for Toxic Substances and Disease Registry. Many of these children are exposed to lead through peeling paint in older homes. Others are exposed through dust or soil that has been contaminated by old paint or past emissions of leaded gasoline. Since children between the ages of 12–36 months are apt to put things in their mouths, they are more likely than older children to take in lead. Pregnant women who come into contact with lead can pass it along to the fetus.

Over 80% of American homes built before 1978 have lead-based paint in them, according to the Centers for Disease Control and Prevention (CDC). The older the home, the more likely it is to contain lead paint, and the higher the concentration of lead in the paint is apt to be. Some homes also have lead in the water pipes or plumbing. People may have lead in the paint, dust, or soil around their homes or in their drinking water without knowing it, since lead can't be seen, smelled, or tasted. Because lead doesn't break down naturally, it can continue to cause problems until it is removed.

Causes and symptoms

Before scientists knew how harmful it could be, lead was widely used in paint, gasoline, water pipes, and many other products. Today house paint is almost lead-free, gasoline is unleaded, and household plumbing is no longer made with lead materials. Still, remnants of the old hazards remain. Following are some sources of lead exposure:

- Lead-based paint. This is the most common source of exposure to large amounts of lead among preschoolers. Children may eat paint chips from older homes that have fallen into disrepair. They may also chew on painted surfaces such as windowsills. In addition, paint may be disturbed during remodeling.

- Dust and soil. These can be contaminated with lead from old paint or past emissions of leaded gasoline. In addition, pollution from operating or abandoned industrial sites and smelters can find its way into the soil, resulting in soil contamination.

- Drinking water. Exposure may come from lead water pipes, found in many homes built before 1930. Even newer copper pipes may have lead solder. Also, some new homes have brass faucets and fittings that can leach lead.

- Jobs and hobbies. A number of activities can expose participants to lead. These include making pottery or stained glass, refinishing furniture, doing home repairs, and using indoor firing ranges. When adults take part in such activities, they may inadvertently expose children to lead residue that is on their clothing or on scrap materials.

- Food. Imported food cans often have lead solder. Lead may also be found in leaded crystal glassware and some imported ceramic or old ceramic dishes (e.g., ceramic dishes from Mexico). A 2003 study of cases of lead poisoning in pregnant women found that 70% of the patients were Hispanics, most of whom had absorbed the lead from their pottery. In addition, food may be contaminated by lead in the water or soil.

- Folk medicines. Certain folk medicines (for example, alarcon, alkohl, azarcon, bali goli, coral, ghasard, greta, liga, pay-loo-ah, and rueda) and traditional cosmetics (kohl, for example) contain large amounts of lead.

- Moonshine whiskey. Lead poisoning from drinking illegally distilled liquor is still a cause of death among adults in the southern United States.

- Gunshot **wounds**. Toxic amounts of lead can be absorbed from bullets or bullet fragments that remain in the body after emergency surgery.

Chronic lead poisoning

New evidence suggests that lead may be harmful to children even at low levels that were once thought to be safe, and the risk of damage rises as blood levels of lead increase. The symptoms of chronic lead poisoning take time to develop, however. Children can appear healthy despite having high levels of lead in their blood. Over time, though, problems such as the following may arise:

- learning disabilities

- hyperactivity

- mental retardation

- slowed growth

- hearing loss

- headaches

It is also known that certain genetic factors increase the harmful effects of lead poisoning in susceptible children; however, these factors are not completely understood as of 2003.

Lead poisoning is also harmful to adults, in whom it can cause high blood pressure, digestive problems, nerve disorders, memory loss, and muscle and joint **pain**. In addition, it can lead to difficulties during **pregnancy**, as well as cause reproductive problems in both men and women.

More recently, chronic exposure to lead in the environment has been found to speed up the progression of kidney disorders in patients without diabetes.

Acute lead poisoning

Acute lead poisoning, while less common, shows up more quickly and can be fatal. Symptoms such as the following may occur:

- severe abdominal pain

- diarrhea

- nausea and **vomiting**

- weakness of the limbs

- seizures

- coma

Diagnosis

A high level of lead in the blood can be detected with a simple blood test. In fact, testing is the only way to know for sure if children without symptoms have been exposed to lead, since they can appear healthy even as long-term damage occurs. The CDC recommends testing all children at 12 months of age and, if possible, again at 24 months. Testing should start at six months for children at risk for lead poisoning. Based on these test results and a child's risk factors, the doctor will then decide whether further testing is needed and how often. In some states, more frequent testing is required by law.

Children at risk

Children with an increased risk of lead poisoning include those who:

- Live in or regularly visit a house built before 1978 in which chipped or peeling paint is present.

- Live in or regularly visit a house that was built before 1978 where remodeling is planned or underway.

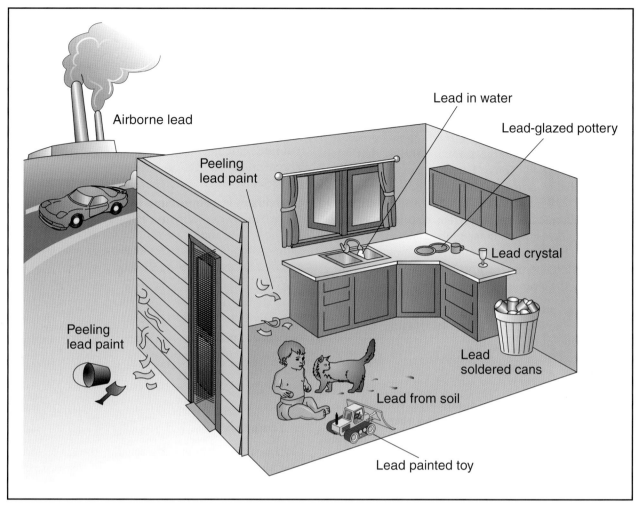

Continuous exposure to lead can damage nearly every system in the human body and is particularly harmful to the developing brain of fetuses and young children. Common sources of lead exposure include lead-based paint, dust and soil, drinking water, food from cans, and eating utensils, such as plates and drinking glasses, that are lead-based. *(Illustration by Electronic Illustrators Group.)*

- Have a brother or sister, housemate, or playmate who has been diagnosed with lead poisoning.

- Have the habit of eating dirt, or have been diagnosed with pica.

- Live with an adult whose job or hobby involves exposure to lead.

- Live near an active lead smelter, battery-recycling plant, or other industry that can create lead pollution.

Adults at risk

Testing is also important for adults whose job or hobby puts them at risk for lead poisoning. This includes people who take part in the following activities:

- glazed pottery or stained glass making
- furniture refinishing
- home renovation
- target shooting at indoor firing ranges
- battery reclamation
- precious metal refining
- radiator repair
- art restoration

Treatment

The first step in treating lead poisoning is to avoid further contact with lead. For adults, this usually means making changes at work or in hobbies. For children, it means finding and removing sources of lead in the home. In most states, the public health department can help assess the home and identify lead sources.

If the problem is lead paint, a professional with special training should remove it. Removal of lead paint is not a do-it-yourself project. Scraping or sanding lead paint creates large amounts of dust that can poison people in the home. This dust can stay around long after the work is completed. In addition, heating lead paint can release lead into the air. For these reasons, lead paint should only be removed by someone who knows how to do the job safely and has the equipment to clean up thoroughly. Occupants, especially children and pregnant women, should leave the home until the cleanup is finished.

Medical professionals should take all necessary steps to remove bullets or bullet fragments from patients with gunshot injuries.

Chelation therapy

If blood levels of lead are high enough, the doctor may also prescribe **chelation therapy**. This refers to treatment with chemicals that bind to the lead and help the body pass it in urine at a faster rate. There are four chemical agents that may be used for this purpose, either alone or in combination. Edetate calcium disodium (EDTA calcium) and dimercaprol (BAL) are given through an intravenous line or in shots, while succimer (Chemet) and penicillamine (Cuprimine, Depen) are taken by mouth. (Although many doctors prescribe penicillamine for lead poisoning, this use of the drug has not been approved by the Food and Drug Administration.)

Alternative treatment

Changes in diet are no substitute for medical treatment. However, getting enough calcium, zinc, and protein may help reduce the amount of lead the body absorbs. Iron is also important, since people who are deficient in this nutrient absorb more lead. Garlic and thiamine, a B-complex vitamin, have been used to treat lead poisoning in animals. However, their usefulness in humans for this purpose has not been proved. Nutritional, botanical, and homeopathic medicines can be administered once the source is removed, to help correct any imbalances brought on by lead toxicity.

KEY TERMS

Chelation therapy—Treatment with chemicals that bind to a poisonous metal and help the body pass it in urine at a faster rate.

Dimercaprol (BAL)—A chemical agent used to remove excess lead from the body.

Edetate calcium disodium (EDTA calcium)—A chemical agent used to remove excess lead from the body.

Penicillamine (Cuprimine, Depen)—A drug used to treat medical problems (such as excess copper in the body and rheumatoid arthritis) and to prevent kidney stones. It is also sometimes prescribed to remove excess lead from the body.

Pica—An abnormal appetite or craving for non-food items, often such substances as chalk, clay, dirt, laundry starch, or charcoal.

Succimer (Chemet)—A drug used to remove excess lead from the body.

Prognosis

If acute lead poisoning reaches the stage of seizures and coma, there is a high risk of death. Even if the person survives, there is a good chance of permanent brain damage. The long-term effects of lower levels of lead can also be permanent and severe. However, if chronic lead poisoning is caught early, these negative effects can be limited by reducing future exposure to lead and getting proper medical treatment.

Prevention

Many cases of lead poisoning can be prevented. These steps can help:

- Keep the areas where children play as clean and dust-free as possible.

- Wash pacifiers and bottles when they fall to the floor, and wash stuffed animals and toys often.

- Make sure children wash their hands before meals and at bedtime.

- Mop floors and wipe windowsills and other chewable surfaces, such as cribs, twice a week with a solution of powdered dishwasher detergent in warm water.

- Plant bushes next to an older home with painted exterior walls to keep children at a distance.

- Plant grass or another ground cover in soil that is likely to be contaminated, such as soil around a home built before 1960 or located near a major highway.

- Have household tap water tested to find out if it contains lead.

- Use only water from the cold-water tap for drinking, cooking, and making baby formula, since hot water is likely to contain higher levels of lead.

- If the cold water hasn't been used for six hours or more, run it for several seconds, until it becomes as cold as it will get, before using it for drinking or cooking. The more time water has been sitting in the pipes, the more lead it may contain.

- If you work with lead in your job or hobby, change your clothes before you go home.

- Do not store food in open cans, especially imported cans.

- Do not store or serve food in pottery meant for decorative use.

Resources

BOOKS

Beers, Mark H., MD, and Robert Berkow, MD., editors. "Poisoning: Lead Poisoning." In *The Merck Manual of Diagnosis and Therapy*. Whitehouse Station, NJ: Merck Research Laboratories, 2004.

PERIODICALS

Gavaghan, Helen. "Lead, Unsafe at Any Level." *Bulletin of the World Health Organization* January 2002: 82.

Kaufmann, R. B., C. J. Staes, and T. D. Matte. "Deaths Related to Lead Poisoning in the United States, 1979-1998." *Environmental Research* 91 (February 2003): 78–84.

Lanphear, B. P., K. N. Dietrich, and O. Berger. "Prevention of Lead Toxicity in US Children." *Ambulatory Pediatrics* 3 (January-February 2003): 27–36.

Lidsky, T. I., and J. S. Schneider. "Lead Neurotoxicity in Children: Basic Mechanisms and Clinical Correlates." *Brain* 126, Part 1 (January 2003): 5–19.

Lin, J. L., D. T. Lin-Tan, K. H. Hsu, and C. C. Yu. "Environmental Lead Exposure and Progression of Chronic Renal Diseases in Patients Without Diabetes." *New England Journal of Medicine* 348 (January 23, 2003): 277–286.

"National Campaign to Promote New 24/7 Poison Hotline." *Medical Letter on the CDC & FDA* March 10, 2002: 12.

Shannon, M. "Severe Lead Poisoning in Pregnancy." *Ambulatory Pediatrics* 3 (January-February 2003): 37–39.

Tarkin, I. S., A. Hatzidakis, S. C. Hoxie, et al. "Arthroscopic Treatment of Gunshot Wounds to the Shoulder." *Arthroscopy* 19 (January 2003): 85–89.

"Tofu May Lower Lead Levels in Blood." *Townsend Letter for Doctors and Patients* February-March 2002: 23.

ORGANIZATIONS

Centers for Disease Control and Prevention. 1600 Clifton Rd., NE, Atlanta, GA 30333. (800) 311-3435, (404) 639-3311. < http://www.cdc.gov >.

National Lead Information Center, National Safety Council. 1025 Connecticut Ave. N.W., Suite 1200, Washington, DC 20036. (800) 532-3394. < http://www.nsc.org/ehc/lead.htm >.

Office of Water Resources Center, Environmental Protection Agency. Mail Code (4100), Room 2615 East Tower Basement, 401 M St. S.W., Washington, DC 20460. (800) 426–4791. < http://www.epa.gov/ow/ >.

Linda Wasmer Smith
Rebecca J. Frey, PhD

Learning disorders

Definition

Learning disorders are academic difficulties experienced by children and adults of average to above-average intelligence. People with learning disorders have difficulty with reading, writing, mathematics, or a combination of the three. These difficulties significantly interfere with academic achievement or daily living.

Description

Learning disorders, or disabilities, affect approximately 2 million children between the ages of six and 17 (5% of public school children), although some experts think the figure may be as high as 15%. These children have specific impairments in acquiring, retaining, and processing information. Standardized tests place them well below their IQ range in their area of difficulty. The three main types of learning disorders are reading disorders, mathematics disorders, and disorders of written expression. The male: female ratio for learning disorders is about 5:1.

Reading disorders

Reading disorders are the most common type of learning disorder. Children with reading disorders have difficulty recognizing and interpreting letters and words (**dyslexia**). They aren't able to recognize and decode the sounds and syllables (phonetic structure) behind written words and language in general. This condition lowers accuracy and comprehension in reading.

Mathematics disorders

Children with mathematics disorders (dyscalculia) have problems recognizing and counting numbers correctly. They have difficulty using numbers in everyday settings. Mathematics disorders are typically diagnosed in the first few years of elementary school when formal teaching of numbers and basic math concepts begins. Children with mathematics disorders usually have a co-existing reading disorder, a disorder of written expression, or both.

Disorders of written expression

Disorders of written expression typically occur in combination with reading disorders or mathematics disorders or both. The condition is characterized by difficulty with written compositions (dysgraphia). Children with this type of learning disorder have problems with spelling, punctuation, grammar, and organizing their thoughts in writing.

Causes and symptoms

Learning disorders are thought to be caused by neurological abnormalities that trigger impairments in the regions of the brain that control visual and language processing and attention and planning. These traits may be genetically linked. Children from families with a history of learning disorders are more likely to develop disorders themselves. In 2003 a team of Finnish researchers reported finding a candidate gene for developmental dyslexia on human chromosome 15q21.

Learning difficulties may also be caused by such medical conditions as a traumatic brain injury or brain infections such as **encephalitis** or **meningitis**.

The defining symptom of a learning disorder is academic performance that is markedly below a child's age and grade capabilities and measured IQ. Children with a reading disorder may confuse or transpose words or letters and omit or add syllables to words. The written homework of children with disorders of written expression is filled with grammatical, spelling, punctuation, and organizational errors. The child's handwriting is often extremely poor. Children with mathematical disorders are often unable to count in the correct sequence, to name numbers, and to understand numerical concepts.

Diagnosis

Problems with vision or hearing, mental disorders (depression, **attention-deficit/hyperactivity disorder**), **mental retardation**, cultural and language differences, and inadequate teaching may be mistaken for learning disorders or complicate a diagnosis. A comprehensive medical, psychological, and educational assessment is critical to making a clear and correct diagnosis.

A child thought to have a learning disorder should undergo a complete medical examination to rule out an organic cause. If none is found, a psychoeducational assessment should be performed by a psychologist, psychiatrist, neurologist, neuropsychologist, or learning specialist. A complete medical, family, social, and educational history is compiled from existing medical and school records and from interviews with the child and the child's parents and teachers. A series of written and verbal tests are then given to the child to evaluate his or her cognitive and intellectual functioning. Commonly used tests include the Wechsler Intelligence Scale for Children (WISC-III), the Woodcock-Johnson Psychoeducational Battery, the Peabody Individual Achievement Test-Revised (PIAT-R) and the California Verbal Learning Test (CVLT). Federal legislation mandates that this testing is free of charge within the public school system.

Treatment

Once a learning disorder has been diagnosed, an individual education plan (IEP) is developed for the child in question. IEPs are based on psychoeducational test findings. They provide for annual retesting to measure a child's progress. Learning-disordered students may receive special instruction within a regular general education class or they may be taught in a special education or learning center for a portion of the day.

Common strategies for the treatment of reading disorders focus first on improving a child's recognition of the sounds of letters and language through phonics training. Later strategies focus on comprehension, retention, and study skills. Students with disorders of written expression are often encouraged to keep journals and to write with a computer keyboard instead of a pencil. Instruction for students with mathematical disorders emphasizes real-world uses of arithmetic, such as balancing a checkbook or comparing prices.

Prognosis

Resources

BOOKS

American Psychiatric Association. *Diagnostic and Statistical Manual of Mental Disorders.* 4th ed., revised. Washington, DC: American Psychiatric Association, 2000.

Beers, Mark H., MD, and Robert Berkow, MD., editors. "Learning Disorders." In *The Merck Manual of Diagnosis and Therapy.* Whitehouse Station, NJ: Merck Research Laboratories, 2004.

PERIODICALS

Galaburda, D. M., and B. C. Duchaine. "Developmental Disorders of Vision." *Neurologic Clinics* 21 (August 2003): 687–707.

Gillberg, C., and H. Soderstrom. "Learning Disability." *Lancet* 362 (September 6, 2003): 811–821.

Taipale, M., N. Kaminen, J. Nopola-Hemmi, et al. "A Candidate Gene for Developmental Dyslexia Encodes a Nuclear Tetratricopeptide Repeat Domain Protein Dynamically Regulated in Brain." *Proceedings of the National Academy of Sciences in the USA* 100 (September 30, 2003): 11553–11558.

Taylor, K. E., and J. Walter. "Occupation Choices of Adults With and Without Symptoms of Dyslexia." *Dyslexia* 9 (August 2003): 177–185.

Witt, W. P., A. W. Riley, and M. J. Coiro. "Childhood Functional Status, Family Stressors, and Psychosocial Adjustment Among School-Aged Children with Disabilities in the United States." *Archives of Pediatric and Adolescent Medicine* 157 (July 2003): 687–695.

ORGANIZATIONS

The Interactive Guide to Learning Disabilities for Parents, Teachers, and Children. < http://www.ldonline.org >.

Learning Disabilities Association of America. 4156 Library Road, Pittsburg, PA 15234. (412) 341-1515. < http://www.ldanatl.org >.

National Center for Learning Disabilities (NCLD). 381 Park Avenue South, Suite 1401, New York, NY 10016. (410) 296-0232. < http://www.ncld.org >.

OTHER

LD Online Page. < http://www.ldonline.org >.

Paula Anne Ford-Martin
Rebecca J. Frey, PhD

Leeches

Definition

Leeches are bloodsucking worms with segmented bodies. They belong to the same large classification of worms as earthworms and certain oceanic worms.

Leeches can primarily be found in freshwater lakes, ponds, or rivers. They range in size from 0.2 in (5 mm) to nearly 18 in (45 cm) and have two characteristic suckers located at either end of their bodies. Leeches consume the blood of a wide variety of animal hosts, ranging from fish to humans. To feed, a leech first attaches itself to the host using the suckers. One of these suckers surrounds the leech's mouth, which contains three sets of jaws that bite into the host's flesh, making a Y-shaped incision. As the leech begins to feed, its saliva releases chemicals that dilate blood vessels, thin the blood, and deaden the **pain** of the bite. Because of the saliva's effects, a person bitten by a leech may not even be aware of it until afterwards, when he or she sees the incision and the trickle of blood that is difficult to stop.

For centuries, leeches were a common tool of doctors, who believed that many diseases were the result of "imbalances" in the body that could be stabilized by releasing blood. For example, leeches were sometimes attached to veins in the temples to treat headaches. Advances in medical knowledge led doctors to abandon bloodletting and the use of leeches in the mid-nineteenth century. In recent years, however, doctors have found a new purpose for leeches–helping to restore blood circulation to grafted or severely injured tissue.

Purpose

There are many occasions in medicine, mostly in surgery and trauma care, when blood accumulates and causes trouble. Leeches can be used to reduce the swelling of any tissue that is holding too much blood. This problem is most likely to occur in two situations:

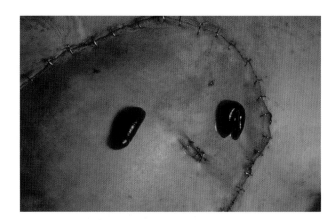

These leeches are being used to reduce venous congestion, or excessive amounts of blood in the blood vessels. *(Photograph by Michael English, M.D., Custom Medical Stock Photo. Reproduced by permission.)*

- Trauma. Large **blood clots** resulting from trauma can threaten tissue survival by their size and pressure. Blood clots can also obstruct the patient's airway.

- Surgical procedures involving reattachment of severed body parts or tissue reconstruction following **burns**. In these situations it is difficult for the surgeon to make a route for blood to leave the affected part and return to the circulation. The hardest part of reattaching severed extremities like fingers, toes and ears is to reconnect the tiny veins. If the veins are not reconnected, blood will accumulate in the injured area. A similar situation occurs when plastic surgeons move large flaps of skin to replace skin lost to burns, trauma or radical surgery. The skin flaps often drain blood poorly, get congested, and begin to die. Leeches have come to the rescue in both situations.

Precautions

It is important to use only leeches that have been raised in the laboratory under sterile conditions in order to protect patients from infection. Therapeutic leeches belong to one of two species–*Hirudo michaelseni* or *Hirudo medicinalis*.

Description

One or more leeches are applied to the swollen area, depending on the size of the graft or injury, and left on for several hours. The benefits of the treatment lie not in the amount of blood that the leeches ingest, but in the anti-bloodclotting (anticoagulant) enzymes in the saliva that allow blood to flow from the bite for up to six hours after the animal is detached, effectively draining away blood that could otherwise accumulate

and cause tissue death. Leech saliva has been described as a better anticoagulant than many currently available to treat strokes and heart attacks. Active investigation of the chemicals in leech saliva is currently under way, and one anticoagulant drug, hirudin, is derived from the tissues of *Hirudo medicinalis*.

Aftercare

The leeches are removed by pulling them off or by loosening their grip with **cocaine**, heat, or acid. The used leeches are then killed by placing them in an alcohol solution and disposed of as a biohazard. Proper care of the patient's sore is important, as is monitoring the rate at which it bleeds after the leech is removed. Any clots that form at the wound site during treatment should be removed to ensure effective blood flow.

Risks

Infection is a constant possibility until the sore heals. It is also necessary to monitor the amount of blood that the leeches have removed from the patient, since a drop in red blood cell counts could occur in rare cases of prolonged bleeding.

Resources

PERIODICALS

Daane, S., et al. "Clinical Use of Leeches in Reconstructive Surgery." *American Journal of Orthopedics* 26, no. 8 (August 1997): 528-532.

J. Ricker Polsdorfer, MD

Legionnaires' disease

Definition

Legionnaires' disease is a type of **pneumonia** caused by *Legionella* bacteria. The bacterial species responsible for Legionnaires' disease is *L. pneumophila*. Major symptoms include **fever**, chills, muscle aches, and a **cough** that is initially nonproductive. Definitive diagnosis relies on specific laboratory tests for the bacteria, bacterial antigens, or antibodies produced by the body's immune system. As with other types of pneumonia, Legionnaires' disease poses the greatest threat to people who are elderly, ill, or immunocompromised.

Description

Legionella bacteria were first identified as a cause of pneumonia in 1976, following an outbreak of pneumonia among people who had attended an American Legion convention in Philadelphia, Pennsylvania. This eponymous outbreak prompted further investigation into *Legionella* and it was discovered that earlier unexplained pneumonia outbreaks were linked to the bacteria. The earliest cases of Legionnaires' disease were shown to have occurred in 1965, but samples of the bacteria exist from 1947.

Exposure to the *Legionella* bacteria doesn't necessarily lead to infection. According to some studies, an estimated 5-10% of the American population show serologic evidence of exposure, the majority of whom do not develop symptoms of an infection. *Legionella* bacteria account for 2-15% of the total number of pneumonia cases requiring hospitalization in the United States.

There are at least 40 types of *Legionella* bacteria, half of which are capable of producing disease in humans. A disease that arises from infection by *Legionella* bacteria is referred to as legionellosis. The *L. pneumophila bacterium*, the root cause of Legionnaires' disease, causes 90% of legionellosis cases. The second most common cause of legionellosis is the *L. micdadei* bacterium, which produces the Philadelphia pneumonia-causing agent.

Approximately 10,000-40,000 people in the United States develop Legionnaires' disease annually. The people who are the most likely to become ill are over age 50. The risk is greater for people who suffer from health conditions such as malignancy, diabetes, lung disease, or **kidney disease**. Other risk factors include immunosuppressive therapy and cigarette **smoking**. Legionnaires' disease has occurred in children, but typically it has been confined to newborns receiving respiratory therapy, children who have had recent operations, and children who are immunosuppressed. People with HIV infection and **AIDS** do not seem to contract Legionnaires' disease with any greater frequency than the rest of the population, however, if contracted, the disease is likely to be more severe compared to other cases.

Cases of Legionnaires' disease that occur in conjunction with an outbreak, or epidemic, are more likely to be diagnosed quickly. Early diagnosis aids effective and successful treatment. During epidemic outbreaks, fatalities have ranged from 5% for previously healthy individuals to 24% for individuals with underlying illnesses. Sporadic cases (that is, cases unrelated to a wider outbreak) are harder to detect and treatment may be delayed pending an accurate diagnosis. The overall fatality rate for sporadic cases ranges from 10-19%. The outlook is bleaker in severe cases that require respiratory support or dialysis. In such cases, fatality may reach 67%.

Causes and symptoms

Legionnaires' disease is caused by inhaling *Legionella* bacteria from the environment. Typically, the bacteria are dispersed in aerosols of contaminated water. These aerosols are produced by devices in which warm water can stagnate, such as air-conditioning cooling towers, humidifiers, shower heads, and faucets. There have also been cases linked to whirlpool spa baths and water misters in grocery store produce departments. Aspiration of contaminated water is also a potential source of infection, particularly in hospital-acquired cases of Legionnaires' disease. There is no evidence of person-to-person transmission of Legionnaires' disease.

Once the bacteria are in the lungs, cellular representatives of the body's immune system (alveolar macrophages) congregate to destroy the invaders. The typical macrophage defense is to phagocytose the invader and demolish it in a process analogous to swallowing and digesting it. However, the *Legionella* bacteria survive being phagocytosed. Instead of being destroyed within the macrophage, they grow and replicate, eventually killing the macrophage. When the macrophage dies, many new *Legionella* bacteria are released into the lungs and worsen the infection.

Legionnaires' disease develops 2-10 days after exposure to the bacteria. Early symptoms include lethargy, headaches, fever, chills, muscle aches, and a lack of appetite. Respiratory symptoms such as coughing or congestion are usually absent. As the disease progresses, a dry, hacking cough develops

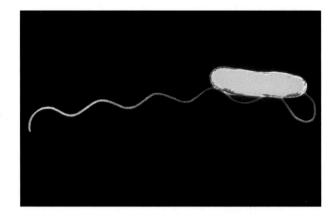

A transmission electron microscopy (TEM) image of *Legionella pneumophila,* the bacteria which causes Legionnaires' disease. *(Custom Medical Stock Photo. Reproduced by permission.)*

and may become productive after a few days. In about a third of Legionnaires' disease cases, blood is present in the sputum. Half of the people who develop Legionnaires' disease suffer **shortness of breath** and a third complain of breathing-related chest **pain**. The fever can become quite high, reaching 104 °F (40 °C) in many cases, and may be accompanied by a decreased heart rate.

Although the pneumonia affects the lungs, Legionnaires' disease is accompanied by symptoms that affect other areas of the body. About half the victims experience **diarrhea** and a quarter have **nausea and vomiting** and abdominal pain. In about 10% of cases, acute renal failure and scanty urine production accompany the disease. Changes in mental status, such as disorientation, confusion, and **hallucinations**, also occur in about a quarter of cases.

In addition to Legionnaires' disease, *L. pneumophila* legionellosis also includes a milder disease, Pontiac fever. Unlike Legionnaires' disease, Pontiac fever does not involve the lower respiratory tract. The symptoms usually appear within 36 hours of exposure and include fever, **headache**, muscle aches, and lethargy. Symptoms last only a few days and medical intervention is not necessary.

Diagnosis

The symptoms of Legionnaires' disease are common to many types of pneumonia and diagnosis of sporadic cases can be difficult. The symptoms and chest x rays that confirm a case of pneumonia are not useful in differentiating between Legionnaires' disease and other pneumonias. If a pneumonia case involves multisystem symptoms, such as diarrhea and

vomiting, and an initially dry cough, laboratory tests are done to definitively identify *L. pneumophila* as the cause of the infection.

If Legionnaires' disease is suspected, several tests are available to reveal or indicate the presence of *L. pneumophila* bacteria in the body. Since the immune system creates antibodies against infectious agents, examining the blood for these indicators is a key test. The level of immunoglobulins, or antibody molecules, in the blood reveals the presence of infection. In microscopic examination of the patient's sputum, a fluorescent stain linked to antibodies against *L. pneumophila* can uncover the presence of the bacteria. Other means of revealing the bacteria's presence from patient sputum samples include isolation of the organism on culture media or detection of the bacteria by DNA probe. Another test detects *L. pneumophila* antigens in the urine.

Treatment

Most cases of *Legionella* pneumonia show improvement within 12-48 hours of starting antibiotic therapy. The antibiotic of choice has been erythromycin, sometimes paired with a second antibiotic, rifampin. Tetracycline, alone or with rifampin, is also used to treat Legionnaires' disease, but has had more mixed success in comparison to erythromycin. Other **antibiotics** that have been used successfully to combat *Legionella* include doxycycline, clarithromycin, fluorinated quinolones, and trimethoprim/ sulfamethoxazole.

The type of antibiotic prescribed by the doctor depends on several factors including the severity of infection, potential **allergies**, and interaction with previously prescribed drugs. For example, erythromycin interacts with warfarin, a blood thinner. Several drugs, such as **penicillins** and **cephalosporins**, are ineffective against the infection. Although they may be deadly to the bacteria in laboratory tests, their chemical structure prevents them from being absorbed into the areas of the lung where the bacteria are present.

In severe cases with complications, antibiotic therapy may be joined by respiratory support. If renal failure occurs, dialysis is required until renal function is recovered.

Prognosis

Appropriate medical treatment has a major impact on recovery from Legionnaires' disease. Outcome is also linked to the victim's general health and absence of complications. If the patient survives the infection, recovery from Legionnaires' disease is complete. Similar to other types of pneumonia, severe cases of Legionnaires' disease may cause scarring in the lung tissue as a result of the infection. Renal failure, if it occurs, is reversible and renal function returns as the patient's health improves. Occasionally, **fatigue** and weakness may linger for several months after the infection has been successfully treated.

Prevention

Since the bacteria thrive in warm stagnant water, regularly disinfecting ductwork, pipes, and other areas that may serve as breeding areas is the best method for preventing outbreaks of Legionnaires' disease. Most outbreaks of Legionnaires' disease can be traced to specific points of exposure, such as hospitals, hotels, and other places where people gather. Sporadic cases

are harder to determine and there is insufficient evidence to point to exposure in individual homes.

Resources

PERIODICALS

Shuman, H. A., et al. "Intracellular Multiplication of Legionella pneumophila: Human Pathogen of Accidental Tourist?" *Current Topics in Microbiology and Immunology* 225 (1998): 99.

Julia Barrett

Leiomyomas *see* **Uterine fibroids**

Leishmaniasis

Definition

Leishmaniasis refers to several different illnesses caused by infection with an organism called a protozoan.

Description

Protozoa are considered to be the most simple organisms in the animal kingdom. They are all single-celled. The types of protozoa that cause leishmaniasis are carried by the blood-sucking sandfly. The sandfly is referred to as the disease vector, simply meaning that the infectious agent (the protozoan) is carried by the sandfly and passed on to other animals or humans in whom the protozoan will set up residence and cause disease. The animal or human in which the protozoan then resides is referred to as the host.

Once the protozoan is within the human host, the human's immune system is activated to try to combat the invader. Specialized immune cells called macrophages work to swallow up the protozoa. Usually, this technique kills a foreign invader, but these protozoa can survive and flourish within macrophages. The protozoa multiply within the macrophages, ultimately causing the macrophage to burst open. The protozoa are released, and take up residence within other neighboring cells.

At this point, the course of the disease caused by the protozoa is dependent on the specific type of protozoa, and on the type of reaction the protozoa elicits from the immune system. There are several types of protozoa that cause leishmaniasis, and they cause different patterns of disease progression.

At any one time, about 20 million people throughout the world are infected with leishmaniasis. Between one million and one and one-half million cases of cutaneous leishmaniasis are reported yearly worldwide. While leishmaniasis exists as a disease in 88 countries on five continents, some countries are hit harder than others. These include Bangladesh, India, Nepal, Sudan, Afghanistan, Brazil, Iran, Peru, Saudi Arabia, and Syria. Other areas that harbor the causative protozoa include China, many countries throughout Africa, Mexico, Central and South America, Turkey, and Greece. Although less frequent, cases have occurred in the United States, in Texas.

As Americans travel to these countries, they will come in contact the protozoa that cause forms of leishmaniasis. Also, physicians were advised in 2004 to suspect cutaneous leishmaniasis in military personnel who were deployed to areas where the infection is present. From August 2002 to February 2004, staff from the U.S. Department of Defense identified 522 confirmed cases of the disease in American military personnel.

In some areas of southern Europe, leishmaniasis is becoming an important disease that infects people with weakened immune systems. In particular, individuals with acquired **immunodeficiency** syndrome (**AIDS**) are at great risk of this infection.

Causes and symptoms

There are a number of types of protozoa that can cause leishmaniasis. Each type exists in specific locations, and there are different patterns to the kind of disease each causes. The overall species name is Leishmania (commonly abbreviated L.). The specific types include: *L. Donovani, L. Infantum, L. Chagasi, L. Mexicana, L. Amazonensis, L. Tropica, L. Major, L. Aethiopica, L. Brasiliensis, L. Guyaensis, L. Panamensis, L. Peruviana.* Some of the names are reflective of the locale in which the specific protozoa is most commonly found, or in which it was first discovered.

Localized cutaneous leishmaniasis

This type of disease occurs most commonly in China, India, Asia Minor, Africa, the Mediterranean Basin, and Central America. It has occurred in an area ranging from northern Argentina all the way up to southern Texas. It is called different names in different locations, including chiclero ulcer, bush **yaws**, uta, oriental sore, Aleppo boil, and Baghdad sore.

This is perhaps the least drastic type of disease caused by any of the Leishmania. Several weeks or months after being bitten by an infected sandfly, the host may notice an itchy bump (lesion) on an arm, leg, or face. Lymph nodes in the area of this bump may be swollen. Within several months, the bump develops a crater (ulceration) in the center, with a raised, reddened ridge around it. There may be several of these lesions near each other, and they may spread into each other to form one large lesion. Although localized cutaneous leishmaniasis usually heals on its own, it may take as long as one year. A depressed, light-colored scar usually remains behind. Some lesions never heal, and may invade and destroy the tissue below. For example, lesions on the ears may slowly, but surely, invade and destroy the cartilage that supports the outer ear.

Diffuse cutaneous leishmaniasis

This type of disease occurs most often in Ethiopia, Brazil, Dominican Republic, and Venezuela.

The lesions of diffuse cutaneous leishmaniasis are very similar to those of localized cutaneous leishmaniasis, except they are spread all over the body. The body's immune system apparently fails to battle the protozoa, which are free to spread throughout. The characteristic lesions resemble those of the dread biblical disease, **leprosy**.

Mucocutaneous leishmaniasis

This form of leishmaniasis occurs primarily in the tropics of South America. The disease begins with the same sores noted in localized cutaneous leishmaniasis. Sometimes these primary lesions heal, other times they spread and become larger. Some years after the first lesion is noted (and sometimes several years after that lesion has totally healed), new lesions appear in the mouth and nose, and occasionally in the area between the genitalia and the anus (the perineum). These new lesions are particularly destructive and painful. They erode underlying tissue and cartilage, frequently eating through the septum (the cartilage that separates the two nostrils). If the lesions spread to the roof of the mouth and the larynx (the part of the wind pipe which contains the vocal cords), they may prevent speech. Other symptoms include **fever**, weight loss, and anemia (low red blood cell count). There is always a large danger of bacteria infecting the already open sores.

Visceral leishmaniasis

This type of leishmaniasis occurs inIndia, China, the southern region of Russia, and throughout Africa,

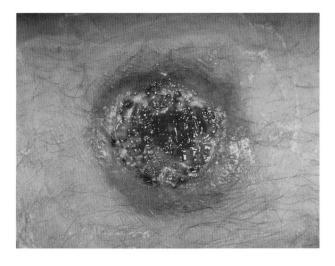

This condition, also called an oriental sore, is caused by the bacterium L. tropica. *(Photograph by Lester V. Bergman, Corbis Images. Reproduced by permission.)*

the Mediterranean, and South and Central America. It /is frequently called Kala-Azar or Dumdum fever.

In this disease, the protozoa use the bloodstream to travel to the liver, spleen, lymph nodes, and bone marrow. Fever may last for as long as eight weeks, disappear, and then reappear again. The lymph nodes, spleen, and liver are often quite enlarged. Weakness, **fatigue**, loss of appetite, **diarrhea**, and weight loss are common. Kala-azar translates to mean "black fever." The name kala-azar comes from a characteristic of this form of leishmaniasis. Individuals with light-colored skin take on a darker, grayish skin tone, particularly of their face and hands. A variety of lesions appear on the skin.

Diagnosis

Diagnosis for each of these types of leishmaniasis involves taking a scraping from a lesion, preparing it in a laboratory, and examining it under a microscope to demonstrate the causative protozoan. Other methods that have been used include culturing a sample piece of tissue in a laboratory to allow the protozoa to multiply for easier microscopic identification; injecting a mouse or hamster with a solution made of scrapings from a patient's lesion to see if the animal develops a leishmaniasis-like disease; and demonstrating the presence in macrophages of the characteristic-appearing protozoan, called Leishman-Donovan bodies.

In some forms of leishmaniasis, a skin test (similar to that given for TB) may be used. In this test, a solution containing a small bit of the protozoan antigen (cell marker that causes the human immune system to react) is injected or scratched into a patient's skin. In a positive reaction, cells from the immune system will race to this spot, causing a characteristic skin lesion. Not all forms of leishmaniasis cause a positive skin test, however.

Treatment

The treatment of choice for all forms of leishmaniasis is a type of drug containing the element antimony. These include sodium sitogluconate, and meglumin antimonate. When these types of drugs do not work, other medications with anti-protozoal activity are utilized, including amphotericin B, pentamidine, flagyl, and allopurinol. In 2004, it was reported that the world's first non-profit drug company was seeking approval in India for a drug to cure visceral leishmaniasis. An estimated 200,000 people die annually from the disease in that country. The company, called OneWorld Health, hoped to offer the drug called paromomycin for a day for a three-week treatment course.

Prognosis

The prognosis for leishmaniasis is quite variable, and depends on the specific strain of infecting protozoan, as well as the individual patient's immune system response to infection. Localized cutaneous leishmaniasis may require no treatment. Although it may take many months, these lesions usually heal themselves completely. Only rarely do these lesions fail to heal and become more destructive.

Disseminated cutaneous leishmaniasis may smolder on for years without treatment, ultimately causing **death** when the large, open lesions become infected with bacteria.

Mucocutaneous leishmaniasis is often relatively resistant to treatment. Untreated visceral leishmaniasis has a 90% death rate, but only a 10% death rate with treatment.

Prevention

Prevention involves protecting against sandfly bites. Insect repellents used around homes, on clothing, on skin, and on bednets (to protect people while sleeping) are effective measures.

Reducing the population of sandflies is also an important preventive measure. In areas where leishmaniasis is very common, recommendations include clearing the land of trees and brush for at least 984 ft

(300 m) around all villages, and regularly spraying the area with insecticides. Because rodents often carry the protozoan that causes leishmaniasis, careful rodent control should be practiced. Dogs, which also carry the protozoan, can be given a simple blood test.

Resources

PERIODICALS

MacReady, Norma. "Leishmaniasis Hits Military Hot Spots." *Internal Medicine News* June 15, 2004: 58.

"Seeking First-time Approval." *Chemist & Druggist* May 8, 2004: 12.

"Treatment of Cutaneous Leishmaniasis Among Travelers Reviewed." *Vaccine Weekly* April 28, 2004: 58.

ORGANIZATIONS

Centers for Disease Control and Prevention. 1600 Clifton Rd., NE, Atlanta, GA 30333. (800) 311-3435, (404) 639-3311. < http://www.cdc.gov >.

Rosalyn Carson-DeWitt, MD
Teresa G. Odle

Leprosy

Definition

Leprosy is a slowly progressing bacterial infection that affects the skin, peripheral nerves in the hands and feet, and mucous membranes of the nose, throat, and eyes. Destruction of the nerve endings causes the the affected areas to lose sensation. Occasionally, because of the loss of feeling, the fingers and toes become mutilated and fall off, causing the deformities that are typically associated with the disease.

Description

Leprosy is also known as Hansen's disease after G. A. Hansen, who in 1878 identified the bacillus *Mycobacterium leprae* that causes the disease.

The infection is characterized by abnormal changes of the skin. These changes, called lesions, are at first flat and red. Upon enlarging, they have irregular shapes and a characteristic appearance. The lesions are typically darker in color around the edges with discolored pale centers. Because the organism grows best at lower temperatures the leprosy bacillus has a preference for the skin, the mucous membranes and the nerves. Infection in and destruction of the nerves leads to sensory loss. The loss of sensation in the fingers and toes increases the risk of injury. Inadequate care causes infection of open **wounds**. **Gangrene** may also follow, causing body tissue to die and become deformed.

Because of the disabling deformities associated with it, leprosy has been considered one of the most dreaded diseases since biblical times, though much of what was called leprosy in the Old Testament most likely was not the same disease. Its victims were often shunned by the community, kept at arm's length, or sent to a leper colony. Many people still have misconceptions about the disease. Contrary to popular belief, it is not highly communicable and is extremely slow to develop. Household contacts of most cases and the medical personnel caring for Hansen's disease patients are not at particular risk. It is very curable, although the treatment is long-term, requiring multiple medications.

The World Health Organization (WHO) puts the number of identified leprosy cases in the world at about 600,000 as of the early 2000s. Seventy percent of all cases are found in just three countries: India, Indonesia, and Myanamar (Burma). The infection can be acquired, however, in the Western Hemisphere as well. There are about 5000 reported cases in the United States as of 2004, almost all of which involve immigrants from developing countries. Cases also occur in some areas of the Caribbean. Although it was thought for many years that only humans are affected by the disease, 15% of wild armadillos in southern Texas and Louisiana have been found to be infected with *M. leprae*.

Causes and symptoms

The organism that causes leprosy is a rod-shaped bacterium called *Mycobacterium leprae*. This bacterium is related to *Mycobacterium tuberculosis*, the causative agent of **tuberculosis**. Because special staining techniques involving acids are required to view these bacteria under the microscope, they are referred to as acid-fast bacilli (AFB).

When *Mycobacterium leprae* invades the body, one of two reactions can take place. In tuberculoid leprosy (TT), the milder form of the disease, the body's immune cells attempt to seal off the infection from the rest of the body by surrounding the offending pathogen. Because this response by the immune system occurs in the deeper layers of the skin, the hair follicles, sweat glands, and nerves can be destroyed. As a result, the skin becomes dry and discolored and loses its sensitivity. Involvement of nerves on the face, arms, or legs can cause them to enlarge and become easily felt by the doctor. This finding is highly suggestive of TT. The scarcity of bacteria in this type of leprosy leads to it being referred to as paucibacillary (PB) leprosy. Seventy to eighty percent of all leprosy cases are of the tuberculoid type.

In lepromatous (LL) leprosy, which is the second and more contagious form of the disease, the body's immune system is unable to mount a strong response to the invading organism. Hence, the organism multiplies freely in the skin. This type of leprosy is also called the multibacillary (MB) leprosy, because of the presence of large numbers of bacteria. The characteristic feature of this disease is the appearance of large nodules or lesions all over the body and face. Occasionally, the mucous membranes of the eyes, nose, and throat may be involved. Facial involvement can produce a lion-like appearance (leonine facies). This type of leprosy can lead to blindness, drastic change in voice, or mutilation of the nose. Leprosy can strike anyone; however, children seem to be more susceptible than adults.

Well-defined **skin lesions** that are numb are the first symptoms of tuberculoid leprosy. Lepromatous leprosy is characterized by a chronic stuffy nose due to invasion of the mucous membranes, and the presence of nodules and lesions all over the body and face.

Although patients with leprosy are commonly thought not to suffer **pain**, neuroapthic pain caused by inflammation of peripheral nerve endings is increasingly recognized as a major complication of the disease in many patients. **Corticosteroids** may be given to reduce the inflammation.

The incubation period of the leprosy bacillus varies anywhere from six months to ten years. On an average, it takes four years for the symptoms of tuberculoid leprosy to develop. Probably because of the slow growth of the bacillus, lepromatous leprosy develops even more slowly, taking an average of eight years for the initial lesions to appear.

It is still not very clear how the leprosy bacillus is transmitted from person to person; about 50% of patients diagnosed with the disease have a history of close contact with an infected family member. Since untreated patients have a large number of *M. leprae* bacilli in their nasal secretions, it is thought that transmission may take place via nasal droplets. The milder tubercular form of leprosy may be transmitted by insect carriers or by contact with infected soil.

The incidence of leprosy is highest in the poverty belt of the globe. Therefore, environmental factors such as unhygienic living conditions, overpopulation, and **malnutrition** may also be contributing factors favoring the infection.

It is also possible that genetic factors are involved in susceptibility to leprosy. In 2003, scientists conducting a genome scan of a large Vietnamese family with many cases of leprosy found that susceptibility to the disease was linked to region q25 on the long arm of chromosome 6. Further study indicated that the leprosy susceptibility gene lies within a region shared by two genes for Parkinson's disease. Further research may confirm that the emergence of leprosy in certain individuals is related to inheritance of genes for Parkinson's disease.

Diagnosis

One of the hallmarks of leprosy is the presence of AFB in smears taken from the skin lesions, nasal scrapings, or tissue secretions. In patients with LL leprosy, the bacilli are easily detected; however, in TT leprosy the bacteria are very few and almost impossible to find. In such cases, a diagnosis is made based on the clinical signs and symptoms, the type and distribution of skin lesions, and history of having lived in an endemic area.

The signs and symptoms characteristic of leprosy can be easily identified by a health worker after a short

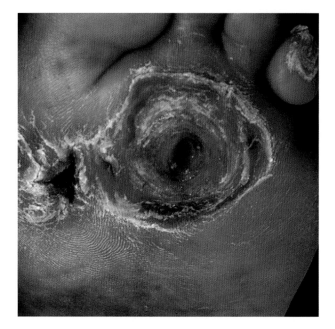

Lesions such as these are characteristic of leprosy.
(Phototake NYC. Reproduced by permission.)

training period. There is no need for a laboratory investigation to confirm a leprosy diagnosis, except in very rare circumstances.

In an endemic area, if smears from an individual show the presence of AFB, or if he has typical skin lesions, he should definitely be regarded as having leprosy. Usually, there is slight discoloration of the skin and loss of skin sensitivity. Thickened nerves accompanied by weakness of muscles supplied by the affected nerve are very typical of the disease. One characteristic occurrence is a foot drop where the foot cannot be flexed upwards, affecting the ability to walk.

Treatment

The most widely used drug for leprosy is dapsone (DDS). However, the emergence of dapsone-resistant strains prompted the introduction of multidrug therapy, or MDT. MDT combines dapsone, rifampin (Rifadin; also known as rifampicin), and clofazimine (Lamprene), all of which are powerful antibacterial drugs. Patients with MB leprosy are usually treated with all three drugs, while patients with PB leprosy are only given rifampin and dapsone. Usually three months after starting treatment, a patient ceases being infectious, though not everyone with this disease is necessarily infectious before treatment. Depending on the type of leprosy, the time required for treatment may vary from six months to two years or more.

Each of the drugs has minor side effects. Dapsone can cause **nausea**, **dizziness**, **palpitations**, **jaundice** and rash. A doctor should be contacted immediately if a rash develops. Dapsone also interacts with the second drug, rifampin. Rifampin increases the metabolizing of dapsone in the body, requiring an adjustment of the dapsone dosage. rifampin may also cause **muscle cramps**, or nausea. If jaundice, flu-like symptoms or a rash appear, a doctor should be contacted immediately. The third drug, clofazimine may cause severe abdominal pain and **diarrhea**, as well as discoloration of the skin. Red to brownish black discoloration of the skin and bodily fluids, including sweat, may persist for months to years after use.

Thalidomide, the most famous agent of **birth defects** in the twentieth century, is now being used to treat complications of leprosy and similar diseases. Thalidomide regulates the immune response by suppressing a protein, tumor necrosis factor alpha.

Leprosy patients should be aware that treatment itself can cause a potentially serious immune system response called a lepra reaction. When **antibiotics** kill *M. leprae*, antigens (the proteins on the surface of the organism that initiate the body's immune system response) are released from the dying bacteria. In some people, when the antigens combine with the antibodies to *M. Leprae* in the bloodstream, a reaction called **erythema nodosum** leprosum may occur, resulting in new lesions and peripheral nerve damage. Cortisone-type medications and, increasingly, thalidomide are used to minimize the effects of lepra reactions.

In some cases, severe ulcers caused by leprosy may be treated surgically with small skin grafts.

Prognosis

Leprosy is curable; however, the deformities and nerve damage associated with leprosy are often irreversible. Preventions or rehabilition of these defects is an integral part of management of the disease. **Reconstructive surgery**, aimed at preventing and correcting deformities, offers the greatest hope for disabled patients. Sometimes, the deformities are such that the patients will not benefit from this type of surgery.

Comprehensive care involves teaching patients to care for themselves. If the patients have significant nerve damage or are at high risk of developing deformities, they must be taught to take care of their insensitive limbs, similar to diabetics with lower leg nerve damage. Lacking the sensation of pain in many cases, the patients should constantly check themselves

KEY TERMS

Endemic area—A geographical area where a particular disease is prevalent.

Gangrene—Death of tissue due to loss of blood supply followed by bacterial invasion and putrefaction.

Incubation period—The time it takes for symptoms to develop after initial exposure to a disease-causing organism.

Lesion—Any visible, local abnormality of the tissues of the skin, such as a wound, sore, rash, or boil.

Mucous membranes—The inner tissue that covers or lines body cavities or canals open to the outside, such as nose and mouth. These membranes secrete mucus and absorb water and salts.

Nasal scraping—Pathological material obtained for clinical study by scratching the inner surface of the nose with a clinical instrument.

Nodules—A small mass of tissue in the form of a protuberance or a knot that is solid and can be detected by touch.

Pathogen—Any disease-producing agent or microorganism.

Smear—A specimen prepared for microscopic study by spreading the material across a slide and treating it with a specific stain.

to identify cuts and **bruises**. If adequate care is not taken, these wounds become festering sores and a source of dangerous infection. Physiotherapy exercises are taught to the patients to maintain a range of movement in finger joints and prevent the deformities from worsening. Prefabricated standardized splints are available and are extremely effective in correcting and preventing certain common deformities in leprosy. Special kinds of footwear have been designed for patients with insensitive feet in order to prevent or minimize the progression of foot ulcers.

Prevention

By early diagnosis and appropriate treatment of infected individuals, even a disease as ancient as leprosy can be controlled. People who are in immediate contact with the leprosy patient should be tested for leprosy. Annual examinations should also be conducted on these people for a period of five years following their last contact with an infectious patient.

Some physicians have advocated dapsone treatment for people in close household contact with leprosy patients.

The WHO Action Program for the Elimination of Leprosy adopted a resolution calling for the elimination of leprosy around the world by the year 2005. This goal is not likely to be reached, however; a computer simulation performed for WHO by a team of Dutch researchers in 2004 indicates that leprosy is likely to persist in some parts of the world until 2020, although its incidence will continue to decline.

Resources

BOOKS

Beers, Mark H., MD, and Robert Berkow, MD., editors. "Infectious Diseases Caused by Mycobacteria." In *The Merck Manual of Diagnosis and Therapy*. Whitehouse Station, NJ: Merck Research Laboratories, 2004.

PERIODICALS

Buschman, E., and E. Skamene. "Linkage of Leprosy Susceptibility to Parkinson's Disease Genes." *International Journal of Leprosy and Other Mycobacterial Diseases* 72 (June 2004): 169–170.

Jayaseelan, A., and W. Aithal. "Pinch Skin Grafting in Non-Healing Leprous Ulcers." *International Journal of Leprosy and Other Mycobacterial Diseases* 72 (June 2004): 139–142.

Meima, A., W. C. Smith, G. J. van Oortmarssen, et al. "The Future Incidence of Leprosy: A Scenario Analysis." *Bulletin of the World Health Organization* 82 (May 2004): 373–380.

Stump, P. R., R. Baccarelli, L. H. Marciano, et al. "Neuropathic Pain in Leprosy Patients." *International Journal of Leprosy and Other Mycobacterial Diseases* 72 (June 2004): 134–148.

ORGANIZATIONS

American Leprosy Missions. 1 ALM Way, Greenville, SC 29601. (1-800-LEPROSY).

British Leprosy Relief Association, LEPRA. Fairfax House, Causton Road, Colchester, Essex CO1 1PU, UK.

INFOLEP, Leprosy Information Services. Postbus 95005,1090 HA, Amsterdam, Netherlands. Infolep@antenna.nl.

WHO/LEP, Action Programme for the Elimination of Leprosy. 20 Avenue Appia CH-1211, Geneva 27, Suisse. < http://www.who.ch/programmes/lep/lep_home.htm >.

OTHER

Cherath, Lata. "Leprosy." *A Healthy Me Page*. < http://www.ahealthyme.com/topic/topic100587076 >.

Lata Cherath, PhD
Rebecca J. Frey, PhD

Leptospirosis

Definition

Leptospirosis is a febrile disease (**fever**) caused by infection with the bacterium *Leptospira interrogans*. *L. interrogans* is sometimes classified as a spirochete because it has a spiral shape. The disease can range from very mild and symptomless to a more serious, even life threatening form, that may be associated with kidney (renal) failure.

Description

An infection by the bacterium *Leptospira interrogans* goes by different names in different regions. Alternate names for leptospirosis include mud fever, swamp fever, cane cutter's fever, rice field fever, Stuttgart disease, swineherd's disease, and Fort Bragg fever. More severe cases of leptospirosis are called Weil's syndrome or icterohemorrhagic fever. This disease is commonly found in tropical and subtropical climates but occurs worldwide.

According to the Centers for Disease Control and Prevention (CDC), between 100 and 200 cases of leptospirosis are reported in the United States each year as of the early 2000s. Almost 75% of cases of leptospirosis in North America occur in males. About 50% of these cases occur in Hawaii, followed by the southern Atlantic, Gulf, and Pacific coastal states. However, because of the nonspecific symptoms of leptospirosis, it is believed that the occurrence in the United States is actually much higher. Leptospirosis occurs year-round in North America, but about half of the cases occur between July and October.

Leptospirosis is called a **zoonosis** because it is a disease of animals that can be transmitted to humans. It can be a very serious problem in the livestock industry. *Leptospira* bacteria have been found in dogs, rats, livestock, mice, voles, rabbits, hedgehogs, skunks, possums, frogs, fish, snakes, and certain birds and insects. Infected animals will pass the bacteria in their urine for months, or even years. In the United States, rats and dogs are more commonly linked with human leptospirosis than other animals.

Humans are considered accidental hosts and become infected with *Leptospira interrogans* by coming into contact with urine from infected animals. Transmission of the organism occurs either through direct contact with urine, or through contact with soil, water, or plants that have been contaminated by animal urine. *Leptospira interrogans* can survive for as long as six months outdoors under favorable conditions. Leptospira bacteria can enter the body through cuts or other skin damage or through mucous membranes (such as the inside of the mouth and nose). It is believed that the bacteria may be able to pass through intact skin, but this is not known.

Once past the skin barrier, the bacteria enter the blood stream and rapidly spread throughout the body. The infection causes damage to the inner lining of blood vessels. The liver, kidneys, heart, lungs, central nervous system, and eyes may be affected.

There are two stages in the disease process. The first stage is during the active Leptospira infection and is called the bacteremic or septicemic phase. The bacteremic phase lasts from three to seven days and presents as typical flu-like symptoms. During this phase, bacteria can be found in the patient's blood and cerebrospinal fluid. The second stage, or immune phase, occurs either immediately after the bacteremic stage or after a 1–3 day symptom-free period. The immune phase can last up to one month. During the immune phase, symptoms are milder but **meningitis** (inflammation of spinal cord and brain tissues) is common. Bacteria can be isolated only from the urine during this second phase.

Causes and symptoms

Leptospirosis is caused by an infection with the bacterium *Leptospira interrogans*. The bacteria are spread through contact with urine from infected animals. Persons at an increased risk for leptospirosis include farmers, miners, animal health care workers, fish farmers and processors, sewage and canal workers, cane harvesters, and soldiers. High-risk activities include care of pets, hunting, trail biking, freshwater swimming, rafting, canoeing, kayaking, and participating in sports in muddy fields. One recent outbreak occurred in Ireland following a canoe competition on a local river.

Symptoms of *Leptospira* infection occur within 7–12 days following exposure to the bacteria. Because the symptoms can be nonspecific, most people who have antibodies to *Leptospira* do not remember having had an illness. Eighty-five to 90% of the cases are not serious and clear up on their own. Symptoms of the first stage of leptospirosis last three to seven days and are: fever (100–105 °F [37.8–40.6 °C]), severe **headache**, muscle **pain**, stomach pain, chills, **nausea**, **vomiting**, back pain, joint pain, neck stiffness, and extreme exhaustion. **Cough** and body rash sometimes occur.

Following the first stage of disease, a brief symptom-free period occurs for most patients. The symptoms of the second stage vary in each patient. Most patients have a low-grade fever, headache, vomiting, and rash. Aseptic meningitis is common in the second stage, symptoms of which include headache and **photosensitivity** (sensitivity of the eye to light). *Leptospira* can affect the eyes and make them cloudy and yellow to orange colored. Vision may be blurred.

Ten percent of the persons infected with *Leptospira* develop a serious disease called Weil's syndrome. The symptoms of Weil's syndrome are more severe than those described above and there is no distinction between the first and second stages of disease. The hallmark of Weil's syndrome is liver, kidney, and blood vessel disease. The signs of severe disease are apparent after 3–7 days of illness. In addition to those listed above, symptoms of Weil's syndrome include **jaundice** (yellow skin and eyes), decreased or no urine output, **hypotension** (low blood pressure), rash, anemia (decreased number of red blood cells), **shock**, and severe mental status changes. Red spots on the skin, "blood shot" eyes, and bloody sputum signal that blood vessel damage and hemorrhage have occurred.

Diagnosis

Leptospirosis can be diagnosed and treated by doctors who specialize in infectious diseases. During the bacteremic phase of the disease, the symptoms are relatively nonspecific. This often causes an initial misdiagnosis because many diseases have similar symptoms to leptospirosis. The later symptoms of jaundice and kidney failure together with the bacteremic phase symptoms suggest leptospirosis. Blood samples will be tested to look for antibodies to *Leptospira interrogans*. Blood samples taken over a period of a few days would show an increase in the number of antibodies. Isolating *Leptospira* bacteria from blood, cerebrospinal fluid (performed by spinal tap), and urine samples is diagnostic of leptospirosis. It may take six weeks for *Leptospira* to grow in laboratory media. Most insurance companies would cover the diagnosis and treatment of this infection.

Several diagnostic tests for leptospirosis have been devised in the early 2000s that are more accurate as well as faster than standard culture. One test uses flow cytometry light scatter analysis; this method can evaluate a sample of infected serum in as little as 90 minutes. A second technique is an IgM-enzyme-linked immunosorbent assay (ELISA), which detects the presence of IgM antibodies to *L. interrogans* in blood serum samples.

Treatment

Leptospirosis is treated with **antibiotics**, penicillin (Bicillin, Wycillin), doxycycline (Monodox), ibramycin, or erythromycin (E-mycin, Ery-Tab). As of the early 2000s, however, many doctors prefer to treat patients with ceftriaxone, which is easier to use than intravenous penicillin. Ciprofloxacin may be combined with other drugs in treating patients who develop **uveitis**. It is generally agreed that antibiotic treatment during the first few days of illness is helpful. However, leptospirosis is often not diagnosed until the later stages of illness. The benefit of antibiotic treatment in the later stages of disease, however, is controversial. A rare complication of antibiotic therapy for leptospirosis is the occurrence of the Jarisch-Herxheimer reaction, which is characterized by fever, chills, headache, and muscle pain.

Patients with severe illness will require hospitalization for treatment and monitoring. Medication or other treatment for pain, fever, vomiting, fluid loss, bleeding, mental changes, and low blood pressure may be provided. Patients with kidney failure will require hemodialysis to remove waste products from the blood.

Prognosis

The majority of patients infected with *Leptospira interrogans* experience a complete recovery. Ten percent of the patients will develop eye inflammation (uveitis) up to one year after the illness. In the United States, about one out of every 100 patients will die from leptospirosis. **Death** is usually caused by kidney failure, but has also been caused by **myocarditis** (inflammation of heart tissue), **septic shock** (reduced blood flow to the organs because of the bacterial infection), organ failure, and/or poorly functioning lungs. Mortality is highest in patients over 60 years of age.

Prevention

Persons who are at an extremely high risk (such as soldiers who are training in wetlands) can be pretreated with 200 mg of doxycycline once a week. As of the early 2000s, there are no vaccines available to prevent leptospirosis in humans, although such vaccines have been formulated by veterinarians for dogs, swine, and cattle.

There are many ways to decrease the chances of being infected by *Leptospira*. These include:

- Avoid swimming or wading in freshwater ponds and slowly moving streams, especially those located near farms.

KEY TERMS

Hemodialysis—The removal of waste products from the blood stream in patients with kidney failure. Blood is removed from a vein, passed through a dialysis machine, and then put back into a vein.

Jarisch-Herxheimer reaction—A rare reaction to the dead bacteria in the blood stream following antibiotic treatment.

Meningitis—Inflammation of tissues in the brain and spinal cord. Aseptic meningitis refers to meningitis with no bacteria present in the cerebral spinal fluid.

Spirochete—Any of a family of spiral- or coil-shaped bacteria known as Spirochetae. *L. interrogans* is a spirochete, as well as the organisms that cause syphilis and relapsing fever.

Zoonosis (plural, zoonoses)—Any disease of animals that can be transmitted to humans. Leptospirosis is an example of a zoonosis.

- Do not conduct canoe or kayak capsizing drills in freshwater ponds. Use a swimming pool instead.

- Boil or chemically treat pond or stream water before drinking it or cooking with it.

- Control rats and mice around the home.

- Have pets and farm animals vaccinated against *Leptospira*.

- Wear protective clothing (gloves, boots, long pants, and long-sleeved shirts) when working with wet soil or plants.

Resources

BOOKS

Beers, Mark H., MD, and Robert Berkow, MD., editors. "Infectious Diseases Caused by Spirochetes." In *The Merck Manual of Diagnosis and Therapy.* Whitehouse Station, NJ: Merck Research Laboratories, 2004.

PERIODICALS

Boland, M., G. Sayers, T. Coleman, et al. "A Cluster of Leptospirosis Cases in Canoeists following a Competition on the River Liffey." *Epidemiology and Infection* 132 (April 2004): 195–200.

Faucher, J. F., B. Hoen, and J. M. Estavoyer. "The Management of Leptospirosis." *Expert Opinion in Pharmacotherapy* 5 (April 2004): 819–827.

Vitale, G., C. La Russa, A. Galioto, et al. "Evaluation of an IgM-ELISA Test for the Diagnosis of Human

Leptospirosis." *New Microbiologica* 27 (April 2004): 149–154.

Yitzhaki, S., A. Barnea, A. Keysary, and E. Zahavy. "New Approach for Serological Testing for Leptospirosis by Using Detection of Leptospira Agglutination by Flow Cytometry Light Scatter Analysis." *Journal of Clinical Microbiology* 42 (April 2004): 1680–1685.

ORGANIZATIONS

American Veterinary Medical Association (AVMA). 1931 North Meacham Road, Suite 100, Schaumburg, IL 60173-4360. < http://www.avma.org >.

Centers for Disease Control and Prevention. 1600 Clifton Rd., NE, Atlanta, GA 30333. (800) 311-3435, (404) 639-3311. < http://www.cdc.gov >.

Belinda Rowland, PhD
Rebecca J. Frey, PhD

Lesch-Nyhan syndrome

Definition

Lesch-Nyhan syndrome, which is also known as HPRT deficiency or Kelley-Seegmiller syndrome, is a rare genetic disorder that affects males. Males with this syndrome develop physical handicaps, **mental retardation**, and kidney problems. It is caused by a total absence of a key enzyme that affects the level of uric acid in the body. Self-injury or **self-mutilation** is a distinctive feature of this genetic disease.

Description

Lesch-Nyhan syndrome was first described in 1964 by Drs. Michael Lesch and William Nyhan. The enzyme deficiency that causes the disorder was discovered in 1967 by a researcher named Seegmiller. The syndrome is caused by a severe change (mutation) in a gene that encodes an enzyme known as hypoxanthine-guanine phosphoribosyl transferase, or HPRT. This gene was identified and sequenced by Friedmann and colleagues in 1985. HPRT catalyzes a reaction that is necessary to prevent the buildup of uric acid, a nitrogenous waste product that is ordinarily excreted from the body through the kidneys. A severe mutation in the HPRT gene leads to an absence of HPRT enzyme activity which, in turn, leads to markedly elevated uric acid levels in the blood (hyperuricemia). This buildup of uric acid is toxic to the body and is related to the symptoms associated with the disease. Absence of the HPRT enzyme activity is also thought to alter the chemistry of certain parts of the brain, such as the basal ganglia, affecting neurotransmitters (chemicals used for communication between nerve cells), acids, and other chemicals. This change in the nervous system is also related to the symptoms associated with Lesch-Nyhan syndrome.

Males with Lesch-Nyhan syndrome develop neurologic problems during infancy. Infants with Lesch-Nyhan syndrome have weak muscle tone (hypotonia) and are unable to develop normally. Affected males develop uncontrollable writhing movements (athetosis) and muscle stiffness (spasticity) over time. Lack of speech is also a common feature of Lesch-Nyhan syndrome. The most dramatic symptom of Lesch-Nyhan syndrome, however, is the compulsive self-injury seen in 85% of affected males. This self-injury involves the biting of their own lips, tongue, and finger tips, as well as head banging. This behavior leads to serious injury and scarring.

Lesch-Nyhan syndrome affects approximately one in 380,000 live births. It occurs evenly among races. Almost always, only male children are affected, although a few cases of the disorder in girls have been reported. Women carriers usually do not have any symptoms. Women carriers can occasionally develop inflammation of the joints (**gout**) as they get older.

Causes and symptoms

Severe changes (mutations) in the HPRT gene completely halt the activity of the enzyme HPRT. There have been many different severe mutations identified in the HPRT gene. These mutations may be different between families. The HPRT gene is located on the X chromosome. Since the HPRT gene is located on the X chromosome, Lesch-Nyhan syndrome is considered X-liked. This means that it only affects males.

A person's sex is determined by their chromosomes. Males have one X chromosome and one Y chromosome. Females, on the other hand, have two X chromosomes. Males who possess a severe mutation in their HPRT gene will develop Lesch-Nyhan syndrome. Females who possess a severe mutation in their HPRT gene will not. They are considered to be carriers. This is because females have another X chromosome without the mutation that prevents them from getting this disease. If a woman is a carrier, she has a 50% risk with any **pregnancy** to pass on her X chromosome with the mutation. Therefore, with every male pregnancy she has a 50% risk to have an affected son, and with every female pregnancy she has a 50% risk to have a daughter who is a carrier.

At birth, males with Lesch-Nyhan syndrome appear completely normal. Development is usually normal for the first few months. Symptoms develop between three to six months of age. Sand-like crystals of uric acid in the diapers may be one of the first symptoms of the disease. The baby may be unusually irritable. Typically, the first sign of nervous system impairment is the inability to lift their head or sit up at an appropriate age. Many patients with Lesch-Nyhan will never learn to walk. By the end of the first year, writhing motions (athetosis), and spasmodic movements of the limbs and facial muscles (chorea) are clear evidence of defective motor development.

The compulsive self-injury associated with Lesch-Nyhan syndrome begins, on average, at three years. The self-injury begins with biting of the lips and tongue. As the disease progresses, affected individuals frequently develop finger biting and head banging. The self-injury can increase during times of **stress**.

Males with Lesch-Nyhan disease may also develop kidney damage due to **kidney stones**. Swollen and tender joints (gout) is another common problem.

Diagnosis

The diagnosis of Lesch-Nyhan syndrome is based initially on the distinctive pattern of the child's symptoms, most commonly involuntary muscle movements or failure to crawl and walk at the usual ages. In some cases the first symptom is related to overproduction of uric acid; the parents notice "orange sand" in the child's diapers. The "sand" is actually crystals of uric acid tinged with blood.

Measuring the amount of uric acid in a person's blood or urine can not definitively diagnose Lesch-Nyhan syndrome. It is diagnosed by measuring the activity of the HPRT enzyme through a blood test. When the activity of the enzyme is very low it is diagnostic of Lesch-Nyhan syndrome. It can also be diagnosed by DNA testing. This is also a blood test. DNA testing checks for changes (mutations) in the HPRT gene. Results from DNA testing are helpful in confirming the diagnosis and also when the child's family is interested in prenatal testing for future pregnancies.

Prenatal diagnosis is possible by DNA testing of fetal tissue drawn by **amniocentesis** or **chorionic villus sampling** (CVS). Fetuses should be tested if the mother is a carrier of a change (mutation) in her HPRT gene. A woman is at risk of being a carrier if she has a son with Lesch-Nyhan syndrome or someone in her family has Lesch-Nyhan syndrome. Any woman at risk of being a carrier should have DNA testing through a blood test.

KEY TERMS

Amniocentesis—A procedure performed at 16-18 weeks of pregnancy in which a needle is inserted through a woman's abdomen into her uterus to draw out a small sample of the amniotic fluid from around the baby. Either the fluid itself or cells from the fluid can be used for a variety of tests to obtain information about genetic disorders and other medical conditions in the fetus.

Athetosis—A condition marked by slow, writhing, involuntary muscle movements.

Basal ganglia—A section of the brain responsible for smooth muscular movement.

Chorea—Involuntary, rapid, jerky movements.

Chorionic villus sampling (CVS)—A procedure used for prenatal diagnosis at 10-12 weeks gestation. Under ultrasound guidance a needle is inserted either through the mother's vagina or abdominal wall and a sample of cells is collected from around the early embryo. These cells are then tested for chromosome abnormalities or other genetic diseases.

Enzyme—A protein that catalyzes a biochemical reaction or change without changing its own structure or function.

Mutation—A permanent change in the genetic material that may alter a trait or characteristic of an individual, or manifest as disease, and can be transmitted to offspring.

Neurotransmitter—Chemical in the brain that transmits information from one nerve cell to another.

Palsy—Uncontrolable tremors.

Spasticity—Increased mucle tone, or stiffness, which leads to uncontrolled, awkward movements.

Treatment

There are no known treatments for the neurological defects of Lesch-Nyhan. Allopurinol (Aloprim, Zyloprim), a drug usually prescribed to lower the risk of gout attacks, can lower blood uric acid levels. This medication is a preventive; it does not correct many of the symptoms of Lesch-Nyhan. Other drugs that are given to manage spasticity include baclofen (Lioresal), which is a muscle relaxant, and benzodiazepine tranquilizers.

Some patients with Lesch-Nyhan syndrome have their teeth removed to prevent self-injury. Restraints may be recommended to reduce self-destructive behaviors, although some patients can be managed with a combination of behavioral modification therapy and medications.

Prognosis

With strong supportive care, infants born with Lesch-Nyhan can live into adulthood with symptoms continuing throughout life. Few live beyond 40, however, with **death** usually resulting either from kidney failure or from aspiration **pneumonia**. Sudden unexpected death from **respiratory failure** is common in these patients.

At present, there are no preventive measures for Lesch-Nyhan syndrome. However, recent studies have indicated that this genetic disorder may be a good candidate for treatment with gene replacement therapy. Unfortunately, the technology necessary to implement this therapy has not yet been perfected.

Resources

BOOKS

Beers, Mark H., MD, and Robert Berkow, MD., editors. "Cerebral Palsy Syndromes." In *The Merck Manual of Diagnosis and Therapy*. Whitehouse Station, NJ: Merck Research Laboratories, 2004.

Jinnah, H. A., and Theodore Friedmann. "Lesch-Nyhan Disease and Its Variants." *The Metabolic and Molecular Bases of Inherited Disease*. New York: McGraw-Hill, 2001.

PERIODICALS

Jinnah, Hyder, MD, PhD. "Lesch-Nyhan Syndrome." *eMedicine* January 25, 2002. < http://www.emedicine.com/neuro/topic630.htm >.

Mak, B. S., et al. "New Mutations of the HPRT Gene in Lesch-Nyhan Syndrome." *Pediatric Neurology* October 2000: 332–335.

Visser, J.E., et al. "Lesch-Nyhan Disease and the Basal Ganglia." *Brain Research Reviews* November 1999: 450–469.

Willers, I. "Germline Mosaicism Complicates Molecular Diagnosis of Lesch-Nyhan Syndrome." *Prenatal Diagnosis* 24 (September 2004): 737–740.

ORGANIZATIONS

Alliance of Genetic Support Groups. 4301 Connecticut Ave. NW, Suite 404, Washington, DC 20008. (202) 966-5557. Fax: (202) 966-8553. < http://www.geneticalliance.org >.

International Lesch-Nyhan Disease Association. 114 Winchester Way, Shamong, NJ 08088-9398. (215) 677-4206.

Lesch-Nyhan Syndrome Registry. New York University School of Medicine, Department of Psychiatry, 550 First Ave., New York, NY 10012. (212) 263-6458.

National Organization for Rare Disorders (NORD). 55 Kenosia Avenue, P. O. Box 1968, Danbury,

CT 06813-1968. (203) 744-0100. Fax: (203) 798-2291.
< http://www.rarediseases.org >.

OTHER

GeneClinics. < http://www.geneclinics.org/profiles/lns/
    details.html >.
Pediatric Database(PEDBASE). < http://www.icondata.
    com/health/pedbase/files/LESCH-NY.HTM >.

Holly Ann Ishmael, M.S.
Rebecca J. Frey, PhD

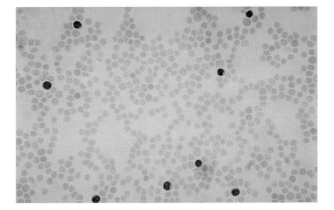

A magnified stain of chronic lymphocytic leukemia cells.
(Custom Medical Stock Photo. Reproduced by permission.)

Leukemia stains

Definition

Leukemia stains are laboratory tests done on bone marrow or blood samples to help diagnose specific types of leukemia.

Purpose

Leukemia stains are done to diagnose and classify leukemia. Blood contains red cells, several varieties of white cells, and platelets. Cancerous overproduction of any one type of cell produces one of many types of leukemia. A patient's specific type of leukemia must be classified in order to provide the best treatment and most accurate prognosis.

The type and maturity of the cells involved are identified by analyzing blood and bone marrow under a microscope. Often, however, the abnormality or immaturity of the cells make it difficult to identify the cell types with certainty. Special leukemia stains help to distinguish one cell type from another.

Description

Special stains are added to bone marrow or blood that has been smeared on a microscope slide. Cell types react differently to the chemicals in the stains.

If the patient has few white cells, a buffy coat smear is made. A tube of blood is spun in a centrifuge. Red cells fall, plasma rises, and white cells settle in a thin middle layer called the buffy coat. The smear is made from this layer.

Sudan black B stain

This stain distinguishes between acute lymphoblastic leukemia (cells stain positive) and acute myeloblastic leukemia (cells stain negative).

Periodic acid-Schiff stain (PAS)

The PAS stain is primarily used to identify erythroleukemia, a leukemia of immature red blood cells. These cells stain a bright fuchsia.

Terminal deoxynucleotidyl transferase stain (TdT)

The TdT stain differentiates between acute lymphoblastic leukemia (cells stain positive) and acute myelogenous leukemia (cells stain negative).

Leukocyte alkaline phosphatase (LAP)

The LAP stain is used to determine if an increase of cells is due to chronic myelogenous leukemia or a noncancerous reaction to an infection or similar conditions. Cells from a noncancerous reaction stain positive with many intense blue granules; cells from chronic myelogenous leukemia have few blue granules.

Tartrate-resistant acid phosphatase stain (TRAP)

The TRAP stain is primarily used to identify **hairy cell leukemia** cells. These cells stain with purple to dark red granules.

Myeloperoxidase stain

The myeloperoxidase stain distinguishes between the immature cells in acute myeloblastic leukemia (cells stain positive) and those in acute lymphoblastic leukemia (cells stain negative).

Leukocyte specific esterase

This stain identifies granulocytes, which show red granules.

KEY TERMS

Bone marrow—The spongy tissue inside large bones where blood cells are formed.

Buffy coat—The thin layer of concentrated white blood cells that forms when a tube of blood is spun in a centrifuge.

Leukemia—Any of several cancers of the bone marrow characterized by the abnormal increase of a type of blood cell.

Leukemia stains—Special stains added to smears of blood or bone marrow, performed to diagnose and classify leukemia.

Leukocyte nonspecific esterase

Nonspecific esterase stain identifies monocytes and immature platelets (megakaryocytes), which show positive black granules.

Preparation

Leukemia stains are done on smears of blood or bone marrow. To collect blood, a healthcare worker draws blood from a vein in the inner elbow region. Collection of the sample takes only a few minutes.

When bone marrow is needed, the person is given **local anesthesia**. Then the physician inserts a needle through the skin and into the bone–usually the breast bone or hip bone–and 0.5-2 mL of bone marrow is withdrawn. This procedure takes approximately 30 minutes.

Aftercare

Patients sometimes feel discomfort or bruising at the puncture site after blood collection. They may also become dizzy or faint. Pressure to the puncture site until the bleeding stops reduces bruising. Warm packs to the puncture site relieve discomfort.

Collection of bone marrow is done under a physician's supervision. The patient is asked to rest after the procedure and is watched for weakness and signs of bleeding.

Normal results

A normal blood or bone marrow smear shows no evidence of leukemic cells. The expected reaction of cells varies with the type of stain.

Abnormal results

Leukemia stain results that help diagnosis and classify leukemia are supported by the results of other laboratory tests and the person's clinical condition.

Resources

BOOKS

Fischbach, Francis. *Manual of Laboratory and Diagnostic Tests.* Philadelphia: Lippincott, 1996.

Nancy J. Nordenson

Leukemias, acute

Definition

Leukemia is a **cancer** that starts in the organs that make blood, namely the bone marrow and the lymph system. Depending on their characteristics, leukemias can be divided into two broad types. Acute leukemias are the rapidly progressing leukemias, while the **chronic leukemias** progress more slowly. The vast majority of the childhood leukemias are of the acute form.

Description

The cells that make up blood are produced in the bone marrow and the lymph system. The bone marrow is the spongy tissue found in the large bones of the body. The lymph system includes the spleen (an organ in the upper abdomen), the thymus (a small organ beneath the breastbone), and the tonsils (an organ in the throat). In addition, the lymph vessels (tiny tubes that branch like blood vessels into all parts of the body) and lymph nodes (pea-shaped organs that are found along the network of lymph vessels) are also part of the lymph system. The lymph is a milky fluid that contains cells. Clusters of lymph nodes are found in the neck, underarm, pelvis, abdomen, and chest.

The cells found in the blood are the red blood cells (RBCs), which carry oxygen and other materials to all tissues of the body; white blood cells (WBCs) that fight infection; and the platelets, which play a part in the clotting of the blood. The white blood cells can be further subdivided into three main types: granulocytes, monocytes, and lymphocytes.

The granulocytes, as their name suggests, have particles (granules) inside them. These granules

CHARLOTTE FRIEND (1921–1987)

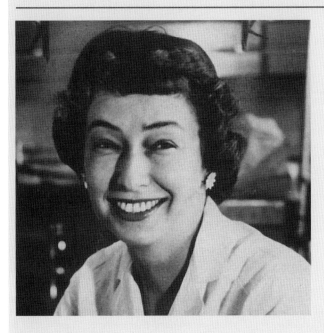

(Library of Congress.)

Charlotte Friend was born to Russian immigrants, Morris Friend and Cecilia (Wolpin), on March 11, 1921, in New York City. At three years of age, her father died of a heart condition. Friend's decision to pursue a career in medicine may well have been influenced by her father's death and by her mother's occupation as a pharmacist. As a child, Friend read books about bacteriologists and, by age ten, she knew that she wanted to study bacteriology. She attended Hunter College, enlisting in the U.S. Navy after her graduation in 1944.

Friend attended Yale University, earning her Ph.D. in bacteriology in 1950. After working for the Memorial Sloan-Kettering Institute for Cancer Research, she became an associate professor at Cornell University in 1952. Friend began researching cancer and became particularly interested in leukemia and its cause. She believed that a virus caused the disease and confirmed this theory by using an electron microscope to photograph the virus in mice. Her findings were initially met with much skepticism but she was able to develop a vaccine that was used successfully with mice, which added credibility to her theory. Her breakthroughs have led medical researchers to new methods of treating cancer and to a greater understanding of the disease.

Friend was a prolific writer who published 113 original papers, 49 abstracts, book chapters, and reviews, many of which she completed individually. She was diagnosed with lymphoma and died on January 13, 1987.

contain special proteins (enzymes) and several other substances that can break down chemicals and destroy microorganisms, such as bacteria. Monocytes are the second type of white blood cell. They are also important in defending the body against pathogens.

The lymphocytes form the third type of white blood cell. There are two main types of lymphocytes: T lymphocytes and B lymphocytes. They have different functions within the immune system. The B cells protect the body by making "antibodies." Antibodies are proteins that can attach to the surfaces of bacteria and viruses. This "attachment" sends signals to many other cell types to come and destroy the antibody-coated organism. The T cells protect the body against viruses. When a virus enters a cell, it produces certain proteins that are projected onto the surface of the infected cell. The T cells recognize these proteins and make certain chemicals that are capable of destroying the virus-infected cells. In addition, the T cells can destroy some types of cancer cells.

The bone marrow makes stem cells, which are the precursors of the different blood cells. These stem cells mature through stages into either RBCs, WBCs, or platelets. In acute leukemias, the maturation process of the white blood cells is interrupted. The immature cells (or "blasts") proliferate rapidly and begin to accumulate in various organs and tissues, thereby affecting their normal function. This uncontrolled proliferation of the immature cells in the bone marrow affects the production of the normal red blood cells and platelets as well.

Acute leukemias are of two types: acute lymphocytic leukemia and acute myelogenous leukemia. Different types of white blood cells are involved in the two leukemias. In acute lymphocytic leukemia (ALL), it is the T or the B lymphocytes that become cancerous. The B cell leukemias are more common than T cell leukemias. Acute myelogenous leukemia, also known as acute nonlymphocytic leukemia (ANLL), is a cancer of the monocytes and/or granulocytes.

Leukemias account for 2% of all cancers. Because leukemia is the most common form of childhood cancer, it is often regarded as a disease of childhood. However, leukemias affect nine times as many adults as children. Half of the cases occur in people who are 60 years of age or older. The incidence of acute and chronic leukemias is about the same. According to the estimates of the American Cancer Society (ACS), approximately 29,000 new cases of leukemia were diagnosed in 1998.

Causes and symptoms

Leukemia strikes both sexes and all ages. The human T-cell leukemia virus (HTLV-I) is believed to be the causative agent for some kinds of leukemias. However, the cause of most leukemias is not known. Acute lymphoid leukemia (ALL) is more common among Caucasians than among African-Americans, while acute myeloid leukemia (AML) affects both races equally. The incidence of acute leukemia is slightly higher among men than women. People with Jewish ancestry have a higher likelihood of getting leukemia. A higher incidence of leukemia has also been observed among persons with **Down syndrome** and some other genetic abnormalities.

Exposure to ionizing radiation and to certain organic chemicals, such as benzene, is believed to increase the risk of getting leukemia. Having a history of diseases that damage the bone marrow, such as **aplastic anemia**, or a history of cancers of the lymphatic system puts people at a high risk for developing acute leukemias. Similarly, the use of anticancer medications, immunosuppressants, and the antibiotic chloramphenicol are also considered risk factors for developing acute leukemias.

The symptoms of leukemia are generally vague and non-specific. A patient may experience all or some of the following symptoms:

- weakness or chronic **fatigue**
- fever of unknown origin
- weight loss that is not due to dieting or **exercise**
- frequent bacterial or viral infections
- headaches
- skin rash
- non-specific bone **pain**
- easy bruising
- bleeding from gums or nose
- blood in urine or stools
- enlarged lymph nodes and/or spleen
- abdominal fullness

Diagnosis

Like all cancers, acute leukemias are best treated when found early. There are no screening tests available.

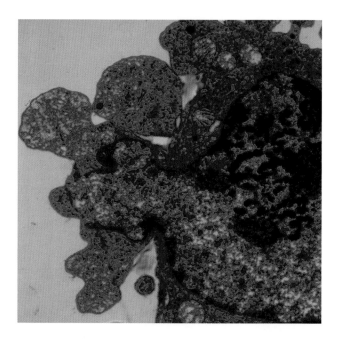

An enhanced transmission electron microscopy (TEM) image of acute myelogenous leukemia cells. *(Photograph by Robert Becker, Ph.D., Custom Medical Stock Photo. Reproduced by permission.)*

If the doctor has reason to suspect leukemia, he or she will conduct a very thorough **physical examination** to look for enlarged lymph nodes in the neck, underarm, and pelvic region. Swollen gums, enlarged liver or spleen, **bruises**, or pinpoint red **rashes** all over the body are some of the signs of leukemia. Urine and blood tests may be ordered to check for microscopic amounts of blood in the urine and to obtain a complete differential **blood count**. This count will give the numbers and percentages of the different cells found in the blood. An abnormal blood test might suggest leukemia; however, the diagnosis has to be confirmed by more specific tests.

The doctor may perform a **bone marrow biopsy** to confirm the diagnosis of leukemia. During the biopsy, a cylindrical piece of bone and marrow is removed. The tissue is generally taken out of the hipbone. These samples are sent to the laboratory for examination. In addition to diagnosis, the biopsy is also repeated during the treatment phase of the disease to see if the leukemia is responding to therapy.

A spinal tap (lumbar puncture) is another procedure that the doctor may order to diagnose leukemia. In this procedure, a small needle is inserted into the spinal cavity in the lower back to withdraw some cerebrospinal fluid and to look for leukemic cells.

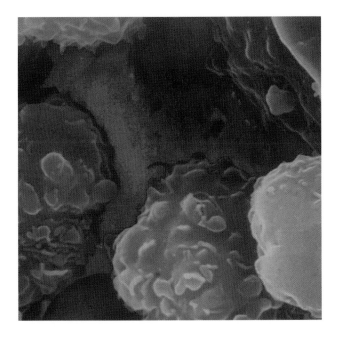

An enhanced scanning electron microscopy (SEM) image of acute myelogenous leukemia cells. *(Photograph by Robert Becker, Ph.D., Custom Medical Stock Photo. Reproduced by permission.)*

Standard imaging tests, such as x rays, **computed tomography scans** (CT scans), and **magnetic resonance imaging** (MRI) may be used to check whether the leukemic cells have invaded other areas of the body, such as the bones, chest, kidneys, abdomen, or brain. A gallium scan or bone scan is a test in which a radioactive chemical is injected into the body. This chemical accumulates in the areas of cancer or infection, allowing them to be viewed with a special camera.

Treatment

There are two phases of treatment for leukemia. The first phase is called "induction therapy." As the name suggests, during this phase, the main aim of the treatment is to reduce the number of leukemic cells as far as possible and induce a remission in the patient. Once the patient shows no obvious signs of leukemia (no leukemic cells are detected in blood tests and bone marrow biopsies), the patient is said to be in remission. The second phase of treatment is then initiated. This is called continuation or maintenance therapy, and the aim in this case is to kill any remaining cells and to maintain the remission for as long as possible.

Chemotherapy is the use of drugs to kill cancer cells. It is usually the treatment of choice and is used to relieve symptoms and achieve long-term remission of the disease. Generally, combination chemotherapy, in which multiple drugs are used, is more efficient than using a single drug for the treatment. Some drugs may be administered intravenously through a vein in the arm; others may be given by mouth in the form of pills. If the cancer cells have invaded the brain, then chemotherapeutic drugs may be put into the fluid that surrounds the brain through a needle in the brain or back. This is known as intrathecal chemotherapy.

Because leukemia cells can spread to all the organs via the blood stream and the lymph vessels, surgery is not considered an option for treating leukemias.

Radiation therapy, which involves the use of x rays or other high-energy rays to kill cancer cells and shrink tumors, may be used in some cases. For acute leukemias, the source of radiation is usually outside the body (external radiation therapy). If the leukemic cells have spread to the brain, radiation therapy can be given to the brain.

Bone marrow transplantation is a process in which the patient's diseased bone marrow is replaced with healthy marrow. There are two ways of doing a bone marrow transplant. In an allogeneic bone marrow transplant, healthy marrow is taken from a donor whose tissue is either the same as or very closely resembles the patient's tissues. The donor may be a twin, a brother or sister (sibling), or a person who is not related at all. First, the patient's bone marrow is destroyed with very high doses of chemotherapy and radiation therapy. Healthy marrow from the donor is then given to the patient through a needle in a vein to replace the destroyed marrow.

In the second type of bone marrow transplant, called an autologous bone marrow transplant, some of the patient's own marrow is taken out and treated with a combination of **anticancer drugs** to kill all the abnormal cells. This marrow is then frozen to save it. The marrow remaining in the patient's body is destroyed with high-dose chemotherapy and radiation therapy. The marrow that was frozen is then thawed and given back to the patient through a needle in a vein. This mode of bone marrow transplant is currently being investigated in clinical trials.

Biological therapy or immunotherapy is a mode of treatment in which the body's own immune system is harnessed to fight the cancer. Substances that are routinely made by the immune system (such as growth factors, hormones, and disease-fighting proteins) are either synthetically made in a laboratory or their effectiveness is boosted and they are then put back into the patient's body. This treatment mode is also being

KEY TERMS

Antibodies—Proteins made by the B lymphocytes in response to the presence of infectious agents, such as bacteria or viruses, in the body.

Biopsy—The surgical removal and microscopic examination of living tissue for diagnostic purposes.

Chemotherapy—Treatment with drugs that act against cancer.

Computerized tomography (CT) scan—A series of x rays put together by a computer in order to form detailed pictures of areas inside the body.

Cytokines—Chemicals made by the cells that act on other cells to stimulate or inhibit their function. Cytokines that stimulate growth are called "growth factors."

Immunotherapy—Treatment of cancer by stimulating the body's immune defense system.

Lumbar puncture—A procedure in which the doctor inserts a small needle into the spinal cavity in the lower back to withdraw some spinal fluid for testing. Also known as a "spinal tap."

Magnetic resonance imaging (MRI)—A medical procedure using a magnet linked to a computer to picture areas inside the body.

Maturation—The process by which stem cells transform from immature cells without a specific function into a particular type of blood cell with defined functions.

Radiation therapy—Treatment using high-energy radiation from x-ray machines, cobalt, radium, or other sources.

Remission—A disappearance of a disease as a result of treatment. Complete remission means that all disease is gone. Partial remission means that the disease is significantly improved by treatment, but residual traces of the disease are still present.

investigated in clinical trials all over the country at major cancer centers.

Prognosis

Like all cancers, the prognosis for leukemia depends on the patient's age and general health. According to statistics, more than 60% of the patients with leukemia survive for at least a year after diagnosis. Acute myelocytic leukemia (AML) has a poorer prognosis rate than acute lymphocytic leukemias

(ALL) and the chronic leukemias. In the last 15 to 20 years, the five-year survival rate for patients with ALL has increased from 38% to 57%.

Interestingly enough, since most childhood leukemias are of the ALL type, chemotherapy has been highly successful in their treatment. This is because chemotherapeutic drugs are most effective against actively growing cells. Due to the new combinations of anticancer drugs being used, the survival rates among children with ALL have improved dramatically. Eighty percent of the children diagnosed with ALL now survive for five years or more, as compared to 50% in the late 1970s.

Prevention

Most cancers can be prevented by changes in lifestyle or diet, which will reduce the risk factors. However, in leukemias, there are no such known risk factors. Therefore, at the present time, no way is known to prevent leukemias from developing. People who are at an increased risk for developing leukemia because of proven exposure to ionizing radiation or exposure to the toxic liquid benzene, and people with Down syndrome, should undergo periodic medical checkups.

Resources

ORGANIZATIONS

American Cancer Society. 1599 Clifton Rd., NE, Atlanta, GA 30329-4251. (800) 227-2345. < http:// www.cancer.org >.

Cancer Research Institute. 681 Fifth Ave., New York, N.Y. 10022. (800) 992-2623. < http:// www.cancerresearch.org >.

Leukemia Society of America, Inc. 600 Third Ave., New York, NY 10016. (800) 955-4572. < http:// www.leukemia.org >.

National Cancer Institute. Building 31, Room 10A31, 31 Center Drive, MSC 2580, Bethesda, MD 20892-2580. (800) 422-6237. < http://www.nci.nih.gov >.

Oncolink. University of Pennsylvania Cancer Center. < http://cancer.med.upenn.edu >.

Lata Cherath, PhD

Leukemias, chronic

Definition

Chronic leukemia is a disease in which too many white blood cells are made in the bone marrow.

Depending on the type of white blood cell that is involved, chronic leukemia can be classified as chronic lymphocytic leukemia or chronic myeloid leukemia.

Description

Chronic leukemia is a **cancer** that starts in the blood cells made in the bone marrow. The bone marrow is the spongy tissue found in the large bones of the body. The bone marrow makes precursor cells called "blasts" or "stem cells" that mature into different types of blood cells. Unlike **acute leukemias**, in which the process of maturation of the blast cells is interrupted, in chronic leukemias, the cells do mature and only a few remain as immature cells. However, even though the cells appear normal, they do not function as normal cells.

The different types of cells that are produced in the bone marrow are red blood cells (RBCs), which carry oxygen and other materials to all tissues of the body; white blood cells (WBCs), which fight infection; and platelets, which play a part in the clotting of the blood. The white blood cells can be further subdivided into three main types: the granulocytes, monocytes, and the lymphocytes.

The granulocytes, as their name suggests, have granules (particles) inside them. These granules contain special proteins (enzymes) and several other substances that can break down chemicals and destroy microorganisms such as bacteria.

Monocytes are the second type of white blood cell. They are also important in defending the body against pathogens.

The lymphocytes form the third type of white blood cell. There are two main types of lymphocytes: T lymphocytes and B lymphocytes. They have different functions within the immune system. The B cells protect the body by making "antibodies." Antibodies are proteins that can attach to the surfaces of bacteria and viruses. This attachment sends signals to many other cell types to come and destroy the antibody-coated organism. The T cell protects the body against viruses. When a virus enters a cell, it produces certain proteins that are projected onto the surface of the infected cell. The T cells can recognize these proteins and produce certain chemicals (cytokines) that are capable of destroying the virus-infected cells. In addition, the T cells can destroy some types of cancer cells.

Chronic leukemias develop very gradually. The abnormal lymphocytes multiply slowly, but in a poorly regulated manner. They live much longer and thus their numbers build up in the body. The two types of chronic leukemias can be easily distinguished under the microscope. Chronic lymphocytic leukemia (CLL) involves the T or B lymphocytes. B cell abnormalities are more common than T cell abnormalities. T cells are affected in only 5% of the patients. The T and B lymphocytes can be differentiated from the other types of white blood cells based on their size and by the absence of granules inside them. In chronic myelogenous leukemia (CML), the cells that are affected are the granulocytes.

Chronic lymphocytic leukemia (CLL) often has no symptoms at first and may remain undetected for a long time. Chronic myelogenous leukemia (CML), on the other hand, may progress to a more acute form.

Chronic leukemias account for 1.2% of all cancers. Because leukemia is the most common form of childhood cancer, it is often regarded as a disease of childhood. However, leukemias affect nine times as many adults as children. In chronic lymphoid leukemia, 90% of the cases are seen in people who are 50 years or older, with the average age at diagnosis being 65. The incidence of the disease increases with age. It is almost never seen in children. Chronic myeloid leukemias are generally seen in people in their mid-40s. It accounts for about 4% of childhood leukemia cases. According to the estimates of the American Cancer Society (ACS), approximately 29,000 new cases of leukemia will be diagnosed in 1998.

Causes and symptoms

Leukemia strikes both sexes and all ages. Although the cause is unknown, chronic leukemia is linked to genetic abnormalities and environmental factors. For example, exposure to ionizing radiation and to certain organic chemicals, such as benzene, is believed to increase the risks for getting leukemia. Chronic leukemia occurs in some people who are infected with two human retroviruses (HTLV-I and HTLV-II). An abnormal chromosome known as the Philadelphia chromosome is seen in 90% of those with CML. The incidence of chronic leukemia is slightly higher among men than women.

The symptoms of chronic leukemia are generally vague and non-specific. In chronic lymphoid leukemia (CLL), a patient may experience all or some of the following symptoms:

- swollen lymph nodes
- an enlarged spleen, which could make the patient complain of abdominal fullness
- chronic **fatigue**

- a general feeling of ill-health
- fever of unknown origin
- night sweats
- weight loss that is not due to dieting or **exercise**
- frequent bacterial or viral infections

In the early stages of chronic myeloid leukemia (CML), the symptoms are more or less similar to CLL. In the later stages of the disease, the patient may experience these symptoms:

- non-specific bone **pain**
- bleeding problems
- mucus membrane irritation
- frequent infections
- a pale color due to a low red blood cell count (anemia)
- swollen lymph glands
- fever
- night sweats

Diagnosis

There are no screening tests available for chronic leukemias. The detection of these diseases may occur by chance during a routine **physical examination**.

If the doctor has reason to suspect leukemia, he or she will conduct a very thorough physical examination to look for enlarged lymph nodes in the neck, under-arm, and pelvic region. Swollen gums, an enlarged liver or spleen, **bruises**, or pinpoint red **rashes** all over the body are some of the signs of leukemia. Urine and blood tests may be ordered to check for microscopic amounts of blood in the urine and to obtain a complete differential **blood count**. This count will give the numbers and percentages of the different cells found in the blood. An abnormal blood test might suggest leukemia; however, the diagnosis has to be confirmed by more specific tests.

The doctor may perform a **bone marrow biopsy** to confirm the diagnosis of leukemia. During the bone marrow biopsy, a cylindrical piece of bone and marrow is removed. The tissue is generally taken out of the hipbone. These samples are sent to the laboratory for examination. In addition to diagnosis, bone marrow biopsy is also done during the treatment phase of the disease to see if the leukemia is responding to therapy.

Standard imaging tests such as x rays, **computed tomography scans** (CT scans), and **magnetic resonance imaging** (MRI) may be used to check whether the leukemic cells have invaded other organs of the body, such as the bones, chest, kidneys, abdomen, or brain.

Treatment

The treatment depends on the specific type of chronic leukemia and its stage. In general, **chemotherapy** is the standard approach to both CLL and CML. **Radiation therapy** is occasionally used. Because leukemia cells can spread to all the organs via the blood stream and the lymph vessels, surgery is not considered an option for treating leukemias.

Bone marrow transplantation (BMT) is becoming the treatment of choice for CML because it has the possibility of curing the illness. BMT is generally not considered an option in treating CLL because CLL primarily affects older people, who are not considered to be good candidates for the procedure.

In BMT, the patient's diseased bone marrow is replaced with healthy marrow. There are two ways of doing a bone marrow transplant. In an allogeneic bone marrow transplant, healthy marrow is taken from another person (donor) whose tissue is either the same or very closely resembles the patient's tissues. The donor may be a twin, a sibling, or a person who is not related at all. First, the patient's bone marrow is destroyed with very high doses of chemotherapy and radiation therapy. To replace the destroyed marrow, healthy marrow from the donor is given to the patient through a needle in the vein.

In the second type of bone marrow transplant, called an autologous bone marrow transplant, some of the patient's own marrow is taken out and treated with a combination of **anticancer drugs** to kill all the abnormal cells. This marrow is then frozen to save it. The marrow remaining in the patient's body is then destroyed with high dose chemotherapy and radiation therapy. Following that, the patient's own marrow that was frozen is thawed and given back to the patient through a needle in the vein. This mode of bone marrow transplant is currently being investigated in clinical trials.

In chronic lymphoid leukemia (CLL), chemotherapy is generally the treatment of choice. Depending on the stage of the disease, single or multiple drugs may be given. Drugs commonly prescribed include steroids, chlorambucil, fludarabine, and cladribine. Low dose radiation therapy may be given to the whole body, or it may be used to alleviate the symptoms and discomfort due to an enlarged spleen and lymph nodes. The spleen may be removed in a procedure called a **splenectomy**.

KEY TERMS

Antibodies—Proteins made by the B lymphocytes in response to the presence of infectious agents, such as bacteria or viruses, in the body.

Biopsy—The surgical removal and microscopic examination of living tissue for diagnostic purposes.

Chemotherapy—Treatment with drugs that act against cancer.

Computerized tomography (CT) scan—A series of x rays put together by a computer in order to form detailed pictures of areas inside the body.

Cytokines—Chemicals made by the cells that act on other cells to stimulate or inhibit their function. Cytokines that stimulate growth are called "growth factors."

Immunotherapy—Treatment of cancer by stimulating the body's immune defense system.

Lumbar puncture—A procedure in which the doctor inserts a small needle into the spinal cavity in the lower back to withdraw some spinal fluid for testing. Also known as a "spinal tap."

Magnetic resonance imaging (MRI)—A medical procedure using a magnet linked to a computer to picture areas inside the body.

Maturation—The process by which stem cells transform from immature cells without a specific function into a particular type of blood cell with defined functions.

Radiation therapy—Treatment using high-energy radiation from x-ray machines, cobalt, radium, or other sources.

Remission—A disappearance of a disease as a result of treatment. Complete remission means that all disease is gone. Partial remission means that the disease is significantly improved by treatment, but residual traces of the disease are still present.

In chronic myeloid leukemia (CML), the treatment of choice is bone marrow transplantation. During the slow progress (chronic phase) of the disease, chemotherapy may be given to try to improve the cell counts. Radiation therapy, which involves the use of x rays or other high-energy rays to kill cancer cells and shrink tumors, may be used in some cases to reduce the discomfort and pain due to an enlarged

spleen. For chronic leukemias, the source of radiation is usually outside the body (external radiation therapy). If the leukemic cells have spread to the brain, radiation therapy can be directed at the brain. As the disease progresses, the spleen may be removed in an attempt to try to control the pain and to improve the blood counts.

In the acute phase of CML, aggressive chemotherapy is given. Combination chemotherapy, in which multiple drugs are used, is more efficient than using a single drug for the treatment. The drugs may either be administered intravenously through a vein in the arm or by mouth in the form of pills. If the cancer cells have invaded the central nervous system (CNS), chemotherapeutic drugs may be put into the fluid that surrounds the brain through a needle in the brain or back. This is known as intrathecal chemotherapy.

Biological therapy or immunotherapy is a mode of treatment in which the body's own immune system is harnessed to fight the cancer. Substances that are routinely made by the immune system (such as growth factors, hormones, and disease-fighting proteins) are either synthetically made in a laboratory, or their effectiveness is boosted and they are then put back into the patient's body. This treatment mode is also being investigated in clinical trials all over the country at major cancer centers.

Prognosis

The prognosis for leukemia depends on the patient's age and general health. According to statistics, in chronic lymphoid leukemia, the overall survival for all stages of the disease is nine years. Most of the deaths in people with CLL are due to infections or other illnesses that occur as a result of the leukemia.

In CML, if bone marrow transplantation is performed within one to three years of diagnosis, 50-60% of the patients survive three years or more. If the disease progresses to the acute phase, the prognosis is poor. Less than 20% of these patients go into remission.

Prevention

Most cancers can be prevented by changes in lifestyle or diet, which will reduce the risk factors. However, in leukemias, there are no known risk factors. Therefore, at the present time, there is no way known to prevent the leukemias from developing. People who are at an increased risk for developing leukemia because of proven exposure to ionizing radiation, the organic liquid benzene, or people who have a history of other cancers of the lymphoid system (Hodgkin's lymphoma) should undergo periodic medical checkups.

Resources

ORGANIZATIONS

American Cancer Society. 1599 Clifton Rd., NE, Atlanta, GA 30329-4251. (800) 227-2345. < http://www.cancer.org >.

Cancer Research Institute. 681 Fifth Ave., New York, N.Y. 10022. (800) 992-2623. < http://www.cancerresearch.org >.

Leukemia Society of America, Inc. 600 Third Ave., New York, NY 10016. (800) 955 4572. < http://www.leukemia.org >.

National Cancer Institute. Building 31, Room 10A31, 31 Center Drive, MSC 2580, Bethesda, MD 20892-2580. (800) 422-6237. < http://www.nci.nih.gov >.

Oncolink. University of Pennsylvania Cancer Center. < http://cancer.med.upenn.edu >.

Lata Cherath, PhD

Leukocytosis

Definition

Leukocytosis is a condition characterized by an elevated number of white cells in the blood.

Description

Leukocytosis is a condition that affects all types of white blood cells. Other illnesses, such as neutrophilia, lymphocytosis, and granulocytosis, target specific types of white blood cells. Normal white blood cell counts are 4,300-10,800 white blood cells per microliter. Leukocyte or white blood cell levels are considered elevated when they are between 15,000-20,000 per microliter. The increased number of leukocytes can occur abnormally as a result of an infection, **cancer**, or drug intake; however, leukocytosis can occur normally after eating a large meal or experiencing **stress**.

Causes and symptoms

Leukemias can cause white blood cell counts to increase to as much as 100,000. Each kind of white cell can produce a leukemia. Apart from leukemias, nearly all leukocytosis is due to one type of white blood cell, the polymorphonuclear leukocyte (PMN). These conditions are more accurately referred to as neutrophilia.

The most common and important cause of neutrophilia is infection, and most infections cause neutrophilia. The degree of elevation often indicates the severity of the infection. Tissue damage from other causes raises the white count for similar reasons. **Burns**, infarction (cutting off the blood supply to a region of the body so that it dies), crush injuries, inflammatory diseases, poisonings, and severe diseases, like kidney failure and **diabetic ketoacidosis**, all cause neutrophilia.

Counts almost as high occur in leukemoid (leukemia-like) reactions caused by infection and non-infectious inflammation.

Drugs can also cause leukocytosis. Cortisone-like drugs (prednisone), lithium, and NSAIDs are the most common offenders.

Non-specific stresses also cause white blood cells to increase in the blood. Extensive testing of medical students reveals that neutrophilia accompanies every examination. Vigorous **exercise** and intense excitement also cause elevated white blood cell counts.

Diagnosis

A complete **blood count** (CBC) is one of the first tests obtained in any medical setting. More than 11,000 white cells in a cubic millimeter of blood is considered high. **Bone marrow biopsy** may help clarify the cause.

Treatment

Relieving the underlying cause returns the count to normal.

Prognosis

By treating the underlying condition, white blood cell counts usually return to normal

Resources

BOOKS

Holland, Steven M., and John I. Gallin. "Disorders of Granulocytes and Monocytes." In *Harrison's Principles of Internal Medicine*, edited by Anthony S. Fauci, et al. New York: McGraw-Hill, 1997.

J. Ricker Polsdorfer, MD

Leukotriene inhibitors

Definition

Leukotriene inhibitors are prescription medications that treat **asthma** and some **allergies** by blocking the formation or activity of leukotrienes—small mediator chemicals produced by cells in the body.

Purpose

More than 50 million Americans suffer from asthma and allergies. Asthma is one of the most prevalent chronic diseases in the United States, affecting 9 million (12.7%) of children. Seasonal allergies affect 20–40 million (20%) of Americans, about 40% of them children. It is estimated that 60–70% of those with asthma also suffer from **allergic rhinitis**, allergies affecting the mucous membranes of the nose.

Asthma, an inflammation of the bronchial airways, and seasonal allergies and allergic **rhinitis** involve several chemical mediators including histamine and leukotrienes. Leukotrienes are a class of unsaturated fatty-acid chains containing 20 carbon atoms.

During an asthma attack or within minutes of exposure to an allergen such as dust or pollen, leukotrienes are released by a type of blood cell in the lungs, causing the following responses:

- contraction of the bronchial airway muscles
- inflammation of the airway linings
- swelling and narrowing of the airways
- production of mucus and fluid
- **wheezing** and shortness of breath
- nasal congestion

Leukotriene inhibitors may decrease the symptoms of mild to moderate allergen-induced asthma, improve nighttime symptoms, and reduce the number of acute asthma attacks. Taken daily on a long-term basis they may help to prevent or control the symptoms of persistent asthma—asthma with symptoms that last at least two days per week or two nights per month. They also are prescribed for children with frequent or more severe asthma attacks and for those who dislike or have difficulty using asthma inhalers. Although leukotriene inhibitors may decrease the need for inhaled beta-agonists or **corticosteroids**, they are not used to treat asthma attacks. Leukotriene inhibitors also may be used to treat symptoms of allergic rhinitis or short-term seasonal allergies, including sneezing, runny nose, **itching**, and wheezing.

Description

Leukotriene inhibitors are often called leukotriene:

- blockers
- modifiers
- antagonists
- pathway modifiers

When they were first introduced in 1996, leukotriene inhibitors represented the first new class of asthma medication in two decades. Classified as anti-inflammatories, they were originally developed to improve lung function in asthmatics by relaxing the smooth muscles around the bronchial airways and by reducing lung inflammation.

Types of leukotriene inhibitors

The available leukotriene inhibitors are: montelukast (Singulair), zafirlukast (Accolate), and zileuton (Zyflo).

Montelukast and zafirlukast are leukotriene-receptor antagonists that prevent leukotriene from binding to cell receptors and initiating the chain of events leading to symptoms of allergy and asthma. Montelukast works rapidly. It is the only leukotriene inhibitor that has been approved by the U.S. Food and Drug Administration (FDA) for use in children as young as two, as well as for the treatment of seasonal allergies.

Zafirlukast is a synthetic peptide that inhibits the receptor binding of three leukotreines (LTC4, LTD4, and LTE4) that cause smooth muscle constriction. It is used for mild to moderate persistent asthma, exercise-induced asthma, and the management of allergic rhinitis in those aged seven and older.

Zileuton is a 5-lipooxygenase pathway inhibitor that interferes with the synthesis of LTA4, LTC4,

LTD4, and LTE4. It is used to treat chronic asthma in adolescents and adults.

Effectiveness

Leukotriene inhibitors may be prescribed along with **inhaled corticosteroids** for control of mild to moderate, persistent asthma. Used alone they are less effective than low-dose inhaled corticosteroids. However, they enable some people to reduce their doses of inhaled corticosteroids. Leukotriene inhibitors may be an option for people with mild asthma who want to avoid corticosteroids, which can cause serious side effects with long-term use. When used in conjunction with beta-agonists, leukotriene inhibitors reduce symptoms and may lower the beta-agonist usage.

Leukotriene inhibitors appear to decrease the symptoms of seasonal allergic rhinitis. Although they may relieve nasal congestion better than **antihistamines**, they are less effective than corticosteroid nasal sprays. A leukotriene inhibitor combined with an antihistamine may be more effective than either drug alone.

Leukotriene inhibitors have helped some children who suffer from nocturnal asthma, exercise- and aspirin-induced asthma, allergic rhinitis, and seasonal allergies.

Clinical studies

Montelukast appears to be an effective asthma controller in about one-third of patients. Another one-third receives no benefit. However, most long-term studies have found that standard inhaled corticosteroids are more effective for controlling asthma than either beta-agonists or leukotriene inhibitors.

A 2003 analysis of 13 clinical studies found that Singulair and Accolate resulted in 60% more asthma flare-ups and other symptoms as compared with traditional asthma treatments. Patients using inhaled corticosteroids had fewer daytime symptoms and night awakenings than those taking Singulair or Accolate. The researchers advised against switching to a leukotriene inhibiter unless the dosage of inhaled medication is less than 400 micrograms per day.

A 2005 study sponsored by Merck, the maker of Singulair, found that a one-year course of Singulair was useful for treating two- to five-year-olds with occasional asthma attacks that were triggered by respiratory infections. Singulair reduced this type of asthma flare-up by 32% as compared with a control group receiving a placebo. Singulair also delayed the onset of the first asthma flare-up and reduced the need for inhaled medication. However, it did not reduce the length or severity of the flare-up once it had begun. The researchers suggested that children with infection-triggered asthma should begin taking a leukotriene inhibitor before the start of the flu season or at the onset of an upper-respiratory-tract infection.

Another 2005 study found that children whose asthma improved with montelukast alone were younger and had had asthma for a shorter period of time as compared with children whose asthma improved only with inhaled corticosteroids. Among the children whose lung function improved by at least 7.5%, 5% took montelukast alone, 23% were on inhaled corticosteroids only, and 17% were on both medications.

Other uses

Leukotriene inhibitors have been used successfully to treat inflammations of the esophagus (esophagitis) or stomach and intestines (**gastroenteritis**) that are caused by white blood cells called eosinophils that are involved in allergic reactions. Montelukast has been used to successfully treat symptoms of interstitial **cystitis**, a chronic inflammation of the bladder.

Recommended dosage

Montelukast is taken once per day in the evening so as to relieve morning allergy symptoms. Although dosing may vary, average daily doses of montelukast for asthma and seasonal allergies are: children aged 1–5: one 4-mg chewable tablet or 4-mg oral granules (one packet), swallowed whole or mixed in a spoonful of soft food; children aged 6–14: one 5-mg chewable tablet; children over 14 and adults: one 10-mg tablet.

The average doses of zafirlukast for children aged 7–11 are 10-mg tablets twice a day. Children aged 12 and older and adults usually take 20-mg tablets twice a day. Zafirlukast is taken one hour before or two hours after a meal, since food reduces its bioavailability by about 49%.

The average dose of zileuton is a 600-mg tablet four times per day for children aged 12 and older and adults.

Leukotriene inhibitors are expensive. Missed doses should be taken as soon as possible unless it is almost time for the next dose, in which case the dose should be skipped.

Precautions

Although leukotriene inhibitors are considered safe, they can raise the levels of liver enzymes. The FDA recommends **liver function tests** monthly for the first three months on medication, followed by quarterly monitoring for the next year, and continued interim testing. Zileuton is contraindicated for those with elevated liver enzymes, active **alcoholism**, or **liver disease**. Increased levels of liver enzymes may be detectable in the blood within two months of starting zileuton. Zileuton can affect liver function and, one rare occasions, can damage the liver.

It is unclear whether leukotriene inhibitors should be taken during **pregnancy**. Zafirlukast and zileuton should not be used by a woman who is breastfeeding. Both medications have been found to increase the risk of mild to moderate respiratory tract infections in patients aged 55 and older.

Medical conditions that may interfere with the use of montelukast include: allergies to **aspirin** or nonsteroidal anti-inflammatories (NSAIDs); liver disease, which can increase the blood levels of the drug; and **phenylketonuria** because chewable tablets may contain aspartame.

A healthcare provider should be contacted if an increased number of short-acting bronchodilator inhalations are needed to relieve an acute asthma attack or if more than the maximum number of daily inhalations are required while using zileuton.

To be effective montelukast and zafirlukast must be taken at the same time every day. Zileuton must be taken at regularly spaced intervals every day, even if asthma symptoms appear to improve. Montelukast should be continued through an acute asthma attack in addition to rescue medication.

Side effects

Although leukotriene inhibitors generally have few side effects and those may subside as the body adjusts to the drug, headaches are common with these medications. Headaches occur in 18–19% of those taking montelukast and in 25% of those taking zileutin. Among 7 to 11 year olds on zanfirlukast, 4.5% suffer from headaches, as do 12.9% of those aged 12 and over.

Other less common side effects of leukotriene inhibitors include:

• rash

• fatigue

• dizziness

• abdominal pain

• nausea and vomiting

• diarrhea

Montelukast appears to cause fewer side effects than other leukotriene inhibitors and is less likely to affect the liver. Side effects occurring in less than 4.2% of patients include:

• heartburn

• weakness

• fever

• nasal congestion

• cough

• dental pain

• rarely, pus in the urine

Rare side effects of zileuton include:

• itching

• flu-like symptoms

• upper right abdominal pain

• yellow eyes or skin (jaundice)

Interactions

Drugs that may interact with montelukast include:

• aspirin

• NSAIDs

• phenobarbital

• rifampin

Zafirlukast and zileuton can raise the blood levels of the asthma medication theophylline (Theo Dur and others) and the blood thinner warfarin (Coumarin). Theophylline levels and blood-clotting times should be monitored frequently.

Medications that may interact with zafirlukast include:

• aspirin

• blood pressure medications

• some seizure medications

Medications that may interact with zileuton include:

• the beta-blocker propanolol

• beta-agonists

• terfenadine (Seldane and others)

Resources

BOOKS

Haughney, John. *Leukotriene Receptor Antagonists: Evidence and Experience Examined.* London: Royal Society of Medicine Press, 2001.

Sampson, A. P., and S. T. Holgate. *Leukotriene Modifiers in Asthma Treatment.* London: Martin Dunitz, 1999.

PERIODICALS

"Asthma: Corticosteroids Are More Effective than Beta-Agonists or Leukotriene Antagonists." *Health & Medicine Week* (December 20, 2004): 77.

"Asthma: Journal Publishes Research on Tailoring Asthma Treatment in Children." *Health & Medicine Week* (February 28, 2005): 75.

Banasiak, Nancy Cantey, and Mikki Meadows-Oliver. "Leukotrienes: Their Role in the Treatment of Asthma and Seasonal Allergic Rhinitis." *Pediatric Nursing* 31, no. 1 (January/February 2005): 35–8.

Ducharme, F. M. "Inhaled Glucocorticoids Versus Leukotriene Receptor Antagonists as Single Agent Asthma Treatment: Systematic Review of Current Evidence." *British Medical Journal* 236, no. 7390 (March 22, 2003): 621–6.

ORGANIZATIONS

American Academy of Allergy, Asthma and Immunology. 555 East Wells Street, Suite 1100, Milwaukee, WI 53202-3823. (800)822-2762. < http://www.aaaai.org >.

Childhood Asthma Research and Education (CARE) Network. National Heart, Lung, and Blood Institute. 6701 Rockledge Drive, MSC 7952, Bethesda, MD 20892-7952. (301) 435-0202. < http://www.asthma-carenet.org >.

OTHER

Lehnert, Paul. "Leukotriene Modifiers for Allergic Rhinitis." *Health Guide A-Z.* WebMD. October 8, 2003 [cited March 14, 2005]. < http://my.webmed.com/hw/allergies/ug2390.asp >.

———. "Leukotriene Pathway Modifiers for Asthma." *Health Guide A-Z.* WebMD. March 5, 2004 [cited March 14, 2005]. < http://my.webmed.com/hw/asthma/hw163553.asp >.

Mayo Clinic Staff. "Medications and Immunotherapy for Asthma." *Asthma Center.* MayoClinic.com. August 13, 2004 [cited March 14, 2005]. < http://www.mayoclinic.com/invoke.cfm?objectid=58BCFCCC-BB00-4E67-A29876A9D30B65ED >.

Margaret Alic, Ph.D.

Levodopa *see* **Antiparkinson drugs**

Levothyroxine *see* **Thyroid hormones**

LGV *see* **Lymphogranuloma venereum**

Lice infestation

Definition

Lice infestations (pediculoses) are infections of the skin, hair, or genital region caused by lice living directly on the body or in hats or other garments. Lice are small wingless insect-like parasites with sucking mouthparts that feed on human blood and lay their eggs on body hairs or in clothing. The name pediculosis comes from the Latin word for louse (singular) or lice (plural). Some anthropologists believe that the different species of head and body lice developed in response to humans' invention and use of clothing about 50,000 years ago.

Description

Lice infestations are not dangerous infections by themselves. It is, however a serious public health problem because some lice can carry organisms that cause other diseases, including **relapsing fever, trench fever**, and epidemic **typhus**. Although trench **fever** is self-limiting, the other two diseases have mortality rates of 5%–10%. Pubic lice are often associated with other **sexually transmitted diseases** (STDs) but do not spread them.

Lice infestations are frequent occurrences in areas of overcrowding or inadequate facilities for bathing and laundry. They are often associated with home-lessness in the general population or with military, refugee, or prisoner camps in war-torn areas. All humans are equally susceptible to louse infestation; the elderly, however, are more vulnerable to typhus and other diseases carried by lice.

Causes and symptoms

The symptoms of lice infestations vary somewhat according to body location, although all are characterized by intense **itching**, usually with injury to the skin caused by scratching or scraping. The itching is an allergic reaction to a toxin in the saliva of the lice. Repeated bites can lead to a generalized skin eruption or inflammation.

Head lice

This type of infestation is caused by *Pediculosis humanus capitis*, the head louse. Head lice can be transmitted from one person to another by the sharing of hats, combs, or hair brushes. Epidemics of head lice are common among school-age children from all class backgrounds in all parts of the United States. The head louse is about 1/16 of an inch in length. The adult form may be visible on the patient's scalp, especially around the ears; or its grayish-white nits (eggs) may be visible at the base of the hairs close to the scalp. It takes between three and 14 days for the nits to hatch. After the nits hatch, the louse must feed on blood within a day or die.

Head lice can spread from the scalp to the eyebrows, eyelashes, and beard in adults, although they are more often limited to the scalp in children. The itching may be intense, and may be followed by bacterial infection of skin that has been scratched open. Another common complication is swelling or inflammation of the neck glands. Head lice do not spread typhus or other systemic diseases.

Body lice

Infestations of body lice are caused by *Pediculosis humanus corporis*, an organism that is similar in size to

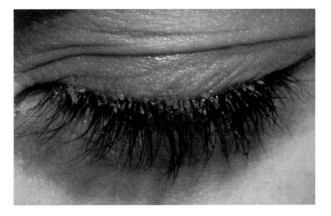

This woman's eyelashes are infested with nits, or eggs, of a body louse. *(Custom Medical Stock Photo. Reproduced by permission.)*

head lice. Body lice, however, are rarely seen on the skin itself because they come to the skin only to feed. They should be looked for in the seams of the patient's clothing. This type of infestation is associated by wearing the same clothing for long periods of time without laundering, as may happen in wartime or in cold climates; or with poor personal hygiene. It can be spread by close personal contact or shared bedding.

Patients with body lice often have intense itching with deep scratches around the upper shoulders, flanks, or neck. The bites first appear as small red pimples but may cause a generalized skin rash. If the infestation is not treated, the patient may develop complications that include **headache**, fever, and bacterial infection with scarring. Body lice can spread systemic typhus or other infections.

Pubic lice

Pubic lice are sometimes called "crabs." This type of infestation is caused by *Phthirus pubis* and is commonly spread by intimate contact. People can also get pubic lice from using the bedding, towels, or clothes of an infected person.

Pubic lice usually appear first on pubic hair, but may spread to other parts of the body, particularly if the patient is very hairy. Pubic lice are also sometimes seen on the eyelashes of children born to infected mothers. It is usually easier for the doctor to see marks from the patient's scratching than the bites from the lice, but pubic lice sometimes produce small bluish spots called maculae ceruleae on the patient's trunk or thighs. Pubic lice also sometimes leave small dark brown specks from their own excreted matter on the parts of the patient's underwear that cover the anal or genital areas.

Diagnosis

Doctors can diagnose lice infestations from looking closely at the parts of the body where the patient has been scratching. Lice are large enough to be easily seen with the naked eye or a magnifying glass. The eggs of pubic lice as well as head lice can often be found by looking at the base of the patient's hairs. Pediatricians are most likely to diagnose lice in school-age children.

It is important for doctors to rule out other diseases that can cause scratching and skin inflammation because the medications used to kill lice are very strong and can have bothersome side effects. The doctor will need to distinguish between head lice and dandruff; between body lice and **scabies** (a disease caused by skin mites); and between pubic lice and eczema. Blood tests or other laboratory tests are not useful in diagnosing lice infestations.

Treatment

Cases of head lice are usually treated with shampoos or rinses containing either lindane (Kwell) or permethrin (Nix). Permethrin is considered preferable, however, because lindane is absorbed through the skin and may produce symptoms of neurotoxicity. The person applying the treatment should wear rubber gloves and rinse the patient's hair or body completely after use. Following the treatment, nits should be removed from the hair with a fine-toothed comb or tweezers. Lindane is also effective for treating infestations of body or pubic lice, but it should not be used by pregnant women. In most cases one treatment is sufficient, but the medication can be reapplied a week later if living lice have reappeared.

Another drug that appears to be effective in treating lice is ivermectin (Stromectol), a strong antiparasite drug that is usually given to treat intestinal worms. Two doses of the drug, however, cured 99% of cases of head lice as well as intestinal worms in a poor population with high rates of infestation with both types of parasites.

Infestations of body lice can also be treated by washing the patient's clothes or bedding in boiling water, ironing seams with an iron on a high setting, or treating the clothes with 1% malathion powder or 10% DDT powder.

If the patient's eyelashes have been infested, the only safe treatments are either a thick coating of petroleum jelly (Vaseline) applied twice daily for eight days, or 1% yellow oxide of mercury applied four times a day for two weeks. Any remaining nits should be removed with tweezers.

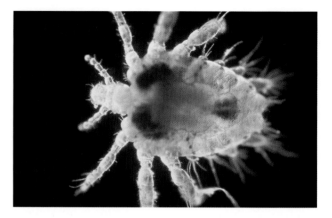

A close-up view of a body louse. (Custom Medical Stock Photo. Reproduced by permission.)

Patients with pubic lice should be examined and tested for other STDs.

Alternative treatment

For pubic lice, some practitioners of **holistic medicine** recommend a mixture of 25% oil of pennyroyal (*Mentha pulegium*), 25% garlic (*Allium sativum*) oil, and 50% distilled water applied three times in a three-day period, followed by removal of dormant eggs to prevent reinfestation.

Another alternative treatment for head lice is tea tree oil, sometimes called melaleuca oil. Tea tree oil appears to work well in treating head lice that have developed resistance to other preparations.

Prognosis

Lice can be successfully eradicated in almost all cases, although a growing number of cases of drug-resistant lice have been reported. As of 2004, some researchers are concerned about the rapid but unpredictable spread of these resistant lice. Ovide, a newer medication containing malathion, appears to be effective in treating patients with permethrin-resistant lice.

In general, patients are more at risk from typhus, trench fever, rickettsial infections, and other diseases spread by lice than from the lice themselves.

Prevention

There are no vaccines or skin treatments that will protect a person against lice prior to contact. In addition, lice infestation does not provide immunity against reinfection; recurrences are in fact quite common.

KEY TERMS

Crabs—An informal or slang term for pubic lice.

Lindane—A benzene compound that is used to kill body and pubic lice. Lindane works by being absorbed into the louse's central nervous system, causing seizures and death.

Maculae ceruleae—Bluish or blue-grey skin eruptions often seen on the trunk or thighs of patients with pubic lice. The Latin words mean blue spots.

Malathion—An insecticide that can be used in 1% powdered form to disinfect the clothes of patients with body lice.

Nits—The eggs produced by head or pubic lice, usually grayish-white in color and visible at the base of hair shafts.

Pediculosis (plural, pediculoses)—The medical term for infestation with lice.

Permethrin—A medication used to rid the scalp of head lice. Permethrin works by paralyzing the lice, so that they cannot feed after hatching within the 24 hours required for survival.

Prevention depends on adequate personal hygiene at the individual level and the following public health measures:

- Teaching school-age children the basics of good personal hygiene, including the importance of not lending or borrowing combs, brushes, or hats.

- Notifying and treating an adult patient's close personal and sexual contacts.

- Examining homeless people, elderly patients incapable of self-care, and other high-risk individuals prior to hospital admission for signs of louse infestation. This measure is necessary to protect other hospitalized people from the spread of lice.

Resources

BOOKS

Beers, Mark H., MD, and Robert Berkow, MD., editors. "Pediculosis." In *The Merck Manual of Diagnosis and Therapy*. Whitehouse Station, NJ: Merck Research Laboratories, 2004.

PERIODICALS

Downs, A. M. "Managing Head Lice in an Era of Increasing Resistance to Insecticides." *American Journal of Clinical Dermatology* 5 (March 2004): 169–177.

Foucault, C., D. Raoult, and P. Brouqui. "Randomized Open Trial of Gentamicin and Doxycycline for Eradication of *Bartonella quintana* from Blood in Patients with Chronic Bacteremia." *Antimicrobial Agents and Chemotherapy* 47 (July 2003): 2204–2207.

Heukelbach, J., and H. Feldmeier. "Ectoparasites—The Underestimated Realm." *Lancet* 363 (March 13, 2004): 889–891.

Heukelbach, J., T. Wilcke, B. Winter, et al. "Efficacy of Ivermectin in a Patient Population Concomitantly Infected with Intestinal Helminths and Ectoparasites." *Arzneimittelforschung* 54 (2004): 416–421.

Hunter, J. A., and S. C. Barker. "Susceptibility of Head Lice (*Pediculus humanus capitis*) to Pediculicides in Australia." *Parasitology Research* 90 (August 2003): 476–478.

Kittler, R., M. Kayser, and M. Stoneking. "Molecular Evolution of *Pediculus humanus* and the Origin of Clothing." *Current Biology* 13 (August 19, 2003): 1414–1417.

Mills, C., B. J. Cleary, J. F. Gilmer, and J. J. Walsh. "Inhibition of Acetylcholinesterase by Tea Tree Oil." *Journal of Pharmacy and Pharmacology* 56 (March 2004): 375–379.

Yoon, K. S., J. R. Gao, S. H. Lee, et al. "Permethrin-Resistant Human Head Lice, *Pediculus capitis*, and Their Treatment." *Archives of Dermatology* 139 (August 2003): 1061–1064.

ORGANIZATIONS

American Academy of Dermatology (AAD). 930 East Woodfield Road, Schaumburg, IL 60173. (847) 330-0230. < http://www.aad.org >.

Rebecca J. Frey, PhD

Lichen planus

Definition

Lichen planus is a skin condition of unknown origin that produces small, shiny, flat-topped, itchy pink or purple raised spots on the wrists, forearms or lower legs, especially in middle-aged patients.

Description

Lichen planus affects between 1-2% of the population, most of whom are middle-aged women. The condition is less common in the very young and the very old. The lesions are found on the skin, genitals, and in the mouth. Most cases resolve spontaneously within two years. Lichen planus is found throughout the world and is equally distributed among races.

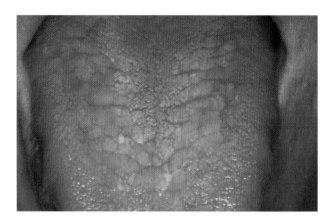

One example of lichen planus on the tongue. *(Custom Medical Stock Photo. Reproduced by permission.)*

Causes and symptoms

No one knows what causes lichen planus, although some experts suspect that it is an abnormal immune reaction following a viral infection, probably aggravated by **stress**. The condition is similar to symptoms caused by exposure to arsenic, bismuth, gold, or developers used in color photography. Occasionally, lichen planus in the mouth appears to be an allergic reaction to medications, filling material, dental hygiene products, chewing gum or candy.

Symptoms can appear suddenly, or they may gradually develop, usually on the arms or legs. The lesions on the skin may be preceded by a dryness and metallic taste or burning in the mouth.

Once the lesions appear, they change over time into flat, glistening, purple lesions marked with white lines or spots. Mild to severe **itching** is common. White, lacy lesions are usually painless, but eroded lesions often burn and can be painful. As the lesions clear up, they usually leave a brown discoloration behind, especially in dark skinned people.

Lichen planus in the mouth occurs in six different forms with a variety of symptoms, appearing as lacy-white streaks, white plaques, or eroded ulcers. Often the gums are affected, so that the surface of the gum peels off, leaving the gums red and raw.

Diagnosis

A doctor can probably diagnose the condition simply from looking at the characteristic lesions, but a **skin biopsy** may be needed to confirm the diagnosis.

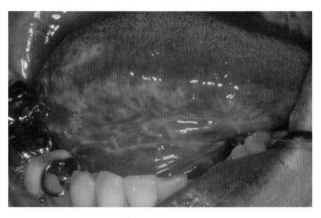

Lichen planus appearing under the tongue. *(Custom Medical Stock Photo. Reproduced by permission.)*

Treatment

Treatment is aimed at easing symptoms. Itching can be treated with steroid creams and oral **antihistamines**. Severe lesions can be treated with **corticosteroids** by mouth, or combinations of photochemotherapy (PUVA) and griseofulvin.

Patients with lesions in the mouth may find that regular professional cleaning of the teeth and conscientious dental care improve the condition. Using milder toothpastes instead of tartar control products also seems to lessen the number of ulcers and makes them less sensitive.

Prognosis

While lichen planus can be annoying, it is usually fairly benign and clears up on its own. It may take months to reach its peak, but it usually clears up within 18 months.

Resources

OTHER

Lichen Planus Self-Help. Baylor College of Dentistry. < http://www.tambcd.edu/lichen >.

Carol A. Turkington

Lichen simplex chronicus

Definition

Lichen simplex chronicus is a chronic inflammation of the skin (**dermatitis**) characterized by small, round itchy spots that thicken and become leathery as a result of scratching.

Description

Also termed neurodermatis, lichen simplex chronicus is the result of chronic skin irritation. It occurs in 4-5 out of every thousand people. Initial irritation causes **itching**, and in turn, itching causes scratching. Scratching leads to further irritation, which damages the skin. The possibility of infection is greatly increased when the outer layer of protective skin is broken. Skin usually repairs itself quickly; however, in the case of lichen simplex chronicus, healing skin causes more itching and more scratching causes a thickening of the skin (lichen). The small skin patches are usually 1–10 in (2.54–25.4 cm) in diameter.

Causes and symptoms

Lichen simplex chronicus is often caused by constant rubbing of the skin. The rubbing begins the chain of events that leads from itching to scratching and then to the presence of leather-like skin patches.

Symptoms are chronic itching which is often accompanied by nervous tension. The appearance of scratch marks and the leathery skin patches can be found anywhere on the body. A prolonged lichen simplex chronicus can result in brown-colored pigmentation at the site of irritation.

Diagnosis

A dermatologist, a physician specializing in the study and treatment of skin disorders, can make a diagnosis after a visual exam.

Treatment

Treatment of the itching is necessary to stop the scratching and resulting skin damage. There are a number of ways to stop itching. Perhaps the most important is to cut fingernails very short. Ice can substitute for the relief of scratching. Heat and fuzzy clothing worsen itching; cold and smooth clothing pacify it. If the itching is persistent, dressings may be applied to the affected areas.

KEY TERMS

Antihistamine—A chemical that interferes with the action of histamine. Histamine is part of an inflammatory response and helps to cause itching.

Callus—Thickened skin due to chronic rubbing or irritation.

Lesion—Abnormal change in tissue caused by localized disease.

Among the topical medications that relieve itching are a number of commercial preparations containing menthol, camphor, eucalyptus oil, and aloe. Topical cortisone is also available without a prescription. Some preparations also contain **antihistamines**, which penetrate intact skin poorly. All these medicines work better under occlusion, which means putting a waterproof barrier like a rubber glove or plastic wrap over them. For broken skin, **topical antibiotics** like bacitracin help prevent infection. These should be used early to forestall further damage to the skin.

Reducing the buildup of thick skin may require medicines that dissolve or melt keratin, the major chemical in skin's outer layer. These keratolytics include urea, lactic acid, and salicylic acid.

Resistant cases of lichen simplex chronicus will often respond to cortisone-like drugs injected directly into the lesions.

Sedatives or tranquilizers may be prescribed to combat the nervous tension and **anxiety** that often accompanies the condition.

Prognosis

Diligent adherence to treatment is usually rewarded with a resolution of the condition. The original cause of itching may be gone, or it may reappear. Preventive treatment in its early stages will arrest the process.

Prevention

Early, gentler substitutes for scratching can entirely prevent lichen simplex chronicus.

Resources

BOOKS

Swerlick, Robert A., and Thomas J. Lawley. "Eczema, Psoriasis, Cutaneous Infections, Acne, and Other

Common Skin Disorders." In *Harrison's Principles of Internal Medicine*, edited by Anthony S. Fauci, et al. New York: McGraw-Hill, 1997.

J. Ricker Polsdorfer, MD

Life support

Definition

Life support refers to a spectrum of techniques used to maintain life after the failure of one or more vital organs.

Purpose

A patient requires life support when one or more vital organs fail, due to causes such as trauma, infection, **cancer**, **heart attack**, or chronic disease. Among the purposes of life support are to:

- Establish and maintain the ABC's of resuscitation—airway, breathing, and circulation.

- Restore the patient's homeostasis—the internal chemical and physical balance of the body.

- Protect the patient from complications of the underlying disease and its treatment.

Precautions

Patients and families need to recognize that life support is an extremely painful, expensive, and emotionally wrenching experience. Life support exposes a patient to vast risks of further medical complications, and offers no guarantee of a positive outcome. Even in successful cases, recovery may be slow and frustrating.

Description

Successful life support begins with establishing the ABC's of resuscitation—airway, breathing, and circulation.

The airway refers to a clear passageway for air to enter the lungs from outside the body. The patient's airway may become blocked by:

- Foreign body obstruction, as by food or dentures

- Injury-related damage and swelling, as from a wound or surgery

- Loss of protective reflexes due to **coma** of any origin

Life support may begin with basic **cardiopulmonary resuscitation (CPR)**, as in cases of cardiac arrest. Thereafter, the most common technique used to create a secure airway is insertion of an endotracheal (ET) tube through the mouth or nose into the windpipe (trachea). An alternative method of securing an airway is by **tracheotomy**, a surgical procedure in which a tube is inserted into the trachea through an incision made in the base of the throat. Of the two options, placement of an ET tube is usually quicker and more convenient, and thus occurs much more commonly. Doctors perform a tracheotomy when they cannot establish an ET airway, or when the patient will require an artificial airway for more than a week or two.

Breathing refers to the movement of air in and out of the lungs. Inadequate breathing may result from:

- Heart disease, as in congestive heart failure

- Primary disease of the lungs, such as **pneumonia**, **asthma**, or emphysema

- Coma of any cause, such as narcotic overdose or stroke

- Muscle **fatigue** or neuromuscular disease (**spinal cord injury** or polio)

- Pain, from rib **fractures** or surgery on the chest

When the patient cannot breathe sufficiently, the physician will use a ventilator, a machine that pumps air in and out of the patient's lungs. For many doctors and members of the public, the term "life support" calls up the image of an ET tube and ventilator.

Circulation refers to the flow of blood around the body from the heart to vital organs. Circulation can fail due to:

- Primary disease of the heart (heart attack)

- Blood loss (trauma or internal bleeding of any cause)

- Severe infection (sepsis)

- Drug reactions or overdoses

- Extreme allergic reaction

- Severe **dehydration** (**gastroenteritis** or heat-related illness)

In order to ensure adequate circulation, the patient will require one or more intravenous (IV) tubes (catheters). The IVs may include both the short needle and tube commonly used in the hand or forearm, and longer catheters inserted into the larger and more central veins of the body. Catheters inserted into these larger veins are known as central lines. Through the IVs the patient receives fluids, drugs, and blood transfusions as needed to support the circulation.

Once the ABC's are secure, life support is directed at maintaining homeostasis, the body's delicate chemical and physical balance. In a healthy person, the body keeps precise control over many components of its makeup, such as its fluids, nutrients, and pressures. When vital organs fail, the body can no longer regulate these components, and the doctor must take steps to restore the normal state.

Preserving the body's internal equilibrium requires careful monitoring of innumerable indicators of the patient's well-being. These indicators include:

- Vital signs (heartbeats per minute, breaths per minute, blood pressure, body temperature, and weight)
- Fluids (input and output of the body)
- Blood cell counts
- Chemical substances of the body (sodium, potassium, sugar, and many others)
- Pressures in the circulation, lungs, and perhaps even the brain
- Presence of germs (bacteria, fungi) causing infection in body systems (lungs, blood, urine)

This intensive monitoring usually takes place in an intensive care unit (ICU) or critical care unit (CCU) and requires:

- Specialized physicians, such as cardiologists, intensivists, and surgeons
- Highly-skilled nursing care, often one nurse per patient around-the-clock
- Extensive support staff, such as respiratory therapists, laboratory technicians, radiology technicians, dieticians, and pharmacists
- Constant measurement of basics such as pulse, heart rhythm, and oxygen level in the blood
- Frequent inspection of the patient's alertness, color, and level of pain
- Use of catheters in the veins and arteries to withdraw blood samples and measure pressures in the circulation
- Use of tubes in the bladder (Foley catheter), stomach (nasogastric tube), and other body cavities
- Frequent laboratory tests on blood, urine, drainage from **wounds**, and other body specimens
- X-ray, ultrasound, computerized tomography (CT), and other imaging procedures
- Electrocardiograms

The treatments of life support include:

- Oxygen
- Intravenous fluids with sugar and basic salts

- Drugs to improve circulation and other body functions
- Antibiotics
- Transfusions
- Surgery
- Nutritional supplements by vein or stomach tube
- Tubes in body cavities (chest or abdomen) to relieve fluid buildup
- Dialysis
- Pacemaker
- Electrical defibrillation
- Various machines to assist heart or lung function
- Transplantation of organs or mechanical substitutes (artificial heart)
- Sedation or even temporary **paralysis** to enable the patient to tolerate these procedures

Preparation

The need for life support may arise suddenly and with little warning. All people should discuss in advance with family and doctor their wishes for the use of life support should a medical crisis develop. The doctor will note the preferences in the patient's record. Patients should sign documents such as an Advance Directive and Durable Power of Attorney for Health Care to express their wishes and designate a surrogate decision-maker in case of incapacitation.

Physicians and medical care providers must anticipate the possibility that a patient will require life support, perhaps suddenly. In preparation, doctors and medical staff must:

- Receive training in resuscitation skills
- Monitor patients carefully
- Maintain proper supplies and equipment
- Discuss in advance with patients and patients' families whether or not to begin life support

Aftercare

If a patient survives life support treatments, doctors will cautiously try to wean the patient from the support systems. Being able to breathe adequately without the ventilator is one major hurdle. Patients commonly fail in their first attempts to breathe on their own, often tiring out after a few hours. Thus, the doctor will reconnect the ventilator, give the patient a rest, and try again in a day or two.

As the patient regains organ function, there is less need for monitors, tests, and treatments that require an intensive care setting. The doctor may transfer the patient to a lower level of hospital care, a skilled nursing facility (SNF), or perhaps directly to home. Physical and occupational therapists may help the patient improve strength and endurance. The patient will receive continuing care from the primary doctor and specialists as needed. The patient may require prescription drugs, assist devices, and psychological therapists.

Risks

The risks and consequences of life support are enormous. These risks include:

- Physical dangers
- Emotional suffering
- Financial costs
- Societal discord

The physical dangers of life support encompass all the hazards of the patient's underlying disease and treatments. Among these risks are:

- Permanent damage to the brain, kidneys, and other vital organs caused by poor circulation or low oxygen content of the blood
- Direct damage to organs from use of medical instruments and procedures
- Infections, often with organisms that are highly resistant to antibiotics
- Abnormal blood clots
- Skin ulcers from lying immobilized for long periods
- Extreme pain
- Exposure of medical personnel to communicable diseases

The emotional consequences of life support touch patients, families, and medical caregivers. These repercussions arise from:

- The frightening environment of an ICU
- The need to make life-and-death decisions
- The anger, guilt, and grief that relate to life-threatening illness
- The fact that many lengthy and difficult treatments will end in failure

The financial costs of life support are huge. A single day of life support costs many thousands of dollars. These expenses fall on individual payers, insurance companies, health plans, and governments.

KEY TERMS

Cardiopulmonary—Relating to the heart and lungs.

Central line—A tube placed by needle into a large, central vein of the body.

Coma—Unconsciousness.

Defibrillation—Use of an electric shock to restore a normal heartbeat.

Endotracheal tube—A tube placed into the windpipe through the nose or mouth.

Foley catheter—A tube that drains urine from the bladder.

Homeostasis—The internal chemical and physical balance of the body.

Nasogastric tube—A tube placed through the nose into the stomach.

Neuromuscular—Relating to nerves and muscles.

Resuscitation—Treatments to restore an adequate airway, breathing, and circulation.

Sepsis—An overwhelming infection with effects throughout the body.

Tracheotomy—A surgical procedure in which a tube is inserted into the trachea through an incision made in the base of the throat.

Trauma—Serious physical injury.

Ventilator—A machine that pumps air in and out of the lungs.

Vital signs—Basic indicators of body function, usually meaning heartbeats per minute, breaths per minute, blood pressure, body temperature, and weight.

All such payers face difficult decisions regarding the allotment of money for such treatment, especially in cases that are likely to be futile.

Society as a whole faces difficult decisions surrounding life support. Some governments have enacted regulations that establish priorities for the spending of health care resources. Patients who do not receive treatment under such rules may feel victimized by society's choices.

Resources

BOOKS

Irwin, Richard S., Frank B. Cerra, and James M. Rippe, editors. *Irwin and Rippe's Intensive Care Medicine.* Philadelphia: Lippincott-Raven, 1999.

Luce, John M., "Approach to the Patient In a Critical Care Setting." In *Textbook of Medicine*, edited by Lee Goldman and J. Claude Bennett, 21st ed. Vol. 1. Philadelphia: W.B. Saunders Company, 2000, pp. 483-4.

Tintinalli, Judith E., et al, editors. *Emergency Medicine: a comprehensive study guide.* New York: McGraw-Hill, 2000.

Isaac R. Berniker

Light sensitivity *see* **Photosensitivity**

Light therapy *see* **Phototherapy**

Light treatment *see* **Ultraviolet light treatment**

Lipase test

Definition

The lipase test is a blood test performed to determine the serum level of a specific protein (enzyme) involved in digestion. Lipase is an enzyme produced by the pancreas, which is a large gland situated near the stomach. Lipase works to break down a certain type of blood lipid (triglycerides) into fatty acids.

Lipase appears in the blood together with another enzyme called amylase following damage to or diseases affecting the pancreas. It was once thought that abnormally high lipase levels were associated only with diseases of the pancreas. Other conditions are now known to be associated with high lipase levels, especially kidney failure and intestinal obstruction. Diseases involving the pancreas, however, produce much higher lipase levels than diseases of other organs. Lipase levels in pancreatic disorders are often 5-10 times higher than normal.

Purpose

The lipase test is most often used in evaluating inflammation of the pancreas (**pancreatitis**), but it is also useful in diagnosing kidney failure, intestinal obstruction, **mumps**, and peptic ulcers. Doctors often order amylase and lipase tests at the same time to help distinguish pancreatitis from ulcers and other disorders in the abdomen. If the patient has acute (sudden onset) pancreatitis, the lipase level usually rises somewhat later than the amylase level—about 24-48 hours after onset of symptoms—and remains abnormally high for 5-7 days. Because the lipase level

---

KEY TERMS

Amylase—A digestive enzyme that breaks down starch.

Lipid—A greasy organic compound that cannot be dissolved in water. Triglycerides, which are broken down by lipase, are one type of blood lipid.

Pancreas—An elongated gland situated across the back of the abdomen behind the stomach. It secretes both digestive enzymes and hormones. Pancreatic hormones regulate the level of sugar in the blood.

Pancreatitis—Inflammation of the pancreas, frequently caused by gallstones, alcohol abuse, viral infection, or injury.

Turbidimetry—A technique of measurement that analyzes the amount of sediment in a liquid.

---

peaks later and remains elevated longer, its determination is more useful in late diagnosis of acute pancreatitis. Conversely, however, lipase levels are not as useful in diagnosing chronic pancreatic disease.

Precautions

Patients should be asked whether they are taking certain prescription drugs that can affect the accuracy of the lipase test. Drugs that can cause elevated lipase levels include bethanechol, cholinergics, codeine, indomethacin, meperidine, methacholine, and morphine. Drugs that may decrease levels include calcium ions.

Description

A lipase test is performed on a sample of the patient's blood, withdrawn from a vein into a vacuum tube. The procedure, which is called a venipuncture, takes about five minutes.

Preparation

The patient should have nothing to eat or drink for 12 hours before the lipase test.

Risks

Risks for this test are minimal, but may include slight bleeding from the puncture site, a small bruise or swelling in the area, **fainting**, or feeling lightheaded.

Normal results

Reference values for lipase determination are laboratory- and method-specific. In general, normal results are usually less than 200 units/L (triolein methods by titration or turbidimetry).

Abnormal results

Increased lipase levels are found in acute pancreatitis, chronic relapsing pancreatitis, and pancreatic **cancer**. High lipase levels also occur in certain liver diseases, kidney failure, bowel obstruction, peptic ulcer disease, and tumors or inflammation of the salivary glands.

Resources

BOOKS

Pagana, Kathleen Deska. *Mosby's Manual of Diagnostic and Laboratory Tests*. St. Louis: Mosby, Inc., 1998.

Janis O. Flores

Lipidoses

Definition

Lipidoses are heredity disorders, passed from parents to their children, characterized by defects of the digestive system that impair the way the body uses fat from the diet. When the body is unable to properly digest fats, lipids accumulate in body tissues in abnormal amounts.

Description

The digestion, storage, and use of fats from foods is a complex process that involves hundreds of chemical reactions in the body. In most people, the body is already programmed by its genetic code to produce all of the enzymes and chemicals necessary to carry out these functions. These genetic instructions are passed from parents to their offspring during reproduction.

People with lipidoses are born without the genetic codes needed to tell their bodies how to complete a particular part of the fat digestion process. In most of these disorders, the body does not produce a certain enzyme or chemical. Over 30 different disorders of fat metabolism are related to genetic defects. Although the defects are passed from parents to children, the parents often do not have the disorders themselves.

The symptoms, available treatments, and long-term consequences of these conditions vary greatly. Some of the conditions become apparent shortly after the infant is born; in others, symptoms may not develop until adulthood. For most of the lipidoses, diagnosis is suspected based on the symptoms and family history. Blood tests, urine tests, and tissue tests can be used to confirm the diagnosis. **Genetic testing** can be used, in some cases, to identify the defective gene. Some of these disorders can be controlled with changes in the diet, medications, or enzyme supplements. For many, no treatment is available. Some may cause **death** in childhood or contribute to a shortened life expectancy. Some of the most common or most serious lipidoses are discussed below.

Fabry's disease

Causes and symptoms

Approximately 1 in every 40,000 males is born with Fabry's disease. This condition has an X-linked, recessive pattern of inheritance, meaning that the defective gene is carried on the X chromosome. A female who carries a defective recessive gene on one of her two X chromosomes has a 50% chance of passing the defective gene to her sons who will develop the disorder associated with the defective gene (a male receives one X chromosome from his mother and one Y chromosome from his father). She also has a 50% chance of passing the defective recessive gene to her daughters who will be carries of the disorder (like their mother). Some female carries of Fabry's disease show mild signs of the disorder, especially cloudiness of the cornea.

The gene that is defective in Fabry's disease causes a deficiency of the enzyme alpha-galactosidase A. Without this enzyme, fatty compounds starts to line the blood vessels. The collection of fatty deposits eventually affects blood vessels in the skin, heart, kidneys, and nervous system. The first symptoms in childhood are **pain** and discomfort in the hands and feet brought on by **exercise**, **fever**, **stress**, or changes in the weather. A raised rash of dark red-purple spots is common, especially on skin between the waistline and the knees. Other symptoms include a decreased ability to sweat and changes in the cornea or outer layer of the eye. Although the disease begins in childhood, it progresses very slowly. Kidney and heart problems develop in adulthood.

Diagnosis

The diagnosis can be confirmed by a blood test to measure for alpha-galactosidase A. Women who are carries of the defective gene can also be identified by a blood test.

Treatment

Treatment focuses on prevention of symptoms and long-term complications. Daily doses of diphenyl-hydantoin (Dilantin) or carbamazapine (Tegretol) can prevent or reduce the severity of pain in the hands and feet associated with the condition. A low sodium, low protein diet may be beneficial to those patients who have some kidney complications. If kidney problems progress, **kidney dialysis** or **kidney transplantation** may be required. Enzyme replacement therapy is currently being explored.

Prognosis

Although patients with Fabry's disease usually survive to adulthood, they are at increased risk for **stroke**, heart attacks, and kidney damage.

Gaucher disease

Causes and symptoms

Gaucher (pronounced go-shay) disease is the most common of the lipid storage disorders. It is found in populations all over the world (20,00 to 40,000 people have a type of the disease), and it occurs with equal frequency in males and females. **Gaucher disease** has a recessive pattern of inheritance, meaning that a person must inherit a copy of the defective gene from both parents in order to have the disease. The genetic defect causes a deficiency of the enzyme glucocerebrosidase that is responsible for breaking down a certain type of fat and releasing it from fat cells. These fat cells begin to crowd out healthy cells in the liver, spleen, bones, and nervous system. Symptoms of Gaucher disease can start in infancy, childhood, or adulthood.

Three types of Gaucher disease have been identified, but there are many variations in how symptoms develop. Type 1 is the most common and affects both children and adults. It occurs much more often in people of Eastern European and Russian Jewish (Ashkenazi) ancestry, affecting 1 out of every 450 live births. The first signs of the disease include an enlarged liver and spleen, causing the abdomen to swell. Children with this condition may be shorter than normal. Other symptoms include tiredness, pain, bone deterioration, broken bones, anemia, and increased bruising. Type 2 Gaucher disease is more serious, beginning within the first few months after birth. Symptoms, which are similar to those in Type 1, progress rapidly, but also include nervous system damage. Symptoms of Type 3 Gaucher disease begin during early childhood with symptoms like Type 1. Unlike Type 2, the progress of the disease is slower, although it also includes nervous system damage.

Diagnosis

Gaucher disease may be suspected based on symptoms and is confirmed with a blood test for levels of the enzyme. Samples of tissue from an affected area may also be used to confirm a diagnosis of the disease.

Treatment

The symptoms of Gaucher disease can be stopped and even reversed by treatment with injections of enzyme replacements. Two enzyme drugs currently available are alglucerase (Ceredase) and imiglucerase (Cerezyme). Other treatments address specific symptoms such as anemia, broken bones, or pain.

Prognosis

The pain and deformities associated with symptoms can make coping with this illness very challenging for individuals and families. With treatment and control of symptoms, people with Type 1 Gaucher disease may lead fairly long and normal lives. Most infants with Type 2 die before the age of 2. Children with Type 3 Gaucher disease may survive to adolescence and early adulthood.

Krabbe's disease

Causes and symptoms

Krabbe's disease is caused by a deficiency of the enzyme galactoside beta-galactosidase. It has a recessive pattern of inheritance and is believed to occur in 1 of 40,000 births in the United States. This condition, which is also called globoid cell leukodystrophy or Krabbe leukodystrophy, is characterized by acute nervous system degeneration. It develops in early infancy with initial symptoms of irritability, **vomiting** and episodes of partial unconsciousness. Symptoms progress rapidly to seizures, difficulty swallowing, blindness, deafness, **mental retardation**, and **paralysis**.

Treatment

No treatment is available.

Prognosis

Children born with Krabbe's disease die in infancy.

Niemann-pick disease

Causes and symptoms

At least five different forms of Niemann-Pick disease (NPD) have been identified. The different types seem to be related to the activity level of the enzyme sphingomyelinase. In patients with Types A and B NPD, there is a build up of sphingomyelin in cells of the brain, liver, spleen, kidney and lung. Type A is the most common form of NPD and the most serious, with death usually occurring by the age of 18 months. Symptoms develop within the first few months of life and include poor appetite, failure to grow, enlarged liver and spleen, and the appearance of cherry red spots in the retina of the eye. Type B develops in infancy or childhood with symptoms of mild liver or spleen enlargement and lung problems. Some adults with this form (Type E) may also show a loss of muscle coordination. Types C or D NPD are related to cholesterol transfer out of cells. Children with Types C or D grow normally in early childhood, but eventually develop difficulty in walking and loss of muscle coordination. Ultimately, the nervous system becomes severely damaged and these patients die. Type C occurs in any population, while Type D has been identified only in patients from Nova Scotia, Canada.

Diagnosis

Diagnosis is confirmed by analyzing a sample of tissue. Prenatal diagnosis of Types A and B of NPD can be done with **amniocentesis** or **chorionic villus sampling**.

Treatment

Treatment consists of supportive care to deal with symptoms and the development of complications. **Bone marrow transplantation** is being investigated as a possible treatment. Low-cholesterol **diets** may be helpful for patients with Types C and D.

Prognosis

Patients with Type A NPD usually die within the first year and a half of life. Type B patients generally live to adulthood but suffer from significant liver and lung problems. With Types C and D NPD, there is significant nervous system damage leading to severe **muscle spasms**, seizures, and eventually, to **coma** and death. Some patients with Types C and D die in childhood, while less severely affected patients may survive to adulthood.

Refsum's disease

Causes and symptoms

Refsum's disease has a recessive pattern of inheritance and affects populations from Northern Europe, particularly Scandinavians most frequently. It is due to a deficiency of phytanic acid hydroxylase, an enzyme that breaks down a fatty acid called phytanic acid. This condition affects the nervous system, eyes, bones, and skin. Symptoms, which usually appear by age 20, include vision problems [retinitis pigmentosa and rhythmic eye movements (nystagmus)], loss of muscle coordination, loss of sense of smell (**anosmia**), pain, **numbness**, and elevated protein in the cerebrospinal fluid.

Treatment

A diet free of phytanic acid (found in dairy products, tuna, cod, haddock, lamb, stewed beef, white bread, white rice, boiled potatoes, and egg yolk) can reduce some of the symptoms. **Plasmapheresis**, a process where whole blood is removed from the body, processed through a filtering system, and then return to the body, may be used to filter phytanic acid from the blood.

Tay-sachs disease

Causes and symptoms

Tay-Sachs disease (TSD) is a fatal condition caused by a deficiency of the enzyme hexosaminidase A (Hex-A). The defective gene that causes this disorder is found in roughly 1 in 250 people in the general population. However, certain populations have significantly higher rates of TSD. French-Canadians living near the St. Lawrence River and in the Cajun regions of Louisiana are at higher risk of having a child with TSD. The highest risk seems to be in people of Eastern European and Russian Jewish (Ashkenazi) descent. Tay-Sachs disease has a recessive pattern of inheritance, and approximately 1 in every 27 people of Jewish ancestry in the United States carries the TSD gene. Symptoms develop in infancy and are due to the accumulation of a fatty acid compound in the nervous system. Early symptoms include loss of vision and physical coordination, seizures, and mental retardation. Eventually, the child develops problems with breathing and swallowing. Blindness, paralysis, and death follow.

Diagnosis

Carriers of the Tay-Sachs related gene can be identified with a blood test. Amniocentesis or chorionic villi sampling can be used to determine if the fetus has Tay-Sachs disease.

Treatment

There is no treatment for Tay-Sachs disease. Parents who are identified as carriers may want to seek **genetic counseling**. If a fetus is identified as having TSD, parents may consider termination of the **pregnancy**.

Prognosis

Children born with Tay-Sachs disease become increasingly debilitated; most die by about age four.

Wolman's disease

Causes and symptoms

Wolman's disease is caused by a genetic defect (with a recessive pattern of inheritance) that results in deficiency of an enzyme that breaks down cholesterol. This causes large amounts of fat to accumulate in body tissues. Symptoms begin in the first few weeks of life and include an enlarged liver and spleen, adrenal calcification (hardening of adrenal tissue due to deposits of calcium salts), and fatty stools.

Treatment

No treatment is currently available.

Prognosis

Death generally occurs before six months of age.

Prevention

Couples who have family histories of genetic defects can undergo genetic testing and counseling to see if they are at risk for having a child with one of the lipidoses disorders. During pregnancy, cell samples can be collected from the fetus using amniocentesis or chorionic villi sampling. The results of these test can indicate if the developing fetus has a lipidosis disorder. Termination of the pregnancy may be considered in some cases.

Resources

ORGANIZATIONS

National Institute of Neurological Disorders and Stroke. P.O. Box 5801, Bethesda, MD 20824. (800) 352-9424. < http://www.ninds.nih.gov/index.htm >.

National Niemann-Pick Foundation. 3734 E. Olive Ave., Gilbert, AZ 85234. (602) 497-6638.

National Organization for Rare Disorders. P.O. Box 8923, New Fairfield, CT 06812-8923. (800) 999-6673. < http://www.rarediseases.org >.

KEY TERMS

Amniocentesis—A procedure where a needle is inserted through the abdomen into the uterus of a pregnant woman to remove a small amount of the fluid that surrounds the developing fetus. This test can be preformed at about week 16 of the pregnancy. Cells from the fetus can be tested for genetic defects.

Chorionic villi sampling—A procedure to remove a small tissue sample of the placenta, the sac that surrounds the developing fetus. This test can be performed as early as week 10 of the pregnancy. The tissue can be tested for genetic defects.

Lipids—Organic compounds not soluble in water, but soluble in fat solvents such as alcohol. Lipids are stored in the body as energy reserves and are also important components of cell membranes.

Recessive—Refers to an inherited characteristic or trait that is expressed only when two copies of the gene responsible for it are present.

X-linked—Refers to a gene carried on the X chromosome, one of the two sex chromosomes.

National Tay-Sachs and Allied Diseases Association. 2001 Beacon St., Suite 204, Brookline, MA 02146. (800) 906-8723. < http://www.ntsad.org >.

OTHER

Gaucher Disease Treatment Program. < http://gaucher.mgh.harvard.edu >.

Rare Genetic Diseases In Children: An Internet Resource Gateway. < http://mcrcr2.med.nyu.edu/murphp01/homenew.htm >.

Altha Roberts Edgren

Lipoproteins test

Definition

Lipoproteins are the "packages" in which cholesterol and triglycerides travel throughout the body. Measuring the amount of cholesterol carried by each type of lipoprotein helps determine a person's risk for cardiovascular disease (disease that affects the heart and blood vessels, also called CVD).

Purpose

Cholesterol and triglycerides are fat-like substances called lipids. Cholesterol is used to build cell membranes and hormones. The body makes cholesterol and gets it from food. Triglycerides provide a major source of energy to the body tissues. Both cholesterol and triglycerides are vital to body function, but an excess of either one, especially cholesterol, puts a person at risk of cardiovascular disease.

Because cholesterol and triglycerides can't dissolve in watery liquid, they must be transported by something that can dissolve in blood serum. Lipoproteins contain cholesterol and triglycerides at the core and an outer layer of protein, called apolipoprotein.

There are four major classes of lipoproteins: chylomicrons, very low-density lipoproteins (VLDL), low-density lipoproteins (LDL), and high-density lipoproteins (HDL). There also are less commonly measured classes such as lipoprotein(a) and subtypes of the main classes. Each lipoprotein has characteristics that make the cholesterol it carries a greater or lesser risk. Measuring each type of lipoprotein helps determine a person's risk for cardiovascular disease more accurately than cholesterol measurement alone. When a person is discovered to be at risk, treatment by diet or medication can be started and his or her response to treatment monitored by repeated testing.

Description

Chylomicrons

Chylomicrons are made in the intestines from the triglycerides in food. They contain very little cholesterol. Chylomicrons circulate in the blood, getting smaller as they deposit the triglycerides in fatty tissue. Twelve hours after a meal, they are gone from circulation. Serum collected from a person directly after eating will form a creamy layer on the top if left undisturbed and refrigerated overnight. This creamy layer is the chylomicrons.

Very low-density lipoproteins (VLDL)

VLDL are formed in the liver by the combination of cholesterol, triglycerides formed from circulating fatty acids, and apolipoprotein. This lipoprotein particle is smaller than a chylomicron, and contains less triglyceride but more cholesterol (10-15% of a person's total cholesterol). As the VLDL circulates in the blood, triglycerides are deposited and the particle gets smaller, eventually becoming a low-density lipoprotein (LDL). Serum from a person with a large amount of VLDL will be cloudy.

Low-density lipoproteins (LDL)

LDL, often called "bad" cholesterol, is formed primarily by the breakdown of VLDL. LDL contains little triglycerides and a large amount of cholesterol (60-70% of a person's total cholesterol). Although the particles are much smaller than chylomicrons and VLDL, LDL particles can vary in size and chemical structure. These variations represent subclasses within the LDL class. Serum from a person with a large amount of LDL will be clear.

LDL carries cholesterol in the blood and deposits it in body tissues and in the walls of blood vessels, a condition known as **atherosclerosis**. The amount of LDL in a person's blood is directly related to his or her risk of cardiovascular disease. The higher the LDL level, the greater the risk. LDL is the lipoprotein class most used to trigger and monitor cholesterol lowering therapy.

High-density lipoproteins (HDL)

HDL is often called "good" cholesterol. HDL removes excess cholesterol from tissues and vessel walls and carries it to the liver, where it is removed from the blood and discarded. The amount of HDL in a person's blood is inversely related to his or her risk of cardiovascular disease. The lower the HDL level, the greater the risk; the higher the level, the lower the risk. The smallest lipoprotein, it contains 20-30% of a person's total cholesterol and can be separated into two major subclasses.

Lipoprotein(a)

Lipoprotein(a) is found in lower concentrations than other lipoproteins, yet it carries a unique and significant risk for cardiovascular disease. Because of its similarity to LDL, test methods often don't measure it separately, but include it within the LDL class. Testing specifically for this class may uncover why a person is not responding to standard cholesterol-lowering treatment. High lipoprotein(a) levels may not respond to treatment aimed at high LDL.

Measurement guidelines

The Expert Panel of the National Cholesterol Education Program (NCEP) sponsored by the National Institutes of Health has published guidelines for the detection of **high cholesterol** in adults. The NCEP panel recommends that adults over the age of 20 be tested for cholesterol and HDL every five years. If the cholesterol is high, the HDL is low (below 35 mg/dl), or other risk factors are present, a complete lipoprotein profile that includes total cholesterol, triglycerides, HDL, and calculated LDL should be done.

Measurement methods

There are a variety of methods to measure the lipoprotein classes. All require separation of the classes before they can be measured. One way to separate them is by spinning serum (the yellow, watery liquid that separates from the cells when **blood clots**) for a long time in a high-speed centrifuge (called ultracentrifugation). The most dense classes will settle toward the bottom, the least dense toward the top. Following centrifugation, the most complete measurement of all the lipoprotein classes is done using electrophoresis. This procedure measures the quantity of each lipoprotein class based on its movement in an electrical field.

In 2003, a new test called the vertical auto profile or VAP, was developed that provides detailed measurements of cholesterol subclasses. These subclasses play important roles in patients later developing heart disease. The new tests were predicted to help identify important, emerging risk factors for heart disease.

Other, less extensive procedures also are used. For example, if only HDL is to be measured, a chemical is added to the serum that will clump the other classes, leaving HDL free in the serum to be measured by a chemical method. LDL often is not measured directly but its level is calculated based on the measurements of total cholesterol, HDL, and triglycerides. The formula is called the Friedewald formula: LDL = total cholesterol - HDL - (triglycerides/5). The calculated result will be inaccurate in a person with high triglycerides. Results usually are available the same or following day.

Preparation

The patient must fast for 12 hours before the test, eating nothing and drinking only water. The person should not have alcohol for 24 hours before the test. There should be a stable diet and no illnesses occurring in the preceding two weeks.

A lipoproteins test requires 5 mL (milliliters) of blood. A person's physical position while having blood collected affects the results. Values from blood drawn while a person is sitting may be different from those while the person is standing. If repeated testing is done, the person should be in the same position each time.

Aftercare

Discomfort or bruising may occur at the puncture site or the person may feel dizzy or faint. Pressure to

---

KEY TERMS

Atherosclerosis—Disease of blood vessels caused by deposits of cholesterol on the inside walls of the vessels.

Cardiovascular disease—Disease that affects the heart and blood vessels.

Cholesterol—A fat-like substance called a lipid. It is used to build cell membranes and hormones. The body makes cholesterol and gets it from food.

Lipoproteins—The packages in which cholesterol and triglycerides travel throughout the body.

---

the puncture site until the bleeding stops reduces bruising. Warm packs to the puncture site relieve discomfort.

Normal results

People with HDL levels between 45 mg/dl and 59 mg/dl carry an average risk for cardiovascular disease. People with HDL levels above 60 mg/dl have a negative risk factor and appear to be protected from cardiovascular disease.

LDL levels below 130 mg/dl are desirable.

Some people have normal variations in their lipoprotein and total cholesterol levels. Repeat testing may be necessary, especially if a value is at a borderline risk category point.

Abnormal results

People with HDL levels 36-44 mg/dl have a moderate risk of cardiovascular disease. HDL levels below 35 mg/dl are a major risk.

LDL levels 130-159 mg/dl place a person at a borderline high risk of cardiovascular disease; levels above 160 mg/dl place a person at high risk. Relative proportions between HDL and LDL are important also. Results of a large clinical trial in 2003 showed that the new VAP cholesterol tests increased lipid-lowering therapy by 59% in high-risk patients with diabetes.

Resources

PERIODICALS

"Doctors Laboratory to Offer VAP Expanded Cholesterol Test." *Heart Diseases Weekly* September 7, 2003: 35.
"Results of a Prospective, Multi-center Study Showed that the Availability of Lipoprotein Subclass Testing

(Vertical Auto profile û VAP û Cholesterol Test)
Increased Use of Lipid-lowering Therapy by 59% in
High-risk Patients with Type 2 Diabetes." *Diagnostics &
Imaging Week* June 19, 2003: 6.

ORGANIZATIONS

American Heart Association. 7320 Greenville Ave. Dallas,
TX 75231. (214) 373-6300. <http://
www.americanheart.org>.

National Heart, Lung and Blood Institute. P.O. Box 30105,
Bethesda, MD 20824-0105. (301) 251-1222. <http://
www.nhlbi.nih.gov>.

Nancy J. Nordenson
Teresa G. Odle

Liposuction

Definition

Liposuction, also known as lipoplasty or suction-assisted lipectomy, is **cosmetic surgery** performed to remove unwanted deposits of fat from under the skin. The doctor sculpts and recontours the patient's body by removing excess fat deposits that have been resistant to reduction by diet or **exercise**. The fat is permanently removed from under the skin with a suction device.

Purpose

Liposuction is intended to reduce and smooth the contours of the body and improve the patient's appearance. Its goal is cosmetic improvement. It is the most commonly performed cosmetic procedure in the United States.

Liposuction does not remove large quantities of fat and is not intended as a weight reduction technique. The average amount of fat removed is about a liter, or a quart. Although liposuction is not intended to remove cellulite (lumpy fat), some doctors believe that it improves the appearance of cellulite areas (thighs, hips, buttocks, abdomen, and chin).

A new technique called liposhaving shows more promise at reducing cellulite.

Precautions

Liposuction is most successful on patients who have firm, elastic skin and concentrated pockets of fat in cellultite areas. To get good results after fat removal, the skin must contract to conform to the

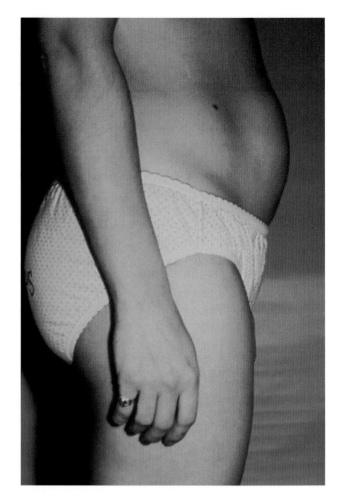

"Before" photo of patient undergoing liposuction. *(Photograph by I. Richard Toranto, M.D., Custom Medical Stock Photo. Reproduced by permission.)*

new contours without sagging. Older patients have less elastic skin and therefore may not be good candidates for this procedure. Patients with generalized fat distribution, rather than localized pockets, are not good candidates.

Patients should be in good general health and free of heart or lung disease. Patients with poor circulation or who have had recent surgery at the intended site of fat reduction are not good candidates.

Description

Most liposuction procedures are performed under **local anesthesia** (loss of sensation without loss of consciousness) by the tumescent or wet technique. In this technique, large volumes of very dilute local anesthetic (a substance that produces anesthesia) are injected under the patient's skin, making the tissue swollen and firm. Epinephrine is added to the solution to

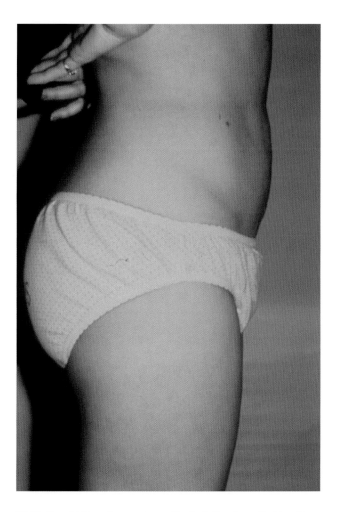

"After" photo of same patient following liposuction. *(Photograph by I. Richard Toranto, M.D., Custom Medical Stock Photo. Reproduced by permission.)*

reduce bleeding, and make possible the removal of larger amounts of fat.

The doctor first numbs the skin with an injection of local anesthetic. After the skin is desensitized, the doctor makes a series of tiny incisions, usually 0.12-0.25 in (3-6 mm) in length. The area is then flooded with a larger amount of local anesthetic. Fat is then extracted with suction through a long, blunt hollow tube called a cannula. The doctor repeatedly pushes the cannula through the fat layers in a radiating pattern creating tunnels, removing fat, and recontouring the area. Large quantities of intravenous fluid (IV) is given during the procedure to replace lost body fluid. Blood transfusions are possible.

Some newer modifications to the procedure involve the use of a cutting cannula called a liposhaver, or the use of ultrasound to help break up the fat deposits. The patient is awake and comfortable during these procedures.

The length of time required to perform the procedure varies with the amount of fat that is to be removed and the number of areas to be treated. Most operations take from 30 minutes to 2 hours, but extensive procedures can take longer. The length of time required also varies with the manner in which the anesthetic is injected.

The cost of liposuction can vary depending upon the standardized fees in the region of the country where it is performed, the extent of the area being treated, and the person performing the procedure. Generally, small areas, such as the chin or knees, can be done for as little as $500, while more extensive treatment, such as when hips, thighs, and abdomen are done simultaneously, can cost as much as $10,000. These procedures are cosmetic and are not covered by most insurance policies.

Preparation

The doctor will do a physical exam and may order blood work to determine clotting time and hemoglobin level for transfusions should the need arise. The patient may be placed on **antibiotics** immediately prior to surgery to ward off infection.

Aftercare

After the surgery, the patient will need to wear a support garment continuously for 2-3 weeks. If ankles or calves were treated, support hose will need to be worn for up to 6 weeks. The support garments can be removed during bathing 24 hours after surgery. A drainage tube, under the skin in the area of the procedure, may be inserted to prevent fluid build-up.

Mild side effects can include a burning sensation at the site of the surgery for up to one month. The patient should be prepared for swelling of the tissues below the operated site for 6-8 weeks after surgery. Wearing the special elastic garments will help reduce this swelling and help to achieve the desired final results.

The incisions involved in this procedure are tiny, but the surgeon may close them with stitches or staples. These will be removed the day after surgery. However, three out of eight doctors use no sutures. Minor bleeding or seepage through the incision site is common after this procedure. Wearing the elastic bandage or support garment helps reduce fluid loss.

This operation is virtually painless. However, for the first postoperative day, there may be some discomfort which will require light **pain** medication. Soreness or aching may persist for several days. The patient can usually return to normal activity within a week.

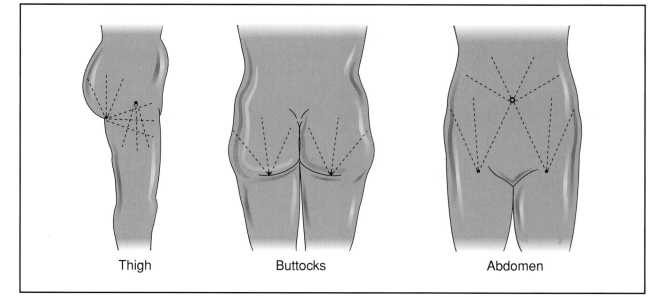

Common entry sites for liposuction procedures. *(Illustration by Electronic Illustrators Group.)*

Postoperative bruising will go away by itself within 10-14 days. Postoperative swelling begins to go down after a week. It may take 3-6 months for the final contour to be reached.

Risks

Liposuction under local anesthesia using the tumescent technique is exceptionally safe. A 1995 study of 15,336 patients showed no serious complications or deaths. Another study showed a 1% risk factor. However, as with any surgery, there are some risks and serious complications. **Death** is possible.

The main hazards associated with this surgery involve migration of a blood clot or fat globule to the heart, brain, or lungs. Such an event can cause a **heart attack**, **stroke**, or serious lung damage. However, this complication is rare and did not occur even once in the study of 15,336 patients. The risk of blood clot formation is reduced with the wearing of special girdle-like compression garments after the surgery, and with the resumption of normal mild activity soon after surgery.

Staying in bed increases the risk of clot formation, but not getting enough rest can result in increased swelling of the surgical area. Such swelling is a result of excess fluid and blood accumulation, and generally comes from not wearing the compression garments. If necessary, this excess fluid can be drained off with a needle in the doctor's office.

Infection is another complication, but this rarely occurs. If the physician is skilled and works in a sterile environment, infection should not be a concern.

If too much fat is removed, the skin may peel in that area. Smokers are at increased risk for shedding skin because their circulation is impaired. Another and more serious hazard of removing too much fat is that the patient may go into **shock**. Fat tissue has an abundant blood supply and removing too much of it at once can cause shock if the fluid is not replaced.

A rare complication is perforation or puncture of an organ. The procedure involves pushing a cannula vigorously through the fat layer. If the doctor pushes too hard or if the tissue gives way too easily under the force, the blunt hollow tube can go too far and injure internal organs.

Liposuction can damage superficial nerves. Some patients lose sensation in the area that has been suctioned, but feeling usually returns with time.

Normal results

The loss of fat cells is permanent, and the patient should have smoother, more pleasing body contours without excessive bulges. However, if the patient overeats, the remaining fat cells will grow in size. Although the patient may gain weight back, the body should retain the new proportions and the suctioned area should remain proportionally smaller.

Tiny **scars** about 0.25-0.5 in (6-12 mm) long at the site of incision are normal. The doctor usually makes the incisions in places where the scars are not likely to show.

In some instances, the skin may appear rippled, wavy, or baggy after surgery. Pigmentation spots may develop. The recontoured area may be uneven. This unevenness is common, occurring in 5-20% of the cases, and can be corrected with a second procedure that is less extensive than the first.

Resources

PERIODICALS

Taylor, Mia, Lloyd A. Hoffman, and Michael Lieberman. "Intestinal Perforation after Suction Lipoplasty: A Case Report and Review of the Literature." *Annals of Plastic Surgery* 38, no. 2: 169-172.

ORGANIZATIONS

American Society of Aesthetic Plastic Surgery. (888) 272-7711.

American Society of Plastic and Reconstructive Surgeons. 44 E. Algonquin Rd., Arlington Heights, IL 60005. (847) 228-9900. < http://www.plasticsurgery.org >.

Lipoplasty Society of North America. (800) 848-1991.

Louann W. Murray, PhD

Listeria monocytogenes infection *see* **Listeriosis**

Listeriosis

Definition

Listeriosis is an illness caused by the bacterium *Listeria monocytogenes* that is acquired by eating contaminated food. The organism can spread to the blood stream and central nervous system. During **pregnancy**, listeriosis often causes **miscarriage** or **stillbirth**.

Description

Listeriosis is caused by an infection with the bacterium *Listeria monocytogenes*. This bacteria can be carried by many animals and birds, and it has been found in soil, water, sewage, and animal feed. Five out of every 100 people carry *Listeria monocytogenes* in their intestines. Listeriosis is considered a "food-borne illness" because most people are probably infected after eating food contaminated with *Listeria monocytogenes*. However, a woman can pass the bacteria to her baby during pregnancy. In addition, there have been a few cases where workers have developed *Listeria* skin infections by touching infected calves or poultry.

In the 1980s, the United States government began taking measures to decrease the occurrence of listeriosis. Processed meats and dairy products are now tested for the presence of *Listeria monocytogenes*. The Food and Drug Administration (FDA) and the Food Safety and Inspection Service (FSIS) can legally prevent food from being shipped, or order food recalls, if they detect any *Listeria* bacteria. These inspections, in combination with the public education regarding the proper handling of uncooked foods, appear to be working. In 1989, there were 1,965 cases of listeriosis with 481 deaths. In 1993, the numbers fell to 1,092 cases with 248 deaths.

In 1996, the Centers for Disease Control and Prevention (CDC) began a nationwide food-borne disease surveillance program called "FoodNet," in which seven states were participating by January 1997. Results from the program indicated that, in 1996, one person out of every 200,000 people got listeriosis. FoodNet also revealed that the hospitalization rate was higher for listeriosis (94%) than for any other food-borne illness. In addition, FoodNet found that the *Listeria* bacteria reached the blood and cerebrospinal fluid in 89% of cases, a higher percentage than in any other food-borne illness.

Persons at particular risk for listeriosis include the elderly, pregnant women, newborns, and those with a weakened immune system (called "immunocompromised"). Risk is increased when a person suffers from diseases such as **AIDS, cancer, kidney disease, diabetes mellitus,** or by the use of certain medications. Infection is most common in babies younger than one month old and adults over 60 years of age. Pregnant women account for 27% of the cases and immunocompromised persons account for almost

70%. Persons with AIDS are 280 times more likely to get listeriosis than others.

Causes and symptoms

As noted, persons become infected with *Listeria monocytogenes* by eating contaminated food. *Listeria* has been found on raw vegetables, fish, poultry, raw (unpasteurized) milk, fresh meat, processed meat (such as deli meat, hot dogs, and canned meat), and certain soft cheeses. Listeriosis outbreaks in the United States since the 1980s have been linked to cole slaw, milk, Mexican-style cheese, undercooked hot dogs, undercooked chicken, and delicatessen foods. Unlike most other bacteria, *Listeria monocytogenes* does not stop growing when food is in the refrigerator – its growth is merely slowed. Fortunately, typical cooking temperatures and the pasteurization process do kill this bacteria.

Listeria bacteria can pass through the wall of the intestines, and from there they can get into the blood stream. Once in the blood stream, they can be transported anywhere in the body, but are commonly found the central nervous system (brain and spinal cord); and in pregnant women they are often found in the placenta (the organ which connects the baby's umbilical cord to the uterus). *Listeria monocytogenes* live inside specific white blood cells called macrophages. Inside macrophages, the bacteria can hide from immune responses and become inaccessible to certain **antibiotics**. *Listeria* bacteria are capable of multiplying within macrophages, and then may spread to other macrophages.

After consuming food contaminated with this bacteria, symptoms of infection may appear anywhere from 11-70 days later. Most people do not get any noticeable symptoms. Scientists are unsure, but they believe that *Listeria monocytogenes* can cause upset stomach and intestinal problems just like other food-borne illnesses. Persons with listeriosis may develop flu-like symptoms such as **fever**, **headache**, **nausea and vomiting**, tiredness, and **diarrhea**.

Pregnant women experience a mild, flu-like illness with fever, muscle aches, upset stomach, and intestinal problems. They recover, but the infection can cause miscarriage, **premature labor**, early rupture of the birth sac, and stillbirth. Unfortunately, half of the newborns infected with *Listeria* will die from the illness.

There are two types of listeriosis in the newborn baby: early-onset disease and late-onset disease. Early-onset disease refers to a serious illness that is present at birth and usually causes the baby to be born prematurely. Babies infected during the pregnancy usually have a blood infection (**sepsis**) and may have a serious, whole body infection called granulomatosis infantisepticum. When a full-term baby becomes infected with *Listeria* during **childbirth**, that situation is called late-onset disease. Commonly, symptoms of late-onset listeriosis appear about two weeks after birth. Babies with late-term disease typically have **meningitis** (inflammation of the brain and spinal tissues); yet they have a better chance of surviving than those with early-onset disease.

Immunocompromised adults are at risk for a serious infection of the blood stream and central nervous system (brain and spinal cord). Meningitis occurs in about half of the cases of adult listeriosis. Symptoms of listerial meningitis occur about four days after the flu-like symptoms and include fever, personality change, uncoordinated muscle movement, **tremors**, muscle contractions, seizures, and slipping in and out of consciousness.

Listeria monocytogenes causes **endocarditis** in about 7.5% of the cases. Endocarditis is an inflammation of heart tissue due to the bacterial infection. Listerial endocarditis causes **death** in about half of the patients. Other diseases which have been caused by *Listeria monocytogenes* include **brain abscess**, eye infection, hepatitis (**liver disease**), **peritonitis** (abdominal infection), lung infection, joint infection, arthritis, heart disease, bone infection, and gallbladder infection.

Diagnosis

Listeriosis may be diagnosed and treated by infectious disease specialists and internal medicine specialists. The diagnosis and treatment of this infection should be covered by most insurance providers.

The only way to diagnose listeriosis is to isolate *Listeria monocytogenes* from blood, cerebrospinal fluid, or stool. A sample of cerebrospinal fluid is removed from the spinal cord using a needle and syringe. This procedure is commonly called a spinal tap. The amniotic fluid (the fluid which bathes the unborn baby) may be tested in pregnant women with listeriosis. This sample is obtained by inserting a needle through the abdomen into the uterus and withdrawing fluid. *Listeria* grows well in laboratory media and test results can be available within a few days.

Treatment

Listeriosis is treated with the antibiotics ampicillin (Omnipen) or sulfamethoxazole-trimethoprim (Bactrim, Septra). Because the bacteria live within macrophage

KEY TERMS

Abscess—An accumulation of pus caused by localized infection in tissues or organs. *Listeria monocytogenes* can cause abscesses in many organs including the brain, spleen, and liver.

Immunocompromised—To have a poor immune system due to disease or medication. Immunocompromised persons are at risk for developing infections because they can't fight off microorganisms like healthy persons can.

Macrophages—White blood cells whose job is to destroy invading microorganisms. *Listeria monocytogenes* avoids being killed and can multiply within the macrophage.

Meningitis—An inflammation of the tissues that surround the brain and spinal cord. It can be caused by a bacterial infection.

Sepsis—The presence of bacteria in the blood stream, a normally sterile environment.

cells, treatment may be difficult and the treatment periods may vary. Usually, pregnant women are treated for two weeks; newborns, two to three weeks; adults with mild disease, two to four weeks; persons with meningitis, three weeks; persons with brain abscesses, six weeks; and persons with endocarditis, four to six weeks.

Patients are often hospitalized for treatment and monitoring. Other drugs may be provided to relieve **pain** and fever and to treat other reactions to the infection.

Prognosis

The overall death rate for listeriosis is 26%. This high death rate is due to the serious illness suffered by newborns, the elderly, and immunocompromised persons. Healthy adults and older children have a low death rate. Complications of *Listeria* infection include: meningitis, sepsis, miscarriage, stillbirth, **pneumonia**, **shock**, endocarditis, **abscess** (localized infection) formation, and eye inflammation.

Prevention

The United States government has already done much to prevent listeriosis. Persons at extremely high risk (pregnant women, immunocompromised persons, etc.) must use extra caution. High risk persons should: avoid soft cheeses, such as Mexican

cheese, feta, Brie, Camembert, and blue cheese (cottage cheese is safe), thoroughly cook leftovers and ready-to-eat foods (such as hot-dogs), and avoid foods from the deli.

For all people, the risk of listeriosis can be reduced by taking these precautions:

- Completely cook all meats and eggs.

- Carefully wash raw vegetables before eating.

- Keep raw meat away from raw vegetables and prepared foods. After cutting raw meat, wash the cutting board with detergent before using it for vegetables.

- Avoid drinking unpasteurized milk or foods made from such milk.

- Wash hands thoroughly after handling raw meat.

- Follow the instructions on food labels. Observe food expiration dates and storage conditions.

Resources

OTHER

"Preventing Foodborne Illness: Listeriosis." *Centers for Disease Control.* < http://www.cdc.gov/ncidad/diseases/foodborn/lister.htm >.

Belinda Rowland, PhD

Lithotripsy

Definition

Lithotripsy is the use of high-energy shock waves to fragment and disintegrate **kidney stones**. The shock wave, created by using a high-voltage spark or an electromagnetic impulse, is focused on the stone. This shock wave shatters the stone and this allows the fragments to pass through the urinary system. Since the shock wave is generated outside the body, the procedure is termed extracorporeal shock wave lithotripsy, or ESWL.

Purpose

ESWL is used when a kidney stone is too large to pass on its own, or when a stone becomes stuck in a ureter (a tube which carries urine from the kidney to the bladder) and will not pass. Kidney stones are extremely painful and can cause serious medical complications if not removed.

Precautions

ESWL should not be considered for patients with severe skeletal deformities, patients weighing over 300 lbs (136 kg), patients with abdominal aortic aneurysms, or patients with uncontrollable bleeding disorders. Patients who are pregnant should not be treated with ESWL. Patients with cardiac **pacemakers** should be evaluated by a cardiologist familiar with ESWL. The cardiologist should be present during the ESWL procedure in the event the pacemaker needs to be overridden.

Description

Lithotripsy uses the technique of focused shock waves to fragment a stone in the kidney or the ureter. The patient is placed in a tub of water or in contact with a water-filled cushion, and a shock wave is created which is focused on the stone. The wave shatters and fragments the stone. The resulting debris, called gravel, then passes through the remainder of the ureter, through the bladder, and through the urethra during urination. There is minimal chance of damage to skin or internal organs because biologic tissues are resilient, not brittle, and because the the shock waves are not focused on them.

Preparation

Prior to the lithotripsy procedure, a complete **physical examination** is done, followed by tests to determine the number, location, and size of the stone or stones. A test called an intravenous pyelogram, or IVP, is used to locate the stones. An IVP involves injecting a dye into a vein in the arm. This dye, which shows up on x ray, travels through the bloodstream and is excreted by the kidneys. The dye then flows down the ureters and into the bladder. The dye surrounds the stones, and x rays are then used to evaluate the stones and the anatomy of the urinary system. (Some people are allergic to the dye material, so it cannot be used. For these people, focused sound waves, called ultrasound, can be used to see where the stones are located.) Blood tests are done to determine if any potential bleeding problems exist. For women of childbearing age, a **pregnancy** test is done to make sure the patient isn't pregnant; and elderly patients have an EKG done to make sure no potential heart problems exist. Some patients may have a stent placed prior to the lithotripsy procedure. A stent is a plastic tube placed in the ureter which allows the passage of gravel and urine after the ESWL procedure is completed.

Aftercare

Most patients have a lot of blood in their urine after the ESWL procedure. This is normal and should clear after several days to a week or so. Lots of fluids should be taken to encourage the flushing of any gravel remaining in the urinary system. The patient should follow up with the urologist in about two weeks to make sure that everything is going as planned. If a stent has been inserted, it is normally removed at this time. Patients may return to work whenever they feel able.

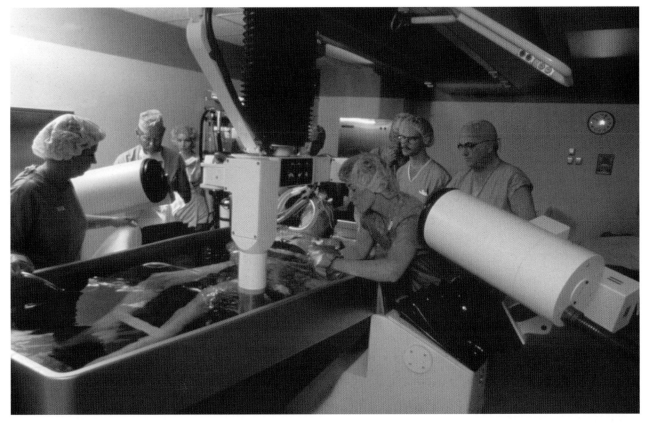

A lithotriptor in use by patient in tub. This noninvasive method crushes kidney stones through shock waves. *(Photo Researchers, Inc. Reproduced by permission.)*

Risks

Abdominal **pain** is not uncommon after ESWL, but it is usually not cause to worry. However, persistent or severe abdominal pain may imply unexpected internal injury. Colicky renal pain is very common as gravel is still passing. Other problems may include perirenal hematomas (**blood clots** near the kidneys) in 66% of the cases; nerve palsies; **pancreatitis** (inflammation of the pancreas); and obstruction by stone fragments. Occasionally, stones may not be completely fragmented during the first ESWL treatment and further ESWL procedures may be required.

Resources

ORGANIZATIONS

American Urological Association. 1120 North Charles St., Baltimore, MD 21201-5559. (410) 727-1100. < http:// www.auanet.org/index_hi.cfm >.

Joseph Knight, PA

Live cell therapy *see* **Cell therapy**

Liver-spleen scan *see* **Liver nuclear medicine scan**

Liver biopsy

Definition

A liver biopsy is a medical procedure performed to obtain a small piece of liver tissue for diagnostic testing. Liver biopsies are sometimes called percutaneous liver biopsies, because the tissue sample is obtained by going through the patient's skin.

Purpose

A liver biopsy is usually done to diagnose a tumor, or to evaluate the extent of damage that has occurred to the liver because of chronic disease. Biopsies are often performed to identify abnormalities in liver tissues after imaging studies have failed to yield clear results.

A liver biopsy may be ordered to evaluate any of the following conditions or disorders:

- Jaundice

- **Cirrhosis**

- Hemochromatosis, which is a condition of excess iron in the liver.

- Repeated abnormal results from liver function tests

- Unexplained swelling or enlargement of the liver

- Primary cancers of the liver, such as hepatomas, cholangiocarcinomas, and angiosarcomas

- Metastatic cancers of the liver.

Precautions

Some patients should not have percutaneous liver biopsies. They include patients with any of the following conditions:

- A **platelet count** below 60,000

- A longer-than-normal **prothrombin time**

- A liver tumor that contains a large number of blood vessels

- A history of unexplained bleeding

- A watery (hydatid) cyst

- An infection in either the cavity around the lungs, or the diaphragm.

Description

Percutaneous liver biopsy is done with a special hollow needle, called a Menghini needle, attached to a suction syringe. Doctors who specialize in the digestive system or liver will sometimes perform liver biopsies. But in most cases, a radiologist (a doctor who specializes in x rays and imaging studies) performs the biopsy. The radiologist will use computed tomography scan (CT scan) or ultrasound to guide the choice of the site for the biopsy.

An hour or so before the biopsy, the patient may be given a sedative to help relaxation. He or she is then asked to lie on the back with the right elbow to the side and the right hand under the head. The patient is instructed to lie as still as possible during the procedure. He or she is warned to expect a sensation resembling a punch in the right shoulder, but to hold still in spite of the momentary feeling.

The doctor marks a spot on the skin where the needle will be inserted and thoroughly cleanses the right side of the upper abdomen with an antiseptic

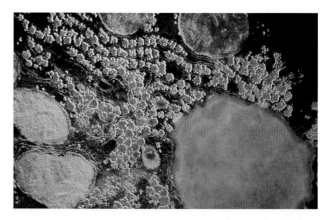

A false color image of hepatocyte cells of the liver that secrete bile. *(Custom Medical Stock Photo. Reproduced by permission.)*

solution. The patient is then given an anesthetic at the biopsy site.

The needle with attached syringe is inserted into the patient's chest wall. The doctor then draws the plunger of the syringe back to create a vacuum. At this point the patient is asked to take a deep breath, exhale the air and hold their breath at the point of complete exhalation. The needle is inserted into the liver and withdrawn quickly, usually within two seconds or less. The negative pressure in the syringe draws or pulls a sample of liver tissue into the biopsy needle. As soon as the needle is withdrawn, the patient can breathe normally. Pressure is applied at the biopsy site to stop any bleeding, and a bandage will be placed over it. The entire procedure takes 10 to 15 minutes. Test results are usually available within a day.

Preparation

Aspirin and non-steroidal anti-inflammatory drugs (NSAIDs) such as ibuprofen are known to thin the blood and interfere with clotting. These medications should be avoided for at least a week before the biopsy. Four to eight hours before the biopsy, patients should stop eating and drinking.

The patient's blood will be tested prior to the biopsy to make sure that it is clotting normally. Tests will include a platelet count and a prothrombin time. Doctors will also ensure that the patient is not taking any other medications, such as blood thinners like Coumadin, that might affect blood clotting.

Aftercare

Liver biopsies are outpatient procedures in most hospitals. After the biopsy, patients are usually

KEY TERMS

Biopsy—A procedure where a piece of tissue is removed from a patient for diagnostic testing.

Menghini needle—A special needle used to obtain a sample of liver tissue.

Percutaneous biopsy—A biopsy in which a needle is inserted and a tissue sample removed through the skin.

Prothrombin time—A blood test that determines how quickly a person's blood will clot.

Vital signs—A person's essential body functions, usually defined as the pulse, body temperature, and breathing rate.

instructed to lie on their right side for about two hours. This provides pressure to the biopsy site and helps prevent bleeding. A nurse will check the patient's vital signs at regular intervals. If there are no complications, the patient is sent home within about four to eight hours.

Patients should arrange to have a friend or relative take them home after discharge. Bed rest for a day is recommended, followed by a week of avoiding heavy work or strenuous **exercise**. The patient can resume eating a normal diet.

Some mild soreness in the area of the biopsy is normal after the anesthetic wears off. Irritation of the muscle that lies over the liver can also cause mild discomfort in the shoulder for some patients. Tylenol can be taken for minor soreness, but aspirin and NSAIDs are best avoided. Patients should call their doctor if they have severe **pain** in the abdomen, chest or shoulder, difficulty breathing, or persistent bleeding. These signs may indicate that there has been leakage of bile into the abdominal cavity, or that air has been introduced into the cavity around the lungs.

Risks

The risks of a liver biopsy are usually very small. When complications do occur, over 90% are apparent within 24 hours after the biopsy. The most significant risk is internal bleeding. Bleeding is most likely to occur in elderly patients, in patients with cirrhosis, or in patients with a tumor that has many blood vessels. Other complications from percutaneous liver biopsies include the leakage of bile or the introduction of air into the chest cavity (**pneumothorax**). There is also a

small chance that an infection may occur, or an internal organ such as the lung, gall bladder, or kidney could be punctured.

Normal results

After the biopsy, the liver sample is sent to the pathology laboratory for study under a microscope. A normal (negative) result would find no evidence of **cancer** or other disease in the tissue sample.

Abnormal results

Changes in liver tissue that are visible under the microscope indicate abnormal results. Possible causes for the abnormality include the presence of a tumor, or a disease such as hepatitis.

Resources

BOOKS

Brown, Kyle E., et al. "Liver Biopsy: Indications, Technique, Complications and Interpretation." In *Liver Disease. Diagnosis and Management*, edited by Bruce R. Bacon and Adrian M. Di Bisceglie. Philadelphia, PA: Churchill Livingstone, 2000.

Reddy, K. Rajender, and Lennox J. Jeffers. "Evaluation of the Liver. Liver Biopsy and Laparoscopy." In *Schiff's Diseases of the Liver*, edited by Eugene R. Schiff, et al. Philadelphia, PA: Lippincott-Raven, 1999.

PERIODICALS

Bravo, Arturo A., et al. "Liver Biopsy" *New England Journal of Medicine* 344, no. 7 (February 15, 2001): 495-500.

Lata Cherath, PhD

Liver cancer

Definition

Liver **cancer** is a relatively rare form of cancer but has a high mortality rate. Liver cancers can be classified into two types. They are either primary, when the cancer starts in the liver itself, or metastatic, when the cancer has spread to the liver from some other part of the body.

Description

Primary liver cancer

Primary liver cancer is a relatively rare disease in the United States, representing about 2% of all malignancies and 4% of newly diagnosed cancers. Hepatocellular carcinoma (HCC) is the fifth most common cancer in the world as of 2004. It is much more common outside the United States, representing 10% to 50% of malignancies in Africa and parts of Asia. Rates of HCC in men are at least two to three times higher than for women. In high–risk areas (East and Southeast Asia, sub-Saharan Africa), men are even more likely to have HCC than women.

According to the American Cancer Society, 18,920 people in the United States will be diagnosed with primary liver cancer in 2004, and 14,270 persons will die from the disease. The incidence of primary liver cancer has been rising in the United States and Canada since the mid-1990s, most likely as a result of the rising rate of **hepatitis C** infections.

TYPES OF PRIMARY LIVER CANCER. In adults, most primary liver cancers belong to one of two types: hepatomas, or hepatocellular carcinomas (HCC), which start in the liver tissue itself; and cholangiomas, or cholangiocarcinomas, which are cancers that develop in the bile ducts inside the liver. About 80% to 90% of primary liver cancers are hepatomas. In the United States, about five persons in every 200,000 will develop a hepatoma (70% to 75% of cases of primary liver cancers are HCC). In Africa and Asia, over 40 persons in 200,000 will develop this form of cancer (more than 90% of cases of primary liver are HCC). Two rare types of primary liver cancer are mixed-cell tumors and Kupffer cell **sarcomas**.

One type of primary liver cancer, called a hepatoblastoma, usually occurs in children younger than four years of age and between the ages of 12 and 15. Unlike liver cancers in adults, hepatoblastomas have a good chance of being treated successfully. Approximately 70% of children with hepatoblastomas experience complete cures. If the tumor is detected early, the survival rate is over 90%.

Metastatic liver cancer

The second major category of liver cancer, metastatic liver cancer, is about 20 times as common in the United States as primary liver cancer. Because blood from all parts of the body must pass through the liver for filtration, cancer cells from other organs and tissues easily reach the liver, where they can lodge and grow into secondary tumors. Primary cancers in the colon, stomach, pancreas, rectum, esophagus, breast, lung, or skin are the most likely to metastasize (spread) to the liver. It is not unusual for the metastatic cancer in the liver to be the first noticeable sign of a cancer that started in another organ. After **cirrhosis**, metastatic liver cancer is the most common cause of fatal **liver disease**.

Causes and symptoms

Risk factors

The exact cause of primary liver cancer is still unknown. In adults, however, certain factors are known to place some individuals at higher risk of developing liver cancer. These factors include:

- Male sex.
- Age over 60 years.
- Ethnicity. Asian Americans with cirrhosis have four times as great a chance of developing liver cancer as Caucasians with cirrhosis, and African Americans have twice the risk of Caucasians. In addition, Asians often develop liver cancer at much younger ages than either African Americans or Caucasians.
- Exposure to substances in the environment that tend to cause cancer (carcinogens). These include: a substance produced by a mold that grows on rice and peanuts (aflatoxin); thorium dioxide, which was once used as a contrast dye for x rays of the liver; vinyl chloride, used in manufacturing plastics; and cigarette smoking.
- Use of oral estrogens for birth control.
- Hereditary **hemochromatosis**. This is a disorder characterized by abnormally high levels of iron storage in the body. It often develops into cirrhosis.
- Cirrhosis. Hepatomas appear to be a frequent complication of cirrhosis of the liver. Between 30% and 70% of hepatoma patients also have cirrhosis. It is estimated that a patient with cirrhosis has 40 times the chance of developing a hepatoma than a person with a healthy liver.
- Exposure to hepatitis viruses: **Hepatitis B** (HBV), Hepatitis C (HCV), **Hepatitis D** (HDV), or **Hepatitis G** (HGV). It is estimated that 80% of worldwide HCC is associated with chronic HBV infection. In Africa and most of Asia, exposure to hepatitis B is an important factor; in Japan and some Western countries, exposure to hepatitis C is connected with a higher risk of developing liver cancer. In the United States, nearly 25% of patients with liver cancer show evidence of HBV infection. Hepatitis is commonly found among intravenous drug abusers. The 70% increase in HCC incidence in the United States is thought to be due to increasing rates of HBV and HCV infections due to increased sexual promiscuity and illicit drug needle sharing.

The association between HDV and HGV and HCC is unclear at this time.

Symptoms of liver cancer

The early symptoms of primary, as well as metastatic, liver cancer are often vague and not unique to liver disorders. The long period between the beginning of the tumor's growth and the first signs of illness is the major reason why the disease has such a high mortality rate. At the time of diagnosis, patients are often fatigued, with **fever**, abdominal **pain**, and loss of appetite. They may look emaciated and generally ill. As the tumor enlarges, it stretches the membrane surrounding the liver (the capsule), causing pain in the upper abdomen on the right side. The pain may extend into the back and shoulder. Some patients develop a collection of fluid, known as **ascites**, in the abdominal cavity. Others may show signs of bleeding into the digestive tract. In addition, the tumor may block the ducts of the liver or the gall bladder, leading to **jaundice**. In patients with jaundice, the whites of the eyes and the skin may turn yellow, and the urine becomes dark–colored.

Diagnosis

Physical examination

If the doctor suspects a diagnosis of liver cancer, he or she will check the patient's history for risk factors and pay close attention to the condition of the patient's abdomen during the **physical examination**. Masses or lumps in the liver and ascites can often be felt while the patient is lying flat on the examination table. The liver is usually swollen and hard in patients with liver cancer; it may be sore when the doctor presses on it. In some cases, the patient's spleen is also enlarged. The doctor may be able to hear an abnormal sound (bruit) or rubbing noise (friction rub) if he or she uses a stethoscope to listen to the blood vessels that lie near the liver. The noises are caused by the pressure of the tumor on the blood vessels.

Laboratory tests

Blood tests may be used to test liver function or to evaluate risk factors in the patient's history. Between 50% and 75% of primary liver cancer patients have abnormally high blood serum levels of a particular protein (alpha-fetoprotein or AFP). The AFP test, however, cannot be used by itself to confirm a diagnosis of liver cancer, because cirrhosis or chronic hepatitis can also produce high alpha–fetoprotein levels. Tests for alkaline phosphatase, bilirubin, lactic dehydrogenase, and other chemicals indicate that the liver is not functioning normally. About 75% of patients with liver cancer show evidence of hepatitis infection. Again, however, abnormal liver function test results are not specific for liver cancer.

Imaging studies

Imaging studies are useful in locating specific areas of abnormal tissue in the liver. Liver tumors as small as an inch across can now be detected by ultrasound or computed tomography scan (CT scan). Imaging studies, however, cannot tell the difference between a hepatoma and other abnormal masses or lumps of tissue (nodules) in the liver. A sample of liver tissue for biopsy is needed to make the definitive diagnosis of a primary liver cancer. CT or ultrasound can be used to guide the doctor in selecting the best location for obtaining the biopsy sample.

Chest x rays may be used to see whether the liver tumor is primary or has metastasized from a primary tumor in the lungs.

Liver biopsy

Liver biopsy is considered to provide the definite diagnosis of liver cancer. A sample of the liver or tissue fluid is removed with a fine needle and is checked under a microscope for the presence of cancer cells. In about 70% of cases, the biopsy is positive for cancer. In most cases, there is little risk to the patient from the biopsy procedure. In about 0.4% of cases, however, the patient develops a fatal hemorrhage from the biopsy because some tumors are supplied with a large number of blood vessels and bleed very easily.

Laparoscopy

The doctor may also perform a **laparoscopy** to help in the diagnosis of liver cancer. First, the doctor makes a small cut in the patient's abdomen and inserts a small, lighted tube called a laparoscope to view the area. A small piece of liver tissue is removed and examined under a microscope for the presence of cancer cells.

Treatment

Treatment of liver cancer is based on several factors, including the type of cancer (primary or metastatic); stage (early or advanced); the location of other primary cancers or metastases in the patient's body; the patient's age; and other coexisting diseases, including cirrhosis. For many patients, treatment of liver cancer is primarily intended to relieve the pain caused by the cancer but cannot cure it.

Surgery

Few liver cancers in adults can be cured by surgery because they are usually too advanced by the time they are discovered. If the cancer is contained within one lobe of the liver, and if the patient does not have either cirrhosis, jaundice, or ascites, surgery is the best treatment option. Patients who can have their entire tumor removed have the best chance for survival. Unfortunately, only about 5% of patients with meta-static cancer (from primary tumors in the colon or rectum) fall into this group. If the entire visible tumor can be removed, about 25% of patients will be cured. The operation that is performed is called a partial hepatectomy, or partial removal of the liver. The surgeon will remove either an entire lobe of the liver (a lobectomy) or cut out the area around the tumor (a wedge resection).

A newer technique that is reported to be safe and effective is laparoscopic radiofrequency ablation (RFA). RFA is a technique in which the surgeon places a special needle electrode in the tumor under guidance from MRI or CT scanning. When the electrode has been properly placed, a radiofrequency current is passed through it, heating the tumor and killing the cancer cells. RFA can be used to treat tumors that are too small or too inaccessible for removal by conventional open surgery.

Chemotherapy

Some patients with metastatic cancer of the liver can have their lives prolonged for a few months by **chemotherapy**, although cure is not possible. If the tumor cannot be removed by surgery, a tube (catheter) can be placed in the main artery of the liver and an implantable infusion pump can be installed. The pump allows much higher concentrations of the cancer drug to be carried to the tumor than is possible with chemotherapy carried through the bloodstream. The drug that is used for infusion pump therapy is usually floxuridine (FUDR), given for 14-day periods alternating with 14-day rests. Systemic chemotherapy can also be used to treat liver cancer. The medications usually used are 5-fluorouracil (Adrucil, Efudex) or methotrexate (MTX, Mexate). Systemic chemotherapy does not, however, significantly lengthen the patient's survival time.

Radiation therapy

Radiation therapy is the use of high-energy rays or x rays to kill cancer cells or to shrink tumors. Its use in liver cancer, however, is only to give short–term relief from some of the symptoms. Liver cancers are not sensitive to radiation, and radiation therapy will not prolong the patient's life.

Liver transplantation

Removal of the entire liver (total hepatectomy) and **liver transplantation** can be used to treat liver cancer. However, there is a high risk of tumor recurrence and metastases after transplantation. In addition, most patients have cancer that is too far advanced at the time of diagnosis to benefit from liver transplantation.

Other therapies

Other therapeutic approaches include:

- Hepatic artery embolization with chemotherapy (chemoembolization).

- Alcohol ablation via ultrasound-guided percutaneous injection.

- Ultrasound-guided cryoablation.

- Immunotherapy with monoclonal antibodies tagged with cytotoxic agents.

- Gene therapy with retroviral vectors containing genes expressing cytotoxic agents.

Alternative treatment

Many patients find that alternative and complementary therapies help to reduce the **stress** associated with illness, improve immune function, and boost spirits. While there is no clinical evidence that these therapies specifically combat disease, activities such as **biofeedback**, relaxation, **therapeutic touch**, **massage therapy** and **guided imagery** have no side effects and have been reported to enhance well–being.

Several other healing therapies are sometimes used as supplemental or replacement cancer treatments, such as antineoplastons, cancell, cartilage (bovine and shark), laetrile, and mistletoe. Many of these therapies have not been the subject of safety and efficacy trials by the National Cancer Institute (NCI). The NCI has conducted trials on cancell, laetrile, and other alternative therapies and found no anticancer activity. These treatments have varying effectiveness and safety considerations. Patients using any alternative remedy should first consult their doctor in order to prevent harmful side effects or interactions with traditional cancer treatment.

KEY TERMS

Aflatoxin—A substance produced by molds that grow on rice and peanuts. Exposure to aflatoxin is thought to explain the high rates of primary liver cancer in Africa and parts of Asia.

Alpha-fetoprotein—A protein in blood serum that is found in abnormally high concentrations in most patients with primary liver cancer.

Cirrhosis—A chronic degenerative disease of the liver, in which normal cells are replaced by fibrous tissue. Cirrhosis is a major risk factor for the later development of liver cancer.

Cryoablation—A technique for removing cancerous tissue by killing it with extreme cold.

Hepatitis—A viral disease characterized by inflammation of the liver cells (hepatocytes). People infected with hepatitis B or hepatitis C virus are at an increased risk for developing liver cancer.

Metastatic cancer—A cancer that has spread to an organ or tissue from a primary cancer located elsewhere in the body.

Radiofrequency ablation—A technique for removing a tumor by heating it with a radiofrequency current passed through a needle electrode.

Prognosis

Liver cancer has a very poor prognosis because it is often not diagnosed until it has metastasized. Fewer than 10% of patients survive three years after the initial diagnosis; the overall five-year survival rate for patients with hepatomas is around 4%. Most patients with primary liver cancer die within six months of diagnosis, usually from liver failure; fewer than 5% are cured of the disease. Patients with liver cancers that metastasized from cancers in the colon live slightly longer than those whose cancers spread from cancers in the stomach or pancreas.

As of 2004, African American and Hispanic patients have much lower 5-year survival rates than Caucasian patients. It is not yet known, however, whether cultural differences as well as biological factors may be partly responsible for the variation in survival rates.

Prevention

There are no useful strategies at present for preventing metastatic cancers of the liver. Primary liver cancers, however, are 75% to 80% preventable.

Current strategies focus on widespread **vaccination** for hepatitis B, early treatment of hereditary hemochromatosis, and screening of high-risk patients with alpha–fetoprotein testing and ultrasound examinations.

Lifestyle factors that can be modified in order to prevent liver cancer include avoidance of exposure to toxic chemicals and foods harboring molds that produce aflatoxin. Most important, however, is avoidance of alcohol and drug **abuse**. Alcohol abuse is responsible for 60% to 75% of cases of cirrhosis, which is a major risk factor for eventual development of primary liver cancer. Hepatitis is a widespread disease among persons who abuse intravenous drugs.

Resources

BOOKS

Beers, Mark H., MD, and Robert Berkow, MD., editors. "Primary Liver Cancer." In *The Merck Manual of Diagnosis and Therapy*. Whitehouse Station, NJ: Merck Research Laboratories, 2004.

PERIODICALS

Berber, E., A. Senagore, F. Remzi, et al. "Laparoscopic Radiofrequency Ablation of Liver Tumors Combined with Colorectal Procedures." *Surgical Laparoscopy, Endoscopy and Percutaneous Techniques* 14 (August 2004): 186–190.

Cahill, B. A., and D. Braccia. "Current Treatment for Hepatocellular Carcinoma." *Clinical Journal of Oncology Nursing* 8 (August 2004): 393–399.

Decadt, B., and A. K. Siriwardena. "Radiofrequency Ablation of Liver Tumours: Systematic Review." *Lancet Oncology* 5 (September 2004): 550–560.

Harrison, L. E., T. Reichman, B. Koneru, et al. "Racial Discrepancies in the Outcome of Patients with Hepatocellular Carcinoma." *Archives of Surgery* 139 (September 2004): 992–996.

Nguyen, M. H., A. S. Whittemore, R. T. Garcia, et al. "Role of Ethnicity in Risk for Hepatocellular Carcinoma in Patients with Chronic Hepatitis C and Cirrhosis." *Clinical Gastroenterology and Hepatology* 2 (September 2004): 820–824.

Stuart, Keith E., MD. "Hepatic Carcinoma, Primary." *eMedicine* July 20, 2004. < http://www.emedicine.com/med/topic2664.htm >.

ORGANIZATIONS

American Cancer Society. 1599 Clifton Rd. NE, Atlanta, GA 30329. (800) 227-2345. < http://www.cancer.org >.

American Institute for Cancer Research (AICR). 1759 R St. NW, Washington, DC 20009. (800) 843-8114. < http://www.aicr.org >.

American Liver Foundation.1425 Pompton Ave., Cedar Grove, NJ 07009. (800) 223-0179. < http://www.liverfoundation.org >.

Cancer Care, Inc. 275 Seventh Ave., New York, NY 10001.(800) 813-HOPE. <http://www.cancercare.org>.

Cancer Hope Network. Suite A., Two North Rd., Chester, NJ 07930. (877) HOPENET. <http://www.cancerhopenetwork.org>.

Hospicelink. Hospice Education Institute, 190 Westbrook Rd., Essex, CT, 06426-1510. (800) 331-1620. <http://www.hospiceworld.com>.

National Cancer Institute (National Institutes of Health). 9000 Rockville Pike, Bethesda, MD 20892. (800) 422-6237. <http://www.nci.nih.gov>.

Wellness Community. Suite 412, 35 E. Seventh St., Cincinnati, OH 45202. (888) 793-9355. <http://www.wellness-community.org>.

OTHER

American Cancer Society (ACS). *Cancer Facts & Figures 2004.* <http://www.cancer.org/downloads/STT/CAFF_finalPWSecured.pdf>.

Rebecca J. Frey, PhD
Laura Ruth, PhD

Liver cirrhosis *see* **Cirrhosis**

Liver disease

Definition

Liver disease is a general term for any damage that reduces the functioning of the liver.

Description

The liver is a large, solid organ located in the upper right-hand side of the abdomen. Most of the liver lies under the rib cage, which helps protect it from physical injury. The liver is made up of two main lobes and two minor lobes and has a total weight in adults of about 3.5 lb (1.6 kg).

Within the liver are tiny ducts (tubes) that collect bile, a product secreted by the liver. Bile is stored in to the gall bladder and then released into the intestines after meals to help in the digestion of fats and the absorption of certain **vitamins**. This system of bile production by the liver, transport through the bile ducts, and storage in the gall bladder is called the biliary system. Damage to this system is called biliary disease.

The liver receives blood that comes directly from the intestines. At any given time the liver contains about 13% of the blood circulating in the body. This blood is rich in nutruents (food, vitamins, and **minerals**) that the body needs to function. Some of the most important functions of the liver are to process these nutrients.

Important functions of the liver include:

- manufacturing and regulating the production of proteins. The most important proteins made in the liver are albumin, which helps maintain blood volume, and clotting factors to help regulate blood clotting.

- making and storing fatty acids and cholesterol.

- forming and releasing bile

- processing and storing sugars in the form of glycogen, which can then be re-converted into energy

- Storing iron, an important element in blood formation

- Breaking down (detoxifying) alcohol, drugs, and environmental poisons so that they can be removed from the body.

- Processing and removing bilirubin, a product released when red blood cells break down, and ammonia, a toxic waste product of protein breakdown.

- Defending against infection by removing bacteria from the blood and making chemicals necessary to the functioning of the immune system.

Although the liver is the only organ that has the capacity to grow back, or regenerate, after injury or damage, sometimes the damage is too great for it to heal. The American Association for the Study of Liver Disease estimates that about 25 million Americans experience a liver-related disease each year. Individuals cannot live without a functioning liver. The ability to transplant livers is improving, **liver transplantation** is not nearly as common or successful as **kidney transplantation**.

Because the liver has many vital functions, there are many types of liver disease. The American Liver Foundation estimates that over 20,000 Americans die of chronic liver disease each year and another 360,000 are hospitalized. Individuals cannot live without a functioning liver.

Congenital Liver Diseases

Congenital liver diseases are disorders that are present at birth. Inherited liver diseases and disorders include:

- Alagile syndrome, a disorder that causes withering of the bile ducts. This disease occurs in less than 1 in 100,000 individuals.

- Alpha 1-antitrypsin deficiency, an inborn error in metabolism and the most common type of genetic liver disease.

- Galactosemia, a hereditary metabolic disease in which the liver is unable to break down the sugar galactose found in milk. It occurs in about one in every 20,000 births.

- Hematochromatosis, a hereditary metabolic disorder in which too much iron is absorbed from the diet and stored in the liver. This disease affects over one million Americans.

- Porphyria, a disorder in which the component of blood that contains iron is not correctly formed.

- Tyrosinemia, a rare inherited error in metabolism that causes severe liver disease in infants and children. It affects fewer than 200,000 individuals in the United States.

- Type I glycogen storage disease, a lack of the enzyme that helps regulate blood glucose (sugar) levels.

- Wilson's disease, an inherited disorder in which copper is accumulated in the liver and nervous system.

Acquired Liver Diseases

Many liver diseases are acquired from infection and exposure of the liver to toxic substances such as alcohol or drugs. In some areas of the world (although not the United States) liver parasites are a common cause of liver disease. In the United States, the most common acquired liver diseases are **hepatitis A**, B, and C and **cirrhosis**. Hepatitis A causes an acute (short-term) illness and is caused by a virus found in food or drinking water contaminated with feces. Hepatitis A infects between 125,000 and 250,000 people in the United States each year and causes about 100 deaths annually.

Hepatitis B is a viral infection spread by blood exchange and sexual contact with an infected person. It can be passed from an infected mother to her fetus. In most people hepatitis B is a short-term illness that causes mild symptoms such as **fatigue**, but in 2–6% of people, the disease lasts a long time and causes permanent liver damage. More than 75,000 people in the United States become infected with hepatitis B each year. Chinese Americans have a hepatitis B infection rate five times that of Caucasian Americans.

Hepatitis C is caused by a virus spread mainly through contact with the blood of an infected person, such as through sharing needles to inject drugs or from a mother to a fetus. Individuals infected with hepatitis C virus may not feel sick or know that they are infected for many years, but the disease can increase the likelihood of developing **liver cancer** of cirrhosis. The

American Liver Foundation estimates that 4 million Americans are infected with hepatitis C, resulting in 10,000–12,000 deaths each year. About 70% of individuals who are infected do not know that they have the virus. African Americans have the highest rate of hepatitis C infections and are twice as likely to be infected with hepatitis C as Caucasian Americans.

Cirrhosis of the liver involves the formation of permanent scar tissue in the liver and loss of liver function. It is often caused by chronic alcohol **abuse** (alcoholic liver disease), but it can also be caused by diseases such as hepatitis. Cirrhosis interferes with blood flow through the liver and can raise pressure in blood vessels supplying the liver and decrease the absorption of nutrients from the blood, leading to **malnutrition**. The liver of individuals with cirrhosis is also less effective in removing toxic wastes from the blood. Cirrhosis can be fatal.

Over 800 over-the-counter and prescription drugs, as well as illicit street drugs, can cause liver damage. One of the most common drugs to cause liver damage is **acetaminophen** (Tylenol) when taken at high doses or by individuals who already have some liver damage. Exposure to toxic chemicals, physical injury, and blockage of the bile ducts call also cause liver damage.

Liver **cancer** can either develop first in the liver (primary liver cancer) or spread there from another site (metastasized cancer). About 16,000 new cases of primary liver cancer are diagnosed each year, most commonly in middle age and older men. Although the cause of liver cancer is unclear, it appears to be associated with chronic infections of hepatitis B and C.

Causes & symptoms

The causes of liver disease are many and varied. Leading causes are viral infection, alcohol abuse, and inherited disease. A common symptoms of liver disease are **jaundice**. With jaundice, the skin and the whites of the eyes take on a yellowish color as a result of the accumulation of bilirubin and bile pigments in the blood. This is a sign that the liver or the biliary system is not functioning properly. Other symptoms of liver disease include an enlarged liver and swollen abdomen, **nausea**, **vomiting**, weight loss, and fatigue. Some infections cause flu-like symptoms of **fever**, **headache**, and weakness.

Diagnosis

Liver function tests, sometimes called a liver panel, measure various enzymes, proteins, and waste products in the blood. These readings can tell a physician whether the liver is damaged and give an idea of how well it is functioning. Liver function tests are the most common way to diagnose liver damage. Based on the results of a liver panel, additional blood tests for infection, a **liver biopsy**, or liver scan may be done to pinpoint the reason for loss of function.

Treatment

Treatments depend on the type of liver disease an individual has. Many liver diseases are treated with altered **diets**, abstinence from alcohol, and medication. Hepatitis can be treated with antiviral medications such as interferon or ribavirin. Liver cancer is treated with **chemotherapy**, radiation, and surgery. As of 2005, over 300 clinical trials were enrolling patients with various types of liver disease in experimental treatment programs. Information on current clinical trials can be found at < http://www.clinicaltrials.gov >.

If the liver fails completely, a liver transplant is possible. About 5,600 liver transplants were performed in the United States in 2003. Donors and recipients are matched on the basis of blood type and must also be about the same weight. There is no machine like a **kidney dialysis** machine to perform the functions of the liver while individuals are awaiting a transplant. In 2003, 1,800 people died awaiting a liver donor, and about 18,000 more are on the waiting list awaiting a donated liver. Livers to be transplanted can come from either a living donor or a deceased donor.

Alternative treatment

A great deal of interest in alternative treatments for hepatitis C has resulted in a review of alternative and complementary treatments by the National Center for Complementary and Alternative Medicine (NCCAM), a division of the United States National Institutes of Health. Although there was in 2003 not enough solid experimental evidence to show that any herbal treatments cured hepatitis C, the most promising herbal treatment was an extract of milk thistle (*Silybum marianum*), a plant in the aster family that has been used for centuries in Europe to treat liver disease and jaundice. Some studies suggested that extracts of milk thistle promoted the growth of certain types of liver cells and acted as an anti-oxidant to protect the liver while producing few unwanted side effects. Other studies showed no protective effects.

Licorice root (*Glycyrrhiza glabra*) was also reviewed by NCCAM. Some studies suggested that

KEY TERMS

Biliary—Relating to the system that produces and transports bile.

Bile—A yellowish-green material secreted by the liver, stored by the gall bladder, and emptied into the small intestine to aid in the digestion and absorption of fats.

Bilirubin—A reddish-yellow substance that results from the breakdown of aging red blood cells. It is found in blood and bile, and if it accumulates in large quantities can cause jaundice.

Biopsy—A diagnostic procedure in which a small sample of tissue is obtained and examined under the microscope to determine they type and stage of a disease.

Congenital—Present at birth.

Feces—Waste products eliminated from the large intestine; excrement.

Jaundice—A yellowish tinge to the skin and whites of the eyes that indicates malfunction of the biliary system and/or liver and build up of bile components in the blood.

licorice root had antiviral properties, however this herb did not reduce the amount of hepatitis C virus circulating in the blood. Long term use of licorice root can have serious, health-threatening side effects.

Other alternative treatments studied by NCCAM include ginseng (*Panax quinquefolius* and *Panax ginseng*), which they concluded might possibly have a positive effect on the liver, especially in the elderly, and schisandra (*Schisandra chinensis* and *Schisandra sphenanthera*) used in Chinese medicine, which seemed to have a liver-protective effect in laboratory animals. Thymus extract and colloidal silver were found to be ineffective in treating liver disease.

Prognosis

The course of liver disease depends on the type of disease. Many individuals recover completely from infections of hepatitis A and B. However, if liver scarring occurs, the effects are irreversible. The initial success rate for liver transplants is good, with about 90% of individuals receiving a liver transplant are alive one year after the transplant operation. However, no alternative treatments produced a better outcome than traditional treatments of hepatitis C.

Prevention

Prevention is an effective way to avoid liver disease. Vaccines exist for hepatitis A and B (but not hepatitis C), although many individuals remain unvaccinated. In addition to **vaccination**, individuals can decrease the likelihood of developing liver disease by

- practicing safe sex

- avoiding sharing needles

- eating a healthy, balanced diet

- taking medications as prescribed

- avoiding drinking alcohol.

Resources

ORGANIZATIONS

American Association for the Study of Liver Disease, 1729 King Street, Suite 200, Alexandria, VA 22314. Telephone: 703-299-9766. < http://www.aasld.org >.

American Liver Foundation, 75 Maiden Lane, Suite 603, New York, NY 10038. Telephone: 800-465-4837 or 888-443-7872. < http://www.liverfoundation.org >.

OTHER

"Hepatitis C and Complementary and Alternative Medicine: 2003 Update" National Center for Complementary and Alternative Medicine. 11 January 2005 [cited 25 March 2005]/ < http://nccam.nih.gov/health/hepatitsc >.

"Liver Disease" *Medline Plus Medical Encyclopedia* 16 July 2004 [cited 25 March 2005]. United States National Library of Medicine and the National Institutes of Health. < http://www.mln.nih.gov/medlineplus/ency/article/000205.htm >.

"Liver Function Test Factsheet" liverfoundation.org. 2003 [cited 23 March 2005]. < http://www.liverfoundation.org/db/articles/1077 >.

Tish Davidson, A.M.

Liver encephalopathy

Definition

Liver encephalopathy is a potentially life-threatening disease in which toxic substances accumulate in the blood. Also known as hepatic encephalopathy or hepatic **coma**, this condition can cause confusion, disorientation, abnormal neurological signs, loss of consciousness, and **death**.

Description

A normally functioning liver metabolizes and detoxifies substances formed in the body during the digestive process. Impaired liver function allows substances like ammonia (formed when the body digests protein), some fatty acids, phenol, and mercaptans to escape into the bloodstream. From there, they may penetrate the blood-brain barrier, affect the central nervous system (CNS), and lead to hepatic coma.

Hepatic coma is most common in patients with chronic **liver disease**. It occurs in 50-70% of all those with **cirrhosis**.

Causes and symptoms

The cause of hepatic coma is unknown, but the condition is frequently associated with the following conditions:

- Acute or chronic liver disease

- Gastrointestinal bleeding

- Azotemia, the accumulation of nitrogen-containing compounds (such as urea) in the blood

- Inherited disorders that disrupt the process by which nitrogen is decomposed and excreted

- The use of shunts (devices implanted in the body to redirect the flow of fluid from one vessel to another)

- Electrolyte imbalances, including low levels of potassium (**hypokalemia**) and abnormally alkaline blood pH (alkalosis). These imbalances may result from the overuse of sedatives, **analgesics**, or **diuretics**; reduced levels of oxygen (hypoxia), or withdrawal of excessive amounts of body fluid (hypovolemia)

- Constipation, which may increase the body's nitrogen load

- Surgery

- Infection

- Acute liver disease.

Binge drinking and acute infection are common causes of hepatic coma in patients with long-standing liver disease.

Symptoms of hepatic encephalopathy range from almost unnoticeable changes in personality, energy levels, and thinking patterns to deep coma.

Inability to reproduce a star or other simple design (**apraxia**) and deterioration of handwriting are common symptoms of early encephalopathy. Decreased brain function can also cause inappropriate behavior, lack of interest in personal grooming, mood swings, and uncharacteristically poor judgment.

The patient may be less alert than usual and develop new sleep patterns. Movement and speech may be slow and labored.

As the disease progresses, patients become confused, drowsy, and disoriented. The breath and urine acquires a sweet, musky odor. The hands shake, the outstretched arms flap (asterixis or "liver flap"), and the patient may lapse into unconsciousness. As coma deepens, reflexes may be heightened (hyperreflexia). The toes sometimes splay when the sole of the foot is stroked (Babinski reflex).

Agitation occasionally occurs in children and in adults who suddenly develop severe symptoms. Seizures are uncommon.

Diagnosis

The absence of sensitive, reliable tests for encephalopathy make the physician's personal observations and professional judgment the most valuable diagnostic tools.

Confusion, disorientation, and other indications of impaired brain function strongly suggest encephalopathy in patients known to have liver disease. CAT scans and examination of spinal fluid don't provide diagnostic clues. Elevated arterial ammonia levels are almost always present in hepatic coma, but levels are not necessarily correlated with the severity or extent of the disease.

Magnetic resonance imaging (MRI) can show severe brain swelling that often occurs prior to coma, and **electroencephalography** (EEG) detects abnormal brain waves even in patients with early, mild symptoms. Blood and urine analyses can provide important information about the cause of encephalopathy in patients suspected of taking large quantities of sedatives or other drugs.

Treatment

This condition may disappear if the cause of symptoms is eliminated. In other cases, treatment is designed to improve liver function as much as possible; remove or relieve factors that worsen symptoms; and decrease the body's production of poisonous substances.

All non-essential medications are discontinued. Soft restraints are recommended in place of sedatives for patients who become agitated.

Enemas or **laxatives** are used to stimulate expulsion of toxic intestinal products. All or most protein is eliminated from the diet, and supplemental feeding may be necessary to replenish lost calories. Regular doses of neomycin (Neobiotic), taken orally or

administered to comatose patients in liquid form through a tube, may be used to decrease production of protein-digesting bacteria in the bowel.

Lactulose, a synthetic sugar, changes the characteristics of intestinal bacteria, decreases the amount of ammonia accumulated in the body, and has laxative properties. The patient is given hourly doses of lactulose syrup until **diarrhea** occurs, then dosage is adjusted to maintain regular bowel function. Lactulose and dietary-protein restrictions may be used to control chronic encephalopathy.

Prognosis

Encephalopathy may be reversible if the responsible factor is identified and removed or treated. Patients whose condition is the result of chronic liver disease may recover completely after the underlying cause is corrected.

Despite intensive treatment, encephalopathy caused by acute liver inflammation (fulminant hepatitis) is fatal for as many as 80% of patients. Those with chronic liver failure often die in hepatic coma.

Resources

ORGANIZATIONS

American Liver Foundation. 1425 Pompton Ave., Cedar Grove, NJ 07009. (800) 223-0179. <http://www.liverfoundation.org>.

Maureen Haggerty

KEY TERMS

Cirrhosis—A serious disease of the liver caused by chronic damage to its cells and the eventual formation of scar tissue (fibrosis).

Coma—A condition of deep unconsciousness from which the person cannot be aroused

Electrolytes—Substances that conduct electricity when they are in solution. In the body, electrolytes in the blood and tissues enable nerve impulses to flow normally.

Encephalopathy—A dysfunction of the brain. Hepatic encephalopathy is brain dysfunction that occurs because the liver isn't removing harmful substances from the blood.

Liver fluke infections *see* **Fluke infections**

Liver function tests

Definition

Liver function tests, or LFTs, include tests for bilirubin, a breakdown product of hemoglobin, and ammonia, a protein byproduct that is normally converted into urea by the liver before being excreted by the kidneys. LFTs also commonly include tests to measure levels of several enzymes, which are special proteins that help the body break down and use (metabolize) other substances. Enzymes that are often measured in LFTs include gamma-glutamyl transferase (GGT); alanine aminotransferase (ALT or SGPT); aspartate aminotransferase (AST or SGOT); and alkaline phosphatase (ALP). LFTs also may include **prothrombin time** (PT), a measure of how long it takes for the blood to clot.

Purpose

Liver function tests are used to aid in the differential diagnosis of **liver disease** and injury, and to help monitor response to treatment.

Precautions

Bilirubin: Drugs that may cause increased blood levels of total bilirubin include anabolic steroids, **antibiotics**, antimalarials, ascorbic acid, Diabinese, codeine, **diuretics**, epinephrine, **oral contraceptives**, and vitamin A.

Ammonia: Muscular exertion can increase ammonia levels, while cigarette **smoking** produces significant increases within one hour of inhalation. Drugs that may cause increased levels include alcohol, **barbiturates**, **narcotics**, and diuretics. Drugs that may decrease levels include broad-spectrum antibiotics, levodopa, lactobacillus, and potassium salts.

ALT: Drugs that may increase ALT levels include **acetaminophen**, ampicillin, codeine, dicumarol, indomethacin, methotrexate, oral contraceptives, **tetracyclines**, and verapamil. Previous intramuscular injections may cause elevated levels.

GGT: Drugs that may cause increased GGT levels include alcohol, phenytoin, and phenobarbital. Drugs that may cause decreased levels include oral contraceptives.

Description

The liver is one of the most important organs in the body. As the body's "chemical factory," it regulates the levels of most of the main blood chemicals and acts with the kidneys to clear the blood of drugs and toxic substances. The liver metabolizes these products, alters their chemical structure, makes them water soluble, and excretes them in bile.

Liver function tests are used to determine if the liver has been damaged or its function impaired. Elevations of certain liver tests in relation to others aids in that determination. For example, aminotransferases (which include ALT and AST) are notably elevated in liver damage caused by liver cell disease (hepatocellular disease). However, in intrahepatic obstructive disease–which may be caused by some drugs or biliary cirrhosis–the alkaline phosphatases are most abnormal.

Alanine aminotransferase

Alanine aminotransferase (ALT), formerly called serum glutamate pyruvate transaminase, or SGPT, is an enzyme necessary for energy production. It is present in a number of tissues, including the liver, heart, and skeletal muscles, but is found in the highest concentration in the liver. Because of this, it is used in conjunction with other liver enzymes to detect liver disease, especially hepatitis or **cirrhosis** without **jaundice**. Additionally, in conjunction with the **aspartate aminotransferase test** (AST), it helps to distinguish between heart damage and liver tissue damage.

Aspartate aminotransferase

Aspartate aminotransferase (AST), formerly called serum glutamic-oxaloacetic transaminase, or SGOT, is another enzyme necessary for energy production. It, too, may be elevated in liver and heart disease. In liver disease, the AST increase is usually less than the ALT increase. However, in liver disease caused by alcohol use, the AST increase may be two or three times greater than the ALT increase.

Alkaline phosphatase

Alkaline phosphatase (ALP) levels usually include two similar enzymes (isoenzymes) that mainly come from the liver and bone and from the placenta in pregnant women. In some cases, doctors may order a test to differentiate between the alkaline phosphatase that originates in the liver and the alkaline phosphatase originating in bone. If a person has elevated ALP, does not have bone disease and is not pregnant, he or she may have a problem with the biliary tract, the system that makes and stores bile. (Bile is made in the liver, then passes through ducts to the gall bladder, where it is stored.)

Gamma-glutamyl transferase

Gamma-glutamyl transferase (GGT), sometimes called gamma-glutamyl transpeptidase (GGPT), is an enzyme that is compared with ALP levels to distinguish between skeletal disease and liver disease. Because GGT is not increased in bone disorders, as is ALP, a normal GGT with an elevated ALP would indicate bone disease. Conversely, because the GGT is more specifically related to the liver, an elevated GGT with an elevated ALP would strengthen the diagnosis of liver or bile-duct disease. The GGT has also been used as an indicator of heavy and chronic alcohol use, but its value in these situations has been questioned recently. It is also commonly elevated in patients with **infectious mononucleosis**.

Bilirubin

Bilirubin, a breakdown product of hemoglobin, is the predominant pigment in a substance produced by the liver called bile. Excess bilirubin causes yellowing of body tissues (jaundice). There are two tests for bilirubin: direct-reacting (conjugated) and indirect-reacting (unconjugated). Differentiating between the two is important diagnostically, as elevated levels of indirect bilirubin are usually caused by liver cell dysfunction (e.g. hepatitis), while elevations of direct bilirubin typically result from obstruction either within the liver (intrahepatic) or a source outside the liver (e.g. **gallstones** or a tumor blocking the bile ducts). Bilirubin measurements are especially valuable in newborns, as extremely elevated levels of unconjugated bilirubin can accumulate in the brain, causing irreparable damage.

Ammonia

Analysis of blood ammonia aids in the diagnosis of severe liver diseases and helps to monitor the course of these diseases. Together with the AST and the ALT, ammonia levels are used to confirm a diagnosis of **Reye's syndrome** (a rare disorder usually seen in children and associated with **aspirin** intake), which is characterized by brain and liver damage following an upper respiratory tract infection, **chickenpox**, or **influenza**. Ammonia levels are also helpful in the diagnosis and treatment of hepatic encephalopathy, a serious brain condition caused by the accumulated toxins that result from liver disease and liver failure.

Preparation

Preparation requirements for all these tests vary from laboratory to laboratory, so it is generally considered best that the patient be in a **fasting** state (nothing to eat or drink) after midnight the day before the test(s).

Aftercare

Because many patients with liver disease have prolonged clotting times, it is important to monitor the puncture site for bleeding after blood is drawn (venipuncture).

Risks

Risks for this test are minimal, but may include slight bleeding from the blood-drawing site, **fainting** or feeling lightheaded after venipuncture, or hematoma (blood accumulating under the puncture site).

Normal results

Reference ranges vary from laboratory to laboratory and also depend upon the method used. However, normal values can generally be found within the following ranges, unless specified differently.

- ALT: 5-35 IU/L (values for the elderly may be slightly higher, and values also may be higher in men and in African-Americans)

- AST: 0-35 IU/L

- ALP: 30-120 IU/L

- GGT: Normal values for this test vary widely, depending on the laboratory performing the test, and the age and sex of the patient. For example, females less than 45 years old have lower values than both males and females over 45 years of age. Values in the newborn can be as much as five times higher than in adults.

- Bilirubin: (Adult, elderly, and child) Total bilirubin: 0.1-1.0 mg/dL; indirect bilirubin: 0.2-0.8 mg/dL; direct bilirubin: 0.1-0.3 mg/dL. (Newborn) Total bilirubin: 1-12 mg/dL. Note: critical values for adult: greater than 1.2 mg/dL. Critical values for newborn (requiring immediate treatment): greater than 15 mg/dL.

- Ammonia: Normal values for this test vary widely, depending upon the laboratory performing the test, the age of the patient, and the type of specimen. For example, values are somewhat higher in arterial than in venous blood.

- PT: 9-12 seconds.

Abnormal results

ALT: Values are significantly increased in cases of hepatitis, and moderately increased in cirrhosis, liver tumor, obstructive jaundice, and severe **burns**. Values are mildly increased in **pancreatitis**, **heart attack**, infectious mononucleosis, and **shock**. Most useful when compared with ALP levels.

KEY TERMS

Cirrhosis—A serious disease of the liver caused by chronic damage to its cells and the eventual formation of scar tissue (fibrosis). The most common symptoms are mild jaundice, fluid collection in the tissues, mental confusion, and vomiting of blood. If left untreated, cirrhosis lead to liver failure and death.

Hemolytic disease of the newborn—Also known as erythroblastosis neonatorum, this is a condition in which a newborn's red blood cells are destroyed by antibodies that have crossed the placenta from the mother's blood. (Hemolytic disease begins in the fetus, in whom the disease is called erythroblastosis fetalis). Severe anemia caused by hemolytic disease is treated in the same way as other anemias, but when jaundice appears due to increased bilirubin, the jaundice is treated by exposing the infant to bright lights. In severe cases, exchange transfusion is required or brain damage may result.

Hepatitis—An inflammation of the liver, with accompanying liver cell damage or cell death, caused most frequently by viral infection, but also by certain drugs, chemicals, or poisons. May be either acute (of limited duration) or chronic

(continuing). Symptoms include jaundice, nausea, vomiting, loss of appetite, tenderness in the right upper abdomen, aching muscles, and joint pain. In severe cases, liver failure may result.

Hepatic encephalopathy—Also called liver encephalopathy or hepatic coma, this is a disorder in which brain function deteriorates because toxic substances, which would normally be removed by the liver, accumulate in the bloodstream due to liver damage or disease. Early symptoms include subtle changes in logical thinking, personality and behavior. As the disorder progresses, signs of drowsiness and confusion increase until eventually the patient loses consciousness and lapses into coma.

Reye's syndrome—A rare disorder characterized by brain and liver damage following an upper respiratory tract infection, chickenpox, or influenza, almost entirely confined to children under age 15, and often related to aspirin ingestion for a viral infection. Symptoms include uncontrollable vomiting, often with lethargy, memory loss, disorientation, or delirium. Swelling of the brain may cause seizures, coma, and in severe cases, death.

- AST: High levels may indicate liver cell damage, hepatitis, heart attack, **heart failure**, or gall stones.
- ALP: Elevated levels occur in diseases that impair bile formation (**cholestasis**). ALP may also be elevated in many other liver disorders, as well as some lung cancers (bronchogenic carcinoma) and Hodgkin's lymphoma. However, elevated ALP levels may also occur in otherwise healthy people, especially among older people.

GGT: Increased levels are diagnostic of hepatitis, cirrhosis, liver tumor or metastasis, as well as injury from drugs toxic to the liver. Although the causes are unclear, GGT levels may increase with alcohol ingestion, heart attack, pancreatitis, infectious mononucleosis, and Reye's syndrome.

Bilirubin: Increased *indirect* or total bilirubin levels can indicate various serious **anemias**, including hemolytic disease of the newborn and **transfusion** reaction. Increased *direct* bilirubin levels can be diagnostic of bile duct obstruction, gallstones, cirrhosis, or hepatitis. It is important to note that if total bilirubin levels in the newborn reach or exceed critical levels, exchange transfusion is necessary to avoid kernicterus, a condition that causes brain damage.

Ammonia: Increased levels are seen in primary liver cell disease, Reye's syndrome, severe heart failure, hemolytic disease of the newborn, and hepatic encephalopathy.

PT: Elevated in acute liver injury, vitamin K deficiencies, and disorders with impair the absorption of vitamin K, including cholestasis.

Resources

BOOKS

Pagana, Kathleen Deska. *Mosby's Manual of Diagnostic and Laboratory Tests.* St. Louis: Mosby, Inc., 1998.

Janis O. Flores

Liver nuclear medicine scan

Definition

A liver scan is a diagnostic procedure to evaluate the liver for suspected disease. A radioactive substance which concentrates in the liver is injected intravenously and the image of its distribution in the body is analyzed to diagnose certain abnormalities.

Purpose

In the past, liver scans were used to evaluate the liver in a wide variety of situations. It was considered a useful study to detect abnormalities, but was often not able to establish a specific diagnosis. In the 1990s, radionuclide imaging of the liver (use of a radioactive form of cobalt or iodine) evolved into a more specialized study, used to identify individual diseases or conditions. This is accomplished by using different radioisotopes precisely designed to further evaluate a particular case. Isotopes are different forms of the same substance, such as radioactive iodine, that are injected into the body. This allows the physician to trace the process of the substance throughout the part of the body that is being tested for disease.

A liver scan is usually ordered after blood studies and other imaging procedures have shown a liver abnormality. It is most often used to further evaluate masses or tumors. These may be benign growths in the liver, or **cancer** which has developed in the liver or has spread (or metastasized) from another organ.

A liver scan may also be helpful in diagnosing specific disorders, by detecting features which are characteristic of a disorder, such as **cirrhosis** of the liver. This study may also be part of the battery of tests used to evaluate potential candidates for liver transplant.

Precautions

Women who are pregnant or breast feeding should not have this test.

Description

This test can be performed in an outpatient setting or a hospital x-ray department. The patient usually lies down while a radioactive substance (radioactive isotope) which accumulates in the liver is injected through a vein in the arm. Scanning times may vary, depending on the specific radioisotope used. It most often begins within minutes after injection. The radionuclide scanner, sometimes called a gamma camera or scintillation camera, is positioned above the upper abdomen and may lightly touch the patient. It is important for the patient to lie quietly. Position changes and brief periods

of breath holding may be required. The test usually takes approximately one hour.

A specialized liver scan used to assess blood flow is frequently used. It may be referred to as a radionuclide blood pool or volume study, a labeled red cell scintigram, or some combination of these terms. Other studies may be named for the radioisotope used. This test may also be called a liver-spleen scan.

Preparation

No physical preparation is required. A liver scan should be performed before doing any study that uses iodinated or barium-containing contrast agents, to prevent inaccurate results.

The patients should understand that there is no danger of radioactive exposure to themselves or others. Only small amounts of radionuclide are used. The total amount of radiation absorbed is often less than the dose received from ordinary x rays. The scanner does not emit any radiation, but detects and records it from the patient.

Aftercare

No special precautions are needed.

Normal results

A normal scan will show a liver of normal size, shape, and position.

Abnormal results

An abnormal liver scan may result from a mass. Depending on the radioisotope and technique used, the scan may identify particular types of tumors or certain cancers. Too much radioisotope in the spleen and bones, compared to the liver, can indicate potential **hypertension** or cirrhosis. Liver diseases such as cirrhosis or hepatitis may also cause an abnormal scan, but are rarely diagnosed from the information revealed by this study alone.

Resources

PERIODICALS

Drane, Walter E. "Scintigraphic Techniques for Hepatic Imaging." *Radiologic Clinics of North America* 36 (March 1998): 309-318.

Ellen S. Weber, MSN

National Transplant Waiting List By Organ Type (June 2000)

Organ Needed	Number Waiting
Kidney	48,349
Liver	15,987
Heart	4,139
Lung	3,695
Kidney-Pancreas	2,437
Pancreas	942
Heart-Lung	212
Intestine	137

Liver transplantation

Definition

Liver transplantation is a surgery that removes a diseased liver and replace it with a healthy donor liver.

Purpose

The liver is the body's principle chemical factory. It receives all nutrients, drugs, and toxins absorbed from the intestines and performs the final stages of digestion, converting food into energy and replacement parts for the body. The liver also filters the blood of all waste products, removes and detoxifies poisons and excretes many of these into the bile. It processes other chemicals for excretion by the kidneys. The liver is also an energy storage organ, changing food energy to a chemical called glycogen that can be rapidly converted to fuel.

As the liver fails, all of its functions diminish. **Nutrition** suffers, toxins build up, and waste products accumulate. Scar tissue builds up on the liver if disease is of long duration. As the liver **scars**, blood flow is progressively restricted in the portal vein, which carries blood from the stomach and abdominal organs to the liver. The resulting high blood pressure (**hypertension**) causes swelling of and bleeding from the blood vessels of the esophagus. Severe **jaundice**, fluid accumulation in the abdomen (**ascites**), and deterioration of mental function, due to the build-up of toxins in the blood (**liver encephalopathy**), eventually occur, leading to **death**.

Among the many causes of liver failure that bring patients to transplant surgery are:

- Progressive hepatitis (mostly due to virus infection) accounts for more than a third.

- Alcohol damage brings in about 20%

- Scarring or abnormality of the biliary system accounts for roughly another 20%.

- The remainder comes from selected cancers, other uncommon diseases, and a situation called fulminant liver failure.

Fulminant liver failure most commonly happens during acute viral hepatitis, but it is also the result of **mushroom poisoning** by *Amanita phalloides* and toxic reactions to some medicines, like an overdose of **acetaminophen**. This is a special category of candidates for liver transplant because of the speed of their disease and the immediate need of treatment.

The first human liver transplant was performed in 1963, and since then, thousands of liver transplants are done every year. Since the introduction of of cyclosporine (a drug that suppresses the immune response that rejects the donor organ), success rates for liver transplantation have reached 85%.

Precautions

Patients with advanced heart and lung disease, who are HIV positive, and who **abuse** drugs and alcohol are poor candidates for liver tranplantation. Their ability to survive the surgery and the difficult recovery period, as well as their longterm prognosis, is hindered by their conditions.

Description

There are three types of liver transplantation methods. They include:

- Orthotopic transplantation is the replacement of a whole diseased liver with a healthy donor liver.

- Heterotopic transplantation is the addition of a donor liver at another site, while the diseased liver is left intact.

- Reduced-size liver transplantation is the replacement of a whole diseased liver with a portion of a healthy

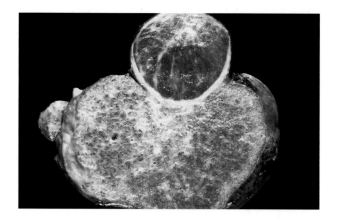

The diseased liver of a patient ready for transplantation.
(Custom Medical Stock Photo. Reproduced by permission.)

donor liver. Reduced-size liver transplants are most often performed on children.

When an orthotopic transplantation is performed, a segment of the inferior vena cava attached to the liver is taken from the donor as well. The same parts are removed from the recipient and replaced by connecting the inferior vena cava, the hepatic artery, the portal vein and the bile ducts.

When there is a possibility that the afflicted liver may recover, a heterotopic tranplantation is performed. The donor liver is placed in a different site, but it still has to have the same connections. It is usually attached very near the original liver, and if the original liver recovers, the donor shrivels away. If the original liver does not recover, it will shrivel, leaving the donor in place.

Reduced-size liver transplantation tranplants part of a donor liver into a patient. It is possible to divide the liver into eight pieces, each supplied by a different set of blood vessels. Two of these pieces have been enough to save a patient in liver failure, especially if the patient is a child. It is therefore possible to transplant one liver into at least two patients and to transplant part of a liver from a living donor and have both donor and recipient survive. Liver tissue grows to accommodate its job so long as there is initially enough of the organ to use. Patients have survived with only 15-20% of their original liver, provided that 15-20% was healthy.

Availability of organs for transplant is a current crisis in the transplantation business. In October 1997, a national distribution system was established that gives priority to the sickest patients closest in location to the donor liver, but makes livers available nationally. It is now possible to preserve a liver out of the body for 10-20 hours by flushing it with cooled solutions of special chemicals and nutrients, so it can be transported across the country.

Preparation

Before transplantation takes place, the patient is first determined to be a good candidate for transplantation by going through rigorous medical examination. A suitable candidate boosts their nutritional intake in order to ensure that they are as healthy as possible before surgery. Drugs are administered that will decrease rejection after surgery. Consultation with the patient, as well as any family, is conducted to explain the surgery and its complications. Psychological counciling is recommended.

Aftercare

In order to prevent organ rejection, immunosuppressive drugs will be taken. Hospitalization ranges from four weeks to five months, depending on the rate of recovery.

Successfully receiving a transplanted liver is only the beginning of a life-long process. Patients with transplanted livers have to stay on **immunosuppressant drugs** for the rest of their lives to prevent organ rejection. Although many can reduce the dosage after the initial few months, virtually none can discontinue drugs altogether. Prednisone, azathioprine, and tacrolimus are often combined with cyclosporine for better results. Newer immunosuppressive agents are coming that promise even better results. In spite of immunosuppressants, rejection occurs most of the time and requires additional medication. In some cases it cannot be reversed, and retransplantation becomes necessary.

Risks

Early failure of the transplant occurs once in four surgeries and has to be repeated. Some transplants never work, some succumb to infection, and some suffer immune rejection. Primary failure is apparent within one or two days. Infections happen in half the patients and often appear during the first week. Rejection usually starts at the end of the first week. The surgery itself may need revision because of narrowing, leaking, or **blood clots** at the connections.

There are potential social and economic problems, psychological problems, and a vast array of possible medical and surgical complications. Close medical surveillance must continue for the rest of the patient's life.

KEY TERMS

Acetaminophen—A common pain reliever (Tylenol).

Antigen—Any chemical that provokes an immune response.

Bile ducts—Tubes carrying bile from the liver to the intestines.

Biliary system—The tree of tubes that carries bile.

Hepatic artery—The blood vessel supplying arterial blood to the liver.

Inferior vena cava—The biggest vein in the body, returning blood to the heart from the lower half of the body.

Leukemia—A cancer of the white blood cells.

Lymphoma—A cancer of lymphatic tissue.

Portal vein—The blood vessel carrying venous blood from the abdominal organs to the liver.

Infections are a constant risk while on immunosuppressive agents, because the immune system is supposed to prevent them. A way has not yet been devised to control rejection without hampering immune defenses against infections. Not only do ordinary infections pose a threat, but because of the impaired immunity, transplant patients are susceptible to the same "opportunistic" infections that threaten **AIDS** patients–pneumocystis **pneumonia**, herpes and cytomegalovirus infections, fungi, and a host of bacteria.

Immunosuppression also hinders the body's ability to resist **cancer**. All the drugs used to prevent rejection increase the risk of leukemias and lymphomas.

There is also a risk of the original disease returning. Hepatitis virus still inhabits the patient, as does the urge to drink alcohol. Newer **antiviral drugs** hold out promise for dealing with hepatitis, and Alcoholics Anonymous (AA) is the most effective treatment known for **alcoholism**.

Drug reactions are also a continuing threat. Every drug used to suppress the immune system has potential problems.

Resources

ORGANIZATIONS

American Liver Foundation. 1425 Pompton Ave., Cedar Grove, NJ 07009. (800) 223-0179. <http://www.liverfoundation.org>.

J. Ricker Polsdorfer, MD

Ller-Christi *see* **Histiocytosis X**

Loaiasis *see* **Filariasis**

Lobectomy *see* **Lung surgery**

Lobotomy *see* **Psychosurgery**

Local anesthetic *see* **Anesthesia, local**

Localized scratch dermatitis *see* **Lichen simplex chronicus**

Lockjaw *see* **Tetanus**

Loperamide *see* **Antidiarrheal drugs**

Loratadine *see* **Antihistamines**

Lou Gehrig's disease *see* **Amyotrophic lateral sclerosis**

Louis-Bar syndrome *see* **Ataxia-telangiectasia**

Low potassium blood level *see* **Hypokalemia**

Low back pain

Definition

Low back **pain** is a common musculoskeletal symptom that may be either acute or chronic. It may be caused by a variety of diseases and disorders that affect the lumbar spine. Low back pain is often accompanied by **sciatica**, which is pain that involves the sciatic nerve and is felt in the lower back, the buttocks, and the backs of the thighs.

Description

Low back pain is a symptom that affects 80% of the general United States population at some point in life with sufficient severity to cause absence from work. It is the second most common reason for visits to primary care doctors, and is estimated to cost the American economy $75 billion every year.

Low back pain may be experienced in several different ways:

- Localized. In localized pain the patient will feel soreness or discomfort when the doctor palpates, or presses on, a specific surface area of the lower back.
- Diffuse. Diffuse pain is spread over a larger area and comes from deep tissue layers.

- Radicular. The pain is caused by irritation of a nerve root. Sciatica is an example of radicular pain.
- Referred. The pain is perceived in the lower back but is caused by inflammation elsewhere– often in the kidneys or lower abdomen.

Causes and Symptoms

Acute pain

Acute pain in the lower back that does not extend to the leg is most commonly caused by a sprain or muscle tear, usually occurring within 24 hours of heavy lifting or overuse of the back muscles. The pain is usually localized, and there may be **muscle spasms** or soreness when the doctor touches the area. The patient usually feels better when resting.

Chronic pain

Chronic low back pain has several different possible causes:

MECHANICAL. Chronic strain on the muscles of the lower back may be caused by **obesity**; **pregnancy**; or job-related stooping, bending, or other stressful postures.

MALIGNANCY. Low back pain at night that is not relieved by lying down may be caused by a tumor in the cauda equina (the roots of the spinal nerves controlling sensation in and movement of the legs), or a **cancer** that has spread to the spine from the prostate, breasts, or lungs. The risk factors for the spread of cancer to the lower back include a history of **smoking**, sudden weight loss, and age over 50.

ANKYLOSING SPONDYLITIS. Ankylosing spondylitis is a form of arthritis that causes chronic pain in the lower back. The pain is made worse by sitting or lying down and improves when the patient gets up. It is most commonly seen in males between 16 and 35. Ankylosing spondylitis is often confused with mechanical back pain in its early stages.

HERNIATED SPINAL DISK. Disk herniation is a disorder in which a spinal disk begins to bulge outward between the vertebrae. Herniated or ruptured disks are a common cause of chronic low back pain in adults.

PSYCHOGENIC. Back pain that is out of proportion to a minor injury, or that is unusually prolonged, may be associated with a somatoform disorder or other psychiatric disturbance.

Low back pain with leg involvement

Low back pain that radiates down the leg usually indicates involvement of the sciatic nerve. The nerve can be pinched or irritated by herniated disks, tumors of the cauda equina, abscesses in the space between the spinal cord and its covering, **spinal stenosis**, and compression **fractures**. Some patients experience **numbness** or weakness of the legs as well as pain.

Diagnosis

The diagnosis of low back pain can be complicated. Most cases are initially evaluated by primary care physicians rather than by specialists.

Initial workup

PATIENT HISTORY. The doctor will ask the patient specific questions about the location of the pain, its characteristics, its onset, and the body positions or activities that make it better or worse. If the doctor suspects that the pain is referred from other organs, he or she will ask about a history of diabetes, peptic ulcers, **kidney stones**, urinary tract infections, or **heart murmurs**.

PHYSICAL EXAMINATION. The doctor will examine the patient's back and hips to check for conditions that require surgery or emergency treatment. The examination includes several tests that involve moving the patient's legs in specific positions to test for nerve root irritation or disk herniation. The flexibility of the lumbar vertebrae may be measured to rule out ankylosing spondylitis.

Imaging studies

Imaging studies are not usually performed on patients whose history and **physical examination** suggest routine muscle strain or overuse. X rays are ordered for patients whose symptoms suggest cancer, infection, inflammation, pelvic or abdominal disease, or bone fractures. MRIs are usually ordered only for patients with certain types of masses or tumors.

It is important to know that the appearance of some abnormalities on imaging studies of the lower back does not necessarily indicate that they cause the pain. Many patients have minor deformities that do not create symptoms. The doctor must compare the results of imaging studies very carefully with information from the patient's history and physical examination.

Treatment

All forms of treatment of low back pain are aimed either at symptom relief or to prevent interference with the processes of healing. None of these methods appear to speed up healing.

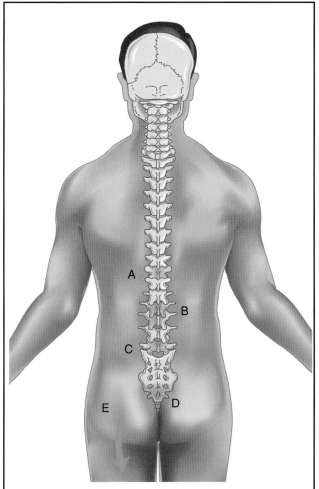

Sites of low back pain. Pain anywhere along the spine (A) can be caused by osteoarthritis. Pain along one or the other side of the spine may be (B) a kidney infection. Trauma to back muscles, joints, or disks (C) causes low back pain. Damage to the coccyx (D) can occur during a fall. Sciatica (E) can cause pain to run down from the back and buttocks area down a leg. *(Illustration by Electronic Illustrators Group.)*

Acute pain

Acute back pain is treated with **nonsteroidal anti-inflammatory drugs** (NSAIDs), such as ibuprofen, **muscle relaxants**, or **aspirin**. Applications of heat or cold compresses are also helpful to most patients. If the patient has not experienced some improvement after several weeks of treatment, the doctor will reinvestigate the cause of the pain.

Chronic pain

Patients with chronic back pain are treated with a combination of medications, physical therapy, and occupational or lifestyle modification. The medications given

are usually NSAIDs, although patients with hypertension, kidney problems, or stomach ulcers should not take these drugs. Patients who take NSAIDs for longer than six weeks should be monitored periodically for complications.

Physical therapy for chronic low back pain usually includes regular **exercise** for fitness and flexibility, and massage or application of heat if necessary.

Lifestyle modifications include giving up smoking, weight reduction (if necessary), and evaluation of the patient's occupation or other customary activities.

Patients with herniated disks are treated surgically if the pain does not respond to medication.

Patients with chronic low back pain sometimes benefit from **pain management** techniques, including **biofeedback**, **acupuncture**, and **chiropractic** manipulation of the spine.

Psychotherapy is recommended for patients whose back pain is associated with a somatoform, **anxiety**, or depressive disorder.

Low back pain with leg involvement

Treatment of sciatica and other disorders that involve the legs may include NSAIDs. Patients with long-standing sciatica or spinal stenosis that do not respond to NSAIDs are treated surgically. Although some doctors use cortisone injections to relieve the pain, this form of treatment is still debated.

Alternative treatment

A thorough differential diagnosis is important before any treatment is considered. There are times when alternative therapies are the most beneficial, and other times when more invasive treatments are needed.

Chiropractic

Chiropractic treats patients by manipulating or adjusting sections of the spine. It is one of the most popular forms of alternative treatment in the United States for relief of back pain caused by straining or lifting injuries. Some osteopathic physicians, physical therapists, and naturopathic physicians also use spinal manipulation to treat patients with low back pain.

Traditional Chinese medicine

Practitioners of **traditional Chinese medicine** treat low back pain with acupuncture, *tui na* (push-and-rub) massage, and the application of herbal poultices.

Herbal medicine

Herbal medicine can utilize a variety of antispasmodic herbs in combination to help relieve low back pain due to spasm. Lobelia (*Lobelia inflata*) and myrrh (*Commiphora molmol*) are two examples of antispasmodic herbs.

Homeopathy

Homeopathic treatment for acute back pain consists of applications of *Arnica* oil to the sore area or oral doses of *Arnica* or *Rhus toxicodendron*. *Bellis perennis* is recommended for deep muscle injuries. Other remedies may be recommended based on the symptoms presented by the patient.

Body work and yoga

Massage and the numerous other body work techniques can be very effective in treating low back pain. **Yoga**, practiced regularly and done properly, can be most useful in preventing future episodes of low back pain.

Prognosis

The prognosis for most patients with acute low back pain is excellent. About 80% of patients recover completely in 4-6 weeks. The prognosis for recovery from chronic pain depends on the underlying cause.

Prevention

Low back pain due to muscle strain can be prevented by lifestyle choices, including regular physical exercise and weight control, avoiding smoking, and learning the proper techniques for lifting and moving heavy objects. Exercises designed to strengthen the muscles of the lower back, and chairs or car seats with lumbar supports are also recommended.

Resources

BOOKS

Hellman, David B. "Arthritis & Musculoskeletal Disorders." In *Current Medical Diagnosis and Treatment, 1998*, edited by Stephen McPhee, et al., 37th ed. Stamford: Appleton & Lange, 1997.

Rebecca J. Frey, PhD

Low blood magnesium *see* **Magnesium imbalance**

Low blood phosphate level *see* **Phosphorus imbalance**

Low blood pressure *see* **Orthostatic hypotension; Hypotension**

Low blood sugar *see* **Hypoglycemia**

Low calcium blood level *see* **Hypocalcemia**

Low sodium blood level *see* **Hyponatremia**

Lower esophageal ring

Definition

Lower esophageal ring is a condition in which there is a ring of tissue inside the lower part of the esophagus (the tube connecting the throat with the stomach). This tissue causes narrowing and partial blockage of the esophagus. Lower esophageal ring can also refer to the ring itself.

Description

Lower esophageal ring (also called Schatzki's ring and B-ring) affects about 10-14% of the population. Normally, the lower part of the esophagus, near where the esophagus meets the stomach, has an inside diameter of 1.5-2 inches. The diameter of this part of the esophagus is less when lower esophageal ring is present, and diameters as small as one-eighth inch have been seen. When the inside diameter is less than about three-fourths of an inch, intermittent difficulty with swallowing can result. About 96% of people with lower esophageal ring have no symptoms.

Causes and symptoms

Causes

Lower esophageal ring seems to result from infoldings of tissue near the bottom of the esophagus, but the underlying cause is unknown. Although some specialists speculate they are due to a congenital defect, most people do not develop symptoms until they reach their forties or later. Although lower esophageal ring is generally associated with hiatal **hernia**, and sometimes with **heartburn**, the cause/effect relationship is unclear.

Symptoms

Intermittent difficulty swallowing solid food is the primary symptom of this condition. The degree of difficulty in swallowing is directly related to the degree the esophagus is narrowed. Certain foods, especially tough or fibrous foods like meat, are more likely to cause swallowing difficulties.

Diagnosis

Gastroenterologists and internists are best equipped to diagnose and treat lower esophageal ring. The diagnosis is based on the patient's history of swallowing difficulties and a barium x ray of the upper gastrointestinal tract. For a barium x ray, the patient swallows a liquid containing barium, a substance that is opaque to x rays. Subsequent x-ray photography reveals the shape of the esophagus and any narrow regions present.

The presence of a lower esophageal ring can also be shown with a test called an esophagoscopy. This procedure visualizes the inside of the esophagus with an inserted, thin, flexible tube. However, this test is less sensitive for lower esophageal ring and costs about five times as much as barium x ray. However, if the findings of a barium x ray are not definitive, esophagoscopy should be done. Biopsies can then be done on questionable areas.

Treatment

Dietary change

Swallowing difficulties due to lower esophageal ring can often be relieved by chewing food more thoroughly. Soft foods and liquids may also be recommended.

Dilation

Lower esophageal rings can be corrected by passing a bougie (a cylindrical, mercury-filled dilator) through the esophagus. This procedure, called bougienage, is effective most of the time, but may need to be repeated every few years. Complications and adverse reactions are extremely rare.

Surgery

If bougienage is unsuccessful, lower esophageal ring tissue can be surgically removed.

Prognosis

The probability of a favorable outcome is high. Swallowing difficulties can be alleviated in almost every case, and the rate of complications from bougienage or surgery is less than 1%.

Prevention

Since the cause of lower esophageal ring is not known, there are no definitive preventive measures. Nevertheless, anyone with lower esophageal ring who also suffers from heartburn would be wise to prevent or treat the heartburn. It is possible that the stomach acid in the esophagus associated with heartburn contributes to esophageal ring.

Resources

ORGANIZATIONS

The American College of Gastroenterology (ACG). P.O. Box 3099, Alexandria, VA 22302. (800) 432-2876. < http://www.healthtouch.com >.

American Gastroenterological Association (AGA). 7910 Woodmont Ave., 7th Floor, Bethesda, MD 20814.

KEY TERMS

Bougie—A mercury-filled dilator in the shape of a cylinder or tapered cylinder. Bougies come in a range of different sizes.

Bougienage—The procedure of dilating tubal organs, like the esophagus, with a bougie or bougies.

Congenital—Existing at birth.

Dysphagia—Difficulty swallowing.

Esophagoscopy (also esophagoendoscopy)—Examination of the inside of the esophagus using a flexible tube that transmits video images.

Esophagus—The tube connecting the throat to the stomach, which is about ten inches long in adults. It is coated with mucus and surrounded by muscles, and pushes food to the stomach by sequential waves of contraction. It functions to transport food from the throat to the stomach and to keep the contents of the stomach in the stomach.

Heartburn—A burning sensation in the chest that can extend to the neck, throat, and face, caused by the movement of stomach acid into the esophagus.

Hiatal hernia—A condition where part of the stomach extends through the diaphragm into the chest cavity.

(310) 654-2055. < aga001@aol.com > < http://www.gastro.org/index.html >.

American Society for Gastrointestinal Endoscopy. 13 Elm St., Manchester, MA 01944. (508) 526-8330. < http://www.asge.org/doc/201 >.

National Digestive Diseases Information Clearinghouse. 2 Information Way, Bethesda, MD 20892-3570. (800) 891-5389. < http://www.niddk.nih.gov/health/digest/nddic.htm >.

Lorraine Lica, PhD

Lumpectomy

Definition

A lumpectomy is a type of surgery used to treat **breast cancer**. It is considered "breast-conserving" surgery because in a lumpectomy, only the malignant tumor and a surrounding margin of normal breast tissue are removed. Lymph nodes in the armpit (axilla) also may be removed. This procedure is called lymph node dissection.

Purpose

Lumpectomy is a surgical treatment for newly diagnosed breast **cancer**. It is estimated that at least 50% of women with breast cancer are good candidates for this procedure. The location, size, and type of tumor are of primary importance when considering breast cancer surgery options. The size of the breast is another factor the surgeon considers when recommending surgery. The patient's psychological outlook, as well as her lifestyle and preferences, should also be taken into account when treatment decisions are made.

The extent and severity of a cancer is evaluated or "staged" according to a fairly complex system. Staging considers the size of the tumor and whether the cancer has spread to other areas, such as the chest wall and the lymph nodes, and/or to distant parts of the body. Women with early stage breast cancers usually are better candidates for lumpectomy. In most cases, a course of **radiation therapy** after surgery is part of the treatment. **Chemotherapy** or antiestrogens also may be prescribed.

Many studies have compared the survival rates of women who have had removal of a breast (**mastectomy**) with those who have undergone lumpectomy and radiation therapy. The data demonstrate that for women with comparable stages of breast cancer, survival rates are similar between the two groups, but the risk of the cancer recurring in the breast is slightly higher with lumpectomy. A 2003 study confirmed that younger women who have lumpectomies have a higher risk of tumor recurrence than those who have mastectomies.

In some instances, women with later stage breast cancer may be able to have lumpectomy. Chemotherapy may be administered before surgery to decrease tumor size and the chance of spread in selected cases.

Precautions

A number of factors may prevent or prohibit a breast cancer patient from having a lumpectomy. The tumor itself may be too large or located in an area where it would be difficult to remove with good cosmetic results. Sometimes several areas of cancer are found in one breast, so the tumor cannot be removed as a single lump. A cancer that has already attached itself to nearby structures, such as the skin or the chest wall, needs more extensive surgery.

Certain medical or physical circumstances also may eliminate lumpectomy as a treatment option. Sometimes lumpectomy may be attempted, but the surgeon is unable to remove the tumor with a sufficient amount of normal tissue surrounding it. This may be termed "persistently positive margins," or "lack of clear margins," referring to the margin of unaffected tissue around the tumor. Lumpectomy is not used for women who have had a previous lumpectomy and have a recurrence of the breast cancer.

The need for radiation therapy after lumpectomy makes this surgery medically unacceptable for some women. For instance, radiation therapy cannot be administered to pregnant women because it may injure the fetus. If, however, delivery would be completed prior to the need for radiation, pregnant women may undergo lumpectomy. Women with collagen vascular disease, such as lupus erythematosus or **scleroderma**, would experience scarring and damage to their connective tissue if exposed to radiation treatments. A woman who has already had therapeutic radiation to the chest area for other reasons cannot have additional exposure for breast cancer therapy.

Some women may choose not to have a lumpectomy for other reasons. They may strongly fear a recurrence of breast cancer, and may consider a lumpectomy too risky. Others feel uncomfortable living with a cancerous breast and experience more peace of mind with the entire breast removed.

The need for radiation therapy also may be a barrier due to non-medical concerns. Some women simply fear this type of treatment and choose more extensive surgery so that radiation will not be required. The commitment of time, usually five days a week for six weeks, may not be acceptable for others. This may be due to financial, personal, or job-related constraints. Finally, in geographically isolated areas, a course of radiation therapy may require lengthy travel, and perhaps unacceptable amounts of time away from family and other responsibilities.

Description

Lumpectomy is an imprecise term. Any amount of tissue, from 1% to 50% of the breast, may be removed and called a lumpectomy. Breast conservation surgery is a frequently-used synonym for lumpectomy. Partial mastectomy, quadrantectomy, segmental excision, wide excision, and tylectomy are other names for this procedure.

A lumpectomy is frequently done in a hospital setting (especially if lymph nodes are to be removed at the same time), but specialized outpatient facilities sometimes are preferred. The surgery is usually done while the patient is under **general anesthesia**. Local anesthetic with additional **sedation** may be used for some patients. The tumor and surrounding margin of tissue is removed and sent to the pathologist. The surgical site is closed.

If axillary lymph nodes were not removed in a prior biopsy, a second incision is made in the armpit. The fat pad that contains lymph nodes is removed from this area and also is sent to the pathologist for analysis. This portion of the procedure is called an axillary lymph node dissection; it is critical for determining the stage of the cancer. Typically, 10 to 15 nodes are removed, but the number may vary. Surgical drains may be left in place in either location to prevent fluid accumulation. The surgery may last from one to three hours.

The patient may stay in the hospital one or two days, or return home the same day. This generally depends on the extent of the surgery and the medical condition of the patient, as well as physician and patient preferences. A woman usually goes home with a small bandage. The inner part of the surgical site usually has dissolvable stitches. The skin may be sutured or stitched; or the skin edges may be held together with steristrips, which are special thin, clear pieces of tape.

Preparation

Routine preoperative preparations, such as having nothing to eat or drink the night before surgery, are typically ordered for a lumpectomy. Information about expected outcomes and potential complications also is part of preparation for lumpectomy, as it is for any surgical procedure. It is especially important that women know about sensations they might experience after the operation, so the sensations are not misinterpreted as signs of further cancer or poor healing.

If the tumor cannot be felt (not palpable), a preoperative localization procedure is needed. A fine wire, or other device is placed at the tumor site, using x ray or ultrasound for guidance. This is usually done in the radiology department of a hospital. The woman is most often sitting up and awake, although some sedation may be administered.

Aftercare

After a lumpectomy, patients are usually cautioned against lifting anything that weighs more than five pounds for several days. Other activities may be restricted (especially if the axillary lymph nodes were removed) according to individual needs. **Pain** is often enough to limit inappropriate motion. Women often are instructed to wear a well-fitting support bra both day and night for approximately one week after surgery.

Pain is usually well controlled with prescribed medication. If it is not, the patient should contact the surgeon, as severe pain may be a sign of a complication that needs medical attention. A return visit to the surgeon normally is scheduled approximately 10 days to two weeks after the operation. Studies have shown that women improve their survival rates after lumpectomy if they stop **smoking**.

Radiation therapy is usually started as soon as feasible after lumpectomy. Other additional treatments, such as chemotherapy or hormone therapy, may also be prescribed. The timing of these is specific to each individual patient.

Risks

The risks are similar to those associated with any surgical procedure. Risks include bleeding, infection, asymmetry, anesthesia reaction, or unexpected scarring. A lumpectomy also may cause loss of sensation in the breast. The size and shape of the breast will be affected by the operation. Fluid can accumulate in the area where tissue was removed, requiring drainage.

If lymph node dissection is performed, there are several potential complications. A woman may experience decreased feeling in the back of her armpit. She also may experience other sensations, including **numbness**, **tingling**, or increased skin sensitivity. An inflammation of the arm vein, called phlebitis, can occur. There may be injury to the nerves controlling arm motion.

Approximately 2% to 10% of patients develop **lymphedema** (swelling of the arm) after axillary lymph node dissection. This swelling of the arm can range from mild to severe. It can be treated with elastic bandages and specialized physical therapy, but it is a chronic condition, requiring continuing care. **Lymphedema** can arise at any time, even years after surgery.

KEY TERMS

Lymph node—A small mass of tissue in the form of a knot or protuberance. Lymph nodes are the primary sources of lymph fluid, which serve in the body's defense by removing toxic fluids and bacteria.

A new technique often eliminates the need to remove many axillary lymph nodes. Sentinel lymph node mapping and biopsy is based on the idea that the condition of the first lymph node in the network, which drains the affected area, can predict whether the cancer may have spread to the rest of the nodes. It is thought that if this first, or sentinel, node is cancer-free, there is no need to look further. Many patients with early-stage breast cancers may be spared the risks and complications of axillary lymph node dissection as the use of this approach continues to increase.

Normal results

When lumpectomy is performed, it is anticipated that it will be the definitive surgical treatment for breast cancer. Other forms of therapy, especially radiation, are often prescribed as part of the total treatment plan. A 2003 study reported that radiation of the entire breast produces better results than radiation of part of the breast. The expected outcome after lumpectomy and radiation is no recurrence of the breast cancer, however, women who have had lumpectomies, particularly those who were young at the time of treatment, should continue to see their physicians for regular breast cancer check-ups, since the cancer can recur.

Abnormal results

An unforeseen outcome of lumpectomy may be recurrence of the breast cancer, either locally or distally (in a part of the body far from the original site). Recurrence may be discovered soon after lumpectomy or years after the procedure. For this reason, it is important for patients to be regularly and closely monitored by their physicians. A 2003 report showed that **magnetic resonance imaging** (MRI) is accurate in detecting any cancer left in the breast after lumpectomy. Women should continue to have regular mammograms. While the scar tissue from lumpectomy and radiation therapy can make mammograms less comfortable, a special cushion was approved by the U.S. Food and Drug Administration in 2003 that reduces discomfort in women who have had breast conserving surgery.

Resources

PERIODICALS

Ford, Steve. "Lumpectomy Associated With Higher Long-term Risk of Recurrence than Mastectomy." *Practice Nurse* November 28, 2003: 50.

Jancin, Bruce. "Cushion Lessens Mammogram Pain After Lumpectomy (Pain Decreased 54%)." *OB GYN News* (February 15, 2003): 9 - 11.

"MR Accurate in Detecting Residual Disease Following Lumpectomy." *Women's Health Weekly* May 29, 2003:14.

Norton, Patrice G.W. "More Data Support Breast Conservation Over Mastectomy (For Phase I or II Cancer)." *Family Practice News* January 15, 2003: 31.

"Smoking Decreases Survival of Patients Treated with Lumpectomy and Radiation." *Cancer Weekly* November 11, 2003: 36.

"Study: Whole-breast Irradiation After Lumpectomy Has Clear Long-term Benefits." *Cancer Weekly* November 11, 2003: 39.

Ellen S. Weber, MSN
Teresa G. Odle

Lumpy breasts *see* **Fibrocystic condition of the breast**

Lumpy jaw *see* **Actinomycosis**

Lung abscess

Definition

Lung **abscess** is an acute or chronic infection of the lung, marked by a localized collection of pus, inflammation, and destruction of tissue.

Description

Lung abscess is the end result of a number of different disease processes ranging from fungal and bacterial infections to **cancer**. It can affect anyone at any age. Patients who are most vulnerable include those weakened by cancer and other chronic diseases; patients with a history of **substance abuse**, diabetes, epilepsy, or poor dental hygiene; patients who have recently had operations under anesthesia; and **stroke** patients. In children, the most vulnerable patients are those with weakened immune systems, **malnutrition**, or blunt injuries to the chest.

Causes and symptoms

The immediate cause of most lung abscesses is infection caused by bacteria. About 65% of these infections are produced by anaerobes, which are bacteria that do not need air or oxygen to live. The remaining cases are caused by a mixture of anaerobic and aerobic (air breathing) bacteria. When the bacteria arrive in the lung, they are engulfed or eaten by special cells called phagocytes. The phagocytes release chemicals that contribute to inflammation and eventual necrosis, or death, of a part of the lung tissue. There are several different ways that bacteria can get into the lung.

Aspiration

Aspiration refers to the accidental inhalation of material from the mouth or throat into the airway and lungs. It is responsible for about 50% of cases of lung abscess. The human mouth and gums contain large numbers of anaerobic bacteria; patients with **periodontal disease** or poor **oral hygiene** have higher concentrations of these organisms. Aspiration is most likely to occur in patients who are unconscious or semiconscious due to anesthesia, seizures, alcohol and drug **abuse**, or stroke. Patients who have problems swallowing or coughing, or who have nasogastric tubes in place are also at risk of aspiration.

Bronchial obstruction

The bronchi are the two branches of the windpipe that lead into the lungs. If they are blocked by tissue swelling, cancerous tumors, or **foreign objects**, a lung abscess may form from infection trapped behind the blockage.

Spread of infection

About 20% of cases of **pneumonia** that cause the death of lung tissue (necrotizing pneumonia) will develop into lung abscess. Lung abscess can also be caused by the spread of other infections from the liver, abdominal cavity, or open chest **wounds**. Rarely, **AIDS** patients can develop lung abscess from *Pneumocystis carinii* and other organisms that take advantage of a weakened immune system.

Lung abscess is usually slow to develop. It may take about two weeks after aspiration or bronchial obstruction for an abscess to produce noticeable symptoms. The patient may be acutely ill for two weeks to three months. In the beginning, the symptoms of lung abscess are difficult to distinguish from those of severe pneumonia. Adults will usually have moderate **fever** (101-102 °F/38-39 °C), chills, chest pain, and general weakness. Children may or may not have chest pain, but usually suffer weight loss and high fevers. As the illness progresses, about 75% of patients will **cough** up foul or musty-smelling sputum; some also cough up blood.

Lung abscess can lead to serious complications, including **emphysema**, spread of the abscess to other parts of the lung, hemorrhage, **adult respiratory distress syndrome**, rupture of the abscess, inflammation of the membrane surrounding the heart, or chronic inflammation of the lung.

Diagnosis

The diagnosis is made on the basis of the patient's medical history (especially recent operations under **general anesthesia**) and general health as well as imaging studies. Smears and cultures taken from the patient's sputum are not usually very helpful because they will be contaminated with bacteria from the mouth. The doctor will first use a bronchoscope (lighted tube inserted into the windpipe) to rule out the possibility of lung cancer. In some cases of serious infection, the doctor can use a fiberoptic bronchoscope with a protected specimen brush to take material directly from the patient's lungs, for identification of the organism. This technique is time- consuming and expensive, and requires the patient to be taken off **antibiotics** for 48 hours. It is usually used only to evaluate severely ill patients with weakened immune systems.

In most cases, the doctor will use the results of a **chest x ray** to help distinguish lung abscess from **empyema**, cancer, **tuberculosis**, or cysts. In patients with lung abscess, the x ray will show a thick-walled unified clear space or cavity surrounded by solid tissue. There is often a visible air-fluid level. The doctor may also order a CT scan of the chest, in order to have a clearer picture of the exact location of the abscess.

Blood tests cannot be used to make a diagnosis of lung abscess, but they can be useful in ruling out other conditions. Patients with lung abscess usually have abnormally high white blood cell counts (**leukocytosis**) when their blood is tested, but this condition is not unique to lung abscess.

Treatment

Lung abscess is treated with a combination of antibiotic drugs, **oxygen therapy**, and surgery. The antibiotics that are usually given for lung abscess are penicillin G, penicillin V, and clindamycin. They are given intravenously until the patient shows signs of improvement, and then continued in oral form. The patient may need to take antibiotics for a month or longer, until the chest x ray indicates that the abscess is healing. Oxygen may be given to patients who are having trouble breathing.

Surgical treatment

Most patients with lung abscess will not need surgery. About 5% of patients–usually those who do not respond to antibiotics or are coughing up large amounts of blood (500 mL or more)–may have emergency surgery for removal of the diseased part of the lung or for insertion of a tube to drain the abscess. Antibiotic treatment is considered to have failed if fever and other symptoms continue after 10-14 days of treatment; if chest x rays indicate that the abscess is not shrinking; or if the patient has pneumonia that is spreading to other parts of the lung.

Supportive care

Because lung abscess is a serious condition, patients need quiet and bed rest. Hospital care usually includes increasing the patient's fluid intake to loosen up the secretions in the lungs, and physical therapy to strengthen the patient's breathing muscles.

Follow-up

Patients with lung abscess need careful follow-up care after the acute infection subsides. Follow-up usually includes a series of chest x rays to make sure that the infection has cleared up. Treatment with antibiotics may continue for as long as four months, to prevent recurrence.

Prognosis

About 95% of lung abscess patients can be treated successfully with antibiotics alone. Patients who need surgical treatment have a mortality rate of 10-15%.

Prevention

Some of the conditions that make people more vulnerable to lung abscess concern long-term lifestyle behaviors, such as substance abuse and lack of dental care. Others, however, are connected with chronic illness and hospitalization. Aspiration can be prevented with proper care of unconscious patients, which includes suctioning of throat secretions and positioning patients to promote drainage. Patients who are conscious can be given physical therapy to help them cough up material in their lungs and airways. Patients

KEY TERMS

Abscess—An area of injured body tissue that fills with pus, as in lung abscess.

Anaerobe—A type of bacterium that does not require air or oxygen to live. Anaerobic bacteria are frequent causes of lung abscess.

Aspiration—Inhalation of fluid or foreign bodies into the airway or lungs. Aspiration often happens after vomiting.

Bronchoscope—A lighted, flexible tube inserted into the windpipe to view the bronchi or withdraw fluid samples for testing. Bronchoscopy with a protected brush can be used in the diagnosis of lung abscess in severely ill patients.

Bronchus—One of the two large tubes connecting the windpipe and the lungs.

Leukocytosis—An increased level of white cells in the blood. Leukocytosis is a common reaction to infections, including lung abscess.

Necrotizing pneumonia—Pneumonia that causes the death of lung tissue. It often precedes the development of lung abscess.

Sputum—The substance that is brought up from the lungs and airway when a person coughs or spits. It is usually a mixture of saliva and mucus, but may contain blood or pus in patients with lung abscess or other diseases of the lungs.

with weakened immune systems can be isolated from patients with pneumonia or fungal infections.

Resources

BOOKS

Stauffer, John L. "Lung." In *Current Medical Diagnosis and Treatment, 1998*, edited by Stephen McPhee, et al., 37th ed. Stamford: Appleton & Lange, 1997.

Rebecca J. Frey, PhD

Lung biopsy

Definition

Lung biopsy is a medical procedure performed to obtain a small piece of lung tissue for examination under a microscope. Biopsy examinations are usually performed by pathologists, who are doctors with special training in tissue abnormalities and other signs of disease.

Purpose

Lung biopsies are useful, first of all, in confirming a diagnosis of **cancer**, especially if malignant cells are detected in the patient's sputum. A lung biopsy may be ordered to examine other abnormalities that appear on chest x rays, such as lumps (nodules). It is also helpful in diagnosing symptoms such as coughing up bloody sputum, **wheezing** in the chest, or difficult breathing. In addition to evaluating lung tumors and their associated symptoms, lung biopsies can be used in the diagnosis of lung infections, especially **tuberculosis**, drug reactions, and such chronic diseases of the lung as **sarcoidosis**.

A lung biopsy can be used for treatment as well as diagnosis. **Bronchoscopy**, which is a type of lung biopsy performed with a long slender instrument called a bronchoscope, can be used to clear a patient's air passages of secretions and to remove blockages from the airways.

Precautions

As with any other biopsy, lung biopsies should not be performed on patients who have problems with blood clotting because of low platelet counts. Platelets are small blood cells that play a role in the blood clotting process. If the patient has a **platelet count** lower than 50,000/cubic mm, he or she can be given a platelet **transfusion** as a temporary relief measure, and a biopsy can then be performed.

Description

Overview

The lungs are a pair of cone-shaped organs that lie in the chest cavity. An area known as the mediastinum separates the right and the left lungs from each other. The heart, the windpipe (trachea), the lymph nodes, and the tube that brings the food to the stomach (the esophagus) lie in this mediastinal cavity. Lung biopsies may involve entering the mediastinum, as well as the lungs themselves.

Types of lung biopsies

Lung biopsies can be performed using a variety of techniques. A bronchoscopy is ordered if a patch that looks suspicious on the x ray seems to be located deep in the chest. If the area lies close to the chest wall, a needle biopsy is often done. If both these methods fail to diagnose the problem, an open surgical biopsy may be carried out. If there are indications that the lung cancer has spread to the lymph nodes in the mediastinum, a **mediastinoscopy** is performed.

NEEDLE BIOPSY. When a needle biopsy is to be done, the patient will be given a sedative about an hour before the procedure, to help relaxation. The patient sits in a chair with arms folded on a table in front of him or her. X rays are then taken to identify the location of the suspicious areas. Small metal markers are placed on the overlying skin to mark the biopsy site. The skin is thoroughly cleansed with an antiseptic solution, and a local anesthetic is injected to numb the area.

The doctor then makes a small cut (incision) about half an inch in length. The patient is asked to take a deep breath and hold it while the doctor inserts the special biopsy needle through the incision into the lung. When enough tissue has been obtained, the needle is withdrawn. Pressure is applied at the biopsy site and a sterile bandage is placed over the cut. The entire procedure takes between 30 and 45 minutes.

The patient may feel a brief sharp **pain** or some pressure as the biopsy needle is inserted. Most patients, however, do not experience severe pain.

OPEN BIOPSY. Open biopsies are performed in a hospital under **general anesthesia**. As with needle biopsies, patients are given sedatives before the procedure. An intravenous line is placed in the arm to give medications or fluids as necessary. A hollow tube, called an endotracheal tube, is passed through the throat, into the airway leading to the lungs. It is used to convey the general anesthetic.

Once the patient is under the influence of the anesthesia, the surgeon makes an incision over the lung area. Some lung tissue is removed and the cut closed with stitches. The entire procedure usually takes about an hour. A chest tube is sometimes placed with one end inside the lung and the other end protruding through the closed incision. Chest tube placement is done to prevent the lungs from collapsing by removing the air from the lungs. The tube is removed a few days after the biopsy.

A **chest x ray** is done following an open biopsy, to check for lung collapse. The patient may experience some grogginess for a few hours after the procedure. He or she may also experience tiredness and muscle aches for a day or two, because of the general anesthesia. The throat may be sore because of the placement of the hollow endotracheal tube. The patient may also

have some pain or discomfort at the incision site, which can be relieved by medication.

MEDIASTINOSCOPY. The preparation for a mediastinoscopy is similar to that for an open biopsy. The patient is sedated and prepared for general anesthesia. The neck and the chest will be cleansed with an antiseptic solution.

After the patient has been put to sleep, an incision about two or three inches long is made at the base of the neck. A thin, hollow, lighted tube, called a mediastinoscope, is inserted through the cut into the space between the right and the left lungs. The doctor examines the space thoroughly and removes any lymph nodes or tissues that look abnormal. The mediastinoscope is then removed, and the incision stitched up and bandaged. A mediastinoscopy takes about an hour.

Preparation

Before scheduling any lung biopsy, the doctor will check to see if the patient is taking any prescription medications, if he or she has any medication **allergies**, and if there is a history of bleeding problems. Blood tests may be performed before the procedure to check for clotting problems and blood type, in case a transfusion becomes necessary.

If an open biopsy or a mediastinoscopy is being performed, the patient will be asked to sign a consent form. Since these procedures are done under general anesthesia, the patient will be asked to refrain from eating or drinking anything for at least 12 hours before the biopsy.

Aftercare

Needle biopsy

Following a needle biopsy, the patient is allowed to rest comfortably. He or she will be checked by a nurse at two-hour intervals. If there are no complications after four hours, the patient can go home. Patients are advised to rest at home for a day or two before resuming regular activities, and to avoid strenuous activities for a week after the biopsy.

Open biopsy or mediastinoscopy

After an open biopsy or a mediastinoscopy, patients are taken to a recovery room for observation. If no other complications develop, they are taken back to the hospital room. Stitches are usually removed after seven to 14 days.

If the patient has extreme pain, light-headedness, difficulty breathing, or develops a blue tinge to the skin after an open biopsy, the doctor should be notified immediately. The sputum may be slightly bloody for a day or two after the procedure. If, however, the bleeding is heavy or persistent, it should be brought to the attention of the doctor.

Risks

Needle biopsy

Needle biopsy is a less risky procedure than an open biopsy, because it does not involve general anesthesia. Very rarely, the lung may collapse because of air that leaks in through the hole made by the biopsy needle. If the lung collapses, a tube will have to be inserted into the chest to remove the air. Some coughing up of blood occurs in 5% of needle biopsies. Prolonged bleeding or infection may also occur, although these are very rare.

Open biopsy

Possible complications of an open biopsy include infection or lung collapse. **Death** occurs in about 1 in 3000 cases. If the patient has very severe breathing problems before the biopsy, breathing may be slightly impaired following the operation. If the person's lungs were functioning normally before the biopsy, the chances of any respiratory problems are very small.

Mediastinoscopy

Complications due to mediastinoscopy are rare; death occurs in fewer than 1 in 3000 cases. More common complications include lung collapse or bleeding caused by damage to the blood vessels near the heart. Injury to the esophagus or voice box (larynx) may sometimes occur. If the nerves leading to the larynx are injured, the patient may be left with a permanently hoarse voice. All of these complications are very rare.

Normal results

Normal results of a needle biopsy and an open biopsy include the absence of any evidence of infection in the lungs. No lumps or nodules will be detected in the lungs and the cells will not show any cancerous abnormalities. Normal results from the mediastinoscopy will show the lymph nodes to be free of cancer.

Abnormal results

Abnormal results may be associated with diseases other than cancer. Nodules in the lungs may

KEY TERMS

Bronchoscopy—A medical test that enables the doctor to see the breathing passages and the lungs through a hollow, lighted tube.

Endotracheal tube—A hollow tube that is inserted into the windpipe to administer anesthesia.

Lymph nodes—Small, bean-shaped structures scattered along the lymphatic vessels which serve as filters. Lymph nodes retain any bacteria or cancer cells that are traveling through the system.

Mediastinoscopy—A medical procedure that allows the doctor to see the organs in the mediastinal space using a thin, lighted, hollow tube (a mediastinoscope).

Mediastinum—The area between the lungs, bounded by the spine, breastbone, and diaphragm.

Sputum—Mucus or phlegm that is coughed up from the passageways (bronchial tubes) in the lungs.

be due to active infections such as tuberculosis, or may be **scars** from a previous infection. The lung cells on microscopic examination do not resemble normal cells, and show certain abnormalities that point to cancer. In a third of biopsies using a mediastinoscope, the lymph nodes that are biopsied prove to be cancerous. Abnormal results should always be considered in the context of the patient's medical history, **physical examination**, and other tests such as sputum examination, chest x rays, etc. before a final diagnosis is made.

Resources

ORGANIZATIONS

American Cancer Society. 1599 Clifton Rd., NE, Atlanta, GA 30329-4251. (800) 227-2345. <http://www.cancer.org>.

American Lung Association. 1740 Broadway, New York, NY 10019. (800) 586-4872. <http://www.lungusa.org>.

Cancer Research Institute. 681 Fifth Ave., New York, N.Y. 10022. (800) 992-2623. <http://www.cancerresearch.org>.

National Cancer Institute. Building 31, Room 10A31, 31 Center Drive, MSC 2580, Bethesda, MD 20892-2580. (800) 422-6237. <http://www.nci.nih.gov>.

Lata Cherath, PhD

Lung cancer, non-small cell

Definition

Non-small cell lung **cancer** (NSCLC) is a disease in which the cells of the lung tissues grow uncontrollably and form tumors.

Description

There are two kinds of lung cancers, primary and secondary. Primary lung cancer starts in the lung itself, and is divided into **small cell lung cancer** and non-small cell lung cancer. Small cell lung cancers are shaped like an oat and called oat-cell cancers; they are aggressive, spread rapidly, and represent 20% of lung cancers. Non-small cell lung cancer represents almost 80% of all primary lung cancers. Secondary lung cancer is cancer that starts somewhere else in the body (for example, the breast or colon) and spreads to the lungs.

The lungs

The lungs are located along with the heart in the chest cavity. The lungs are not simply hollow balloons but have a very organized structure consisting of hollow tubes, blood vessels and elastic tissue. The hollow tubes, called bronchi, are highly branched, becoming smaller and more numerous at each branching. They end in tiny, blind sacs made of elastic tissue called alveoli. These sacs are where the oxygen a person breathes in is taken up into the blood, and where carbon dioxide moves out of the blood to be breathed out.

Normal healthy lungs are continually secreting mucus that not only keeps the lungs moist, but also protects the lungs by trapping foreign particles like dust and dirt in breathed air. The inside of the lungs is covered with small hairlike structures called cilia. The cilia move in such a way that mucus is swept up out of the lungs and into the throat.

Lung cancer

Most lung cancers start in the cells that line the bronchi, and can take years to develop. As they grow larger they prevent the lungs from functioning normally. The tumor can reduce the capacity of the lungs, or block the movement of air through the bronchi in the lungs. As a result, less oxygen gets into the blood and patients feel short of breath. Tumors may also block the normal movement of mucus up into the throat. As a result, mucus builds up in the lungs and infection may develop behind the tumor. Once lung cancer has developed it frequently spreads to other parts of the body.

The speed at which non-small cell tumors grow depends on the type of cells that make up the tumor. The following three types account for the vast majority of non-small cell tumors:

- Adenocarcinomas are the most common and often cause no symptoms. Frequently they are not found until they are advanced.

- Squamous cell carcinomas usually produce symptoms because they are centrally located and block the lungs.

- Undifferentiated large cell and giant cell carcinomas tend to grow rapidly, and spread quickly to other parts of the body.

Worldwide, lung cancer is the most common cancer in males, and the fifth most common cancer in women. The worldwide mortality rate for patients with lung cancer is 86%. In the United States, lung cancer is the leading cause of **death** from cancer among both men and women. The World Health Organization estimates that the worldwide mortality from lung cancer will increase to three million by the year 2025. Of those three million deaths, almost two and a half million will result from non-small cell lung cancer.

The American Cancer Society (ACS) estimates that 173,770 Americans will develop lung cancer in 2004, 93,110 men and 80,660 women. Of these patients, 160,440 will die of the disease.

The incidence of lung cancer is beginning to fall in developed countries. This may be a result of antismoking campaigns. In developing countries, however, rates continue to rise, which may be a consequence of both industrialization and the increasing use of tobacco products.

Causes and symptoms

Causes

Tobacco **smoking** accounts for 87% of all lung cancers. Giving up tobacco can prevent most lung cancers. Smoking **marijuana** cigarettes is considered another risk factor for cancer of the lung. Second hand smoke also contributes to the development of lung cancer among nonsmokers.

Certain hazardous materials that people may be exposed to in their jobs have been shown to cause lung cancer. These include asbestos, coal products, and radioactive substances. Air pollution may also be a contributing factor. Exposure to radon, a colorless, odorless gas that sometimes accumulates in the basement of homes, may cause lung cancer in a tiny minority of patients. In addition, patients whose lungs are scarred from other lung conditions may have an increased risk of developing lung cancer.

Symptoms

Lung cancers tend to spread very early, and only 15% are detected in their early stages. The chances of early detection, however, can be improved by seeking medical care at once if any of the following symptoms appear:

- a **cough** that does not go away
- chest **pain**
- **shortness of breath**
- recurrent lung infections, such as **bronchitis** or pneumonia
- bloody or brown-colored spit or phlegm (sputum)
- persistent hoarseness
- significant weight loss that is not due to dieting or vigorous **exercise**; **fatigue** and loss of appetite
- unexplained fever

Although these symptoms may be caused by diseases other than lung cancer, it is important to consult a doctor to rule out the possibility of lung cancer.

If lung cancer has spread to other organs, the patient may have other symptoms such as headaches, bone **fractures**, pain, bleeding, or **blood clots**.

Diagnosis

Physical examination and diagnostic tests

The doctor will first take a detailed medical history and assess risk factors. During a complete **physical examination** the doctor will examine the patient's throat to rule out other possible causes of hoarseness or coughing, and will listen to the patient's breathing and chest sounds.

If the doctor has reason to suspect lung cancer, particularly if the patient has a history of heavy smoking or occupational exposure to irritating substances, a **chest x ray** may be ordered to see if there are any masses in the lungs. Special imaging techniques, such as computed tomography (CT) scans or **magnetic resonance imaging** (MRI), may provide more precise information about the size, shape, and location of any tumors.

Sputum analysis

Sputum analysis is a noninvasive test that involves microscopic examination of cells that are coughed up from the lungs. This test can diagnose at least 30% of lung cancers, even if tumors are not visible on chest x rays. In addition, the test can detect cancer in its very early stages, before it spreads to other regions. The sputum test does not provide any information about the location of the tumor.

Lung biopsy

Lung biopsy is the most definitive diagnostic tool for cancer. It can be performed in three different ways. **Bronchoscopy** involves the insertion of a slender, lighted tube, called a bronchoscope, down the patient's throat and into the lungs. This test allows the doctor to see the tubes inside the lungs, and to obtain samples of lung tissue. If a needle biopsy is to be performed, the location of the tumor is first identified using a computerized tomography (CT) scan or magnetic resonance imaging (MRI). The doctor then inserts a needle through the chest wall and collects a sample of tissue from the tumor. In the third procedure, known as surgical biopsy, the chest wall is opened up and a part of the tumor, or all of it, is removed. A doctor who specializes in the study of diseased tissue (a pathologist) examines the tumor to identify the cancer's type and stage.

Treatment

Staging

Treatment for non-small cell lung cancer depends primarily on the stage of the cancer. Staging is a process that tells the doctor if the cancer has spread and the extent of its spread. The most commonly used treatments are surgery, **radiation therapy**, and **chemotherapy**.

Non-small cell lung cancer has six stages:

- Occult carcinoma. Cancer cells have been found in the sputum, but no tumor has yet been found.
- Stage 0. A small group of cancerous cells have been found in one location.
- Stage I. The cancer is only in the lung and has not spread anywhere else.
- Stage II. The cancer has spread to nearby lymph nodes.
- Stage III. The cancer has spread to more distant lymph nodes, and/or other parts of the chest like the diaphragm.
- Stage IV. The cancer has spread to other parts of the body.

Surgery

Surgery is the standard treatment for the earlier stages of non-small cell lung cancer. The surgeon will decide on the type of surgery, depending on how much of the lung is affected. There are three different types of surgical procedures:

- Wedge resection is the removal of a small part of the lung.
- Lobectomy is the removal of one lobe of the lung. (The right lung has three lobes and the left lung has two lobes.)
- Pneumonectomy is the removal of an entire lung.

Lung surgery is a major procedure and patients can expect to experience pain, weakness in the chest, and shortness of breath. Air and fluid collect in the chest after surgery. As a result, patients will need help to turn over, cough, and breath deeply. Patients should be encouraged to perform these activities because they help get rid of the air and fluid and speed up recovery. It can take patients several months before they regain their energy and strength.

Radiotherapy

Patients whose cancer has progressed too far for surgery (Stages III and IV) may receive radiotherapy. Radiotherapy involves the use of high-energy rays to kill cancer cells. It is used either by itself or in combination with surgery or chemotherapy. The amount of radiation used depends on the size and the location of the tumor.

Radiation therapy may produce such side effects as tiredness, skin **rashes**, upset stomach, and **diarrhea**. Dry or sore throats, difficulty in swallowing, and loss of hair in the treated area are all minor side effects of radiation. These may disappear either during the course of the treatment or after the treatment is over.

Chemotherapy

Chemotherapy is also given to patients whose cancer has progressed too far for surgery. Chemotherapy is medication that is usually given intravenously to kill cancer cells. These drugs enter the bloodstream and travel to all parts of the body, killing cancer cells that have spread to different organs. Chemotherapy is used as the primary treatment for cancers that have spread beyond the lung and cannot be removed by surgery. It can also be used in addition to surgery or radiation therapy.

Chemotherapy for NSCLC has made significant advances since the early 1980s in improving the patient's quality of life as well as length of survival. Newer cytotoxic (cell-killing) agents developed in the 1990s, such as the taxanes, are typically combined with either cisplatin or carboplatin as first-line therapy for non-small cell lung cancer.

Newer drugs for lung cancer developed since 2000 include gefinitib (Iressa) and pemetrexed (Alimta). The FDA approved gefinitib in May 2003 as a treatment for patients with NSCLC who have not responded to platinum-based or taxane chemotherapy. It is taken by mouth and works by inhibiting an enzyme involved in the growth of tumor cells. Pemetrexed, which is given by injection, was approved by the FDA in February 2004 for the treatment of **mesothelioma**, a type of lung cancer caused by exposure to asbestos fibers. However, the drug appears to be effective in treating other types of lung cancer as well.

Chemotherapy is also used as palliative treatment for non-small cell lung cancer. Palliative refers to any type of therapy that is given to relieve the symptoms of a disease but not to cure it.

Chemotherapy for non-small cell lung cancer often has severe side effects, including **nausea and vomiting**, hair loss, anemia, weakening of the immune system, and sometimes **infertility**. Most of these side effects end when the treatment is over. Other medications can be given to lessen the unpleasant side effects of chemotherapy.

Alternative treatment

Because non-small cell lung cancer has a poor prognosis with conventional medical treatment, many patients are willing to try complementary and alternative therapies. These therapies are used to try to reduce **stress**, ease side effects and symptoms, or control disease. Two treatments sometimes used are shark cartilage and mistletoe. Although shark cartilage is thought to interfere with the tumor's blood supply, clinical trials have so far been inconclusive. Mistletoe is a poisonous plant that has been shown to kill cancer cells in the laboratory. Again, however, clinical trials with cancer patients have been inconclusive.

Patients who decide to try complementary and alternative therapies should tell their doctor. Some of these therapies may interfere with conventional treatment.

Prognosis

The prognosis for non-small cell lung cancer is better if the disease is found early, and removed

KEY TERMS

Bronchi—The tubes that carry air into the lungs.

Lymph—Clear fluid containing white blood cells that is collected from the tissues of the body and flows in vessels called the lymphatic system.

Lymph node—Small oval-shaped filters in the lymphatic system that trap bacteria and other unwanted particles to ensure their removal from the body.

Palliative—Referring to any type of treatment that is given to relieve the symptoms of a disease rather than to cure it.

Respiratory distress—A condition in which patients with lung disease are not able to get enough oxygen.

surgically. For patients whose disease is caught in Stage I, the survival rate five years after surgery ranges from 60% to 80%. Up to 55% of Stage II patients are alive after five years, but only about 30% of Stage III patients make it to five years. Unfortunately, 85% of patients already have at least Stage III cancer by the time they are diagnosed. Many of these patients have disease that is too advanced for surgery. Despite treatment with radiotherapy and chemotherapy, the five-year survival for patients with inoperable disease is extremely low.

Prevention

The best way to prevent lung cancer is not to start smoking or to quit smoking. Secondhand smoke from other people's tobacco should also be avoided. Appropriate precautions should be taken when working with cancer-causing substances (carcinogens). Testing houses for the presence of radon gas, and removing asbestos from buildings have also been suggested as preventive strategies.

Resources

BOOKS

Beers, Mark H., MD, and Robert Berkow, MD., editors. "Bronchogenic Carcinoma." In *The Merck Manual of Diagnosis and Therapy*. Whitehouse Station, NJ: Merck Research Laboratories, 2004.

Brambilla, Christian, and Elisabeth Brambilla, editors. *Lung Tumors. Fundamental Biology and Clinical Management*. New York: Marcel Dekker, 1999.

Skarin, Harry S., editor. *Multimodality Treatment of Lung Cancer*. New York: Marcel Dekker, 2000.

PERIODICALS

Carney, Desmond N., and Heine H. Hansen. "Non-Small-Cell Lung Cancer: Stalemate or Progress?" *New England Journal of Medicine* 343, no. 17 (26 October 2000): 1261–3.

Cohen, M. H., G. A. Williams, R. Sridhara, et al. "United States Food and Drug Administration Drug Approval Summary: Gefitinib (ZD1839; Iressa) Tablets." *Clinical Cancer Research* 10 (February 15, 2004): 1212–1218.

Deslauriers, Jean, and Jocelyn Gregoire. "Clinical and Surgical Staging of Non-Small Cell Lung Cancer." *Chest* 117, no. 4, Supplement 1 (April 2000): 96S–103S.

Fossella, F. V. "Pemetrexed for Treatment of Advanced Non-Small Cell Lung Cancer." *Seminars in Oncology* 31 (February 2004): 100–105.

Frampton, J. E., and S. E. Easthope. "Gefitinib: A Review of Its Use in the Management of Advanced Non-Small-Cell Lung Cancer." *Drugs* 64 (2004): 2475–2492.

Johnson, David H. "Locally Advanced, Unresectable Non-Small Cell Lung Cancer. New Treatment Strategies." *Chest* 117, no.4, Supplement 1 (April 2000): 123S–126S.

Ramalingam, S., and C. P. Belani. "State-of-the-Art Chemotherapy for Advanced Non-Small Cell Lung Cancer." *Seminars in Oncology* 31 (February 2004): 68–74.

Rigas, J. R. "Taxane-Platinum Combinations in Advanced Non-Small Cell Lung Cancer: A Review." *Oncologist* 9, Supplement 2 (2004): 16–23.

ORGANIZATIONS

Alliance for Lung Cancer Advocacy, Support and Education. PO Box 849 Vancouver, WA 98666. (800) 298-2436. < http://www.alcase.org >.

American Lung Association. 1740 Broadway New York, NY 10019. (212) 315-8700. < http://www.lungusa.org >.

National Cancer Institute (National Institutes of Health). 9000 Rockville Pike, Bethesda, MD 20892. (800) 422-6237. < http://www.nci.nih.gov >.

National Center for Complementary and Alternative Medicine (National Institutes of Health). PO Box 8218, Silver Spring, MD 20907-8218. (888) 644-6226. < http://nccam.nih.gov >.

OTHER

American Cancer Society (ACS). *Cancer Facts & Figures 2004*. < http://www.cancer.org/downloads/STT/CAFF_finalPWSecured.pdf >.

FDA News, February 5, 2004. "FDA Approves First Drug for Rare Type of Cancer." < http://www.fda.gov/bbs/topics/NEWS/2004/NEW01018.html >.

Lata Cherath, PhD
Alison McTavish, M.Sc.
Rebecca J. Frey, PhD

Lung cancer, small cell

Definition

Small cell lung **cancer** is a disease in which the cells of the lung tissues grow uncontrollably and form tumors.

Description

Lung cancer is divided into two main types: small cell and non-small cell. Small cell lung cancer is the least common of the two, accounting for only about 20% of all lung cancers. In the past, the disease was called oat cell cancer because, when viewed under a microscope, the cancer cells resemble oats. This type of lung cancer grows quickly and is more likely to spread to other organs in the body.

The lungs are located along with the heart in the chest cavity. The lungs are not simply hollow balloons, but have a very organized structure consisting of hollow tubes, blood vessels, and elastic tissue. The hollow tubes, called bronchi, are multi-branched, becoming smaller and more numerous at each branching. They end in tiny, blind sacs made of elastic tissue called alveoli. These sacs are where the oxygen a person breathes in is taken up into the blood, and where carbon dioxide moves out of the blood to be breathed out.

Normal, healthy lungs are continually secreting mucus that not only keeps the lungs moist, but also protects the lungs by trapping foreign particles like dust and dirt in breathed air. The inside of the lungs is covered with small, hair-like structures called cilia. The cilia move in such a way that mucus is swept up out of the lungs and into the throat.

Small cell lung tumors usually start to develop in the central bronchi. They grow quickly and prevent the lungs from functioning at their full capacity. Tumors may block the movement of air through the bronchi in the lungs. As a result, less oxygen gets into the blood and patients feel short of breath. Tumors may also block the normal movement of mucus into the throat. As a result, mucus builds up in the lungs and infection may develop behind the tumor.

Lung cancer is a growing global epidemic. Worldwide, lung cancer is the second most common cancer among both men and women and is the leading cause of cancer **death** in both sexes. The worldwide mortality rate for patients with lung cancer is 86%. Of the 160,000 deaths from lung cancer that occur annually in the United States, about 40,000 are caused by small cell lung cancer. Although there are differences in mortality rates between ethnic groups, this is mainly due to differences in **smoking** habits.

Causes and symptoms

Causes

Tobacco smoking accounts for nearly 90% of all lung cancers. The risk of developing lung cancer is increased for smokers who start at a young age, and for those who have smoked for a long time. The risk also increases as more cigarettes are smoked, and when cigarettes with higher tar content are smoked. Smoking **marijuana** cigarettes is also a risk factor for lung cancer. These cigarettes have a higher tar content than tobacco cigarettes.

Certain hazardous materials that people may be exposed to in their jobs have been shown to cause lung cancer. These include asbestos, coal products, and radioactive substances. Air pollution may also be a contributing factor. Exposure to radon, a colorless, odorless gas that sometimes accumulates in the basement of homes, may cause lung cancer in some patients. In addition, patients whose lungs are scarred from other lung conditions may have an increased risk of developing lung cancer.

Although the exact cause of lung cancer is not known, people with a family history of lung cancer appear to have a slightly higher risk of contracting the disease.

Symptoms

Small cell lung cancer is an aggressive disease that spreads quickly. Symptoms depend on the tumor's location within the lung, and on whether the cancer has spread to other parts of the body. More than 80% of small cell lung cancer patients have symptoms for only three months or less, and few cases are detected early. The following symptoms are the most commonly reported by small cell lung cancer patients at the time of their diagnosis:

- a persistent **cough**
- chest **pain**
- **shortness of breath** and wheezing
- persistent hoarseness
- fatigue and loss of appetite

Although some patients may experience bloody spit or phlegm, this symptom is more commonly seen in patients with other types of lung cancer.

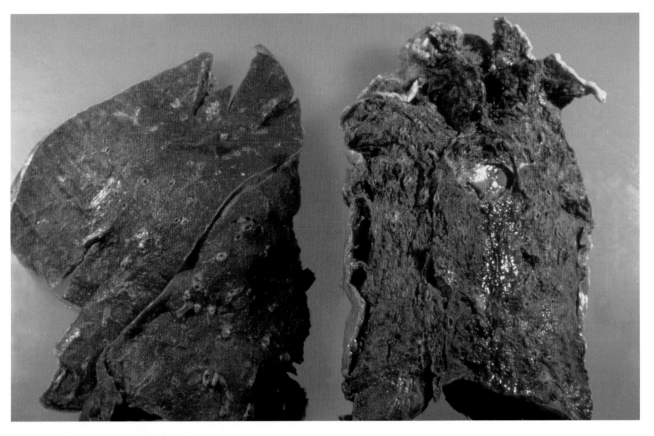

A normal lung (left) and the lung of a cigarette smoker (right). *(Photograph by A. Glauberman, Photo Researchers, Inc. Reproduced by permission.)*

Small cell tumors often press against a large blood vessel near the lungs called the superior vena cava (SVC), causing a condition known as SCV syndrome. This condition may cause patients to retain water, cough, and have shortness of breath. Because small cell lung cancer often spreads quickly to the bones and central nervous system, patients may also have bone pain, headaches, and seizures.

Diagnosis

If lung cancer is suspected, the doctor will take a detailed medical history that checks both symptoms and risk factors. During a complete **physical examination**, the doctor will examine the patient's throat to rule out other possible causes of hoarseness or coughing, and listen to the patient's breathing and the sounds made when the patient's chest and upper back are tapped. A **chest x ray** may be ordered to check for masses in the lungs. Special imaging techniques, such as computed tomography (CT) scans or **magnetic resonance imaging** (MRI), may provide more precise information about the size, shape, and location of any tumors.

Sputum analysis involves microscopic examination of the cells that are either coughed up from the lungs, or are collected through a special instrument called a bronchoscope. The sputum test does not, however, provide any information about the location of the tumor and must be followed by other tests.

Lung biopsy is the most definitive diagnostic tool for cancer. It can be performed in several different ways. The doctor can perform a **bronchoscopy**, which involves the insertion of a slender, lighted tube, called a bronchoscope, down the patient's throat and into the lungs. In addition to viewing the passageways of the lungs, the doctor can use the bronchoscope to obtain samples of the lung tissue. In another procedure known as a needle biopsy, the location of the tumor is first identified using a CT scan or MRI. The doctor then inserts a needle through the chest wall and collects a sample of tissue from the tumor. In the third procedure, known as surgical biopsy, the chest wall is opened up and a part of the tumor, or all of it, is removed for examination.

Treatment

Staging

Staging procedures are important in lung cancer because they tell doctors whether patients have disease only in their lungs, or whether the cancer has spread to other parts of the body. To establish the cancer stage, doctors have to perform various tests. These may include **bone marrow aspiration and biopsy**, CT scans of the chest and abdomen, MRI scans of the brain, and radionuclide bone scans. All of these tests determine the extent to which the cancer has spread. Once the stage is determined, doctors can decide on a course of treatment, and can have a better idea of the patient's prognosis.

Unlike other types of lung cancer, the staging of small cell lung cancer is relatively simple. This is because approximately 70% of patients already have metastatic disease when they are diagnosed, and small differences in the amount of tumor found in the lungs do not change the prognosis. Small cell lung cancer is usually divided into three stages:

• Limited stage: The cancer is found only in one lung and in lymph nodes close to the lung.

• Extensive stage: The cancer has spread beyond the lungs to other parts of the body.

• Recurrent stage: The cancer has returned following treatment.

Without treatment, small cell lung cancer has the most aggressive clinical course of any type of pulmonary tumor, with median survival from diagnosis of only 2–4 months. Compared with other cell types of lung cancer, small cell lung cancer has a greater tendency to be widely disseminated by the time of diagnosis, but is much more responsive to **chemotherapy** and irradiation.

Treatment of small cell lung cancer depends on whether the patient has limited, extensive, or recurrent disease. Treatment usually involves radiotherapy and chemotherapy. Surgery is rarely used for this type of lung cancer because the tumor is usually too advanced.

Patients with limited-stage disease are usually treated with chemotherapy. Combinations of two or more drugs have a better effect than treatment with a single drug. Up to 90% of patients with this stage of disease will respond to chemotherapy. The chemotherapy most commonly prescribed is a combination of the drugs etoposide (Vepesid) and cisplatin (Platinol). Combining chemotherapy with chest radiotherapy and/or occasionally surgery has also prolonged survival for limited-stage patients.

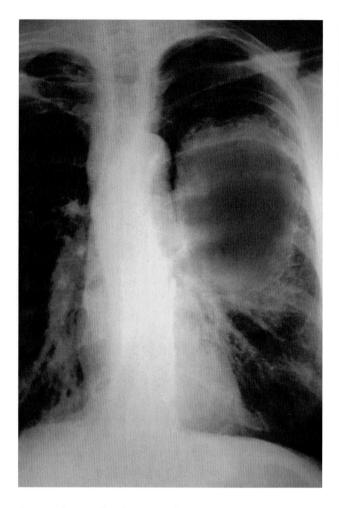

An x-ray image showing an oval-shaped carcinoma in the left lung (right of image). *(Custom Medical Stock Photo. Reproduced by permission.)*

In addition to chest radiotherapy, some patients are also treated with **radiation therapy** to the brain, even if no cancer is found there. This treatment, called prophylactic cranial irradiation (PCI), is given to prevent tumors from forming in the brain. The combination of etoposide and cisplatin chemotherapy with chest radiation therapy and PCI has increased the two-year survival of limited-stage small cell lung cancer patients to almost 50%.

Combinations of different chemotherapy agents are also used for treating extensive-stage small cell lung cancer. However, compared with limited-stage patients, the percentage of extensive-stage patients who respond to therapy is lower. Commonly used drug combinations include cyclophosphamide (Cytoxan), doxorubicin (Adriamycin), and vincristine (Oncovin), or etoposide and cisplatin. The addition of radiation therapy to chemotherapy does not improve

KEY TERMS

Bronchi—Hollow tubes that carry air into the lungs.

PCI—A type of radiotherapy that is used to prevent tumors from growing in the brain.

Radionuclide bone scan—A test that tells if cancer has spread to the bones.

Superior vena cava (SVC) syndrome—A condition seen in lung cancer patients where the tumor presses against a large blood vessel and causes various symptoms.

survival in these patients. However, radiation therapy is used for the palliative (pain relief) treatment of symptoms of metastatic lung cancer, particularly brain and bone tumors.

Patients who have recurrent small cell lung cancer often become resistant to chemotherapy. These patients are treated with palliative radiotherapy. Their doctor may also recommend that they take part in a clinical trial of a new therapy. Patients whose relapse occurs more than six months after their initial treatment, however, may still respond to traditional chemotherapy.

Alternative treatment

Many cancer patients have tried using shark cartilage to treat their disease. Shark cartilage is thought to interfere with the tumor's blood supply. A clinical trial using this treatment in lung cancer patients is ongoing. Information on this and other alternative treatments is available on the Internet from the National Center for Complementary and Alternative Medicine.

Patients who decide to try complementary and alternative therapies should tell their doctor. Some of these therapies may interfere with conventional treatment.

Prognosis

Small cell lung cancer is a very aggressive disease. Without treatment, limited-stage patients will survive for three to six months, while extensive-stage patients will survive six to 12 weeks. However, small cell lung cancer is much more responsive to chemotherapy and radiation therapy than other types of lung cancer. Among patients treated with chemotherapy, 70–90% have a major response to treatment.

Survival in patients responding to therapy is four to five times longer than in patients without treatment. In addition, two years after the start of therapy, about 10% of patients remain free of disease. In general, women tend to have a better prognosis than men. Patients whose disease has spread to the central nervous system or liver have a much worse prognosis. Although the overall survival at five years is 5% to 10%, survival is higher in patients with limited stage disease. About 70% of patients who are disease free after two years do not relapse. After five to 10 disease-free years, relapses are rare.

Prevention

The best way to prevent lung cancer is either not start smoking, or quit smoking. Secondhand smoke from other people's tobacco should also be avoided. Appropriate precautions should be taken when working with substances that can cause cancer (carcinogens). Testing houses for the presence of radon gas, and removing asbestos from buildings have also been suggested as preventive strategies.

Resources

BOOKS

Pass, Harvey I., et al. *Lung Cancer Principles and Practice.* Philadelphia: Lippincott Williams and Wilkins, 2000.

PERIODICALS

Adjei, Alex A., et al. "Current Guidelines for the Management of Small Cell Lung Cancer." *Mayo Clinic Proceedings* 74 (August 1999): 809-16.

Sandler, Alan. "Extensive Small Cell Lung Cancer: A Treatment Overview." *Oncology* 14, no. 7, Supplement 5 (July 2000): 49-55.

Tamura, Tomohide. "New State of the Art in Small Cell Lung Cancer." *Oncology* 15, no. 1, Supplement 1 (January 2001): 8-10.

ORGANIZATIONS

Alliance for Lung Cancer Advocacy, Support, and Education. P.O. Box 849, Vancouver, WA 98666. (800) 298-2436. < http://www.alcase.org >.

American Lung Association.1740 Broadway New York, NY 10019. (212) 315-8700. < http://www.lungusa.org >.

National Cancer Institute (National Institutes of Health). 9000 Rockville Pike, Bethesda, MD 20892. (800) 422-6237. < http://www.nci.nih.gov >.

National Center for Complementary and Alternative Medicine (National Institutes of Health). P.O. Box 8218, Silver Spring, MD 20907-8218. (888) 644-6226. < http://nccam.nih.gov >.

Lata Cherath, PhD
Alison McTavish, MSc

Lung diseases due to gas or chemical exposure

Definition

Lung diseases due to gas or chemical exposure are conditions that can be acquired from indoor and outdoor air pollution and from ingesting tobacco smoke.

Description

The lungs are susceptible to many airborne poisons and irritants. Mucus present in the airways blocks foreign particles of a certain size, however it is unable to filter all airborne particulates. There are hundreds of substances that can pollute air and harm lungs. Harmful gases and chemicals are just one type of airborne pollutant that can adversely affect the lungs. They include:

- Vehicle exhaust
- Localized pollutants such as arsenic, asbestos, lead, and mercury
- Outdoor pollutants caused by industry and intensified by weather conditions
- Household heating, such as wood-burning stoves
- Household chemical products
- Tobacco smoke.

Lungs respond to irritants in four ways, each of which can occur separately or, more often, trigger other responses.

- **Asthma** occurs when irritation causes the smooth muscles surrounding the airways to constrict.
- Increased mucus comes from irritated mucus glands lining the airway. Excess mucus clogs the airway and prevents air from circulating.
- Constriction of the lungs results from scarring when the supporting tissues are damaged.
- **Cancer** is caused by certain irritants, such as asbestos and tobacco smoke.

The major categories that airborne irritants fall into are allergic, organic, inorganic, and poisonous, with many agents occupying more than one category.

- Allergic irritants bother only people who are sensitive to them. Cat hair, insect parts, and pollen are common allergens. Chemicals called sulfites, which are widely used as food preservatives, also cause asthma.

- There are many organic dusts that irritate the lungs. Most of them occur on the job and cause occupational lung disease. Grain dust causes silo filler's disease. Cotton and other textile dusts cause **byssinosis**. Mold spores in hay cause farmer's lung.
- Inorganic dusts and aerosolized chemicals also are found mostly on the job. Classic among them are asbestos and coal dust. Many metals (cadmium, arsenic, chromium, and phosphorus), various other fine particles (cement, mica, rock), acid fumes, ammonia, ozone, and automobile and industrial emissions are part of a very long list.
- While tobacco smoke is a culprit in many smokers, a 2003 report found that those who work in the tobacco industry experience higher incidence of lung disease from tobacco dust in their work environment.
- Most intentional poisons (cyanide, nerve gas) that enter through the lungs pass through and damage other parts of the body. Mustard gas, used during World War I and banned since, directly and immediately destroys lungs.
- Tobacco use **scars** the lungs and causes **emphysema** and lung cancer.

Causes and symptoms

Lung disease generates three major symptoms–coughing, **wheezing**, and **shortness of breath**. It also predisposes the lungs to infections such as **bronchitis** and **pneumonia**. Cancer is a late effect, requiring prolonged exposure to an irritant. In the case of tobacco, an average of a pack of cigarettes a day for forty years, or two packs a day for twenty years, will greatly increase the risk of lung cancer.

Diagnosis

A history of exposure combined with a **chest x ray** and lung function studies completes the diagnostic evaluation in most cases. Lung function measures the amount of air breathed in and out, the speed it moves, and the effectiveness of oxygen exchange with the blood. If the cause still is unclear, a **lung biopsy** aids diagnosis.

Treatment

Eliminating the offending irritant and early **antibiotics** for infection are primary. There are many techniques available to remove excess mucus from the lungs. Respiratory therapists are trained in these methods. Finally, there are several machines available to enrich the oxygen content of breathed air.

A surgical treatment called lung reduction volume surgery is emerging as a treatment for certain people over age 65 with severe emphysema. It promises substantial return of lung function for selected patients by cutting away diseased parts of the lungs so that healthy tissue functions better. In the fall of 2003, Medicare announced that it would begin paying for the surgery.

Prognosis

Many of these diseases are progressive, because the irritants stay in the lungs forever. Others remain stable after the offensive agents are removed from the environment. Lungs do not heal from destructive damage, but they can clean out infection and excess mucus, and function better.

Prevention

Industrial air filters, adequate ventilation, and respirators in polluted work sites now are mandatory. Tobacco smoke is the world's leading cause of lung disease and many other afflictions. **Smoking** cessation programs are widely available.

Resources

PERIODICALS

"Medicare Will Cover Lung Volume Reduction Surgery for Certain Patients." *Health & Medicine Week* October 20, 2003: 245.

Mustajbegovic, Jadranka, et al. "Respiratory Findings in Tobacco Workers." *Chest* May 2003: 1740-1749.

ORGANIZATIONS

American Lung Association. 1740 Broadway, New York, NY 10019. (800) 586-4872. <http://www.lungusa.org>.

J. Ricker Polsdorfer, MD
Teresa G. Odle

Lung fluke infections *see* **Fluke infections**

Lung function tests *see* **Pulmonary function test**

Lung perfusion and ventilation scan

Definition

A lung perfusion scan is a nuclear medicine test that produces a picture of blood flow to the lungs. A lung ventilation scan measures the ability of the lungs to take in air and uses radiopharmaceuticals to produce a picture of how air is distributed in the lungs.

Purpose

Lung perfusion scans and lung ventilation scans are usually performed in the same session. They are done to detect pulmonary embolisms, determine how much blood is flowing to lungs, determine which areas of the lungs are capable of ventilation, and assess how well the lungs are functioning after surgery. These tests are called by different names, including perfusion lung scan, aerosol lung scan, radionucleotide ventilation lung scan, ventilation lung scan, xenon lung scan, ventilation/perfusion scanning (VPS), pulmonary scintiphotography, or, most commonly, V/Q scan.

Precautions

The amount of radioactivity a person is exposed to during these tests is very low and is not harmful. However, if the patient has had other recent radio-nuclear tests, it may be necessary to wait until other radiopharmaceuticals have been cleared from the body so that they do not interfere with these tests.

Description

In a lung perfusion scan, a small amount of the protein labeled with a radioisotope is injected into the patient's hand or arm vein. The patient is positioned under a special camera that can detect radioactive material, and a series of photographs are made of the chest. When these images are projected onto a screen (oscilloscope), they show how the radioactive protein has been distributed by the blood vessels running through the lungs.

In a lung ventilation scan, a mask is placed over the nose and mouth, and the patient is asked to inhale and exhale a combination of air and radioactive gas. Pictures are then taken that show the distribution of the gas in the lungs. Each test takes 15-30 minutes.

Preparation

There is little preparation needed for these tests. The patient may eat and drink normally before the procedure. Tests to check for **pulmonary embolism** are often performed on an emergency basis.

Aftercare

No special aftercare is needed. The patient may resume normal activities immediately.

Risks

There are practically no risks associated with these tests.

Normal results

Normal results in both tests show an even distribution of radioactive material in all parts of the lungs.

Abnormal results

In the lung perfusion scan, an absence of radioactive marker material suggests decreased blood flow to that part of the lung, and possibly a pulmonary **embolism**. However, **pneumonia**, **emphysema**, or lung tumors can create readings on the lung perfusion scan that falsely suggest a pulmonary embolism is present.

In the lung ventilation scan, absence of marker material when the lung perfusion scan for the area is normal suggests lung disease.

Certain combinations of abnormalities in lung perfusion and ventilation scans suggest pulmonary embolism.

Resources

BOOKS

Pagana, Kathleen Deska. *Mosby's Manual of Diagnostic and Laboratory Tests.* St. Louis: Mosby, Inc., 1998.

Tish Davidson, A.M.

Lung surgery

Definition

Lung surgery includes a variety of procedures used to diagnose or treat diseases of the lungs. Biopsies are performed to extract a small amount of tissue for diagnosis, resections remove a portion of lung tissue, and other surgeries are aimed at reducing the volume of the lungs, removing cancerous tumors, or improving lung function.

Purpose

The type of lung surgery performed will depend upon the underlying disease or condition, as well as other factors.

- Pneumonectomy usually refers to the removal of a lung, or sometimes one or more lobes (sections containing lung tissue, air sacs, ducts, and respiratory bronchiole). It is most commonly indicated in certain forms and stages of lung **cancer**.

- Thoracotomy, or surgical incision of the chest wall, is used primarily as a diagnostic tool when other procedures have failed to provide adequate diagnostic information.

- Lobectomy is the term used to describe removal of one lobe of a lung. It is most commonly indicated for lung cancer, but may also be used for **cystic fibrosis** patients if other treatments have failed.

- Other surgical procedures include segmental resection or wedge resection. A resection is the removal of a part of the lung, often in order to remove a tumor. Wedge resection is removal of a wedge-shaped portion of lung tissue.

- Volume reduction surgery is a newer surgery used to help relieve **shortness of breath** and increase tolerance for **exercise** in patients with chronic obstructive pulmonary disease, such as **emphysema**.

- Other surgeries are continuously improved upon to make biopsy less invasive and surgery more effective, such as video-assisted lobectomy. Other purposes for lung surgery may include severe **abscess**, areas of long-term infection, or permanently enlarged or collapsed lung tissue.

Precautions

Thoracotomy should not be performed on patients whose general health status will not tolerate major surgery. Any surgery carries with it risks associated with **general anesthesia** and possibility of infection. Patients whose risk for these complications outweighs benefit may not be considered candidates for lung surgery. Each individual patient's condition will be reviewed prior to the treatment decision.

Description

Lung surgery procedures will vary depending on the underlying cause of the surgical test or intervention. A patient will be placed under general anesthesia during the surgery. An incision is made to examine the lungs. Diseased tissue is removed and may be sent for biopsy. Following the surgery, drainage tubes may be placed in the chest to drain fluids, blood, and air from the chest cavity. Tubes will most likely remain in place for one to two days, depending on the surgery and the patient's condition. The chest cavity, ribs, and skin are closed and the incision will be sutured. Hospital stay averages from three to 10 days.

Pneumonectomy consists of removal of all of one lung. It may often be indicated only when a lobectomy does not successfully remove the cancerous or damaged tissue. Thoracotomy consists of reaching the lung tissue through incision and obtaining tissue for a biopsy. The biopsy is used to diagnose or stage cancer, and thoracotomy may be avoided until other less invasive methods have failed. Volume reduction surgery involves incision and removal of those parts of the lung or lungs which are the most destroyed, in order to allow for full function of the remaining lung structure. This procedure is still being studied.

Lobectomy is performed in the same general manner as other lung surgeries, but will involve removal of an entire lobe of the lung. Most patients with Stage I or II **non-small cell lung cancer** will receive this treatment for their disease, or a less extensive resection. Lobectomy may only be performed if a wedge or segmental resection is ineffective, but is generally preferred as treatment for primary lung cancer in any patient who can tolerate the procedure. Wedge and segmental resections are still major surgery, but remove less tissue and may be the first choice for some patients, such as those with Stage I and Stage

II non-small cell lung cancer. Patients who do not have enough pulmonary function to undergo a lobectomy will receive a wedge or segmental resection instead. This may lead to a higher recurrence rate of cancer. In general, the surgery method chosen will depend on specific circumstances and consideration of benefit versus risk.

Preparation

Preparation for lung surgery is much like that for any major surgery. Patients will receive instructions from a physician concerning limit of food or water intake prior to the surgery, as well as risks and expected recovery. Patients should continue to follow treatment for the underlying condition, unless instructed otherwise by the physician, and should discuss medications and changes in condition with their physician prior to the surgery.

Aftercare

The chest tube inserted at the end of surgery will remain in place until the lung has fully expanded. Patients will be carefully monitored in the hospital for complications and infection. Deep breathing is recommended to help lessen the risk of **pneumonia** and infection. Breathing exercises will also help expand the lung. After discharge from the hospital, the patient may still receive some **pain** or infection-fighting medications and should recover within one to three months of the operation.

Risks

Risks of lung surgery follows those of any major surgery involving general anesthesia. These risks include reactions to anesthetics or medications, bleeding, infection, and problems restoring breathing. Lung surgery, in particular, offers the risk of pneumonia and **blood clots**. Thoracotomy, as a biopsy procedure, offers greater risk than most biopsy procedures.

Normal results

Outcome for any lung surgery depends on many factors and the severity of disease. In general, the predicted benefits, which justified the surgery, are normal expected results. Thoracotomy results in a definitive diagnosis in more than 90% of patients. Volume reduction surgery has been shown to result in relief of some symptoms and improvement in quality of life for selected patients with severe emphysema and have shown short-term promise.

Mortality from lung surgery improves as procedures move from the more complete pneumonectomy to lobectomy, and the lowest rate for segmental resection.

Resources

ORGANIZATIONS

American Cancer Society. 1599 Clifton Rd., NE, Atlanta, GA 30329-4251. (800) 227-2345. < http://www.cancer.org >.

American Lung Association. 1740 Broadway, New York, NY 10019. (800) 586-4872. < http://www.lungusa.org >.

National Heart, Lung and Blood Institute. P.O. Box 30105, Bethesda, MD 20824-0105. (301) 251-1222. < http://www.nhlbi.nih.gov >.

Teresa Odle

Lung transplantation

Definition

Lung transplantation involves removal of one or both diseased lungs from a patient and the replacement of the lungs with healthy organs from a donor. Lung transplantation may refer to single, double, or even heart-lung transplantation.

Purpose

The purpose of lung transplantation is to replace a lung that no longer functions, or is cancerous, with a healthy lung. In order to qualify for lung transplantation, a patient must suffer from severe lung disease which limits activities of daily living. There should be potential for rehabilitated breathing function. Attempts at other medical treatments should be exhausted before transplantion is considered. Many candidates for this procedure have end-stage fibrotic lung disease, are dependent on **oxygen therapy**, and are likely to die of their disease in 12-18 months.

Patients with **emphysema** or chronic obstructive pulmonary disease (COPD) should be under 60 years of age, have a life expectancy without transplantation of two years or less, progressive deterioration, and emotional stability in order to be considered for lung transplantation. Young patients with end-stage **silicosis** (a progressive lung disease) may be candidates for lung or heart-lung transplantation. Patients with Stage III or Stage IV **sarcoidosis** (a chronic lung

National Transplant Waiting List By Organ Type (June 2000)	
Organ Needed	**Number Waiting**
Kidney	48,349
Liver	15,987
Heart	4,139
Lung	3,695
Kidney-Pancreas	2,437
Pancreas	942
Heart-Lung	212
Intestine	137

disease) with **cor pulmonale** should be considered as early as possible for lung transplantation. Other indicators of lung transplantation include pulmonary vascular disease and chronic pulmonary infection.

Precautions

Patients who have diseases or conditions which may make them more susceptible to organ rejection should not receive a lung transplant. This includes patients who are acutely ill and unstable; who have uncontrolled or untreatable pulmonary infection; significant dysfunction of other organs, particularly the liver, kidney, or central nervous system; and those with significant coronary disease or left ventricular dysfunction. Patients who actively smoke cigarettes or are dependent on drugs or alcohol may not be selected. There are a variety of protocols that are used to determine if a patient will be placed on a transplant recipient list, and criteria may vary depending on location.

Description

Once a patient has been selected as a possible organ recipient, the process of waiting for a donor organ match begins. The donor organ must meet clear requirements for tissue match in order to reduce the chance of organ rejection. It is estimated that it takes an average of one to two years to receive a suitable donor lung, and the wait is made less predictable by the necessity for tissue match. Patients on a recipient list must be available and ready to come to the hospital immediately when a donor match is found, since the life of the lungs outside the body is brief.

Single lung transplantation is performed via a standard thoracotomy (incision in the chest wall) with the patient under **general anesthesia**. Cardiopulmonary bypass (diversion of blood flow from the heart) is not always necessary for a single lung transplant. If bypass is necessary, it involves re-routing of the blood through tubes to a heart-lung bypass machine. Double lung transplantation involves implanting the lungs as two separate lungs, and cardiopulmonary bypass is usually required. The patient's lung or lungs are removed and the donor lungs are stitched into place. Drainage tubes are inserted into the chest area to help drain fluid, blood, and air out of the chest. They may remain in place for several days. Transplantation requires a long hospital stay and recovery can last up to six months.

Heart-lung transplants always require the use of cardiopulmonary bypass. An incision is made through the middle of the sternum. The heart, lung, and supporting structures are transplanted into the recipient at the same time.

Preparation

In addition to tests and criteria for selection as a candidate for transplantation, patients will be prepared by discussing the procedure, risks, and expected prognosis at length with their doctor. Patients should continue to follow all therapies and medications for treatment of the underlying disease unless otherwise instructed by their physician. Since lung transplantation takes place under general anesthesia, normal surgical and anesthesia preparation should be taken when possible. These include no food or drink from midnight before the surgery, discussion of current medications with the physician, and informing the physician of any changes in condition while on the recipient waiting list.

Aftercare

Careful monitoring will take place in a recovery room immediately following the surgery and in the patient's hospital room. Patients must take immunosuppression, or anti-rejection, drugs to reduce the risk of rejection of the transplanted organ. The body considers the new organ an invader and will fight its presence. The **anti-rejection drugs** lower the body's immune function in order to improve acceptance of the new organs. This also makes the patient more susceptible to infection.

Frequent check-ups with a physician, including x ray and blood tests, will be necessary following surgery, probably for a period of several years.

Risks

Lung transplantation is a complicated and risky procedure, partly because of the organs and systems involved, and also because of the risk of rejection by

---

KEY TERMS

Pulmonary—Refers to the respiratory system, or breathing function and system.

Sarcoidosis—A chronic disease with unknown cause that involves formation of nodules in bones, skin, lymph nodes, and lungs.

Silicosis—A progressive disease that results in impairment of lung function and is caused by inhalation of dust containing silica.

---

the recipient's body. Acute rejection most often occurs within the first four months following surgery, but may occur years later. Infection is a substantial risk for organ recipients. An early complication of the surgery can be poor healing of the bronchial and tracheal openings created during the surgery. A late complication and risk is chronic rejection. This can result in inflammation of the bronchial tubes or in late infection from the prolonged use of **immunosuppressant drugs** to fight rejection. Overall, lung transplant recipients have demonstrated average one and two-year survival rates of more than 70%.

Normal results

The outcome of lung transplantation can be measured in survival rates, and also in improved quality of life for recipients. Studies have reported improved quality of life after lung and heart-lung transplants. One study showed that at the two-year follow-up period, 86% of studied recipients reported no limitation to their activity. Demonstration of normal results for patients may include quality of life measurements, as well as testing to ensure lack of infection and rejection.

Resources

ORGANIZATIONS

Children's Organ Transplant Association, Inc. 2501 COTA Drive, Bloomington, IN 47403. (800) 366-2682. < http://www.cota.org >.

Second Wind Lung Transplant Association, Inc. 9030 West Lakeview Court, Crystal River, FL 34428. (888) 222-2690. < http://www.arthouse.com/secondwind >.

Teresa Odle

Lupus erythematosus *see* **Systemic lupus erythematosus**

Luque rod *see* **Spinal instrumentation**

Luteinizing hormone test

Definition

The luteinizing hormone (LH) test is a test of the blood or urine to measure the level of luteinizing hormone (lutropin). This hormone level is highest immediately before a woman ovulates during her menstrual cycle.

Purpose

The LH test is frequently used to determine the timing of ovulation. Couples who are trying to become pregnant may use information about the timing of ovulation to improve their chance of conception. The LH test and other hormone tests may be used during **infertility** screening to chart a woman's menstrual cycle. It may also be used during preparation for **in vitro fertilization**, to determine when eggs are mature and ready to be removed from the ovary.

Description

Lutenizing hormone is a hormone released by the pituitary gland, a small gland at the base of the brain. The hormone stimulates the ovaries to produce and release eggs each month during the menstrual cycle. The level of LH in the blood is highest before ovulation. This increase in hormone level is sometimes called a "surge." A urine or blood sample can be analyzed by a laboratory for the level of LH present. An LH test may be used as part of an infertility screening to determine if there is a hormonal imbalance that might make it difficult to become pregnant. If fertility drugs are given to stimulate ovulation, an LH test can help determine the best time for sexual intercourse. The LH test may also be used to determine when eggs are mature enough to be surgically removed from the ovary as part of the in vitro fertilization process. LH tests may also aid in the diagnoses of polycystic ovary disease, premature ovarian failure, and **menopause**.

A urine LH detection kit is also available for use at home. These are sometimes called "ovulation tests" and are similar to home **pregnancy** test kits. A sample of the woman's first morning urine is tested with the materials provided in the kit. These home tests are often used by women who want to become pregnant. By monitoring levels of LH and watching for the "surge," they can time sexual intercourse to coincide with ovulation, increasing the chance that the egg will be fertilized.

Preparation

If a blood sample is taken, the skin around the vein where the needle will be inserted is swabbed with an antiseptic. No special preparation is necessary for collection of a urine sample.

Aftercare

No special aftercare is required. If the blood is tested, as with any blood sampling, the area where the needle was inserted should be kept clean.

Risks

There are no significant risks associated with either the blood or urine test for LH.

Normal results

The level of LH in the blood or urine will vary depending on when the sample was taken during the menstrual cycle. LH levels will be highest around the time of ovulation, about halfway between a woman's menstrual periods. Levels will be lower during the rest of the month. Women who have already experienced menopause will normally have lower LH levels.

Abnormal results

LH levels that remain low throughout the menstrual cycle may indicate a hormonal imbalance that could prevent ovulation. Additional testing may be required if this test is done as part of an infertility screening.

Resources

BOOKS

Zaret, Barry L., et al., editors. *The Patient's Guide to Medical Tests.* Boston: Houghton Mifflin, 1997.

Altha Roberts Edgren

Lyme borreliosis *see* **Lyme disease**

Lyme disease

Definition

Lyme disease is an infection transmitted by the bite of ticks carrying the spiral-shaped bacterium *Borrelia burgdorferi*. The disease was named for Lyme, Connecticut, the town where it was first diagnosed in 1975 after a puzzling outbreak of arthritis. The organism was named for its discoverer, Willy Burgdorfer. The effects of this disease can be long-term and disabling unless it is recognized and treated properly with **antibiotics**.

Description

Lyme disease, which is also called Lyme borreliosis, is a vector-borne disease. This term means that it is delivered from one host to another. It is also classified as a **zoonosis**, which means that it is a disease of animals that can be transmitted to humans under natural conditions. In this case, a tick bearing the *Borrelia burgdorferi* organism literally inserts it into a host's bloodstream when it bites the host to feed on its blood. It is important to note that neither *Borrelia burgdorferi* nor Lyme disease can be transmitted directly from one person to another, or from pets to humans.

Controversy clouds the true incidence of Lyme disease because no test is definitively diagnostic for the disease, and many of its symptoms mimic those of so many other diseases. Cases of Lyme disease have been reported in 49 of the 50 states; however, 92% of the 17,730 cases reported to the Centers for Disease Control and Prevention (CDC) in 2000 were from only nine states (Connecticut, Rhode Island, New York, Pennsylvania, Delaware, New Jersey, Maryland, Massachusetts, and Wisconsin). The disease is also found in Scandinavia, continental Europe, the countries of the former Soviet Union, Japan, and China; in addition, it is possible that it has spread to Australia.

In the United States, Lyme disease accounts for more than 90% of all reported vector-borne illnesses. It is a significant public health problem and continues to be diagnosed in increasing numbers. The Centers for Disease Control and Prevention (CDC) attributes this increase to the growing size of the deer herd and the geographical spread of infected ticks rather than to improved diagnosis. In addition, some epidemiologists believe that the actual incidence of Lyme disease in the United States may be 5–10 times greater than that reported by the CDC. The reasons for this difference include the narrowness of the CDC's case definition as well as frequent misdiagnoses of the disease.

The risk for acquiring Lyme disease varies, depending on what stage in its life cycle a tick has reached. A tick passes through three stages of development—larva, nymph, and adult—each of which is dependent on a live host for food. In the United States, *Borrelia burgdorferi* is borne by ticks of several species in the genus *Ixodes*, which usually feed on the white-footed mouse and deer (and are often called deer ticks). In the summer, the larval ticks hatch from eggs laid in the ground and feed by attaching themselves to small animals and birds. At this stage they are not a problem for humans. It is the next stage—the nymph—that causes most cases of Lyme disease. Nymphs are very active from spring through early summer, at the height of outdoor activity for most people. Because they are still quite small (less than 2 mm), they are difficult to spot, giving them ample opportunity to transmit *Borrelia burgdorferi* while feeding. Although far more adult ticks than nymphs carry *Borrelia burgdorferi*, the adult ticks are much larger, more easily noticed, and more likely to be removed before the 24 hours or more of continuous feeding needed to transmit *Borrelia burgdorferi*.

Causes and symptoms

Lyme disease is caused by *Borrelia burgdorferi*. Once *Borrelia burgdorferi* gains entry to the body through a tick bite, it can move through the bloodstream quickly. Only 12 hours after entering the bloodstream, *Borrelia burgdorferi* can be found in cerebrospinal fluid (which means it can affect the nervous system). Treating Lyme disease early and thoroughly is important because Lyme disease can hide for long periods within the body in a clinically latent state. That ability explains why symptoms can recur in cycles and can flare up after months or years, even over decades. It is important to note, however, that not many people who are exposed to *Borrelia burgdorferi* develops the disease.

Lyme disease is usually described in terms of length of infection (time since the person was bitten by a tick infected with Lyme disease) and whether *Borrelia burgdorferi* is localized or disseminated (spread through the body by fluids and cells carrying *Borrelia burgdorferi*). Furthermore, when and how symptoms of Lyme disease appear can vary widely from patient to patient. People who experience

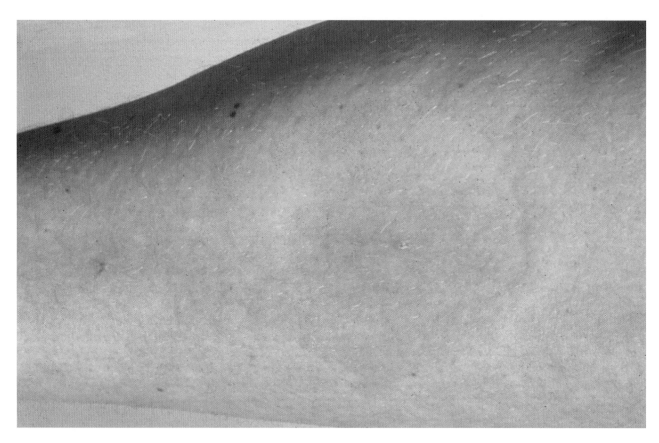

The first sign of Lyme disease is usually an itchy rash around the site of the tick bite. *(Science Photo Library. Custom Medical Stock Photo. Reproduced by permission.)*

recurrent bouts of symptoms over time are said to have chronic Lyme disease.

Early localized Lyme disease

The most recognizable indicator of Lyme disease is a rash around the site of the tick bite. Often, the tick exposure has not been recognized. The eruption might be warm or itch. The rash—erythema migrans (EM)-generally develops within 3-30 days and usually begins as a round, red patch that expands outward. About 75% of patients with Lyme disease develop EM. Clearing may take place from the center out, leaving a bull's-eye effect; in some cases, the center gets redder instead of clearing. The rash may look like a bruise on people with dark skin. Of those who develop Lyme disease, about 50% notice flu-like symptoms, including **fatigue**, **headache**, chills and **fever**, muscle and joint **pain**, and lymph node swelling. However, a rash at the site can also be an allergic reaction to the tick saliva rather than an indicator of Lyme disease, particularly if the rash appears in *less* than three days and disappears only days later.

Late disseminated disease and chronic Lyme disease

Weeks, months, or even years after an untreated tick bite, symptoms can appear in several forms, including:

- Fatigue, forgetfulness, confusion, mood swings, irritability, numbness.

- Neurologic problems, such as pain (unexplained and not triggered by an injury), Bell's palsy (facial **paralysis**, usually one-sided but may be on both sides), and a mimicking of the inflammation of brain membranes known as **meningitis**; (fever, severe headache).

- Arthritis (short episodes of pain and swelling in joints) and other musculoskeletal complaints. Arthritis eventually develops in about 60% of patients with untreated Lyme disease.

Less common effects of Lyme disease are heart abnormalities (such as irregular rhythm or cardiac block) and eye abnormalities (such as swelling of the cornea, tissue, or eye muscles and nerves).

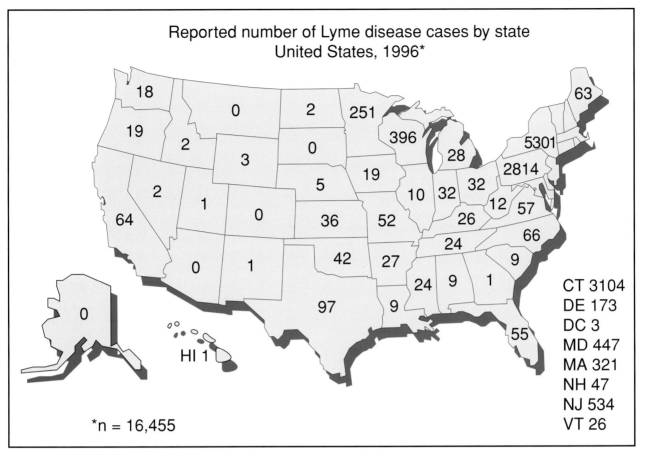

Reported number of Lyme disease cases by state
United States, 1996*

CT 3104
DE 173
DC 3
MD 447
MA 321
NH 47
NJ 534
VT 26

*n = 16,455

Lyme disease accounts for more than 90% of all reported vector-borne illnesses in the United States. It is caused by an infection transmitted by the bite of ticks carrying the *Borrelia burgdorferi* bacterium. *(Data taken from the Centers for Disease Control. Illustration by Electronic Illustrators Group.)*

Diagnosis

A clear diagnosis of Lyme disease can be difficult, and relies on information the patient provides and the doctor's clinical judgment, particularly through elimination of other possible causes of the symptoms. Lyme disease may mimic other conditions, including **chronic fatigue syndrome** (CFS), **multiple sclerosis** (MS), and other diseases with many symptoms involving multiple body systems. Differential diagnosis (distinguishing kyme disease from other diseases) is based on clinical evaluation with laboratory tests used for clarification when necessary. A two-test approach is common to confirm the results. Because of the potential for misleading results (false-positive and false-negative), laboratory tests alone cannot establish the diagnosis.

In February 1999 the Food and Drug Administration (FDA) approved a new blood test for Lyme disease called PreVue. The test, which searches for antigens (substances that stimulate the production of antibodies) produced by *Borrelia burgdorferi*, gives results within one hour in the doctor's office. A positive result from the PreVue test is confirmed by a second blood test known as the Western blot, which must be done in a laboratory.

Doctors generally know which disease-causing organisms are common in their geographic area. The most helpful piece of information is whether a tick bite or rash was noticed and whether it happened locally or while traveling. Doctors may not consider Lyme disease if it is rare locally, but will take it into account if a patient mentions vacationing in an area where the disease is commonly found.

Treatment

The treatment for Lyme disease is antibiotic therapy; however, overprescribing of antibiotics can lead to serious problems, so the decision to treat must be made with care. Disease organisms can develop resistance to families of medications over time, rendering the drugs useless. Furthermore, testing and treatments can be expensive. If a patient has strong indications of Lyme disease (symptoms and medical history), the doctor will probably begin treatment on the presumption of this disease. The American College of Physicians recommends treatment for a patient with a rash resembling EM or who has arthritis, a history of an EM-type rash, and a previous tick bite.

The benefits of treating early must be weighed against the risks of over treatment. The longer a patient is ill with Lyme disease before treatment, the longer the course of therapy must be, and the more aggressive the treatment. The development of opportunistic organisms may produce other symptoms. For example, after long-term antibiotic therapy, patients can become more susceptible to yeast infections. Treatment may also be associated with adverse drug reactions.

For most patients, oral antibiotics (doxycycline or amoxicillin) are prescribed for 21 days. When symptoms indicate nervous system involvement or a severe episode of Lyme disease, intravenous antibiotic (ceftriaxone) may be given for 14-30 days. Some physicians consider intravenous ceftriaxone the best therapy for any late manifestation of disease, but treatments for late Lyme disease are still controversial as of 2003. **Corticosteroids** (oral) may be prescribed if eye abnormalities occur, but they should not be used without first consulting an eye doctor.

The doctor may have to adjust the treatment regimen or change medications based on the patient's response. Treatment can be difficult because *Borrelia burgdorferi* comes in several strains (some may react to different antibiotics than others) and may even have the ability to switch forms during the course of infection. Also, *Borrelia burgdorferi* can shut itself up in cell niches, allowing it to hide from antibiotics. Finally, antibiotics can kill *Borrelia burgdorferi* only while it is active rather than dormant.

Alternative treatment

Supportive therapies may minimize symptoms of LD or improve the immune response. These include vitamin and **nutritional supplements**, mostly for chronic fatigue and increased susceptibility to infection. For example, yogurt and *Lactobacillus acidophilus* preparations help fight yeast infections, which are common in people on long-term antibiotic therapy. In addition, botanical medicine and homeopathy can be considered to help bring the body's systems back to a state of health and well being. A Western herb,

spilanthes (*Spilanthes* spp.), may be effective in treating diseases like LD that are caused by spirochetes (spiral-shaped bacteria).

Prognosis

If aggressive antibiotic therapy is given early, and the patient cooperates fully and sticks to the medication schedule, recovery should be complete. Only a small percentage of Lyme disease patients fail to respond or relapse (have recurring episodes). Most long-term effects of the disease result when diagnosis and treatment is delayed or missed. Co-infection with other infectious organisms spread by ticks in the same areas as *Borrelia burgdorferi* (**babesiosis** and **ehrlichiosis**, for instance) may be responsible for treatment failures or more severe symptoms. Most fatalities reported with Lyme disease involved patients coinfected with babesiosis.

Prevention

Update on vaccination

A vaccine for Lyme disease known as LYMErix was available from 1998 to 2002, when it was removed from the United States market. The decision was influenced by reports that LYMErix may be responsible for neurologic complications in vaccinated patients. Researchers from Cornell-New York Hospital presented a paper at the annual meeting of the American Neurological Association in October 2002 that identified nine patients with neuropathies linked to **vaccination** with LYMErix. In April 2003, the National Institute of Allergy and Infectious Diseases (NIAID) awarded a federal grant to researchers at Yale University School of Medicine to develop a new vaccine against Lyme disease. As of late 2003, the best prevention strategy is through minimizing risk of exposure to ticks and using personal protection precautions.

Minimizing risk of exposure

Precautions to avoid contact with ticks include moving leaves and brush away from living quarters. Most important are personal protection techniques when outdoors, such as:

• Spraying tick repellent on clothing and exposed skin.

• Wearing light-colored clothing to maximize ability to see ticks.

• Tucking pant legs into socks or boot top.

• Checking children and pets frequently for ticks.

KEY TERMS

Babesiosis—A disease caused by protozoa of the genus *Babesia* characterized by a malaria-like fever, anemia, vomiting, muscle pain, and enlargement of the spleen. Babesiosis, like Lyme disease, is carried by a tick.

Bell's palsy—Facial paralysis or weakness with a sudden onset, caused by swelling or inflammation of the seventh cranial nerve, which controls the facial muscles. Disseminated Lyme disease sometimes causes Bell's palsy.

Blood-brain barrier—A blockade of cells separating the circulating blood from elements of the central nervous system (CNS); it acts as a filter, preventing many substances from entering the central nervous system.

Cerebrospinal fluid—Clear fluid found around the brain and spinal cord and in the ventricles of the brain.

Disseminated—Scattered or distributed throughout the body. Lyme disease that has progressed beyond the stage of localized EM is said to be disseminated.

Erythema migrans (EM)—A red skin rash that is one of the first signs of Lyme disease in about 75% of patients.

Lyme borreliosis—Another name for Lyme disease.

Spirochete—A spiral-shaped bacterium. The bacteria that cause Lyme disease and syphilis, for example, are spirochetes.

Vector—An animal carrier that transfers an infectious organism from one host to another. The vector that transmits Lyme disease from wildlife to humans is the deer tick or black-legged tick.

Zoonosis (plural, zoonoses)—Any disease of animals that can be transmitted to humans under natural conditions. Lyme disease and babesiosis are examples of zoonoses.

In highly tick-populated areas, each individual should be inspected at the end of the day to look for ticks.

Minimizing risk of disease

The two most important factors are removing the tick quickly and carefully, and seeking a doctor's evaluation at the first sign of symptoms of Lyme disease. When in an area that may be tick-populated:

- Check for ticks, particularly in the area of the groin, underarm, behind ears, and on the scalp.
- Stay calm and grasp the tick as near to the skin as possible, using a tweezer.
- To minimize the risk of squeezing more bacteria into the bite, pull straight back steadily and slowly.
- Do not try to remove the tick by using petroleum jelly, alcohol, or a lit match.
- Place the tick in a closed container (for species identification later, should symptoms develop) or dispose of it by flushing.
- See a physician for any sort of rash or patchy discoloration that appears three to 30 days after a tick bite.

Resources

BOOKS

Beers, Mark H., MD, and Robert Berkow, MD., editors. "Bacterial Diseases Caused by Spirochetes: Lyme Disease (Lyme Borreliosis)." In *The Merck Manual of Diagnosis and Therapy*. Whitehouse Station, NJ: Merck Research Laboratories, 2004.

PERIODICALS

Edlow, Jonathan A., MD. "Tick-Borne Diseases, Lyme." *eMedicine* December 13, 2002. < http://www.emedicine.com/emerg/topic588.htm >.

Krupp, L. B., L. G. Hyman, R. Grimson, et al. "Study and Treatment of Post Lyme Disease (STOP-LD): A Randomized Double Masked Clinical Trial." *Neurology* 60 (June 24, 2003): 1923–1930.

Nachman, S. A., and L. Pontrelli. "Central Nervous System Lyme Disease." *Seminars in Pediatric Infectious Diseases* 14 (April 2003): 123–130.

Pavia, C. S. "Current and Novel Therapies for Lyme Disease." *Expert Opinion on Investigational Drugs* 12 (June 2003): 1003–1016.

Susman, Ed. "ANA: Neurological Impairment Seen in Patients Given LYMErix Lyme Disease Vaccine." *Doctor's Guide* October 16, 2002. < http://www.plsgroup.com/dg/220652.htm >.

Wormser, G. P., R. Ramanathan, J. Nowakowski, et al. "Duration of Antibiotic Therapy for Early Lyme Disease. A Randomized, Double-Blind, Placebo-Controlled Trial." *Annals of Internal Medicine* 138 (May 6, 2003): 697–704.

ORGANIZATIONS

Centers for Disease Control and Prevention. 1600 Clifton Rd., NE, Atlanta, GA 30333. (800) 311-3435, (404) 639-3311. < http://www.cdc.gov >.

Lyme Disease Foundation. One Financial Plaza, Hartford, CT, 06103. (800) 886-LYME. < http://www.lyme.org >.

Lyme Disease Network of NJ, Inc. 43 Winton Road, East Brunswick, NJ 08816. < http://www.lymenet.org >.

National Institute of Allergy and Infectious Diseases (NIAID). 31 Center Drive, Room 7A50 MSC 2520, Bethesda, MD, 20892. (301) 496-5717. < http:// www.niaid.nih.gov >.

OTHER

Centers for Disease Control and Prevention, Division of Vector-Borne Infectious Diseases. *CDC Lyme Disease Home Page.* < http://www.cdc.gov/ncidod/dvbid/ lyme/ >.

National Institute of Neurological Disorders and Stroke (NINDS) Fact Sheet. *Bell's Palsy.* Bethesda, MD: NINDS, 2003.

NINDS Information Page. *Neurological Complications of Lyme Disease.* Bethesda, MD: NINDS, 2003.

Rebecca J. Frey, PhD

Lymph node angiogram *see*
Lymphangiography

Lymph node biopsy

Definition

A lymph node biopsy is a procedure in which all or part of a lymph node is removed and examined to determine if there is **cancer** within the node.

Purpose

The lymph system is the body's primary defense against infection. It consists of the spleen, tonsils, thymus, lymph nodes, lymph vessels, and the clear, slightly yellow fluid called lymph. These components produce and transport white blood cells called lymphocytes and macrophages that rid the body of infection. The lymph system is also involved in the production of antibodies. Antibodies are proteins that fight bacteria, viruses, and other foreign materials that enter the body.

The lymph vessels are similar to veins, only instead of carrying blood as veins do, they circulate lymph to most tissues in the body. Lymph nodes are about 600 small, bean-shaped collections of tissue found along the lymph vessel. They produce cells and proteins that fight infection, and clean and filter lymph. Lymph nodes are sometimes called lymph glands, although they are not true glands. When someone talks about having swollen glands, they are actually referring to lymph nodes.

Normal lymph glands are no larger than 0.5 in (1.3 cm) in diameter and are difficult to feel. However, lymph nodes can enlarge to greater than 2.5 in (6 cm) and can become sore. Most often the swelling is caused by an infection, but it can also be caused by cancer.

Cancers can metastasize (spread) through the lymph system from the site of the original tumor to distant parts of the body where secondary tumors are formed. The purpose of a lymph node biopsy is to determine the cause of the swelling and/or to see if cancer has begun to spread through the lymph system. This information is important in staging the cancer and devising a treatment plan.

Precautions

Women who are pregnant should inform their doctor before a lymph node biopsy, although **pregnancy** will not affect the results.

Description

There are three kinds of lymph node biopsy. Sentinel lymph node mapping and biopsy is a promising new technique that is discussed in its own entry. Fine needle aspiration (FNA) biopsy, often just called needle biopsy, is done when the lymph node of interest is near the surface of the body. A hematologist (a doctor who specializes in blood diseases) usually performs the test. In FNA biopsy, a needle is inserted through the skin and into the lymph node, and a sample of tissue is drawn out of the node. This material is preserved and sent to the laboratory for examination.

Advantages of a needle biopsy are that the test is minimally invasive. Only a local anesthetic is used, the procedure generally takes less than half an hour, and there is little **pain** afterwards. The disadvantage is that cancer may not be detected in the small sample of cells removed by the needle.

Open lymph node biopsy is a surgical procedure. It is done by a surgeon under **general anesthesia** on lymph nodes in the interior of the body and under **local anesthesia** on surface lymph nodes where FNA biopsy is considered inadequate. Once there is adequate anesthesia, the surgeon makes a small cut and removes either the entire lymph node or a slice of tissue that is then sent to the laboratory for examination. Results in both kinds of biopsies take one to three days.

Open biopsy can be advantageous in that it is easier to detect and identify the type of cancer in a large piece of tissue. Also, lymph nodes deep in the body can be sampled. Disadvantages include a longer recovery time,

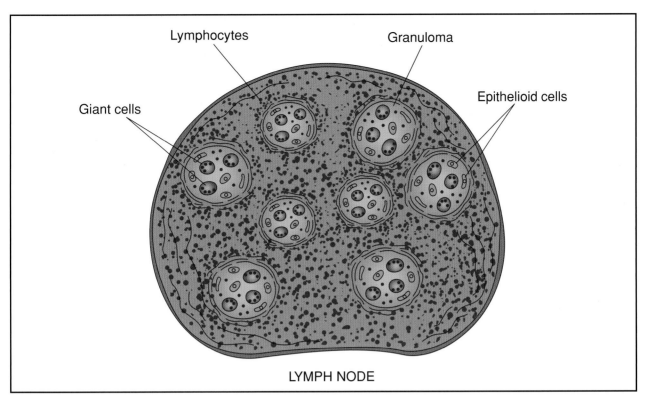

Lymph node biopsy is a procedure in which a sample of lymph node tissue is removed for laboratory analysis. It is generally performed on an outpatient basis. *(Illustration by Electronic Illustrators Group.)*

soreness at the biopsy site for several days, and the use of deeper anesthesia, increasing the risks to the patient. The procedure is done in a hospital or outpatient surgery center and takes about an hour, with additional time to recover from general anesthesia.

Preparation

No particular preparation is necessary for a needle biopsy. For an open biopsy, patients need standard pre-operative blood tests and other tests to evaluate general health. The doctor should be informed about any medications (prescription, non-prescription, or herbal) the patient is taking, as well as past bleeding problems or **allergies** to medication or anesthesia.

Aftercare

Little aftercare is needed in a needle biopsy other than a bandage to keep the biopsy site clean. Patients who have general anesthesia for an open biopsy often feel drowsy and tired for several days following the procedure, and should not plan to drive home after biopsy. The incision site must be kept clean and dry, and a follow-up visit to check on healing is usually necessary.

Risks

There are few risks associated with lymph node biopsy. The main risks are excessive bleeding (usually only in people with blood disorders) and allergic reaction to general anesthesia (rare). Occasionally the biopsy site becomes infected.

Normal results

Normal lymph nodes are small and flat. When examined under the microscope, they show no signs of cancer or infection.

Abnormal results

Abnormal lymph nodes are usually enlarged and contain cancerous (malignant) cells and/or show signs of infection.

Resources

ORGANIZATIONS

American Cancer Society. 1599 Clifton Road NE, Atlanta, GA 30329. 800(ACS)-2345. < http:// www.cancer.org >.

KEY TERMS

Lymph nodes—Small, bean-shaped organs located throughout the lymphatic system. The lymph nodes store special cells that can trap cancer cells or bacteria that are traveling through the body in lymph. Also called lymph glands.

Lymphocytes—Small white blood cells that bear the major responsibility for carrying out the activities of the immune system; they number about 1 trillion.

Malignant—Cancerous. Cells tend to reproduce without normal controls on growth and form tumors or invade other tissues.

Spleen—An organ located at the left side of the stomach that acts as a reservoir for blood cells and produces lymphocytes and other products involved in fighting infection.

Thymus—An organ near the base of the neck that produces cells that fight infection. It is at its largest at puberty, then declines in size and function during adult life.

Tonsils—Small masses of tissue at the back of the throat.

Cancer Information Service. National Cancer Institute. Building 31, Room 10A19, 9000 Rockville Pike, Bethesda, MD 20892. (800)4-CANCER. <http://www.nci.nih.gov/cancerinfo>.

OTHER

ThriveOnline June 12, 2001. <http://thriveonline.oxygen.com/medical/library/article/003933.html>.

Tish Davidson, A.M.

Lymphadenitis

Definition

Lymphadenitis is the inflammation of a lymph node. It is often a complication of a bacterial infection of a wound, although it can also be caused by viruses or other disease agents. Lymphadenitis may be either generalized, involving a number of lymph nodes; or limited to a few nodes in the area of a localized infection. Lymphadenitis is sometimes accompanied by lymphangitis, which is the inflammation of the lymphatic vessels that connect the lymph nodes.

Description

Lymphadenitis is marked by swollen lymph nodes that are painful, in most cases, when the doctor touches them. If the lymphadenitis is related to an infected wound, the skin over the nodes may be red and warm to the touch. If the lymphatic vessels are also infected, there will be red streaks extending from the wound in the direction of the lymph nodes. In most cases, the infectious organisms are hemolytic *Streptococci* or *Staphylococci*. Hemolytic means that the bacteria produce a toxin that destroys red blood cells.

The extensive network of lymphatic vessels throughout the body and their relation to the lymph nodes helps to explain why bacterial infection of the nodes can spread rapidly to or from other parts of the body. Lymphadenitis in children often occurs in the neck area because these lymph nodes are close to the ears and throat, which are frequent locations of bacterial infections in children.

Causes and symptoms

Streptococcal and staphylococcal bacteria are the most common causes of lymphadenitis, although viruses, protozoa, rickettsiae, fungi, and the **tuberculosis** bacillus can also infect the lymph nodes. Diseases or disorders that involve lymph nodes in specific areas of the body include rabbit **fever (tularemia)**, **catscratch disease**, **lymphogranuloma venereum**, **chancroid**, **genital herpes**, infected **acne**, dental abscesses, and bubonic **plague**. In children, **tonsillitis** or bacterial sore throats are the most common causes of lymphadenitis in the neck area. Diseases that involve lymph nodes throughout the body include mononucleosis, **cytomegalovirus infection**, **toxoplasmosis**, and **brucellosis**.

The early symptoms of lymphadenitis are swelling of the nodes caused by a buildup of tissue fluid and an increased number of white blood cells resulting from the body's response to the infection. Further developments include fever, often as high as 101-102 °F (38-39 °C) together with chills, loss of appetite, heavy perspiration, a rapid pulse, and general weakness.

Diagnosis

Physical examination

The diagnosis of lymphadenitis is usually based on a combination of the patient's history, the external symptoms, and laboratory cultures. The doctor will press (palpate) the affected lymph nodes to see if they

2288

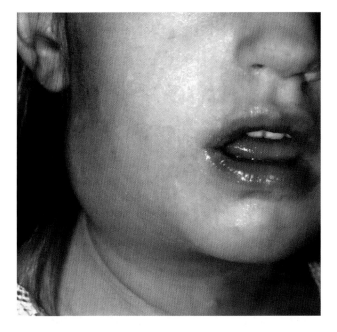

Swollen lymph node glands in a young girl's neck. *(Custom Medical Stock Photo. Reproduced by permission.)*

are sore or tender. Swollen nodes without soreness are often caused by cat-scratch disease. In children, the doctor will need to rule out **mumps**, tumors in the neck region, and congenital cysts that resemble swollen lymph nodes.

Although lymphadenitis is usually diagnosed in lymph nodes in the neck, arms, or legs, it can also occur in lymph nodes in the chest or abdomen. If the patient has acutely swollen lymph nodes in the groin, the doctor will need to rule out a **hernia** in the groin that has failed to reduce (incarcerated inguinal hernia). Hernias occur in 1% of the general population; 85% of patients with hernias are male.

Laboratory tests

The most significant tests are a white blood cell count (WBC) and a **blood culture** to identify the organism. A high proportion of immature white blood cells indicates a bacterial infection. Blood cultures may be positive, most often for a species of staphylococcus or streptococcus. In some cases, the doctor may order a biopsy of the lymph node.

Treatment

Medications

The medications given for lymphadenitis vary according to the bacterium or virus that is causing it. If the patient also has lymphangitis, he or she will be treated with **antibiotics**, usually penicillin G (Pfizerpen, Pentids), nafcillin (Nafcil, Unipen), or **cephalosporins**. Erythromycin (Eryc, E-Mycin, Erythrocin) is given to patients who are allergic to penicillin.

Supportive care

Supportive care of lymphadenitis includes resting the affected limb and treating the area with hot moist compresses.

Surgery

Cellulitis associated with lymphadenitis should *not* be treated surgically because of the risk of spreading the infection. Pus is drained only if there is an **abscess** and usually after the patient has been started on antibiotic treatment. In some cases, a biopsy of an inflamed lymph node is necessary if no diagnosis has been made and no response to treatment has occurred.

Prognosis

The prognosis for recovery is good if the patient is treated promptly with antibiotics. In most cases, the infection can be brought under control in three or four days. Patients with untreated lymphadenitis may develop blood **poisoning** (septicemia), which is sometimes fatal.

Prevention

Prevention of lymphadenitis depends on prompt treatment of bacterial and viral infections.

Resources

BOOKS

McPhee, Stephen, et al., editors. "Blood Vessels & Lymphatics." In *Current Medical Diagnosis and Treatment, 1998.* 37th ed. Stamford: Appleton & Lange, 1997.

Rebecca J. Frey, PhD

Lymphangiography

Definition

Lymphangiography, or lymph node angiogram, is a test which utilizes x-ray technology, along with the injection of a contrast agent, to view lymphatic circulation and lymph nodes for diagnostic purposes.

Purpose

The lymphatic system is a one way circulation that channels tissue fluid back into the heart. The watery fluid called lymph seeps out of the blood into tissues, and while journeying back to the heart, it picks up germs, **cancer** cells, and some waste products. Lymph passes through the lymph nodes, which are major arsenals of immune defense that attack germs carried in the lymph. Cancer cells are also subject to attack in lymph nodes.

Cancers of the lymph system, such as **Hodgkin's disease** and non-Hodgkin's lymphomas, spread throughout the body. Treatment often depends upon finding all the disease and directing radiation to each location. Planning other kinds of treatment, such as surgery or **chemotherapy**, may also require that the full extent of the disease be known.

The lymphatic circulation may become clogged by infection, injury, or several other types of cancer that

have spread through lymphatic channels. Swelling, sometimes massive, can result from blocked lymphatics. The most outstanding example of this is the tropical disease **filariasis**, which results in the swelling of the legs termed elephangiasis.

Lymphangiography gives precise information on the extent and location of lymph vessels and lymph nodes. Oftentimes, it is performed to evaluate the extent of a lymphatic cancer. Rarely, it is a tool, which aids surgeons attempting to reconstruct the lymphatics.

Precautions

Lymphangiography should not be performed on patients with dye or shellfish **allergies** or on patients with chronic lung disease, **kidney disease**, heart disease, or **liver disease**.

Description

A lymphangiogram begins by injecting a blue dye into a hand or foot. The lymph system picks up dye, which in turn will highlight the lymph vessels. This process may take a full day. When the lymphatic channel is clearly visible, the radiologist will insert an even tinier needle into that vessel and inject a contrast agent. X rays outline the journey of the contrast agent as it travels to the heart through lymph vessels and nodes.

Preparation

Unless a dye allergy is suspected, no special preparation is need. If an allergy is suspected, a non-ionic contrast agent can be administered instead.

Aftercare

Prior to suture removal seven to 10 days after the procedure, the patient should watch for any sign of infection around the site.

Risks

Lipid **pneumonia** can occur if the contrast agent penetrates the thoracic duct. An allergic reaction to the contrast agent is possible, causing a range of symptoms that can range from innocuous to life threatening.

Resources

BOOKS

Merrill, Vinta. "Lymphangiography." In *Atlas of Roentgenographic Positions and Standard Radiologic Procedures.* Saint Louis: The C. V. Mosby Co., 1975.

J. Ricker Polsdorfer, MD

Lymphedema

Description

Lymphedema involves blockage of the lymph vessels, with a resulting accumulation of lymphatic fluid in the interstitial tissues of the body. The lymphatic system consists of lymph vessels and lymph nodes throughout the body. The lymph vessels collect lymphatic fluid, which consists of protein, water, fats, and wastes from cells. The lymph vessels transport the fluid to the lymph nodes, where waste materials and foreign materials are filtered out from the fluid. The fluid is then returned to the blood. When the vessels are damaged or missing, the lymph fluid cannot move freely throughout the system but accumulates. This accumulation of fluid results in abnormal swelling of the arm(s) or leg(s), and occasionally swelling in other parts of the body.

Lymphedema is a very serious condition. There is no cure for lymphedema and once it develops, it can be a long-term, uncomfortable, and sometimes painful condition requiring daily treatment. When lymphedema is not treated, the protein-rich fluid continues to accumulate, leading to even more swelling and hardening (referred to as fibrosis) of the tissues. This fluid is a good culture medium for bacteria, thus resulting in reoccurring infections when there are injuries to the skin, decrease or loss of functioning of the affected limbs, and skin breakdown. Infections, referred to lymphangitis, can affect the connective tissue under the skin. Repeated infections may result in scarring, which in turn makes the tissue susceptible to more swelling and infection. Over time, these infections result in tissue hardening (i.e., fibrosis), which is a characteristic of advanced chronic lymphedema. In very severe cases, untreated lymphedema may even result in a rare form of lymphatic **cancer** called lymphangiosarcoma.

Lymphedema affects approximately 100 million people worldwide, including at least 3 million people in the United States.

Symptoms of lymphedema include:

- swelling of an affected limb, which may develop gradually or suddenly
- tightness of the skin and a feeling of heaviness in the affected area
- discomfort or a feeling of "pins and needles" in the affected area
- pitting **edema**, which can be identified by observing a temporary indentation in the swollen area when pressure is placed on the affected area
- aching in the adjacent shoulder or hip due to the increasing weight of the swelling limb
- tight fitting of a ring, wristwatch, or bracelet, without a gain in weight.

In 90% of the cases, lymphedema is diagnosed through observations, measurements, and symptoms. The remaining 10% require the use of more complex diagnostic tests such as lymphoscintigraphy. Lymphoscintigraphy is a technique in which a radioactive substance that concentrates in the lymphatic vessels is injected into the affected tissue and is mapped using a gamma camera, which images the location of the radioactive tracer. **Magnetic resonance imaging** (MRI), computed tomography (CT) scanning, and duplex ultrasound are imaging techniques that are also sometimes used as diagnostic tools for lymphedema.

There are three stages of lymphedema:

- Stage 1 (spontaneously reversible) - tissue is still at the pitting stage and soft to the touch. Upon waking in the morning, the limbs or affected areas are of normal or almost normal size
- Stage 2 (spontaneously irreversible) - tissue is nonpitting and no longer soft to the touch, fibrosis begins to form, and the limbs increase in size
- Stage 3 (lymphostatic **elephantiasis**) - swelling is irreversible and the affected areas are very swollen. The skin hardens and begins to break down, fibrosis is more extensive, and patients may need surgery to remove some of the swollen tissues.

Causes

Primary lymphedema is an inherited condition, where the patient is born without lymph vessels and nodes. The swelling associated with primary lymphedema usually occurs during adolescence and affects the foot or calf. A rare form of primary lymphedema, called Milroy's Disease, occurs in **pregnancy**. However, secondary lymphedema, or acquired lymphedema, develops as a result of an injury to the lymph system. Specific causes include surgical treatments for certain types of cancers, especially those cancers that currently require the removal of lymph nodes. Radiation treatment for cancer or for some AIDs-related diseases such as Kaposi-Sarcoma may also result in lymphedema, as radiation may damage or destroy lymph nodes or cause the formation of scar tissue that can interrupt the normal flow of the lymphatic fluid. Specific cancers and their treatment that may result in lymphedema include **malignant melanoma**, breast (in both women and men), gynecological, head and neck, prostate, testicular, bladder, and **colon cancer**. Other causes of lymphedema include trauma to the lymphatic system from **burns**, **liposuction**, tattooing, injuries, surgery, radiation, **obesity**, heart or circulatory disease, and **multiple sclerosis**. Lymphedema in people at risk may not develop the condition immediately, but develop the condition weeks, months, or even years later. Aircraft travel has been linked to the development of lymphedema in patients after cancer surgery, possible due to the decreased cabin pressure.

In Western countries, one of the most common causes of lymphedema is **mastectomy** with axillary dissection (removal of the breast and underarm lymph tissue for treatment of **breast cancer**), which may result in lymphedema of the breast, underarm, or arm on the side of the surgery in 10-20% of patients. This occurs because the lymphatic drainage of the arm passes through the axilla (armpit), and tissue in the axilla is removed during the mastectomy. To reduce the risk of developing lymphedema after breast cancer treatment, there is an alternative treatment that avoids axillary lymph node dissection. Sentinel **lymph node biopsy** is a new diagnostic procedure used to determine whether the breast cancer has spread (metastasized) to axillary lymph nodes. A sentinel lymph node biopsy requires the removal of only one to three lymph nodes for close review by a pathologist. If the sentinel nodes do not contain tumor (cancer) cells, this may eliminate the need to remove additional lymph nodes in the axillary area. Early research on this technique indicates that sentinel lymph node biopsy may be associated with less pain and fewer complications than standard axillary dissection. Because the procedure is so new, long term data are not yet available. However, there is still a risk for developing lymphedema because of follow-up radiation treatments or **chemotherapy**, which may also damage the lymph nodes.

Persons who have developed lymphedema after cancer treatment should be checked for a possible reoccurrence of cancer if they experience a sudden increase of swelling, for the tumor growth may be responsible for blocking lymphatic flow.

Treatments

Lymphedema is a chronic condition that cannot be cured, but it can be improved with treatment. There are several major components of a lymphedema treatment program, which should be administered by the health care provider in cooperation with a physical therapist trained in lymphedema treatment. Complete Decongestive Therapy (CDT; also referred to as Complex Decongestive Therapy (CDT) or as Complete Decongestive Physiotherapy (CDP)) combines manual lymph drainage (MLD) with compression techniques and with patient education on self-care needs. The goals of the treatment program are to:

- remove the stagnant lymph fluids out of the tissues
- reduce and help control swelling
- soften fibrotic tissue
- improve the overall health of the patient.

However, some lymphedema specialists feel that lymphedema patients with metastatic cancer should not be treated with CDT, to prevent the spreading of the cancer.

MLD was developed in 1932 in Denmark by a doctor and his wife. It was widely used in Europe and now is accepted as a therapy for lymphedema patients in the United States. In MLD a series of rhythmic, light strokes are made in a specific sequence along the lymphatic vessels and the adjoining tissues. These movements remove the lymph fluids from the tissues and return them to the circulatory system, thus reducing swelling in the affected area.

Compression techniques include the use of compression garments, compression aids, and compression bandages. These techniques encourage natural drainage and prevent swelling by supporting tissues in a way that aids in drainage. Compression garments are knit, stretch sleeves or stockings. Compression aids are custom-fitted sleeves, stockings, or pads made of fabric-covered foam. Bandages are an effective and flexible means of compression. They work when the patient is active or is resting and can easily be adjusted to fit changing limb sizes. However, the bandage should be a special type of short-stretch bandage and not the long-stretch bandage that is commonly known as Ace bandages. Only persons who are trained in lymphedema therapy should tape or wrap swollen areas.

Self-care techniques are practiced by the patient or his or her caregiver at home, between visits to the therapist. Self-care techniques include self-massage, skin care to maintain healthy tissue, nutritious diet, and **exercise** to increase lymph flow, increase mobility, and to improve the patient's general health.

Exposure to extreme heat has the potential to increase lymphedema swelling, so an affected person or a person at risk of developing lymphedema should avoid hot tubs, saunas, and steam rooms.

To keep the affected extremities as healthy as possible, a person with lymphedema should keep the swollen areas clean and avoid heavy lifting and pulling as well as avoid any type of trauma, such as cuts, **bruises**, **sunburn** or other burns, injections, **sports injuries**, insect bites, or cat scratches. Some doctors and lymphedema therapists recommend that a person with lymphedema use a preventative course of **antibiotics** when having dental treatment, that is, starting antibiotics several days before the appointment and continuing several days afterwards. A person at risk of developing lymphedema (for example, a woman who has been treated for breast cancer) should also observe the same type of precautions to prevent the development of the condition.

If infections occur, then all treatments for lymphedema should be discontinued while the infection is present, and the infection treated with antibiotics.

Surgery is sometimes used to remove excess tissue ("debulking") if the swollen limb becomes so large and heavy as to interfere with movement.

Exercise is important for a person with lymphedema, but only in moderation. If the extremity starts to ache, the person should lie down and elevate the swollen limb. Recommended exercises include walking, swimming, light aerobics, bike riding, and **yoga**.

Persons with lymphedema should wear a lymphedema alert bracelet or necklace for safety during a medical emergency, explaining the risk of infections. They may also benefit from counseling and membership in support groups to deal with the psychological impact of the disease. Sometimes patients with lymphedema will be denied insurance coverage for treatment; as a result patient advocacy groups in 2005 are attempting to get a law passed through the U.S. Congress guaranteeing insurance coverage for lymphedema.

Alternative and complementary therapies

The use of clinical **aromatherapy** in conjunction with CDT may improve the quality of life for persons with lymphedema. Clinical aromatherapy involves the use of essential oils to improve the functioning of the immune system, for the immune system is closely associated with the lymphatic system. Also a massage oil comprised of a blend of frankincense, grapefruit, hyssop, and lavender, may be used to soften scarred and fibrotic tissues. Radiation treatments can cause skin **contractures**, which can be helped by massage with a blend of cajeput, frankincense, hyssop, lavender, sage, and tea tree. Radiation can also have adverse effects on the bowel, resulting in poor bowel functioning, scarring, and activity restrictions. Massaging the abdomen with a blend of grapefruit, fennel, helichrysum, lavender, myrrh, and sage may improve intestinal functions. When compression techniques are used, the underlying skin can be treated with a blend of bay laurel, chamomile, geranium, helchrysum, lavender, patchouli, and vetiver in a combination of castor oil, safflower oil, and grapeseed oil as carrier oils. Good skin care is important in preventing infections. Body oils that contain cajeput, cypress, lavender, marjoram, and rosewood can be applied after bathing to keep the skin moist and healthy. Finger nail beds can be a portal of entry for infections, so can be kept moist with an essential oil blend of chamomile, geranium, lavender, lemon, sage, tea tree, and ylang ylang.

Resources

BOOKS

Burt, Jeannie, and White, Gwen. *Lymphedema: A Breast Cancer Patient's Guide to Prevention and Healing.* Berkeley, CA: Publisher's Group West, 1999.

French, Ramona Moody. *Milady's Guide to Lymph Drainage Massage.* Clifton Park, NY: Milady Publishing, 2003.

Kelly, Deborah G. *A Primer on Lymphedema.* Essex, United Kingdom: Pearson Education, 2001.

Parker, James N. and Parker, Philip M. . San Diego, CA: Icon Health Publications, 2004.

PERIODICALS

Heckathorn, Peg. *"Use of Aromatherapy in Lymphedema Management."* Lymph Link. Oct-Dec. 2003, Vol. 15, No. 4, 6-12

Axillary nodes—Lymph nodes found in the armpit that drain the lymph channels from the breast.

Clinical aromatherapy—Aromatherapy is the therapeutic use of plant-derived, aromatic essential oils to promote physical and psychological well-being. It is sometimes used in combination with massage and other therapeutic techniques as part of a holistic treatment approach.

Debulking—General term used for surgeries in which subcutaneous tissue is removed from lymphodemous limb.

Fibrosis—Formation of fibrous tissue as a reaction or as a repair process; may occur due to treatment and/or disease. in lymphedema condition known as hardening of the limb with resulting restriction of circulatory flow, increased infection, and weeping sores.

Fibrotic—Pertaining to or characterized by fibrosis. In dermatological description, "fibrotic" would be used to describe leathery, bound-down, or thickened, scarred skin.

Interstitial fluid—The fluid between cells in tissues. Referred to as the liquid subtance of the body.

Interstitial space—The fluid filled areas that surround the cells of a given tissue; also known as tissue space.

Long-stretch bandages—Specialized bandages, similar to an Ace bandage, that have 100 to 200% stretch.

Low-stretch bandage—Specialized bandages, with 30 to 90% stretch, that are used to obtain the correct compression during the treatment of lymphedema; also known as short-stretch bandages.

Lymph—The almost colourless fluid that bathes body tissues and is found in the lymphatic vessels that drain the tissues of the fluid that filters across the blood vessel walls from blood. Lymph carries antibodies and lymphocytes (white blood cells that help fight infection) that have entered the lymph nodes from the blood.

Lymph nodes—Small bean-shaped organs of the immune system, distributed widely throughout the body and linked by lymphatic vessels. Lymph nodes are garrisons of B, T, and other immune cells.

Lymph System—When sickness or infection invades the body, the immune system is the first line of defense. A big part of that defense is the lymph system. Lymph is carried through the body by lymph vessels that have valves and muscles to help move the fluid. Along the route are lymph nodes that serve as filters for harmful substances. This network of vessels and nodes together is called the lymph system.

Lymphatic fluid—The clear fluid found outside the cells which bathes the tissues. It is collected, filtered, and transported by the lymphatic system from around the tissues to the blood circulatory system. Fluid that collects as a result of lymphedema.

Nail beds—The underlying connective tissue that nourishes the finger and toenails.

Pitting edema—When a swollen area is pressed, the pressure leaves an indentation (pit) that takes time to fill back in.

Sentinel node biopsy—A newer procedure performed in order to determine whether breast cancer has spread to auxiliary (underarm) lymph nodes. A blue radioactive tracer and/or blue dye is injected into the area of the breast tumor. The lymphatic vessels carry the dye or radioactive material, to a "sentinel node". This sentinel node is thought to be the first lymph node receiving fluid from the tumor and the one most likely to contain cancer cells if the cancer has spread. Only if the sentinel node contains cancer cells are more lymph nodes removed.

Skin contracture—A permanent tightening of the skin that prevents normal movement of the associated body part and that can cause permanent deformity. A contracture develops when the normally elastic connective tissues are replaced by inelastic fibrous tissue. This makes the affected area resistant to stretching and prevents normal movement.

OTHER

Lymph Notes, an online information resource and support group for those with lymphedema and for the family, friends, and therapists who care for them. Web site: < www.lymphnotes.com/index.php >

National Lymphedema Network, Latham Square Building, Suite 1111, 1611 Telegraph Avenue, Oakland, CA 94612-2138. Telephone: (800) 541-3259. Fax: (510) 208-3110. Web site: < www.lymphnet.org >

Lymphedema People. Web site: < www.lymphedemapeople.com/ >

Lymphatic Research Foundation. < http:// www.lymphaticresearch.org >

Lymphedema Awareness Foundation. < http:// www.elymphnotes.com/ >

Judith Sims

Lymphocyte typing

Definition

Lymphocyte typing focuses on identifying the numbers and relative percentages of lymphocytes in an individual's bloodstream. Lymphocytes, primarily T cells and B cells, are types of white blood cells, the underlying supports of the immune system in the bloodstream.

Purpose

Determining the numbers and relative percentages of T cells and B cells provides information on the state of a person's immune system. By comparing these values to normal numbers and percentages, the presence of disease and the side effects of certain drugs can be revealed. Lymphocyte typing can also show whether a person has been exposed to certain poisonous substances.

Description

To do a white blood cell count, a small amount of blood is drawn from a vein. The total number of white blood cells is calculated, either through microscopic examination of a blood smear or by using automated counting equipment. For a white blood cell count with differential, 100 white blood cells are counted and the proportion of each type is calculated. Since T cells and B cells have similar appearances, a differential can only give the proportion of lymphocytes in the blood, not the proportion of specific lymphocyte types.

For more specific information on B cells and T cells, it is necessary to divide the blood into its separate components. In this procedure, a tube of blood is placed in a centrifuge, a piece of equipment that spins the tube in circles at high speed. The force generated by the spinning causes the various elements in the bloodstream to settle at different levels of the tube.

The lymphocytes are extracted from the tube and treated with special dyes, or stains. Each stain is equipped with an antibody portion that adheres to a specific type of lymphocyte, such as a B cell or a T cell. The stains make the cells visible to an automated counting machine, called a flow cytometer. Based on the number of times the machine detects a particular stain, it can calculate the number of the associated cell type. This procedure can also be used to classify T cells and B cells into their subtypes.

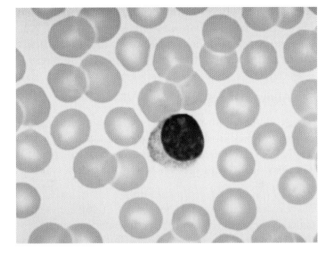

A lymphocyte cell. (Photograph by Lester V. Bergman, Corbis Images. Reproduced by permission.)

KEY TERMS

Immune system—The body's system of defenses against infectious diseases.

Lymphocytosis—A condition in which the number of lymphocytes increases above normal levels.

Lymphopenia—A condition in which the number of lymphocytes falls below normal levels.

White blood cell—A class of cells in the blood that form the foundation of the body's immune system.

Preparation

If possible, a person should avoid eating a heavy meal within hours of the test or engaging in strenuous **exercise** for the 24 hours preceding the blood test.

Normal results

In general, normal levels of white blood cells vary slightly by age and gender. Normal values are lower in children under the age of 15 and in young adults between the ages of 20 and 30. After age 30, men have slightly higher levels of white blood cells than women.

Normal adult levels of white blood cells are 4,500-11,000 cells per microliter of blood. Lymphocytes account for approximately 25-45% of the total white blood cell count; the normal range is 1,000-4,800 lymphocytes per microliter of blood. Of the total lymphocytes, 60-80% are T cells and approximately 15% are B cells. (There are two other types of lymphocytes; natural killer and K-type; that constitute a minor proportion of the total lymphocyte numbers.)

Abnormal results

A higher-than-normal level of lymphocytes is called lymphocytosis. Lymphocytosis occurs if a person has a viral, bacterial, or other type of infection. It can also occur with certain blood disorders, such as leukemia.

Lower-than-normal levels of lymphocytes is called lymphopenia. Lymphopenia can be an indicator of certain cancers, bone marrow failure, or immune system deficiency. Medical treatments, such as **chemotherapy** and **radiation therapy**, can also deplete the body's supply of lymphocytes, as can exposure to poisonous substances.

Resources

BOOKS

Corbett, Jane Vincent. *Laboratory Tests & Diagnostic Procedures with Nursing Diagnoses.* 4th ed. Stamford: Appleton & Lange, 1996.

Turgeon, Mary Louise. *Immunology & Serology in Laboratory Medicine.* St. Louis: Mosby-Year Book, Inc., 1996.

Julia Barrett

Lymphocytic choriomeningitis

Definition

Lymphocytic choriomeningitis (LCM) is a viral infection of the membranes surrounding the brain and spinal cord and of the cerebrospinal fluid.

Description

Lymphocytic choriomeningitis virus infection is relatively rare and recovery usually occurs spontaneously within a couple of weeks. Many cases are probably not even identified because the symptoms range from extremely mild to those resembling severe flu. A few patients develop symptoms of **meningitis**. In some rare cases, the LCM viral infection can spread throughout the central nervous system, and may even be fatal.

Causes and symptoms

LCM is caused by an arenavirus, which is an RNA virus and is a mild cousin in the family containing the much more threatening arenaviruses that cause hemmorrhagic **fever**. Humans acquire LCM virus from infected rodents by coming in contact with the animals or their excretions. Exposure to the virus is not as unlikely to occur as it seems, because the viral hosts can be common house mice and even pets, such as hamsters and chinchillas. Most cases of LCM occur in fall and winter, when mice seek warmth inside dwellings. Food and dust can become contaminated by the excretions of rodents infected with LCM virus. In 1997, French scientists alerted physicians to suspect LCM viral infection in people who had contact with Syrian hamsters.

The symptoms of LCM occur in two phases. The first (prodrome) stage can produce fever, chills, muscle aches, **cough**, and **vomiting**. In the second phase, characteristic meningitis symptoms of **headache**, stiff neck, listlessness, and **nausea and vomiting** may occur. In adults, complications are rare and recovery may even occur before the second phase.

The virus is not spread from person to person, except through **pregnancy**. LCM virus is one of the few viruses that can cross the placenta from mother to child during pregnancy and may be an underrecognized cause of congenital infection in newborns. Infection with cytomegalovirus, *Toxoplasma gondii,* or LCM virus can appear similar enough in infants to be confused when diagnosed. In cases that have been recognized among infants, LCM viral infection has a high mortality rate (about one-third of the babies studied died).

Diagnosis

LCM can be distinguished from bacterial meningitis by the history of prodrome symptoms and the period of time before meningitis symptoms begin, which is about 15-21 days for LCM.

Treatment

No antiviral agents exist for LCM virus. Treatment consists of supporting the patient and treating the symptoms until the infection subsides, generally within a few weeks.

Jill S. Lasker

Lymphocytic leukemia, acute *see* **Leukemias, acute**

Lymphocytic leukemia, chronic *see* **Leukemias, chronic**

Lymphocytopenia

Definition

Lymphocytopenia is a condition marked by an abnormally low level of lymphocytes in the blood. Lymphocytes are a specific type of white blood cell with important functions in the immune system.

Description

Lymphocytes normally account for 15–40% of all white cells in the bloodstream. They help to protect the body from infections caused by viruses or fungi. They also coordinate the activities of other cells in the immune system. In addition, lymphocytes fight **cancer** and develop into antibody-producing cells that neutralize the effect of foreign substances in the blood.

Lymphocytopenia is the result of abnormalities in the way lymphocytes are produced, make their way through the bloodstream, or are lost or destroyed. These conditions can result from congenital or drug-induced decreases in the body's ability to recognize and attack invaders.

Causes and symptoms

Lymphocytopenia has a wide range of possible causes:

- **AIDS** and other viral, bacterial, and fungal infections

- Chronic failure of the right ventricle of the heart. This chamber of the heart pumps blood to the lungs.

- Hodgkin's disease and cancers of the lymphatic system

- A leak or rupture in the thoracic duct. The thoracic duct removes lymphatic fluid from the legs and abdomen.

- Leukemia

- Side effects of prescription medications

- Malnutrition. **Diets** that are low in protein and overall calorie intake may cause lymphocytopenia.

- Radiation therapy

- High **stress** levels

- Trauma.

The symptoms of lymphocytopenia vary. Lymphocytes constitute only a fraction of the body's white blood cells, and a decline in their number may not produce any symptoms. A patient who has lymphocytopenia may have symptoms of the condition responsible for the depressed level of lymphocytes.

Diagnosis

Lymphocytopenia is most often detected when blood tests are performed to diagnose other diseases.

Treatment

Treatment for lymphocytopenia is designed to identify and correct the underlying cause of the condition.

Drug-depressed lymphocyte levels usually return to normal a few days after the patient stops taking the medication.

A deficiency of B lymphocytes, which mature into antibody-producing plasma cells, can result in abnormally low lymphocyte levels. When the number of B lymphocytes is low, the patient may be treated with **antibiotics**, antifungal medications, antiviral agents, or a substance containing a high concentration of antibodies (gamma globulin) to prevent infection.

It is not usually possible to restore normal lymphocyte levels in AIDS patients. Drugs like AZT (azidothymidine, sold under the trade name Retrovir) can increase the number of helper T cells, which help other cells wipe out disease organisms.

Prognosis

Very low levels of lymphocytes make patients vulnerable to life-threatening infection. Researchers are studying the effectiveness of transplanting bone marrow and other cells to restore normal lymphocyte levels. **Gene therapy**, which uses the body's own resources or artificial substances to counter diseases or disorders, is also being evaluated as a treatment for lymphocytopenia.

Resources

BOOKS

Berktow, Robert, et al., editors. *Merck Manual of Medical Information: Home Edition.* Whitehouse Station, NJ: Merck Research Laboratories, 1997.

Maureen Haggerty

Lymphogranuloma venereum

Definition

Lymphogranuloma venereum (LGV) is a sexually transmitted systemic disease (STD) caused by a parasitic organism closely related to certain types of bacteria. It affects the lymph nodes and rectal area, as well as the genitals, in humans. The name comes from two Latin words that mean a swelling of granulation tissue in the lymph nodes resulting from sexual intercourse. Granulation tissue is tissue that forms during wound or ulcer healing that has a rough or lumpy surface.

Description

Although LGV is easily treated in its early stages, it can produce serious complications in its later stages. LGV is most likely to occur among people living in tropical or subtropical countries and among military personnel or tourists in countries or large cities with high rates of the disease. Prostitutes play a major role in carrying and transmitting LGV, as was documented during an outbreak in Florida in the late 1980s. There are about 1000 documented cases of LGV in the United States in an average year.

Causes and symptoms

LGV is caused by *Chlamydia trachomatis*, a globe-shaped parasitic organism that reproduces only inside of living cells. *C. trachomatis* has 17 subtypes and is responsible for a wide range of infections in both men and women; however, only subtypes L1, L2, and L3 cause lymphogranuloma venereum. The parasite has a two-part lifecycle. In the first stage, it is inert and can survive outside of cells. In its second stage, it lacks a cell wall and actively reproduces after gaining entry to a cell. As the chlamydia organism reproduces inside the cell, it pushes the nucleus aside and forms an inclusion that can be identified with tissue staining. LGV differs from other diseases caused by *C. trachomatis* in that it affects the body's lymphatic system and not just the moist tissues of the genital region. In humans, the chlamydia organism is transmitted through vaginal or anal intercourse, oral sex, or contact with fluid from open ulcers or infected tissues.

Lymphogranuloma venereum has three stages. In its primary stage, the disease is more likely to be detected in men; it may go unnoticed in women. After an incubation period of four to 30 days, a small painless ulcer or blister develops in the genital area. Second-stage LGV develops between one and six weeks later. In this stage, the infection spreads to the lymphatic system, forming buboes (swellings) in the lymph nodes of the groin area. The buboes often merge, soften, and rupture, forming sinuses and fistulas (hollow passages and ducts) that carry an infectious bloody discharge to the outside of the body. Patients with second-stage LGV may also have **fever**, **nausea**, headaches, pains in their joints, skin **rashes**, and enlargement of the spleen or liver. Third-stage LGV, which is sometimes called anogenitorectal syndrome, develops in about 25% of patients. In men, this stage is usually seen in homosexuals. Third-stage LGV is marked by rectal **pain**, **constipation**, a discharge containing pus or bloody mucus, and the development of strictures (narrowing or tightening of a body passage) in the rectum or vagina.

LGV can have a number of serious complications. *C. trachomatis* infections of any subtype are associated with long-term fertility problems in women. Strictures in the rectum can completely close off the lower bowel, producing eventual rupture of the bowel and inflammation of the abdominal cavity. The patient can develop chronic abscesses or fistulae in the anal area or in the vagina in women. Long-term blockages in the lymph nodes can produce **elephantiasis**, a condition in which the patient's upper legs and groin area become greatly enlarged. Patients with chronic LGV infection

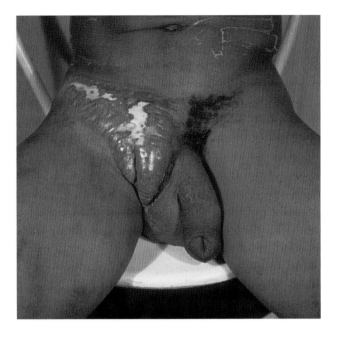

This man suffers from lymphogranuloma venereum, a vener-eal disease that is caused by the bacterium *Chlamydia tracho-matis.* (Photograph by Milton Reisch, M.D., Corbis Images. Reproduced by permission.)

have a higher risk of developing **cancer** in the inflamed areas.

Chronic LGV can be reactivated in patients who become infected with the **AIDS** virus. These patients develop open ulcers in the groin that are difficult to treat.

Diagnosis

The diagnosis of LGV is usually made on the basis of the patient's history, careful examination of the genital area and lymph nodes, and blood tests or cultures to confirm the diagnosis. In the early stages of the disease, the doctor will need to distinguish between LGV and such other STDs as **syphilis** and herpes. If the patient has developed buboes, the doctor will need to rule out **tuberculosis, cat-scratch disease,** bubonic **plague,** or **tularemia** (a disease similar to plague that is carried by rabbits and squirrels). If the patient has developed rectal strictures, the doctor will need to rule out tumors or colitis.

There are several blood tests that can be used to confirm the diagnosis of LGV. The most commonly used are the complement fixation (CF) test and the microimmunofluorescence (micro-IF) tests. Although the micro-IF test is considered more sensitive than the CF test, it is less widely available. An antibody titer (concentration) of 1:64 or greater on the CF test or

1:512 or greater on the micro-IF test is needed to make the diagnosis of LGV. In some cases, the diagnosis can be made from culturing *C. trachomatis* taken from samples of tissue fluid from ulcers or buboes, or from a tissue sample from the patient's rectum.

Treatment

LGV is treated with oral **antibiotics,** usually tetra-cycline or doxycycline for 10-20 days, or erythromycin or trimethoprim sulfamethoxazole for 14 days. Pregnant women are usually treated with erythromy-cin rather than the **tetracyclines,** because this class of medications can harm the fetus.

Patients who have developed second- and third-stage complications may need surgical treatment. The doctor can treat buboes by withdrawing fluid from them through a hollow needle into a suction syringe. This procedure is called aspiration. Fistulas and abscesses also can be treated surgically. Patients who develop elephantiasis are usually treated by plastic surgeons. Patients with rectal strictures may need surgery to prevent bowel obstruction and rupture into the abdomen.

Prognosis

The prognosis for recovery for most patients is good, with the exception of AIDS patients. Prompt treatment of the early stages of LGV is essential to prevent transmission of the disease as well as fertility problems and other serious complications of the later stages.

Prevention

Prevention of lymphogranuloma venereum has four important aspects:

- Avoidance of casual sexual contacts, particularly with prostitutes, in countries with high rates of the disease.

- Observance of proper safeguards by health professionals. Doctors and other healthcare workers should wear gloves when touching infected areas of the patient's body or handling soiled dressings and other contaminated items. All contaminated materials and instruments should be double-bagged before disposing.

- Tracing and examination of an infected person's recent sexual contacts.

- Monitoring the patient for recurring symptoms for a period of six months after antibiotic treatment.

Resources

BOOKS

Chambers, Henry F. "Infectious Diseases: Bacterial & Chlamydial." In *Current Medical Diagnosis and Treatment, 1998*, edited by Stephen McPhee, et al., 37th ed. Stamford: Appleton & Lange, 1997.

Rebecca J. Frey, PhD

Lymphomas *see* **Hodgkin's disease**

Lymphopenia *see* **Lymphocytopenia**

Lymphosarcomas *see* **Malignant lymphomas**

Lysergic acid diethylamide (LSD)

Definition

Lysergic acid diethylamide (LSD), also known as "acid," belongs to a class of drugs known as hallucinogens, which distort perceptions of reality. LSD is the most potent mood- and perception-altering drug known: doses as small as 30 micrograms can produce effects lasting six to 12 hours.

Purpose

In the United States, LSD has no accepted medical use and its manufacture is illegal.

Description

LSD is produced synthetically from a fungus that grows on rye grass. This odorless, colorless, and slightly bitter-tasting chemical is generally ingested orally and absorbed from the gastrointestinal system. Manufacturers commonly distribute LSD in small squares of absorbent paper soaked with the drug, which users chew and swallow. Use of LSD and other hallucinogens by secondary school students has decreased since 1998, but has increased among older teens and young adults attending dance clubs and all-night raves, according to the National Institute on Drug **Abuse**.

LSD alters perceptions by disrupting the action of the neurotransmitter serotonin, although precisely how it does this is unclear. Studies suggest LSD acts on certain groups of serotonin receptors, and that its effects are most prominent in two brain regions: the cerebral cortex and the locus ceruleus. The cerebral cortex is involved in mood and perception, and the locus ceruleus receives sensory signals from all areas of the body. Natural hallucinogens resembling LSD, such as mescaline and psilocybin, have been used in social and religious rituals for thousands of years.

After its discovery in 1938, LSD was used experimentally to treat neuroses, narcotic **addiction**, **autism**, **alcoholism**, and terminally ill **cancer** patients, and to study the mechanisms of psychotic diseases like **schizophrenia**. Nearly 30 years after its discovery, manufacture, possession, sale, and use of LSD was restricted in the United States under the Drug Abuse Control Amendment of 1965.

LSD's effects generally begin within an hour of taking the drug and last for up to 12 hours. The drug is absorbed from the gastrointestinal tract, and circulated throughout the body and to the brain. It is metabolized in the liver and excreted in the urine about 24 hours after ingestion. Physical effects of LSD may include loss of appetite, sleeplessness, pupil dilation, **dry mouth**, salivation, **palpitations**, perspiration, **nausea**, **dizziness**, blurred vision, and **anxiety**, as well as increased body temperature, heartbeat, blood pressure, and blood sugar.

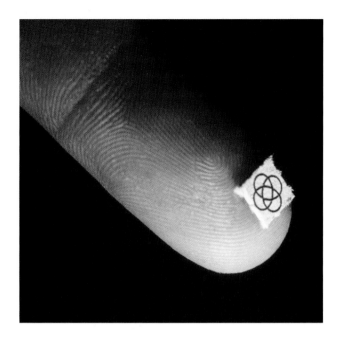

LSD on blotter paper. *(Custom Medical Stoch Photo Inc. Reproduced by permission)*

The major effects of LSD are emotional and sensory. Emotions may shift instantaneously from euphoria to confusion and despair, and users may feel as if they are experiencing several emotions simultaneously. Colors, smells, and sounds may be highly intensified, and time may appear to move very slowly. Sensory perceptions may blend in a phenomenon known as synesthesia, in which a person sees sounds, or smells colors, for example. Users may have out-of-body sensations, or may perceive their body has changed shape or merged with another person or object.

Precautions

Unlike **cocaine**, amphetamines, heroin, alcohol, and nicotine, LSD is not considered addictive, but it is considered dangerous; users are at risk for several short- and long-term side effects. LSD's effects are unpredictable and may vary with the amount ingested and the user's personality, mood, expectations, and surroundings. Users may experience enjoyable sensations on some "trips," and terrifying feelings of anxiety and despair on others. Most LSD-related deaths stem not from the LSD's physical effects on the body, but from the panicked reactions ensuing from intense LSD-triggered illusions.

Side Effects

Two long-term effects are associated with LSD use: **psychosis**, and hallucinogen persisting perception disorder (HPPD), also known as "flashbacks." The exact causes of these effects, including the mechanism by which LSD may cause them, is unknown. Chronic hallucinogen users or individuals with underlying personality problems are most vulnerable to these effects, but individuals with no history of psychological disorders have also experienced them. LSD-induced psychosis may include dramatic mood swings, loss of cognitive and communication skills, and **hallucinations**. Flashbacks generally involve seeing bright flashes, or halos or trails attached to moving objects after the LSD "trip" has ended. Flashbacks can last a few seconds or even several hours.

According to the Drug Abuse Warning Network (DAWN), the number of LSD-related hospital emergencies is low compared to those related to cocaine, heroin, **marijuana**, methamphetamine, and other illicit drugs. One reason for this trend may be that LSD currently sold on the black market is less potent than in the past. LSD dose strengths tend to range from 20 to 80 micrograms today, compared to 100 to 200 micrograms reported during the 1960s and early 1970s.

Interactions

LSD flashbacks can be spurred by use of drugs such as marijuana. Preliminary evidence suggests serotonin reuptake inhibitors like Prozac and Zoloft may also exacerbate the LSD flashback syndrome.

Resources

PERIODICALS

Aghajanian, G. K. and G. J. Marek. "Serotonin and Hallucinogens." *Neuropsychopharmacology* 1999: 16S-23S

ORGANIZATIONS

National Clearinghouse for Alcohol and Drug Information. 11426 Rockville Pike, Suite 200, Rockville, MD. 20852. (800) 729-6686. < http:\\www.health.org >.

National Institute on Drug Abuse. P.O. Box 30652, Bethesda, MD. 20824-0652. (888) 644-6432. < http:\\www.drugabuse.gov >.

U.S. Department of Justice, Drug Enforcement Administration. 2401 Jefferson Davis Highway, Alexandria, VA 22301. (888) 644-6432. < http:\\www.usdoj.gov/dea >.

Ann Quigley

M

Macular degeneration

Definition

Macular degeneration is the progressive deterioration of a critical region of the retina called the macula. The macula is a 3-5 mm area in the retina that is responsible for central vision. This disorder leads to irreversible loss of central vision, although peripheral vision is retained. In the early stages, vision may be gray, hazy, or distorted.

Description

Macular degeneration is the most common cause of legal blindness in people over 60, and accounts for approximately 11.7% of blindness in the United States. About 28% of the population over age 74 is affected by this disease.

Age-related macular degeneration (ARMD) is the most common form of macular degeneration. It is also known as age-related maculopathy (ARM), aged macular degeneration, and senile macular degeneration. Approximately 10 million Americans have some vision loss that is due to ARMD.

ARMD is subdivided into a dry (atrophic) and a wet (exudative) form. The dry form is more common and accounts for 70-90% of cases of ARMD. It progresses more slowly than the wet form and vision loss is less severe. In the dry form, the macula thins over time as part of the **aging** process and the pigmented retinal epithelium (a dark-colored cell layer at the back of the eye) is gradually lost. Words may appear blurred or hazy and colors may appear dim or gray.

In the wet form of ARMD, new blood vessels grow underneath the retina and distort the retina. These blood vessels can leak, causing scar tissue to form on the retina. The wet form may cause visual distortion and make straight lines appear wavy. A central blind spot develops. The wet type progresses more rapidly and vision loss is more pronounced. Treatments are available for some, but not most, cases of the wet form.

Other less common forms of macular degeneration include:

- Cystoid macular degeneration. Loss of vision in the macula due to fluid-filled areas (cysts) in the macular region. This may be a result of other disorders, such as aging, inflammation, or high myopia.

- Diabetic macular degeneration. Deterioration of the macula due to diabetes.

- Senile disciform degeneration (also known as Kuhnt-Junius macular degeneration). A specific and severe type of the wet form of ARMD that involves leaking blood vessels (hemorrhaging) in the macular region. It usually occurs in people over 40 years old.

Causes and symptoms

Age-related macular degeneration is part of the aging process. There may be a hereditary component. Having a family member with ARMD increases a person's risk for developing it. There is a slightly higher incidence in females. Whites and Asians are more susceptible to developing ARMD than blacks, in whom the disorder is rare.

ARMD is thought to be caused by hardening and blocking of the arteries (arteriosclerosis) in the blood vessels supplying the retina. Some of the same things that are bad for the heart are thought to contribute to the development of macular degeneration. These risk factors include **smoking** and a diet that is rich in saturated fat. Smokers have a risk of developing ARMD that is approximately 2.4-3 times that of non-smokers. Smoking increases the risk of developing wet-type ARMD, and may increase the risk of developing dry-type as well. Dietary fat also increase the risk. In one study of older (age 45-84) Americans, signs of early ARMD were 80% more common in the group who ate the most saturated fat compared to those who ate the least. Low consumption of antioxidants, such as foods rich in vitamin A, is associated with a higher risk for developing ARMD. Consumption of moderate amounts of red wine and foods rich in vitamin A is associated with a lower risk. It is generally believed that exposure to ultraviolet (UV) light may contribute to disease development, but this has not been proven.

The main symptom of macular degeneration is a change in central vision. The patient may notice blurred central vision or a blank spot on the page when reading. The patient may notice visual distortion such as bending of straight lines. Images may appear smaller. Some patients notice a change in color perception and some experience abnormal light sensations. These symptoms may come on suddenly and become progressively more troublesome. Sudden onset of symptoms, particularly vision distortion, is an indication for immediate evaluation by an ophthalmologist.

Diagnosis

To make the diagnosis of macular degeneration, the doctor dilates the pupil with eye drops and examines the interior of the eye, looking at the retina for the presence of yellow bumps called drusen and for gross changes in the macula such as thinning. The doctor also administers a visual field test, looking for blank spots in the central vision. The doctor may call for fluorescein **angiography** (intravenous injection of fluorescent dye followed by visual examination and photography of the back of the eye) to determine if blood vessels in the retina are leaking.

A central visual field test called an Amsler grid is usually given to patients who are suspected of having ARMD. It is a grid printed on a sheet of paper (so it is easy to take home). When looking at a central dot on the page, the patient should call the doctor right away if any of the lines appear to be wavy or missing. This may be an indication of fluid and the onset of wet ARMD. Patients may also be asked to come in for more frequent checkups.

Treatment

While loss of vision cannot be reversed, early detection is important because treatments are available that may halt or slow the progression of the wet form of ARMD. Treatment for the dry form is not available as of 1998, but cell transplantation studies are under study.

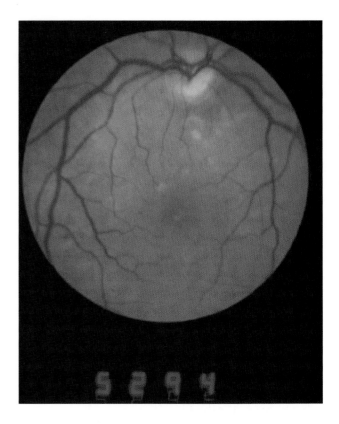

A slit-lamp view showing macular degeneration of the eye. *(Custom Medical Stock Photo. Reproduced by permission.)*

In wet-type ARMD and in senile disciform macular degeneration, new capillaries grow in the macular region and leak. This leaking of blood and fluid causes a portion of the retina to detach. Blood vessel growth, called neovascularization, can be treated with laser photocoagulation in some cases, depending upon the location and extent of the growth. Argon or krypton lasers can destroy the new tissue and flatten the retina. This treatment is effective in about half the cases but results may be temporary. A concern with laser therapy is that the laser also destroys the photoreceptors in the treated area. If the blood vessels have grown into the fovea (a region of the macula responsible for fine vision), treatment may not be possible. Because capillaries can grow very quickly, this form of macular degeneration should be handled as an emergency and treated quickly. Patients who are experiencing visual distortion should seek help immediately.

Another form of treatment for the wet form of ARMD is **radiation therapy** with either x rays or a proton beam. Blood vessels that are proliferating (growing) are sensitive to treatment with low doses of ionizing radiation. Nerve cells in the retina are not growing and are insensitive, so they are not harmed by this treatment. External beam radiation treatment has shown promising results at slowing progression in limited, early trials. An alternative treatment is internal beam radiation therapy. For this treatment, the patient is given a local anesthetic and an applicator containing strontium 90 is inserted into the affected eye. This brief and localized radiation therapy prevents the growth of blood vessels.

Other therapies that are under study include treatment with alpha-interferon, thalidomide, and other drugs that slow the growth of blood vessels. Subretinal surgery also has shown promise in rapid-onset cases of wet ARMD. This surgery carries the risk of **retinal detachment**, hemorrhage, and acceleration of cataract formation. Other experimental treatments include photodynamic therapy (PDT). For this treatment, a photosensitizing dye is injected, followed by irradiation of the area of new blood vessel growth with a special, low-intensity diode laser. This treatment damages the cells in the blood vessel walls and causes them to stop growing.

A controversial treatment called rheotherapy involves pumping the patient's blood through a device that removes some proteins and fats. As of 1998, this had not been proven to be safe or effective.

Alternative treatment

Consumption of a diet rich in antioxidants (beta carotene and the mixed carotenoids that are precursors of vitamin A, **vitamins** C and E, selenium, and zinc), or taking antioxidant **nutritional supplements**, may help prevent macular degeneration, particularly if started early in life. Good dietary sources of antioxidants include citrus fruits, cauliflower, broccoli, nuts, seeds, orange and yellow vegetables, cherries, blackberries, and blueberries. Research has shown that nutritional therapy can prevent ARMD or slow its progression once established. Some doctors recommend taking beta carotene and zinc as a precautionary measure. Some vitamins are marketed specifically for the eyes.

Prognosis

The dry form of ARMD is self-limiting and eventually stabilizes. The loss of vision is permanent. The vision of patients with the wet form of ARMD often stabilizes or improves even without treatment, at least temporarily. However, after a few years, patients with the wet form of ARMD are usually left with only coarse peripheral vision remaining.

Many patients with macular degeneration lose their central vision permanently and may become

---

KEY TERMS

Drusen—Tiny yellow dots on the retina that can be soft or hard and that usually do not interfere with vision.

Fovea—A tiny pit in the macula that is responsible for sharp vision.

Neovascularization—Growth of new capillaries.

Photoreceptors—Specialized nerve cells (rods and cones) in the retina that are responsible for vision.

Retina—The light-sensitive membrane at the back of the eye that images are focused on. The retina sends the images to the brain via the optic nerve.

---

legally blind. However, macular degeneration rarely causes total loss of vision. Peripheral vision is retained. The patient can compensate, to some extent, for the loss of central vision, even though macular degeneration may render them legally blind. Improved lighting and special low-vision aids may help even if sharpness of vision (visual acuity) is poor. Vision aids include special magnifiers that allow the patient to read and telescopic aids for long-distance vision. The use of these visual aids plus the retained peripheral vision usually allow the patient to remain independent. Registration as a legally blind person will enable a patient to obtain special services and considerations.

Prevention

Avoiding the risk factors for macular degeneration may help prevent it. This includes avoiding tobacco smoke and eating a diet low in saturated fat. Some other behaviors that may help reduce the risk of wet-type ARMD are eating a diet rich in green, leafy vegetables and yellow vegetables such as carrots, sweet potatoes, and winter squash; drinking moderate amounts of alcohol, such as one or two glasses of red wine a day; and taking an antioxidant vitamin supplement, especially vitamin A. Some vitamins may be toxic in large doses, so patients should speak with their doctors. Vitamins C and E have not been shown to reduce risk, nor did selenium in one large study. The use of zinc is controversial: some studies showed a benefit, others showed no benefit, and one actually showed an increased risk of ARMD with increased levels of zinc in the blood. Some doctors suggest that wearing UV-blocking sunglasses reduces risk. Use of estrogen in postmenopausal women is associated with a lower risk of developing ARMD.

Resources

ORGANIZATIONS

American Academy of Ophthalmology. 655 Beach Street, P.O. Box 7424, San Francisco, CA 94120-7424. < http://www.eyenet.org >.

American Optometric Association. 243 North Lindbergh Blvd., St. Louis, MO 63141. (314) 991-4100. < http://www.aoanet.org >.

Prevent Blindness America. 500 East Remington Road, Schaumburg, IL 60173. (800) 331-2020. < http://www.preventblindness.org >.

Louann W. Murray, PhD

Macule *see* **Skin lesions**

Mad cow disease *see* **Creutzfeldt-Jakob disease**

Madura foot *see* **Mycetoma**

Maduromycosis *see* **Mycetoma**

Magnesium hydroxide *see* **Antacids**

▌ Magnesium imbalance

Definition

A mineral found in the fluid that surrounds cells, magnesium (Mg) is an essential component of more than 300 enzymes that regulate many body functions. Imbalances occur when the blood contains more or less magnesium than it should.

Description

Magnesium is necessary for the formation and functioning of healthy bones, teeth, muscles, and nerves. It converts food into energy, builds proteins, and is instrumental in maintaining adequate levels of calcium in the blood. Magnesium helps prevent cardiovascular disease and irregular heartbeat, reduces the risk of bone loss (**osteoporosis**), and increases an individual's chance of surviving a **heart attack**. It may also help prevent **stroke** and lessen the effects of existing osteoporosis.

Fish, dairy products, leafy green vegetables, legumes, nuts, seeds, and grains are especially good sources of magnesium, but varying amounts of this mineral are found in all foods. Some is stored in the kidneys, and excess amounts are excreted in the urine or stools.

Magnesium deficiency (hypomagnesemia) or excess (hypermagnesemia) is rare, but either condition can be serious.

Causes and symptoms

Hypomagnesemia

Magnesium deficiency most often occurs in people who have been fed intravenously for a long time, whose diet does not contain enough magnesium, or who are unable to absorb and excrete the mineral properly.

Secreting too much aldosterone (the hormone that regulates the body's salt-fluid balance), ADH (a hormone that inhibits urine production), or thyroid hormone can cause hypomagnesemia.

Other factors associated with hypomagnesemia include:

- Loss of body fluids as a result of stomach suctioning or chronic **diarrhea**
- Cisplatin (a **chemotherapy** drug)
- Long-term diuretic therapy
- Hypercalcemia (abnormally high levels of calcium in the blood)
- Diabetic acidosis (a condition in which the body's tissues have a higher-than-normal acid content)
- Complications of bowel surgery
- Chronic **alcoholism**
- Malnutrition
- Starvation
- Severe **dehydration**.

People who have hypomagnesemia usually experience loss of weight and appetite, bloating, and muscle **pain**, and they pass stools that have a high fat content. Also, they may be listless, disoriented, confused, and very irritable. Other symptoms of hypomagnesemia are:

- Nausea
- Vomiting
- Muscle weakness
- Tremor
- Irregular heart beat
- Delusions and **hallucinations**
- Leg and foot cramps
- Muscle twitches
- Changes in blood pressure.

Severe magnesium deficiency can cause seizures, especially in children.

Neonatal hypomagnesemia can occur in premature babies and in infants who have genetic parathyroid disorders or who have had blood transfusions. This condition also occurs in babies born to magnesium-deficient mothers or to women who have:

- Diabetes mellitus
- Hyperparathyroidism (overactive parathyroid glands)
- Toxemia (a pregnancy-related condition characterized by high blood pressure and fluid retention).

Hypermagnesemia

Hypermagnesemia is most common in patients whose kidneys cannot excrete the magnesium they derive from food or take as medication. This condition can also develop in patients who take magnesium salts, or in healthy people who use large quantities of magnesium-containing **antacids**, **laxatives**, or **analgesics** (pain relievers).

Magnesium **poisoning** can cause severe diarrhea in young people, and mask the symptoms of other illnesses. Very high overdoses can lead to **coma**. The risk of complications of magnesium poisoning is greatest for:

- Elderly people with inefficient kidney function
- Patients with kidney problems or intestinal disorders
- People who use **antihistamines**, **muscle relaxants**, or narcotics.

Severe dehydration or an overdose of supplements taken to counteract hypomagnesemia can also cause this condition.

People who have hypermagnesemia may feel flushed and drowsy, perspire heavily, and have diarrhea. Breathing becomes shallow, reflexes diminish, and the patient becomes unresponsive. Muscle weakness and hallucinations are common. The patient's heart beat slows dramatically and blood pressure plummets. Extreme toxicity, which can lead to coma and cardiac arrest, can be fatal.

Diagnosis

Blood tests are used to measure magnesium levels.

Treatment

The goal of treatment is to identify and correct the cause of the imbalance. Oral magnesium supplements

---

> ## KEY TERMS
>
> **Hypermagnesemia**—An abnormally high concentration of magnesium in the blood.
>
> **Hypomagnesemia**—An abnormally low concentration of magnesium in the blood.

---

or injections are usually prescribed to correct mild magnesium deficiency. If the deficiency is more severe or does not respond to treatment, magnesium sulfate or magnesium chloride may be administered intravenously.

Doctors usually prescribe **diuretics** (urine-producing drugs) for patients with hypermagnesemia and advise them to drink more fluids to flush the excess mineral from the body. Patients whose magnesium levels are extremely high may need mechanical support to breathe and to circulate blood throughout their bodies.

Intravenously administered calcium gluconate may reverse damage caused by excess magnesium. Intravenous furosemide (Lasix) or ethacrynic acid (Edecrin) can increase magnesium excretion in patients who get enough fluids and whose kidneys are functioning properly.

In an emergency, dialysis can provide temporary relief for patients whose kidney function is poor or who are unable to excrete excess **minerals**.

Prognosis

Because imbalances may recur if the underlying condition is not eliminated, monitoring of magnesium levels should continue after treatment has been completed.

Prevention

Most people consume adequate amounts of magnesium in the food they eat. Dietary supplements can be used safely, but should only be used under a doctor's supervision.

Resources

OTHER

"Mineral Guide." *CNN Page.* May 2, 1998. <http://www.cnn.com/HEALTH>.

Maureen Haggerty

Magnetic field therapy

Definition

Magnetic therapy is the use of magnets to relieve **pain** in various areas of the body.

Purpose

Some of the benefits that magnetic therapy claims to provide include:

- pain relief
- reduction of swelling
- improved tissue alkalinization
- more restful sleep
- increased tissue oxygenation
- relief of stress
- increased levels of cellular oxygen
- improved blood circulation
- anti-infective activity

Description

Origins

Magnetic therapy dates as far back as the ancient Egyptians. Magnets have long been believed to have healing powers associated with muscle pain and stiffness. Chinese healers as early as 200 B.C. were said to use magnetic lodestones on the body to correct unhealthy imbalances in the flow of *qi,* or energy. The ancient Chinese medical text known as *The Yellow Emperor's Canon of Internal Medicine* describes this procedure. The *Vedas,* or ancient Hindu scriptures, also mention the treatment of diseases with lodestones. The word "lodestone" or leading stone, came from the use of these stones as compasses. The word "magnet" probably stems from the Greek *Magnes lithos,* or "stone from Magnesia," a region of Greece rich in magnetic stones. The Greek phrase later became *magneta* in Latin.

Sir William Gilbert's 1600 treatise, *De Magnete,* was the first scholarly attempt to explain the nature of magnetism and how it differed from the attractive force of static electricity. Gilbert allegedly used magnets to relieve the arthritic pains of Queen Elizabeth I. Contemporary American interest in magnetic therapy began in the 1990s, as several professional golfers and football players offered testimony that the devices seemed to cure their nagging aches and injuries.

Many centuries ago, the earth was surrounded by a much stronger magnetic field than it is today. Over the past 155 years, scientists have been studying the decline of this magnetic field and the effects it has had on human health. When the first cosmonauts and astronauts were going into space, physicians noted that they experienced bone calcium loss and **muscle cramps** when they were out of the Earth's magnetic field for any extended period of time. After this discovery was made, artificial magnetic fields were placed in the space capsules.

There are two theories that are used to explain magnetic therapy. One theory maintains that magnets produce a slight electrical current. When magnets are applied to a painful area of the body, the nerves in that area are stimulated, thus releasing the body's natural painkillers. The other theory maintains that when magnets are applied to a painful area of the body, all the cells in that area react to increase blood circulation, ion exchange, and oxygen flow to the area. Magnetic fields attract and repel charged particles in the bloodstream, increasing blood flow and producing heat. Increased oxygen in the tissues and blood stream is thought to make a considerable difference in the speed of healing.

Preparations

There are no special preparations for using magnetic therapy other than purchasing a product that is specific for the painful area being treated. Products available in a range of prices include necklaces and bracelets; knee, back, shoulder and wrist braces; mattress pads; gloves; shoe inserts; and more.

Precautions

The primary precaution involved with magnetic therapy is to recognize the expense of this therapy. Magnets have become big business; they can be found in mail-order catalogs and stores ranging from upscale department stores to specialty stores. As is the case with many popular self-administered therapies, many far-fetched claims are being made about the effectiveness of magnetic therapy. Consumers should adopt a "let the buyer beware" approach to magnetic therapy. Persons who are interested in this form of treatment should try out a small, inexpensive item to see if it works for them before investing in the more expensive products.

Side effects

There are very few side effects from using magnetic therapy. Generally, patients using this therapy find that it either works for them or it does not. Patients using transcranial magnetic stimulation for the treatment of depression reported mild **headache** as their only side effect.

Research and general acceptance

Magnetic therapy is becoming more and more widely accepted as an alternative method of pain relief. Since the late 1950s, hundreds of studies have demonstrated the effectiveness of magnetic therapy. In 1997, a group of physicians at Baylor College of Medicine in Houston, Texas studied the use of magnetic therapy in 50 patients who had developed **polio** earlier in life. These patients had muscle and joint pain that standard treatments failed to manage. In this study, 29 of the patients wore a magnet taped over a trouble spot, and 21 others wore a nonmagnetic device. Neither the researchers nor the patients were told which treatment they were receiving (magnetic or nonmagnetic). As is the case with most studies involving a placebo, some of the patients responded to the nonmagnetic therapy, but 75% of those using the magnetic therapy reported feeling much better.

In another study at New York Medical College in Valhalla, New York, a neurologist tested magnetic therapy on a group of 19 men and women complaining of moderate to severe burning, **tingling**, or **numbness** in their feet. Their problems were caused by diabetes or other conditions present such as **alcoholism**. This group of patients wore a magnetic insole inside one of their socks or shoes for 24 hours a day over a two-month period, except while bathing. They wore a nonmagnetic insert in their other sock or shoe. Then for two months they wore magnetic inserts on both feet. By the end of the study, nine out of ten of the diabetic patients reported relief, while only three of nine non-diabetic patients reported relief. The neurologist in charge of the study believes that this study opens the door to additional research into magnetic therapy for diabetic patients. He plans a larger follow-up study in the near future.

As of 2000, a federally funded study is underway at the University of Virginia. This study is evaluating the effectiveness of magnetic mattress pads in easing the muscle pain, stiffness and **fatigue** associated with **fibromyalgia**.

Magnetic therapy is also being studied in the treatment of depression in patients with **bipolar disorder**. A procedure called repeated transcranial magnetic stimulation has shown promise in treating this condition. In this particular study, patients with depression had a lower relapse rate than did those

KEY TERMS

Fibromyalgia—A chronic syndrome characterized by fatigue, widespread muscular pain, and pain at specific points on the body.

Lodestone—A variety of magnetite that possesses magnetic polarity.

Transcranial magnetic stimulation—A procedure used to treat patients with depression.

using **electroconvulsive therapy**. Unlike electroconvulsive therapy, patients using magnetic therapy did not suffer from seizures, memory lapses, or impaired thinking.

Resources

PERIODICALS

"Magnets for Pain Relief: Attractive but Unproven." *Tufts University Health and Nutrition Letter* 1999: 3.

Vallbona, C. "Evolution of Magnetic Therapy from Alternative to Traditional Medicine." *Physical Medicine Rehabilitation Clinics of North America* 1999: 729-54.

Kim A. Sharp, M.Ln.

Magnetic resonance imaging

Definition

Magnetic resonance imaging (MRI) is the newest, and perhaps most versatile, medical imaging technology available. Doctors can get highly refined images of the body's interior without surgery, using MRI. By using strong magnets and pulses of radio waves to manipulate the natural magnetic properties in the body, this technique makes better images of organs and soft tissues than those of other scanning technologies. MRI is particularly useful for imaging the brain and spine, as well as the soft tissues of joints and the interior structure of bones. The entire body is visible to the technique, which poses few known health risks.

Purpose

MRI was developed in the 1980s. The latest additions to MRI technology are **angiography** (MRA) and spectroscopy (MRS). MRA was developed to study blood flow, while MRS can identify the chemical composition of diseased tissue and produce color images of brain function. The many advantages of MRI include:

- Detail. MRI creates precise images of the body based on the varying proportions of magnetic elements in different tissues. Very minor fluctuations in chemical composition can be determined. MRI images have greater natural contrast than standard x rays, computed tomography scan (CT scan), or ultrasound, all of which depend on the differing physical properties of tissues. This sensitivity lets MRI distinguish fine variations in tissues deep within the body. It also is particularly useful for spotting and distinguishing diseased tissues (tumors and other lesions) early in their development. Often, doctors prescribe an MRI scan to more fully investigate earlier findings of the other imaging techniques.

- Scope. The entire body can be scanned, from head to toe and from the skin to the deepest recesses of the brain. Moreover, MRI scans are not obstructed by bone, gas, or body waste, which can hinder other imaging techniques. (Although the scans can be degraded by motion such as breathing, heartbeat, and normal bowel activity.) The MRI process produces cross-sectional images of the body that are as sharp in the middle as on the edges, even of the brain through the skull. A close series of these two-dimensional images can provide a three-dimensional view of a targeted area.

- Safety. MRI does not depend on potentially harmful ionizing radiation, as do standard x-ray and CT scans. There are no known risks specific to the procedure, other than for people who might have metal objects in their bodies.

MRI is being used increasingly during operations, particularly those involving very small structures in the head and neck, as well as for preoperative assessment and planning. Intraoperative MRIs have shown themselves to be safe as well as feasible, and to improve the surgeon's ability to remove the entire tumor or other abnormality.

Given all the advantages, doctors would undoubtedly prescribe MRI as frequently as ultrasound scanning, but the MRI process is complex and costly. The process requires large, expensive, and complicated equipment; a highly trained operator; and a doctor specializing in radiology. Generally, MRI is prescribed only when serious symptoms and/or negative results from other tests indicate a need. Many times another test is appropriate for the type of diagnosis needed.

Doctors may prescribe an MRI scan of different areas of the body.

- Brain and head. MRI technology was developed because of the need for brain imaging. It is one of the few imaging tools that can see through bone (the skull) and deliver high quality pictures of the brain's delicate soft tissue structures. MRI may be needed for patients with symptoms of a **brain tumor**, **stroke**, or infection (like **meningitis**). MRI also may be needed when cognitive and/or psychological symptoms suggest brain disease (like Alzheimer's or Huntington's diseases, or **multiple sclerosis**), or when developmental retardation suggests a birth defect. MRI can also provide pictures of the sinuses and other areas of the head beneath the face. Recent refinements in MRI technology may make this form of diagnostic imaging even more useful in evaluating patients with brain **cancer**, stroke, **schizophrenia**, or epilepsy. In particular, a new 3-D approach to MRI imaging known as diffusion tensor imaging, or DTI, measures the flow of water within brain tissue, allowing the radiologist to tell where the normal flow of fluid is disrupted, and to distinguish more clearly between cancerous and normal brain tissue. The introduction of DTI has led to a technique known as fiber tracking, which allows the neurosurgeon to tell whether a space-occupying brain tumor has damaged or displaced the nerve pathways in the white matter of the brain. This information in turn improves the surgeon's accuracy during the actual operation.

- Spine. Spinal problems can create a host of seemingly unrelated symptoms. MRI is particularly useful for identifying and evaluating degenerated or herniated spinal discs. It can also be used to determine the condition of nerve tissue within the spinal cord.

- Joint. MRI scanning is most commonly used to diagnose and assess joint problems. MRI can provide clear images of the bone, cartilage, ligament, and tendon that comprise a joint. MRI can be used to diagnose joint injuries due to sports, advancing age, or arthritis. MRI can also be used to diagnose shoulder problems, like a torn rotator cuff. MRI can also detect the presence of an otherwise hidden tumor or infection in a joint, and can be used to diagnose the nature of developmental joint abnormalities in children.

- Skeleton. The properties of MRI that allow it to see through the skull also allow it to view the inside of bones. It can be used to detect bone cancer, inspect the marrow for leukemia and other diseases, assess bone loss (**osteoporosis**), and examine complex **fractures**.

- The rest of the body. While CT and ultrasound satisfy most chest, abdominal, and general body imaging needs, MRI may be needed in certain circumstances to provide better pictures or when repeated scanning is required. The progress of some therapies, like **liver cancer** therapy, needs to be monitored, and the effect of repeated x-ray exposure is a concern.

Precautions

MRI scanning should not be used when there is the potential for an interaction between the strong MRI magnet and metal objects that might be imbedded in a patient's body. The force of magnetic attraction on certain types of metal objects (including surgical steel) could move them within the body and cause serious injury. Metal may be imbedded in a person's body for several reasons.

- Medical. People with implanted cardiac **pacemakers**, metal aneurysm clips, or who have had broken bones repaired with metal pins, screws, rods, or plates must tell their radiologist prior to having an MRI scan. In some cases (like a metal rod in a reconstructed leg) the difficulty may be overcome.

- Injury. Patients must tell their doctors if they have bullet fragments or other metal pieces in their body from old **wounds**. The suspected presence of metal, whether from an old or recent wound, should be confirmed before scanning.

- Occupational. People with significant work exposure to metal particles (working with a metal grinder, for example) should discuss this with their doctor and radiologist. The patient may need prescan testing–usually a single, regular x ray of the eyes to see if any metal is present.

Chemical agents designed to improve the picture and/or allow for the imaging of blood or other fluid flow during MRA may be injected. In rare cases, patients may be allergic to or intolerant of these agents, and these patients should not receive them. If these chemical agents are to be used, patients should discuss any concerns they have with their doctor and radiologist.

The potential side effects of magnetic and electric fields on human health remain a source of debate. In particular, the possible effects on an unborn baby are not well known. Any woman who is, or may be, pregnant should carefully discuss this issue with her doctor and radiologist before undergoing a scan.

As with all medical imaging techniques, **obesity** greatly interferes with the quality of MRI.

Description

In essence, MRI produces a map of hydrogen distribution in the body. Hydrogen is the simplest element known, the most abundant in biological tissue, and one that can be magnetized. It will align itself within a strong magnetic field, like the needle of a compass. The earth's magnetic field is not strong enough to keep a person's hydrogen atoms pointing in the same direction, but the superconducting magnet of an MRI machine can. This comprises the "magnetic" part of MRI.

Once a patient's hydrogen atoms have been aligned in the magnet, pulses of very specific radio wave frequencies are used to knock them back out of alignment. The hydrogen atoms alternately absorb and emit radio wave energy, vibrating back and forth between their resting (magnetized) state and their agitated (radio pulse) state. This comprises the "resonance" part of MRI.

The MRI equipment records the duration, strength, and source location of the signals emitted by the atoms as they relax and translates the data into an image on a television monitor. The state of hydrogen in diseased tissue differs from healthy tissue of the same type, making MRI particularly good at identifying tumors and other lesions. In some cases, chemical agents such as gadolinium can be injected to improve the contrast between healthy and diseased tissue.

A single MRI exposure produces a two-dimensional image of a slice through the entire target area. A series of these image slices closely spaced (usually less than half an inch) makes a virtual three-dimensional view of the area.

Magnetic resonance spectroscopy (MRS) is different from MRI because MRS uses a continuous band of radio wave frequencies to excite hydrogen atoms in a variety of chemical compounds other than water. These compounds absorb and emit radio energy at characteristic frequencies, or spectra, which can be used to identify them. Generally, a color image is created by assigning a color to each distinctive spectral emission. This comprises the "spectroscopy" part of MRS. MRS is still experimental and is available in only a few research centers.

Doctors primarily use MRS to study the brain and disorders, like epilepsy, **Alzheimer's disease**, brain tumors, and the effects of drugs on brain growth and metabolism. The technique is also useful in evaluating metabolic disorders of the muscles and nervous system.

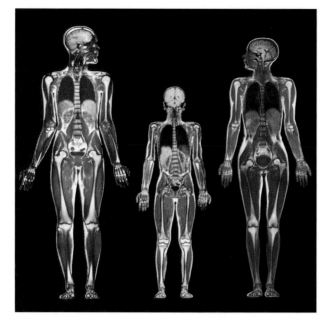

MRI body scans of a man, woman, and child. *(Simon Fraser, Photo Researchers. Reproduced by permission.)*

Magnetic resonance angiography (MRA) is another variation on standard MRI. MRA, like other types of angiography, looks specifically at fluid flow within the blood (vascular) system, but does so without the injection of dyes or radioactive tracers. Standard MRI cannot make a good picture of flowing blood, but MRA uses specific radio pulse sequences to capture usable signals. The technique is generally used in combination with MRI to obtain images that show both vascular structure and flow within the brain and head in cases of stroke, or when a blood clot or aneurysm is suspected.

Regardless of the exact type of MRI planned, or area of the body targeted, the procedure involved is basically the same and occurs in a special MRI suite. The patient lies back on a narrow table and is made as comfortable as possible. Transmitters are positioned on the body and the cushioned table that the patient is lying on moves into a long tube that houses the magnet. The tube is as long as an average adult lying down, and the tube is narrow and open at both ends. Once the area to be examined has been properly positioned, a radio pulse is applied. Then a two-dimensional image corresponding to one slice through the area is made. The table then moves a fraction of an inch and the next image is made. Each image exposure takes several seconds and the entire exam will last anywhere from 30-90 minutes. During this time, the patient is not allowed to move. If the patient moves during the scan, the picture will not be clear.

Depending on the area to be imaged, the radio-wave transmitters will be positioned in different locations.

- For the head and neck, a helmet-like hat is worn.
- For the spine, chest, and abdomen, the patient will be lying on the transmitters.
- For the knee, shoulder, or other joint, the transmitters will be applied directly to the joint.

Additional probes will monitor vital signs (like pulse, respiration, etc.).

The process is very noisy and confining. The patient hears a thumping sound for the duration of the procedure. Since the procedure is noisy, music supplied via earphones is often provided. Some patients get anxious or panic because they are in the small, enclosed tube. This is why vital signs are monitored and the patient and medical team can communicate between each other. If the chest or abdomen are to be imaged, the patient will be asked to hold his/her breath as each exposure is made. Other instructions may be given to the patient, as needed. In many cases, the entire examination will be performed by an MRI operator who is not a doctor. However, the supervising radiologist should be available to consult as necessary during the exam, and will view and interpret the results sometime later.

Preparation

In some cases (such as for MRI brain scanning or an MRA), a chemical designed to increase image contrast may be given by the radiologist immediately before the exam. If a patient suffers from **anxiety** or claustrophobia, drugs may be given to help the patient relax.

The patient must remove all metal objects (watches, jewelry, eye glasses, hair clips, etc). Any magnetized objects (like credit and bank machine cards, audio tapes, etc.) should be kept far away from the MRI equipment because they can be erased. The patient cannnot bring their wallet or keys into the MRI machine. The patient may be asked to wear clothing without metal snaps, buckles, or zippers, unless a medical gown is worn during the procedure. The patient may be asked to remove any hair spray, hair gel, or cosmetics that may interfere with the scan.

Aftercare

No aftercare is necessary, unless the patient received medication or had a reaction to a contrast agent. Normally, patients can immediately return to their daily activities. If the exam reveals a serious

KEY TERMS

Angiography—Any of the different methods for investigating the condition of blood vessels, usually via a combination of radiological imaging and injections of chemical tracing and contrasting agents.

Diffusion tensor imaging (DTI)—A refinement of magnetic resonance imaging that allows the doctor to measure the flow of water and track the pathways of white matter in the brain. DTI is able to detect abnormalities in the brain that do not show up on standard MRI scans.

Gadolinium—A very rare metallic element useful for its sensitivity to electromagnetic resonance, among other things. Traces of it can be injected into the body to enhance the MRI pictures.

Hydrogen—The simplest, most common element known in the universe. It is composed of a single electron (negatively charged particle) circling a nucleus consisting of a single proton (positively charged particle). It is the nuclear proton of hydrogen that makes MRI possible by reacting resonantly to radio waves while aligned in a magnetic field.

Ionizing radiation—Electromagnetic radiation that can damage living tissue by disrupting and destroying individual cells. All types of nuclear decay radiation (including x rays) are potentially ionizing. Radio waves do not damage organic tissues they pass through.

Magnetic field—The three-dimensional area surrounding a magnet, in which its force is active. During MRI, the patient's body is permeated by the force field of a superconducting magnet.

Radio waves— Electromagnetic energy of the frequency range corresponding to that used in radio communications, usually 10,000 cycles per second to 300 billion cycles per second. Radio waves are the same as visible light, x rays, and all other types of electromagnetic radiation, but are of a higher frequency.

condition that requires more testing and/or treatment, appropriate information and counseling will be needed.

Risks

MRI poses no known health risks to the patient and produces no physical side effects. Again, the potential effects of MRI on an unborn baby are not well known. Any woman who is, or may be, pregnant, should carefully discuss this issue with her doctor and radiologist before undergoing a scan.

Normal results

A normal MRI, MRA, or MRS result is one that shows the patient's physical condition to fall within normal ranges for the target area scanned.

Abnormal results

Generally, MRI is prescribed only when serious symptoms and/or negative results from other tests indicate a need. There often exists strong evidence of a condition that the scan is designed to detect and assess. Thus, the results will often be abnormal, confirming the earlier diagnosis. At that point, further testing and appropriate medical treatment is needed. For example, if the MRI indicates the presence of a brain tumor, an MRS may be prescribed to determine the type of tumor so that aggressive treatment can begin immediately without the need for a surgical biopsy.

Resources

PERIODICALS

Clark, C. A., T. R. Barrick, M. M. Murphy, and B. A. Bell. "White Matter Fiber Tracking in Patients with Space-Occupying Lesions of the Brain: A New Technique for Neurosurgical Planning?" *Neuroimage* 20 (November 2003): 1601–1608.

Hendler, T., P. Pianka, M. Sigal, et al. "Delineating Gray and White Matter Involvement in Brain Lesions: Three-dimensional Alignment of Functional Magnetic Resonance and Diffusion-Tensor Imaging." *Journal of Neurosurgery* 99 (December 2003): 1018–1027.

Kubicki, M., C. F. Westin, P. G. Nestor, et al. "Cingulate Fasciculus Integrity Disruption in Schizophrenia: A Magnetic Resonance Diffusion Tensor Imaging Study." *Biological Psychiatry* 54 (December 1, 2003): 1171–1180.

Mahmoud-Ghoneim, D., G. Toussaint, J. M. Constans, and J. D. de Certaines. "Three-Dimensional Texture Analysis in MRI: A Preliminary Evaluation in Gliomas." *Magnetic Resonance Imaging* 21 (November 2003): 983–987.

Rees, J. "Advances in Magnetic Resonance Imaging of Brain Tumours." *Current Opinion in Neurology* 16 (December 2003): 643–650.

Satoh, T., K. Onoda, and S. Tsuchimoto. "Intraoperative Evaluation of Aneurysmal Architecture: Comparative Study with Transluminal Images of 3D MR and CT Angiograms." *American Journal of Neuroradiology* 24 (November-December 2003): 1975–1981.

ORGANIZATIONS

American College of Radiology. 1891 Preston White Drive, Reston, VA 22091. (800) 227-5463. < http://www.acr.org >.

American Society of Radiologic Technologists. 15000 Central Ave. SE, Albuquerque, NM 87123-3917. (505) 298-4500. < http://www.asrt.org >.

Center for Devices and Radiological Health. United States Food and Drug Administration. 1901 Chapman Ave., Rockville, MD 20857. (301) 443-4109. < http://www.fda.gov/cdrh >.

Kurt Richard Sternlof
Rebecca J. Frey, PhD

Magnetic resonance spectroscopy *see*
Magnetic resonance imaging

Major depression *see* **Depressive disorders**

Major tranquilizers *see* **Antipsychotic drugs**

Malabsorption syndrome

Definition

Malabsorption syndrome is an alteration in the ability of the intestine to absorb nutrients adequately into the bloodstream. It may refer to malabsorption of one specific nutrient or for specific carbohydrates, fats, or trace elements (micronutrients).

Causes and symptoms

Protein, fats, and carbohydrates (macronutrients) normally are absorbed in the small intestine; the small bowel also absorbs about 80% of the eight to ten liters of fluid ingested daily. There are many different conditions that affect fluid and nutrient absorption by the intestine. A fault in the digestive process may result from failure of the body to produce the enzymes needed to digest certain foods. Congenital structural defects or diseases of the pancreas, gall bladder, or liver may alter the digestive process. Inflammation, infection, injury, or surgical removal of portions of the intestine may also result in absorption problems; reduced length or surface area of intestine available for fluid and nutrient absorption can result in malabsorption. **Radiation therapy** may injure the mucosal lining of the intestine, resulting in **diarrhea** that may not become evident until several years later. The use of some **antibiotics** can also affect the bacteria that normally live in the intestine and affect intestinal function.

Risk factors for malabsorption syndrome include:

- premature birth
- family history of malabsorption or **cystic fibrosis**
- use of certain drugs, such as mineral oil or other **laxatives**
- travel to foreign countries
- intestinal surgery, including bowel transplantation
- excess alcohol consumption.

The most common symptoms of malabsorption include:

- Anemia, with weakness and **fatigue** due to inadequate absorption of vitamin B_{12}, iron, and **folic acid**
- Diarrhea, steatorrhea (excessive amount of fat in the stool), and abdominal distention with cramps, bloating, and gas due to impaired water and carbohydrate absorption, and irritation from unabsorbed fatty acids. The individual may also report explosive diarrhea with greasy, foul-smelling stools.
- **Edema** (fluid retention in the body's tissues) due to decreased protein absorption
- Malnutrition and weight loss due to decreased fat, carbohydrate, and protein absorption. Weight may be 80–90% of usual weight despite increased oral intake of nutrients.
- Muscle cramping due to decreased vitamin D, calcium, and potassium levels
- Muscle wasting and atrophy due to decreased protein absorption and metabolism
- Perianal skin burning, **itching**, or soreness due to frequent loose stools.

Irregular heart rhythms may also result from inadequate levels of potassium and other electrolytes. Blood clotting disorders may occur due to a **vitamin K deficiency**. Children with malabsorption syndrome often exhibit a failure to grow and thrive.

Several disorders can lead to malabsorption syndrome, including cystic fibrosis, chronic **pancreatitis**, **lactose intolerance**, and gluten enteropathy (nontropical sprue.)

Tropical sprue is a malabsorptive disorder that is uncommon in the United States, but seen more often in people from the Caribbean, India, or southeast Asia. Although its cause is unknown, it is thought to be related to environmental factors, including infection, intestinal parasites, or possibly the consumption of certain food toxins. Symptoms often include a sore tongue, anemia, weight loss, along with diarrhea and passage of fatty stools.

Whipple's disease is a relatively rare malabsorptive disorder, affecting mostly middle-aged men. The cause is thought to be related to bacterial infection, resulting in nutritional deficiencies, chronic low-grade **fever**, diarrhea, joint **pain**, weight loss, and darkening of the skin's pigmentation. Other organs of the body may be affected, including the brain, heart, lungs, and eyes.

Short bowel syndromes—which may be present at birth (congenital) or the result of surgery—reduce the surface area of the bowel available to absorb nutrients and can also result in malabsorption syndrome. Congenital short bowel syndrome occurs in about 24 out of 100,000 live births and has a high mortality rate (about 38%).

Diagnosis

The diagnosis of malabsorption syndrome and identification of the underlying cause can require extensive diagnostic testing. The first phase involves a thorough medical history and **physical examination** by a physician, who will then determine the appropriate laboratory studies and x rays to assist in diagnosis. A 72-hour stool collection may be ordered for fecal fat measurement; increased fecal fat in the stool collected indicates malabsorption. A biopsy of the small intestine may be done to assist in differentiating between malabsorption syndrome and small bowel disease. Ultrasound, computed tomography scan (CT scan), **magnetic resonance imaging** (MRI), **barium enema**, or other x rays to identify abnormalities of the gastrointestinal tract and pancreas may also be ordered.

A newer method of obtaining diagnostic information about the small intestine was approved by the Food and Drug Administration (FDA) in 2001. Known as the M2A Imaging System, the device was developed by a company in Atlanta, Georgia. The M2A system consists of an imaging capsule, a portable belt-pack image receiver and recorder, and a specially modified computer. The patient swallows the capsule, which is the size of a large pill. A miniature lens in the capsule transmits images through an antenna/transmitter to the belt-pack receiver, which the patient wears under ordinary clothing as he or she goes about daily activities. The belt-pack recording device is returned after seven or eight hours to the doctor, who then examines the images recorded as a digital video. The capsule itself is simply allowed to pass through the digestive tract.

Preparation requires only **fasting** the night before the M2A examination and taking nothing but clear liquids for two hours after swallowing the capsule.

After four hours the patient can eat food without interfering with the test. As of the early 2000s, the M2A system is used to evaluate gastrointestinal bleeding from unknown causes, inflammatory bowel disease, some malabsorption syndromes, and to monitor surgical patients following small-bowel transplantation.

Laboratory studies of the blood may include:

- Serum cholesterol. May be low due to decreased fat absorption and digestion.
- Serum sodium, potassium, and chloride. May be low due to electrolyte losses with diarrhea.
- Serum calcium. May be low due to vitamin D and amino acid malabsorption.
- Serum protein and albumin. May be low due to protein losses.
- Serum vitamin A and carotene. May be low due to bile salt deficiency and impaired fat absorption.
- D-xylose test. Decreased excretion may indicate malabsorption.
- Schilling test. May indicate malabsorption of vitamin B_{12}.

Treatment

Fluid and nutrient monitoring and replacement is essential for any individual with malabsorption syndrome. Hospitalization may be required when severe fluid and electrolyte imbalances occur. Consultation with a dietitian to assist with nutritional support and meal planning is helpful. If the patient is able to eat, the diet and supplements should provide bulk and be rich in carbohydrates, proteins, fats, **minerals**, and **vitamins**. The patient should be encouraged to eat several small, frequent meals throughout the day, avoiding fluids and foods that promote diarrhea. Intake and output should be monitored, along with the number, color, and consistency of stools.

The individual with malabsorption syndrome must be monitored for **dehydration**, including dry tongue, mouth and skin; increased thirst; low, concentrated urine output; or feeling weak or dizzy when standing. Pulse and blood pressure should be monitored, observing for increased or irregular pulse rate, or **hypotension** (low blood pressure). The individual should also be alert for signs of nutrient, vitamin, and mineral depletion, including **nausea** or **vomiting**; fissures at corner of mouth; fatigue or weakness; dry, pluckable hair; easy bruising; **tingling** in fingers or toes; and **numbness** or burning sensation in legs or feet. Fluid volume excess, as a result of diminished

KEY TERMS

Anemia—A decrease in the number of red blood cells in the bloodstream, characterized by pallor, loss of energy, and generalized weakness.

Atrophy—A wasting away of a tissue or organ, often because of insufficient nutrition.

Biopsy—A tissue sample removed from the body for examination under the microscope.

Cystic fibrosis—A hereditary genetic disorder that occurs most often in Caucasians. Thick, sticky secretions from mucus-producing glands cause blockages in the pancreatic ducts and the airways.

Edema—From the Greek word meaning swelling, an excessive accumulation of fluid in the tissue spaces. Excessive generalized edema may also be referred to as ascites.

Gluten enteropathy—A hereditary malabsorption disorder caused by sensitivity to gluten, a protein found in wheat, rye, barley, and oats. Also called non-tropical sprue or celiac disease.

Intestines—The intestines, also known as the bowels, are divided into the large and small intestines. They extend from the stomach to the anus.

Short bowel syndrome—A condition in which the bowel is not as long as normal, either because of surgery or because of a congenital defect. Because the bowel has less surface area to absorb nutrients, it can result in malabsorption syndrome.

Steatorrhea—An excessive amount of fat in the stool.

Trace elements—A group of elements that are present in the human body in very small amounts but are nonetheless important to good health. They include chromium, copper, cobalt, iodine, iron, selenium, and zinc. Trace elements are also called micronutrients.

protein stores, may require fluid intake restrictions. The physician should also be notified of any **shortness of breath**.

Other specific medical management for malabsorption syndrome is dependent upon the cause. Treatment for tropical sprue consists of folic acid supplements and long-term antibiotics. Depending on the severity of the disorder, this treatment may be continued for six months or longer. Whipple's disease also may require long-term use of antibiotics, such as tetracycline.

Management of some individuals with malabsorption syndrome may require injections of vitamin B_{12} and oral iron supplements. The doctor may also prescribe enzymes to replace missing intestinal enzymes, or antispasmodics to reduce abdominal cramping and associated diarrhea. People with cystic fibrosis and chronic pancreatitis require pancreatic supplements. Those with lactose intolerance or gluten enteropathy (nontropical sprue) will have to modify their **diets** to avoid foods that they cannot properly digest.

Prognosis

The expected course for the individual with malabsorption syndrome varies depending on the cause. The onset of symptoms may be slow and difficult to diagnose. Treatment may be long, complicated, and changed often for optimal effectiveness. Patience and a positive attitude are important in controlling or curing the disorder. Careful monitoring is necessary to prevent additional illnesses cause by nutritional deficiencies.

Resources

BOOKS

Beers, Mark H., MD, and Robert Berkow, MD, editors. "Malabsorption Syndromes." Section 3, Chapter 30. In *The Merck Manual of Diagnosis and Therapy.* Whitehouse Station, NJ: Merck Research Laboratories, 2004.

PERIODICALS

Adler, Douglas J., MD, and Christopher J. Gostout, MD. "Wireless Capsule Endoscopy." *Hospital Physician* May 2003: 17–22.

Forsberg, G., A. Fahlgren, P. Horstedt, et al. "Presence of Bacteria and Innate Immunity of Intestinal Epithelium in Childhood Celiac Disease." *American Journal of Gastroenterology* 99 (May 2004): 905–906.

Kumar, N., and P. A. Low. "Myeloneuropathy and Anemia Due to Copper Malabsorption." *Journal of Neurology* 251 (June 2004): 747–749.

Sabharwal, G., P. J. Strouse, S. Islam, and N. Zoubi. "Congenital Short-Gut Syndrome." *Pediatric Radiology* 34 (May 2004): 424–427.

Thompson, B. F., L. C. Fry, C. D. Wells, et al. "The Spectrum of GI Strongyloidiasis: An Endoscopic-Pathologic Study." *Gastrointestinal Endoscopy* 59 (June 2004): 906–910.

Wales, P. W., N. de Silva, J. Kim, et al. "Neonatal Short Bowel Syndrome: Population-Based Estimates of Incidence and Mortality Rates." *Journal of Pediatric Surgery* 39 (May 2004): 690–695.

ORGANIZATIONS

National Digestive Diseases Information Clearinghouse. 2 Information Way, Bethesda, MD 20892-3570.

(800) 891-5389. Fax: (703) 738-4929. <http://digestive.niddk.nih.gov>.

Kathleen D. Wright, RN
Rebecca J. Frey, PhD

Malaria

Definition

Malaria is a serious infectious disease spread by certain mosquitoes. It is most common in tropical climates. It is characterized by recurrent symptoms of chills, **fever**, and an enlarged spleen. The disease can be treated with medication, but it often recurs. Malaria is endemic (occurs frequently in a particular locality) in many third world countries. Isolated, small outbreaks sometimes occur within the boundaries of the United States.

Description

Malaria is a growing problem in the United States. Although only about 1400 new cases were reported in the United States and its territories in 2000, many involved returning travelers. In addition, locally transmitted malaria has occurred in California, Florida, Texas, Michigan, New Jersey, and New York City. While malaria can be transmitted in blood, the American blood supply is not screened for malaria. Widespread malarial epidemics are far less likely to occur in the United States, but small localized epidemics could return to the Western world. As of late 2002, primary care physicians are being advised to screen returning travelers with fever for malaria, and a team of public health doctors in Minnesota is recommending screening immigrants, refugees, and international adoptees for the disease—particularly those from high-risk areas.

The picture is far more bleak, however, outside the territorial boundaries of the United States. A recent government panel warned that disaster looms over Africa from the disease. Malaria infects between 300 and 500 million people every year in Africa, India, southeast Asia, the Middle East, Oceania, and Central and South America. A 2002 report stated that malaria kills 2.7 million people each year, more than 75 percent of them African children under the age of five. It is predicted that within five years, malaria will kill about as many people as does **AIDS**. As many as half a billion people worldwide are left with chronic anemia

due to malaria infection. In some parts of Africa, people battle up to 40 or more separate episodes of malaria in their lifetimes. The spread of malaria is becoming even more serious as the parasites that cause malaria develop resistance to the drugs used to treat the condition. In late 2002, a group of public health researchers in Thailand reported that a combination treatment regimen involving two drugs known as dihydroartemisinin and azithromycin shows promise in treating multidrug-resistant malaria in southeast Asia.

Causes and symptoms

Human malaria is caused by four different species of a parasite belonging to genus *Plasmodium*: *Plasmodium falciparum* (the most deadly), *Plasmodium vivax*, *Plasmodium malariae*, and *Plasmodium ovale*. The last two are fairly uncommon. Many animals can get malaria, but human malaria does not spread to animals. In turn, animal malaria does not spread to humans.

A person gets malaria when bitten by a female mosquito who is looking for a blood meal and is infected with the malaria parasite. The parasites enter the blood stream and travel to the liver, where they multiply. When they re-emerge into the blood, symptoms appear. By the time a patient shows symptoms, the parasites have reproduced very rapidly, clogging blood vessels and rupturing blood cells.

Malaria cannot be casually transmitted directly from one person to another. Instead, a mosquito bites an infected person and then passes the infection on to the next human it bites. It is also possible to spread malaria via contaminated needles or in blood transfusions. This is why all blood donors are carefully screened with questionnaires for possible exposure to malaria.

It is possible to contract malaria in non-endemic areas, although such cases are rare. Nevertheless, at least 89 cases of so-called airport malaria, in which travelers contract malaria while passing through crowded airport terminals, have been identified since 1969.

The amount of time between the mosquito bite and the appearance of symptoms varies, depending on the strain of parasite involved. The incubation period is usually between 8 and 12 days for falciparum malaria, but it can be as long as a month for the other types. Symptoms from some strains of *P.vivax* may not appear until 8–10 months after the mosquito bite occurred.

The primary symptom of all types of malaria is the "malaria ague" (chills and fever). In most cases, the fever has three stages, beginning with uncontrollable shivering for an hour or two, followed by a rapid spike in temperature (as high as 106°F), which lasts three to six hours. Then, just as suddenly, the patient begins to sweat profusely, which will quickly bring down the fever. Other symptoms may include **fatigue**, severe **headache**, or **nausea and vomiting**. As the sweating subsides, the patient typically feels exhausted and falls asleep. In many cases, this cycle of chills, fever, and sweating occurs every other day, or every third day, and may last for between a week and a month. Those with the chronic form of malaria may have a relapse as long as 50 years after the initial infection.

Falciparum malaria is far more severe than other types of malaria because the parasite attacks all red blood cells, not just the young or old cells, as do other types. It causes the red blood cells to become very "sticky." A patient with this type of malaria can die within hours of the first symptoms. The fever is prolonged. So many red blood cells are destroyed that they block the blood vessels in vital organs (especially the kidneys), and the spleen becomes enlarged. There may be brain damage, leading to **coma** and convulsions. The kidneys and liver may fail.

Malaria in **pregnancy** can lead to premature delivery, **miscarriage**, or **stillbirth**.

Certain kinds of mosquitoes (called anopheles) can pick up the parasite by biting an infected human. (The more common kinds of mosquitoes in the United States do not transmit the infection.) This is true for as long as that human has parasites in his/her blood. Since strains of malaria do not protect against each other, it is possible to be reinfected with the parasites again and again. It is also possible to develop a chronic infection without developing an effective immune response.

Diagnosis

Malaria is diagnosed by examining blood under a microscope. The parasite can be seen in the blood smears on a slide. These blood smears may need to be repeated over a 72-hour period in order to make a diagnosis. Antibody tests are not usually helpful because many people developed antibodies from past infections, and the tests may not be readily available. A new laser test to detect the presence of malaria parasites in the blood was developed in 2002, but is still under clinical study.

Two new techniques to speed the laboratory diagnosis of malaria show promise as of late 2002. The first is acridine orange (AO), a staining agent that works much faster (3–10 min) than the traditional Giemsa stain (45–60 min) in making the malaria parasites visible under a microscope. The second is a bioassay technique that measures the amount of a substance called histadine-rich protein II (HRP2) in the patient's blood. It allows for a very accurate estimation of parasite development. A dip strip that tests for the presence of HRP2 in blood samples appears to be more accurate in diagnosing malaria than standard microscopic analysis.

Anyone who becomes ill with chills and fever after being in an area where malaria exists must see a doctor and mention their recent travel to endemic areas. A person with the above symptoms who has been in a high-risk area should insist on a blood test for malaria. The doctor may believe the symptoms are just the common flu virus. Malaria is often misdiagnosed by North American doctors who are not used to seeing the disease. Delaying treatment of falciparum malaria can be fatal.

Treatment

Falciparum malaria is a medical emergency that must be treated in the hospital. The type of drugs, the method of giving them, and the length of the treatment depend on where the malaria was contracted and how sick the patient is.

For all strains except falciparum, the treatment for malaria is usually chloroquine (Aralen) by mouth for three days. Those falciparum strains suspected to be resistant to chloroquine are usually treated with a combination of quinine and tetracycline. In countries where quinine resistance is developing, other treatments may include clindamycin (Cleocin), mefloquin (Lariam), or sulfadoxone/pyrimethamine (Fansidar). Most patients receive an antibiotic for seven days. Those who are very ill may need intensive care and intravenous (IV) malaria treatment for the first three days.

Anyone who acquired falciparum malaria in the Dominican Republic, Haiti, Central America west of the Panama Canal, the Middle East, or Egypt can still be cured with chloroquine. Almost all strains of falciparum malaria in Africa, South Africa, India, and southeast Asia are now resistant to chloroquine. In Thailand and Cambodia, there are strains of falciparum malaria that have some resistance to almost all known drugs.

A patient with falciparum malaria needs to be hospitalized and given **antimalarial drugs** in different

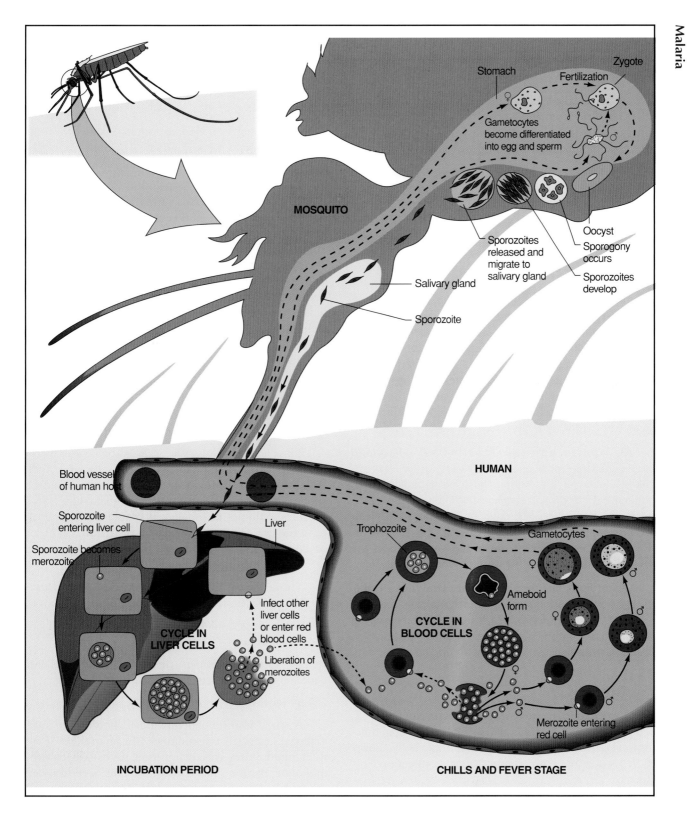

The life cycle of *Plasmodium vivax,* the parasite that causes malaria. *(Illustration by Hans & Cassady.)*

combinations and doses depending on the resistance of the strain. The patient may need IV fluids, red blood cell transfusions, **kidney dialysis**, and assistance breathing.

A drug called primaquine may prevent relapses after recovery from *P. vivax* or *P. ovale*. These relapses are caused by a form of the parasite that remains in the liver and can reactivate months or years later.

Another new drug, halofantrine, is available abroad. While it is licensed in the United States, it is not marketed in this country and it is not recommended by the Centers for Disease Control and Prevention in Atlanta.

Alternative treatments

The Chinese herb qiinghaosu (the Western name is artemisinin) has been used in China and southeast Asia to fight severe malaria, and became available in Europe in 1994. Because this treatment often fails, it is usually combined with another antimalarial drug (mefloquine) to boost its effectiveness. It is not available in the United States and other parts of the developed world due to fears of its toxicity, in addition to licensing and other issues.

A Western herb called wormwood (*Artemesia annua*) that is taken as a daily dose can be effective against malaria. Protecting the liver with herbs like goldenseal (*Hydrastis canadensis*), Chinese goldenthread (*Coptis chinensis*), and milk thistle (*Silybum marianum*) can be used as preventive treatment. Preventing mosquitoes from biting you while in the tropics is another possible way to avoid malaria.

As of late 2002, researchers are studying a traditional African herbal remedy against malaria. Extracts from *Microglossa pyrifolia*, a trailing shrub belonging to the daisy family (Asteraceae), show promise in treating drug-resistant strains of *P. falciparum*.

Prognosis

If treated in the early stages, malaria can be cured. Those who live in areas where malaria is epidemic, however, can contract the disease repeatedly, never fully recovering between bouts of acute infection.

Prevention

Several researchers are currently working on a malarial vaccine, but the complex life cycle of the malaria parasite makes it difficult. A parasite has much more genetic material than a virus or bacterium.

For this reason, a successful vaccine has not yet been developed.

Malaria is an especially difficult disease to prevent by **vaccination** because the parasite goes through several separate stages. One recent promising vaccine appears to have protected up to 60% of people exposed to malaria. This was evident during field trials for the drug that were conducted in South America and Africa. It is not yet commercially available.

The World Health Association (WHO) has been trying to eliminate malaria for the past 30 years by controlling mosquitoes. Their efforts were successful as long as the pesticide DDT killed mosquitoes and antimalarial drugs cured those who were infected. Today, however, the problem has returned a hundredfold, especially in Africa. Because both the mosquito and parasite are now extremely resistant to the insecticides designed to kill them, governments are now trying to teach people to take antimalarial drugs as a preventive medicine and avoid getting bitten by mosquitoes.

A newer strategy as of late 2002 involves the development of genetically modified non-biting mosquitoes. A research team in Italy is studying the feasibility of this means of controlling malaria.

Travelers to high-risk areas should use insect repellant containing DEET for exposed skin. Because DEET is toxic in large amounts, children should not use a concentration higher than 35%. DEET should not be inhaled. It should not be rubbed onto the eye area, on any broken or irritated skin, or on children's hands. It should be thoroughly washed off after coming indoors.

Those who use the following preventive measures get fewer infections than those who do not:

- Between dusk and dawn, remain indoors in well-screened areas.
- Sleep inside pyrethrin or permethrin repellent-soaked mosquito nets.
- Wear clothes over the entire body.

Anyone visiting endemic areas should take antimalarial drugs starting a day or two before they leave the United States. The drugs used are usually chloroquine or mefloquine. This treatment is continued through at least four weeks after leaving the endemic area. However, even those who take antimalarial drugs and are careful to avoid mosquito bites can still contract malaria.

International travelers are at risk for becoming infected. Most Americans who have acquired

KEY TERMS

Arteminisinins—A family of antimalarial products derived from an ancient Chinese herbal remedy. Two of the most popular varieties are artemether and artesunate, used mainly in southeast Asia in combination with mefloquine.

Chloroquine—An antimalarial drug that was first used in the 1940s, until the first evidence of quinine resistance appeared in the 1960s. It is now ineffective against falciparum malaria almost everywhere. However, because it is inexpensive, it is still the antimalarial drug most widely used in Africa. Native individuals with partial immunity may have better results with chloroquine than a traveler with no previous exposure.

Mefloquine—An antimalarial drug that was developed by the United States Army in the early 1980s. Today, malaria resistance to this drug has become a problem in some parts of Asia (especially Thailand and Cambodia).

Mefloquine—An antimalarial drug that was developed by the United States Army in the early 1980s. Today, malaria resistance to this drug has become a problem in some parts of Asia (especially Thailand and Cambodia).

Quinine— One of the first treatments for malaria, quinine is a natural product made from the bark of the Cinchona tree. It was popular until being superseded by the development of chloroquine in the 1940s. In the wake of widespread chloroquine resistance, however, it has become popular again. Quinine, or its close relative quinidine, can be given intravenously to treat severe *Falciparum* malaria.

Sulfadoxone/pyrimethamine (Fansidar)—An antimalarial drug developed in the 1960s. It is the first drug tried in some parts of the world where chloroquine resistance is widespread. It has been associated with severe allergic reactions due to its sulfa component.

falciparum malaria were visiting sub-Saharan Africa; travelers in Asia and South America are less at risk. Travelers who stay in air conditioned hotels on tourist itineraries in urban or resort areas are at lower risk than backpackers, missionaries, and Peace Corps volunteers. Some people in western cities where malaria does not usually exist may acquire the infection from a mosquito carried onto a jet. This is called airport or runway malaria.

Resources

BOOKS

Beers, Mark H., MD, and Robert Berkow, MD, editors. "Extraintestinal Protozoa: Malaria." Section 13, Chapter 161. In *The Merck Manual of Diagnosis and Therapy*. Whitehouse Station, NJ: Merck Research Laboratories, 2004.

PERIODICALS

Causer, Louise M, et al. "Malaria Surveillance—United States, 2000." *Morbidity and Mortality Weekly Report* July 12, 2002: 9–15. Abstract.

Coluzzi, M., and C. Costantini. "An Alternative Focus in Strategic Research on Disease Vectors: The Potential of Genetically Modified Non-Biting Mosquitoes." *Parassitologia* 44 (December 2002): 131–135.

"Combination Approach Results in Significant Drop in Malaria Rates in Viet Nam." *TB & Outbreaks Week* Abstract (September 24, 2002): 17.

Devi, G., V. A. Indumathi, D. Sridharan, et al. "Evaluation of ParaHITf Strip Test for Diagnosis of Malarial Infection." *Indian Journal of Medical Science* 56 (October 2002): 489–494.

Keiser, J., J. Utzinger, Z. Premji, et al. "Acridine Orange for Malaria Diagnosis: Its Diagnostic Performance, Its Promotion and Implementation in Tanzania, and the Implications for Malaria Control." *Annals of Tropical Medicine and Parasitology* 96 (October 2002): 643–654.

Kohler, I., K. Jenett-Siems, C. Kraft, et al. "Herbal Remedies Traditionally Used Against Malaria in Ghana: Bioassay-Guided Fractionation of *Microglossa pyrifolia* (Asteraceae)." *Zur Naturforschung* 57 (November-December 2002): 1022–1027.

Krudsood, S., K. Buchachart, K. Chalermrut, et al. "A Comparative Clinical Trial of Combinations of Dihydroartemisinin Plus Azithromycin and Dihydroartemisinin Plus Mefloquine for Treatment of Multidrug-Resistant *Falciparum* Malaria." *Southeast Asian Journal of Tropical Medicine and Public Health* 33 (September 2002): 525–531.

"Laser-based Malaria Test could be Valuable." *Medical Devices & Surgical Technology Week* September 22, 2002: 4.

McClellan, S. L. "Evaluation of Fever in the Returned Traveler." *Primary Care* 29 (December 2002): 947–969.

"Multilateral Initiative on Malaria to Move to Sweden." *TB & Outbreaks Week* September 24, 2002: 17.

Noedl, H., C. Wongsrichanalai, R. S. Miller, et al. "*Plasmodium falciparum*: Effect of Anti-Malarial Drugs on the Production and Secretion Characteristics of Histidine-Rich Protein II." *Experimental Parasitology* 102 (November-December 2002): 157–163.

"Promising Vaccine May Provide Long-Lasting Protection." *Medical Letter on the CDC & FDA* September 15, 2002: 14.

Stauffer, W. M., D. Kamat, and P. F. Walker. "Screening of International Immigrants, Refugees, and Adoptees." *Primary Care* 29 (December 2002): 879–905.

Thang, H. D., R. M. Elsas, and J. Veenstra. "Airport Malaria: Report of a Case and a Brief Review of the Literature." *Netherlands Journal of Medicine* 60 (December 2002): 441–443.

ORGANIZATIONS

Centers for Disease Control Malaria Hotline. (770) 332-4555.
Centers for Disease Control Travelers Hotline. (770) 332-4559.

OTHER

Malaria Foundation Page. < http://www.malaria.org >.

Carol A. Turkington
Rebecca J. Frey, PhD

Malaya *see* **Elephantiasis**

Male breast enlargement *see* **Gynecomastia**

Male condom *see* **Condom**

Male infertility *see* **Infertility**

Male pattern baldness *see* **Alopecia**

Malignant lymphomas

Definition

Lymphomas are a group of cancers in which cells of the lymphatic system become abnormal and start to grow uncontrollably. Because there is lymph tissue in many parts of the body, lymphomas can start in almost any organ of the body.

Description

The lymph system is made up of ducts or tubules that carry lymph to all parts of the body. Lymph is a milky fluid that contains the lymphocytes or white blood cells. These are the infection-fighting cells of the blood. Small pea-shaped organs are found along the network of lymph vessels. These are called the lymph nodes, and their main function is to make and store the lymphocytes. Clusters of lymph nodes are found in the pelvis region, underarm, neck, chest, and abdomen. The spleen (an organ in the upper abdomen), the tonsils, and the thymus (a small organ found beneath the breastbone) are part of the lymphatic system.

The lymphocyte is the main cell of the lymphoid tissue. There are two main types of lymphocytes: the T lymphocyte and the B lymphocyte. Lymphomas develop from these two cell types. B cell lymphomas are more common among adults, while among children, the incidence of T and B cell lymphomas are almost equal.

The T and the B cell perform different jobs within the immune system. When an infectious bacterium enters the body, the B cell makes proteins called "antibodies." These antibodies attach themselves to the bacteria, and flag them for destruction by other immune cells. The T cells help protect the body against viruses. When a virus enters the cell, it generally produces certain proteins that are projected on the surface of the infected cell. T cells recognize these proteins and produce certain substances (cytokines) that destroy the infected cells. Some of the cytokines made by the T cells attract other cell types, which are capable of digesting the virus-infected cell. The T cells can also destroy some types of cancerous cells.

Lymphomas can be divided into two main types: Hodgkin's lymphoma or **Hodgkin's disease**, and non-Hodgkin's lymphomas. There are at least 10 types of non-Hodgkin's lymphomas. They are grouped (staged) by how aggressively they grow; slow growing (low grade), intermediate growing, and rapidly growing (high grade); and how far they spread.

A majority of non-Hodgkin's lymphomas begin in the lymph nodes. About 20% start in other organs, such as the lungs, liver or the gastrointestinal tract. Malignant lymphocytes multiply uncontrollably and do not perform their normal functions. Hence, the body's ability to fight infections is affected. In addition, these malignant cells may crowd the bone marrow, and, depending on the stage, prevent the production of normal red blood cells, white blood cells, and platelets. A low red blood cell count causes anemia, while a reduction in the number of platelets makes the person susceptible to excessive bleeding. Cancerous cells can also invade other organs through the circulatory system of the lymph, causing those organs to malfunction.

Causes and symptoms

The exact cause of non-Hodgkin's lymphomas is not known. However, the incidence has increased significantly in the recent years. Part of the increase is due to the **AIDS** epidemic. Individuals infected with the AIDS virus have a higher likelihood of developing non-Hodgkin's lymphomas. In general, males are at a higher risk for having non-Hodgkin's lymphomas than are females. The risk increases with age. Though it can strike people as young as 40, people between the ages of 60 and 69 are at the highest risk.

People exposed to certain pesticides and ionizing radiation have a higher than average chance of developing this disease. For example, an increased incidence of lymphomas has been seen in survivors of the atomic bomb explosion in Hiroshima, and in people who have undergone aggressive **radiation therapy**. People who suffer from immune-deficient disorders, as well as those who have been treated with immune suppressive drugs for heart or kidney transplants, and for conditions such as **rheumatoid arthritis** and autoimmune diseases, are at an increased risk for this disease.

There have been some studies that have shown a loose association between retroviruses, such as HTLV-I, and some rare forms of lymphoma. The Epstein-Barr virus has been linked to Burkitt's lymphoma in African countries. However, a direct cause-and-effect relationship has not been established.

The symptoms of lymphomas are often vague and non-specific. Patients may experience loss of appetite, weight loss, **nausea**, **vomiting**, abdominal discomfort, and **indigestion**. The patient may complain of a feeling of fullness, which is a result of enlarged lymph nodes in the abdomen. Pressure or **pain** in the lower back is another symptom. In the advanced stages, the patient may have bone pain, headaches, constant coughing, and abnormal pressure and congestion in the face, neck, and upper chest. Some may have fevers and night sweats. In most cases, patients go to the doctor because of the presence of swollen glands in the neck, armpits, or groin area. Since all the symptoms are common to many other illnesses, it is essential to seek medical attention if any of the conditions persist for two weeks or more. Only a qualified physician can correctly diagnose if the symptoms are due to lymphoma or some other ailment.

Diagnosis

Like all cancers, lymphomas are best treated when found early. However, it is often difficult to diagnose lymphomas. There are no screening tests available, and, since the symptoms are non-specific, lymphomas are rarely recognized in their early stages. Detection often occurs by chance during a routine **physical examination**.

When the doctor suspects lymphoma, a complete medical history is taken, and a thorough physical examination is performed. Enlargement of the lymph nodes, liver, or spleen may suggest lymphomas. Blood tests will determine the cell counts and obtain information on how well the organs, such as the kidney and liver, are functioning.

A biopsy of the enlarged lymph node is the most definitive diagnostic tool for staging purposes. The

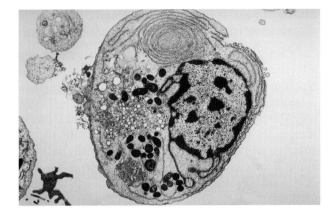

A malignant lymph cell. *(Custom Medical Stock Photo. Reproduced by permission.)*

doctor may perform a **bone marrow biopsy**. During the biopsy, a cylindrical piece of bone and marrow fluid is removed. They are generally taken out of the hipbone. These samples are sent to the laboratory for examination. In addition to diagnosis, the biopsy may also be repeated during the treatment phase of the disease to see if the lymphoma is responding to therapy.

Once the exact form of lymphoma is known, it is then staged to determine how aggressive it is, and how far it has spread. Staging is necessary to plan appropriate treatment.

Conventional imaging tests, such as x rays, **computed tomography scans** (CT scans), **magnetic resonance imaging**, and abdominal sonograms, are used to determine the extent of spread of the disease.

Lymphangiograms are x rays of the lymphatic system. In this procedure, a special dye is injected into the lymphatic channels through a small cut (incision) made in each foot. The dye is injected slowly over a period of three to four hours. This dye clearly outlines the lymphatic system and allows it to stand out. Multiple x rays are then taken and any abnormality, if present, is revealed.

Rarely, a lumbar puncture or a spinal tap is performed to check if malignant cells are present in the fluid surrounding the brain. In this test, the physician inserts a needle into the epidural space at the base of the spine and collects a small amount of spinal fluid for microscopic examination.

Treatment

Treatment options for lymphomas depend on the type of lymphoma and its present stage. In most cases, treatment consists of **chemotherapy**, radiotherapy, or a combination of the two methods.

Chemotherapy is the use of anti-cancer drugs to kill **cancer** cells. In non-Hodgkin's lymphomas, combination therapy, which involves the use of multiple drugs, has been found more effective than single drug use. The treatment may last about six months, but in some cases may last as long as a year. The drugs may either be administered intravenously (through a vein) in the arm or given orally in the form of pills. If cancer cells have invaded the central nervous system, then chemotherapeutic drugs may be instilled, through a needle in the brain or back, into the fluid that surrounds the brain. This procedure is known as intrathecal chemotherapy.

Radiation therapy, where high-energy ionizing rays are directed at specific portions of the body, such as the upper chest, abdomen, pelvis, or neck, is often used for treatment of lymphomas. External radiation therapy, where the rays are directed from a source outside the body, is the most common mode of radiation treatment.

Bone marrow transplantation is used in cases where the lymphomas do not respond to conventional therapy, or in cases where the patient has had a relapse or suffers from recurrent lymphomas.

There are two ways of doing bone marrow transplantation. In a procedure called "allogeneic bone marrow transplant," a donor is found whose marrow matches that of the patient. The donor can be a twin (best match), a sibling, or a person who is not related at all. High-dose chemotherapy or radiation therapy is given to eradicate the lymphoma. The donor marrow is then given to replace the marrow destroyed by the therapy.

In "autologous bone marrow transplantation," some of the patient's own bone marrow is harvested, chemically purged, and frozen. High-dose chemotherapy and radiation therapy are given. The marrow that was harvested, purged, and frozen is then thawed and put back into the patient's body to replace the destroyed marrow.

A new treatment option for patients with lymphoma is known as "peripheral stem cell transplantation." In this treatment approach, cells that normally circulate in the blood are collected when the patient has normal blood counts taken, and these cells are saved via a process called "pheresis." Researchers are exploring whether these cells can be used to restore the normal function and development of blood cells, rather than using a bone marrow transplant.

KEY TERMS

Antibodies—Proteins made by the B lymphocytes in response to the presence of infectious agents such as bacteria or viruses in the body.

Biopsy—The surgical removal and microscopic examination of living tissue for diagnostic purposes.

Growth factors (cytokines)—Chemicals made by the cells that act on other cells to stimulate or inhibit their function. Cytokines that stimulate growth are called "growth factors."

Prognosis

Like all cancers, the prognosis for lymphoma depends on the stage of the cancer, and the patient's age and general health. When all the different types and stages of lymphoma are considered together, only 50% of patients survive 5 years or more after initial diagnosis. This is because some types of lymphoma are more aggressive than others.

The survival rate among children is definitely better than among older people. About 90% of the children diagnosed with early stage disease survive 5 years or more, while only 60-70% of adults diagnosed with low grade lymphomas survive for 5 years or more. The survival rate for children with the more advanced stages is about 75-85%, while among adults it is 40-60%.

Prevention

Although many cancers may be prevented by making diet and life style changes which reduce risk factors, there is currently no known way to prevent lymphomas. Protecting oneself from developing AIDS, which may be a risk factor for lymphomas, is the only preventive measure that can be practiced.

At present, there are no special tests that are available for early detection of non-Hodgkin's lymphomas. Paying prompt attention to the signs and symptoms of this disease, and seeing a doctor if the symptoms persist, are the best strategies for an early diagnosis of lymphoma. Early detection affords the best chance for a cure.

Resources

ORGANIZATIONS

American Cancer Society. 1599 Clifton Rd., NE, Atlanta, GA 30329-4251. (800) 227-2345. < http:// www.cancer.org >.

Cancer Research Institute. 681 Fifth Ave., New York, N.Y. 10022. (800) 992-2623. <http://www.cancerresearch.org>.

Leukemia Society of America, Inc. 600 Third Ave., New York, NY 10016. (800) 955 4572. <http://www.leukemia.org>.

Lymphoma Research Foundation. 8800 Venice Boulevard, Suite 207, Los Angeles, CA 90034. (310) 204 7040.

National Cancer Institute. Building 31, Room 10A31, 31 Center Drive, MSC 2580, Bethesda, MD 20892-2580. (800) 422-6237. <http://www.nci.nih.gov>.

Oncolink. University of Pennsylvania Cancer Center. <http://cancer.med.upenn.edu>.

OTHER

"Adults Non-Hodgkin's Lymphoma." *National Cancer Institute Page.* <http://www.nci.nih.gov>.

"Childhood Non-Hodgkin's Lymphoma." *National Cancer Institute Page.* <http://www.nci.nih.gov>.

"Hodgkin's Disease" and Non-Hodgkin's Lymphoma." *The Leukemia Society.* <http://www.leukemia-lymphoma.org/hm_lls>.

Lata Cherath, PhD

Malignant melanoma

Definition

Malignant melanoma is a type of **cancer** arising from the melanocyte cells of the skin. Melanocytes are cells in the skin that produce a pigment called melanin. Malignant melanoma develops when the melanocytes no longer respond to normal control mechanisms of cellular growth. They may then invade nearby structures or spread to other organs in the body (metastasis), where again they invade and compromise the function of that organ.

Description

Melanocytes are derived from a structure in the human embryo called the neural crest. They are distributed in the epidermis and thus are found throughout the skin. They produce a brown pigment known as melanin and are responsible for racial variation in skin color as well as the color of **moles**. Malignant degeneration of the melanocyte gives rise to the tumor known as melanoma, which has four subtypes. These are: superficial spreading, nodular, lentigo maligna, and acral lentiginous melanomas, accounting for 70%, 15% to 30%, 4% to 10%, and 2% to 8% of cases, respectively. Malignant melanoma may develop anywhere on the body. In men, it is most common on the trunk. In women, it is most common on the back or legs. The subtype also may influence where the tumor develops; lentigo melanoma is more common on the face while acral lentiginous melanoma is more common on the palms of the hand, soles of the feet, or in the nail beds.

The locally invasive characteristic of this tumor involves vertical penetration through the skin and into the dermis and subcutaneous (under-the-skin) tissues of the malignant melanocytes. With the exception of the nodular variety of melanoma, there is often a phase of radial or lateral growth associated with these tumors. Since it is the vertical growth that characterizes the malignancy, the nodular variant of melanoma carries the worst prognosis. Fortunately, the superficial spreading type is most common.

The primary tumor begins in the skin, often from the melanocytes of a pre-existing mole. Once it becomes invasive, it may progress beyond the site of origin to the regional lymph nodes or travel to other organ systems in the body and become systemic in nature.

Lymph is the clear, protein-rich fluid that bathes the cells throughout our body. Lymph will work its way back to the bloodstream via small channels known as lymphatics. Along the way, the lymph is filtered through cellular stations known as nodes, thus they are called lymph nodes. Nearly all organs in the body have a primary lymph node group filtering the tissue fluid, or lymph, that comes from that organ. Different areas of the skin have different primary nodal stations. For the leg, they are in the groin. For the arm, the armpit or axilla. For the face, it is the neck. Depending where on the torso the tumor develops, it may drain into one groin or armpit, or both.

Cancer, as it invades in its place of origin, may also work its way into blood vessels. If this occurs, it provides yet another route for the cancer to spread to other organs of the body. When the cancer spreads elsewhere in the body, it has become systemic in extent and the tumor growing elsewhere is known as a metastasis.

Untreated malignant melanoma follows a classic progression. It begins and grows locally, penetrating vertically. It may be carried via the lymph to the regional nodes, known as regional metastasis. It may go from the lymph to the bloodstream or penetrate blood vessels, directly allowing it a route to go elsewhere in the body. When systemic disease or distant metastasis occur, melanoma commonly involves the lung, brain, liver, or occasionally bone. The malignancy causes **death** when its uncontrolled growth compromises vital organ function.

Of the anticipated new cases of cancer for the year 2003 in the United States, malignant melanoma will account for 5% of malignancies in men and 4% in women, being the sixth most common cancer in men and the seventh in women. It is estimated there will be 553,400 total cancer deaths in the United States in 2001. Malignant melanoma will account for 7,800 of these deaths, for an incidence of 1.5% of total deaths related to cancer.

The incidence of primary cutaneous malignant melanoma has been steadily increasing, possibly related to increase of sun exposure. Currently, the risk is about 13 per 100,000 of the population. It affects all age groups but is most commonly seen in patients between 30 and 60 years of age.

Sun exposure definitely increases the risk of developing melanoma, particularly in older males. The melanocytes are part of the integument's photoprotective mechanism; in response to sunlight, they produce melanin that has a protective role from the sun's ultraviolet rays. For Caucasians, the amount of melanin present in the skin is directly related to sun exposure. However, it is not so much the total sun exposure that seems important, rather it is the history of **sunburn**, (especially if severe or at an early age), that correlates with the increased risk. On this basis populations of fair-skinned people living in areas of high sun exposure such as the southwest United States or Australia are subject to increased risk. Malignant melanoma also affects non-Caucasians—though sun exposure probably does not play a role—at a rate of 10% that of Caucasians. The most common form of melanoma in African Americans is acral lentiginous melanoma.

Malignant melanoma may arise in the skin anywhere on the body. It is estimated that 50%–70% develop spontaneously while the remainder start in a pre-existing mole.

Causes and symptoms

The predisposing causes to the development of malignant melanoma are environmental and genetic. The environmental factor is excessive sun exposure. There are also genetically transmitted familial syndromes with alterations in the CDKN2A gene, which encodes for the tumor-suppressing proteins p16 and p19. In 2003 a group of Swedish researchers reported that 63 out of a group of 71 melanoma patients, or 89% of the group, had mutations in either the NRAS or the BRAF gene. The researchers found that these

mutations occur at an early point in the development of melanoma and remain as the tumor progresses.

As of early 2003, some researchers think there may be two pathways to malignant melanoma, one involving exposure to sunlight and the other with melanocyte proliferation triggered by other factors. This hypothesis is based on the difference in distribution of moles on the body between patients who develop melanomas on the face and neck, and those who develop melanomas on the trunk.

A small percentage of melanomas arise within burn scar tissue. As of 2003, researchers do not fully understand the relationship between deep **burns** and an increased risk of skin cancer.

As mentioned previously, melanin production in fair-skinned people is induced by sun exposure. An exposure substantial enough to result in a mild sunburn will be followed by melanin producing a tan that may last a few weeks. Both ultraviolet radiation and damaging oxygen radicals caused by sun exposure may damage cells, particularly their DNA. It is suspected that this damage induces mutations that result in the development of malignant melanoma. Though these mutations are alterations of the genome causing the melanoma, they are environmentally induced and account for sporadic or spontaneous cases of this disease.

A positive family history of one or two first-degree relatives having had melanoma substantially increases the risk on a genetic basis. A family tendency is observed in 8% to 12% of patients. There is a syndrome known as the dysplastic (atypical) nevus syndrome that is characterized by atypical moles with bothersome clinical features in children under age 10. Such individuals have to be observed closely for the development of malignant melanoma. Chromosome 9p has been identified as being involved in familial predisposition. There are mutations in up to 50% of familial melanoma patients of the tumor-suppressing gene CDKN2A. The actual number of moles increases risk, but the size of the moles needs be considered. Those with 10 larger moles of over 1 cm (0.4 in.) are at more risk than those with a higher number (50-99) of smaller moles. Finally, when a child is born with a large congenital mole, careful observation for change is appropriate because of increased risk.

An excellent way of identifying changes of significance in a mole is the ABCDE rule:

• Asymmetry

• Border irregularity

• Color variegation

- Diameter greater than 6 mm (0.24 in)
- Elevation above surrounding tissue.

Notice that three of the criteria refer to variability of the lesion (color variegation refers to areas of light color and black scattered within the mole). Thus small, uniform regular lesions have less cause for concern. It is important to realize that change in a mole or the rapid development of a new one are very important symptoms.

Another summary of important changes in a mole is the Glasgow 7-point scale. The symptoms and signs below can occur anywhere on the skin, including the palms of the hands, soles of the feet, and also the nail beds:

- Change in size
- Change in shape
- Change in color
- Inflammation
- Crusting and bleeding
- Sensory change
- Diameter greater than 7 mm (0.28 in.)

In this scheme, change is emphasized along with size. Bleeding and sensory changes are relatively late symptoms.

Symptoms related to the presence of regional disease are mostly those of nodules or lumps in the areas containing the lymph nodes draining the area. Thus nodularity can be found in the armpit, the groin, or the neck if regional nodes are involved. There is also a special type of metastasis that can occur regionally with malignant melanoma; it is known as an in-transit metastasis. If the melanoma is spreading through the lymph system, some of the tumor may grow there, resulting in a nodule part way between the primary site and the original lymph node. These in-transit metastasis are seen both at the time of original presentation or later after primary treatment has been rendered, the latter being a type of recurrence.

Finally, in those who either present with or progress to widespread or systemic disease, symptoms and signs are related to the affected organ. Thus neurologic problems, lung problems, or liver problems develop depending on the organ involved.

Diagnosis

None of the clinical signs or symptoms discussed above are absolute indications that a patient has malignant melanoma. The actual diagnosis is

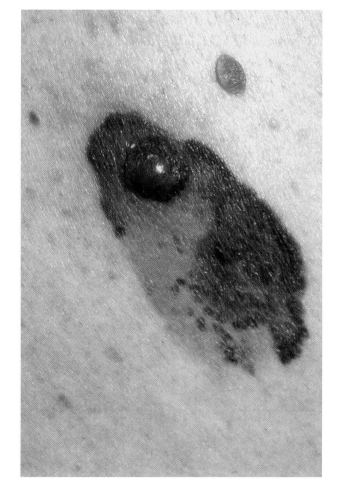

A close-up image of a malignant melanoma on a patient's back. *(Custom Medical Stock Photo. Reproduced by permission.)*

accomplished by biopsy, a procedure that removes tissue to examine under a microscope. It is important that the signs and symptoms are used to develop a suspicion of the diagnosis because the way the biopsy is performed for melanoma may be different than for other lesions of the skin.

The doctor may also use a dermatoscope to examine the mole prior to removal. The dermatoscope, which can be used to distinguish between benign moles and melanomas, is an instrument that resembles an ophthalmoscope. An immersion oil is first applied to the mole to make the outer layers of skin transparent.

When dealing with an early malignant melanoma, it is very important to establish the exact thickness of penetration of the primary tumor. Any biopsy that does not remove the full vertical extent of the primary is inadequate. Therefore, if a skin lesion is suspicious, full thickness excisional biopsy is the approach recommended. Shave biopsies and biopsies that remove only a portion of the suspect area are inappropriate. Often, in an early case, the excision involves just the suspicious lesion with minimal normal skin, but it should be a full vertical excision of the skin. If a melanoma is diagnosed, further treatment of this area will often be necessary but does not compromise outcome (prognosis). In some special areas of the body, minor modifications may be necessary about initial total excision, but full thickness excision should always be the goal. (See staging, below.)

Once the diagnosis is obtained, careful examination of the patient for regional lymph node involvement should be done. A careful review to uncover any symptoms of widespread disease is also appropriate.

The more common patient has an early melanoma, and extensive testing is not usually warranted. Routine testing in this situation involves a complete **blood count**, a **chest x ray**, and determinations of blood enzymes including lactic dehydrogenase and alkaline phosphatase.

If the patient has signs or symptoms of more advanced disease, or if the lesion's depth of penetration is sizeable, further imaging studies may be appropriate. These would involve CAT scans of the abdomen, the chest, or regional nodal areas, or a CT or MRI of the brain.

Treatment

The key to successful treatment is early diagnosis. Patients identified with localized, thin, small lesions (typified by superficial spreading subtype) nearly always survive. For those with advanced lesions, the outcome is poor in spite of progress in systemic therapy.

Clinical staging

Malignant melanoma is locally staged based on the depth of penetration through the skin and its appendages. There are two ways of looking at the depth of penetration. The Clarke system utilizes the layers of the dermis and the skin appendages present at that layer to identify the depth of penetration. The Breslow system uses the absolute measurement of depth. Though useful conceptually, the Clarke system is used less frequently because of the fact that skin is of different thickness in different regions of the body. The depth of penetration is much greater when the tumor reaches the subcutaneous fat when the skin involved is the back as opposed to the face. It turns out that the Breslow measurement is more reproducible and thus more useful; therefore, for purposes here, depth of penetration by absolute measurement (Breslow) is used in local staging.

Stage I and stage II have no involvement of the regional lymph nodes and are thus localized to the site of origin. These stages are subdivided on the basis of penetration. Stage Ia is 0.75 mm or less (1 mm = 0.04 in), and Stage Ib is 0.75–1.5 mm penetration. Stage IIa is 1.5–4.0 mm and Stage IIb is over 4.0 mm or into the subcutaneous fat. In stage III and IV, there is disease beyond the primary site. Stage III is defined by the presence of in-transit or regional nodal metastasis or both. Stage IV is defined by the presence of distant metastasis.

Once the diagnosis of malignant melanoma has been established by biopsy and the stage has been identified using the results of the examination and studies, a treatment plan is developed. Melanoma is not cured unless it is diagnosed at a stage when it can be isolated and removed surgically. Considerations revolve around the extent of the local and regional nodal surgery for stages I through III. For stage IV patients, or those that are treated and then develop recurrence at distant sites, **chemotherapy** or immunotherapy is planned. Studies are in progress to improve the results from traditional chemotherapeutic regimens. Adjuvant therapy (auxiliary drug treatment used to make possibility of relapse less for those at high risk) is also considered.

Surgical therapy for the primary site is that of wide local removal of the skin including subcutaneous tissue surrounding the lesion. In the past, wide excisions were large and encompassed 2 in. of tissue in all directions wherever feasible. It has been shown that such wide local excisions are not necessary and the issue has become: how wide is enough? Studies from the World Health Organization Melanoma Group and by the Melanoma Intergroup Committee in the United States have provided general guidelines based on the depth of penetration of the melanoma. These guidelines and anatomic considerations need to be kept in mind by the surgeon.

The next issue in primary management is whether the patient should have the regional lymph nodes removed in addition to treatment of the primary tumor. The problems associated with the resection of regional lymph nodes are those of lifelong **edema** or swelling in the extremity. Though it does not occur in all patients (5% to 20%, depending on the extremity and extent of the dissection), it can be a disabling symptom. Certainly, if it could be ascertained that there was disease in the nodes, resection (removal) would be appropriate. However, if there was no disease, the risk of edema should be avoided. In patients with no signs of regional disease, depth of penetration of the primary tumor helps guide the decision. If the tumor penetrates less than 1mm, dissection is not usually done. If it is 1-2 mm, node dissection may be done at the time of primary treatment or the patient may be observed and only undergo lymph node dissection if the area later shows signs of disease. If the patient has enlarged lymph nodes or the depth of the tumor has led to the evaluation by CAT scan showing enlarged nodes, resection of the nodes will be considered. In the latter case, more extensive imaging of the lung, liver, or brain may be appropriate to be sure the patient does not already have stage IV disease.

Questions related to which patients should have resection of regional lymph nodes have led to an intermediary procedure known as sentinel node mapping and biopsy. Intermediate thickness melanomas between 1 and 4 mm deep (0.04 and 0.16 in.) may have nodal involvement even if the examination and any other studies done are normal. If a radioisotope tracer or blue dye is injected into the area of the primary tumor, very shortly it will travel to the lymph nodes draining that area. These sentinel nodes are thus identifiable and are the most likely to harbor any regional metastatic disease. If these nodes alone are biopsied and are normal, the rest of the lymph node group can be spared. If they show microscopic deposits of tumor, then the full resection of the lymph node group may be completed. This procedure allows selection of those patients with intermediate thickness melanoma who will benefit from the regional lymph node dissection.

Patients with metastatic melanoma who do not respond well to other therapies may be candidates for treatment with aldesleukin. Aldesleukin is a form of interleukin, a specific kind of biological response modifier that promotes the development of T-cells. These cells are part of the lymphatic system and can directly interact with and fight cancer cells. Although aldesleukin is produced naturally in the body, its therapeutic form is developed via biotechnology in a laboratory setting. Treatment is considered palliative, which means that it provides comfort but does not produce a cure. Side effects, however, can be severe, and range from flu-like symptoms to whole-body infection (**sepsis**) and **coma**.

Some patients, such as those with IIb or stage III melanoma, are at high risk for the development of recurrence after treatment. Although these patients are clinically free of disease after undergoing primary treatment, they are more likely to have some microscopic disease in the body that studies have not yet been able to identify. In an effort to decrease the rate of relapse, adjuvant therapy may be considered. Interferon alpha 2a is an agent that stimulates the immune system. This adjuvant therapy may slightly increase the duration of a patient's disease-free state and lengthen overall survival. However, interferon alpha 2a has high toxicity and patients may not tolerate the side effects.

Unfortunately, treatment for those patients who present with or go on to develop systemic disease usually fails; melanoma that has metastasized to the brain is particularly difficult to treat. The chemotherapeutic agent dacarbazine, or DTIC, seems to be the most active agent. Overall responses are noted in about 20% of patients, and they last only two to six months. Combination therapy may be an option. The regimen of DTIC + BCNU (carmustine) + cisplatin + tamoxifen delivers a response rate of 40%. Combining biologic or immunologic agents such as interferon with standard chemotherapeutic agents is under study and showing improved response rates, though toxicity is substantial and only the healthier, younger patients tolerate the treatment.

Some researchers are investigating the reasons why melanomas are so resistant to chemotherapy. One suggestion as of late 2003 is that the genes ordinarily responsible for apoptosis (cell self-destruction) do not function normally in melanomas. The development of new drugs to treat melanoma depends on a better understanding of the complex processes involved in apoptosis.

Alternative treatment

Though **radiation therapy** has a minimal role in the primary treatment of malignant melanoma, for patients who have metastatic disease, radiation may be helpful. This is true in patients who have developed tumor deposits in such areas as the brain or bone.

Prognosis

Almost all patients survive stage Ia malignant melanoma, and the suvivorship for stage I overall is more than 90%. Survival drops in stage IIa to about 65% at five years and is worse yet for stage IIb at slightly over 50%. Stage III has a survival rate at 5 years of 10%–47%, depending on the size and number of regional nodes involved. Stage IV malignant melanoma is almost always a fatal disease.

KEY TERMS

Adjuvant therapy—Treatment given to patients who are at risk of having microscopic untreated disease present but have no obvious symptoms.

Dermis—The deeper portion or layer of the skin beneath the epidermis.

Dysplastic nevus syndrome—A familial syndrome characterized by the presence of multiple atypical appearing moles, often at a young age.

Epidermis—The uppermost layer of skin cells.

Genome—The genetic makeup of a cell, composed of DNA.

Immunotherapy—A form of treatment that uses biologic agents to enhance or stimulate normal immune function.

Integument—The medical name for the skin.

Lymph node dissection—Surgical removal of a group of lymph nodes.

Lymphedema—Swelling of an arm or leg following surgical removal of the lymph nodes that drain the limb.

Melanocytes—Skin cells derived from the neural crest that produce the protein pigment melanin.

Metastasis (plural, metastases)—A tumor growth or deposit that has spread via lymph or blood to an area of the body remote from the primary tumor.

Nevus (plural, nevi)—A medical term for mole.

Resection—The act of removing something surgically.

Skin appendages—Structures related to the integument such as hair follicles and sweat glands.

Variegation—Patchy variation in color.

Coping with cancer treatment

For those with familial tendencies for malignant melanoma, **genetic counseling** may be appropriate. Psychological counseling may be appropriate for anyone having trouble coping with a potentially fatal disease. Local cancer support groups may be helpful and are often identified by contacting local hospitals or the American Cancer Society.

Prevention

Though it is difficult to prove that **sunscreens** statistically reduce the frequency of malignant melanoma at this time, most authorities recommend their use as protection from ultraviolet light (considered a major factor in the development of melanoma.) Avoidance of severe sunburns is recommended.

Resources

BOOKS

Abeloff, Armitage, Lichter, and Niederhuber. *Clinical Oncology Library*. 2nd ed. London: Churchill Livingstone, 1999.

Beers, Mark H., MD, and Robert Berkow, MD, editors. "Dermatologic Disorders: Malignant Tumors." Section 10, Chapter 126. In *The Merck Manual of Diagnosis and Therapy*. Whitehouse Station, NJ: Merck Research Laboratories, 2004.

Beers, Mark H., MD, and Robert Berkow, MD, editors. "Dermatologic Disorders: Moles." Section 10, Chapter 125 In *The Merck Manual of Diagnosis and Therapy*. Whitehouse Station, NJ: Merck Research Laboratories, 2004.

Beers, Mark H., MD, and Robert Berkow, MD, editors. "Dermatologic Disorders: Reactions to Sunlight." Section 10, Chapter 119. In *The Merck Manual of Diagnosis and Therapy*. Whitehouse Station, NJ: Merck Research Laboratories, 2004.

PERIODICALS

Brown, C. K., and J. M. Kirkwood. "Medical Management of Melanoma." *Surgical Clinics of North America* 83 (April 2003): 283–322.

Carlson, J. A., A. Slominski, G. P. Linette, et al. "Malignant Melanoma 2003: Predisposition, Diagnosis, Prognosis, and Staging." *American Journal of Clinical Pathology* 120 , Supplement (December 2003): S101–S127.

Eigentler, T. K., U. M. Caroli, P. Radny, and C. Garbe. "Palliative Therapy of Disseminated Malignant Melanoma: A Systematic Review of 41 Randomised Clinical Trials." *Lancet Oncology* 4 (December 2003): 748–759.

Halder, R. M., and C. J. Ara. "Skin Cancer and Photoaging in Ethnic Skin." *Dermatologic Clinics* 21 (October 2003): 725–732.

Horig, H., and H. L. Kaufman. "Local Delivery of Poxvirus Vaccines for Melanoma." *Seminars in Cancer Biology* 13 (December 2003): 417–422.

Jellouli-Elloumi, A., L. Kochbati, S. Dhraief, et al. "Cancers Arising from Burn Scars: 62 Cases." [in French] *Annales de dermatologie et de venereologie* 130 (April 2003): 413–416.

McWilliams, R. R., P. D. Brown, J. C. Buckner, et al. "Treatment of Brain Metastases from Melanoma." *Mayo Clinic Proceedings* 78 (December 2003): 1529–1536.

Omholt, K., A. Platz, L. Kanter, et al. "NRAS and BRAF Mutations Arise Early During Melanoma Pathogenesis and Are Preserved Throughout Tumor Progression."

Clinical Cancer Research 9 (December 15, 2003): 6483–6488.

Rockmann, H., and D. Schadendorf. "Drug Resistance in Human Melanoma: Mechanisms and Therapeutic Opportunities" Onkologie 26 (December 2003): 581–587.

Weinstock, Martin A. "Early Detection of Melanoma." JAMA, The Journal of the American Medical Association 284 (August 16, 2000): 886.

Whiteman, D. C., P. Watt, D. M. Purdie, et al. "Melanocytic Nevi, Solar Keratoses, and Divergent Pathways to Cutaneous Melanoma." Journal of the National Cancer Institute 95 (June 4, 2003): 806–812.

ORGANIZATIONS

American Academy of Dermatology. 930 N. Meacham Road, P.O. Box 4014, Schaumburg, IL 60168-4014. (847) 330-0230. Fax: (847) 330-0050. <http://www.aad.org>.

American Cancer Society. 1599 Clifton Road NE, Atlanta, GA 30329. (800) ACS-2345.

National Cancer Institute (NCI). NCI Public Inquiries Office, Suite 3036A, 6116 Executive Boulevard, MSC8332, Bethesda, MD 20892-8322. (800) 4-CANCER or (800) 332-8615 (TTY). <http://www.nci.nih.gov>.

OTHER

Cancer Resource Center. American Cancer Society. June 20, 2001. <http://www3.cancer.org/cancerinfo>.

Melanoma Patient's Information Page. June 20, 2001. <http://www.mpip.org>.

National Cancer Institute. June 13, 2001. <http://rex.nci.nih.gov/PATIENTS/INFO_PEOPL_DOC.html>.

Richard A. McCartney, MD
Rebecca J. Frey, PhD

Malignant plasmacytoma see **Multiple myeloma**

Malingering

Definition

In the context of medicine, malingering is the act of intentionally feigning or exaggerating physical or psychological symptoms for personal gain.

Description

People may feign physical or psychological illness for any number of reasons. Faked illness can get them out of work, military duty, or criminal prosecution. It can also help them obtain financial compensation through insurance claims, lawsuits, or workers' compensation. Feigned symptoms may also be a way of getting the doctor to prescribe certain drugs.

According to the American Psychiatric Association, patients who malinger are different from people who invent symptoms for sympathy (factitious diseases). Patients who malinger clearly have something tangible to gain. People with factitious diseases appear to have a need to play the "sick" role. They may feign illness for attention or sympathy.

Malingering may take the form of complaints of chronic **whiplash pain** from automobile accidents. Whiplash claims are controversial. Although some people clearly do suffer from whiplash injury, others may be exaggerating the pain for insurance claims or lawsuits. Some intriguing scientific studies have shown that chronic whiplash pain after automobile accidents is almost nonexistent in Lithuania and Greece. In these countries, the legal systems do not encourage personal injury lawsuits or financial settlements. The psychological symptoms experienced by survivors of disaster (**post-traumatic stress disorder**) are also faked by malingerers.

Causes and symptoms

People malinger for personal gain. The symptoms may vary. Generally malingerers complain of psychological disorders such as **anxiety**. They may also complain of chronic pain for which objective tests such as x rays can find no physical cause. Because it is often impossible to determine who is malingering and who is not, it is impossible to know how frequently malingering occurs.

Diagnosis

Malingering may be suspected:

- When a patient is referred for examination by an attorney
- When the onset of illness coincides with a large financial incentive, such as a new disability policy
- When objective medical tests do not confirm the patient's complaints
- When the patient does not cooperate with the diagnostic work-up or prescribed treatment
- When the patient has antisocial attitudes and behaviors (antisocial personality).

The diagnosis of malingering is a challenge for doctors. On the one hand, the doctor does not

GALE ENCYCLOPEDIA OF MEDICINE

2331

want to overlook a treatable disease. On the other hand, he or she does not want to continue ordering tests and treatments if the symptoms are faked. Malingering is difficult to distinguish from certain legitimate **personality disorders**, such as factitious diseases or post-traumatic distress syndrome. In legal cases, malingering patients may be referred to a psychiatrist. Psychiatrists use certain written tests to try to determine whether the patient is faking the symptoms.

Treatment

In a sense, malingering cannot be treated because the American Psychiatric Association does not recognize it as a personality disorder. Patients who are purposefully faking symptoms for gain do not want to be cured. Often, the malingering patient fails to report any improvement with treatment, and the doctor may try many treatments without success.

Resources

ORGANIZATIONS

American Psychiatric Association. 1400 K Street NW, Washington DC 20005. (888) 357-7924. <http://www.psych.org>.

Robert Scott Dinsmoor

Mallet finger

Definition

Mallet finger refers to the involuntary flexion of the distal phalanx of a finger caused by the disruption or tearing of its extensor tendon.

Description

Tendons are the strong "cables" between muscles and bones that help control movements of the body. They consist of white, glistening, fibrous cords, of various length and thickness, either round or flattened, and lacking in elasticity. In mallet finger, which often occurs as a sports-related injury, the tendon on the back of the finger becomes damaged or torn near the outermost joint. Without the support provided by the tendon, the short bone at the tip of the finger drops downward at an awkward angle. This bone, referred to as the "distal phalanx" of a finger, is the one furthest from the palm. In addition to tendon damage, mallet finger may involve a fracture of the distal phalanx. Mallet finger is sometimes called baseball finger.

Causes and symptoms

Mallet finger usually occurs while playing a sport that involves a ball—for example, reaching out to catch a hard pass in basketball or bare-handing a baseball. Instead of landing on the palm of the hand, the ball accidentally hits the tip of an extended (or partially extended) finger. This straight-on impact causes instantaneous stretch of the tendon, which may overextend or tear away. Mallet finger can also result from hitting the hand against a hard object or receiving a cut from a sharp edge such as a knife.

Symptoms of mallet finger include **pain** and swelling around the top part of the finger, near the outermost joint. These symptoms occur right after the injury. Redness and swelling develop soon afterward. The tip of the finger has an abnormal-looking downward droop, and it may be difficult to fully extend the finger.

Diagnosis

Mallet finger is usually diagnosed after a relatively brief **physical examination** conducted by an emergency care physician or by an orthopedist, the type of doctor who specializes in such injuries. The downward droop of the fingertip is the major indication of mallet finger, along with the tenderness and pain that occurs in the

KEY TERMS

Distal Phalanx—The outermost bone of any finger or toe.

Fracture—A break in bone.

Orthopedist—A doctor who specializes in disorders of the musculoskeletal system.

Phalanx—Any of the digital bones of the hand or foot. Humans have three phalanges to each finger and toe with the exception of the thumb and big toe which have only two each.

Tendon—A tough cord of dense white fibrous connective tissue that connects a muscle with some other part, especially a bone, and transmits the force which the muscle exerts.

affected area. X rays will be taken to determine if the bone at the top of the finger has been fractured. Mallet finger is typically covered by medical insurance.

Treatment

If symptoms of mallet finger appear, the affected individual should consult a physician or seek emergency care. In the meantime, ice (wrapped in a towel or cloth) can be applied to the affected area to help reduce swelling and alleviate pain.

Treatment usually involves wearing a splint around the top of the affected finger in order to keep it extended and allow the injury to heal. The splint must be worn at all times for six to eight weeks, though it may be briefly removed to wash the finger, but with extreme care so as not to allow the fingertip to bend. For the next six to eight weeks after that, the splint need only be worn during sleep or athletic activities.

If the bone at the top of the finger has sustained a large fracture, surgery may necessary. If the tendon was damaged due to a cut, stitches may be required both to repair the tendon and to adequately close the wound.

Over-the-counter (OTC) or prescription pain medication can be used to alleviate pain.

Alternative treatment

Acupuncture, therapeutic massage, and **yoga** are believed by some practitioners of alternative medicine to have generalized pain-relieving effects. Any of these therapies may provide additional comfort while the finger heals.

Prognosis

With proper treatment, most people regain full use of the affected finger.

Prevention

Caution should be used when playing ball sports or using knives or other sharp implements.

Resources

BOOKS

Brukner, Peter, et al. *Clinical Sports Medicine*: McGraw-Hill, 2000.

PERIODICALS

Lester, B., et al. "A simple effective splinting technique for the mallet finger." *American Journal of Orthopedics* March 2000: 202-6.

Takami H, et al. "Operative treatment of mallet finger due to intra-articular fracture of the distal phalanx." *Archives of Orthopaedic and Trauma Surgery* 120 (2000): 9-13.

ORGANIZATIONS

American Academy of Orthopaedic Surgeons. 6300 North River Road, Rosemont, IL 60018-4262. (800) 346-AAOS. <http://www.aaos.org>.

Greg Annussek

Mallory-Weiss syndrome

Definition

Mallory-Weiss syndrome is bleeding from an arterial blood vessel in the upper gastrointestinal tract, caused by a mucosal gastric tear at or near the point where the esophagus and stomach join.

Description

Mallory-Weiss syndrome causes about 5% of all upper gastrointestinal bleeding. The condition was originally diagnosed in alcoholics and is associated with heavy alcohol use, although it can also be found in patients who are not alcoholics. Earlier episodes of heavy hiccupping, **vomiting**, and retching are reported by about half the patients who are diagnosed with Mallory-Weiss syndrome. It is thought that the tear or laceration occurs when there is a sudden increase in intra-abdominal pressure. Patients with increased pressure in the vein leading into the liver (portal **hypertension**) are more likely to bleed heavily from an

KEY TERMS

Electrolytes—Salts and minerals that can conduct electrical impulses in the body. Common human electrolytes are sodium chloride, potassium, calcium, and sodium bicarbonate. Electrolytes control the fluid balance of the body and are important in muscle contraction, energy generation, and almost every major biochemical reaction in the body.

Endoscopy—A procedure in which an instrument containing a camera and a light source is inserted into the gastrointestinal tract so that the doctor can visually inspect the gastrointestinal system.

Esophageal varix—An enlarged vein of the esophagus. (Plural: esophageal varices.)

Portal hypertension—High blood pressure in the portal vein, which carries blood from the abdominal organs to the liver.

esophageal laceration than those whose blood pressure is normal.

Causes and symptoms

In Mallory-Weiss syndrome, a tear occurs in the gastric mucosa, near where the esophagus and stomach join. About 10% of the tears are in the esophagus. Most are either right at the junction of the esophagus and stomach or in the stomach just slightly below the junction.

Bleeding from the tear causes a disruption in fluid and electrolyte balance of the body. The patient often produces vomit tinged with either fresh blood or older, blackish blood. Blood loss can be considerable.

Diagnosis

A Mallory-Weiss syndrome tear is not visible on standard upper gastrointestinal x rays. A tear about one-eighth to one and one-half inches long (0.5–4 cm) is revealed by endoscopy. Endoscopy also shows that in 35% of patients there is another potential cause for gastrointestinal bleeding, such as peptic ulcer, erosive **gastritis**, or esophageal varices.

Treatment

The patient is resuscitated and stabilized with blood transfusions and intravenous fluids to restore the fluid and electrolyte balance. Most of the time,

esophageal bleeding stops spontaneously. When bleeding does not stop, patients are treated with an injection of epinephrine (adrenaline) and/or the bleeding artery is cauterized with heat. If these treatments fail, surgery is performed to stop the bleeding.

Prognosis

In 90-95% of patients whose bleeding does not stop spontaneously, cauterization without surgery will stop the bleeding. Patients at highest risk for a recurrence of bleeding are those with portal hypertension.

Prevention

Mallory-Weiss syndrome is associated with **alcoholism**. Limiting alcohol intake may help prevent the disorder.

Resources

BOOKS

"Mallory-Weiss Syndrome." In *Current Medical Diagnosis and Treatment, 1998.* edited by Stephen McPhee, et al., 37th ed. Stamford: Appleton & Lange, 1997.

Tish Davidson, A.M.

Malnutrition

Definition

Malnutrition is the condition that develops when the body does not get the right amount of the **vitamins**, **minerals**, and other nutrients it needs to maintain healthy tissues and organ function.

Description

Undernutrition

Malnutrition occurs in people who are either undernourished or overnourished. Undernutrition is a consequence of consuming too few essential nutrients or using or excreting them more rapidly than they can be replaced.

Infants, young children, and teenagers need additional nutrients. So do women who are pregnant or breastfeeding. Nutrient loss can be accelerated by **diarrhea**, excessive sweating, heavy bleeding (hemorrhage), or kidney failure. Nutrient intake can be restricted by age-related illnesses and conditions, excessive dieting, **food allergies**, severe injury, serious illness, a lengthy hospitalization, or **substance abuse**.

The leading cause of **death** in children in developing countries is **protein-energy malnutrition**. This type of malnutrition is the result of inadequate intake of calories from proteins, vitamins, and minerals. Children who are already undernourished can suffer from protein-energy malnutrition (PEM) when rapid growth, infection, or disease increases the need for protein and essential minerals. These essential minerals are known as micronutrients or trace elements.

Two types of protein-energy malnutrition have been described—kwashiorkor and marasmus. Kwashiorkor occurs with fair or adequate calorie intake but inadequate protein intake, while marasmus occurs when the diet is inadequate in both calories and protein.

About 1% of children in the United States suffer from chronic malnutrition, in comparison to 50% of children in southeast Asia. About two-thirds of all the malnourished children in the world are in Asia, with another one-fourth in Africa.

Overnutrition

In the United States, nutritional deficiencies have generally been replaced by dietary imbalances or excesses associated with many of the leading causes of death and disability. Overnutrition results from eating too much, eating too many of the wrong things, not exercising enough, or taking too many vitamins or other dietary replacements.

Risk of overnutrition is also increased by being more than 20% overweight, consuming a diet high in fat and salt, and taking high doses of:

- Nicotinic acid (niacin) to lower elevated cholesterol levels
- Vitamin B_6 to relieve **premenstrual syndrome**
- Vitamin A to clear up skin problems
- Iron or other trace minerals not prescribed by a doctor.

Nutritional disorders can affect any system in the body and the senses of sight, taste, and smell. They may also produce **anxiety**, changes in mood, and other psychiatric symptoms. Malnutrition begins with changes in nutrient levels in blood and tissues. Alterations in enzyme levels, tissue abnormalities, and organ malfunction may be followed by illness and death.

Causes and symptoms

Causes

Poverty and lack of food are the primary reasons why malnutrition occurs in the United States. Ten percent of all members of low income households do not always have enough healthful food to eat. Protein-energy malnutrition occurs in 50% of surgical patients and in 48% of all other hospital patients.

Loss of appetite associated with the **aging** process. Malnutrition affects one in four elderly Americans, in part because they may lose interest in eating. In addition, such dementing illnesses as **Alzheimer's disease** may cause elderly persons to forget to eat.

There is an increased risk of malnutrition associated with chronic diseases, especially disease of the intestinal tract, kidneys, and liver. Patients with chronic diseases like **cancer**, **AIDS**, intestinal parasites, and other gastric disorders may lose weight rapidly and become susceptible to undernourishment because they cannot absorb valuable vitamins, calories, and iron.

People with drug or alcohol dependencies are also at increased risk of malnutrition. These people tend to maintain inadequate **diets** for long periods of time and their ability to absorb nutrients is impaired by the alcohol or drug's affect on body tissues, particularly the liver, pancreas, and brain.

Eating disorders. People with anorexia or bulimia may restrict their food intake to such extremes that they become malnourished.

Food **allergies**. Some people with food allergies may find it difficult to obtain food that they can digest. In addition, people with food allergies often need additional calorie intake to maintain their weight.

Failure to absorb nutrients in food following bariatric (weight loss) surgery. **Bariatric surgery** includes such techniques as stomach stapling (gastroplasty) and various intestinal bypass procedures to help people eat less and lose weight. Malnutrition is, however, a possible side effect of bariatric surgery.

Symptoms

Unintentionally losing 10 pounds or more may be a sign of malnutrition. People who are malnourished may be skinny or bloated. Their skin is pale, thick, dry, and **bruises** easily. **Rashes** and changes in pigmentation are common.

Hair is thin, tightly curled, and pulls out easily. Joints ache and bones are soft and tender. The gums bleed easily. The tongue may be swollen or shriveled and cracked. Visual disturbances include night blindness and increased sensitivity to light and glare.

Other symptoms of malnutrition include:

- anemia
- diarrhea
- disorientation
- night blindness
- irritability, anxiety, and attention deficits
- goiter (enlarged thyroid gland)
- loss of reflexes and lack of muscular coordination
- muscle twitches
- amenorrhea (cessation of menstrual periods)
- scaling and cracking of the lips and mouth.

Malnourished children may be short for their age, thin, listless, and have weakened immune systems.

Diagnosis

Overall appearance, behavior, body-fat distribution, and organ function can alert a family physician, internist, or **nutrition** specialist to the presence of malnutrition. Patients may be asked to record what they eat during a specific period. X rays can determine bone density and reveal gastrointestinal disturbances, and heart and lung damage.

Blood and urine tests are used to measure the patient's levels of vitamins, minerals, and waste products. Nutritional status can also be determined by:

- Comparing a patient's weight to standardized charts
- Calculating body mass index (BMI) according to a formula that divides height into weight
- Measuring skinfold thickness or the circumference of the upper arm.

Treatment

Normalizing nutritional status starts with a nutritional assessment. This process enables a clinical nutritionist or registered dietician to confirm the presence of malnutrition, assess the effects of the disorder, and formulate diets that will restore adequate nutrition.

Patients who cannot or will not eat, or who are unable to absorb nutrients taken by mouth, may be fed intravenously (parenteral nutrition) or through a tube inserted into the gastrointestinal (GI) tract (enteral nutrition).

Tube feeding is often used to provide nutrients to patients who have suffered **burns** or who have

inflammatory bowel disease. This procedure involves inserting a thin tube through the nose and carefully guiding it along the throat until it reaches the stomach or small intestine. If long-term tube feeding is necessary, the tube may be placed directly into the stomach or small intestine through an incision in the abdomen.

Tube feeding cannot always deliver adequate nutrients to patients who:

- Are severely malnourished
- Require surgery
- Are undergoing **chemotherapy** or radiation treatments
- Have been seriously burned
- Have persistent diarrhea or **vomiting**
- Whose gastrointestinal tract is paralyzed.

Intravenous feeding can supply some or all of the nutrients these patients need.

Prognosis

Up to 10% of a person's body weight can be lost without side effects, but if more than 40% is lost, the situation is almost always fatal. Death usually results from **heart failure**, electrolyte imbalance, or low body temperature. Patients with semiconsciousness, persistent diarrhea, **jaundice**, or low blood sodium levels have a poorer prognosis.

Some children with protein-energy malnutrition recover completely. Others have many health problems throughout life, including **mental retardation** and the inability to absorb nutrients through the intestinal tract. Prognosis for all patients with malnutrition seems to be dependent on the age of the patient, and the length and severity of the malnutrition, with young children and the elderly having the highest rate of long-term complications and death.

Prevention

Breastfeeding a baby for at least six months is considered the best way to prevent early-childhood malnutrition. The United States Department of Agriculture and Health and Human Service recommend that all Americans over the age of two:

- Consume plenty of fruits, grains, and vegetables
- Eat a variety of foods that are low in fats and cholesterols and contain only moderate amounts of salt, sugars, and sodium
- Engage in moderate physical activity for at least 30 minutes, at least several times a week

KEY TERMS

Anemia—Not enough red blood cells in the blood.

Anorexia nervosa—Eating disorder marked by malnutrition and weight loss commonly occurring in young women.

Bariatric—Pertaining to the study, prevention, or treatment of overweight.

Calorie—A unit of heat measurement used in nutrition to measure the energy value of foods. A calorie is the amount of heat energy needed to raise the temperature of 1 kilogram of water 1°C.

Kwashiorkor—Severe malnutrition in children primarily caused by a protein-poor diet, characterized by growth retardation.

Marasmus—Severe malnutrition in children caused by a diet lacking in calories as well as protein. Marasmus may also be caused by disease and parasitic infection.

Micronutrients—Essential dietary elements that are needed only in very small quantities. Micronutrients are also known as trace elements. They include copper, zinc, selenium, iodine, magnesium, iron, cobalt, and chromium.

- Achieve or maintain their ideal weight

- Use alcohol sparingly or avoid it altogether.

Every patient admitted to a hospital should be screened for the presence of illnesses and conditions that could lead to protein-energy malnutrition. Patients with higher-than-average risk for malnutrition should be more closely assessed and reevaluated often during long-term hospitalization or nursing-home care.

Resources

BOOKS

Beers, Mark H., MD, and Robert Berkow, MD, editors. "Malnutrition." Section 1, Chapter 2. In *The Merck Manual of Diagnosis and Therapy*.Whitehouse Station, NJ: Merck Research Laboratories, 2004.

Flancbaum, Louis, MD, with Erica Manfred and Deborah Biskin. *The Doctor's Guide to Weight Loss Surgery*. West Hurley, NY: Fredonia Communications, 2001.

PERIODICALS

Alvarez-Leite, J. I. "Nutrient Deficiencies Secondary to Bariatric Surgery." *Current Opinion in Clinical Nutrition and Metabolic Care* 7 (September 2004): 569–575.

Amella, E. J. "Feeding and Hydration Issues for Older Adults with Dementia." *Nursing Clinics of North America* 39 (September 2004): 607–623.

Bryan, J., S. Osendorp, D. Hughes, et al. "Nutrients for Cognitive Development in School-Aged Children." *Nutrition Reviews* 62 (August 2004): 295–306.

Grigsby, Donna G., MD. "Malnutrition." *eMedicine* December 18, 2003. < http://www.emedicine.com/ped/topic1360.htm >.

Gums, J. G. "Magnesium in Cardiovascular and Other Disorders." *American Journal of Health-System Pharmacy* 61 (August 1, 2004): 1569–1576.

Halsted, G. H. "Nutrition and Alcoholic Liver Disease." *Seminars in Liver Disease* 24 (August 2004): 289–304.

Reid, C. L. "Nutritional Requirements of Surgical and Critically-Ill Patients: Do We Really Know What They Need?" *Proceedings of the Nutrition Society* 63 (August 2004): 467–472.

ORGANIZATIONS

American College of Nutrition. 722 Robert E. Lee Drive, Wilmington, NC 20412-0927. (919) 452-1222.

American Institute of Nutrition. 9650 Rockville Pike, Bethesda, MD 20814-3990. (301) 530-7050.

Food and Nutrition Information Center. 10301 Baltimore Boulevard, Room 304, Beltsville, MD 20705-2351. < http://www.nalusda.gov/fnic >.

OTHER

World Health Organization (WHO) Nutrition web site. < http://www.who.int/nut/index.htm >.

Mary K. Fyke
Rebecca J. Frey, PhD

Malocclusion

Definition

Malocclusion is a problem in the way the upper and lower teeth fit together in biting or chewing. The word malocclusion literally means "bad bite." The condition may also be referred to as an irregular bite, crossbite, or overbite.

Description

Malocclusion may be seen as crooked, crowded, or protruding teeth. It may affect a person's appearance, speech, and/or ability to eat.

Causes and symptoms

Malocclusions are most often inherited, but may be acquired. Inherited conditions include too many or too few teeth, too much or too little space between teeth, irregular mouth and jaw size and shape, and atypical formations of the jaws and face, such as a **cleft palate**. Malocclusions may be acquired from habits like finger or thumb sucking, tongue thrusting, premature loss of teeth from an accident or dental disease, and medical conditions such as enlarged tonsils and adenoids that lead to mouth breathing.

Malocclusions may be symptomless or they may produce **pain** from increased **stress** on the oral structures. Teeth may show abnormal signs of wear on the chewing surfaces or decay in areas of tight overlap. Chewing may be difficult.

Diagnosis

Malocclusion is most often found during a routine dental examination. A dentist will check a patient's occlusion by watching how the teeth make contact when the patient bites down normally. The dentist may ask the patient to bite down with a piece of coated paper between the upper and lower teeth; this paper will leave colored marks at the points of contact. When malocclusion is suspected, photographs and x rays of the face and mouth may be taken for further study. To confirm the presence and extent of malocclusion, the dentist makes plaster, plastic, or artificial stone models of the patient's teeth from impressions. These models duplicate the fit of the teeth and are very useful in treatment planning.

Treatment

Malocclusion may be remedied by orthodontic treatment; orthodontics is a specialty of dentistry that manages the growth and correction of dental and facial structures. Braces are the most commonly used orthodontic appliances in the treatment of malocclusion. At any given time, approximately 4 million people in the United States are wearing braces, including 800,000 adults.

Braces apply constant gentle force to slowly change the position of the teeth, straightening them and properly aligning them with the opposing teeth. Braces consist of brackets cemented to the surface of each tooth and wires of stainless steel or nickel titanium alloy. When the wires are threaded through the brackets, they exert pressure against the teeth, causing them to move gradually.

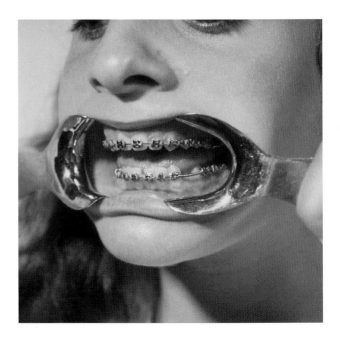

Orthodontia treatments usually include the use of braces and retainers. *(Photograph by Lester V. Bergman, Corbis Images. Reproduced by permission).*

Braces are not removable for daily tooth brushing, so the patient must be especially diligent about keeping the mouth clean and removing food particles which become easily trapped, to prevent **tooth decay**. Foods that are crunchy should be avoided to minimize the risk of breaking the appliance. Hard fruits, vegetables, and breads must be cut into bite-sized pieces before eating. Foods that are sticky, including chewing gum, should be avoided because they may pull off the brackets or weaken the cement. Carbonated beverages may also weaken the cement, as well as contribute to tooth decay. Teeth should be brushed immediately after eating sweet foods. Special floss threaders are available to make flossing easier.

If overcrowding is creating malocclusion, one or more teeth may be extracted (surgically removed), giving the others room to move. If a tooth has not yet erupted or is prematurely lost, the orthodontist may insert an appliance called a space maintainer to keep the other teeth from moving out of their natural position. In severe cases of malocclusion, surgery may be necessary and the patient would be referred to yet another specialist, an oral or maxillofacial surgeon.

Once the teeth have been moved into their new position, the braces are removed and a retainer is worn until the teeth stabilize in that position. Retainers do not move teeth, they only hold them in place.

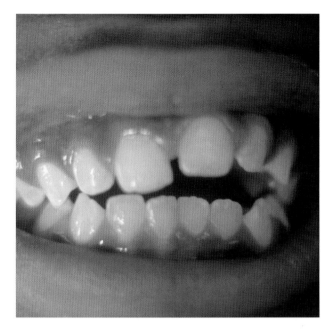

This patient's teeth are misarranged because of excessive thumb sucking. (Custom Medical Stock Photo. Reproduced by permission.)

Orthodontic treatment is the only effective treatment for malocclusion not requiring surgery. However, depending on the cause and severity of the condition, an orthodontist may be able to suggest other appliances as alternatives to braces.

Alternative treatment

There are some techniques of **craniosacral therapy** that can alter structure. This therapy may allow correction of some cases of malocclusion. If surgery is required, pre- and post-surgical care with homeopathic remedies, as well as vitamin and mineral supplements, can enhance recovery. Night guards are sometimes recommended to ease the strain on the jaw and to limit teeth grinding.

Prognosis

Depending on the cause and severity of the malocclusion and the appliance used in treatment, a patient may expect correction of the condition to take 2 or more years. Patients typically wear braces 18-24 months and a retainer for another year. Treatment is faster and more successful in children and teens whose teeth and bones are still developing. The length of treatment time is also affected by how well the patient follows orthodontic instructions.

Prevention

In general, malocclusion is not preventable. It may be minimized by controlling habits such as finger or thumb sucking. An initial consultation with an orthodontist before a child is 7 years old may lead to appropriate management of the growth and development of the child's dental and facial structures, circumventing many of the factors contributing to malocclusion.

Resources

ORGANIZATIONS

American Association of Oral and Maxillofacial Surgeons. 9700 West Bryn Mawr Ave., Rosemont, IL 60018-5701. (847) 678-6200. < http://www.aaoms.org >.

American Association of Orthodontists. 401 North Lindbergh Boulevard, St. Louis, MO 63141-7816. (314) 993-1700. < http://www.aaortho.org >.

Bethany Thivierge

MALT lymphoma

Definition

MALT lymphomas are solid tumors that originate from cancerous growth of immune cells that are recruited to secretory tissue such as the gastrointestinal tract, salivary glands, lungs, and the thyroid gland.

Description

The digestive tract is generally not associated with lymphoid tissue, with the exception of small collections of lymphocytes such as Peyer's patches. A specific kind of white blood cell, B-lymphocytes, can accumulate in response to infections of the digestive tract and other secretory tissues, or as a result of autoimmune conditions such as Sjgren's syndrome. When the growth of these lymphocytes is maintained through continued infection or autoimmune disease, a malignant cell can arise and replace the normal lymphocytes. These lymphomas, derived from mucosa-associated lymphoid tissue (MALT), most commonly arise in the stomach. Their growth seems to be dependent upon continuous stimulation of the immune system by an infectious agent, such as H. pylori, or some other entity, termed an antigen, that the body recognizes as foreign. This antigen-driven growth permits these tumors to be treated by eliminating the stimulus that generated the original, normal immune response. In the stomach they are associated, in greater than 90% of all cases, with the bacteria called Helicobacter pylori (H. pylori). This bacteria is also associated with peptic stomach irritation, ulcers, and gastric **cancer**. MALT lymphomas are generally indolent, that is, they grow slowly and cause little in the way of symptoms. Those MALT lymphomas that arise in the stomach in response to H. pylori infections are generally successfully treated with **antibiotics**, which eliminate the bacteria.

Demographics

MALT lymphomas occur at a frequency of about 1.5 per 100,000 people per year in the United States and account for about 10% of all non-Hodgkin's lymphomas. The frequency varies among different populations. For example, in parts of Italy the frequency of MALT lymphomas is as high as 13 per 100,000 people per year. This can in part be attributed to different rates of infection with H. pylori. However, other hereditary, dietary, or environmental factors are almost certainly involved.

Causes and symptoms

The majority of MALT lymphomas appear to be the result of infectious agents, most commonly H. pylori in the stomach. It is not known if infectious agents also cause MALT lymphomas outside of the stomach. In some cases, such as in the thyroid, MALT lymphomas seem to arise in patients who have autoimmune diseases, which make their immune systems treat their own tissue as foreign or antigenic. It is believed that there must be additional factors, in addition to infection or autoimmunity, that influence the development of MALT lymphomas. For example, in the United States, where infections with H. pylori are quite common, less than 1 in 30,000 people who have H. pylori in their stomachs develop MALT lymphomas. In addition, individuals who develop MALT lymphomas are more likely to develop other forms of cancer. This would suggest that there might be genetic factors predisposing individuals to develop MALT lymphomas or other tumors in response to environmental or infectious agents.

In general, patients have stomach **pain**, ulcers, or other localized symptoms, but rarely do they suffer from systemic complaints such as **fatigue** or **fever**.

Diagnosis

The indolent nature of most MALT lymphomas means that the majority of patients are diagnosed at early stages with relatively nonspecific symptoms. In the case of gastric MALT lymphomas, the physician will then have a gastroenterologist perform an endoscopy to examine the interior of the stomach. MALT lymphomas are then recognized as areas of inflammation or ulceration within the stomach. It is unusual for masses recognizable as tumors to be seen upon examination. Definitive diagnosis of MALT lymphoma requires a biopsy, in which a bit of tissue is removed from the stomach or other involved site. Examination of this tissue by a pathologist is the first step in distinguishing among the possible diagnoses of inflammation, indolent lymphoma, or a more aggressive form of cancer, such as gastric cancer or a rapidly growing non-Hodgkin's lymphoma. The pathologist evaluates the type of lymphoid cells that are present in the biopsy to establish the nature of the lesion. In addition, it is essential that the pathologist determine whether or not the lymphoma has grown beyond the borders of the mucosa, which lines the stomach or other gland.

Treatment

The best staging system to employ for MALT lymphomas is still the subject of discussion. However, it is standard practice that patients presenting with MALT lymphomas should be evaluated in a similar manner to individuals with nodal lymphomas, the more common type of lymphoma that originates at sites within the lymphoid system. These procedures include a complete history and physical, blood tests, chest x rays, and **bone marrow biopsy**. This evaluation will permit the oncologist to determine if the disease is localized or if it has spread to other sites within the body.

In general, the prognosis for patients with MALT lymphomas is good, with overall five-year survival rates that are greater than 80%. The features that are most closely related to the outlook for newly diagnosed individual patients are: whether the primary site is in the stomach or is extra-gastric; if the disease has spread beyond the initial location; and whether the histologic evaluation of the initial tumor biopsies is consistent with a low-grade, slowly growing lesion, as compared to a high-grade lesion that is more rapidly growing. In general, the histologic grade is the most important feature, with high-grade lesions requiring the most aggressive treatment.

Treatment of MALT lymphomas differs from that of most lymphomas. In the most common type of MALT lymphomas—low-grade lesions originating in the stomach—treatment with antibiotics to eliminate H. pylori leads to complete remissions in the majority of patients. The effectiveness of this treatment is indistinguishable from surgery, **chemotherapy**, **radiation therapy**, or a combination of surgery with drugs or irradiation. Approximately one-third of patients in this group have evidence of disseminated disease, where lymphoma cells are detected at sites in addition to the gastric mucosa. The response of these patients to antibiotic treatment is not significantly different from that for individuals with localized disease. For both groups a complete remission is achieved in about 75% of patients, who remain, on average, free of disease for about 5 years.

Prognosis

Patients with MALT lymphomas arising outside of the digestive tract also have good prognoses. Effective treatment for these lymphomas has been achieved with local radiation, chemotherapy, and/or interferon. Surgery followed by chemotherapy or radiation is also effective with nongastrointestinal MALT lymphomas. Overall these patients have five-year survival rates greater than 90%.

While the outlook for patients with MALT lymphomas is good, difficulties in diagnosis and staging have left the optimal treatment a matter of continued study. This is an especially open question for those patients who fail to respond to antibiotic therapy, or

> **KEY TERMS**
>
> **Antigen**—A foreign substance that leads to an immune response, including the production of antibodies by B cells.
>
> **Autoimmune disease**—A condition in which an individual's immune system reacts to their own tissues, viewing self components as if they were foreign antigens.
>
> **Bone marrow biopsy**—A procedure in which cellular material is removed from the pelvis or breastbone and examined under a microscope to look for the presence of abnormal blood cells characteristic of specific forms of leukemia and lymphoma.
>
> **Indolent lymphoma (also called low-grade)**—Cancerous growths of lymphoid tissue that progress slowly to more aggressive forms of cancer.
>
> **Lymphoid tissue**—Sites within the body that produce cells of the immune system, including lymph nodes, bone marrow, and the thymus.

whose disease recurs. It may be the case that in these patients, the MALT lymphoma may have already progressed to a point where high-grade lesions, not observed in the original biopsies, were resistant to the initial treatment. The best treatment for these patients remains to be established. IN general, these patients are treated with chemotherapy in a similar manner to patients with other types of lymphoma. Given the success of antibiotics, and the good prognosis for gastric MALT lymphomas in general, no sufficient body of evidence exists to determine the best chemotherapy for patients who fail to achieve a complete and lasting remission upon initial treatment. At present, a chemotherapeutic regime designated CHOP includes the anti-cancer drugs cyclophosphamide, doxorubicin, vincristine, and prednisone. Similar drug combinations are being used for patients whose MALT lymphomas do not respond to antibiotic treatment.

Clinical trials are underway and mostly concentrate upon optimizing treatment of gastric MALT lymphomas that involve H. pylori. The aspects of treatment being addressed are the most effective antibiotics and the use of **antacids** to modulate irritation in the stomach. These protocols have been designed to follow the natural history of gastric lymphomas and to establish the biological features that predict treatment response to antibiotics and duration of remission.

Prevention

There are currently no commonly accepted means to prevent MALT lymphomas. While the H. pylori infections are associated with this and other gastric disease, the eradication of H pylori in asymptomatic individuals is not currently recommended for prevention of MALT lymphomas or gastric cancer.

Resources

PERIODICALS

Thieblemont, C., et al. "Mucosa-associated Lymphoid Tissue Lymphoma is a Disseminated Disease in One-third of 158 Patients Analyzed." *Blood* 95 (February 2000): 802-6.

Zucca, E., et al. "The Gastric Marginal Zone Lymphoma of MALT Type." *Blood* 96 (July 2000): 410-19.

OTHER

"Low-Grade Non-Hodgkin's Lymphoma: A Year 2000 Perspective." *Medscape*. June 2000. < http://www.medscape.com/medscape/oncology/clinicalmgmt/CM.v03/public/index-CM.v03.html >.

Warren Maltzman, Ph.D.

Malta fever *see* **Brucellosis**

Mammogram screening *see* **Mammography**

Mammography

Definition

Mammography is the study of the breast using x ray. The actual test is called a mammogram. There are two types of mammograms. A screening mammogram is ordered for women who have no problems with their breasts. It consists of two x-ray views of each breast. A diagnostic mammogram is for evaluation of new abnormalities or of patients with a past abnormality requiring follow-up (i.e., a woman with **breast cancer** treated with **lumpectomy**). Additional x rays from other angles or special views of certain areas are taken.

Purpose

The purpose of screening mammography is breast **cancer** detection. A screening test, by definition, is used for patients without any signs or symptoms in order to detect disease as early as possible. Many studies have shown that having regular mammograms increases a woman's chances of finding breast cancer in an early stage, when it is more likely to be curable. It

has been estimated that a mammogram may find a cancer as much as two years before it can be felt. The American Cancer Society, American College of Radiology, American College of Surgeons and American Medical Association recommend annual mammograms for every woman beginning at age 40.

Screening mammograms usually are not recommended for women under age 40 who have no special risk factors and a normal physical breast examination. Below age 40, breasts tend to be "radiographically dense," which means it is difficult to see many details. In 2003, a new technique that introduces radiographic contrast into digital mammograms was proving useful at improving visibility of breast cancer in younger women. Screening mammograms can detect cancers in their earliest stages and greatly reduce mortality, particularly among women age 40 to 69. In fact, a study in 2003 found that women age 40 and older who had annual screening mammograms had better breast cancer prognoses because their cancers were diagnosed at earlier stages than women who had mammograms less often.

Some women are at increased risk for developing breast cancer, such as those with two or more relatives who have the disease. The 2003 American Cancer Society guidelines stated that women at increased risk might benefit from earlier screening mammograms and more frequent intervals for screening. However, the society suggested that evidence was not strong enough at that time to support making specific recommendations concerning screening examinations.

Diagnostic mammography is used to evaluate an existing problem, such as a lump, discharge from the nipple, or unusual tenderness in one area. The cause of the problem may be definitively diagnosed from this study, but further investigation using other methods often is necessary. This exam also is used to evaluate findings from screening mammography.

Description

A mammogram may be offered in a variety of settings. Hospitals, outpatient clinics, physicians' offices, or other facilities may have mammography equipment. In the United States, since October 1, 1994, only places certified by the U.S. Food and Drug Administration (FDA) are legally permitted to perform, interpret, or develop mammograms under the Mammography Quality Standards Act (MQSA).

In addition to the usual paperwork, a woman will be asked to fill out a form seeking information relevant to her risk of breast cancer and special

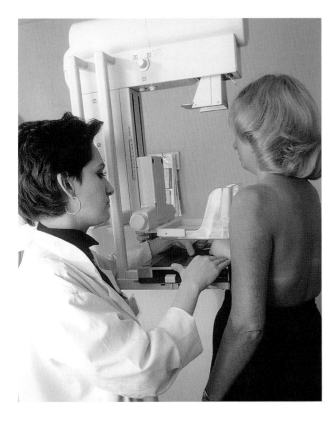

A person undergoing a mammography. *(Custom Medical Stoch Photo Inc. Reproduced by permission)*

mammography needs. The woman is asked about personal and family history of cancer, details about menstruation, child bearing, birth control, **breast implants**, other breast surgery, age, and **hormone replacement therapy**. Information about Breast Self Examination (BSE) and other breast health issues usually are available at no charge.

At some centers, a technologist may perform a **physical examination** of the breasts before the mammogram. Whether or not this is done, it is essential for the patient to tell the technologist about any lumps, nipple discharge, breast **pain**, or other concerns.

Clothing from the waist up is removed and a hospital gown or similar covering is put on. The woman stands facing the mammography machine. The technologist exposes one breast and places it on a plastic or metal film holder about the size of a placemat. The breast is compressed as flat as possible between the film holder and a rectangle of plastic (called a paddle), which presses down onto the breast from above. The compression should only last a few seconds, just enough to take the x ray. Good compression can be uncomfortable, but it is necessary to ensure the clearest view of all breast tissues.

Next, the woman is positioned with her side toward the mammography unit. The film holder is tilted so the outside of the breast rests against it, and a corner touches the armpit. The paddle again holds the breast firmly as the x ray is taken. This procedure is repeated for the other breast. A total of four x rays, two of each breast, are taken for a screening mammogram. Additional x rays, using special paddles, different breast positions, or other techniques are usually taken for a diagnostic mammogram.

The mammogram may be seen and interpreted by a radiologist right away, or it may not be reviewed until later. If there are any questionable areas or an abnormality, extra x rays may be recommended. These may be taken during the same appointment. More commonly, especially for screening mammograms, the woman is called back on another day for these additional films.

A screening mammogram usually takes approximately 15 to 30 minutes. A woman having a diagnostic mammogram can expect to spend up to an hour at the mammography facility.

The cost of mammography varies widely. Many mammography facilities accept "self referral." This means women can schedule themselves without a physician's referral. However, some insurance policies require a doctor's prescription to ensure payment. Medicare will pay for annual screening mammograms for all women with Medicare who are age 40 or older and a baseline mammogram for those age 35 to 39.

A digital mammogram is performed in the same way as a traditional exam, but the image is viewed on a computer monitor, stored as a digital file, and can be printed on film. Medicare now pays a small additional fee for digital mammography.

Preparation

The compression or squeezing of the breast for a mammogram is a concern for some women, but necessary to render a quality image. Even with concerns about pain, a 2003 study said that three-fourths of women reported the pain associated with a mammogram as four on a 10-point scale. Mammograms should be scheduled when a woman's breasts are least likely to be tender. One week after the menstrual period is usually best. The MQSA regulates equipment compression for consistency and performance.

Women should not put deodorant, powder, or lotion on their upper body on the day the mammogram is performed. Particles from these products can get on the breast or film holder and may look like abnormalities on the mammogram film.

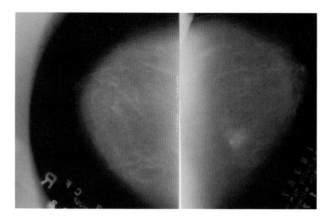

Comparison of two mammograms—cancerous tissue is shown on left and normal tissue on right. (Custom Medical Stock Photo. Reproduced by permission.)

Aftercare

No special aftercare is required.

Risks

The risk of radiation exposure from a mammogram is considered virtually nonexistent. Experts are unanimous that any negligible risk is far outweighed by the potential benefits of mammography.

Some breast cancers do not show up on mammograms, or "hide" in dense breast tissue. A normal (or negative) study is not a guarantee that a woman is cancer-free. Mammograms find about 85% to 90% of breast cancers.

"False positive" readings also are possible, and 5% to 10% of mammogram results indicate the need for additional testing, most of which confirm that no cancer is present.

Normal results

A mammography report describes details about the x ray appearance of the breasts. It also rates the mammogram according to standardized categories, as part of the Breast Imaging Reporting and Data System (BIRADS) created by the American College of Radiology (ACR). A normal mammogram may be rated as BIRADS 1 or negative, which means no abnormalities were seen. A normal mammogram may also be rated as BIRADS 2 or benign findings. This means that one or more abnormalities were found but are clearly benign (not cancerous), or variations of normal. Some kinds of calcification, lymph nodes, or implants in the breast might generate a BIRADS 2 rating. A BIRADS 0 rating indicates that

KEY TERMS

Breast biopsy—A procedure in which suspicious tissue is removed and examined by a pathologist for cancer or other disease. The breast tissue may be obtained by open surgery or through a needle.

Radiographically dense—Difficult to see details of breast tissue on x ray.

the mammogram is incomplete and requires further assessment.

Abnormal results

Many mammograms are considered borderline or indeterminate in their findings. BIRADS 3 means an abnormality is present and probably (but not definitely) benign. A follow-up mammogram within a short interval of six months is suggested. This helps to ensure that the abnormality is not changing, or is "stable." This stability in the abnormality indicates that a cancer is probably not present. If the abnormality is cancerous, it will likely grow and change in the time between mammograms. Some women are uncomfortable or anxious about waiting and may want to consult with their doctor about having a biopsy. BIRADS 4 means suspicious for cancer. A biopsy is usually recommended in this case. BIRADS 5 means an abnormality is highly suggestive of cancer. The suspicious area should be biopsied.

Often, screening mammograms are followed up with additional imaging. The reasons are numerous; they may mot mean the radiologist suspects a cancerous lesion, only that he or she cannot make a clear diagnosis from the screening mammogram views. The most common imaging methods are additional views on the mammogram, sometimes called magnification views, and ultrasound. In recent years, some patients have received **magnetic resonance imaging** (MRI) of the breast. A new technique called dual-energy contrast enhanced digital subtraction mammography is reported to find cancers that may be missed by conventional mammography. It may be ordered in the future as a follow-up study.

Resources

BOOKS

Henderson, Craig. *Mammography & Beyond. Developing Technologies for the Early Detection of Breast Cancer: A Non-technical Summary.* Washington, DC: National Academy Press, 2001.

Love, Susan M., with Karen Lindsey. *Dr. Susan Love's Breast Book*. 3rd ed. Boulder, CO: Perseus Book Group, 2000.

PERIODICALS

"Contrast Mammography Reveals Hard-to-find Cancers." *Cancer Weekly* October 14, 2003: 34.

"Mammography in Women Over Forty Catches Disease Earlier." *Women's Health Weekly* August 14, 2003: 14.

"New Digital Technique Improves Mammography Results." *Women's Health Weekly* September 18, 2003: 28.

Smith, Robert A., et al. "American Cancer Society Guidelines for Breast Cancer Screening: Update 2003." *Cancer* May-June 2003: 141-170.

"Stress—Not Pain— Is Major Barrier to Mammography." *Contemporary OB/GYN* July 2003: 17.

ORGANIZATIONS

American Cancer Society. 1599 Clifton Rd., Atlanta, GA 30329. (800) ACS-2345. < http://www.cancer.org >.

National Cancer Institute. Office of Cancer Communications, Bldg. 31, Room 10A31, Bethesda, MD 20892. NCI/Cancer Information Service: (800) 4-CANCER. < http://cancernet.nci.nih.gov >.

U.S. Food and Drug Administration. 5600 Fishers Lane, Rockville, MD 20857. (800) 532-4440. < http://www.fda.gov >.

Ellen S. Weber, MSN
Teresa G. Odle

Manganese excess *see* **Mineral toxicity**

Mania

Definition

Mania is an abnormally elated mental state, typically characterized by feelings of euphoria, lack of inhibitions, racing thoughts, diminished need for sleep, talkativeness, risk taking, and irritability. In extreme cases, mania can induce **hallucinations** and other psychotic symptoms.

Description

Mania typically occurs as a symptom of **bipolar disorder** (a mood disorder characterized by both manic and depressive episodes). Individuals experiencing a manic episode often have feelings of self-importance, elation, talkativeness, sociability, and a desire to embark on goal-oriented activities, coupled with the less desirable characteristics of irritability, impatience, impulsiveness, hyperactivity, and a decreased need for

sleep. (Note: Hypomania is a term applied to a condition resembling mania. It is characterized by persistent or elevated expansive mood, hyperactivity, inflated self esteem, etc., but of less intensity than mania.) Severe mania may have psychotic features.

Causes and symptoms

Mania can be induced by the use or **abuse** of stimulant drugs such as **cocaine** and amphetamines. It is also the predominant feature of bipolar disorder, or manic depression, an affective mental illness that causes radical emotional changes and mood swings.

The Diagnostic and Statistical Manual of Mental Disorders, Fourth Edition (*DSM-IV*), the diagnostic standard for mental health professionals in the U.S., describes a manic episode as an abnormally elevated mood lasting at least one week that is distinguished by at least three of the following symptoms: inflated self-esteem, decreased need for sleep, talkativeness, racing thoughts, distractibility, increase in goal-directed activity, or excessive involvement in pleasurable activities that have a high potential for painful consequences. If the mood of the patient is irritable and not elevated, four of these symptoms are required.

Diagnosis

Mania is usually diagnosed and treated by a psychiatrist and/or a psychologist in an outpatient setting. However, most severely manic patients require hospitalization. In addition to an interview, several clinical inventories or scales may be used to assess the patient's mental status and determine the presence and severity of mania. An assessment commonly includes the Young Mania Rating Scale (YMRS). The Mini-Mental State Examination (MMSE) may also be given to screen out other illnesses such as **dementia**.

Treatment

Mania is primarily treated with drugs. The following mood-stabilizing agents are commonly prescribed to regulate manic episodes:

• Lithium (Cibalith-S, Eskalith, Lithane) is one of the oldest and most frequently prescribed drugs available for the treatment of mania. Because the drug takes four to seven days to reach a therapeutic level in the bloodstream, it is sometimes prescribed in conjunction with neuroleptics (**antipsychotic drugs**) and/or **benzodiazepines** (tranquilizers) to provide more immediate relief of mania.

• Carbamazepine (Tegretol, Atretol) is an anticonvulsant drug usually prescribed in conjunction with other mood-stabilizing agents. The drug is often used to treat bipolar patients who have not responded well to lithium therapy. As of early 1998, carbamazepine was not approved for the treatment of mania by the FDA.

• Valproate (divalproex sodium, or Depakote; valproic acid, or Depakene) is an anticonvulsant drug prescribed alone or in combination with carbamazepine and/or lithium. For patients experiencing "mixed mania," or mania with features of depression, valproate is preferred over lithium.

Clozapine (Clozaril) is an atypical antipsychotic medication used to control manic episodes in patients who have not responded to typical mood-stabilizing agents. The drug has also been a useful preventative treatment in some bipolar patients. Other new anticonvulsants (lamotrigine, gubapentin) are being investigated for treatment of mania and bipolar disorder.

Prognosis

Patients experiencing mania as a result of bipolar disorder will require long-term care to prevent recurrence; bipolar disorder is a chronic condition that requires lifelong observation and treatment after diagnosis. Data show that almost 90% of patients who experience one manic episode will go on to have another.

Prevention

Mania as a result of bipolar disorder can only be prevented through ongoing pharmacologic treatment. Patient education in the form of therapy or self-help groups is crucial for training patients to recognize signs of mania and to take an active part in their treatment program. Psychotherapy is an important adjunctive treatment for patients with bipolar disorder.

Resources

ORGANIZATIONS

American Psychiatric Association. 1400 K Street NW, Washington, DC 20005. (888) 357-7924. < http://www.psych.org >.

National Alliance for the Mentally Ill (NAMI). Colonial Place Three, 2107 Wilson Blvd., Ste. 300, Arlington, VA 22201-3042. (800) 950-6264. < http://www.nami.org >.

National Depressive and Manic-Depressive Association (NDMDA). 730 N. Franklin St., Suite 501, Chicago, IL 60610. (800) 826-3632. < http://www.ndmda.org >.

National Institute of Mental Health. Mental Health Public Inquiries, 5600 Fishers Lane, Room 15C-05, Rockville, MD 20857. (888) 826-9438. < http://www.nimh.nih.gov >.

Paula Anne Ford-Martin

Manic depression *see* **Bipolar disorder**

Manic episode *see* **Mania**

MAO inhibitors *see* **Monoamine oxidase inhibitors**

Marasmus *see* **Protein-energy malnutrition**

Marble bones *see* **Osteopetroses**

Marburg virus infection *see* **Hemorrhagic fevers**

Marfan syndrome

Definition

Marfan syndrome is an inherited disorder of the connective tissue that causes abnormalities of the patient's eyes, cardiovascular system, and musculoskeletal system. It is named for the French pediatrician, Antoine Marfan (1858-1942), who first described it in 1896. Marfan syndrome is sometimes called arachnodactyly, which means "spider-like fingers" in Greek, since one of the characteristic signs of the disease is disproportionately long fingers and toes. It is estimated that one person in every 3000-5000 has Marfan syndrome, or about 50,000 people in the United States. Marfan syndrome is one of the more common inheritable disorders.

Description

Marfan syndrome affects three major organ systems of the body: the heart and circulatory system, the bones and muscles, and the eyes. The genetic mutation responsible for Marfan was discovered in 1991. It affects the body's production of fibrillin, which is a protein that is an important part of connective tissue. Fibrillin is the primary component of the microfibrils that allow tissues to stretch repeatedly without weakening. Because the patient's fibrillin is abnormal, his or her connective tissues are looser than usual, which weakens or damages the support structures of the entire body.

The most common external signs associated with Marfan syndrome include excessively long arms and legs, with the patient's arm span being greater than his or her height. The fingers and toes may be long and slender, with loose joints that can be bent beyond their normal limits. This unusual flexibility is called hypermobility. The patient's face may also be long and narrow, and he or she may have a noticeable curvature of the spine. It is important to note, however, that Marfan patients vary widely in the external signs of their disorder and in their severity; even two patients from the same family may look quite different. Most of the external features of Marfan syndrome become more pronounced as the patient gets older, so that diagnosis of the disorder is often easier in adults than in children. In many cases, the patient may have few or very minor outward signs of the disorder, and the diagnosis may be missed until the patient develops vision problems or cardiac symptoms.

Marfan syndrome by itself does not affect a person's intelligence or ability to learn. There is, however, some clinical evidence that children with Marfan have a slightly higher rate of hyperactivity and attention-deficit disorder (ADD) than the general population. In addition, a child with undiagnosed nearsightedness related to Marfan may have difficulty seeing the blackboard or reading printed materials, and thus do poorly in school.

Marfan syndrome affects males and females equally, and appears to be distributed equally among all races and ethnic groups. The rate of mutation of the fibrillin gene, however, appears to be related to the age of the patient's father; older fathers are more likely to have new mutations appear in chromosome 15.

Causes and symptoms

Marfan syndrome is caused by a single gene for fibrillin on chromosome 15, which is inherited in most cases from an affected parent. Between 15 and 25% of cases result from spontaneous mutations. Mutations of the fibrillin gene (FBNI) are unique to each family affected by Marfan, which makes rapid genetic diagnosis impossible, given present technology. The syndrome is an autosomal dominant disorder, which means that someone who has it has a 50% chance of passing it on to any offspring.

Another important genetic characteristic of Marfan syndrome is variable expression. This term means that the mutated fibrillin gene can produce a variety of symptoms of very different degrees of severity, even in members of the same family.

Cardiac and circulatory abnormalities

The most important complications of Marfan are those affecting the heart and major blood vessels; some are potentially life-threatening. About 90% of Marfan patients will develop cardiac complications.

- Aortic enlargement. This is the most serious potential complication of Marfan syndrome. Because of the abnormalities of the patient's fibrillin, the walls of the aorta (the large blood vessel that carries blood away from the heart) are weaker than normal and tend to stretch and bulge out of shape. This stretching increases the likelihood of an **aortic dissection**, which is a tear or separation between the layers of tissue that make up the aorta. An aortic dissection usually causes severe **pain** in the abdomen, back, or chest, depending on the section of the aorta that is affected. Rupture of the aorta is a medical emergency requiring immediate surgery and medication.

- Aortic regurgitation. A weakened and enlarged aorta may allow some blood to leak back into the heart during each heartbeat; this condition is called aortic regurgitation. Aortic regurgitation occasionally causes **shortness of breath** during normal activity. In serious cases, it causes the left ventricle of the heart to enlarge and may eventually lead to heart failure.

- **Mitral valve prolapse**. Between 75 and 85% of Marfan patients have loose or "floppy" mitral valves, which are the valves that separate the chambers of the heart. When these valves do not cover the opening between the chambers completely, the condition is called mitral valve prolapse. Complications of mitral valve prolapse include **heart murmurs** and **arrhythmias**. In rare cases, mitral valve prolapse can cause sudden death.

- Infective **endocarditis**. Infective endocarditis is an infection of the endothelium, the tissue that lines the heart. In patients with Marfan, it is the abnormal mitral valve that is most likely to become infected.

- Other complications. Some patients with Marfan develop cystic disease of the lungs or recurrent spontaneous **pneumothorax**, which is a condition in which air accumulates in the space around the lungs. Many will also eventually develop **emphysema**.

Musculoskeletal abnormalities

Marfan syndrome causes an increase in the length of the patient's bones, with decreased support from the ligaments that hold the bones together. As a result, the patient may develop various deformities of the skeleton or disorders related to the relative looseness of the ligaments.

Disorders of the spine

- **Scoliosis**. Scoliosis, or curvature of the spine, is a disorder in which the vertebrae that make up the spine twist out of line from side to side into an S-shape or a spiral. It is caused by a combination of the rapid growth of children with Marfan, and the looseness of the ligaments that help the spine to keep its shape.

- **Kyphosis** is an abnormal outward curvature of the spine at the back, sometimes called hunch back when it occurs in the upper back. Marfan patients may develop kyphosis either in the upper (thoracic) spine or the lower (lumbar) spine.

- Spondylolisthesis. Spondylolisthesis is the medical term for a forward slippage of one vertebra on the one below it. It produces an ache or stiffness in the lower back.

- Dural ectasia. The dura is the tough, fibrous outermost membrane covering the brain and the spinal cord. The weak dura in Marfan patients swells or bulges under the pressure of the spinal fluid. This swelling is called ectasia. In most cases, dural ectasia occurs in the lower spine, producing low back ache, a burning feeling, or **numbness** or weakness in the legs.

Disorders of the chest and lower body

- Pectus excavatum. Pectus excavatum is a malformation of the chest in which the patient's breastbone, or sternum, is sunken inward. It can cause difficulties in breathing, especially if the heart, spine, and lung have been affected by Marfan. It also usually causes concerns about appearance.

- Pectus carinatum. In other patients with Marfan the sternum is pushed outward and narrowed. Although pectus carinatum does not cause breathing difficulties, it can cause embarassment about appearance. A few patients with Marfan may have a pectus excavatum on one side of their chest and a pectus carinatum on the other.

- Foot disorders. Patients with Marfan are more likely to develop pes planus (flat feet) or so-called "claw" or "hammer" toes than people in the general population. They are also more likely to suffer from chronic pain in their feet.

- Protrusio acetabulae. The acetabulum is the socket of the hip joint. In patient's with Marfan, the acetabulum becomes deeper than normal during growth, for reasons that are not yet understood. Although protrusio acetabulae does not cause problems during childhood and adolescence, it can lead to a painful form of arthritis in adult life.

Disorders of the eyes and face

Although the visual problems that are related to Marfan syndrome are rarely life-threatening, they are important in that they may be the patient's first indication of the disorder. Eye disorders related to the syndrome include the following:

- Myopia (nearsightedness). Most patients with Marfan develop nearsightedness, usually in childhood.

- Ectopia lentis. Ectopia lentis is the medical term for dislocation of the lens of the eye. Between 65 and 75% of Marfan patients have dislocated lenses. This condition is an important indication for diagnosis of the syndrome because there are relatively few other disorders that produce it.

- **Glaucoma**. This condition is much more prevalent in patients with Marfan syndrome than in the general population.

- **Cataracts**. Patients with Marfan are more likely to develop cataracts, and to develop them much earlier in life, sometimes as early as 40 years of age.

- **Retinal detachment**. Patients with Marfan are more vulnerable to this disorder because of the weakness of their connective tissues. Untreated retinal detachment can cause blindness. The danger of retinal detachment is an important reason for patients to avoid contact sports or other activities that could cause a blow on the head or being knocked to the ground.

- Other facial problems. Patients with Marfan sometimes develop dental problems related to crowding of the teeth caused by a high-arched palate and a narrow jaw.

Other disorders

- Striae. Striae are stretch marks in the skin caused by rapid weight gain or growth; they frequently occur in pregnant women, for example. Marfan patients often develop striae over the shoulders, hips, and lower back at an early age because of rapid bone growth. Although the patient may be self-conscious about the striae, they are not a danger to health.

- Obstructive **sleep apnea**. Obstructive sleep apnea refers to partial obstruction of the airway during sleep, causing irregular breathing and sometimes **snoring**. In patients with Marfan, obstructive sleep apnea is caused by the unusual flexibility of the tissues lining the patient's airway. This disturbed breathing pattern increases the risk of aortic dissection.

Diagnosis

Presently, there is no objective diagnostic test for Marfan syndrome, in part because the disorder does not produce any measurable biochemical changes in the patient's blood or body fluids, or cellular changes that could be detected from a tissue sample. Although researchers in molecular biology are currently investigating the FBNI gene through a process called mutational analysis, it is presently not useful as a diagnostic test because there is evidence that there can be mutations in the fibrillin gene that do not produce Marfan. Similarly, there is no reliable prenatal test, although some physicians have used ultrasound to try to determine the length of fetal limbs in at-risk pregnancies.

The diagnosis is made by taking a family history and a thorough examination of the patient's eyes, heart, and bone structure. The examination should include an echocardiogram taken by a cardiologist, a slit-lamp **eye examination** by an ophthalmologist, and a work-up of the patient's spinal column by an orthopedic specialist. In terms of the cardiac examination, a standard electrocardiogram (EKG) is not sufficient for diagnosis; only the echocardiogram can detect possible enlargement of the aorta. The importance of the slit-lamp examination is that it allows the doctor to detect a dislocated lens, which is a significant indication of the syndrome.

The symptoms of Marfan syndrome in some patients resemble the symptoms of homocystinuria, which is an inherited disorder marked by extremely high levels of homocystine in the patient's blood and urine. This possibility can be excluded by a urine test.

In other cases, the diagnosis remains uncertain because of the mildness of the patient's symptoms, the absence of a family history of the syndrome, and other variables. These borderline conditions are sometimes referred to as marfanoid syndromes.

Treatment

The treatment and management of Marfan is tailored to the specific symptoms of each patient. Some patients find that the syndrome has little impact on their overall lifestyle; others have found their lives centered on the disorder.

Cardiovascular system

After a person has been diagnosed with Marfan, he or she should be monitored with an echocardiogram every six months until it is clear that the aorta is not growing larger. After that, the patient should have an echocardiogram once a year. If the echocardiogram does not allow the physician to visualize all portions of the aorta, CT (computed tomography) or MRI (**magnetic resonance imaging**) may be used. In cases involving a possible aortic dissection, the patient may be given a TEE (transesophageal echocardiogram).

Medications. A Marfan patient may be given drugs called beta-blockers to slow down the rate of aortic enlargement and decrease the risk of dissection by lowering the blood pressure and decreasing the forcefulness of the heartbeat. The most commonly used beta-blockers in Marfan patients are propranolol (Inderal) and atenolol (Tenormin). Patients who are allergic to beta-blockers may be given a calcium blocker such as verapamil.

Because Marfan patients are at increased risk for infective endocarditis, they must take a prophylactic dose of an antibiotic before having dental work or minor surgery, as these procedures may allow bacteria to enter the bloodstream. Penicillin and amoxicillin are the **antibiotics** most often used.

Surgical treatment. Surgery may be necessary if the width of the patient's aorta increases rapidly or reaches a critical size (about 2 inches). As of 2000, the most common surgical treatment involves replacing the patient's aortic valve and several inches of the aorta itself with a composite graft, which is a prosthetic heart valve sewn into one end of a Dacron tube. This surgery has been performed widely since about 1985; most patients who have had a composite graft have not needed additional surgery.

Patients who have had a valve replaced must take an anticoagulant medication, usually warfarin (Coumadin), in order to minimize the possibility of a clot forming on the prosthetic valve.

Musculoskeletal system

Children diagnosed with Marfan should be checked for scoliosis by their pediatricians at each annual **physical examination**. The doctor simply asks the child to bend forward while the back is examined for changes in the curvature. In addition, the child's spine should be x rayed in order to measure the extent of scoliosis or kyphosis. The curve is measured in degrees by the angle between the vertebrae as seen on the x ray. Curves of 20° or less are not likely to become worse. Curves between 20 and 40 degrees are likely to increase in children or adolescents. Curves of 40 degrees or more are highly likely to worsen, even in an adult, because the spine is so badly imbalanced that the force of gravity will increase the curvature.

Scoliosis between 20 and 40 degrees in children is usually treated with a back brace. The child must wear this appliance about 23 hours a day until growth is complete. If the spinal curvature increases to 40 or 50 degrees, the patient may require surgery in order to prevent lung problems, back pain, and further deformity. Surgical treatment of scoliosis involves straightening the spine with metal rods and fusing the vertebrae in the straightened position.

Spondylolisthesis is treated with a brace in mild cases. If the slippage is more than 30 degree, the slipped vertebra may require surgical realignment.

Dural ectasia can be distinguished from other causes of back pain on an MRI. Mild cases are usually not treated. Medication or spinal shunting to remove some of the spinal fluid are used to treat severe cases.

Pectus excavatum and pectus carinatum can be treated by surgery. In pectus excavatum, the deformed breastbone and ribs are raised and straightened by a metal bar. After four to six months, the bar is removed in an outpatient procedure.

Protrusio acetabulae may require surgery in adult life to provide the patient with an artificial hip joint, if the arthritic pains are severe.

Pain in the feet or limbs is usually treated with a mild analgesic such as **acetaminophen**. Patients with Marfan should consider wearing shoes with low heels, special cushions, or orthotic inserts. Foot surgery is rarely necessary.

Visual and dental concerns

Patients with Marfan should have a thorough eye examination, including a slit-lamp examination, to test for dislocation of the lens as well as nearsightedness. Dislocation can be treated by a combination of special glasses and daily use of one percent atropine sulfate ophthalmic drops, or by surgery.

Because patients with Marfan are at increased risk of glaucoma, they should have the fluid pressure inside the eye measured every year as part of an eye examination. Glaucoma can be treated with medications or with surgery.

Cataracts are treated with increasing success by implant surgery. It is important, however, to seek treatment at medical centers with eye surgeons familiar with the possible complications of **cataract surgery** in patients with Marfan syndrome.

All persons with Marfan should be taught to recognize the signs of retinal detachment (sudden blurring of vision in one eye becoming progressively worse without pain or redness) and to seek professional help immediately.

Children with Marfan should be evaluated by their dentist at each checkup for crowding of the teeth and possible misalignment, and referred to an orthodontist if necessary.

Athletic activities and occupational choice. People with Marfan should avoid sports or occupations that require heavy weight lifting, rough physical contact, or rapid changes in atmospheric pressure (e.g., scuba diving). Weight lifting increases blood pressure, which in turn may enlarge the aorta. Rough physical contact may cause retinal detachment. Sudden changes in air pressure may produce pneumothorax. Regular noncompetitive physical **exercise**, however, is beneficial for Marfan patients. Good choices include brisk walking, shooting baskets, and slow-paced tennis.

Social and lifestyle issues

Smoking. Smoking is particularly harmful for Marfan patients because it increases their risk of emphysema.

Pregnancy. Until very recently, women with Marfan were advised not to become pregnant because of the risk of aortic enlargement or dissection. The development of beta-blockers and echocardiograms, however, allows doctors now to monitor patients throughout pregnancy. It is recommended that patients have an echocardiogram during each of the three trimesters of pregnancy. Normal, vaginal delivery is not necessarily more stressful than a Caesarian section, but patients in prolonged labor may be given a Caesarian to reduce strain on the heart. A pregnant woman with Marfan should also receive **genetic counseling** regarding the 50% risk of having a child with the syndrome.

Appearance and Social Concerns. Children and adolescents with Marfan may benefit from supportive counseling regarding appearance, particularly if their symptoms are severe and causing them to withdraw from social activities. In addition, families may wish to seek counseling regarding the effects of the syndrome on relationships within the family. Many people respond with guilt, fear, or blame when a genetic disorder is diagnosed in the family, or they may overprotect the affected member. Support groups are often good sources of information about Marfan; they can

KEY TERMS

Arachnodactyly—A condition characterized by abnormally long and slender fingers and toes.

Ectopia lentis—Dislocation of the lens of the eye. It is one of the most important single indicators in diagnosing Marfan syndrome.

Fibrillin—A protein that is an important part of the structure of the body's connective tissue. In Marfan's syndrome, the gene responsible for fibrillin has mutated, causing the body to produce a defective protein.

Hypermobility—Unusual flexibility of the joints, allowing them to be bent or moved beyond their normal range of motion.

Kyphosis—An abnormal outward curvature of the spine, with a hump at the upper back.

Pectus carinatum—An abnormality of the chest in which the sternum (breastbone) is pushed outward. It is sometimes called "pigeon breast."

Pectus excavatum—An abnormality of the chest in which the sternum (breastbone) sinks inward; sometimes called "funnel chest."

Scoliosis—An abnormal, side-to-side curvature of the spine.

offer helpful suggestions about living with it as well as emotional support.

Prognosis

The prognosis for patient's with Marfan has improved markedly in recent years. As of 1995, the life expectancy of people with the syndrome has increased to 72 years, up from 48 years in 1972. This dramatic improvement is attributed to new surgical techniques, improved diagnosis, and new techniques of medical treatment.

The most important single factor in improving the patient's prognosis is early diagnosis. The earlier that a patient can benefit from the new techniques and lifestyle modifications, the more likely he or she is to have a longer life expectancy.

Resources

BOOKS

Beers, Mark H., and Robert Berkow, editors. *Pediatrics.* Whitehouse Station, NJ: Merck Research Laboratories, 1999.

Pyeritz, Reed E., and Cheryll Gasner. *The Marfan Syndrome.* New York: National Marfan Syndrome, 1999.

Rebecca J. Frey, PhD

Marie-Strümpell disease *see* **Ankylosing spondylitis**

Marijuana

Definition

Marijuana (marihuana) *Cannabis sativa L.*, also known as Indian hemp, is a member of the Cannabaceae or hemp family, thought to have originated in the mountainous districts of India, north of the Himalayan mountains.

Description

The herb was referred to as "hempe" in A.D. 1000 and listed in a dictionary under that English name. Supporters of the notorious Pancho Villa first used the name marijuana in 1895 in Sonora, Mexico. They called the mood-altering herb they smoked marijuana. The term hashish, is derived from the name for the Saracen soldiers, called *hashashins*, who ingested the highly potent cannabis resin before being sent out to assassinate enemies.

Two related species of cannabis are *C. ruderalis*, and *C. indica*, a variety known as Indian hemp. Indian hemp grows to a height of about 4 ft (1.2 m) and the seed coats have a marbled appearance.

The species *C. sativa L.* has many variations, depending on the soil, temperature, and light conditions, and the origin of the parent seed. These factors also affect the relative amounts of THC (tetra-hydro-cannabinol) and cannabidiol, the chemicals present in varying amounts in cannabis that determine if the plant is primarily a fiber type or an intoxicant. Generally the species grown at higher elevations and in hotter climates exudes more of the resin and is more medicinally potent.

Marijuana is a somewhat weedy plant and may grow as high as 18 ft (5.4 m). The hairy leaves are arranged opposite one another on the erect and branching stem. Leaves are palmate and compound, deeply divided into five to seven narrow, toothed and pointed leaflets. Male and female flowers are small and greenish in color and grow on separate plants.

Male flowers grow in the leaf axils in elongated clusters. The female flowers grow in spike-like clusters. The resinous blossoms have five sepals and five petals. The male and female blossoms can be distinguished at maturity. The male plant matures first, shedding its pollen and dying after flowering. Female plants die after dropping the mature seeds. Marijuana produces an abundance of quickly germinating seeds. This hardy annual is wind pollinated and has escaped from cultivation to grow wild along roadsides, trails, stream banks, and in wayside places throughout the world. The plant matures within three to five months after the seed has been sown.

History

Marijuana has been cultivated for thousands of years. Cannabis was first described for its therapeutic use in the first known Chinese pharmacopoeia, the *Pen Ts'ao.* (A pharmacopoeia is a book containing a list of medicinal drugs, and their descriptions of preparation and use.) Cannabis was called a "superior" herb by the Emperor Shen-Nung (2737-2697 B.C.), who is believed to have authored the work. Cannabis was recommended as a treatment for numerous common ailments. Around that same period in Egypt, cannabis was used as a treatment for sore eyes. The herb was used in India in cultural and religious ceremonies, and recorded in Sanskrit scriptural texts around 1,400 B.C. Cannabis was considered a holy herb and was characterized as the "soother of grief," "the sky flyer," and "the poor man's heaven." Centuries later, around 700 B.C., the Assyrian people used the herb they called *Qunnabu,* for incense. The ancient Greeks used cannabis as a remedy to treat inflammation, earache, and **edema** (swelling of a body part due to collection of fluids). Shortly after 500 B.C. the historian and geographer Herodotus recorded that the peoples known as Scythians used cannabis to produce fine linens. They called the herb *kannabis* and inhaled the "intoxicating vapor" that resulted when it was burned. By the year 100 B.C. the Chinese were using cannabis to make paper.

Cannabis use and cultivation migrated with the movement of various traders and travelers, and knowledge of the herb's value spread throughout the Middle East, Eastern Europe, and Africa. Around 100, Dioscorides, a surgeon in the Roman Legions under the Emperor Nero, named the herb *Cannabis sativa* and recorded numerous medicinal uses. In the second century, the Chinese physician Hoa-Tho, used cannabis in surgical procedures, relying on its analgesic properties. In ancient India, around 600, Sanskrit writers recorded a recipe for "pills of gaiety," a combination of hemp and sugar. By 1150, Moslems were using cannabis fiber in Europe's first paper production. This use of cannabis as a durable and renewable source of paper fiber continued for the next 750 years.

By the 1300s, government and religious authorities, concerned about the psychoactive effects on citizens consuming the herb, were placing harsh restrictions on its use. The Emir Soudon Sheikhouni of Joneima outlawed cannabis use among the poor. He destroyed the crops and ordered that offenders' teeth be pulled out. In 1484, Pope Innocent VIII outlawed the use of hashish, a concentrated form of cannabis. Cannabis cultivation continued, however, because of its economic value. A little more than a century later, the English Queen Elizabeth I issued a decree commanding that landowners holding sixty acres or more must grow hemp or pay a fine. Commerce in hemp, which was primarily valued for the strength and versatility of its fibers, was profitable and thriving. Hemp ropes and sails were crossing the sea to North America with the explorers. By 1621, the British were growing cannabis in Virginia where cultivation of hemp was mandatory. In 1776, the Declaration of Independence was drafted on hemp paper. Both President George Washington and President Thomas Jefferson were advocates of hemp as a valuable cash crop. Jefferson urged farmers to grow the crop in lieu of tobacco. By the 1850s, hemp had become the third largest agricultural crop grown in North America. The U. S. Census of that year recorded 8,327 hemp plantations, each with 2,000 or more acres in cultivation. But the invention of the cotton gin was already bringing many changes, and cotton was becoming a prime and profitable textile fiber. More change came with the introduction of the sulfite and chlorine processes used to turn trees into paper. Restrictions on the personal use of cannabis as a mood-altering, psychoactive herb, were soon to come.

Controversy

The 1856 edition of the *Encyclopedia Britannica*, in its lengthy entry on hemp, noted that the herb "produces inebriation and **delirium** of decidedly hilarious character, inducing violent laughter, jumping and dancing." This inebriating effect of marijuana use has fueled the controversy and led to restrictions that have surrounded marijuana use throughout history in many cultures and regions of the world. Cannabis use has been criminalized in some parts of the United States since 1915. Utah was the first state to criminalize it, then California and Texas. By 1923, Louisiana, Nevada, Oregon, and Washington had legal restrictions on the herb. New York prohibited cannabis use in 1927.

Despite the restrictions, cannabis use was woven into the cultural and social fabric in some communities, and widespread use persisted, particularly among the Mexican, Asian, and African American populations.

In 1937, the federal government passed the Marihuana Tax Act, prohibiting the cultivation and farming of marijuana. This bill was introduced to Congress by then Secretary of the Treasury Andrew Mellon, who was also a banker for the DuPont Corporation. That same year, the DuPont Chemical Company filed a patent for nylon, plastics, and a new bleaching process for paper. The 1937 Marijuana Transfer Tax Bill prohibited industrial and medical use of marijuana and classified the flowering tops as narcotic, and restrictions on the cultivation and use of cannabis continued. Marijuana was categorized as an illegal narcotic, in the company of **LSD** and heroin, **cocaine**, and morphine. Illegal use continued. The FBI publication, *Uniform Crime Reports for The United States, 1966* reported that 641,642 Americans were arrested for marijuana offenses that year, with as many as 85% of these arrests for simple possession, rather than cultivation or commerce.

In a reversal of the state-by-state progression of criminalizing marijuana that led to the 1937 Marijuana Transfer Tax Bill, there is a movement underway, state by state, to endorse the legalized use of medical marijuana. By 1992, 35 states in the U. S. had endorsed referenda for medical marijuana. A growing body of scientific research and many thousands of years of folk use support the importance of medical marijuana in treatment of a variety of illnesses, and the economic value of hemp in the textile, paper, and cordage industries has a long history.

The controversy and misinformation persists around this relatively safe and non-toxic herb. The World Health Organization, in a 1998 study, stated that the risks from cannabis use were unlikely to seriously compare to the public health risks of the legal drugs, alcohol and tobacco. And despite thousands of years of human consumption, not one **death** has been directly attributed to cannabis use. According to Lester Grinspoon, MD, and James B. Bakalar, JD, in a 1995 *Journal of the American Medical Association* article, "Marihuana is also far less addictive and far less subject to **abuse** than many drugs now used as **muscle relaxants**, hypnotics, and **analgesics**. The chief legitimate concern is the effect of **smoking** on the lungs. Cannabis smoke carries even more tars and other particulate matter than tobacco smoke. But the amount smoked is much less, especially in medical use, and once marihuana is an openly recognized medicine, solutions may be found."

Purpose

The whole cannabis plant, including buds, leaves, seeds, and root, have all been utilized throughout the long history of this controversial herb. Despite persistent legal restrictions and severe criminal penalties for illicit use, marijuana continues to be widely used in the United States, and throughout the world, both for its mood-altering properties and its proven medicinal applications. The conflicting opinions on the safety and effectiveness of cannabis in a climate of prohibition make any discussion of its beneficial uses politically charged. Marijuana has analgesic, antiemetic, anti-inflammatory, sedative, anticonvulsive, and laxative actions. Clinical studies have demonstrated its effectiveness in relieving **nausea and vomiting** following **chemotherapy** treatments for **cancer**. The herb has also been shown to reduce intra-ocular pressure in the eye by as much as 45%, a beneficial action in the treatment for **glaucoma**. Cannabis has proven anticonvulsive action, and may be helpful in treating epilepsy. Other research has documented an in-vitro tumor inhibiting effect of THC. Marijuana also increases appetite and reduces **nausea** and has been used with **AIDS** patients to counter weight loss and "wasting" that may result from the disease. Several chemical constituents of cannabis displayed antimicrobial action and antibacterial effects in research studies. The components CBC and d-9-tetrahydrocannabinol have been shown to destroy and inhibit the growth of streptococci and staphylococci bacteria.

Cannabis contains chemical compounds known as cannabinoids. Different cannabinoids seem to exert different effects on the body after ingestion. Scientific research indicates that these substances have potential therapeutic value for **pain** relief, control of nausea and **vomiting**, and appetite stimulation. The primary active agent identified to date is 9-tetrahydrocannabinol, known as THC. This chemical may constitute as much as 12% of the active chemicals in the herb, and is said to be responsible for as much as 70–100% of the euphoric action, or "high," experienced when ingesting the herb. The predominance of this mental lightness or "euphoria" depends on the balance of other active ingredients and the freshness of the herb. THC degrades into a component known as cannabinol, or CBN. This relatively inactive chemical predominates in marijuana that has been stored too long prior to use. Another chemical component, cannabidiol, known as CBD, has a sedative and mildly analgesic effect, and contributes to a somatic heaviness sometimes experienced by marijuana users.

Before prohibition, cannabis was recommended for treatment of **gonorrhea**, **angina** pectoris (constricting pain in the chest due to insufficient blood to the heart), and **choking** fits. It was also used for **insomnia**, **neuralgia**, rheumatism, gastrointestinal disorders, **cholera**, **tetanus**, epilepsy, strychnine **poisoning**, **bronchitis**, **whooping cough**, and **asthma**. Other phytotherapeutic (plant-based therapeutic) uses include treatment of ulcers, cancer, **emphysema**, migraine, Lou Gehrig's disease, HIV infection, and **multiple sclerosis**.

The United States federal government policy prohibits physicians from prescribing marijuana, even for seriously ill patients because of possible adverse effects, and the disputed belief that cannabis is dangerously addictive. U. S. Attorney General Janet Reno warned that physicians in any state who prescribed marijuana could lose the privilege of writing prescriptions, be excluded from Medicare and Medicaid reimbursement, and even be prosecuted for a federal crime, according to a 1997 editorial in the *New England Journal of Medicine*.

Preparations

Cannabis extracts, prepared for medicinal application, are prohibited in the United States. Marijuana is ingested by smoking, which quickly delivers the active ingredients to the blood system. The dried herb can also be prepared for eating in cookies or other baked goods. The essential oil consists of beta caryophyllenes, humules, caryophyllene oxide, alpha-pinenes, beta-pinenes, limonene, myrcene, and betaocimene. The oil expressed from the seeds is used for massage and in making salves used to relieve muscle strain.

Precautions

Marijauna is considered a Class I narcotic and its use has been restricted by federal law since 1937. Penalties include fines and imprisonment. The National Commission on Marihuana and Drug Abuse concluded in 1972 that "A careful search of the literature and testimony of the nation's health officials has not revealed a single human fatality in the United States proven to have resulted solely from ingestion of marihuana."

Research has shown that cannabis acts to increase heart frequency by as much as 40 beats per minute. A study reported by The American Heart Association in February 2000, concluded that smoking marijuana can precipitate a **heart attack** in persons with pre-existing heart conditions. One hour after smoking marijuana, the likelihood of having a heart attack is four and one-half times greater than if the person had not smoked, according to the research.

An additional health concern is the effect that marijuana smoking has on the lungs. Cannabis smoke carries more tars and other particulate matter than tobacco smoke.

Although marijuana is less likely than some other drugs to lead to dependence, heavy users may suffer a withdrawal syndrome characterized by **anxiety**, irritability, chills, and **muscle cramps** if they stop usage abruptly.

More seriously, marijuana has been linked to the onset or worsening of certain psychiatric conditions, including **panic disorder**, **schizophrenia**, and depersonalization disorder. Persons diagnosed with or at risk for these conditions should not use marijuana.

Side effects

The *PDR For Herbal Medicine* reports, "No health hazards or side effects are known in conjunction with the proper administration of designated therapeutic dosages." Smoking the herb, however, " . . . leads almost at once to euphoric states (pronounced gaiety, laughing fits)," according to the PDR, while "long term usage leads to a clear increase in tolerance for most of the pharmacological effects." The ability to safely operate automobiles and machinery can be impaired for up to eight hours after ingesting the herb. Chronic abuse results in "laryngitis, bronchitis, apathy, psychic decline and disturbances of genital functions," according to the PDR.

Some people may be hypersensitive to marijuana. They may be allergic or hypersensitive to the plant. Chronic sinus fungal infections have been linked to chronic marijuana smoking.

A team of German researchers reported in early 2004 that marijuana appears to speed up the progression of cancer. If this finding is replicated by other researchers, it would limit the usefulness of marijuana in treating pain and depression in cancer patients.

Interactions

Marijauna use may mask the perceived effects of alcohol and cocaine when the drugs are consumed together. Marijuana is said to exert a synergistic effect with other medicinal agents. When used with nitrous oxide it may enhance the effect.

Resources

BOOKS

Beers, Mark H., MD, and Robert Berkow, MD, editors. "Cannabis (Marijuana) Dependence." Section 15, Chapter 195. In *The Merck Manual of Diagnosis and Therapy.* Whitehouse Station, NJ: Merck Research Laboratories, 2004.

PERIODICALS

Amtmann, D., P. Weydt, K. L. Johnson, et al. "Survey of Cannabis Use in Patients with Amyotrophic Lateral Sclerosis." *American Journal of Hospice and Palliative Care* 21 (March-April 2004): 95–104.

Arsenault, L., M. Cannon, J. Witton, and R. M. Murray. "Causal Association between Cannabis and Psychosis: Examination of the Evidence." *British Journal of Psychiatry* 184 (February 2004): 110–117.

Dannon, P. N., K. Lowengrub, R. Amiaz, et al. "Comorbid Cannabis Use and Panic Disorder: Short Term and Long Term Follow-Up Study." *Human Psychopharmacology* 19 (March 2004): 97–101.

Haney, M., C. L. Hart, S. K. Vosburg, et al. "Marijuana Withdrawal in Humans: Effects of Oral THC or Divalproex." *Neuropsychopharmacology* 29 (January 2004): 158–170.

Hart, S., O. O. Fischer, and A. Ullrich. "Cannabinoids Induce Cancer Cell Proliferation Via Tumor Necrosis Factor Alpha-Converting Enzyme (TACE/ADAM17)-Mediated Transactivation of the Epidermal Growth Factor Receptor." *Cancer Research* 64 (March 15, 2004): 1943–1950.

Simeon, D. "Depersonalisation Disorder: A Contemporary Overview." *CNS Drugs* 18 (2004): 343–354.

OTHER

Campaign to Legalise Cannabis International Association. *Cannabis Campaigner's Guide, Up-to-Date Chronology of Cannabis Hemp.* < http://www.paston.co.uk/users/webbooks/chronol.html >.

Center for Cardiovascular Education, Inc. *Smoking Marijuana Increases Heart Attack Risk.* Heart Information Network. June 14, 2000. < http://www.heartinfo.org/news2000/marijuana061400.htm >.

Deerman, Dixie, RN. *The Best Herb You're Not Using That Could Add Years to Your Life!* North Carolina: Community of Compassion, 2000.

Goddard, Ian Williams. *Proven: Cannabis Is Safe Medicine.* < http://sers.erols.com/igoddard/hempsafe.htm >.

Lewin, Louis. *Phantastica, Hallucinating Substances, Indian Hemp: Cannabis Indica.* < http://users.lycaeum.org/~sputnik/Ludlow/Texts/phantastica.html >.

Taima in Japan. *Drug War Facts: Marijuana.* < http://taima.org/drugfacts/mj.htm >.

Clare Hanrahan
Rebecca J. Frey, PhD

Marriage counseling

Definition

Marriage counseling is a type of psychotherapy for a married couple or established partners that tries to resolve problems in the relationship. Typically, two people attend counseling sessions together to discuss specific issues.

Purpose

Marriage counseling is based on research that shows that individuals and their problems are best handled within the context of their relationships. Marriage counselors are trained in psychotherapy and family systems, and focus on understanding their clients' symptoms and the way their interactions contribute to problems in the relationship.

Description

Marriage counseling is usually a short-term therapy that may take only a few sessions to work out problems in the relationship. Typically, marriage counselors ask questions about the couple's roles, patterns, rules, goals, and beliefs. Therapy often begins as the couple analyzes the good and bad aspects of the relationship. The marriage counselor then works with the couple to help them understand that, in most cases, both partners are contributing to problems in the relationship. When this is understood, the two can then learn to change how they interact with each other to solve problems. The partners may be encouraged to draw up a contract in which each partner describes the behavior he or she will be trying to maintain.

Marriage is not a requirement for two people to get help from a marriage counselor. Anyone person wishing to improve his or her relationships can get help with behavioral problems, relationship issues, or with mental or emotional disorders. Marriage counselors also offer treatment for couples before they get married to help them understand potential problem areas. A third type of marriage counseling involves postmarital therapy, in which divorcing couples who share children seek help in working out their differences. Couples in the midst of a divorce find that marriage therapy during separation can help them find a common ground as they negotiate interpersonal issues and child custody.

Choosing a therapist

A marriage counselor is trained to use different types of therapy in work with individuals, couples, and groups. American Association of Marriage and Family Therapy (AAMFT) training includes supervision by experienced therapists, a minimum of a master's degree (including specific training in marriage and family therapy), and specific graduate training in marriage and **family therapy**.

When looking for a marriage counselor, a couple should find out the counselor's training and educational background, professional associations, such as AAMFT, and state licensure, and whether the person has experience in treating particular kinds of problem. Also, questions should be asked concerning fees, insurance coverage, the average length of therapy, and so on.

Normal results

Marriage counseling helps couples learn to deal more effectively with problems, and can help prevent small problems from becoming serious. Research shows that marriage counseling, when effective, tends to improve a person's physical as well as mental health, in addition to improving the relationship.

Resources

ORGANIZATIONS

American Association for Marriage and Family Therapy. 1133 15th St., NW Suite 300, Washington, DC 20005-2710. (202) 452-0109. <http://www.aamft.org>.

American Psychological Association (APA). 750 First St. NE, Washington, DC 20002-4242. (202) 336-5700. <http://www.apa.org>.

Carol A. Turkington

Marshall-Marchetti-Krantz procedure

Definition

The Marshall-Marchetti-Krantz procedure surgically reinforces the bladder neck in order to prevent unintentional urine loss.

Purpose

The Marshall-Marchetti-Krantz procedure is performed to correct **stress** incontinence in women, a common result of **childbirth** and/or **menopause**. Incontinence also occurs when an individual involuntarily loses urine after pressure is placed on the abdomen (like during **exercise**, sexual activity, sneezing, coughing, laughing, or hugging).

Precautions

In some women, stress incontinence may be controlled through nonsurgical means, such as:

- Kegel exercises (exercises that tighten pelvic muscles)
- Biofeedback (monitors temperature and muscle contractions in the vagina to help incontinent patients control their pelvic muscles)
- **Bladder training** (behavioral modification program used to treat stress incontinence)
- Medication
- Inserted incontinence devices.

Each patient should undergo a full diagnostic workup to determine the best course of treatment.

Description

The Marshall-Marchetti-Krantz procedure, also known as retropubic suspension or bladder neck suspension surgery, is performed by a surgeon in a hospital setting. The patient is placed under **general anesthesia**, and a long, thin, flexible tube (catheter) is inserted into the bladder through the narrow tube (urethra) that drains the body's urine. An incision is made across the abdomen, and the bladder is exposed. The bladder is separated from surrounding tissues. Stitches (sutures) are placed in these tissues near the bladder neck and urethra. The urethra is then lifted, and the sutures are attached to the pubic bone itself, or to tissue (fascia) behind the pubic bone. The sutures support the bladder neck, helping the patient gain control over urine flow.

Preparation

A complete evaluation to determine the cause of incontinence is critical to proper treatment. A thorough medical history and general **physical examination** should be performed on candidates for the Marshall-Marchetti-Krantz procedure. Diagnostic testing may include x rays, ultrasound, urine tests, and examination of the pelvis. It may also include a series of urodynamic testing exams that measure bladder pressure and capacity, and urinary flow.

Patients undergoing a Marshall-Marchetti-Krantz procedure must not eat or drink for eight hours prior to the surgery.

Aftercare

Recovery from a Marshall-Marchetti-Krantz procedure requires two to six days of hospitalization. The catheter will be removed from the patient's bladder once normal bladder function resumes. Patients are advised to refrain from heavy lifting for four to six weeks after the procedure.

Patients should contact their physician immediately if they experience **fever**, **dizziness**, or extreme **nausea**, or if their incision site becomes swollen, red, or hard.

Risks

The Marshall-Marchetti-Krantz procedure is an invasive surgical procedure and, as such, it carries risks of infection, internal bleeding, and hemorrhage. There is also a possibility of permanent damage to the bladder or urethra. The urethra may become scarred, causing a permanent narrowing, or stricture.

Normal results

Approximately 85% of women who undergo the Marshall-Marchetti-Krantz procedure are cured of their stress incontinence.

Resources

ORGANIZATIONS

American Foundation for Urologic Disease. 1128 North Charles St., Baltimore, MD 21201. (800) 242-2383. <http://www.afud.org>.

National Association for Continence. P.O. Box 8310, Spartanburg, SC 29305-8310. (800) 252-3337. <http://www.nafc.org>.

Paula Anne Ford-Martin

Massage therapy

Definition

Massage therapy is the scientific manipulation of the soft tissues of the body for the purpose of normalizing those tissues and consists of manual techniques that include applying fixed or movable pressure, holding, and/or causing movement of or to the body.

Purpose

Generally, massage is known to affect the circulation of blood and the flow of blood and lymph, reduce muscular tension or flaccidity, affect the nervous system through stimulation or **sedation**, and enhance tissue healing. These effects provide a number of benefits:

- reduction of muscle tension and stiffness
- relief of muscle spasms
- greater flexibility and range of motion
- increase of the ease and efficiency of movement
- relief of **stress** and aide of relaxation
- promotion of deeper and easier breathing
- improvement of the circulation of blood and movement of lymph

- relief of tension-related conditions, such as headaches and eyestrain
- promotion of faster healing of soft tissue injuries, such as pulled muscles and sprained ligaments, and reduction in **pain** and swelling related to such injuries
- reduction in the formation of excessive scar tissue following soft tissue injuries
- enhancement in the health and nourishment of skin
- improvement in posture through changing tension patterns that affect posture
- reduction in stress and an excellent stress management tool
- creation of a feeling of well-being
- reduction in levels of **anxiety**
- increase in awareness of the mind-body connection
- promotion of a relaxed state of mental awareness

Massage therapy also has a number of documented clinical benefits. For example, massage can reduce anxiety, improve pulmonary function in young **asthma** patients, reduce psycho-emotional distress in persons suffering from chronic inflammatory bowel disease, increase weight and improve motor development in premature infants, and may enhance immune system functioning. Some medical conditions that massage therapy can help are: **allergies**, anxiety and stress, arthritis, asthma and **bronchitis**, **carpal tunnel syndrome** and other repetitive motion injuries, chronic and temporary pain, circulatory problems, depression, digestive disorders, **tension headache**, **insomnia**, myofascial pain, **sports injuries**, and temporomandibular joint dysfunction.

Description

Origins

Massage therapy is one of the oldest health care practices known to history. References to massage are found in Chinese medical texts more than 4,000 years old. Massage has been advocated in Western health care practices at least since the time of Hippocrates, the "Father of Medicine." In the fourth century B.C. Hippocrates wrote, "The physician must be acquainted with many things and assuredly with rubbing" (the ancient Greek term for massage was rubbing).

The roots of modern, scientific massage therapy go back to Per Henrik Ling (1776–1839), a Swede, who developed an integrated system consisting of massage and active and passive exercises. Ling established the Royal Central Gymnastic Institute in Sweden in 1813 to teach his methods.

Modern, scientific massage therapy was introduced in the United States in the 1850s by two New York physicians, brothers George and Charles Taylor, who had studied in Sweden. The first clinics for massage therapy in the United States were opened by two Swedish physicians after the Civil War period. Doctor Baron Nils Posse operated the Posse Institute in Boston and Doctor Hartwig Nissen opened the Swedish Health Institute near the Capitol in Washington, D.C.

Although there were periods when massage fell out of favor, in the 1960s it made a comeback in a different way as a tool for relaxation, communication, and alternative healing. Today, massage is one of the most popular healing modalities. It is used by conventional, as well as alternative, medical communities and is now covered by some health insurance plans.

Massage therapy is the scientific manipulation of the soft tissues of the body for the purpose of normalizing those tissues and consists of a group of manual techniques that include applying fixed or movable pressure, holding, and/or causing movement of or to the body. While massage therapy is applied primarily with the hands, sometimes the forearms or elbows are used. These techniques affect the muscular, skeletal, circulatory, lymphatic, nervous, and other systems of the body. The basic philosophy of massage therapy embraces the concept of *vis Medicatrix naturae*, which is aiding the ability of the body to heal itself, and is aimed at achieving or increasing health and well-being.

Touch is the fundamental medium of massage therapy. While massage can be described in terms of the type of techniques performed, touch is not used solely in a mechanistic way in massage therapy. One could look at a diagram or photo of a massage technique that depicts where to place one's hands and what direction the **stroke** should go, but this would not convey everything that is important for giving a good massage. Massage also has an artistic component.

Because massage usually involves applying touch with some degree of pressure and movement, the massage therapist must use touch with sensitivity in order to determine the optimal amount of pressure to use for each person. For example, using too much pressure may cause the body to tense up, while using too little may not have enough effect. Touch used with sensitivity also allows the massage therapist to receive useful information via his or her hands about the client's body, such as locating areas of muscle tension and other soft tissue problems. Because touch is also a form of communication, sensitive touch can convey a sense of caring—an essential element in the therapeutic relationship—to the person receiving massage.

In practice, many massage therapists use more than one technique or method in their work and sometimes combine several. Effective massage therapists ascertain each person's needs and then use the techniques that will meet those needs best.

Swedish massage uses a system of long gliding strokes, kneading, and friction techniques on the more superficial layers of muscles, generally in the direction of blood flow toward the heart, and sometimes combined with active and passive movements of the joints. It is used to promote general relaxation, improve circulation and range of motion, and relieve muscle tension. Swedish massage is the most commonly used form of massage.

Deep tissue massage is used to release chronic patterns of muscular tension using slow strokes, direct pressure, or friction directed across the grain of the muscles. It is applied with greater pressure and to deeper layers of muscle than Swedish, which is why it is called deep tissue and is effective for chronic muscular tension.

Sports massage uses techniques that are similar to Swedish and deep tissue, but are specially adapted to deal with the effects of athletic performance on the body and the needs of athletes regarding training, performing, and recovery from injury.

Neuromuscular massage is a form of deep massage that is applied to individual muscles. It is used primarily to release trigger points (intense knots of muscle tension that refer pain to other parts of the body), and also to increase blood flow. It is often used to reduce pain. Trigger point massage and myotherapy are similar forms.

Acupressure applies finger or thumb pressure to specific points located on the **acupuncture** meridians (channels of energy flow identified in Asian concepts of anatomy) in order to release blocked energy along these meridians that causes physical discomforts, and re-balance the energy flow. **Shiatsu** is a Japanese form of acupressure.

The cost of massage therapy varies according to geographic location, experience of the massage therapist, and length of the massage. In the United States, the average range is from $35-60 for a one hour session. Massage therapy sessions at a client's home or office may cost more due to travel time for the massage therapist. Most sessions are one hour. Frequency of massage sessions can vary widely. If a person is receiving massage for a specific problem, frequency can vary widely based on the condition, though it usually will be once a week. Some people incorporate massage into their regular personal health and fitness program. They will go for massage on a regular basis, varying from once a week to once a month.

The first appointment generally begins with information gathering, such as the reason for getting massage therapy, physical condition and medical history, and other areas. The client is asked to remove clothing to one's level of comfort. Undressing takes place in private, and a sheet or towel is provided for draping. The massage therapist will undrape only the part of the body being massaged. The client's modesty is respected at all times. The massage therapist may use an oil or cream, which will be absorbed into the skin in a short time.

To receive the most benefit from a massage, generally the person being massaged should give the therapist accurate health information, report discomfort of any kind (whether it is from the massage itself or due to the room temperature or any other distractions), and be as receptive and open to the process as possible.

Insurance coverage for massage therapy varies widely. There tends to be greater coverage in states that license massage therapy. In most cases, a physician's prescription for massage therapy is needed. Once massage therapy is prescribed, authorization from the insurer may be needed if coverage is not clearly spelled out in one's policy or plan.

Preparations

Going for a massage requires little in the way of preparation. Generally, one should be clean and should not eat just before a massage. One should not be under the influence of alcohol or non-medicinal drugs. Massage therapists generally work by appointment and usually will provide information about how to prepare for an appointment at the time of making the appointment.

Precautions

Massage is comparatively safe; however it is generally contraindicated, i.e., it should not be used, if a person has one of the following conditions: advanced heart diseases, **hypertension** (high blood pressure), phlebitis, thrombosis, **embolism**, kidney failure, **cancer** if massage would accelerate metastasis (i.e., spread a tumor) or damage tissue that is fragile due to **chemotherapy** or other treatment, infectious diseases, contagious skin conditions, acute inflammation, infected injuries, unhealed **fractures**, **dislocations**, **frostbite**, large hernias, torn ligaments, conditions prone to hemorrhage, and **psychosis**.

Massage should not be used locally on affected areas (i.e., avoid using massage on the specific areas of the body that are affected by the condition) for the following conditions: **rheumatoid arthritis** flare up, eczema, **goiter**, and open **skin lesions**. Massage may be used on the areas of the body that are not affected by these conditions.

In some cases, precautions should be taken before using massage for the following conditions: **pregnancy**, high fevers, **osteoporosis**, diabetes, recent postoperative cases in which pain and muscular splinting (i.e., tightening as a protective reaction) would be increased, apprehension, and mental conditions that may impair communication or perception. In such cases, massage may or may not be appropriate. The decision on whether to use massage must be based on whether it may cause harm. For example, if someone has osteoporosis, the concern is whether bones are strong enough to withstand the pressure applied. If one has a health condition and has any hesitation about whether massage therapy would be appropriate, a physician should be consulted.

Side effects

Massage therapy does not have side effects. Sometimes people are concerned that massage may leave them too relaxed or too mentally unfocused. To the contrary, massage tends to leave people feeling more relaxed and alert.

Research and general acceptance

Before 1939, more than 600 research studies on massage appeared in the main journals of medicine in English. However, the pace of research was slowed by medicine's disinterest in massage therapy.

Massage therapy research picked up again in the 1980s, as the growing popularity of massage paralleled the growing interest in complementary and alternative medicine. Well designed studies have documented the benefits of massage therapy for the treatment of acute and chronic pain, acute and chronic inflammation, chronic **lymphedema**, **nausea**, muscle spasm, various soft tissue dysfunctions, anxiety, depression, insomnia, and psycho-emotional stress, which may aggravate mental illness.

Premature infants treated with daily massage therapy gain more weight and have shorter hospital stays than infants who are not massaged. A study of 40 low-birth-weight babies found that the 20 massaged babies had a 47% greater weight gain per day and stayed in the hospital an average of six days less than 20 infants who did not receive massage, resulting a cost savings of approximately $3,000 per infant. Cocaine-exposed, preterm infants given massage three times daily for a 10 day period showed significant improvement. Results indicated that massaged infants had fewer postnatal complications and exhibited fewer stress behaviors during the 10 day period, had a 28% greater daily weight gain, and demonstrated more mature motor behaviors.

A study comparing 52 hospitalized depressed and adjustment disorder children and adolescents with a control group that viewed relaxation videotapes, found massage therapy subjects were less depressed and anxious, and had lower saliva cortisol levels (an indicator of less depression).

Another study showed massage therapy produced relaxation in 18 elderly subjects, demonstrated in measures such as decreased blood pressure and heart rate and increased skin temperature.

A combination of massage techniques for 52 subjects with traumatically induced spinal pain led to significant improvements in acute and chronic pain and increased muscle flexibility and tone. This study also found massage therapy to be extremely cost effective, with cost savings ranging from 15-50%. Massage has also been shown to stimulate the body's ability to naturally control pain by stimulating the brain to produce endorphins. **Fibromyalgia** is an example of a condition that may be favorably affected by this effect.

A pilot study of five subjects with symptoms of tension and anxiety found a significant response to massage therapy in one or more psycho-physiological parameters of heart rate, frontalis and forearm extensor electromyograms (EMGs) and skin resistance, which demonstrate relaxation of muscle tension and reduced anxiety.

Lymph drainage massage has been shown to be more effective than mechanized methods or diuretic drugs to control **lymphedema** secondary to radical **mastectomy**, consequently using massage to control lymphedema would significantly lower treatment costs. A study found that massage therapy can have a powerful effect upon psycho-emotional distress in persons suffering from chronic inflammatory bowel disease. Massage therapy was effective in reducing the frequency of episodes of pain and disability in these patients.

Massage may enhance the immune system. A study suggests an increase in cytotoxic capacity associated with massage. A study of **chronic fatigue syndrome** subjects found that a group receiving massage therapy had lower depression, emotional distress, and somatic symptom scores, more hours of sleep, and lower epinephrine and cortisol levels than a control group.

Resources

ORGANIZATIONS

American Massage Therapy Association. 820 Davis Street, Suite 100, Evanston, IL. <http://www.amtamassage.org>.

Elliot Greene

Mastectomy

Definition

Mastectomy is the surgical removal of the breast for the treatment or prevention of **breast cancer**.

Purpose

Mastectomy is performed as a surgical treatment for breast **cancer**. The severity of a breast cancer is evaluated according to a complex system called staging. This takes into account the size of the tumor and whether it has spread to the lymph nodes, adjacent tissues, and/or distant parts of the body. A mastectomy usually is the recommended surgery for more advanced breast cancers. Women with earlier stage breast cancers, who might also have breast-conserving surgery (**lumpectomy**), may choose to have a mastectomy. In the United States, approximately 50,000 women a year undergo mastectomy.

The size, location, and type of tumor are important considerations when choosing the best surgery to treat breast cancer. The size of the breast also is an important factor. A woman's psychological concerns and lifestyle choices also should be considered when making a decision.

There are many factors that may make a mastectomy the treatment of choice for a patient. Large tumors are difficult to remove with good cosmetic results. This is especially true if the woman has small breasts. Sometimes multiple areas of cancer are found in one breast, making removal of the whole breast necessary. The surgeon sometimes is unable to remove the tumor with a sufficient amount, or margin, of normal tissue surrounding it. In this situation, the entire breast needs to be removed. Recurrence of breast cancer after a lumpectomy is another indication for mastectomy.

Radiation therapy is almost always recommended following a lumpectomy. If a woman is unable to have radiation, a mastectomy is the treatment of choice. Pregnant women cannot have radiation therapy for fear of harming the fetus. A woman with certain collagen vascular diseases, such as **systemic lupus erythematosus** or **scleroderma**, would experience unacceptable scarring and damage to her connective tissue from radiation exposure. Any woman who has had therapeutic radiation to the chest area for other reasons cannot tolerate additional exposure for breast cancer therapy.

The need for radiation therapy after breast conserving surgery may make mastectomy more appealing for nonmedical reasons. Some women fear radiation and choose the more extensive surgery so radiation treatment will not be required. The commitment of time, usually five days a week for six weeks, may not be acceptable for other women. This may be due to financial, personal, or job-related factors. In geographically isolated areas, a course of radiation therapy may require lengthy travel and perhaps unacceptable amounts of time away from family or other responsibilities.

Some women choose mastectomy because they strongly fear recurrence of the breast cancer, and lumpectomy seems too risky. Keeping a breast that has contained cancer may feel uncomfortable for some patients. They prefer mastectomy, so the entire breast will be removed. However, studies have shown that survival rates for women choosing mastectomy and those undergoing breast-conserving surgery have been the same.

The issue of prophylactic or preventive mastectomy, or removal of the breast to prevent future breast cancer, is controversial. Women with a strong family history of breast cancer and/or who test positive for a known cancer-causing gene may choose to have both breasts removed. Patients who have had certain types of breast cancers that are more likely to recur may elect to have the unaffected breast removed. Although there is some evidence that this procedure can decrease the chances of developing breast cancer, it is not a guarantee. It is not possible to guarantee that all breast tissue has been removed. There have been cases of breast cancers occurring after both breasts have been removed.

Studies have shown that women who choose preventive mastectomy generally are satisfied with their choice, but also believe they lacked enough information before deciding, particularly about the surgery, **genetic testing**, and **breast reconstruction**. A study

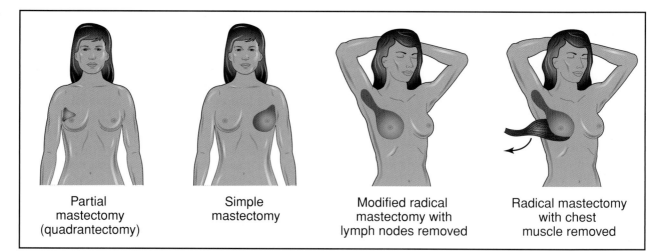

Partial
mastectomy
(quadrantectomy)

Simple
mastectomy

Modified radical
mastectomy with
lymph nodes removed

Radical mastectomy
with chest
muscle removed

There are four types of mastectomies: partial mastectomy, or lumpectomy, in which the tumor and surrounding tissue is removed; simple mastectomy, where the entire breast and some axillary lymph nodes are removed; modified radical mastectomy, in which the entire breast and all axillary lymph nodes are removed; and the radical mastectomy, where the entire breast, axillary lymph nodes, and chest muscles are removed. *(Illustration by Electronic Illustrators Group.)*

released in 2003 concerning women who underwent radical mastectomy of one breast and chose surgical removal of the other breast as a preventive measure found that 83% were highly satisfied with their decision.

Precautions

The decision to have mastectomy or lumpectomy should be carefully considered. It is important that the woman be fully informed of all the potential risks and benefits of each surgical treatment before making a choice.

Description

There are several types of mastectomies. The radical mastectomy, also called the Halsted mastectomy, is rarely performed today. It was developed in the late 1800s, when it was thought that more extensive surgery was most likely to cure cancer. A radical mastectomy involves removal of the breast, all surrounding lymph nodes up to the collarbone, and the underlying chest muscle. Women often were left disfigured and disabled, with a large defect in the chest wall requiring **skin grafting**, and significantly decreased arm sensation and motion. Unfortunately, and inaccurately, it still is the operation many women picture when the word mastectomy is mentioned.

Surgery that removes breast tissue, nipple, an ellipse of skin, and some axillary or underarm lymph nodes, but leaves the chest muscle intact, usually is

called a modified radical mastectomy. This is the most common type of mastectomy performed today. The surgery leaves a woman with a more normal chest shape than the older radical mastectomy procedure, and a scar that is not visible in most clothing. It also allows for immediate or delayed breast reconstruction.

In a simple mastectomy, only the breast tissue, nipple, and a small piece of overlying skin are removed. If a few of the axillary lymph nodes closest to the breast also are taken out, the surgery may be called an extended simple mastectomy.

There are other variations on the term mastectomy. A skin-sparing mastectomy uses special techniques that preserve the patient's breast skin for use in reconstruction, although the nipple still is removed. Total mastectomy is a confusing expression, as it may be used to refer to a modified radical mastectomy or a simple mastectomy. In 2003, surgeons reported on a new technique that spared the nipple in many women with early stage breast cancer.

Many women choose to have breast reconstruction performed in conjunction with the mastectomy. The reconstruction can be done using a woman's own abdominal tissue, or using saline-filled artificial expanders, which leave the breast relatively flat but partially reconstructed. Additionally, there are psychological benefits to coming out of the surgery with the first step to a reconstructed breast. Immediate reconstruction will add time and cost to the mastectomy procedure, but the patient can avoid the physical impact of a later surgery.

A mastectomy typically is performed in a hospital setting, but specialized outpatient facilities sometimes are used. The surgery is done under **general anesthesia**. The type and location of the incision may vary according to plans for reconstruction or other factors, such as old **scars**. As much breast tissue as possible is removed. Approximately 10 to 20 axillary lymph nodes usually are removed. All tissue is sent to the pathology laboratory for analysis. If no immediate reconstruction is planned, surgical drains are left in place to prevent fluid accumulation. The skin is sutured and bandages are applied.

The surgery may take from two to five hours. Patients usually stay at least one night in the hospital, although outpatient mastectomy is increasingly performed for about 10% of all patients. Insurance usually covers the cost of mastectomy. If immediate reconstruction is performed, the length of stay, recovery period, insurance reimbursement, and fees will vary. In 1998, the Women's Health and Cancer Rights Act required insurance plans to cover the cost of breast reconstruction in conjunction with a mastectomy procedure.

Preparation

Routine preoperative preparations, such as not eating or drinking the night before surgery, typically are ordered for a mastectomy. On rare occasions, the patient also may be asked to donate blood in case a blood **transfusion** is required during surgery. The patient should advise the surgeon of any medications she is taking. Information regarding expected outcomes and potential complications also should be part of preparation for a mastectomy, as for any surgical procedure. It is especially important that women know about sensations they might experience after surgery, so they are not misinterpreted as a sign of poor wound healing or recurrent cancer.

Aftercare

In the past, women often stayed in the hospital at least several days. Now many patients go home the same day or within a day or two after their mastectomies. Visits from home care nurses can sometimes be arranged, but patients need to learn how to care for themselves before discharge from the hospital. Patients may need to learn to change bandages and/or care for the incision. The surgical drains must be attended to properly; this includes emptying the drain, measuring fluid output, moving clots through the drain, and identifying problems that need attention from the doctor or nurse. If the drain becomes

blocked, fluid or blood may collect at the surgical site. Left untreated, this accumulation may cause infection and/or delayed wound healing.

After a mastectomy, activities such as driving may be restricted according to individual needs. **Pain** is usually well controlled with prescribed medication. Severe pain may be a sign of complications, and should be reported to the physician. A return visit to the surgeon is usually scheduled 7 to 10 days after the procedure.

Exercises to maintain shoulder and arm mobility may be prescribed as early as 24 hours after surgery. These are very important in restoring strength and promoting good circulation. However, intense **exercise** should be avoided for a time after surgery in order to prevent injury. The specific exercises suggested by the physician will change as healing progresses. Physical therapy is an integral part of care after a mastectomy, aiding in the overall recovery process.

Emotional care is another important aspect of recovery from a mastectomy. A mastectomy patient may feel a range of emotions including depression, negative self-image, grief, fear and **anxiety** about possible recurrence of the cancer, anger, or guilt. Patients are advised to seek counseling and/or support groups and to express their emotions to others, whether family, friends, or therapists. Assistance in dealing with the psychological effects of the breast cancer diagnosis, as well as the surgery, can be invaluable for women.

Measures to prevent injury or infection to the affected arm should be taken, especially if axillary lymph nodes were removed. There are a number of specific instructions directed toward avoiding pressure or constriction of the arm. Extra care must be exercised to avoid injury, to treat it properly if it occurs, and to seek medical attention promptly when appropriate.

Additional treatment for breast cancer may be necessary after a mastectomy. Depending on the type of tumor, lymph node status, and other factors, **chemotherapy**, radiation therapy, and/or hormone therapy may be prescribed.

Risks

Risks that are common to any surgical procedure include bleeding, infection, anesthesia reaction, or unexpected scarring. After mastectomy and axillary lymph node dissection, a number of complications are possible. A woman may experience decreased feeling in the back of her armpit or other sensations including **numbness**, **tingling**, or increased skin sensitivity. Some women report phantom breast symptoms, experiencing **itching**, aching, or other sensations in the breast that has been removed. There may be scarring around where the lymph nodes were removed, resulting in decreased arm mobility and requiring more intense physical therapy.

Approximately 10% to 20% of patients develop **lymphedema** after axillary lymph node removal. This swelling of the arm, caused by faulty lymph drainage, can range from mild to severe. It can be treated with elevation, elastic bandages, and specialized physical therapy. **Lymphedema** is a chronic condition that requires continuing treatment. This complication can arise at any time, even years after surgery. A new technique called sentinel lymph node mapping and biopsy often eliminates the need for removing some or all lymph nodes by testing the first lymph node for cancer.

Normal results

A mastectomy is performed as the definitive surgical treatment for breast cancer. The goal of the procedure is that the breast cancer is completely removed and does not recur.

Abnormal results

An abnormal result of a mastectomy is the incomplete removal of the breast cancer or a recurrence of the cancer. Other abnormal results include long-lasting (chronic) pain or impairment that does not improve after several months of physical therapy.

Resources

PERIODICALS

"American Women Still Having Too Many Mastectomies." *Women's Health Weekly* February 6, 2003: 10.

Frost, Marlene, et al. "Long-term Satisfaction and Psychological and Social Function Following Bilateral Prophylactic Mastectomy." *Journal of the American Medical Association* July 20, 2000: 319-24.

"Majority Satisfied with Prophylactic Mastectomy Decision." *AORN Journal* November 2003: 773.

"Studies Compare Mastectomy, Lumpectomy Survival Rates." *Clinican Reviews* January 2003: 24.

ORGANIZATIONS

American Cancer Society. 1599 Clifton Rd., NE, Atlanta, GA 30329-4251. (800) 227-2345. < http://www.cancer.org >.

National Lymphedema Network. 2211 Post St., Suite 404, San Francisco, CA 94115-3427. (800) 541-3259 or (415) 921-1306. < http://www.wenet.net/~lymphnet/ >.

Y-ME National Organization for Breast Cancer Information and Support. 18220 Harwood Ave., Homewood, IL 60430. 24-hour hotlines: (800) 221-2141 or (708) 799-8228.

OTHER

ibreast.org April 15, 2001. [cited June 12, 2001]. < http://www.breastcancer.org >.

Living Beyond Breast Cancer April 15, 2001. [cited June 12, 2001]. < http://www.lbbc.org >.

Ellen S. Weber, MSN
Teresa G. Odle

Mastitis

Definition

Mastitis is an infection of the breast. It usually only occurs in women who are breastfeeding their babies.

Description

Breastfeeding is the act of allowing a baby to suckle at the breast to drink the mother's milk. In the process, unaccustomed to the vigorous pull and tug of the infant's suck, the nipples may become sore, cracked, or irritated. This creates a tiny opening in the breast, through which bacteria can enter. The presence of milk, with high sugar content, gives the bacteria an excellent source of **nutrition**. Under these conditions, the bacteria are able to multiply, until they are plentiful enough to cause an infection within the breast.

Mastitis usually begins more than two to four weeks after delivery of the baby. It is a relatively uncommon complication of breastfeeding mothers, occurring in only approximately 3% to 5% of nursing women.

Causes and symptoms

The most common bacteria causing mastitis is called *Staphylococcus aureus*. In 25-30% of people, this bacteria is present on the skin lining normal, uninfected nostrils. It is probably this bacteria, clinging to the baby's nostrils, that is available to create infection when an opportunity (crack in the nipple) presents itself.

Usually, only one breast is involved. An area of the affected breast becomes swollen, red, hard, and painful. Other symptoms of mastitis include **fever**, chills, and increased heart rate.

Diagnosis

Diagnosis involves obtaining a sample of breast milk from the infected breast. The milk is cultured, allowing colonies of bacteria to grow. The causative bacteria then can be specially prepared for identification under a microscope. At the same time, tests can be performed to determine what type of antibiotic would be most effective against that particular bacteria. Sometimes, women and their physicians confuse mastitis with breast engorgement, or the tenderness and redness that appears when milk builds up in the breasts. Mastitis often can be distinguished if symptoms are accompanied by fever.

Treatment

A number of **antibiotics** are used to treat mastitis, including cephalexin, amoxicillin, azithromycin, dicloxacillin, and clindamycin. Breastfeeding usually should be continued, because the rate of **abscess** formation (an abscess is a persistent pocket of pus) in the infected breast goes up steeply among women who stop breastfeeding during a bout with mastitis. Most practitioners allow women to take **acetaminophen** while nursing, to relieve both fever and **pain**. As always, breastfeeding women need to make sure that any medication they take is also safe for the baby, since almost all drugs they take

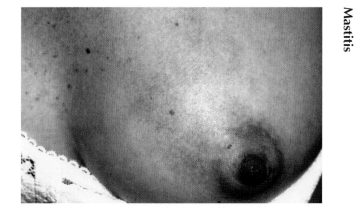

Mastitis is usually caused by a bacterial infection through a nipple damaged during breastfeeding. *(Photograph by Dr. P. Marazzi, Photo Researchers, Inc. Reproduced by permission.)*

appear in the breastmilk. Warm compresses applied to the affected breast can be soothing.

Prognosis

Prognosis for uncomplicated mastitis is excellent. About 10% of women with mastitis will end up with an abscess within the affected breast. An abscess is a collection of pus within the breast. This complication will require a surgical procedure to drain the pus.

Prevention

The most important aspect of prevention involves good handwashing to try to prevent the infant from acquiring the *Staphylococcus aureus* bacteria in the first place. Keeping the breast clean before breastfeeding also helps prevent infection. Keeping the breasts from becoming engorged may help prevent mastitis by preventing plugging of milk ducts.

Resources

PERIODICALS

Hager, W. David. "Managing Mastitis: Antibiotics Can Prove Invaluable in the Treatment of Mastitis, but Before You Prescribe Them, It's Important to Distinguish Breast Engorgement from Infectious Mastitis." *Contemporary OB/GYN* January 2004: 32–41.

ORGANIZATIONS

La Leche League International. 1400 N. Meacham Rd., Schaumburg, IL 60173-4048. (800) 525-3243. < http://www.lalecheleague.org >.

Rosalyn Carson-DeWitt, MD
Teresa G. Odle

Mastocytosis

Definition

Mastocytosis is a disease characterized by the presence of too many mast cells in various organs and tissues.

Description

The body has a variety of free-roaming cell populations that function as immunogenic agents. Most immunogenic cells fall into the category of white blood cells, but some remain in tissues and are not found in the blood. Mast cells are such a group.

Mast cells are found primarily in the skin and digestive system, including the liver and spleen, and produce histamine, a chemical most famous for its ability to cause **itching**. Histamine also causes acid **indigestion**, **diarrhea**, flushing, heart pounding, headaches, and can even cause the blood pressure to drop suddenly.

Mastocytosis comes in three forms. Most cases produce symptoms but do not shorten life expectancy. The three forms are:

- Mastocytoma, a benign skin tumor.
- Urticaria pigmentosa, small collections of mast cells in the skin that manifest as salmon or brown-colored patches.
- Systemic mastocytosis, the collection of mast cells in the skin, lymph nodes, liver, spleen, gastrointestinal tract, and bones.

Causes and symptoms

The cause of mastocytosis is unknown. People with systemic mastocytosis have bone and joint **pain**. Peptic ulcers are frequent because of the increased stomach acid stimulated by histamine. Many patients with systemic mastocytosis also develop urticaria pigmentosa. These **skin lesions** itch when stroked and may become fluid-filled.

Diagnosis

A biopsy of the skin patches aids diagnosis. An elevated level of histamine in the urine or blood is also indicative of mastocytosis.

Treatment

Mastocytoma usually occurs in childhood and clears-up on its own. Urticaria pigmentosa (present

---

KEY TERMS

Non-steroidal anti-inflammatory drugs (NSAIDs)—Aspirin, ibuprofen, naproxen, and many others.

Peptic ulcer—Ulcers in the stomach and upper duodenum (first portion of the small intestine) caused by stomach acid and a bacterium called *Helicobacter pylori*.

---

alone without systemic disease) also dramatically clears or improves as adolescence approaches.

Several medications are helpful in relieving symptoms of systemic mastocytosis. **Antihistamines** and drugs that reduce stomach acid are frequently needed. Headaches respond to migraine treatment. A medicine called cromolyn helps with the bowel symptoms. Several other standard and experimental medications have been used.

Prognosis

Mastocytoma and urticaria pigmentosa rarely if ever, develop into systemic mastocytosis, and both spontaneously improve over time. Systemic mastocytosis is only symptomatically treated. There is no known treatment that decreases the number of mast cells within tissue.

Resources

BOOKS

Austen, K. Frank. "Diseases of Immediate Type Hypersensitivity." In *Harrison's Principles of Internal Medicine*, edited by Anthony S. Fauci, et al. New York: McGraw-Hill, 1997.

J. Ricker Polsdorfer, MD

Mastoid tympanoplasty *see* **Mastoidectomy**

Mastoidectomy

Definition

Mastoidectomy is a surgical procedure to remove an infected portion of the bone behind the ear when

---

medical treatment is not effective. This surgery is rarely needed today because of the widespread use of **antibiotics**.

Purpose

Mastoidectomy is performed to remove infected air cells within the mastoid bone caused by **mastoiditis**, ear infection, or an inflammatory disease of the middle ear (cholesteatoma). The cells are open spaces containing air that are located throughout the mastoid bone. They are connected to a cavity in the upper part of the bone, which is in turn connected to the middle ear. As a result, infections in the middle ear can sometimes spread through the mastoid bone. When antibiotics cannot clear this infection, it may be necessary to remove the infected air cells by surgery. Mastoidectomies are also performed sometimes to repair paralyzed facial nerves.

Description

Mastoidectomy is performed less often today because of the widespread use of antibiotics to treat ear infections.

There are several different types of mastoidectomy:

- Simple (or closed). The operation is performed through the ear or through a cut (incision) behind the ear. The surgeon opens the mastoid bone and removes the infected air cells. The eardrum is cut (incised) to drain the middle ear. **Topical antibiotics** are then placed in the ear.

- Radical mastoidectomy. The eardrum and most middle ear structures are removed, but the innermost small bone (the stapes) is left behind so that a hearing aid can be used later to offset the **hearing loss**.

- Modified radical mastoidectomy. The eardrum and the middle ear structures are saved, which allows for better hearing than is possible after a radical operation.

The wound is then stitched up around a drainage tube, which is removed a day or two later. The procedure usually takes between two and three hours.

Preparation

The doctor will give the patient a thorough ear, nose, and throat examination as well as a detailed hearing test before surgery. Patients are given an injection before surgery to make them drowsy.

Aftercare

Painkillers are usually needed for the first day or two after the operation. The patient should drink fluids freely. After the stitches are removed, the bulky mastoid dressing can be replaced with a smaller dressing if the ear is still draining. The patient is given antibiotics for several days.

The patient should tell the doctor if any of the following symptoms occur:

- Bright red blood on the dressing.
- Stiff neck or disorientation. These may be signs of **meningitis**.
- Facial **paralysis**, drooping mouth, or problems swallowing.

Risks

Complications do not often occur, but they may include:

- Persistent ear drainage.
- Infections, including meningitis or brain abscesses.
- Hearing loss.
- Facial nerve injury. This is a rare complication.
- Temporary **dizziness**.
- Temporary loss of taste on the side of the tongue.

Resources

ORGANIZATIONS

American Academy of Otolaryngology-Head and Neck Surgery, Inc. One Prince St., Alexandria VA 22314-3357. (703) 836-4444. < http://www.entnet.org >.

American Hearing Research Foundation. 55 E. Washington St., Suite 2022, Chicago, IL 60602. (312) 726-9670. < http://www.american-hearing.org/ >.

Better Hearing Institute. 515 King Street, Suite 420, Alexandria, VA 22314. (703) 684-3391.

Carol A. Turkington

Mastoiditis

Definition

Mastoiditis is an infection of the spaces within the mastoid bone. It is almost always associated with **otitis media**, an infection of the middle ear. In the most serious cases, the bone itself becomes infected.

Description

The mastoid is a part of the side (temporal bone) of the skull. It can be felt as a bony bump just behind and slightly above the level of the earlobe. The mastoid has been described as resembling a "honeycomb" of tiny partitioned-off airspaces. The mastoid is connected with the middle ear, so that when there is a collection of fluid in the middle ear, there is usually also a slight collection of fluid within the airspaces of the mastoid.

Mastoiditis can range from a simple case of some fluid escaping into the mastoid air cells during a middle ear infection, to a more complex infection which penetrates through to the lining of the mastoid bone, to a very severe and destructive infection of the mastoid bone itself.

Causes and symptoms

Mastoiditis is caused by the same types of bacteria which cause middle ear infections (*Streptococcus pneumoniae* and *Haemophilus influenzae*), as well as by a variety of other bacteria (*Staphylococcus aureus*, *Pseuodomonas aeruginosa*, *Klebsiella*, **Escherichia coli**, *Proteus*, *Prevotella*, *Fusobacterium*, *Porphyromonas*, and *Bacteroides*). Mastoiditis may occur due to the progression of an untreated, or undertreated, middle ear infection.

Symptoms of mastoiditis may at first be the same as symptoms of an early middle ear infection. With progression, however, the swollen mastoid may push the outer ear slightly forward and away from the head. The area behind the ear will appear red and swollen, and will be very sore. There may be drainage of pus from the infected ear. In some cases, the skin over the

---

mastoid may develop an opening through which pus drains. **Fever** is common.

Diagnosis

Mastoiditis is usually suspected when a severe middle ear infection is accompanied by redness, swelling, and **pain** in the mastoid area. A computed tomography scan (CT scan) will show inflammation and fluid within the airspaces of the mastoid, as well as the erosion of the little walls of bone that should separate the air spaces. If there is any fluid draining from the ear or mastoid, this can be collected and processed in a laboratory to allow identification of the causative organism. If there is no fluid available, a tiny needle can be used to obtain a sample of the fluid which has accumulated behind the eardrum.

Treatment

Identification of the causative organism guides the practitioner's choice of antibiotic. Depending on the severity of the infection, the antibiotic can be given initially through a needle in the vein (intravenously or IV), and then (as the patient improves) by mouth.

In the case of a very severe infection of the mastoid bone itself, with a collection of pus (**abscess**), an operation to remove the mastoid part of the temporal bone is often necessary (**mastoidectomy**).

Prognosis

With early identification of mastoiditis, the prognosis is very good. When symptoms are not caught early enough, however, a number of complications can occur. These include an infection of the tissues covering the brain and spinal cord (**meningitis**), a pocket of infection within the brain (abscess), or an abscess within the muscles of the neck. All of these complications have potentially more serious prognoses.

Prevention

Prevention of mastoiditis involves careful and complete treatment of any middle ear infections.

Resources

ORGANIZATIONS

American Academy of Otolaryngology-Head and Neck Surgery, Inc. One Prince St., Alexandria VA 22314-3357. (703) 836-4444. <http://www.entnet.org>.

Rosalyn Carson-DeWitt, MD

Maternal serum alpha-fetoprotein test *see* **Alpha-fetoprotein test**

Maternal to fetal infections

Definition

Maternal to fetal infections are transmitted from the mother to her fetus, either across the placenta during fetal development (prenatal) or during labor and passage through the birth canal (perinatal).

Description

Antibodies in the maternal blood prevent most infections from being transmitted to the fetus. However some maternal-to-fetal infections, particularly in the first trimester of **pregnancy**, can cause **miscarriage** or severe **birth defects**. Other infections can cause preterm labor, fetal or neonatal **death**, or serious illness in newborns. Perinatal transmissions infect the fetus after its protective membranes rupture—the waters break—and during labor and delivery when the fetus is exposed to maternal blood. Perinatal transmission is more likely if the waters break prematurely.

Toxoplasmosis

Up to one-third of all people are infected with **toxoplasmosis**. The U.S. Centers for Disease Control and Prevention (CDC) estimate that 25–45% of women of childbearing age carry the parasite *Toxoplasma gondii* that causes toxoplasmosis. Very few infected people have symptoms and most pregnant women have antibodies that protect the fetus from infection. However in one-third of women who are infected for the first time during pregnancy, the parasite infects the placenta and enters the fetal circulation. Congenital (present at birth) infection occurs in one out of every 800–1,400 infants born to infected mothers. The fetal infection rate is above 60% if maternal infection occurs during the third trimester, but the most severe fetal complications occur with first-trimester infection.

Viral respiratory infections

Cytomegalovirus (CMV) is the most common infection that can be transmitted to a fetus. From 50–80% of childbearing-age women have been infected by CMV prior to pregnancy. However about 1–3% of women have their first or primary CMV infection during pregnancy and about one-third of these infections are transmitted to fetuses. Although most infants with congenital CMV have no problems, infection in early pregnancy can cause miscarriage or birth defects and CMV is a leading cause of congenital deafness. In later pregnancy CMV infection may cause preterm labor, **stillbirth**, or serious newborn illness. In the United States about 8,000 infants annually are born with potentially fatal CMV-related birth defects.

Fifth disease, caused by the parvovirus B19, is very common among children. About one-half of all adults are susceptible. About one-third of infants whose mothers contract fifth disease during pregnancy show signs of infection at birth. Although not usually dangerous, fifth disease contracted early in pregnancy can cause miscarriage or severe fetal anemia (low **blood count**) that can lead to congestive **heart failure**.

A fetus infected from its mother by *Varicella zoster* virus may develop pocks that can cause limb deformities early in development. If a woman contracts varicella (**chickenpox**) during the first 20 weeks of pregnancy, there is a 2% chance that her newborn will have varicella syndrome. However the greatest risk from varicella is if the mother contracts the virus just before delivery when she has not yet produced antibodies to protect the newborn.

In the past **rubella** was a common cause of birth defects. However routine vaccinations have made prenatal infection rare in the developed world. Rubella infection during the first 10 weeks of pregnancy may cause fetal death and more than 50% of newborns have severe birth defects. Infections contracted later in pregnancy do not cause congenital defects, although the newborn may become seriously ill and eventually develop **diabetes mellitus**.

Bacterial infections

Invasive group B streptococcal (GBS) disease is the most common cause of life-threatening infection in newborns. Up to 20% of pregnant women carry GBS in their vaginas during the last trimester, with the potential of infecting the fetus during birth. Although premature infants are more susceptible to GBS, 75% of infected infants are full-term. During the 1970s GBS emerged as the most common cause of newborn **sepsis**, or blood infection, and meningitis—infection of the fluid and lining surrounding the brain. GBS also is a frequent cause of newborn **pneumonia**. Maternal infection at conception or within the first two weeks of pregnancy may lead to hearing and vision loss and **mental retardation**. Between 1993 and 2002 congenital GBS infection in the United States decreased from 1.7 per 1,000 live births to 0.4 per 1,000 due to the use of **antibiotics** during delivery.

The food-borne bacterial infections listeriosis—caused by *Listeria monocytogenes*—and salmonellosis or food poisoning—caused by *Salmonella* bacteria—can be transmitted to a fetus. *Listeria monocytogenes* is ubiquitous in soil and groundwater, on plants, and in animals. Most human infections result from ingesting contaminated foods. Hormonal changes make pregnant women about 20 times more likely than other healthy adults to contract **listeriosis** and about one-third of all cases occur in pregnant women. Listeriosis can cause miscarriage, fetal or newborn death, premature delivery, or severe illness in the mother and infant.

Each year an estimated 8,000 pregnant women in the United States are infected with **syphilis** caused by the spirochete *Treponema pallidum*. Rising rates of syphilis among pregnant women are increasing the number of infants born with congenital syphilis. Congenital syphilis is a severe, disabling, and often life-threatening disease that can cause facial deformity, blindness, and deafness.

Every year in the United States an estimated 40,000 pregnant women are infected with gonorrhea—caused by *Neisseria gonorrhoeae*—and an estimated 200,000 are infected with chlamydia—caused by *Chlamydia trachomatis*. Chlamydia can cause premature membrane rupture and labor. Both infections can cause newborn conjunctivitis—a discharge of pus from the eyes.

Sexually transmitted viral infections

Each year an estimated 8,000 pregnant American women are infected with HIV, the human **immunodeficiency** virus that causes acquired immune deficiency syndrome (**AIDS**). About 20–25% of pregnant women with untreated HIV transmit it to their fetuses. In developed countries widespread HIV testing and antiretroviral therapy have reduced maternal-fetal transmission dramatically.

Genital herpes are caused by herpes simplex virus (HSV) type-2 and, less frequently, by HSV type-1 that usually causes cold sores. About 25% of American adults are infected with HSV-2, affecting one in 1,800–5,000 live births. There is little risk of fetal transmission if the mother is infected before the third trimester and has no genital sores at the time of delivery. However infection during the third trimester—when the virus is likely to be active and the mother has not yet made sufficient antibodies to protect her fetus—may lead to congenital HSV infection. This can seriously damage the newborn's eyes, central nervous system, and internal organs, lead to mental retardation and, rarely, death.

Genital or venereal **warts** are caused by some types of human papillomavirus (HPV). At least 20 million Americans are infected and about 5.5 million new cases are reported annually. **Genital warts** are highly infectious and tend to grow faster during pregnancy. If vaginal warts are very large they may interfere with the infant's passage through the birth canal, necessitating a **cesarean section** (C-section).

An estimated 8,000 pregnant women are infected with **hepatitis B** in the United States every year. They are at risk for premature delivery and, if untreated, newborns may develop chronic **liver disease**.

Causes and symptoms

Toxoplasmosis

The single-celled protozoan *Toxoplasma gondii* produces eggs in cat intestines. The eggs shed in cat feces and can survive for up to 18 months in the soil. Human infection occurs from handling contaminated soil or feces or by ingesting raw or undercooked meat from infected animals.

Although the symptoms of toxoplasmosis usually are very mild or absent, infection occurring early in fetal development can cause:

- premature birth and low birth weight—under 5 lb (2.3 kg)
- slow growth
- **fever**
- skin **rashes**
- easy bruising
- anemia
- a small or large head (microcephaly or macrocephaly)
- fluid in the cavities of the brain (hydrocephaly)

- inflammation of the brain, heart, or lungs
- severe or prolonged jaundice
- an enlarged liver and spleen
- an eye inflammation called choriorectinitis which can lead to blindness
- severe illness or death shortly after birth

Symptoms of congenital toxoplasmosis may appear months or years after birth and may include:

- seizures or other neurological problems
- visual impairment
- hearing loss
- mental retardation

Viral respiratory infections

Although most CMV-infected newborns have no symptoms, 10–15% may exhibit:

- low birth weight
- rashes
- small bruises
- jaundice
- enlarged liver and spleen
- hernias in the groin
- microcephaly or hydrocephaly
- respiratory problems
- brain damage

From 0.5–15% of CMV-infected infants develop hearing, vision, or neurological problems over several years. In addition to crossing the placenta, there is a 1% risk of perinatal CMV transmission.

Symptoms of congenital fifth disease include:

- bright red rash on the cheeks
- lacy, red rash on the neck, trunk, and legs
- joint pain
- fatigue
- malaise

Varicella syndrome in a newborn is characterized by:

- abnormally small limbs and head
- scarring of the skin
- eye defects
- mental retardation

In addition to various birth defects, newborns infected with rubella early in the pregnancy may have:

- low birth weight
- bruising
- bluish-red skin lesions
- enlarged lymph nodes
- enlarged liver and spleen
- brain inflammation
- pneumonia

Bacterial infections

Although most GBS carriers have no symptoms, GBS in pregnant women may cause:

- bladder or urinary tract infections
- infection of the womb
- stillbirth

Pregnant women are more likely to transmit GBS to their fetuses if they:

- previously delivered a GBS-infected baby
- have a urinary tract infection caused by GBS
- carry GBS late in pregnancy
- begin labor or membrane rupture before 37 weeks of gestation
- have membrane rupture 18 hours or more before delivery
- experience fever during labor

Symptoms of congenital GBS infection include:

- breathing difficulties
- shock
- sepsis
- pneumonia
- meningitis

Listeriosis may cause flu-like symptoms and the infection can be transmitted prenatally even if the mother has no symptoms.

Symptoms of salmonellosis can be severe in pregnant women and newborns and may include:

- **diarrhea**
- fever
- abdominal cramps
- rarely, meningitis

Syphilis can be transmitted to a fetus either prenatally or perinatally if the mother is infected during pregnancy or was inadequately treated for a past infection. In adults syphilis usually causes genital lesions 10–90 days after exposure, with a rash developing six weeks later. Symptoms may go unnoticed. Congenital syphilis can cause premature birth or stillbirth.

A surviving newborn with untreated congenital syphilis may have no initial symptoms but may gain little weight and, during the first month of life, develop:

- rash or small fluid-filled blisters on the palms and soles of the feet
- raised bumps around the nose, mouth, and diaper region
- cracks around the mouth
- nasal discharge of mucus, pus, or blood
- enlarged lymph nodes, liver, and spleen
- bone inflammation
- rarely, meningitis

Early-stage symptoms of congenital syphilis include:

- failure to thrive
- fever
- severe congenital pneumonia
- rash and lesions around the mouth, genitalia, and anus
- bone lesions
- nose cartilage infection or saddle nose (lacking a bridge)

Symptoms of late-stage congenital syphilis include:

- copper-colored rashes on the face, palms, and soles
- scarring around earlier lesions
- gray patches on the anus or outer vagina
- notched or peg-shaped teeth
- joint swelling
- bone pain
- abnormalities in the lower leg bones
- neurological conditions
- visual loss or blindness
- hearing loss or deafness

Both **gonorrhea** and chlamydia can be transmitted perinatally. **Conjunctivitis** caused by gonorrhea usually appears two to seven days after birth. Conjunctivitis caused by chlamydia usually appears 5–12 days after birth, although sometimes it takes six weeks to develop.

Symptoms of gonorrhea in women, if present, may include:

- bleeding during vaginal intercourse
- pain or burning with urination
- yellow or bloody vaginal discharge
- pelvic inflammatory disease

Sexually transmitted viral infections

HIV can be transmitted through the placenta, during labor and delivery, and through breast milk. HIV-infected infants do not have symptoms at birth, although about 15% develop serious symptoms or die within the first year. Almost one-half die by the age of 10.

Factors that may increase the risk of maternal HIV transmission include:

- the mother's viral load—the amount of HIV in her blood
- use of illicit drugs
- severe inflammation of the fetal membranes
- a prolonged period between membrane rupture and delivery

Most women carrying HSV never have recognizable symptoms; however a first episode of genital herpes during pregnancy can be passed to the fetus and may cause premature birth. Both HSV-1 and HSV-2 can be transmitted during birth if the mother has active genital sores, causing facial or genital herpes in the newborn.

Initial symptoms of congenital herpes usually appear within four weeks of birth and may be quite mild:

- blisters on the skin
- fever
- tiredness
- loss of appetite

More serious symptoms of congenital HSV infection include:

- a skin rash with small fluid-filled blisters
- chronic or recurring eye and skin infections
- cataracts
- widespread infection affecting many organs including the lungs and liver
- a life-threatening brain infection called herpes encephalitis

Nearly 50% of women infected with HPV have no symptoms although genital warts may appear weeks or months after infection. They can become larger during pregnancy causing difficulty with urination. Vaginal warts can reduce the elasticity of the vagina and cause obstruction during delivery. Symptoms of congenital HPV infection may include lung infection and obstructed air passages from warts inside the windpipe.

Although hepatitis B can be transmitted to the fetus through the placenta, most often it is transmitted perinatally. Since the virus is thought to pass through the umbilical cord, C-sections do not prevent transmission. Congenital hepatitis B can cause chronic liver infection, although symptoms usually do not become apparent until young adulthood.

Diagnosis

Diagnosis of maternal, fetal, or congenital infection can be difficult. An obstetrician may diagnose a maternal infection based on the woman's symptoms and blood tests. Sometimes a fetal infection can be diagnosed using ultrasound. Diagnosis of congenital infections in newborns may be based on a **physical examination**, symptoms, and blood or urine tests. Ultrasound scanning may be used to image the newborn's brain and **echocardiography** may be used to diagnose heart problems.

Toxoplasmosis

Prenatal tests for toxoplasmosis include:

- a blood test for maternal antibodies
- testing of the amniotic fluid and fetal blood
- fetal ultrasound

Postnatal diagnosis for congenital toxoplasmosis may include:

- antibody tests of the cord blood and cerebrospinal fluid
- an ophthalmologic examination
- neurological examinations
- a computed axial tomography (CT or CAT) scan

A 2005 study advised that all pregnant women and newborns have blood screenings for toxoplasmosis

Viral and bacterial infections

Diagnostic procedures include:

- blood tests for maternal antibodies against CMV or fifth disease

- ultrasound for fetal fifth disease
- bacterial cultures from blood, spinal fluid, skin, the vagina, or rectum for GBS
- a maternal blood test for listeriosis

Sexually transmitted infections (STIs)

The CDC recommends that all pregnant women be screened on their first prenatal visit for syphilis, gonorrhea, chlamydia, HIV, hepatitis B, and **hepatitis** C.

Infants are tested for syphilis at birth. Syphilis in an older infant may be diagnosed by a blood test, a lumbar puncture to look for signs of syphilis in the brain and central nervous system, an ophthalmologic examination, dark-field microscopy to visualize the spirochete, or **bone x rays**.

Maternal gonorrhea can be diagnosed by staining or culturing a cervical smear or testing for the bacterial DNA in a urine or cervical sample.

Women who were not screened for HIV during pregnancy may be screened during labor or delivery with a rapid test. The most common screening for HIV tests for antibodies in the blood; however most infants born to infected mothers test positive for 6–18 months because of the presence of maternal antibodies. An HIV blood test performed within 48 hours of birth detects only about 40% of infections, so testing is repeated at one and six months.

An HSV culture from an affected genital site— preferably on the first day of the outbreak—can test for herpes simplex. A blood test can show if a person has ever been infected with HSV and may distinguish between HSV-1 and HSV-2 and old or recently acquired infections. An examination or test can indicate whether a pregnant woman has active genital herpes near the time of delivery.

Genital warts are diagnosed visually. Vinegar may whiten infected areas to make them more visible. Cervical warts can be diagnosed by removing a piece of tissue for microscopic examination.

Treatment

Infants born with serious infections are treated in the neonatal care unit with intravenous drugs. Infants born to infected mothers may be treated with medications even if they show few or no signs of infection.

Toxoplasmosis

Maternal toxoplasmosis is treated with spiramycin during the first and early second trimesters of pregnancy. Fetal toxoplasmosis may be treated by giving the mother pyrimethamine and **sulfonamides** such as sulfadiazine during the later second and third trimesters.

Newborns with symptoms of toxoplasmosis are treated with pyrimethamine and sulfadiazine for one year; leucovorin for one year to protect the bone marrow from pyrimethamine toxicity; **corticosteroids** for heart, lung, or eye inflammations; clindamycin; and a corticosteroid to reduce the inflammation of chorioretinitis.

Viral respiratory infections

There is no effective treatment for CMV, although ganciclovir may be used to treat some symptoms.

Fetal anemia caused by fifth disease may resolve on its own. If the fetus is at risk for heart failure, a fetal blood **transfusion** may be performed. The mother also may receive medication that passes through the placenta to the fetus.

Exposure to chickenpox or rubella by a non-immune pregnant woman may be treated with an injection of immune globulin to help prevent fetal transmission. Congenital chickenpox is treated immediately to prevent serious complications or death. There is no specific treatment for rubella infection.

Bacterial infections

Pregnant women with GBS in their urine are treated with penicillin. Most GBS-carriers are treated with intravenous antibiotics—from membrane rupture through labor—to prevent fetal transmission. Infants born with congenital GBS infections are treated immediately with intravenous antibiotics.

Maternal and congenital listeriosis and syphilis are treated with antibiotics.

Maternal gonorrhea may be treated with cefixime, ceftriaxone, or levofloxacin. Since women often are infected with both gonorrhea and chlamydia, a combination of antibiotics such as ceftriaxone and doxycycline or azithromycin are used to treat both infections.

An antibiotic ointment such as silver nitrate is placed under the eyelids of all newborns as preventative treatment for gonorrhea. An infant born to a gonorrhea-infected mother is treated with penicillin. Conjunctivitis caused by gonorrhea is treated with an eye ointment containing polymyxin and bacitracin, erythromycin, or tetracycline. An antibiotic such as ceftriaxone is given intravenously. Congenital

chlamydia is treated with erythromycin eye ointment and oral tablets.

Viral STIs

Women who are being treated for HIV with combination drugs may stop treatment for the first trimester of pregnancy to avoid the risk of birth defects and to avoid missing doses due to **vomiting**, which can cause the growth of drug-resistant HIV strains. Although the side effects of the anti-retroviral drugs may worsen during pregnancy, stopping treatment can worsen a woman's condition.

Zidovudine (ZDV, AZT, Retrovir) is the only drug that has been proven to help prevent fetal HIV infection. HIV-positive pregnant women usually take ZDV from 14–34 weeks of gestation. During delivery the mother receives ZDV intravenously. The newborn is given liquid ZDV every six hours for six weeks. A 2004 study of HIV-positive Thai women found that oral ZDV beginning at 28 weeks of gestation, with a single dose of nevirapine during labor, greatly reduces HIV transmission.

Pneumonia caused by *Pneumocystis carinii* often is the first AIDS-related illness to appear in HIV-infected infants and is a major cause of death during the first year. The CDC recommends that all babies born to HIV-infected mothers be treated with anti-pneumonia drugs beginning at four–six weeks and continuing until the infant is found to be HIV-negative.

Although there is no cure for genital herpes, outbreaks just prior to delivery may be prevented by acyclovir (Zovirax), famciclovir (Famvir), or valacyclover (Valtrex). An HSV-infected newborn is treated immediately with intravenous **antiviral drugs** such as acyclovir. Eye infections are treated with trifluridine drops.

There is no cure for HPV and treatment during pregnancy often is ineffective, although it may include:

- Imiquimod cream
- 5% 5-fluorouracil cream
- trichloroacetic acid
- freezing or burning the warts with a laser
- surgical removal
- alpha interferon injected into the wart

HPV infection in newborns is treated by surgically removing the warts. If the warts obstruct breathing passages, frequent **laser surgery** is required. Interferon may be used to reduce the likelihood of recurrence.

Non-infected pregnant women may begin the hepatitis B vaccine series if they are at high-risk for infection. Infants born to mothers infected with hepatitis B are given both the first dose of hepatitis B vaccine and hepatitis B immune globulin within 12 hours of birth. The second and third doses of vaccine are given at one month and six months of age.

Prognosis

Maternal treatment with spiramycin for toxoplasmosis infection occurring within the first two weeks of pregnancy prevents transmission to the fetus. The prognosis for congenital toxoplasmosis depends on its severity.

With treatment most infants with congenital CMV survive, although almost all suffer from its effects.

A GBS-carrier's risk of delivering an infected child decreases from one in 200 to one in 4,000 if she is treated with antibiotics. GBS-infected mothers are less likely to infect their newborns if treated with antibiotics during labor. Although immediate penicillin treatment for GBS-infected newborns is very effective, about 5% of GBS-infected newborns die.

Many fetuses infected with syphilis early in gestation are stillborn. Nearly 50% of untreated fetuses die shortly before or after birth. However the fetus is at minimal risk if the mother receives adequate treatment with penicillin during pregnancy.

Pregnant women on combined antiretroviral therapy are at a 1–2% risk of transmitting HIV to the fetus. If the mother's viral load is under 1,000 and she is treated with ZDV, the risk of transmission is almost zero. Mothers with a high viral load may reduce the risk of transmission by having a C-section before labor begins and the membranes rupture. Congenital HIV infection that is treated with combination drugs, including **protease inhibitors**, may reduce the risk of death by 67%.

Women with an active HSV infection can reduce the risk of fetal transmission with a C-section. Although immediate medication for the newborn may prevent or reduce the damage from HSV, one-half of infants born with widespread HSV infections die and the other one-half may have brain damage.

Infants born to hepatitis B-infected mothers have a greater-than-95% chance of being protected against the virus if they receive the first dose of vaccine and immune globulin within 12 hours of birth.

Prevention

General advice for preventing infection during pregnancy includes:

- good hygiene—including frequent thorough hand washing and not sharing food or drinks—particularly for mothers who have or work with young children and may be at risk for CMV
- vaccinations several months before a planned pregnancy
- appropriate vaccinations after the first trimester of pregnancy
- contacting a healthcare provider immediately upon being exposed to a transmittable infection

To avoid *Taxoplasma* during pregnancy women should:

- keep cats indoors
- avoid handling cat litter without rubber gloves and wash thoroughly
- disinfect the cat box with boiling water for five minutes
- cover sandboxes
- wear gloves for gardening and wash afterwards
- avoid insects that may have been exposed to cat feces
- wash after handling cats, raw meat or poultry, soil, or sand
- avoid raw or undercooked meat and poultry, unwashed fruits and vegetables, raw eggs, and unpasteurized milk
- kill *Taxoplasma* by freezing food or cooking it thoroughly

All non-immune women of childbearing age should be vaccinated against rubella and chickenpox before pregnancy. Pregnant women should be tested for immunity to rubella at their first prenatal visit.

Women should be tested for GBS between 35 and 37 weeks of pregnancy to determine whether the bacteria are likely to be present at delivery.

Since *Listeria* can grow at temperatures below 40°F (4°C), pregnant women should handle food cautiously and avoid:

- hot dogs and luncheon and deli meats unless they are reheated to steaming
- soft cheeses
- refrigerated meat spreads
- refrigerated smoked seafood unless it is in a cooked dish
- raw unpasteurized milk

KEY TERMS

Antibody—A blood protein produced in response to a specific foreign substance including bacteria, viruses, and parasites; the antibody destroys the organism, providing protection against disease.

Cesarean section; C-section—Incision through the abdominal and uterine walls to deliver the fetus.

Conjunctivitis—An inflammation of the eye that can be caused by gonorrhea or chlamydia.

Cytomegalovirus; CMV—A common human herpes virus that is normally not harmful but may cause severe complications if transmitted to a fetus.

Fifth disease—Erythema infectiosum; a common respiratory infection among children caused by parvovirus B19 that usually is not serious but can cause fetal complications.

Group B streptococcal (GBS) disease—A common bacterial infection that is potentially life-threatening if transmitted to a fetus during early pregnancy or birth.

Herpes simplex virus; HSV—A very common sexually transmitted infection; Type-2 HSV causes genital herpes and type-1 HSV usually causes cold sores but also can cause genital herpes; congenital HSV can be transmitted to the fetus during birth if the mother has an active infection.

Human papillomavirus (HPV)—A large family of viruses, some of which cause genital warts; HPV can be transmitted to a fetus during birth.

Immune globulin—Serum containing antibodies against a specific infection.

Listeriosis—A food-borne bacterial infection caused by *Listeria monocytogenes* to which pregnant women are particularly susceptible.

Meningitis—An inflammation of the membranes covering the brain and spinal cord that can be caused by various congenital infections.

Perinatal infection—A maternal infection that is transmitted to the fetus after membrane rupture or during labor or delivery.

Placenta—The uterine organ that provides nourishment to the fetus.

Prenatal infection—A maternal infection that is transmitted to the fetus through the placenta.

Rubella—German measles; three-day measles; a viral infection that causes death or severe birth defects if transmitted to the fetus during the first 10 weeks of gestation.

Salmonellosis—Food poisoning; an infection by bacteria of the genus *Salmonella* that usually causes severe diarrhea and may be transmitted to the fetus.

Sepsis—A systemic or body-wide response to infection.

Sexually transmitted infection; STI—An infectious disease that is transmitted through sexual activity.

Ultrasound—High-frequency sound waves that are used to visualize parts of the body or a fetus in the womb.

Varicella—Chickenpox; a disease caused by the *Varicella zoster* virus—human herpes virus 3—that can cause severe birth defects if transmitted to the fetus during the first 20 weeks of pregnancy and newborn complications if it is transmitted perinatally.

Pregnant women should use precooked or ready-to-eat perishables immediately, clean the refrigerator regularly, and keep the refrigerator at or below 40°F (4°C).

Salmonellosis may be prevented by:

- cooking all meat, poultry, seafood, and eggs thoroughly

- avoiding sushi containing raw fish

- washing raw vegetables thoroughly

- avoiding unpasteurized milk, soft cheeses, and alfalfa sprouts

Prevention of STIs includes:

- abstaining from sexual contact outside of a mutually monogamous relationship

- using latex condoms correctly and consistently

- avoiding blood-contaminated needles, razors, or other items

Precautions for preventing fetal exposure to HIV-infected maternal blood include avoiding: **amniocentesis**, fetal scalp blood sampling, premature rupturing of the fetal membranes.

Prevention of maternal-to-fetal HSV transmission includes:

- abstaining from sexual activity during the last trimester of pregnancy or if there are signs of an outbreak or visible sores

- using a **condom** even if no symptoms are present

- postponing membrane rupture

- avoiding a fetal monitor that makes tiny punctures in the scalp
- avoiding vacuum or forceps deliveries which cause breaks in the infant's scalp

Resources

BOOKS

Creasy, Robert K., et al. *Maternal-Fetal Medicine: Principles and Practices.* 5th ed. London: W. B. Saunders, 2003.

MacLean, Allan, et al., editors. *Infection and Pregnancy.* London: Royal College of Obstetricians and Gynaecologists, 2001.

PERIODICALS

"Cytomegalovirus; Advances Made in Diagnosis of Maternal CMV Infection." *Women's Health Weekly* September 2, 2004: 51.

Lallemant, M., et al. "Single-dose Prenatal Nevirapine plus Standard Zidovudine to Prevent Mother-to-Child Transmission of HIV-1 in Thailand." *New England Journal of Medicine* 351, no. 3 (July 15, 2004): 217–28.

Montoya, J. G., and O. Liesenfeld. "Toxoplasmosis." *Lancet* 363, no. 9425 (June 12, 2004): 1965-76.

"Parasitology; Preventive Practices Eliminate the Risk for Congenital Toxoplasmosis." *Health & Medicine Week* May 3, 2004: 715.

ORGANIZATIONS

American College of Obstetricians and Gynecologists. 409 12th St. SW, PO Box 96920, Washington, DC 20080-6920. 202-863-2518. < http://www.acog.org >.

American Social Health Association. PO Box 13827, Research Triangle Park, NC 27709-3827. 800-783-9877. < http://www.ashastd.org >.

Association of Women's Health, Obstetric and Neonatal Nurses. 2000 L Street NW, Suite 740, Washington, DC 20036. 800-673-8499. 202-261-2400. < http://www.awhonn.org >.

Centers for Disease Control and Prevention. 1600 Clifton Road, Atlanta, GA 30333. 888-232-3228. < http://www.cdc.gov >.

Hepatitis B Foundation. 700 East Butler Avenue, Doylestown, PA 18901-3697. 215-489-4900. < http://www.hepb.org >.

March of Dimes Birth Defects Foundation. 1275 Mamaroneck Avenue, White Plains, NY 10605. < http://www.marchofdimes.com >.

OTHER

Barss, Vanessa A. *Patient Information: Avoiding Infections in Pregnancy.* UpToDate Patient Information. January 11, 2002 [cited March 15, 2005]. < http://patients.uptodate.com/ topic.asp?file = pregnan/2251 >.

Cytomegalovirus (CMV) Infection. National Center for Infectious Diseases, CDC. October 26, 2002 [cited February 21, 2005]. < http://www.cdc.gov/ncidod/ diseases/cmv.htm >.

"Genital Herpes." *Health Matters.* NIAID Fact Sheet. September 2003 [cited February 21, 2005]. < http://www.niaid.nih.gov/factsheets/ stdherp.htm >.

"Gonorrhea." *Health Matters.* NIAID Fact Sheet. October 2004 [cited February 21, 2005]. < http://www.niaid.nih.gov/factsheets/stdgon.htm >.

"Group B Streptococcal Disease (GBS)." *Disease Information.* Division of Bacterial and Mycotic Diseases, CDC. February 11, 2004 [cited February 21, 2005]. < http://www.cdc.gov/ncidod/dbmd/ diseaseinfo/groupbstrep_g.htm >.

Herpes Simplex and Pregnancy. International Herpes Alliance. [Cited February 21, 2005]. < http:// www.herpesalliance.org/resources—04.htm >.

"HIV and AIDS in Pregnancy." *Professionals & Researchers.* March of Dimes. November 2002 [cited February 22, 2005]. < http://www.marchofdimes.com/professionals/ 681_1223.asp >.

"HIV and Pregnancy." *AIDSinfo.* Health Information for Patients, U.S. Department of Health and Human Services. October 2004 [cited February 22, 2005]. < http://aidsinfo.nih.gov/other/cbrochure/English/ 11_en.html >.

"Human Papillomavirus and Genital Warts." *Health Matters.* NIAID Fact Sheet. July 2004 [cited February 21, 2005]. < http://www.niaid.nih.gov/factsheets/ stdhpv.htm >.

Listeriosis and Pregnancy: What is Your Risk? Food Safety and Inspection Service, U.S. Department of Agriculture. September 2001 [cited March 16, 2005]. < http://www.fsis.usda.gov/OA/pubs/ lm_tearsheet.htm >.

"Mother-To-Infant Transmission." *Science.* HIV Prevention Site, Division of AIDS, NIAID. May 21, 2002 [cited February 22, 2005]. < http://www.niaid. nih.gov/daids/prevention/infant.htm >.

Pregnancy and HIV. AIDS InfoNet. May 2, 2004 [cited March 16, 2005]. < http://www.aidsinfonet.org/en/doc/ 611.doc >.

Pregnant Women and Hepatitis B. Hepatitis B Foundation. [Cited February 22, 2005]. < http://www.hepb.org/02-0068.hepb >.

"STDs & Pregnancy." *STD Prevention.* National Center for HIV, SID and TB Prevention, CDC. [Cited February 22, 2005]. < http://www.cdc.gov/STDFact-STDs&Pregnancy.htm >.

Margaret Alic, Ph.D.

Mathematics disorder *see* **Learning disorders**

Maxillofacial trauma

Definition

Maxillofacial trauma refers to any injury to the face or jaw caused by physical force, **foreign objects**, or **burns**.

Description

Maxillofacial trauma includes injuries to any of the bony or fleshy structures of the face.

Any part of the face may be affected. Teeth may be knocked out or loosened. The eyes and their muscles, nerves, and blood vessels may be injured as well as the eye socket (orbit), which can be fractured by a forceful blow. The lower jaw (mandible) may be dislocated by force. Although anchored by strong muscles for chewing, the jaw is unstable in comparison with other bones and is easily dislocated from the temporomandibular joints that attach it to the skull. A fractured nose or jaw may affect the ability to breathe or eat. Any maxillofacial trauma may also prevent the passage of air or be severe enough to cause a **concussion** or more serious brain injury.

Athletes are particularly at risk of maxillofacial injuries. Boxers suffer repeated blows to the face and occasional knockouts (traumatic brain injury). Football, basketball, hockey, and soccer players, and many other athletes are at risk for milder forms of brain injury called concussions. There are an estimated 300,000 cases every year. Overall, there are one million new traumatic brain injuries every year, causing 50,000 deaths. Of the rest, 7–9% are left with long-term disability.

Burns to the face are also categorized as maxillofacial trauma.

Causes and symptoms

There are no reliable statistics on the incidence of maxillofacial trauma because there are so many types and many are not reported. Automobile accidents are a major cause, as well as participation in sports, fights, and other violent acts, and being hit by an object accidentally, for instance being hit by a baseball while watching a game. People most at risk are athletes, anyone who drives a vehicle or rides in one, and those who do dangerous work or engage in aggressive types of behavior.

One study reported in August 2000 that 42% of all facial **fractures** resulted from sports activity.

The major symptoms of most facial injuries are **pain**, swelling, bleeding, and bruising, although a fractured jaw also prevents the person from working his jaw properly, and symptoms of a fractured nose also include black eyes and possible blockage of the airway due to swelling and bleeding.

Symptoms of eye injury or orbital fracture can include blurred or double vision, decreased mobility of the eye, and **numbness** in the area of the eye. In severe injuries there can be temporary or permanent loss of vision.

Burn symptoms are pain, redness, and possibly blisters, **fever**, and **headache**. Extensive burns can cause the victim to go into **shock**. In that situation, he will have low blood pressure and a rapid pulse.

Symptoms of traumatic brain injury include problems with thinking, memory, and judgement as well as mood swings, and difficulty with coordination and balance. These symptoms linger for weeks or months, and in severe cases can be permanent. Double vision for months after the injury is not uncommon.

Diagnosis

Trauma is usually diagnosed in an emergency room or physician's office by **physical examination** and/or x ray. Some injuries require diagnosis by a specialist. A detailed report of how the injury occurred is also taken. In some cases, diagnosis cannot be made until swelling subsides.

Treatment

Treatment varies, depending on the type and extent of the injury.

Dislocation of the jaw can be treated by a primary care physician by exerting pressure in the proper manner. If muscle spasm prevents the jaw from moving back into alignment, a sedative is administered intravenously (IV) to relax the muscles. Afterward, the patient must avoid opening the jaw wide as he will be prone to repeat **dislocations**.

A jaw fracture may be minor enough to heal with simple limitation of movement and time. More serious fractures require complicated, multi-step treatment. The jaw must be surgically immobilized by a qualified oral or maxillofacial surgeon or an otolaryngologist. The jaw is properly aligned and secured with metal pins and wires. Proper alignment is necessary to ensure that the bite is correct. If the bite is off, the patient may develop a painful disorder called temporomandibular joint syndrome.

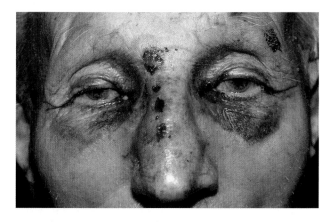

Face of an elderly woman suffering from maxillofacial trauma. *(Photo Researchers. Reproduced by permission.)*

During the weeks of healing the patient is limited to a liquid diet sipped through a straw and must be careful not to choke or vomit since he cannot open his mouth to expel the vomitus. The surgeon will prescribe pain relievers and perhaps **muscle relaxants**. Healing time varies according to the patient's overall health, but will take at least several weeks.

Another common maxillofacial fracture is a broken nose. The bones that form the bridge of the nose may be fractured, but cartilage may also be damaged, particularly the nasal septum which divides the nose. If hit from the side, the bones and cartilage are displaced to the side, but if hit from the front, they are splayed out. Severe swelling can inhibit diagnosis and treatment. Mild trauma to the nose can sometimes heal without the person being aware of the fracture unless there is obvious deformity. The nose will be tender for at least three weeks.

Either before the swelling begins or after it subsides, some 10 days after the injury, the doctor can assess the extent of the damage. Physical examination of the inside using a speculum and the outside, in addition to a detailed history of how the injury occurred will determine appropriate treatment. The doctor should be informed of any previous nasal fractures, nasal surgery, or chronic disease such as **osteoporosis**. Sometimes an x ray is useful, but it is not always required.

A primary care physician may treat a nasal fracture himself, but if there is extensive damage or the air passage is blocked, he will refer the patient to an otolaryngologist or a plastic surgeon for treatment. Initially the nose may be packed to control bleeding and hold the shape. It is reset under anesthesia. A protective shield or bandage may be placed over it while the fracture heals.

In the case of orbital fractures, there is great danger of permanent damage to vision. Double vision and decreased mobility of the eye are common complications. Surgical reconstruction may be required if the fracture changes the position of the eye or there is other facial deformity. Treatment requires a maxillofacial surgeon.

When the eyes have been exposed to chemicals, they must be washed out for 15 minutes with clear water. Contact lenses may be removed only after rinsing the eyes. The eyes should then be kept covered until the person can be evaluated by a primary care physician or ophthalmologist.

When a foreign object is lodged in the eye, the person should not rub the eye or put pressure on it which would further injure the eyeball. The eye should be covered to protect it until medical attention can be obtained.

Several kinds of traumatic injuries can occur to the mouth. A person can suffer a laceration (cut) to the lips or tongue, or loosening of teeth, or have teeth knocked out. Such injuries often accompany a jaw fracture or other facial injury. **Wounds** to the soft tissues of the mouth bleed freely, but the plentiful blood supply that leads to this heavy bleeding also helps healing. It is important to clean the wound thoroughly with salt water or hydrogen peroxide rinse to prevent infection. Large cuts may require sutures, and should be done by a maxillofacial surgeon for a good cosmetic result, particularly when the laceration is on the edge of the lip line (vermilion). The doctor will prescribe an antibiotic because there is normally a large amount of bacteria present in the mouth.

Any injury to the teeth should be evaluated by a dentist for treatment and prevention of infection. Implantation of a tooth is sometimes possible if it has been handled carefully and protected. The tooth should be held by the crown, not the root, and kept in milk, saline, or contact lens fluid. The patient's dentist can refer him to a specialist in this field.

For first degree burns, put a cold-water compress on the area or run cold water on it. Put a clean bandage on it for protection. Second and third degree burn victims must be taken to the hospital for treatment.

Fluids are replaced there through an IV. This is vital since a patient in shock will die unless those lost fluids are replaced quickly. **Antibiotics** are given to combat infection since the burns make the body vulnerable to infection.

Treatment for a **head injury** requires examination by a primary care physician unless symptoms point to a more serious injury. In that case, the victim must seek emergency care. A concussion is treated with rest and avoidance of contact sports. Very often athletes who have suffered a concussion are allowed to play again too soon, perhaps in the mistaken impression that the injury is not so bad if the player did not lose consciousness. Anyone who has had one concussion is at increased risk of another one.

Danger signs that the injury is more serious include worsening headaches, **vomiting**, weakness, numbness, unsteadiness, change in the appearance of the eyes, seizures, slurred speech, confusion, agitation, or the victim won't wake up. These signs require immediate transport to the hospital. A neurologist will evaluate the situation, usually with a CT scan. A stay in a **rehabilitation** facility may become necessary.

Alternative treatments

Fractures, burns, and deep lacerations require treatment by a doctor but alternative treatments can help the body withstand injury and assist the healing process. Calcium, **minerals**, **vitamins**, all part of a balanced and nutrient-rich diet, as well as regular **exercise**, build strong bones that can withstand force well. After an injury, **craniosacral therapy** may help healing and ease the headaches that follow a concussion or other head trauma. A physical therapist can offer ultrasound that raises temperature to ease pain, or **biofeedback** in which the patient learns how to tense and relax muscles to relieve pain. **Hydrotherapy** may ease the **stress** of recovering from trauma. Chinese medicine seeks to reconnect the chi along the body's meridians and thus aid healing. Homeopathic physicians may prescribe natural medicines such as Arnica or Symphytum to enhance healing.

Prognosis

When appropriate treatment is obtained quickly after an injury, the prognosis can be excellent. However, if the victim of trauma has osteoporosis or a debilitating chronic disease, healing is more problematic. Healing also depends upon the extent of the injury. An automobile accident or a gunshot wound, for example, can cause severe facial trauma that may require multiple surgical procedures and a considerable amount of time to heal. Burns and lacerations cause scarring that might be improved by **plastic surgery**.

Prevention

Safety equipment is vital to preventing maxillofacial trauma from automobile accidents and sports.

KEY TERMS

Corneal abrasion—A scratch on the surface of the eyeball.

Mandible—The lower jaw, a U-shaped bone attached to the skull at the temporomandibular joints.

Maxilla—The bone of the upper jaw which serves as a foundation of the face and supports the orbits.

Orbit—The eye socket which contains the eyeball, muscles, nerves, and blood vessels that serve the eye.

Otolaryngologist—Ear, nose and throat specialist.

Shock—A reduction of blood flow in the body caused by loss of blood and/or fluids. Can be fatal if not treated quickly.

Temporomandibular joint—The mandible attaches to the temporal bone of the skull and works like a hinge.

Temporomandibular joint syndrome—TMJ Syndrome refers to an incorrect alignment of the lower jaw to the skull which causes the bite to be off line. It causes chronic headaches, nausea, and other symtoms.

Nasal septum—The cartilage which divides the nose in half.

Vermilion border—The line between the lip and the skin.

Here is a partial list of equipment people should always use:

- seatbelts
- automobile air bags
- approved child safety seats
- helmets for riding motorcycles or bicycles, skateboarding, snowboarding, and other sports
- safety glasses for the job, yard work, sports
- other approved safety equipment for sports such as mouthguards, masks, and goggles

Resources

PERIODICALS

Perkins, Stephen W. "The Incidence of Sports-Related Facial Trauma in Children." *Ear, Nose and Throat Journal* August 2000.

Roberts, Graham. "Dental Emergencies (ABC of Oral Health)." *British Medical Journal* September 2, 2000.

ORGANIZATIONS

American Association of Oral & Maxillofacial Surgeons. 9700 W. Bryn Mawr Ave., Rosemont, IL 60018. (847) 678-6200.

Brain Injury Association, Inc. 105 N. Alfred St., Alexandria, VA 22314. (703) 236-6000. < http:// www.biausa.org. >.

OTHER

"Broken Nose." < http://www.intelihealth.com >.

"Burns: Take Them Seriously." Virtual Hospital. < http://www.vh.org/Patients/IHB/HealthProse/ Family medicine/burns.html >.

"Fractured Jaw." < http://www.cbshealthwatch.com/cx/ viewarticle/150454 >.

"Major Domains of Complementary & Alternative Medicine." National Institutes of Health. < http://nccam.nih.gov/fcp/classify/ >.

Barbara J. Mitchell

MCS syndrome *see* **Multiple chemical sensitivity**

MD *see* **Muscular dystrophy**

Measles

Definition

Measles is an infection caused by a virus, which causes an illness displaying a characteristic skin rash known as an exanthem. Measles is also sometimes called rubeola, 5-day measles, or hard measles.

Description

Measles infections appear all over the world. Prior to the current effective immunization program, large-scale measles outbreaks occurred on a two to three-year cycle, usually in the winter and spring. Smaller outbreaks occurred during the off-years. Babies up to about eight months of age are usually protected from contracting measles, due to immune cells they receive from their mothers in the uterus. Once someone has had measles infection, he or she can never get it again.

Causes and symptoms

Measles is caused by a type of virus called a para-myxovirus. It is an extremely contagious infection, spread through the tiny droplets that may spray into the air when an individual carrying the virus sneezes or coughs. About 85% of those people exposed to the

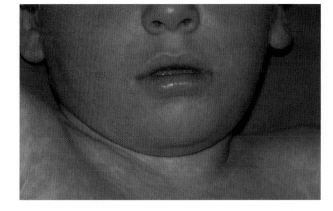

Measles on child's face. *(Custom Medical Stock Photo. Reproduced by permission.)*

virus will become infected with it. About 95% of those people infected with the virus will develop the illness called measles. Once someone is infected with the virus, it takes about 7–18 days before he or she actually becomes ill. The most contagious time period is the three to five days before symptoms begin through about four days after the characteristic measles rash has begun to appear.

The first signs of measles infection are **fever**, extremely runny nose, red, runny eyes, and a **cough**. A few days later, a rash appears in the mouth, particularly on the mucous membrane which lines the cheeks. This rash consists of tiny white dots (like grains of salt or sand) on a reddish bump. These are called Koplik's spots, and are unique to measles infection. The throat becomes red, swollen, and sore.

A couple of days after the appearance of the Koplik's spots, the measles rash begins. It appears in a characteristic progression, from the head, face, and neck, to the trunk, then abdomen, and next out along the arms and legs. The rash starts out as flat, red patches, but eventually develops some bumps. The rash may be somewhat itchy. When the rash begins to appear, the fever usually climbs higher, sometimes reaching as high as 105°F (40.5°C). There may be **nausea**, **vomiting**, **diarrhea**, and multiple swollen lymph nodes. The cough is usually more problematic at this point, and the patient feels awful. The rash usually lasts about five days. As it fades, it turns a brownish color, and eventually the affected skin becomes dry and flaky.

Many patients (about 5–15%) develop other complications. Bacterial infections, such as ear infections, sinus infections, and **pneumonia** are common, especially in children. Other viral infections may also strike the patient, including **croup**, **bronchitis**, **laryngitis**, or

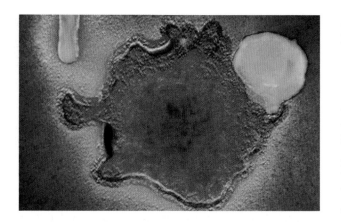

A transmission electron microscopy (TEM) image of a single measles virion. *(Custom Medical Stock Photo. Reproduced by permission.)*

viral pneumonia. Inflammation of the liver, appendix, intestine, or lymph nodes within the abdomen may cause other complications. Rarely, inflammations of the heart or kidneys, a drop in **platelet count** (causing episodes of difficult-to-control bleeding), or reactivation of an old **tuberculosis** infection can occur.

An extremely serious complication of measles infection is swelling of the brain. Called **encephalitis**, this can occur up to several weeks after the basic measles symptoms have resolved. About one out of every thousand patients develops this complication, and about 10-15% of these patients die. Symptoms include fever, **headache**, sleepiness, seizures, and **coma**. Long-term problems following recovery from measles encephalitis may include seizures and **mental retardation**.

A very rare complication of measles can occur up to 10 years following the initial infection. Called **subacute sclerosing panencephalitis**, this is a slowly progressing, smoldering swelling and destruction of the entire brain. It is most common among people who had measles infection prior to the age of two years. Symptoms include changes in personality, decreased intelligence with accompanying school problems, decreased coordination, involuntary jerks and movements of the body. The disease progresses so that the individual becomes increasingly dependent, ultimately becoming bedridden and unaware of his or her surroundings. Blindness may develop, and the temperature may spike (rise rapidly) and fall unpredictably as the brain structures responsible for temperature regulation are affected. **Death** is inevitable.

Measles during **pregnancy** is a serious disease, leading to increased risk of a **miscarriage** or **stillbirth**.

In addition, the mother's illness may progress to pneumonia.

Diagnosis

Measles infection is almost always diagnosed based on its characteristic symptoms, including Koplik's spots, and a rash which spreads from central body structures out towards the arms and legs. If there is any doubt as to the diagnosis, then a specimen of body fluids (mucus, urine) can be collected and combined with fluorescent-tagged measles virus antibodies. Antibodies are produced by the body's immune cells that can recognize and bind to markers (antigens) on the outside of specific organisms, in this case the measles virus. Once the fluorescent antibodies have attached themselves to the measles antigens in the specimen, the specimen can be viewed under a special microscope to verify the presence of measles virus.

Treatment

There are no treatments available to stop measles infection. Treatment is primarily aimed at helping the patient to be as comfortable as possible, and watching carefully so that **antibiotics** can be started promptly if a bacterial infection develops. Fever and discomfort can be treated with **acetaminophen**. Children with measles should never be given **aspirin**, as this has caused the fatal disease **Reye's syndrome** in the past. A cool-mist vaporizer may help decrease the cough. Patients should be given a lot of liquids to drink, in order to avoid **dehydration** from the fever.

Some studies have shown that children with measles encephalitis benefit from relatively large doses of vitamin A.

Alternative treatment

Botanical immune enhancement (with **echinacea**, for example) can assist the body in working through this viral infection. Homeopathic support also can be effective throughout the course of the illness. Some specific alternative treatments to soothe patients with measles include the Chinese herbs bupleurum (*Bupleurum chinense*) and peppermint (*Mentha piperita*), as well as a preparation made from empty cicada (*Cryptotympana atrata*) shells. The itchiness of the rash can be relieved with witch hazel (*Hamamelis virginiana*), chickweed (*Stellaria media*), or oatmeal baths. The eyes can be soothed with an eyewash made from the herb eyebright (*Euphrasia officinalis*). Practitioners of **ayurvedic medicine** recommend ginger or clove tea.

KEY TERMS

Antibodies—Cells made by the immune system which have the ability to recognize foreign invaders (bacteria, viruses), and thus stimulate the immune system to kill them.

Antigens—Markers on the outside of such organisms as bacteria and viruses, which allow antibodies to recognize foreign invaders.

Encephalitis—Swelling, inflammation of the brain.

Exanthem (plural, exanthems or exanthemata)—A skin eruption regarded as a characteristic sign of such diseases as measles, German measles, and scarlet fever.

Koplik's spots—Tiny spots occurring inside the mouth, especially on the inside of the cheek. These spots consist of minuscule white dots (like grains of salt or sand) set onto a reddened bump. Unique to measles.

Prognosis

The prognosis for an otherwise healthy, well-nourished child who contracts measles is usually quite good. In developing countries, however, death rates may reach 15–25%. Adolescents and adults usually have a more difficult course. Women who contract the disease while pregnant may give birth to a baby with hearing impairment. Although only 1 in 1,000 patients with measles will develop encephalitis, 10–15% of those who do will die, and about another 25% will be left with permanent brain damage.

Prevention

Measles is a highly preventable infection. A very effective vaccine exists, made of live measles viruses which have been treated so that they cannot cause actual infection. The important markers on the viruses are intact, however, which causes an individual's immune system to react. Immune cells called antibodies are produced, which in the event of a future infection with measles virus will quickly recognize the organism, and kill it off. Measles vaccines are usually given at about 15 months of age; because prior to that age, the baby's immune system is not mature enough to initiate a reaction strong enough to insure long-term protection from the virus. A repeat injection should be given at about 10 or 11 years of age. Outbreaks on college campuses have occurred among unimmunized or incorrectly immunized students.

Measles vaccine should not be given to a pregnant woman, however, in spite of the seriousness of gestational measles. The reason for not giving this particular vaccine during pregnancy is the risk of transmitting measles to the unborn child.

Surprisingly, new cases of measles began being reported in some countries—including Great Britain—in 2001 because of parents' fears about vaccine safety. The combined vaccine for measles, **mumps**, and **rubella** (MMR) was claimed to cause **autism** or bowel disorders in some children. However, the World Health Organization (WHO) says there is no scientific merit to these claims. The United Nations expressed concern that unwarranted fear of the vaccine would begin spreading the disease in developing countries, and ultimately in developed countries as well. Parents in Britain began demanding the measles vaccine as a separate dose and scientists were exploring that option as an alternative to the combined MMR vaccine. Unfortunately, several children died during an outbreak of measles in Dublin because they had not received the vaccine. Child mortality due to measles is considered largely preventable, and making the MMR vaccine widely available in developing countries is part of WHO's strategy to reduce child mortality by two-thirds by the year 2015.

Resources

BOOKS

Beers, Mark H., MD, and Robert Berkow, MD, editors. "Viral Infections: Measles." Section 19, Chapter 265. In *The Merck Manual of Diagnosis and Therapy*. Whitehouse Station, NJ: Merck Research Laboratories, 2004.

PERIODICALS

Chiba, M. E., M. Saito, N. Suzuki, et al. "Measles Infection in Pregnancy." *Journal of Infection* 47 (July 2003): 40–44.

Jones, G., R. W. Steketee, R. E. Black, et al. "How Many Child Deaths Can We Prevent This Year?" *Lancet* 362 (July 5, 2003): 65–71.

McBrien, J., J. Murphy, D. Gill, et al. "Measles Outbreak in Dublin, 2000." *Pediatric Infectious Disease Journal* 22 (July 2003): 580–584.

"Measles—United States, 2000. (From the Centers for Disease Control and Prevention)." *Journal of the American Medical Association* 287, no. 9 (March 6, 2002): 1105–1112.

Scott, L. A., and M. S. Stone. "Viral Exanthems." *Dermatology Online Journal* 9 (August 2003): 4.

Sur, D. K., D. H. Wallis, and T. X. O'Connell. "Vaccinations in Pregnancy." *American Family Physician* 68 (July 15, 2003): 299–304.

"WHO: Vaccine Fears Could Lead to Unnecessary Deaths." *Medical Letter on the CDC & FDA* March 17, 2002: 11.

ORGANIZATIONS

American Academy of Pediatrics (AAP). 141 Northwest Point Boulevard, Elk Grove Village, IL 60007. (847) 434-4000. < http://www.aap.org >.

Centers for Disease Control and Prevention. 1600 Clifton Rd., NE, Atlanta, GA 30333. (800) 311-3435, (404) 639-3311. < http://www.cdc.gov >.

Rosalyn Carson-DeWitt, MD
Rebecca J. Frey, PhD

Mebendazole *see* **Antihelminthic drugs**

Mechanical debridement *see* **Debridement**

Mechanical ventilation *see* **Inhalation therapies**

Meckel's diverticulum

Definition

Meckel's diverticulum is a congenital pouch (diverticulum) approximately two inches in length and located at the lower (distal) end of the small intestine. It was named for Johann F. Meckel, a German anatomist who first described the structure.

Description

The diverticulum is most easily described as a blind pouch that is a remnant of the omphalomesenteric duct or yolk sac that nourished the early embryo. It contains all layers of the intestine and may have ectopic tissue present from either the pancreas or stomach.

The rule of 2s is the classical description. It is located about 2 ft from the end of the small intestine, is often about 2 in in length, occurs in about 2% of the population, is twice as common in males as females, and can contain two types of ectopic tissue—stomach or pancreas. Many who have a Meckel's diverticulum never have trouble but those that do present in the first two decades of life and often in the first two years.

There are three major complications that may result from the development of Meckel's diverticulum. The most common problem is inflammation or infection that mimics **appendicitis**. This diagnosis is defined at the time of surgery for suspected appendicitis.

Bleeding caused by ectopic stomach tissue that results in a bleeding ulcer is the second most frequent problem. Bleeding may be brisk or massive. The third potential complication is obstruction due to **intussusception**, or a twist around a persistent connection to the abdominal wall. This problem presents as a small bowel obstruction, however, the true cause is identified at the time of surgical exploration.

Meckel's diverticulum is a developmental defect that is present in about 2% of people, but does not always cause symptoms. Meckel's diverticula (plural of diverticulum) are found twice as frequently in men as in women. Complications occur three to five times more frequently in males.

Causes and symptoms

Meckel's diverticulum is not hereditary. It is a vestigial remnant of the omphalomesenteric duct, an embryonic structure that becomes the intestine. As such, there is no genetic defect or abnormality.

Symptoms usually occur in children under 10 years of age. There may be bleeding from the rectum, **pain** and **vomiting**, or simply tiredness and weakness from unnoticed blood loss. It is common for a Meckel's diverticulum to be mistaken for the much more common disease appendicitis. If there is obstruction, the abdomen will distend and there will be cramping pain and vomiting.

Diagnosis

The situation may be so acute that surgery is needed on an emergency basis. This is often the case with bowel obstruction. With heavy bleeding or severe pain, whatever the cause, surgery is required. The finer points of diagnosis can be accomplished when the abdomen is open for inspection during a surgical procedure. This situation is called an acute abdomen.

If there is more time (not an emergency situation), the best way to diagnose Meckel's diverticulum is with a nuclear scan. A radioactive isotope injected into the bloodstream will accumulate at sites of bleeding or in stomach tissue. If a piece of stomach tissue or a pool of blood shows up in the lower intestine, Meckel's diverticulum is indicated.

Treatment

A Meckel's diverticulum that is causing discomfort, bleeding, or obstruction must be surgically removed. This procedure is very similar to an **appendectomy**.

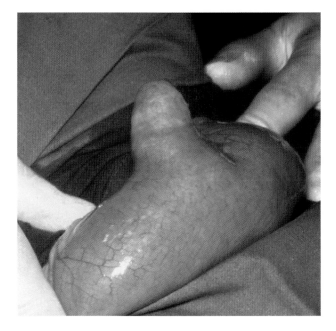

A close-up image of a patient's small intestine with a protruding sac. This condition, called Meckel's diverticulum, is a congenital abnormality occurring in 2% of the population, usually males. *(Custom Medical Stock Photo. Reproduced by permission.)*

KEY TERMS

Appendectomy—The procedure to surgically remove an appendix.

Appendicitis—Inflammation of the appendix.

Appendix—A portion of intestine attached to the cecum.

Cecum—The first part of the large bowel.

Congenital—Refers to a disorder which is present at birth.

Distal—Away from the point of origin.

Ectopic—Tissue found in an abnormal location.

Intussusception—One piece of bowel inside another, causing obstruction.

Isotope—Any of two or more species of atoms of a chemical element with the same atomic number and nearly identical chemical behavior but with differing atomic mass and physical properties.

Peptic ulcer—A wound in the bowel that can be caused by stomach acid or a bacterium called *Helicobacter pylori*.

Volvulus—A twisted loop of bowel, causing obstruction.

Prognosis

The outcome after surgery is usually excellent. The source of bleeding, pain, or obstruction is removed so the symptoms also disappear. A Meckel's diverticulum will not return.

Resources

BOOKS

Aspinall, Richard J., and Simon T. Taylor-Robinson. *Mosby's Color Atlas & Text of Gastroenterology.* St. Louis: Mosby-Year Book, 2001.

Cousins, Claire, and Ralph Boulton. *A Color Handbook of Gastroenterology.* New York: McGraw-Hill, 1999.

Lipsky, Martin S., and Richard Sadovsky. *Gastrointestinal Problems.* Philadelphia: Lippincott Williams & Wilkins Publishers, 2000.

Sanderson, Ian R., and W. Allan Walker. *Development of the Gastrointestinal Tract.* Hamilton, Ontario, Canada: B. C. Decker, 1999.

Stringer, David A., and Paul S. Babyn. *Pediatric Gastrointestinal Imaging and Intervention.* 2nd ed. Hamilton, Ontario, Canada: B. C. Decker, 2000.

PERIODICALS

al Mahmeed, T., J. K. MacFarlane, and D. Filipenko. "Ischemic Meckel's diverticulum and acute appendicitis." *Canadian Journal of Surgery* 43, no. 2 (2000): 146-47.

Arnio, P., and I. S. Salonen. "Abdominal disorders arising from 71 Meckel's diverticulum." *Annals of Surgery and Gynecology* 89, no. 4 (2000): 281-84.

Heider, R., D. M. Warshauer, and K. E. Behrns. "Inverted Meckel's diverticulum as a source of chronic gastrointestinal blood loss." *Surgery* 128, no. 1 (2000): 107-08.

Martin, J. P., P. D. Connor, and K. Charles. "Meckel's diverticulum." *American Family Physician* 61, no. 4 (2000): 1037-42.

Nagler, J., J. L. Clarke, and S. A. Albert. "Meckel's diverticulitis in an elderly man diagnosed by computed tomography." *Journal of Clinical Gastroenterology* 30, no. (2000): 87-88.

ORGANIZATIONS

American Academy of Family Physicians. 11400 Tomahawk Creek Parkway, Leawood, KS 66211-2672. (913) 906-6000. fp@aafp.org. < http://www.aafp.org/ >.

American Academy of Pediatrics. 141 Northwest Point Boulevard, Elk Grove Village, IL 60007-1098. (847) 434-4000. Fax: (847) 434-8000. kidsdoc@aap.org. < http://www.aap.org/default.htm >.

American College of Gastroenterology. 4900 B South 31st Street, Arlington, VA 22206. (703) 820-7400. Fax: (703) 931-4520. < http://www.acg.gi.org >.

American College of Surgeons. 633 North St. Clair St., Chicago, IL 60611-32311. (312) 202-5000. Fax: (312)

202-5001. postmaster@facs.org. <http://www.facs.org/>.

American Medical Association. 515 N. State Street, Chicago, IL 60610. (312) 464-5000. <http://www.ama-assn.org/>.

OTHER

American Academy of Family Physicians.
<http://www.aafp.org/afp/20000215/1037.html>.
"Meckel's Diverticulum." *Merck Manual.*
<http://www.merck.com/pubs/mmanual/section19/chapter268/268d.htm>.

L. Fleming Fallon, Jr., MD, DrPH

Median nerve entrapment *see* **Carpal tunnel syndrome**

Mediastinoscopy

Definition

Mediastinoscopy is a surgical procedure that allows physicians to view areas of the mediastinum, the cavity behind the breastbone that lies between the lungs. The organs in the mediastinum include the heart and its vessels, the lymph nodes, trachea, esophagus, and thymus.

Mediastinoscopy is most commonly used to detect or stage **cancer**. It is also ordered to detect infection, and to confirm diagnosis of certain conditions and diseases of the respiratory organs. The procedure involves insertion of an endotracheal (within the trachea) tube, followed by a small incision in the chest. A mediastinoscope is inserted through the incision. The purpose of this equipment is to allow the physician to directly see the organs inside the mediastinum, and to collect tissue samples for laboratory study.

Purpose

Mediastinoscopy is often the diagnostic method of choice for detecting lymphoma, including Hodgkin's disease. The diagnosis of **sarcoidosis** (a chronic lung disease) and the staging of lung cancer can also be accomplished through mediastinoscopy. Lung cancer staging involves the placement of the cancer's progression into stages, or levels. These stages help a physician study cancer and provide consistent definition levels of cancer and corresponding treatments. The lymph nodes in the mediastinum are likely to show if lung cancer has spread beyond the lungs. Mediastinoscopy allows a physician to observe and extract a sample from the nodes for further study. Involvement of these lymph nodes indicates diagnosis and stages of lung cancer.

Mediastinoscopy may also be ordered to verify a diagnosis that was not clearly confirmed by other methods, such as certain radiographic and laboratory studies. Mediastinoscopy may also aid in certain surgical biopsies of nodes or cancerous tissue in the mediastinum. In fact, the surgeon may immediately perform a surgical procedure if a malignant tumor is confirmed while the patient is undergoing mediastinoscopy, thus combining the diagnostic exam and surgical procedure into one operation when possible.

Although still performed in 2001, advancements in computed tomography (CT) and **magnetic resonance imaging** (MRI) techniques, as well as the new developments in ultrasonography, have led to a decline in the use of mediastinoscopy. In addition, better results of fine-needle aspiration (drawing out fluid by suction) and core-needle biopsy (using a needle to obtain a small tissue sample) investigations, along with new techniques in **thoracoscopy** (examination of the thoracic cavity with a lighted instrument called a thoracoscope) offer additional options in examining mediastinal masses. Mediastinoscopy may be required, however, when these other methods cannot be used or when the results they provide are inconclusive.

Precautions

Because mediastinoscopy is a surgical procedure, it should only be performed when the benefits of the exam's findings outweigh the risks of surgery and anesthesia. Patients who previously had mediastinoscopy should not receive it again if there is scarring present from the first exam.

Several other medical conditions, such as impaired cerebral circulation, obstruction or distortion of the upper airway, or thoracic **aortic aneurysm** (abnormal dilation of the thoracic aorta) may also preclude mediastinoscopy. Anatomic structures that can be compressed by the mediastinoscope may complicate these pre-existing medical conditions.

Description

Mediastinoscopy is usually performed in a hospital under **general anesthesia**. An endotracheal tube is inserted first, after **local anesthesia** is applied to the throat. Once the patient is under general anesthesia, a small incision is made usually just below the neck or at the notch at the top of the breastbone. The surgeon may clear a path and feel the patient's lymph nodes first to evaluate any abnormalities within the nodes. Next, the physician will insert the mediastinoscope through the incision. The scope is a narrow, hollow tube with an attached light that allows the surgeon to see inside the area. The surgeon can insert tools through the hollow tube to help perform biopsies. A sample of tissue from the lymph nodes or a mass can be extracted and sent for study under a microscope or on to a laboratory for further testing.

In some cases, analysis of the tissue sample which shows malignancy will suggest the need for immediate surgery while the patient is already prepared and under anesthesia. In other cases, the surgeon will complete the visual study and tissue extraction and stitch the small incision closed. The patient will remain in the surgery recovery area until it is determined that the effects of anesthesia have lessened and it is safe for the patient to leave the area. The entire procedure should take about an hour, not counting preparation and recovery time. Studies have shown that mediastinoscopy is a safe, thorough, and cost-effective diagnostic tool with less risk than some other procedures.

Preparation

Patients are asked to sign a consent form after having reviewed the risks of mediastinoscopy and known risks or reactions to anesthesia. The physician will normally instruct the patient to fast from midnight before the test until after the procedure is completed. A physician may also prescribe a sedative the night before the exam and before the procedure. Often a local anesthetic will be applied to the throat to prevent discomfort during placement of the endotracheal tube.

Aftercare

Following mediastinoscopy, patients will be carefully monitored to watch for changes in vital signs or indications of complications of the procedure or the anesthesia. A patient may have a **sore throat** from the endotracheal tube, temporary chest **pain**, and soreness or tenderness at the site of incision.

Risks

Complications from the actual mediastinoscopy procedure are relatively rare—the overall complication rate in various studies has been 1.3–3.0%. However, the following complications, in decreasing order of frequency, have been reported:

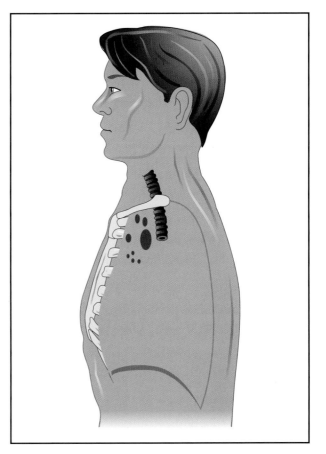

Mediastinoscopy is a surgical procedure used to detect or stage lymphoma or lung cancer. In this procedure, the surgeon makes an incision below the neck and inserts a mediastinoscope (a narrow, hollow tube with an attached light) through it to reach the area behind the breastbone. The surgeon can then insert tools through the scope to collect tissue for laboratory analysis. *(Illustration by Electronic Illustrators Group.)*

- hemorrhage
- pneumothorax (air in the pleural space)
- recurrent laryngeal nerve injury, causing hoarseness
- infection
- tumor implantation in the wound
- phrenic nerve injury (injury to a thoracic nerve)
- esophageal injury
- chylothorax (chyle—a milky lymphatic fluid—in the pleural space)
- air **embolism** (air bubble)
- transient hemiparesis (**paralysis** on one side of the body)

The usual risks associated with general anesthesia also apply to this procedure.

KEY TERMS

Endotracheal—Placed within the trachea, also known as the windpipe.

Hodgkin's disease—A malignancy of lymphoid tissue found in the lymph nodes, spleen, liver, and bone marrow.

Lymph nodes—Small round structures located throughout the body; contain cells that fight infections.

Pleural space—Space between the layers of the pleura (membrane lining the lungs and thorax).

Sarcoidosis—A chronic disease characterized by nodules in the lungs, skin, lymph nodes and bones; however, any tissue or organ in the body may be affected.

Thymus—An unpaired organ in the mediastinal cavity that is important in the body's immune response.

Normal results

In the majority of procedures performed to diagnose cancer, a normal result involves evidence of small, smooth, normal-appearing lymph nodes and no abnormal tissue, growths, or signs of infection. In the case of lung cancer staging, results are related to the severity and progression of the cancer.

Abnormal results

Abnormal findings may indicate lung cancer, **tuberculosis**, the spread of disease from one body part to another, sarcoidosis (a disease that causes nodules, usually affecting the lungs), lymphoma (abnormalities in the lymph tissues), and Hodgkin's disease.

Resources

BOOKS

Fischbach, Frances Talaska. *A Manual of Laboratory and Diagnostic Tests.* 6th ed. Philadelphia: Lippincott Williams and Wilkins, 2000.

Pagana, Kathleen Deska, and Timothy James Pagana. *Mosby's Manual of Diagnostic and Laboratory Tests.* St. Louis, MO: Mosby, 1998.

PERIODICALS

Deslauriers, Jean, and Jocelyn Gregoire. "Clinical and Surgical Staging of Non-Small Cell Lung Cancer." *Chest,* Supplement (April 2000): 96S–103S.

Tahara R. W., et al. "Is There a Role for Routine Mediastinoscopy in Patients With Peripheral T1 Lung Cancers?" *American Journal of Surgery* December 2000: 488–491.

ORGANIZATIONS

Alliance for Lung Cancer Advocacy, Support, and Education. P.O. Box 849, Vancouver, WA 98666. (800) 298-2436. < http://www.alcase.org >.

American Cancer Society. 1599 Clifton Rd. NE, Atlanta, GA 30329. 800–ACS–2345 < http://www.cancer.org >.

American Lung Association. 1740 Broadway, New York, NY 10019-4374. 800-LUNG-USA (800-586-4872). < http://www.lungusa.org >.

Teresa Odle

Meditation

Definition

Meditation is a practice of concentrated focus upon a sound, object, visualization, the breath, movement, or attention itself in order to increase awareness of the present moment, reduce **stress**, promote relaxation, and enhance personal and spiritual growth.

Purpose

Meditation benefits people with or without acute medical illness or stress. People who meditate regularly have been shown to feel less **anxiety** and depression. They also report that they experience more enjoyment and appreciation of life and that their relationships with others are improved. Meditation produces a state of deep relaxation and a sense of balance or equanimity. According to Michael J. Baime, "Meditation cultivates an emotional stability that allows the meditator to experience intense emotions fully while simultaneously maintaining perspective on them." Out of this experience of emotional stability, one may gain greater insight and understanding about one's thoughts, feelings, and actions. This insight in turn offers the possibility to feel more confident and in control of life. Meditation facilitates a greater sense of calmness, empathy, and acceptance of self and others.

Meditation can be used with other forms of medical treatment and is an important complementary therapy for both the treatment and prevention of many stress-related conditions. Regular meditation can reduce the number of symptoms experienced by patients with a wide range of illnesses and disorders.

MAHARISHI MAHESH YOGI (1911–)

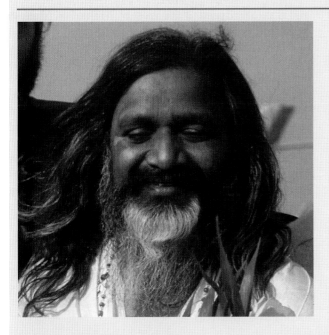

(Archive. Reproduced by permission.)

Maharishi Mahesh Yogi is one of the most recognized spiritual leaders of the world. Almost single-handedly, the Maharishi (meaning great sage) brought Eastern culture into Western consciousness. He emerged in the late 1950s in London and the United States as a missionary in the cause of Hinduism, the philosophy of which is called Vedanta—a belief that "holds that God is to be found in every creature and object, that the purpose of human life is to realize the godliness in oneself and that religious truths are universal."

By 1967, the Maharishi became a leader among flower-children and an anti-drug advocate. The Maharishi's sudden popularity was helped along by such early fans as the Beatles, Mia Farrow, and Shirley MacLaine. These people, and many others, practiced Transcendental Meditation (TM), a Hindu-influenced procedure that endures in America to this day.

When the 1960s drew to a close, the Maharishi began to fade from public view. The guru still had enough followers, though, to people the Maharishi International University, founded in 1971. One of the main draws of Maharishi International University was the study of TM-Sidha, an exotic form of Transcendental Meditation. Sidhas believe that group meditation can elicit the maharishi effect—a force strong enough to conjure world peace.

Based upon clinical evidence as well as theoretical understanding, meditation is considered to be one of the better therapies for **panic disorder**, **generalized anxiety disorder**, **substance dependence** and **abuse**, ulcers, colitis, chronic **pain**, **psoriasis**, and dysthymic disorder. It is considered to be a valuable adjunctive therapy for moderate **hypertension** (high blood pressure), prevention of cardiac arrest (**heart attack**), prevention of **atherosclerosis** (hardening of arteries), arthritis (including **fibromyalgia**), **cancer**, **insomnia**, migraine, and prevention of **stroke**. Meditation may also be a valuable complementary therapy for **allergies** and **asthma** because of the role stress plays in these conditions. Meditative practices have been reported to improve function or reduce symptoms in patients with some neurological disorders as well. These include people with Parkinson's disease, people who experience **fatigue** with **multiple sclerosis**, and people with epilepsy who are resistant to standard treatment.

Overall, a 1995 report to the National Institutes of Health on alternative medicine concluded that, "More than 30 years of research, as well as the experience of a large and growing number of individuals and health care providers, suggests that meditation and similar forms of relaxation can lead to better health, higher quality of life, and lowered health care costs..."

Description

Origins

Meditation techniques have been practiced for millennia. Originally, they were intended to develop spiritual understanding, awareness, and direct experience of ultimate reality. The many different religious traditions in the world have given rise to a rich variety of meditative practices. These include the contemplative practices of Christian religious orders, the Buddhist practice of sitting meditation, and the whirling movements of the Sufi dervishes. Although meditation is an important spiritual practice in many religious and spiritual traditions, it can be practiced by anyone regardless of their religious or cultural background to relieve stress and pain.

As Western medical practitioners begin to understand the mind's role in health and disease, there has been more interest in the use of meditation in medicine. Meditative practices are increasingly offered in medical clinics and hospitals as a tool for improving health and quality of life. Meditation has been used as the primary therapy for treating certain diseases; as an additional therapy in a comprehensive treatment plan; and as a means of improving the quality of life of people with debilitating, chronic, or terminal illnesses.

Sitting meditation is generally done in an upright seated position, either in a chair or cross-legged on a cushion on the floor. The spine is straight yet relaxed. Sometimes the eyes are closed. Other times the eyes are open and gazing softly into the distance or at an object. Depending on the type of meditation, the meditator may be concentrating on the sensation of the movement of the breath, counting the breath, silently repeating a sound, chanting, visualizing an image, focusing awareness on the center of the body, opening to all sensory experiences including thoughts, or performing stylized ritual movements with the hands.

Movement meditation can be spontaneous and free-form or involve highly structured, choreographed, repetitive patterns. Movement meditation is particularly helpful for those people who find it difficult to remain still.

Generally speaking, there are two main types of meditation. These types are concentration meditation and mindfulness meditation. Concentration meditation practices involve focusing attention on a single object. Objects of meditation can include the breath, an inner or external image, a movement pattern (as in **tai chi** or **yoga**), or a sound, word, or phrase that is repeated silently (mantra). The purpose of concentrative practices is to learn to focus one's attention or develop concentration. When thoughts or emotions arise, the meditator gently directs the mind back to the original object of concentration.

Mindfulness meditation practices involve becoming aware of the entire field of attention. The meditator is instructed to be aware of all thoughts, feelings, perceptions or sensations as they arise in each moment. Mindfulness meditation practices are enhanced by the meditator's ability to focus and quiet the mind. Many meditation practices are a blend of these two forms.

The study and application of meditation to health care has focused on three specific approaches: 1. transcendental meditation (TM); 2. The "relaxation response," a general approach to meditation developed by Dr. Herbert Benson; and 3. mindfulness meditation, specifically the program of mindfulness-based **stress reduction** (MBSR) developed by Jon Kabat-Zinn.

Transcendental meditation

TM has its origins in the Vedic tradition of India and was introduced to the West by **Maharishi Mahesh Yogi**. TM has been taught to somewhere between two and four million people. It is one of the most widely practiced forms of meditation in the West. TM has been studied many times; these studies have produced much of the information about the physiology of meditation. In TM, the meditator sits with closed eyes and concentrates on a single syllable or word (mantra) for 20 minutes at a time, twice a day. When thoughts or feelings arise, the attention is brought back to the mantra. According to Charles Alexander, an important TM researcher, "During TM, ordinary waking mental activity is said to settle down, until even the subtlest thought is transcended and a completely unified wholeness of awareness . . . is experienced. In this silent, self-referential state of pure wakefulness, consciousness is fully awake to itself alone. . . ." TM supporters believe that TM practices are more beneficial than other meditation practices.

The relaxation response

The relaxation response involves a similar form of mental focusing. Dr. Herbert Benson, one of the first Western doctors to conduct research on the effects of meditation, developed this approach after observing the profound health benefits of a state of bodily calm he calls "the relaxation response." In order to elicit this response in the body, he teaches patients to focus upon the repetition of a word, sound, prayer, phrase, or movement activity (including swimming, jogging, yoga, and even knitting) for 10–20 minutes at a time, twice a day. Patients are also taught not to pay attention to distracting thoughts and to return their focus to the original repetition. The choice of the focused repetition is up to the individual. Instead of Sanskrit terms, the meditator can choose what is personally meaningful, such as a phrase from a Christian or Jewish prayer.

Mindfulness meditation

Mindfulness meditation comes out of traditional Buddhist meditation practices. Psychologist Jon Kabat-Zinn has been instrumental in bringing this form of meditation into medical settings. In formal mindfulness practice, the meditator sits with eyes closed, focusing the attention on the sensations and movement of the breath for approximately 45–60 minutes at a time, at least once a day. Informal mindfulness practice involves bringing awareness to every

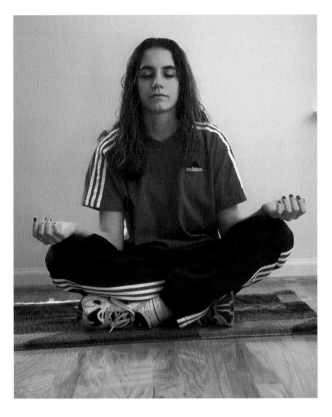

Girl in meditation. *(Photograph by Robert J. Huffman. Field Mark Publications. Reproduced by permission.)*

Dervish—A member of the Sufi order. Their practice of meditation involves whirling ecstatic dance.

Mantra—A sacred word or formula repeated over and over to concentrate the mind.

Transcendental meditation (TM)—A meditation technique based on Hindu practices that involves the repetition of a mantra.

activity in daily life. Wandering thoughts or distracting feelings are simply noticed without resisting or reacting to them. The essence of mindfulness meditation is not what one focuses on but rather the quality of awareness the meditator brings to each moment. According to Kabat-Zinn, "It is this investigative, discerning observation of whatever comes up in the present moment that is the hallmark of mindfulness and differentiates it most from other forms of meditation. The goal of mindfulness is for you to be more aware, more in touch with life and whatever is happening in your own body and mind at the time it is happening—that is, the present moment." The MBSR program consists of a series of classes involving meditation, movement, and group process. There are over 240 MBSR programs offered in health care settings around the world.

Meditation is not considered a medical procedure or intervention by most insurers. Many patients pay for meditation training themselves. Frequently, religious groups or meditation centers offer meditation instruction free of charge or for a nominal donation. Hospitals may offer MBSR classes at a reduced rate for their patients and a slightly higher rate for the general public.

Precautions

Meditation appears to be safe for most people. There are, however, case reports and studies noting some adverse effects. Thirty-three to 50% of the people participating in long silent meditation retreats (two weeks to three months) reported increased tension, anxiety, confusion, and depression. On the other hand, most of these same people also reported very positive effects from their meditation practice. Kabat-Zinn notes that these studies fail to differentiate between serious psychiatric disturbances and normal emotional mood swings. These studies do suggest, however, that meditation may not be recommended for people with psychotic disorders, severe depression, and other severe **personality disorders** unless they are also receiving psychological or medical treatment.

Side effects

There are no reported side effects from meditation except for positive benefits.

Research and general acceptance

The scientific study of the physiological effects of meditation began in the early 1960s. These studies prove that meditation affects metabolism, the endocrine system, the central nervous system, and the autonomic nervous system. In one study, three advanced practitioners of Tibetan Buddhist meditation practices demonstrated the ability to increase "inner heat" as much as 61%. During a different meditative practice they were able to dramatically slow down the rate at which their bodies consumed oxygen. Preliminary research shows that mindfulness meditation is associated with increased levels of melatonin. These findings suggest a potential role for meditation in the treatment and prevention of breast and prostrate cancer.

Despite the inherent difficulties in designing research studies, there is a large amount of evidence of the medical benefits of meditation. Meditation is particularly effective as a treatment for chronic pain. Studies have shown meditation reduces symptoms of pain and pain-related drug use. In a four-year follow-up study, the majority of patients in a MBSR program reported "moderate to great improvement" in pain as a result of participation in the program.

Meditation has long been recommended as a treatment for high blood pressure; however, there is a debate over the amount of benefit that meditation offers. Although most studies show a reduction in blood pressure with meditation, medication is still more effective at lowering high blood pressure.

Meditation may also be an effective treatment for **coronary artery disease**. A study of 21 patients practicing TM for eight months showed increases in their amount of **exercise** tolerance, amount of workload, and a delay in the onset of ST-segment depression. Meditation is also an important part of Dean Ornish's program, which has been proven to reverse coronary artery disease.

Research also suggests that meditation is effective in the treatment of chemical dependency. Gelderloos and others reviewed 24 studies and reported that all of them showed that TM is helpful in programs to stop **smoking** and also in programs for drug and alcohol abuse.

Studies also imply that meditation is helpful in reducing symptoms of anxiety and in treating anxiety-related disorders. Furthermore, a study in 1998 of 37 psoriasis patients showed that those practicing mindfulness meditation had more rapid clearing of their skin condition, with standard UV light treatment, than the control subjects. Another study found that meditation decreased the symptoms of fibromyalgia; over half of the patients reported significant improvement. Meditation was one of several stress management techniques used in a small study of HIV-positive men. The study showed improvements in the T-cell counts of the men, as well as in several psychological measures of well-being.

Resources

BOOKS

Astin, John A., et al. "Meditation" in *Clinician's Complete Reference to Complementary and Alternative Medicine*, edited by Donald Novey. St. Louis, MO: Mosby, 2000.

Baime, Michael J. "Meditation and Mindfulness" in *Essentials of Complementary and Alternative Medicine*, edited Wayne B. Jonas and Jeffrey S. Levin. New York: Lippencott, Williams and Wilkins, 1999.

ORGANIZATIONS

Insight Meditation Society. 1230 Pleasant, St. Barre, MA 01005. (978) 355-4378. FAX: (978) 355-6398. < http://www.dharma.org >.

Mind-Body Medical Institute. Beth Israel Deaconess Medical Center. One Deaconess Road, Boston, MA 02215. (617) 632-9525. < http://www.mindbody.harvard.edu >.

OTHER

Videos are available from the organizations listed above.

Linda Chrisman

Medullary sponge kidney

Definition

Medullary sponge kidney is a congenital defect of the kidneys where the kidneys fill with pools of urine.

Description

One of every 100 to 200 people have some form of this disease. The kidneys filter urine from the blood and direct it down tiny collecting tubes toward the ureters (ducts that carry urine from the kidney to the bladder). These tiny tubes gradually join together until they reach the renal pelvis, where the ureters begin. As the tubes join, they are supposed to get progressively bigger as they get fewer in number. In medullary sponge kidney, the tubes are irregular in diameter, forming pools of urine along the way. These pools encourage stone formation and infection.

Causes and symptoms

Although some cases of this disorder seem to be inherited, usually the cause is not known.

The symptoms associated with medullary sponge kidney are those related to infection and stone passage. Infection causes **fever**; back and flank **pain**; cloudy, frequent, and burning urine; and general discomfort. Stones cause pain in the flank or groin as they pass. They usually cause some bleeding. The bleeding may not be visible in the urine, but it is apparent under a microscope.

Diagnosis

Recurring kidney infections, bleeding, or stones will prompt x rays of the kidneys. The appearance

KEY TERMS

Congenital—Present at birth.

Intravenous pyelogram—X rays of the upper urinary system using a contrast agent that is excreted by the kidneys into the urine.

Thiazide diuretic—A particular class of medication that encourages urine production.

of medullary sponge kidney on an intravenous pyelogram (x rays of the upper urinary system) is characteristic.

Treatment

Many people never have trouble with this disorder. For those that do, infections and stones will need periodic treatment. Infections should be treated with **antibiotics** early in order to prevent kidney damage. Stones may need to be surgically removed. Often, removal can be accomplished without an incision but rather by reaching up with instruments through the lower urinary tract to grab the stones. There is also a new method of stone treatment called shock wave **lithotripsy**. A special machine delivers a focused blast of shock waves that breaks stones into sand so that they will pass out naturally. It is considered reasonably safe and usually effective.

Prognosis

Ignoring symptoms can result in progressive damage to the kidneys and ultimate kidney failure, but attentive early treatment will preserve kidney function.

Prevention

Diligent monitoring for infection at regular intervals and at the first symptom will give the best long-term results. By drinking extra liquids, most stones can be prevented. The most common kind of stones, calcium stones, can be deterred by regularly taking a medication that encourages urine production (thiazide diuretic).

Resources

ORGANIZATIONS

American Association of Kidney Patients. 100 S. Ashley Dr., #280, Tampa, FL 33602. (800) 749-2257. < http://www.aakp.org >.

American Kidney Foundation. 6110 Executive Boulevard, #1010, Rockville, M D 20852. 800-638-8299.
National Kidney Foundation. 30 East 33rd St., New York, NY 10016. (800) 622-9010. < http://www.kidney.org >.

J. Ricker Polsdorfer, MD

Medulloblastoma *see* **Brain tumor**

Mefloquine *see* **Antimalarial drugs**

Megalencephaly *see* **Congenital brain defects**

Melanoma *see* **Malignant melanoma**

Melioidosis

Definition

Melioidosis is an infectious disease of humans and animals caused by a gram-negative bacillus found in soil and water. It has both acute and chronic forms.

Description

Melioidosis, which is sometimes called *Pseudomonas pseudomallei* infection, is endemic (occurring naturally and consistently) in Southeast Asia, Australia, and parts of Africa. It was rare in the United States prior to recent immigration from Southeast Asia. Melioidosis is presently a public health concern because it is most common in **AIDS** patients and intravenous drug users.

Causes and symptoms

Melioidosis is caused by *Pseudomonas pseudomallei,* a bacillus that can cause disease in sheep, goats, pigs, horses, and other animals, as well as in humans. The organism enters the body through skin abrasions, **burns,** or **wounds** infected by contaminated soil; inhalation of dust; or by eating food contaminated with *P. pseudomallei*. Person-to-person transmission is unusual. Drug addicts acquire the disease from shared needles. The incubation period is two to three days.

Chronic melioidosis is characterized by **osteomyelitis** (inflammation of the bone) and pus-filled abscesses in the skin, lungs, or other organs. Acute melioidosis takes one of three forms: a localized skin infection that may spread to nearby lymph nodes; an infection of the lungs associated with high **fever** (102°F/38.9°C), **headache**, chest **pain**, and coughing;

and septicemia (blood **poisoning**) characterized by disorientation, difficulty breathing, severe headache, and an eruption of pimples on the head or trunk. The third form is most common among drug addicts and may be rapidly fatal.

Diagnosis

Melioidosis is usually suspected based on the patient's history, especially travel, occupational exposure to infected animals, or a history of intravenous drug. Diagnosis must then be confirmed through laboratory tests. *P. pseudomallei* can be cultured from samples of the patient's sputum, blood, or tissue fluid from abscesses. Blood tests, including complement fixation (CF) tests and hemagglutination tests, also help to confirm the diagnosis. In acute infections, chest x rays and **liver function tests** are usually abnormal.

Treatment

Patients with mild or moderate infections are given a course of trimethoprim-sulfamethoxazole (TMP/SMX) and ceftazidime by mouth. Patients with acute melioidosis are given a lengthy course of ceftazidime followed by TMP/SMX. In patients with acute septicemia, a combination of **antibiotics** is administered intravenously, usually tetracycline, chloramphenicol, and TMP/SMX.

Prognosis

The mortality rate in acute cases of pulmonary melioidosis is about 10%; the mortality rate for the septicemic form is significantly higher (slightly above 50%). The prognosis for recovery from mild infections is excellent.

Prevention

There is no form of immunization for melioidosis. Prevention requires prompt cleansing of scrapes, burns, or other open wounds in areas where the disease is common and avoidance of needle sharing among drug addicts.

Resources

BOOKS

Pollock, Matthew. "Infections Due to Pseudomonas Species and Related Organisms." In *Harrison's Principles of Internal Medicine*, edited by Anthony S. Fauci, et al. New York: McGraw-Hill, 1997.

Rebecca J. Frey, PhD

Membranous glomerulopathy *see* **Nephrotic syndrome**

Memory loss *see* **Amnesia**

Ménière's disease

Definition

Ménière's disease is a condition characterized by recurrent vertigo (**dizziness**), **hearing loss**, and **tinnitus** (a roaring, buzzing or ringing sound in the ears).

Description

Ménière's disease was named for the French physician Prosper Ménière, who first described the illness in 1861. It is an abnormality within the inner ear. A fluid called endolymph moves in the membranous labyrinth or semicircular canals within the bony labyrinth inside the inner ear. When the head or body moves, the endolymph moves, causing nerve receptors in the membranous labyrinth to send signals to the brain about the body's motion. A change in the volume of the endolymph fluid, or swelling or rupture of the membranous labyrinth, is thought to result in Ménière's disease symptoms.

Causes and symptoms

Causes

The cause of Ménière's disease is unknown as of 2002; however, scientists are studying several possible causes, including noise pollution, viral infections, or alterations in the patterns of blood flow in the structures of the inner ear. Since Ménière's disease sometimes runs in families, researchers are also looking into genetic factors as possible causes of the disorder.

One area of research that shows promise is the possible relationship between Ménière's disease and **migraine headache**. Dr. Ménière himself suggested the possibility of a link, but early studies yielded conflicting results. A rigorous German study published in late 2002 reported that the lifetime prevalence of migraine was 56% in patients diagnosed with Ménière's disease as compared to 25% for controls. The researchers noted that further work is necessary to determine the exact nature of the relationship between the two disorders.

A study published in late 2002 reported that there is a significant increase in the number of CD4 cells in the blood of patients having an acute attack of Ménière's disease. CD4 cells are a subtype of T cells, which are produced in the thymus gland and regulate the immune system's response to infected or malignant cells. Further research is needed to clarify the role of these cells in Ménière's disease.

Another possible factor in the development of Ménière's disease is the loss of myelin from the cells surrounding the vestibular nerve fibers. Myelin is a whitish fatty material in the cell membrane of the Schwann cells that form a sheath around certain nerve cells. It acts like an electrical insulator. A team of researchers at the University of Virginia reported in 2002 that the vestibular nerve cells in patients with unilateral Ménière's disease are demyelinated; that is, they have lost their protective "insulation." The researchers are investigating the possibility that a viral disease or disorder of the immune system is responsible for the demyelination of the vestibular nerve cells.

Symptoms

The symptoms of Ménière's disease are associated with a change in fluid volume within the labyrinth of the inner ear. Symptoms include severe dizziness or vertigo, tinnitus, hearing loss, and the sensation of **pain** or pressure in the affected ear. Symptoms appear suddenly, last up to several hours, and can occur as often as daily to as infrequently as once a year. A typical attack includes vertigo, tinnitus, and hearing loss; however, some individuals with Ménière's disease may experience a single symptom, like an occasional bout of slight dizziness or periodic, intense ringing in the ear. Attacks of severe vertigo can force the sufferer to have to sit or lie down, and may be accompanied by **headache**, **nausea**, **vomiting**, or **diarrhea**. Hearing tends to recover between attacks, but becomes progressively worse over time.

Ménière's disease usually starts between the ages of 20 and 50 years; however, it is not uncommon for elderly people to develop the disease without a previous history of symptoms. Ménière's disease affects men and women in equal numbers. In most patients only one ear is affected but in about 15% both ears are involved.

Diagnosis

An estimated 3–5 million people in the United States have Ménière's disease, and almost 100,000 new cases are diagnosed each year. Diagnosis is based on medical history, **physical examination**, hearing and balance tests, and medical imaging with **magnetic resonance imaging** (MRI).

Several types of tests may be used to diagnose the disease and to evaluation the extent of hearing loss. In patients with Ménière's disease, audiometric tests (hearing tests) usually indicate a sensory type of hearing loss in the affected ear. Speech discrimination or the ability to distinguish between words that sound alike is often diminished. In about 50% of patients, the balance function is reduced in the affected ear. An electronystagnograph (ENG) may be used to evaluate balance. Since the eyes and ears work together through the nervous system to coordinate balance, measurement of eye movements can be used to test the balance system. For this test, the patient is seated in a darkened room and recording electrodes, similar to those used with a heart monitor, are placed near the eyes. Warm and cool water or air are gently introduced into the each ear canal and eye movements are recorded.

Another test that may be used is an electrocochleograph (EcoG), which can measure increased inner ear fluid pressure.

Treatment

There is no cure for Ménière's disease, but medication, surgery, and dietary and behavioral changes, can help control or improve the symptoms.

Medications

Symptoms of Ménière's disease may be treated with a variety of oral medicine or through injections. **Antihistamines**, like diphenhydramine, meclizine, and cyclizine can be prescribed to sedate the vestibular system. A barbiturate medication like pentobarbital may be used to completely sedate the patient and relieve the vertigo. Anticholinergic drugs, like atropine or scopolamine, can help minimize **nausea and vomiting**. Diazepam has been found to be particularly effective for relief of vertigo and nausea in Ménière's disease. There have been some reports of successful control of vertigo after **antibiotics** (gentamicin or streptomycin) or a steroid medication (dexamethasone) are injected directly into the inner ear. Some researchers have found that gentamicin is effective in relieving tinnitus as well as vertigo.

A newer medication that appears to be effective in treating the vertigo associated with Méniere's disease is flunarizine, which is sold under the trade name Sibelium. Flunarizine is a calcium channel blocker and anticonvulsant that is presently used to treat Parkinson's disease, migraine headache, and other circulatory disorders that affect the brain.

Surgical procedures

Surgical procedures may be recommended if the vertigo attacks are frequent, severe, or disabling and cannot be controlled by other treatments. The most common surgical treatment is insertion of a small tube or shunt to drain some of the fluid from the canal. This treatment usually preserves hearing and controls vertigo in about one-half to two-thirds of cases, but it is not a permanent cure in all patients.

The vestibular nerve leads from the inner ear to the brain and is responsible for conducting nerve impulses related to balance. A vestibular neurectomy is a procedure where this nerve is cut so the distorted impulses causing dizziness no longer reach the brain. This procedure permanently cures the majority of patients and hearing is preserved in most cases. There is a slight risk that hearing or facial muscle control will be affected.

A labyrinthectomy is a surgical procedure in which the balance and hearing mechanism in the inner ear are destroyed on one side. This procedure is considered when the patient has poor hearing in the affected ear. Labyrinthectomy results in the highest rates of control of vertigo attacks, however, it also causes complete deafness in the affected ear.

Alternative treatment

Changes in diet and behavior are sometimes recommended. Eliminating **caffeine**, alcohol, and salt may relieve the frequency and intensity of attacks in some people with Méniere's disease. Reducing **stress** levels and eliminating tobacco use may also help.

Acupuncture is an alternative treatment that has been shown to help patients with Méniere's disease. The World Health Organization (WHO) lists Méniere's disease as one of 104 conditions that can be treated effectively with acupuncture.

KEY TERMS

Myelin—A whitish fatty substance that acts like an electrical insulator around certain nerves in the peripheral nervous system. It is thought that the loss of the myelin surrounding the vestibular nerves may influence the development of Méniere's disease.

T cell—A type of white blood cell produced in the thymus gland that regulates the immune system's response to diseased or malignant cells. It is possible that a subcategory of T cells known as CD4 cells plays a role in Méniere's disease.

Tinnitus—A roaring, buzzing or ringing sound in the ears.

Transcutaneous electrical nerve stimulation (TENS)—A treatment in which a mild electrical current is passed through electrodes on the skin to stimulate nerves and block pain signals.

Vertigo—The medical term for dizziness or a spinning sensation.

Prognosis

Méniere's disease is a complex and unpredictable condition for which there is no cure. The vertigo associated with the disease can generally be managed or eliminated with medications and surgery. Hearing tends to become worse over time, and some of the surgical procedures recommended, in fact, cause deafness.

Prevention

Since the cause of Méniere's disease is unknown as of 2002, there are no current strategies for its prevention. Research continues on the environmental and biological factors that may cause Méniere's disease or induce an attack, as well as on the physiological components of the fluid and labyrinth system involved in hearing and balance. Preventive strategies and more effective treatment should become evident once these mechanisms are better understood.

Resources

BOOKS

Beers, Mark H., MD, and Robert Berkow, MD, editors. *The Merck Manual of Diagnosis and Therapy.* Whitehouse Station, NJ: Merck Research Laboratories, 2004.

Pelletier, Kenneth R., MD. *The Best Alternative Medicine,* Part II. "CAM Therapies for Specific Conditions: Ménière's Disease." New York: Simon & Schuster, 2002.

PERIODICALS

Ballester, M., P. Liard, D. Vibert, and R. Hausler. "Ménière's Disease in the Elderly." *Otology and Neurotology* 23 (January 2002): 73–78.

Corvera, J., G. Corvera-Behar, V. Lapilover, and A. Ysunza. "Objective Evaluation of the Effect of Flunarizine on Vestibular Neuritis." *Otology and Neurotology* 23 (November 2002): 933–937.

Friberg, U., and H. Rask-Andersen. "Vascular Occlusion in the Endolymphatic Sac in Ménière's Disease." *Annals of Otology, Rhinology, and Laryngology* 111 (March 2002): 237–245.

Fung, K., Y. Xie, S. F. Hall, et al. "Genetic Basis of Familial Ménière's Disease." *Journal of Otolaryngology* 31 (February 2002): 1–4.

Ghosh, S., A. K. Gupta, and S. S. Mann. "Can Electrocochleography in Ménière's Disease Be Noninvasive?" *Journal of Otolaryngology* 31 (December 2002): 371–375.

Mamikoglu, B., R. J. Wiet, T. Hain, and I. J. Check. "Increased CD4 + T cells During Acute Attack of Ménière's Disease." *Acta Otolaryngologica* 122 (December 2002): 857–860.

Radtke, A., T. Lempert, M. A. Gresty, et al. "Migraine and Ménière's Disease: Is There a Link?" *Neurology* 59 (December 10, 2002): 1700–1704.

Spencer, R. F., A. Sismanis, J. K. Kilpatrick, and W. T. Shaia. "Demyelination of Vestibular Nerve Axons in Unilateral Ménière's Disease." *Ear, Nose and Throat Journal* 81 (November 2002): 785–789.

Steenerson, Ronald L., and Gaye W. Cronin. "Treatment of Tinnitus with Electrical Stimulation." *Otolaryngology-Head and Neck Surgery* 121 (November 1999): 511–513.

Yetiser, S., and M. Kertmen. "Intratympanic Gentamicin in Ménière's Disease: The Impact on Tinnitus." *International Journal of Audiology* 41 (September 2002): 363–370.

ORGANIZATIONS

American Academy of Otolaryngology-Head and Neck Surgery, Inc. One Prince St., Alexandria VA 22314-3357. (703) 836-4444. < http://www.entnet.org >.

Ménière's Network. 2000 Church St., P.O. Box 111, Nashville, TN 37236. (800) 545-4327. < http://www.healthy.net/pan/cso/cioi/mn.htm >.

On-Balance, A Support Group for People with Ménière's Disease. < http://www.midwestear.com/onbal.htm >.

Vestibular Disorders Association. P.O. Box 4467, Portland, OR 97208-4467. (800) 837-8428.

Altha Roberts Edgren
Rebecca J. Frey, PhD

Meningioma *see* **Brain tumor**

Meningitis

Definition

Meningitis is a serious inflammation of the meninges, the thin, membranous covering of the brain and the spinal cord. Meningitis is most commonly caused by infection (by bacteria, viruses, or fungi), although it can also be caused by bleeding into the meninges, **cancer**, diseases of the immune system, and an inflammatory response to certain types of **chemotherapy** or other chemical agents. The most serious and difficult-to-treat types of meningitis tend to be those caused by bacteria. In some cases, meningitis can be a potentially fatal condition.

Description

Meningitis is a particularly dangerous infection because of the very delicate nature of the brain. Brain cells are some of the only cells in the body that, once killed, will not regenerate themselves. Therefore, if enough brain tissue is damaged by an infection, serious, life-long handicaps will remain.

In order to learn about meningitis, it is important to have a basic understanding of the anatomy of the brain. The meninges are three separate membranes, layered together, which encase the brain and spinal cord:

- The dura is the toughest, outermost layer, and is closely attached to the inside of the skull.

- The middle layer, the arachnoid, is important because of its involvement in the normal flow of the cerebrospinal fluid (CSF), a lubricating and nutritive fluid that bathes both the brain and the spinal cord.

- The innermost layer, the pia, helps direct blood vessels into the brain.

- The space between the arachnoid and the pia contains CSF, which helps insulate the brain from trauma. Many blood vessels course through this space.

CSF, produced within specialized chambers deep inside the brain, flows over the surface of the brain and spinal cord. This fluid serves to cushion these relatively delicate structures, as well as supplying important nutrients for brain cells. CSF is reabsorbed by blood vessels located within the meninges. A careful balance between CSF production and reabsorption is important to avoid the accumulation of too much CSF.

Because the brain is enclosed in the hard, bony case of the skull, any disease that produces swelling

HATTIE ALEXANDER (1901–1968)

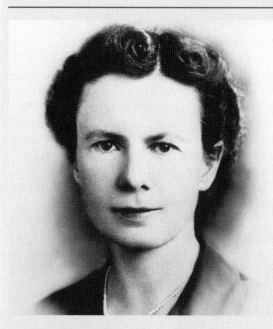

(Betmann/CORBIS. Reproduced by permission.)

Hattie Alexander, a dedicated pediatrician, medical educator, and researcher in microbiology, won international recognition for deriving a serum to combat influenzal meningitis, a common disease that previously had been nearly always fatal to infants and young children. Alexander subsequently investigated microbiological genetics and the processes whereby bacteria, through genetic mutation, acquire resistance to antibiotics. In 1964, as president of the American Pediatric Society, she became one of the first women to head a national medical association.

As an intern at the Harriet Lane Home of Johns Hopkins Hospital from 1930 to 1931, Alexander became interested in influenzal meningitis. The source of the disease was *Hemophilus influenzae*, a bacteria that causes inflammation of the meninges, the membranes surrounding the brain and spinal cord. In 1931, Alexander began a second internship at the Babies Hospital of the Columbia-Presbyterian Medical Center in New York City. There, she witnessed first-hand the futility of medical efforts to save babies who had contracted influenzal meningitis.

Alexander's early research focused on deriving a serum (the liquid component of blood, in which antibodies are contained) that would be effective against influenzal meningitis. Serums derived from animals that have been exposed to a specific disease-producing bacterium often contain antibodies against the disease and can be developed for use in immunizing humans against it. Alexander knew that the Rockefeller Institute in New York City, however, had been able to prepare a rabbit serum for the treatment of pneumonia, another bacterial disease. Alexander therefore experimented with rabbit serums, and by 1939 was able to announce the development of a rabbit serum effective in curing infants of influenzal meningitis.

In the early 1940s, Alexander experimented with the use of drugs in combination with rabbit serum in the treatment of influenzal meningitis. Within the next two years, she saw infant deaths due to the disease drop by eighty percent.

will be damaging to the brain. The skull cannot expand at all, so when the swollen brain tissue pushes up against the skull's hard bone, the brain tissue becomes damaged and may ultimately die. Furthermore, swelling on the right side of the brain will not only cause pressure and damage to that side of the brain, but by taking up precious space within the tight confines of the skull, the left side of the brain will also be pushed up against the hard surface of the skull, causing damage to the left side of the brain as well.

Another way that infections injure the brain involves the way in which the chemical environment of the brain changes in response to the presence of an infection. The cells of the brain require a very well-regulated environment. Careful balance of oxygen, carbon dioxide, sugar (glucose), sodium, calcium, potassium, and other substances must be maintained in order to avoid damage to brain tissue. An infection upsets this balance, and brain damage can occur when the cells of the brain are either deprived of important nutrients or exposed to toxic levels of particular substances.

The cells lining the brain's tiny blood vessels (capillaries) are specifically designed to prevent many substances from passing into brain tissue. This is commonly referred to as the blood-brain barrier. The blood-brain barrier prevents various substances that could be poisonous to brain tissue (toxins), as well as many agents of infection, from crossing from the blood stream into the brain tissue. While this barrier is obviously an important protective feature for the brain, it also serves to complicate treatment in the case of an infection by making it difficult for medications to pass out of the blood and into the brain tissue where the infection is located.

Causes and symptoms

The most common infectious causes of meningitis vary according to an individual's age, habits, living environment, and health status. While nonbacterial types of meningitis are more common, bacterial meningitis is the more potentially life-threatening. Three bacterial agents are responsible for about 80% of all bacterial meningitis cases. These bacteria are *Haemophilus influenzae* type b, *Neisseria meningitidis* (causing meningococcal meningitis), and *Streptococcus pneumoniae* (causing pneumococcal meningitis).

In newborns, the most common agents of meningitis are those that are contracted from the newborn's mother, including Group B streptococci (becoming an increasingly common infecting organism in the newborn period), *Escherichia coli*, and *Listeria monocytogenes*. The highest incidence of meningitis occurs in babies under a month old, with an increased risk of meningitis continuing through about two years of age.

Older children are more frequently infected by the bacteria *Haemophilus influenzae*, *Neisseria meningitidis*, and *Streptococci pneumoniae*.

Adults are most commonly infected by either *S. pneumoniae* or *N. meningitidis*, with pneumococcal meningitis the more common. Certain conditions predispose to this type of meningitis, including **alcoholism** and chronic upper respiratory tract infections (especially of the middle ear, sinuses, and mastoids).

N. meningitidis is the only organism that can cause epidemics of meningitis. In particular, these have occurred when a child in a crowded day-care situation or a military recruit in a crowded training camp has fallen ill with meningococcal meningitis.

Viral causes of meningitis include the herpes simplex virus, the **mumps** and **measles** viruses (against which most children are protected due to mass immunization programs), the virus that causes chicken pox, the **rabies** virus, and a number of viruses that are acquired through the bites of infected mosquitoes.

A number of medical conditions predispose individuals to meningitis caused by specific organisms. Patients with **AIDS** (acquired immune deficiency syndrome) are more prone to getting meningitis from fungi, as well as from the agent that causes **tuberculosis**. Patients who have had their spleens removed, or whose spleens are no longer functional (as in the case of patients with **sickle cell disease**) are more susceptible to other infections, including meningococcal and pneumococcal meningitis.

The majority of meningitis infections are acquired by blood-borne spread. A person may have another type of infection (of the lungs, throat, or tissues of the heart) caused by an organism that can also cause meningitis. If this initial infection is not properly treated, the organism will continue to multiply, find its way into the blood stream, and be delivered in sufficient quantities to invade past the blood brain barrier. Direct spread occurs when an organism spreads to the meninges from infected tissue next to or very near the meninges. This can occur, for example, with a severe, poorly treated ear or sinus infection.

Patients who suffer from skull **fractures** possess abnormal openings to the sinuses, nasal passages, and middle ears. Organisms that usually live in the human respiratory system without causing disease can pass through openings caused by such fractures, reach the meninges, and cause infection. Similarly, patients who undergo surgical procedures or who have had foreign bodies surgically placed within their skulls (such as tubes to drain abnormal amounts of accumulated CSF) have an increased risk of meningitis.

Organisms can also reach the meninges via an uncommon but interesting method called intraneural spread. This involves an organism invading the body at a considerable distance away from the head, spreading along a nerve, and using that nerve as a kind of ladder into the skull, where the organism can multiply and cause meningitis. Herpes simplex virus is known to use this type of spread, as is the rabies virus.

The most classic symptoms of meningitis (particularly of bacterial meningitis) include **fever**, **headache**, **vomiting**, sensitivity to light (photophobia), irritability, severe **fatigue** (lethargy), stiff neck, and a reddish purple rash on the skin. Untreated, the disease progresses with seizures, confusion, and eventually **coma**.

A very young infant may not show the classic signs of meningitis. Early in infancy, a baby's immune system is not yet developed enough to mount a fever in response to infection, so fever may be absent. Some infants with meningitis have seizures as their only identifiable symptom. Similarly, debilitated elderly patients may not have fever or other identifiable symptoms of meningitis.

Damage due to meningitis occurs from a variety of phenomena. The action of infectious agents on the brain tissue is one direct cause of damage. Other types of damage may be due to the mechanical effects of swelling and compression of brain tissue against the bony surface of the skull. Swelling of the meninges may interfere with the normal absorption of CSF by blood vessels, causing accumulation of CSF and damage from the resulting pressure on the brain.

Interference with the brain's carefully regulated chemical environment may cause damaging amounts of normally present substances (carbon dioxide, potassium) to accumulate. Inflammation may cause the blood-brain barrier to become less effective at preventing the passage of toxic substances into brain tissue.

Diagnosis

A number of techniques are used when examining a patient suspected of having meningitis to verify the diagnosis. Certain manipulations of the head (lowering the head, chin towards chest, for example) are difficult to perform and painful for a patient with meningitis.

The most important test used to diagnose meningitis is the lumbar puncture (commonly called a spinal tap). Lumbar puncture (LP) involves the insertion of a thin needle into a space between the vertebrae in the lower back and the withdrawal of a small amount of CSF. The CSF is then examined under a microscope to look for bacteria or fungi. Normal CSF contains set percentages of glucose and protein. These percentages will vary with bacterial, viral, or other causes of meningitis. For example, bacterial meningitis causes a greatly lower than normal percentage of glucose to be present in CSF, as the bacteria are essentially "eating" the host's glucose, and using it for their own **nutrition** and energy production. Normal CSF should contain no infection-fighting cells (white blood cells), so the presence of white blood cells in CSF is another indication of meningitis. Some of the withdrawn CSF is also put into special lab dishes to allow growth of the infecting organism, which can then be identified more easily. Special immunologic and serologic tests may also be used to help identify the infectious agent.

In rare instances, CSF from a lumbar puncture cannot be examined because the amount of swelling within the skull is so great that the pressure within the skull (intracranial pressure) is extremely high. This pressure is always measured immediately upon insertion of the LP needle. If it is found to be very high, no fluid is withdrawn because doing so could cause herniation of the brain stem. Herniation of the brain stem occurs when the part of the brain connecting to the spinal cord is thrust through the opening at the base of the skull into the spinal canal. Such herniation will cause compression of those structures within the brain stem that control the most vital functions of the body (breathing, heart beat, consciousness). **Death** or permanent debilitation follows herniation of the brain stem.

KEY TERMS

Blood-brain barrier—An arrangement of cells within the blood vessels of the brain that prevents the passage of toxic substances, including infectious agents, from the blood and into the brain. It also makes it difficult for certain medications to pass into brain tissue.

Cerebrospinal fluid (CSF)—Fluid made in chambers within the brain which then flows over the surface of the brain and spinal cord. CSF provides nutrition to cells of the nervous system, as well as providing a cushion for the nervous system structures. It may accumulate abnormally in some disease processes, causing pressure on and damage to brain structures.

Lumbar puncture (LP)—A medical test in which a very narrow needle is inserted into a specific space between the vertebrae of the lower back in order to draw off a sample of CSF for further examination.

Meninges—The three-layer membranous covering of the brain and spinal cord, composed of the dura, arachnoid, and pia. It provides protection for the brain and spinal cord, as well as housing many blood vessels and participating in the appropriate flow of CSF.

Treatment

Antibiotic medications (forms of penicillin and **cephalosporins**, for example) are the most important element of treatment against bacterial agents of meningitis. Because of the effectiveness of the blood-brain barrier in preventing the passage of substances into the brain, medications must be delivered directly into the patient's veins (intravenously, or by IV), at very high doses. **Antiviral drugs** (acyclovir) may be helpful in shortening the course of viral meningitis, and antifungal medications are available as well.

Other treatments for meningitis involve decreasing inflammation (with steroid preparations) and paying careful attention to the balance of fluids, glucose, sodium, potassium, oxygen, and carbon dioxide in the patient's system. Patients who develop seizures will require medications to halt the seizures and prevent their return.

Prognosis

Viral meningitis is the least severe type of meningitis, and patients usually recover with no long-term effects from the infection. Bacterial infections, however, are much more severe, and progress rapidly. Without very rapid treatment with the appropriate antibiotic, the infection can swiftly lead to coma and death in less than a day's time. While death rates from meningitis vary depending on the specific infecting organism, the overall death rate is just under 20%.

The most frequent long-term effects of meningitis include deafness and blindness, which may be caused by the compression of specific nerves and brain areas responsible for the senses of hearing and sight. Some patients develop permanent seizure disorders, requiring life-long treatment with anti-seizure medications. Scarring of the meninges may result in obstruction of the normal flow of CSF, causing abnormal accumulation of CSF. This may be a chronic problem for some patients, requiring the installation of shunt tubes to drain the accumulation regularly.

Prevention

Prevention of meningitis primarily involves the appropriate treatment of other infections an individual may acquire, particularly those that have a track record of seeding to the meninges (such as ear and sinus infections). Preventive treatment with **antibiotics** is sometimes recommended for the close contacts of an individual who is ill with meningococcal or *H. influenzae* type b meningitis. A meningococcal vaccine exists, and is sometimes recommended to individuals who are traveling to very high risk areas. A vaccine for *H. influenzae* type b is now given to babies as part of the standard array of childhood immunizations.

Resources

ORGANIZATIONS

American Academy of Neurology. 1080 Montreal Ave., St. Paul, MN 55116. (612) 695-1940. < http://www.aan.com >.

Meningitis Foundation of America. 7155 Shadeland Station, Suite 190, Indianapolis, IN 46256-3922. (800) 668-1129. < http://www.musa.org/welcome.htm >.

Rosalyn Carson-DeWitt, MD

Meningocele *see* **Spina bifida**

Meningococcemia

Definition

Meningococcemia is the presence of meningococcus in the bloodstream. Meningococcus, a bacteria formally called *Neisseria meningitidis*, can be one of the most dramatic and rapidly fatal of all infectious diseases.

Causes and symptoms

Meningococcemia, a relatively uncommon infection, occurs most commonly in children and young adults. In susceptible people, it may cause a very severe illness that can produce **death** within hours. The bacteria, which can spread from person to person, usually first causes a colonization in the upper airway, but without symptoms. From there, it can penetrate into the bloodstream to the central nervous system and cause **meningitis** or develop into a full-blown bloodstream infection (meningococcemia). Fortunately in most colonized people, this does not happen and the result of this colonization is long-lasting immunity against the particular strain.

After colonization is established, symptoms can develop within one day to one to two weeks. After a short period of time (one hour up to one to two days) when the patient complains of **fever** and muscle aches, more severe symptoms can develop. Unfortunately during this early stage, a doctor cannot tell this illness from any other illness, such as a viral infection like **influenza**. Unless the case is occurring in a person known to have been exposed to or in the midst of an epidemic of meningococcal disease, there may be no specific symptoms or signs found that help the doctor diagnose the problem. Rarely, a low-grade bloodstream infection called chronic meningococcemia can occur.

After this initial period, the patient will often complain of continued fever, shaking chills, overwhelming weakness, and even a feeling of impending doom. The organism is multiplying in the bloodstream, unchecked by the immune system. The severity of the illness and its dire complications are caused by the damage the organism does to the small blood vessel walls. This damage is called a **vasculitis**, an inflammation of a blood vessel. Damage to the small vessels causes them to become leaky. The first signs of the infection's severity are small bleeding spots seen on the skin (petechiae). A doctor should always suspect meningococcemia when he/she finds an acutely ill patient with fever, chills, and petechiae.

Quickly (within hours), the blood vessel damage increases and large bleeding areas on the skin (purpura) are seen. The same changes are taking place in the affected person's internal organs. The blood pressure is often low and there may be signs of bleeding from other organs (like coughing up

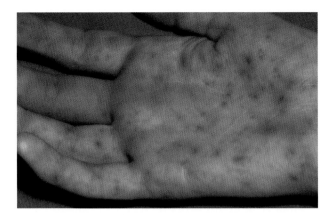

A close-up image of a person's hand with meningococcemia. This disease is caused by the presence of meningococcus (*Neisseria meningitidis*) in the bloodstream. The organism can cause multiple illnesses and can damage small blood vessels. (*Custom Medical Stock Photo. Reproduced by permission.*)

blood, nose bleeds, blood in the urine). The organism not only damages the blood vessels by causing them to leak, but also causes clotting inside the vessels. If this clotting occurs in the larger arteries, it results in major tissue damage. Essentially, large areas of skin, muscle, and internal organs die from lack of blood and oxygen. Even if the disease is quickly diagnosed and treated, the patient has a high risk of dying.

Diagnosis

The diagnosis of meningococcemia can be made by the growth of the organism from blood cultures. Treatment should begin when the diagnosis is suspected and should not be delayed waiting for positive cultures. Obtaining fluid from a petechial spot and staining it in the laboratory can assist in quickly seeing the organism.

Treatment

Immediate treatment of a suspected case of meningococcemia begins with **antibiotics** that work against the organism. Possible choices include penicillin G, ceftriaxone (Rocephin), cefotaxime (Claforan), or trimethoprim/sulfamethoxazole (Bactrim, Septra). If the patient is diagnosed in a doctor's office, antibiotics should be given immediately if possible, even before transfer to the hospital and even if cultures cannot be obtained before treatment. It is most likely that the speed of initial treatment will affect the ultimate outcome.

Prognosis

As many as 15-20% of patients with meningococcemia will die as a result of the acute infection. A significant percentage of the survivors will have tissue damage that requires surgical treatment. This treatment may consist of skin grafts, or even partial or full amputations of an arm or leg. Certain people with immune system defects (particularly those with defects in the complement system) may have recurrent episodes of meningococcemia. These patients, however, seem to have a less serious outcome.

Prevention

Although a vaccine is available for meningococcus, it is still difficult at this time to produce a vaccine for the type B organism, the most common one in the United States. Because of this and the short time that the vaccine seems to offer protection, the product has not been routinely used in the United States. It can be used for travelers going to areas where meningococcal disease is more common or is epidemic. Recently, the vaccine has been suggested for use in incoming college freshman, particularly those living in dormitories. These students appear to have a somewhat higher risk of meningococcal infections.

It is, however, recommended that all people take certain antibiotics if they have had contact (like at home or in a daycare) with a person who has meningococcal infection. The most common antibiotics given are rifampin (Rifadin) or ciprofloxacin (Cipro). These medicines are usually taken by mouth twice a day for two days. This treatment will decrease the risk of infection in these people who have been exposed. However, the overall risk to people who have been exposed, even without antibiotic use, is probably no more than 1-2%.

Resources

PERIODICALS

Salzman, Mark B., and Lorry G. Rubin. "Meningococcemia." *Infectious Disease Clinics of North America* 10 (December 1996): 709-725.

Larry I. Lutwick, MD

Meningomyelocele *see* **Spina bifida**

Menkes' syndrome *see* **Mineral deficiency**

Menopause

Definition

Menopause represents the end of menstruation. While technically it refers to the final period, it is not an abrupt event, but a gradual process. Menopause is not a disease that needs to be cured, but a natural life-stage transition. However, women have to make important decisions about "treatment," including the use of **hormone replacement therapy** (HRT).

Description

Many women have irregular periods and other problems of "pre-menopause" for years. It is not easy to predict when menopause begins, although doctors agree it is complete when a woman has not had a period for a year. Eight out of every 100 women stop menstruating before age 40. At the other end of the spectrum, five out of every 100 continue to have periods until they are almost 60. The average age of menopause is 51.

There is no mathematical formula to figure out when the ovaries will begin to scale back either, but a woman can get a general idea based on her family history, body type, and lifestyle. Women who began menstruating early will not necessarily stop having periods early as well. It is true that a woman will likely enter menopause at about the same age as her mother. Menopause may occur later than average among smokers.

Causes and symptoms

Once a woman enters **puberty**, each month her body releases one of the more than 400,000 eggs that are stored in her ovaries, and the lining of the womb (uterus) thickens in anticipation of receiving a fertilized egg. If the egg is not fertilized, progesterone levels drop and the uterine lining sheds and bleeds.

By the time a woman reaches her late 30s or 40s, her ovaries begin to shut down, producing less estrogen and progesterone and releasing eggs less often. The gradual decline of estrogen causes a wide variety of changes in tissues that respond to estrogen—including the vagina, vulva, uterus, bladder, urethra, breasts, bones, heart, blood vessels, brain, skin, hair, and mucous membranes. Over the long run, the lack of estrogen can make a woman more vulnerable to **osteoporosis** (which can begin in the 40s) and heart disease.

As the levels of hormones fluctuate, the menstrual cycle begins to change. Some women may have longer periods with heavy flow followed by shorter cycles and hardly any bleeding. Others will begin to miss periods completely. During this time, a woman also becomes less able to get pregnant.

The most common symptom of menopause is a change in the menstrual cycle, but there are a variety of other symptoms as well, including:

- hot flashes
- night sweats
- **insomnia**
- mood swings/irritability
- memory or concentration problems
- vaginal dryness
- heavy bleeding
- **fatigue**
- depression
- hair changes
- headaches
- heart **palpitations**
- sexual disinterest
- urinary changes
- weight gain

Diagnosis

The clearest indication of menopause is the absence of a period for one year. It is also possible to diagnose menopause by testing hormone levels. One important test measures the levels of follicle-stimulating hormone (FSH), which steadily increases as a woman ages.

However, as a woman first enters menopause, her hormones often fluctuate wildly from day to day. For example, if a woman's estrogen levels are high and progesterone is low, she may have mood swings, irritability, and other symptoms similar to **premenstrual syndrome** (PMS). As hormone levels shift and estrogen level falls, hot flashes occur. Because of these fluctuations, a normal hormone level when the blood is tested may not necessarily mean the levels were normal the day before or will be the day after.

If it has been at least three months since a woman's last period, an FSH test might be more helpful in determining whether menopause has occurred. Most doctors believe that the FSH test alone cannot be used as proof that a woman has entered early menopause. A better measure of menopause is a test that checks the levels of estrogen, progesterone, testosterone and other hormones at mid-cycle, in addition to FSH.

Treatment

When a woman enters menopause, her levels of estrogen drop and symptoms (such as hot flashes and vaginal dryness) begin. Hormone replacement therapy can treat these symptoms by boosting the estrogen levels enough to suppress symptoms while also providing protection against heart disease and osteoporosis, which causes the bones to weaken. Experts disagree on whether HRT increases or decreases the risk of developing **breast cancer**. A Harvard study concluded that short-term use of hormones carries little risk, while HRT used for more than five years among women 55 and over seems to increase the risk of breast **cancer**.

There are two types of hormone treatments: hormone replacement therapy (HRT) and estrogen replacement therapy (ERT). HRT is the administration of estrogen and progesterone; ERT is the administration of estrogen alone. Only women who have had a **hysterectomy** (removal of the uterus) can take estrogen alone, since taking this "unopposed" estrogen can cause uterine cancer. The combination of progesterone and estrogen in HRT eliminates the risk of uterine cancer.

Most physicians do not recommend HRT until a woman's periods have stopped completely for one year. This is because women in early menopause who still have an occasional period are still producing estrogen; HRT would then provide far too much estrogen.

Most doctors believe that every woman (except those with certain cancers) should take hormones as they approach menopause because of the protection against heart disease, osteoporosis, and uterine cancer and the relatively low risk of breast cancer. Heart disease and osteoporosis are two of the leading causes of disability and **death** among post-menopausal women.

Critics say the benefit of taking hormonal drugs to ease symptoms is not worth the risk of breast cancer. Since menopause is not a disease, many argue that women should not take hormones to cure what is actually a natural process of **aging**. Advocates of HRT contend that the purpose of taking hormones is not to "treat" menopause but to prevent the development of other diseases.

There are risks with HRT and there are risks without it. In order to decide whether to take HRT, a woman should balance her risk of getting breast cancer against her risk of getting heart disease, and decide how bad her menopause symptoms are. Most doctors agree that short-term use of estrogen for those women with symptoms of hot flashes or night sweats is a sensible choice as long as they do not have a history of breast cancer.

For a woman who has no family history of cancer and a high risk of dying from heart disease, for example, the low risk of cancer might be worth the protective benefit of avoiding heart disease. Certainly, for Caucasian women aged 50 to 94, the risk of dying from heart disease is far greater than the risk of dying of breast cancer.

Women are poor candidates for hormone replacement therapy if they have:

- had breast or **endometrial cancer**
- a close relative (mother, sister, grandmother) who died of breast cancer or have two relatives who developed breast cancer before age 40
- had endometrial cancer
- had gallbladder or **liver disease**
- blood clots or phlebitis

Some women with liver or gallbladder disease, or who have clotting problems, may be able to go on HRT if they use a patch to administer the hormones through the skin, bypassing the liver.

Women would make a good candidate for HRT if they:

- need to prevent osteoporosis
- have had their ovaries removed

• need to prevent heart disease

• have significant symptoms.

Taking hormones can almost immediately eliminate hot flashes, vaginal dryness, **urinary incontinence** (depending on the cause), insomnia, moodiness, memory problems, heavy irregular periods, and concentration problems. Side effects of treatment include bloating, breakthrough bleeding, headaches, vaginal discharge, fluid retention, swollen breasts, or **nausea**. Up to 20% of women who try hormone replacement stop within nine months because of these side effects. However, some side effects can be lessened or prevented by changing the HRT regimen.

The decision should be made by a woman and her doctor after taking into consideration her medical history and situation. Women who choose to take hormones should have an annual mammogram, breast exam, and **pelvic exam** and should report any unusual vaginal bleeding or spotting (a sign of possible uterine cancer).

Anti-estrogens

A new type of hormone therapy offers some of the same protection against heart disease and bone loss as estrogen, but without the increased risk of breast cancer. This new class of drugs are known as anti-estrogens. The best known of these anti-estrogens is raloxifene, which mimics the effects of estrogen in the bones and blood, but blocks some of its negative effects elsewhere. It is called an anti-estrogen because for a long time these drugs had been used to counter the harmful effects of estrogen that caused breast cancer. Oddly enough, in other parts of the body these drugs mimic estrogen, protecting against heart disease and osteoporosis without putting a woman at risk for breast cancer.

Like estrogen, raloxifene works by attaching to an estrogen "receptor," much like a key fits into a lock. When raloxifene clicks into the estrogen receptors in the breast and uterus, it blocks estrogen at these sites. This is the secret of its cancer-fighting property. Many tumors in the breast are fueled by estrogen; if the estrogen cannot get in the cell, then the cancer stops growing.

Women may prefer to take raloxifene instead of hormone replacement because the new drug does not boost the breast cancer risk and does not have side effects like uterine bleeding, bloating, or breast soreness. Unfortunately, the drug may worsen hot flashes. Raloxifene is basically a treatment to prevent osteoporosis. It does not help with common symptoms and

it is unclear if it has the same protective effect against heart disease as estrogen does.

Testosterone replacement

The ovaries also produce a small amount of male hormones, which decreases slightly as a woman enters menopause. The vast majority of women never need testosterone replacement, but it can be important if a woman has declining interest in sex. Testosterone can improve the libido, and decrease **anxiety** and depression; adding testosterone especially helps women who have had hysterectomies. Testosterone also eases breast tenderness and helps prevent bone loss. However, testosterone does have side effects. Some women experience mild **acne** and some facial hair growth, but because only small amounts of testosterone are prescribed, most women do not appear to have extreme masculine changes.

Birth control pills

Women who are still having periods but who have annoying menopausal symptoms may take low-dose birth control pills to ease the problems; this treatment has been approved by the FDA for perimenopausal symptoms in women under age 55. HRT is the preferred treatment for menopause, however, because it uses lower doses of estrogen.

Alternative treatment

Some women also report success in using natural remedies to treat the unpleasant symptoms of menopause. Not all women need estrogen and some women cannot take it. Many doctors don't want to give hormones to women who are still having their periods, however erratically. Indeed, only a third of menopausal women in the United States try HRT and of those who do, eventually half of them drop the therapy. Some are worried about breast cancer, some cannot tolerate the side effects, some do not want to medicate what they consider to be a natural occurrence.

Herbs

Herbs have been used to relieve menopausal symptoms for centuries. In general, most herbs are considered safe, and there is no substantial evidence that herbal products are a major source of toxic reactions. But because herbal products are not regulated in the United States, contamination or accidental overdose is possible. Herbs should be bought from a recognized company or through a qualified herbal practitioner.

Women who choose to take herbs for menopausal symptoms should learn as much as possible about herbs and work with a qualified practitioner (an herbalist, a traditional Chinese doctor, or a naturopathic physician). Pregnant women should avoid herbs because of unknown effects on a developing fetus.

The following list of herbs include those that herbalists most often prescribe to treat menstrual complaints:

- Black cohosh (*Cimicifuga racemosa*): hot flashes and other menstrual complaints

- Black currant: breast tenderness

- Chaste tree/chasteberry (*Vitex agnus-castus*): hot flashes, excessive menstrual bleeding, fibroids, and moodiness

- Evening primrose oil (*Oenothera biennis*): mood swings, irritability, and breast tenderness

- Fennel (*Foeniculum vulgare*): hot flashes, digestive gas, and bloating

- Flaxseed (linseed): excessive menstrual bleeding, breast tenderness, and other symptoms, including dry skin and vaginal dryness

- Gingko (*Gingko biloba*): memory problems

- Ginseng (*Panax ginseng*): hot flashes, fatigue and vaginal thinning.

- Hawthorn (*Crataegus laevigata*): memory problems, fuzzy thinking

- Lady's mantle: excessive menstrual bleeding

- Mexican wild yam (*Dioscorea villosa*) root: vaginal dryness, hot flashes and general menopause symptoms

- Motherwort (*Leonurus cardiaca*): night sweats, hot flashes

- Oat (*Avena sativa*) straw: mood swings, anxiety

- Red clover (*Trifolium pratense*): hot flashes

- Sage (*Salvia officinalis*): mood swings, headaches, night sweats

- Valerian (*Valeriana officinalis*): insomnia.

Natural estrogens (phytoestrogens)

Proponents of plant estrogens (including soy products) believe that plant estrogens are better than synthetic estrogen, but science has not yet proven this. The results of smaller preliminary trials suggest that the estrogen compounds in soy products can indeed relieve the severity of hot flashes and lower cholesterol. But no one yet has proven that soy can provide all the benefits of synthetic estrogen without its negative effects.

It is true that people in other countries who eat foods high in plant estrogens (especially soy products) have lower rates of breast cancer and report fewer "symptoms" of menopause. While up to 80% of menopausal women in the United States complain of hot flashes, night sweats, and vaginal dryness, only 15% of Japanese women have similar complaints. When all other things are equal, a soy-based diet may make a difference (and soy is very high in plant estrogens).

The study of phytoestrogens is so new that there are not very many recommendations on how much a woman can consume. Herbal practitioners recommend a dose based on a woman's history, body size, lifestyle, diet, and reported symptoms. Research has indicated that some women were able to ease their symptoms by eating a large amount of fruits, vegetables, and whole grains, together with four ounces of tofu four times a week.

What concerns some critics of other alternative remedies is that many women think that "natural" or "plant-based" means "harmless." In large doses, phytoestrogens can promote the abnormal growth of cells in the uterine lining. Unopposed estrogen of any type can lead to endometrial cancer, which is why women on conventional estrogen-replacement therapy usually take progesterone (progestin) along with their estrogen. However, a plant-based progesterone product can sometimes be effective alone, without estrogen, in assisting the menopausal woman in rebalancing her hormonal action throughout this transition time.

Yoga

Many women find that **yoga** (the ancient meditation/exercise developed in India 5,000 years ago) can ease menopausal symptoms. Yoga focuses on helping women unite the mind, body, and spirit to create balance. Because yoga has been shown to balance the endocrine system, some experts believe it may affect hormone-related problems. Studies have found that yoga can reduce **stress**, improve mood, boost a sluggish metabolism, and slow the heart rate. Specific yoga positions deal with particular problems, such as hot flashes, mood swings, vaginal and urinary problems, and other pains.

Exercise

Exercise helps ease hot flashes by lowering the amount of circulating FSH and LH and by raising endorphin levels that drop while having a hot flash. Even exercising 20 minutes three times a week can significantly reduce hot flashes.

KEY TERMS

Endometrium—The lining of the uterus that is shed with each menstrual period.

Estrogen—Female hormone produced by the ovaries and released by the follicles as they mature. Responsible for female sexual characteristics, estrogen stimulates and triggers a response from at least 300 tissues, and may help some types of breast cancer to grow. After menopause, the production of the hormone gradually stops.

Estrogen replacement therapy (ERT)—A treatment for menopause in which estrogen is given in pill, patch, or cream form.

Follicle-stimulating hormone (FSH)—The pituitary hormone that stimulates the ovary to mature egg capsules (follicles). It is linked with rising estrogen production throughout the cycle. An elevated FSH (above 40) indicates menopause.

Hormone—A chemical messenger secreted by a gland that is released into the blood, and that travels to distant cells where it exerts an effect.

Hormone replacement therapy (HRT)—The use of estrogen and progesterone to replace hormones that the ovary no longer supplies.

Hot flash—A wave of heat that is one of the most common perimenopausal symptoms, triggered by the hypothalamus' response to estrogen withdrawal.

Hysterectomy—Surgical removal of the uterus.

Ovary—One of the two almond-shaped glands in the female reproductive system responsible for producing eggs and the hormones estrogen and progesterone.

Ovulation—The monthly release of an egg from the ovary.

Pituitary gland—The "master gland" at the base of the brain that secretes a number of hormones responsible for growth, reproduction, and other activities. Pituitary hormones stimulate the ovaries to release estrogen and progesterone.

Progesterone—The hormone that is produced by the ovary after ovulation to prepare the uterine lining for a fertilized egg.

Testosterone—Male hormone produced by the testes and (in small amounts) in the ovaries. Testosterone is responsible for some masculine secondary sex characteristics such as growth of body hair and deepening voice.

Uterus—The female reproductive organ that contains and nourishes a fetus from implantation until birth. Also known as the womb.

Vagina—The tube-like passage from the vulva (a woman's external genital structures) to the cervix (the portion of the uterus that projects into the vagina).

Elimination

Regular, daily bowel movements to eliminate waste products from the body can be crucial in maintaining balance through menopause. The bowels are where circulating hormones are gathered and eliminated, keeping the body from recycling them and causing an imbalance.

Acupuncture

This ancient Asian art involves placing very thin needles into different parts of the body to stimulate the system and unblock energy. It is usually painless and has been used for many menopausal symptoms, including insomnia, hot flashes, and irregular periods. Practitioners believe that **acupuncture** can facilitate the opening of blocked energy channels, allowing the life force energy (chi) to flow freely. This allows the menopausal woman to keep her energy moving. Blocked energy usually increases the symptoms of menopause.

Acupressure and massage

Therapeutic massage involving **acupressure** can bring relief from a wide range of menopause symptoms by placing finger pressure at the same meridian points on the body that are used in acupuncture. There are more than 80 different types of massage, including foot **reflexology**, **Shiatsu** massage, or Swedish massage, but they are all based on the idea that boosting the circulation of blood and lymph benefits health.

Biofeedback

Some women have been able to control hot flashes through **biofeedback**, a painless technique that helps a person train her mind to control her body. A biofeedback machine provides information about body processes (such as heart rate) as the woman relaxes her body. Using this technique, it is possible to control the body's temperature, heart rate, and breathing.

Prognosis

Menopause is a natural condition of aging. Some women have no problems at all with menopause, while others notice significant unpleasant symptoms. A wide array of treatments, from natural to hormone replacement, mean that no woman needs to suffer through this time of her life.

Prevention

Menopause is a natural part of the aging process and not a disease that needs to be prevented. Most doctors recommend HRT for almost all post-menopausal women, usually for a few years. When HRT is then stopped, symptoms should be mild or non existent. But HRT is not only useful in lessening the symptoms of menopause; it also protects against heart disease and osteoporosis.

Resources

BOOKS

Goldman, Lee, et al., editors. *Cecil Textbook of Medicine.* 21st ed. W. B. Saunders, 2000.
Goroll, Allan H., et al. *Primary Care Medicine.* 4th ed. Lippincott Williams &Wilkins, 2000.

OTHER

Menopause Online Page. < http://www.menopause-online .com/links.htm >.
Menopause Page. < http://www.howdyneighbor.com/ menopaus >.
Meno Times Online. < http://www.aimnet.com/~hyperion/ meno/menotimes.index.html >.

Laith Farid Gulli, M.D.

Menorrhagia *see* **Dysfunctional uterine bleeding**

▌Men's health

Definition

Men's health is concerned with identifying, preventing, and treating conditions that are most common or specific to men.

Purpose

Men live on average seven years less than women; life expectancy in the United States is 72 years for men and 79 years for women. The reasons for this discrepancy are not completely understood. Men may have some genetic predisposition for lower life expectancy, as women tend to outlive men in most areas throughout the world. But men also have different lifestyle patterns that increase the wear and tear on their bodies. Studies have shown that men tend to drink and smoke more than women, men obtain medical care less frequently than women, and men generally have more stressful habits. It is clear to health professionals that men can benefit from increased knowledge of male medical issues and by understanding how lifestyle choices impact health.

According to the Centers for Disease Control (CDC), the 10 leading causes of **death** for men in the United States are:

- heart disease
- **cancer**
- **stroke**
- accidents
- lung disease (including **emphysema** and chronic bronchitis)
- pneumonia
- diabetes
- **suicide**
- liver disease
- homicides

Men also suffer regularly from conditions as diverse as **sexually transmitted diseases** (STDs), mental illness, arthritis, urinary tract infections, athletic injuries, hair and skin problems, and digestive disorders. The field of men's health strives to reduce the risks and incidence of men's conditions by researching preventive practices, designing testing procedures for early detection, and recommending specialized courses of treatment.

Description

Prevention

Preventive practices for men's health emphasize diet, **exercise** and **stress** management, as well as the elimination of risky behaviors such as **smoking** and excessive drinking. Four of the leading causes of death for American men are related to diet—heart disease, cancer, stroke, and diabetes. In addition men are more likely than women to suffer from diet-related conditions including **high cholesterol**, high blood pressure, and **obesity**, all of which increase the risk of certain diseases and premature death.

For American men, dietary problems are usually not the result of getting too little nourishment but of eating too much fat, sugar, and overall calories. The dietary change most likely to improve the health of males is reduced intake of fats, particularly cholesterol and saturated fats. Cholesterol and saturated fats are found mainly in meat and dairy products. Calories from fat should amount to no more than 30% of total daily calories. Eating adequate protein is generally not a problem for American men, so replacing some dairy and meat consumption with high fiber vegetable proteins such as beans and soy would be beneficial. Complex carbohydrates should provide the bulk of daily calories, such as those from whole grains and legumes, while sugar intake such as in soft drinks, desserts and processed foods, should be significantly reduced. Increasing dietary fiber is recommended by eating plenty of fresh fruits, vegetables, whole grains, and legumes. Other principles of a healthy diet are avoiding artificial and processed foods, eating food that is as fresh and natural as possible, drinking plenty of water, and avoiding hydrogenated or partially hydrogenated oils, which contain unhealthy substances called trans-fatty acids. Overeating should be avoided as should snacking between meals, and alcohol intake should be limited to one or two glasses per day.

Exercise

The health of men has been affected as work patterns have shifted. Physical labor has been replaced by machines and office work. Studies have estimated that more than 30% of Americans are now obese, which means that nearly one out of three people is significantly overweight. Obesity poses many risks including increased chance of heart disease, diabetes, and some cancers. Effective exercise programs help men control weight, reduce stress, increase energy levels, improve self-esteem, reduce **pain** and injuries, and improve sleep. Exercise programs should emphasize flexibility and stretching as well as plenty of aerobic activities, such as running and swimming. These activities exercise the heart and lungs and burn excess calories. Men may also choose anaerobic activities such as weight training to add muscles and increase strength. Routines should begin with warm-ups to reduce the chances of injuries and end with cool-down exercises to speed recovery.

Stress reduction

Stress is a silent killer; chronic (long-term) stress is a risk factor in many of the major diseases affecting men's mortality rates. Prolonged stress also may cause ulcers, **sleep disorders**, addictions, depression, **anxiety**, and other conditions. Reduction of stress may require changes in both activities and attitudes. Exercise is recommended, as is reducing dependence on alcohol and nicotine. Men with extreme job-related stress may choose to spend more time with their families or in enjoyable activities. Men with stress levels that lead to destructive behaviors may need to pursue psychotherapy or significant lifestyle changes. **Nutrition**, social support, and healthy sleep patterns also reduce stress.

Alternative therapies may help with **stress reduction**. Their use has been adopted by many leading health centers. **Biofeedback** utilizes machines that monitor users' stress levels, helping people learn to control them. **Meditation** and other mind/body techniques are taught to enable the relaxation response, which has the opposite effects of stress in the body.

Testing

Routine physical examinations performed by physicians are recommended every three years for men in their twenties and thirties, every two years for men in their forties, and every year for men over 50. Physicians may order several screening tests as well, depending on the age and condition of the patient. Blood tests screen for diabetes, high cholesterol, cancer, infections, and HIV. The prostate-specific antigen (PSA) test is a blood screen for **prostate cancer**. The digital rectal exam is used to manually check the prostate gland for enlargement or irregularities. Urine tests check for infections, kidney problems, and diabetes. The **fecal occult blood test** examines the stool for indications of ulcers or cancer. A **sigmoidoscopy** checks the health of the rectum and lower colon. Electrocardiograms (ECGs) check the status of the heart. Older men may consult an ophthalmologist (eye specialist) every two years for vision and **glaucoma** testing.

Men may perform self-tests as preventative measures. During a skin cancer self-exam, the entire skin is checked closely for irregular or changing **moles**, lesions, or blemishes, usually red, white or blue in color. Abnormal findings should be reported to a physician. Like some forms of skin cancer, **testicular cancer** tends to spread rapidly and early detection is crucial. The testicular self-exam is best performed in the shower or bath, because warm water relaxes the scrotum. The testicles are gently rolled and massaged between the fingers and thumb to feel for bumps, swelling, tenderness, or irregularities. Some self-test kits are available in pharmacies, including kits for blood pressure, high cholesterol, colorectal cancer, and blood glucose (diabetes). These do not take the place of proper medical care, and physicians should be consulted before their use.

Heart disease

Heart disease is the major cause of death among men. It claims nearly 500,000 lives each year in the United States and is more likely in men than women. Heart disease can take several forms but the most prevalent is coronary heart disease, in which the blood vessels that supply the heart with oxygen become blocked and the heart muscle becomes increasingly stressed. Arteriosclerosis, a major factor, is the hardening of arteries due to the accumulation of fatty materials. **Hypertension**, or high blood pressure, also poses major risks for both heart disease and stroke. **Angina** pectoris is the chest pain associated with the early stages of heart disease; more than three million American men suffer from it. When the blockage of blood supply to the heart becomes severe, a myocardial infarction (**heart attack**) may occur, which can be fatal.

The main symptom of angina pectoris is sharp pain on the left side of the chest that may radiate throughout the upper body. Other symptoms include **shortness of breath**, **dizziness**, **fatigue**, and swelling in the legs and ankles. Angina may be triggered by physical or emotional stress and lasts up to 30 minutes. Heart attacks have similar symptoms but with longer and more intense pain in the chest and upper body and may be accompanied by cold sweats and **vomiting**.

The American Heart Association lists the main risk factors for heart disease as being male, old age, having family history of the disease, smoking, high cholesterol, high blood pressure, diabetes, **alcoholism**, obesity, physical inactivity and stress. Clearly, lifestyle habits such as diet, exercise and stress control play major roles in the development and prevention of heart disease in men.

Cancer

The American Cancer Society (ACS) estimates that more than 1.2 million cases of cancer were reported in 2000. Men have a slightly higher risk for cancer than women. The World Health Organization (WHO) estimates that the number of cancer cases in most countries will double in the next 25 years, while men's prostate cancer is expected to go up 40% worldwide. The most common cancers in men are skin, prostate, lung, colorectal (colon and rectum), lymphoma (lymph glands), oral (mouth and throat), and

testicular cancer. The ACS lists seven warning signs of cancer:

- Unusual bleeding or discharge
- Changes in bowel or bladder patterns
- Persistent sores
- Lumps or irregularities on the body
- Difficulty swallowing or indigestion
- Changes in **warts** or moles
- Persistent **cough** or hoarseness in the throat

Although the causes of cancer are incompletely understood, there are several risk factors that increase its chances: family history of cancer, smoking, poor diet (high in fat, low in fiber), excessive alcohol consumption, skin damage from sunlight, and exposure to radiation, chemicals, and environmental pollutants.

The prostate gland is a walnut-sized organ in the male reproductive system, located near the rectum below the bladder. The ACS reported that nearly 232,000 new cases of prostate cancer would be diagnosed in 2005, causing more than 30,000 deaths, making prostate cancer the second most fatal cancer for men behind lung cancer. Worldwide studies have shown that about 12% of men in Western countries get prostate cancer, while 50% have enlarged prostates. Benign prostatic hyperplasia (BPH) is the enlargement of the prostate gland, called benign when it is non-cancerous although growth can be rapid.

With early detection, 98% of men with prostate cancer survive for five years. Symptoms of prostate cancer include difficulty in stopping or starting urination, frequent nighttime urination (nocturia), weak urine flow, and blood in the urine or semen.

Testicular cancer is most common in men between the ages of 15 and 34. The ACS estimated that there would be about 8,100 new cases of testicular cancer in 2005 in the United States. A 2004 study showed that cigarette smoking increased risk of testicular cancer and quitting smoking did not reduce the risk.

Stroke

Strokes occur when the blood supply to the brain is interrupted and brain function becomes impaired due to lack of oxygen. Ischemic strokes occur due to blood vessels becoming blocked while hemorrhagic strokes are the result of broken blood vessels in or near the brain. Ischemic strokes account for about 80% of all strokes. The American Heart Association estimates that more than 600,000 Americans suffer from strokes each year, with men having a 20% higher risk of stroke than women, although more women die from strokes. Other risk factors are hypertension (high blood pressure), previous heart attacks, age, family history, high cholesterol, smoking, obesity, alcoholism, and physical inactivity. African Americans have 60% greater chances for strokes than whites.

Symptoms of strokes include sudden weakness or **numbness**, blurring or loss of vision, difficulty speaking or understanding, sudden severe **headache**, and dizziness or falling. Stroke victims should receive immediate emergency care.

Male urinary tract problems

The urinary system includes the kidneys and bladder, the ureters between the kidneys and bladder, and the urethra, the tube through which urine flows from the bladder. Symptoms of urinary tract problems include frequent urination, excessive urination at night, painful or burning urination, weak urination, blood in the urine, or incontinence (involuntary loss of urine). **Urethritis** is infection of the urethra, which is a major symptom of sexually transmitted diseases (STDs). **Kidney stones** (nephrolithiasis) are the most common urinary tract problems, accounting for nearly one out of every 100 hospital admissions in the United States. Eighty percent of kidney stone patients are men. About 12% of American men will develop kidney stones during their lifetimes. Kidney stones cause extreme pain when they move from the kidneys into the ureters. Ten percent of kidney stone cases require surgery. The best prevention for kidney stones is drinking plenty of fluids daily.

The male reproductive system

The male reproductive system includes the penis, testicles, scrotum, prostate and other organs. Problems include **orchitis**, or infection of the testicles, and hydrocele, the buildup of fluid on the testicles. **Epididymitis** is inflammation of the tube that transports sperm from the testicles, and can cause severe pain, swelling, and **fever**. A varicocele is a group of **varicose veins** in the scrotum that can cause swelling and damage sperm. **Peyronie's disease** is the abnormal curvature of the penis caused by accumulated scar tissue. **Testicular torsion** is considered a medical emergency, when a testicle becomes twisted and blood supply is cut off. This condition can lead to permanent damage if not treated quickly. It is most common in males between the ages of 12 and 18. **Prostatitis** is infection or inflammation of the prostate gland.

Sexually transmitted diseases include **genital warts**, chlamydia, **gonorrhea**, **syphilis**, **genital herpes**, hepatitis and HIV (human **immunodeficiency** virus). HIV is the leading cause of death for American men between the ages of 25 and 45. Symptoms of STDs include discharge of fluid from the penis; painful urination; sores, lesions, **itching**, or **rashes** in the genital area; and swelling of the lymph nodes in the groin. Prevention of STDs begins with safe sexual behavior: wearing condoms, limiting the number of sexual partners, not mixing sexual encounters with alcohol, and avoiding sexual contact with infected people, prostitutes and intravenous drug users. Men who engage in risky behaviors should have frequent HIV tests and medical examinations.

Male sexual health

Erectile dysfunction (ED), also called **impotence**, is a man's inability to maintain an erection for sexual intercourse. It affects nearly one in every 10 American men. Incidence of ED increases with age, but the problem can occur at any age. Up to 80% of ED is caused by physical problems, while 20% of cases are psychogenic, or psychological in origin. Causes of ED include hormonal problems, injuries, nerve damage, diseases, infections, diabetes, stress, depression, anxiety, drug **abuse**, and interactions with prescription drugs. ED also may be the first indication of circulation problems due to diabetes, high blood pressure, or **coronary artery disease**.

A self-test men can perform to determine whether ED is physical or psychological is the stamp test, or nocturnal penile tumescence test. Physically healthy men experience several prolonged erections during sleep. The stamp test is done by attaching a strip of stamps around the penis before bedtime; if the stamps are torn in the morning, it generally indicates that nocturnal (nightly) erections have occurred and thus ED is not physiological. Men with ED should see a urologist for further diagnosis and discussion of the several treatment options available including drugs, hormone injections, and surgical repair or implants. Several new prescription drugs have become available in recent years.

Infertility occurs when men lack an adequate supply of sperm to cause **pregnancy**. As many as 15% of American couples, or more than 5 million Americans, are affected by infertility in one or both partners. A World Health Organization (WHO) project found that in about 20% of infertile couples, the problem was due to the man, while in another 27% of couples both partners had infertility problems. Injuries, **birth defects**, infections, environmental pollutants, chronic stress, drug abuse, and hormonal problems may account for male infertility, while one in four cases has no apparent cause and is termed idiopathic infertility. Declining sperm counts have been observed in industrialized countries, and possible explanations for this decrease are as diverse as increased environmental pollutants to the use of plastic diapers, which a German study claims damages infant testicles by keeping in excess heat. Male infertility can be diagnosed by sperm analysis, blood tests, radiographic scans of the testicles, and other tests.

Other types of **sexual dysfunction** include **premature ejaculation**, in which men cannot sustain intercourse long enough to bring their partners to climax, and retarded ejaculation (also called male orgasmic disorder) when male orgasm becomes difficult. Some men have periods of inadequate sexual desire (hypoactive sexual desire disorder), while sexual aversion disorder (SAD) is fear and repulsion of sexual activity. Dyspareunia is painful intercourse, and should be reported to physicians as it may indicate STDs or infections. In addition to medical care, sexual dysfunction may be treated by **sex therapy** or psychotherapy depending on its causes.

Vasectomies, a form of male birth control, are surgical operations that sever the tubes that transport sperm from the testicles. Vasectomies can be reversed but 10% of men become infertile due to the surgery. **Circumcision** is the surgical removal of the foreskin of the penis, for religious and medical reasons, performed on 60% of newborn males in the United States. Increasing controversy surrounds this procedure. Advocates of circumcision claim it prevents infections (called **balanitis**) on the head of the penis and reduces chances of **penile cancer**. Opponents of circumcision claim that the outdated procedure affords no medical benefits, that it causes unnecessary pain for infants, and that the lack of a foreskin may reduce sexual pleasure and performance.

Men's emotional health

Depression is a mood disorder marked by sadness, emotional pain, and the inability to feel pleasure. At least 10% of men will experience an episode of major depression at least once in their lives. Men with depression are five times more likely to commit suicide, a major cause of mortality in men. Men are half as likely to seek psychological help than women. Men may suffer depression and emotional problems between the ages of 50 and 65, called the midlife crisis as men face the major transition into retirement and older age.

Panic attacks have symptoms of overwhelming fear, chest pain, shortness of breath, numbness, and increased heart rate. Men may mistake them as heart attacks. Men also are plagued by addictions to nicotine, alcohol, and other drugs, which are often the unhealthy escape routes from deeper emotional issues. Studies have estimated that as many as one-third of Americans have suffered from sleep disorders, which may be psychological in origin and related to anxiety, stress and lifestyle.

Mental illness can be particularly difficult for men because in our society men are taught to withhold rather than express emotions and feelings. Emotional problems can be strong signals for men to communicate and confront deeper issues. Help can be found from physicians, psychotherapists, and spiritual or religious counselors.

Osteoporosis

Osteoporosis often is thought of as disease more prevalent in women, but more than two million men have the disease characterized by decrease in bone mass and density. It develops about 10 to 15 years later in life in men than in women and risk of **fractures** from the disease can be greater in men. Men can decrease their risk by increasing calcium and vitamin D.

Resources

PERIODICALS

"Cigarette Smoking Influences Testicular Cancer Risk." *Medical Devices & Surgical Technology Week* March 28, 2004: 218.

"Men's Health: Erectile Dysfunction." *Medical Update* January 2004: 2.

"Osteoporosis Develops Later in Men, Hits Harder." *Internal Medicine News* March 15, 2004: 30.

ORGANIZATIONS

American Foundation for Urologic Disease. 1128 N. Charles St., Baltimore, MD 21201. (401) 468-1800. < http://www.afud.org >.

Center for Holistic Urology. 161 Fort Washington Ave., New York, NY 10032. (212) 305-0347. < http://www.holisticurology.com >.

OTHER

A Man's Life Online Magazine. < http://www.manslife.com >.

The Prostate Cancer Infolink. < http://www.comed.com/prostate >.

Douglas Dupler, MA
Teresa G. Odle

Menstrual disorders

Definition

A menstrual disorder is a physical or emotional problem that interferes with the normal menstrual cycle, causing **pain**, unusually heavy or light bleeding, delayed menarche, or missed periods.

Description

Typically, a woman of childbearing age should menstruate every 28 days or so unless she is pregnant or moving into **menopause**. But numerous things can go wrong with the normal menstrual cycle, some the result of physical causes, others emotional. These include **amenorrhea**, or the cessation of menstruation, menorrhagia, or heavy bleeding, and **dysmenorrhea**, or severe menstrual cramps. Nearly every woman will experience one or more of these menstrual irregularities at some time in her life.

Amenorrhea

There are two types of amenorrhea: primary and secondary. Overall, they affect 2–5% of childbearing women, a number that is considerably higher among female athletes (possibly as high as 66%).

Primary amenorrhea occurs when a girl at least 16 years old is not menstruating. Young girls may not have regular periods for their first year or two, or their periods may be very light, a condition known as **oligomenorrhea**. A light flow is nothing to worry about. But if the period has not begun at all by age 16, there may be something wrong. Amenorrhea is most common in girls who are severely underweight and/or **exercise** intensely, both of which affect the amount of body fat necessary to trigger the release of hormones that, in turn, begins **puberty**.

Secondary amenorrhea occurs in women of childbearing age after a period of normal menstruation and is diagnosed when menstruation has stopped for three months. It can occur in women of any age.

Dysmenorrhea

Characterized by menstrual cramps or painful periods, dysmenorrhea, which comes from the Greek words for "painful flow," affects nearly every woman at some point in her life. It is the most common reproductive problem in women, resulting in numerous days absent from school, work, and other activities. There are two types: primary and secondary.

Primary, or normal cramps, affects up to 90% of all women, usually occurring in women about three years after they start menstruating and continuing through their mid-twenties or until they have a child. About 10% of women who have this type of dysmenorrhea cannot work, attend school, or participate in their normal activities. It may be accompanied by backache, **dizziness, headache, nausea, vomiting, diarrhea** and tenseness. The symptoms typically start a day or two before menstruation, usually ending when menstruation actually begins.

Secondary dysmenorrhea has an underlying physical cause and primarily affects older women, although it may also occur immediately after a woman begins menstruation.

Menorrhagia

Menorrhagia, or heavy bleeding, most commonly occurs in the years just before menopause or just after women start menstruating. It occurs in 15–20% of American women.

Premenstrual dysphoric disorder (PMDD)

The fourth edition of the *Diagnostic and Statistical Manual of Mental Disorders*, or DSM-IV, lists **premenstrual dysphoric disorder** (PMDD) in an appendix of criteria sets for further study. To meet full criteria for PMDD, a patient must have at least five out of 11 emotional or physical symptoms during the week preceding the menses for most menstrual cycles over the previous 12 months. Although the DSM-IV definition of PMDD as a mental disorder is controversial because of fear that it could be used to justify prejudice or job discrimination against women, there is evidence that a significant proportion of pre-menopausal women suffer emotional distress or impairment in job functioning in the week before their menstrual period. One group of researchers estimates that 3–8% of women of childbearing age meet the strict DSM-IV criteria for PMDD, with another 13–18% having symptoms severe enough to interfere with their normal activities.

Causes and symptoms

Amenorrhea

The only symptom of primary amenorrhea is delayed menstruation. In addition to low body weight or excessive exercise, other causes of primary amenorrhea include Turner's syndrome, a birth defect related to the reproductive system, or ovarian problems. In 2003, a group of researchers reported on a new genetic mutation associated with primary amenorrhea. In secondary amenorrhea, the primary symptom is the ceasing of menstruation for at least three months. Causes include **pregnancy** or breast-feeding, sudden weight loss or gain, intense exercise, **stress**, endocrine disorders affecting the thyroid, pituitary or adrenal glands, including **Cushing's Syndrome** and **hyperthyroidism**, problems with or surgery on the ovaries, including removal of the ovaries, cysts or ovarian tumors.

Amenorrhea in athletes or dancers is frequently associated with two other disorders—osteopenia, or reduced bone mass, and eating disorders. This combination is sometimes called the female athlete triad. Osteopenia is of concern because it can lead to premature **osteoporosis**.

Dysmenorrhea

Primary dysmenorrhea is related to the production of prostaglandins, natural chemicals the body makes that cause an inflammatory reaction. They also cause the muscles of the uterus to contract, thus helping the uterus shed the lining built up during the first part of a woman's cycle. Women with severe menstrual pain have higher levels of prostaglandin in their menstrual blood than women who do not have such pain. In some women, prostaglandins can cause some of the smooth muscles in the gastrointestinal tract to contract, resulting in the nausea, vomiting and diarrhea some women experience. Prostaglandins also cause the arteries and veins to expand, so that blood collects in them rather than flowing freely through them, causing pain and heaviness. Yet another reason for severe cramps,

particularly in women who have not yet had a baby, is that the flow of the blood and clots through the tiny cervical opening is painful. After a woman has a baby, however, the cervix opening is larger.

Secondary dysmenorrhea is more serious and is related to some underlying cause. The pain may feel like regular menstrual cramps, but may last longer than normal and occur throughout the month. It may be stronger on one side of the body than the other. Possible causes include:

- A tipped uterus
- Endometriosis, a condition in which the same type of tissue found in the lining of the uterus occurs outside the uterus, usually elsewhere in the pelvic cavity
- Adenomyosis, a condition in which the endometrial lining grows into the muscle of the uterus
- Fibroids
- **Pelvic inflammatory disease** (PID)
- An **IUD**
- A uterine, ovarian, bowel or bladder tumor
- Uterine polyps
- Inflammatory bowel disease
- Scarring or **adhesions** from earlier surgery

Menorrhagia

Heavy bleeding during menstruation is usually related to a hormonal imbalance, although other causes include fibroids, cervical or endometrial polyps, the autoimmune disease lupus, pelvic inflammatory disease (PID), blood platelet disorder, a hereditary blood factor deficiency, or, possibly, some reproductive cancers. Thus, menorrhagia is actually a symptom of an underlying condition rather than a disease itself. It may also be related to the use of an IUD.

Women with menorrhagia experience not only significant inconvenience, but may feel very tired due to the loss of iron-rich blood. It is usually diagnosed when a woman soaks through a tampon or pad every hour for several hours or has a period lasting more than 7 days. Clots are not related to menorrhagia, although women with heavy cycles may pass clots. They are typically a normal part of menstruation, more common when a woman has been sitting or in a stationary position for a while

Diagnosis

Women should seek care from a gynecologist, family practitioner or internist for menstrual irregularities. Depending on the problem, various tests and procedures will be performed, but the one common to any menstrual problem is a **pelvic exam**. This should be scheduled when women are not menstruating, simply for conveniencee.

Male doctors typically have a female nurse or assistant in the room. The examination begins by checking the external genitalia for any sores or irregularities. Then the doctor inserts a speculum (a metal duckbill-shaped device that holds open the vagina) into the vagina and peers throughout the opening to evaluate the health of the cervix (opening of the uterus), and inside the vagina, looking for growths or any other abnormalities.

The doctor will also manually examine the woman, inserting two fingers into the vagina while pressing on the abdomen, again feeling for any lumps or other abnormalities, checking the size and shape of the reproductive organs, and watching for any signs of infection, such as tenderness or pain. The exam is typically covered by insurance and takes about 10 minutes.

Other tests that will be done for menstrual irregularities include:

- A pregnancy test. The nurse takes some blood from a woman's arm and it is tested for the presence of certain hormones that indicate a pregnancy has occurred.

- Ultrasound. Typically performed by a trained ultrasound technologist, it involves using sound waves to get an image of the reproductive system. It is used to look for fibroids and other ovarian abnormalities that may cause heavy bleeding or cramps. Typically, the technologist will smear a jelly over the woman's stomach, then place a probe on her stomach and watch the images appear on a computer screen. It is painless. Women may be asked not to urinate for several hours prior to the test, as a full bladder makes it easier to see the other internal organs. The test takes about 20 minutes.

- Endometrial biopsy. Used to check the health of uterine tissue in women who have unusually heavy bleeding, this test should be performed by the physician. Women should take a pain reliever such as ibuprofen or naproxen prior to the procedure, as there may be some cramping. The woman lies back on the table with her feet in stirrups and the doctor inserts a speculum, then opens the cervix slightly with an instrument called a tenaculum. Then the doctor slides a small, hollow catheter into the uterus and sucks out a small piece of tissue from the uterine lining. The tissue is then examined for any

abnormalities in a laboratory. The test takes about 30 minutes and is typically covered by insurance. Some bleeding may result afterwards.

- Blood, stool and urine tests may also be conducted to check for levels of various hormones, blood cells, and other chemicals.

- Dilation and curettage (D&C): During this minor surgical procedure, the cervix is opened and the lining of the uterus scraped for a tissue sample.

- Laparascopy and **hysteroscopy**: in some instances, these surgical procedures, in which a small camera is inserted into the woman to view the inside of the pelvis, abdomen or uterus.

Treatment

Amenorrhea

For primary amenorrhea with no underlying problem, no treatment is necessary, and a wait-and-see approach is often adopted. If women have genetic or hormonal abnormalities, amenorrhea is often treated with **oral contraceptives** that contain combinations of estrogen and progestin. Side effects include bloating, weight gain and **acne**, although some birth control pills actually improve acne. Progestins, or synthetic progesterone, are also used alone to "jump start" a woman's period. They include medroxyprogesterone (Provera, Amen, **Depo-Provera**), norethindrone acetate (Aygestin, Norlutate), and norgestrel (Ovrel). If the amenorrhia is due to a physical problem, such as a closed vagina, surgery may be required.

With secondary amenorrhia, treatment depends on the cause. Hormonal imbalances are treated with supplemental hormones. Tumors or cysts may require surgery. **Obesity** may require a diet and exercise regimen, while amenorrhia resulting from too much dieting or exercise necessitates lifestyle changes.

Dysmenorrhea

Primary dysmenorrhea is typically treated with nonsteroidal anti-inflammatory medications like ibuprofen and naproxen, which studies show help 64 to 100% of women. Birth control pills relieve pain and symptoms in about 90% of women by suppressing ovulation and reducing the amount of menstrual blood. It may take up to three cycles before a woman feels relief. Heat from a heating pad or hot bath, can also help relieve pain.

Treatment for secondary dysmenorrhea depends on the underlying cause of the condition.

Menorrhagia

If there are no other problems, and the bleeding is due to hormonal imbalances, birth control pills are often prescribed to bring the bleeding under control and regulate menstruation. Such medications as ibuprofen and naproxen can also help reduce the bleeding and any cramping associated with it. In severe cases, doctors may recommend removing the uterus during a **hysterectomy**, or performing some form of endometrial ablation, which removes the lining of the uterus. These procedures are typically only offered to women who have completed their families. A recent British study reported, however, that many women prefer endometrial ablation to hysterectomy because it is less invasive and safer. A new treatment that involves intrauterine hormonal therapy is gaining acceptance, but had not been approved by the FDA as of spring 2004.

Premenstrual dysphoric disorder (PMDD)

Medications that have been reported to be effective in treating PMDD include the **tricyclic antidepressants** and the **selective serotonin reuptake inhibitors** (SSRIs). Effective treatments other than medications include cognitive behavioral therapy (CBT), aerobic exercise, and dietary supplements containing calcium, magnesium, and vitamin B_6.

Alternative treatment

Amenorrhea

There are several herbal remedies that can bring on menstruation, including: black cohosh, cramp bark, chasteberry, celery, turmeric, and marsh mallow. Numerous relaxation techniques, such as **meditation**, deep breathing, and **yoga** can help reduce stress and its affects on menstruation.

Dysmenorrhea

Numerous alternative treatments may help relieve the menstrual pain. These include:

- Transcutaneous **electrical nerve stimulation** (TENS), which several studies found, relieved pain in 42–60% of participants, working faster than naproxen in one study.

- **Acupuncture**: One study of 43 patients followed for a year found that 90% of those who had acupuncture once a week for three menstrual cycles had less pain, and 43% used less pain medication.

- **Omega-3 fatty acids**: Often sold as fish oil supplements, they are a known anti-inflammatory, working against the effects of prostaglandins. Studies found that women with low amounts of omega-3 fatty acids in their **diets** were more likely to have menstrual cramps; those who took supplements had less pain.

- Vitamin B-1: One large study found that symptoms disappeared in 87% of women who took 100 mg a day for 90 days.

- Magnesium supplements: One study of 30 women who took 4.5 milligrams of oral magnesium three times daily for part of the month decreased their symptoms up to 84%.

Menorrhagia

Herbs used to treat menorrhagia include yarrow, nettles and shepherd's purse, as well as agrimony, particularly used in Chinese medicine, ladies mantle, vervain and red raspberry, which are thought to strengthen the uterus. Vitex is another herb recommended for a variety of menstrual disorders ranging from menorrhagia to PMS. Women may want to make sure they are taking an iron supplement to replace the iron lost during the heavy bleeding, although they should check with their doctor to make sure they do not suffer from a condition of having too much iron. Helpful **vitamins** include vitamin A, because women with heavy bleeding typically have lower levels of Vitamin A, K, which aids in clotting, and C and bioflavinoids which help strengthen veins and capillaries. Zinc may also help.

Prognosis

The prognosis for all menstrual irregularities is good once treatment is initiated.

Prevention

Amenorrhea

Simply following a healthy exercise and nutritional program can help prevent amenorrhea, as can reducing stress and learning relaxation techniques. Also, avoiding excessive alcohol intake and quitting **smoking** may prevent missed periods.

Dysmenorrhea

Prevention includes certain dietary supplements and vitamins described above. Exercise may also help.

Menorrhagia

There is little women can do to prevent this menstrual irregularity other than discovering the root

KEY TERMS

Adenomyosis—Uterine thickening caused when endometrial tissue, which normally lines the uterus, extends outward into the fibrous and muscular tissue of the uterus.

Cervical polyps—Growths originating from the surface of the cervix or endocervical canal. These small, fragile growths hang from a stalk and protrude through the cervical opening (the os).

Cushing's syndrome—A group of conditions caused by increased production of cortisol hormones or by the administration of glucocorticoid hormones (cortisone-like hormones).

Endometriosis—A condition in which the tissue that normally lines the uterus (endometrium) grows in other areas of the body, causing pain, irregular bleeding, and frequently, infertility.

Fibroids—Benign tumors of muscle and connective tissue that develop within or are attached to the uterine wall.

Hyperthyroidism—An imbalance in metabolism that occurs from overproduction of thyroid hormone.

Inflammatory bowel disease—A chronic inflammatory disease that can affect any part of the gastrointestinal tract but most commonly affects the ileum.

Lupus (systemic lupus erythematosus or SLE)—A chronic inflammatory autoimmune disorder that may affect many organ systems including the skin, joints, and internal organs.

Menarche—The first menstrual period or the establishment of the menstrual function.

Osteopenia—Reduction in bone mass, usually caused by a lowered rate of formation of new bone that is insufficient to keep up with the rate of bone destruction. Osteopenia often occurs together with amenorrhea and eating disorders in female athletes. It can lead to premature osteoporosis if left untreated.

Pelvic inflammatory disease (PID)—A general term referring to infection involving the lining of the uterus, the Fallopian tubes, or the ovaries.

Turner's syndrome—A disorder in women caused by an inherited chromosomal defect. This disorder inhibits sexual development and causes infertility. A symptom is absence of menstruation.

cause. One thing they can do, however, is stop using an IUD, which can often cause heavier bleeding.

Resources

BOOKS

American Psychiatric Association. *Diagnostic and Statistical Manual of Mental Disorders.* 4th ed., revised. Washington, DC: American Psychiatric Association, 2000.

Beers, Mark H., MD, and Robert Berkow, MD, editors. "Menstrual Abnormalities and Abnormal Uterine Bleeding." Section 18, Chapter 235. In *The Merck Manual of Diagnosis and Therapy.* Whitehouse Station, NJ: Merck Research Laboratories, 2004.

Pelletier, Kenneth R., MD. *The Best Alternative Medicine,* Part II. "CAM Therapies for Specific Conditions: Menstrual Symptoms, Menopause, and PMS." New York: Simon & Schuster, 2002.

PERIODICALS

Aegerter, Ch., D. Friess, and L. Alberio. "Menorrhagia Caused by Severe Hereditary Factor VII Deficiency. Case 1." *Hämostaseologie* 23 (August 2003): 99–102.

Donaldson, M. L. "The Female Athlete Triad. A Growing Health Concern." *Orthopedic Nursing* 22 (September-October 2003): 322–324.

Halbreich, U., J. Borenstein, T. Pearlstein, and L. S. Kahn. "The Prevalence, Impairment, Impact, and Burden of Premenstrual Dysphoric Disorder (PMS/PMDD)." *Psychoneuroendocrinology* 28, Supplement 3 (August 2003): 1–23.

Meduri, G., P. Touraine, I. Beau, et al. "Delayed Puberty and Primary Amenorrhea Associated with a Novel Mutation of the Human Follicle-Stimulating Hormone Receptor: Clinical, Histological, and Molecular Studies." *Journal of Clinical Endocrinology and Metabolism* 88 (August 2003): 3491–3498.

Paddison, K. "Menorrhagia: Endometrial Ablation or Hysterectomy?" *Nursing Standard* 18 (September 17–23): 33–37.

Rapkin, A. "A Review of Treatment of Premenstrual Syndrome and Premenstrual Dysphoric Disorder." *Psychoneuroendocrinology* 28, Supplement 3 (August 2003): 39–53.

"Research Eyes IUS Use for Menstrual Bleeding." *Contraceptive Technology Update* Supplement 3 (June 2004): 67–69.

ORGANIZATIONS

Advancement of Women's Health Research. 1828 L Street, N.W., Suite 625 Washington, DC 20036. 202-223-8224. < http://www.womens-health.org >.

American College of Obstetricians and Gynecologists (ACOG). 409 12th Street, SW, P. O. Box 96920, Washington, DC 20090-6920. < http://www.acog.org >.

American Psychiatric Association (APA). 1400 K Street, NW, Washington, DC 20005. (888) 357-7924. < http://www.psych.org >.

National Women's Health Resource Center. 120 Albany Street Suite 820, New Brunswick, NJ 08901. (877) 986-9472. <www.healthywomen.org>.

Debra Gordon
Rebecca J. Frey, PhD
Teresa G. Odle

Menstrual pain *see* **Dysmenorrhea**

Mental retardation

Definition

Mental retardation is a developmental disability that first appears in children under the age of 18. It is defined as an intellectual functioning level (as measured by standard tests for intelligence quotient) that is well below average and significant limitations in daily living skills (adaptive functioning).

Description

Mental retardation occurs in 2.5–3% of the general population. About 6–7.5 million mentally retarded individuals live in the United States alone. Mental retardation begins in childhood or adolescence before the age of 18. In most cases, it persists throughout adulthood. A diagnosis of mental retardation is made if an individual has an intellectual functioning level well below average and significant limitations in two or more adaptive skill areas. Intellectual functioning level is defined by standardized tests that measure the ability to reason in terms of mental age (intelligence quotient or IQ). Mental retardation is defined as IQ score below 70–75. Adaptive skills are the skills needed for daily life. Such skills include the ability to produce and understand language (communication); home-living skills; use of community resources; health, safety, leisure, self-care, and social skills; self-direction; functional academic skills (reading, writing, and arithmetic); and work skills.

In general, mentally retarded children reach developmental milestones such as walking and talking much later than the general population. Symptoms of mental retardation may appear at birth or later in childhood. Time of onset depends on the suspected cause of the disability. Some cases of mild mental retardation are not diagnosed before the child enters preschool. These children typically have difficulties with social, communication, and functional academic skills. Children who have a neurological disorder or illness such as **encephalitis** or **meningitis** may suddenly show signs of cognitive impairment and adaptive difficulties.

Mental retardation varies in severity. *The Diagnostic and Statistical Manual of Mental Disorders, Fourth Edition* (*DSM-IV*) is the diagnostic standard for mental healthcare professionals in the United States. The *DSM-IV* classifies four different degrees of mental retardation: *mild, moderate, severe,* and *profound*. These categories are based on the functioning level of the individual.

Mild mental retardation

Approximately 85% of the mentally retarded population is in the mildly retarded category. Their IQ score ranges from 50–75, and they can often acquire academic skills up to the 6th grade level. They can become fairly self-sufficient and in some cases live independently, with community and social support.

Moderate mental retardation

About 10% of the mentally retarded population is considered moderately retarded. Moderately retarded individuals have IQ scores ranging from 35–55. They can carry out work and self-care tasks with moderate supervision. They typically acquire communication skills in childhood and are able to live and function successfully within the community in a supervised environment such as a group home.

Severe mental retardation

About 3–4% of the mentally retarded population is severely retarded. Severely retarded individuals have IQ scores of 20–40. They may master very basic self-care skills and some communication skills. Many severely retarded individuals are able to live in a group home.

Profound mental retardation

Only 1–2% of the mentally retarded population is classified as profoundly retarded. Profoundly retarded individuals have IQ scores under 20–25. They may be able to develop basic self-care and communication skills with appropriate support and training. Their retardation is often caused by an accompanying neurological disorder. The profoundly retarded need a high level of structure and supervision.

The American Association on Mental Retardation (AAMR) has developed another widely accepted diagnostic classification system for mental retardation. The AAMR classification system focuses on the capabilities of the retarded individual rather than on the limitations. The categories describe the level of support required. They are: *intermittent support, limited support, extensive support*, and *pervasive support*. To some extent, the AAMR classification mirrors the *DSM-IV* classification. Intermittent support, for example, is support needed only occasionally, perhaps during times of **stress** or crisis. It is the type of support typically required for most mildly retarded individuals. At the other end of the spectrum, pervasive support, or life-long, daily support for most adaptive areas, would be required for profoundly retarded individuals.

Causes and symptoms

Low IQ scores and limitations in adaptive skills are the hallmarks of mental retardation. Aggression, self-injury, and **mood disorders** are sometimes associated with the disability. The severity of the symptoms and the age at which they first appear depend on the cause. Children who are mentally retarded reach developmental milestones significantly later than expected, if at all. If retardation is caused by chromosomal or other genetic disorders, it is often apparent from infancy. If retardation is caused by childhood illnesses or injuries, learning and adaptive skills that were once easy may suddenly become difficult or impossible to master.

In about 35% of cases, the cause of mental retardation cannot be found. Biological and environmental factors that can cause mental retardation include:

Genetics

About 5% of mental retardation is caused by hereditary factors. Mental retardation may be caused by an inherited abnormality of the genes, such as **fragile X syndrome**. Fragile X, a defect in the chromosome that determines sex, is the most common inherited cause of mental retardation. Single gene defects such as **phenylketonuria (PKU)** and other inborn errors of metabolism may also cause mental retardation if they are not found and treated early. An accident or mutation in genetic development may also cause retardation. Examples of such accidents are development of an extra chromosome 18 (trisomy 18) and **Down syndrome**.

Down syndrome, also called mongolism or trisomy 21, is caused by an abnormality in the development of chromosome 21. It is the most common genetic cause of mental retardation.

Prenatal illnesses and issues

Fetal alcohol syndrome affects one in 600 children in the United States. It is caused by excessive alcohol intake in the first twelve weeks (trimester) of **pregnancy**. Some studies have shown that even moderate alcohol use during pregnancy may cause learning disabilities in children. Drug **abuse** and cigarette **smoking** during pregnancy have also been linked to mental retardation.

Maternal infections and illnesses such as glandular disorders, **rubella**, **toxoplasmosis**, and **cytomegalovirus infection** may cause mental retardation. When the mother has high blood pressure (**hypertension**) or blood **poisoning** (toxemia), the flow of oxygen to the fetus may be reduced, causing brain damage and mental retardation.

Birth defects that cause physical deformities of the head, brain, and central nervous system frequently cause mental retardation. Neural tube defect, for example, is a birth defect in which the neural tube that forms the spinal cord does not close completely. This defect may cause children to develop an accumulation of cerebrospinal fluid on the brain (**hydrocephalus**). Hydrocephalus can cause learning impairment by putting pressure on the brain.

Childhood illnesses and injuries

Hyperthyroidism, **whooping cough**, **chickenpox**, **measles**, and Hib disease (a bacterial infection) may cause mental retardation if they are not treated adequately. An infection of the membrane covering the brain (meningitis) or an inflammation of the brain itself (encephalitis) cause swelling that in turn may cause brain damage and mental retardation. Traumatic brain injury caused by a blow or a violent shake to the head may also cause brain damage and mental retardation in children.

Environmental factors

Ignored or neglected infants who are not provided the mental and physical stimulation required for normal development may suffer irreversible learning impairments. Children who live in poverty and suffer from **malnutrition**, unhealthy living conditions, and improper or inadequate medical care are at a higher risk. Exposure to lead can also cause mental retardation. Many children have developed **lead poisoning** by eating the flaking lead-based paint often found in older buildings.

Diagnosis

If mental retardation is suspected, a comprehensive **physical examination** and medical history should be done immediately to discover any organic cause of symptoms. Conditions such as hyperthyroidism and PKU are treatable. If these conditions are discovered early, the progression of retardation can be stopped and, in some cases, partially reversed. If a neurological cause such as brain injury is suspected, the child may be referred to a neurologist or neuropsychologist for testing.

A complete medical, family, social, and educational history is compiled from existing medical and school records (if applicable) and from interviews with parents. Children are given intelligence tests to measure their learning abilities and intellectual functioning. Such tests include the Stanford-Binet Intelligence Scale, the Wechsler Intelligence Scales, the Wechsler Preschool and Primary Scale of Intelligence, and the Kaufmann Assessment Battery for Children. For infants, the Bayley Scales of Infant Development may be used to assess motor, language, and problem-solving skills. Interviews with parents or other caregivers are used to assess the child's daily living, muscle control, communication, and social skills. The Woodcock-Johnson Scales of Independent Behavior and the Vineland Adaptive Behavior Scale (VABS) are frequently used to test these skills.

Treatment

Federal legislation entitles mentally retarded children to free testing and appropriate, individualized education and skills training within the school system from ages 3–21. For children under the age of three, many states have established early intervention programs that assess, recommend, and begin treatment programs. Many day schools are available to help train retarded children in basic skills such as bathing and feeding themselves. Extracurricular activities and social programs are also important in helping retarded children and adolescents gain self-esteem.

Training in independent living and job skills is often begun in early adulthood. The level of training depends on the degree of retardation. Mildly retarded individuals can often acquire the skills needed to live independently and hold an outside job. Moderate to profoundly retarded individuals usually require supervised community living.

Family therapy can help relatives of the mentally retarded develop coping skills. It can also help parents deal with feelings of guilt or anger. A supportive, warm home environment is essential to help the mentally retarded reach their full potential.

Prognosis

Individuals with mild to moderate mental retardation are frequently able to achieve some self-sufficiency and to lead happy and fulfilling lives. To reach these goals, they need appropriate and consistent educational, community, social, family, and vocational supports. The outlook is less promising for those with severe to profound retardation. Studies have shown that these individuals have a shortened life expectancy. The diseases that are usually associated with severe retardation may cause the shorter life span. People with Down syndrome will develop the brain changes that characterize **Alzheimer's disease** in later life and may develop the clinical symptoms of this disease as well.

Prevention

Immunization against diseases such as measles and Hib prevents many of the illnesses that can cause mental retardation. In addition, all children should undergo routine developmental screening as part of their pediatric care. Screening is particularly critical for those children who may be neglected or undernourished or may live in disease-producing conditions. Newborn screening and immediate treatment for PKU and hyperthyroidism can usually catch these disorders early enough to prevent retardation.

Good prenatal care can also help prevent retardation. Pregnant women should be educated about the risks of drinking and the need to maintain good **nutrition** during pregnancy. Tests such as **amniocentesis** and ultrasonography can determine whether a fetus is developing normally in the womb.

Resources

ORGANIZATIONS

American Association on Mental Retardation (AAMR). 444 North Capitol St., NW, Suite 846, Washington, D.C. 20001-1512. (800) 424-3688. < http:// www.aamr.org >.

The Arc. 900 Varnum Street NE, Washington, D.C. 20017. (202) 636-2950. < http://thearc.org >.

Amniocentesis—A test usually done between 16 and 20 weeks of pregnancy to detect any abnormalities in the development of the fetus. A small amount of the fluid surrounding the fetus (amniotic fluid) is drawn out through a needle inserted into the mother's womb. Laboratory analysis of this fluid can detect various genetic defects, such as Down syndrome, or neural tube defects.

Developmental delay—The failure to meet certain developmental milestones, such as sitting, walking, and talking, at the average age. Developmental delay may indicate a problem in development of the central nervous system.

Down syndrome—A disorder caused by an abnormality at the 21st chromosome. One symptom of Down syndrome is mental retardation.

Extensive support—Ongoing daily support required to assist an individual in a specific adaptive area, such as daily help with preparing meals.

Hib disease—An infection caused by *Haemophilus influenza* type b (Hib). This disease mainly affects children under the age of five. In that age group, it is the leading cause of bacterial meningitis, pneumonia, joint and bone infections, and throat inflammations.

Inborn error of metabolism—A rare enzyme deficiency; children with inborn errors of metabolism do not have certain enzymes that the body requires to maintain organ functions. Inborn errors of metabolism can cause brain damage and mental retardation if left untreated. Phenylketonuria is an inborn error of metabolism.

Limited support—A predetermined period of assistance required to deal with a specific event, such as training for a new job.

Phenylketonuria (PKU)—An inborn error in metabolism that prevents the body from using phenylalanine, an amino acid necessary for normal growth and development.

Trisomy—An abnormality in chromosomal development. Chromosomes are the structures within a cell that carry its genetic information. They are organized in pairs. Humans have 23 pairs of chromosomes. In a trisomy syndrome, an extra chromosome is present so that the individual has three of a particular chromosome instead of the normal pair. An extra chromosome 18 (trisomy 18) causes mental retardation.

Ultrasonography—A process that uses the reflection of high-frequency sound waves to make an image of structures deep within the body. Ultrasonography is routinely used to detect fetal abnormalities.

OTHER

Americans With Disabilities Act (ADA) Page. < http://www.usdoj.gov/crt/ada/adahom1.htm >.

Paula Anne Ford-Martin

Mental status examination

Definition

A mental status examination (MSE) is an assessment of a patient's level of cognitive (knowledge-related) ability, appearance, emotional mood, and speech and thought patterns at the time of evaluation. It is one part of a full neurologic (nervous system) examination and includes the examiner's observations about the patient's attitude and cooperativeness as well as the patient's answers to specific questions.

The most commonly used test of cognitive functioning per se is the so-called Folstein Mini-Mental Status Examination (MMSE), developed in 1975.

Purpose

The purpose of a mental status examination is to assess the presence and extent of a person's mental impairment. The cognitive functions that are measured during the MSE include the person's sense of time, place, and personal identity; memory; speech; general intellectual level; mathematical ability; insight or judgment; and reasoning or problem-solving ability. Complete MSEs are most commonly given to elderly people and to other patients being evaluated for **dementia** (including AIDS-related dementia). Dementia is an overall decline in a person's intellectual function—including difficulties with language, simple calculations, planning or decision-making, and motor (muscular movement) skills as well as loss of memory. The MSE is an important part of the differential diagnosis of dementia and other psychiatric symptoms or disorders. The MSE results may suggest specific areas for further testing or specific types of required tests. A mental status examination can also be given repeatedly to monitor or document changes in a patient's condition.

Precautions

The MSE cannot be given to a patient who cannot pay attention to the examiner, for example as a result of being in a **coma** or unconscious; or is completely unable to speak (aphasic); or is not fluent in the language of the examiner.

Description

The MMSE of Folstein evaluates five areas of mental status, namely, orientation, registration, attention and calculation, recall and language. A complete MSE is more comprehensive and evaluates the following ten areas of functioning:

- Appearance. The examiner notes the person's age, race, sex, civil status, and overall appearance. These features are significant because poor personal hygiene or grooming may reflect a loss of interest in self-care or physical inability to bathe or dress oneself.

- Movement and behavior. The examiner observes the person's gait (manner of walking), posture, coordination, eye contact, facial expressions, and similar behaviors. Problems with walking or coordination may reflect a disorder of the central nervous system.

- Affect. Affect refers to a person's outwardly observable emotional reactions. It may include either a lack of emotional response to an event or an overreaction.

- Mood. Mood refers to the underlying emotional "atmosphere" or tone of the person's answers.

- Speech. The examiner evaluates the volume of the person's voice, the rate or speed of speech, the length of answers to questions, the appropriateness and clarity of the answers, and similar characteristics.

- Thought content. The examiner assesses what the patient is saying for indications of **hallucinations**, **delusions**, obsessions, symptoms of dissociation, or thoughts of **suicide**. Dissociation refers to the splitting-off of certain memories or mental processes from conscious awareness. Dissociative symptoms include feelings of unreality, depersonalization, and confusion about one's identity.

- Thought process. Thought process refers to the logical connections between thoughts and their relevance to the main thread of conversation. Irrelevant detail, repeated words and phrases, interrupted thinking (thought blocking), and loose, illogical connections between thoughts, may be signs of a thought disorder.

- Cognition. Cognition refers to the act or condition of knowing. The evaluation assesses the person's orientation (ability to locate himself or herself) with regard to time, place, and personal identity; long- and short-term memory; ability to perform simple arithmetic (counting backward by threes or sevens); general intellectual level or fund of knowledge (identifying the last five Presidents, or similar questions); ability to think abstractly (explaining a proverb); ability to name specified objects and read or write complete sentences; ability to understand and perform a task (showing the examiner how to comb one's hair or throw a ball); ability to draw a simple map or copy a design or geometrical figure; ability to distinguish between right and left.

- Judgment. The examiner asks the person what he or she would do about a commonsense problem, such as running out of a prescription medication.

- Insight. Insight refers to a person's ability to recognize a problem and understand its nature and severity.

The length of time required for a mental status examination depends on the patient's condition. It may take as little as five minutes to examine a healthy person. Patients with speech problems or intellectual impairments, dementia, or other organic brain disorders may require fifteen or twenty minutes. The examiner may choose to spend more time on certain portions of the MSE and less time on others, depending on the patient's condition and answers.

Preparation

Preparation for a mental status examination includes a careful medical and psychiatric history of the patient. The history helps the examiner to interpret the patient's appearance and answers with greater accuracy, because some physical illnesses may produce psychiatric symptoms or require medications that influence the patient's mood or attentiveness. The psychiatric history should include a family history as well as the patient's personal history of development, behavior patterns, and previous treatment for mental disorders (if any). Symptoms of dissociation, for example, often point to a history of childhood abuse, **rape**, or other severe emotional traumas in adult life. The examiner should also include information about the patient's occupation, level of education, marital status, and right- or left-handedness. Information about occupation and education helps in evaluating the patient's use of language, extent of memory loss, reasoning ability, and similar functions. Handedness is important in determining which half of the patient's brain is involved in writing, picking up a pencil, or other similar tasks that he or she may be asked to perform during the examination.

Aftercare

Depending on the examiner's specific observations, the patient may be given additional tests for follow-up. These tests might include blood or urine samples to test for drug or alcohol abuse, anemia, diabetes, disorders of the liver or kidneys, vitamin or thyroid deficiencies, medication side effects, or **syphilis** and **AIDS**. Brain imaging (CT, MRI, or **PET** scans) may be used to look for signs of seizures, strokes, head trauma, brain tumors, or other evidence of damage to specific parts of the brain. A spinal tap may be performed if the doctor thinks the patient may have an infection of the central nervous system.

Normal results

Normal results for a mental status examination depend to some extent on the patient's history, level of education, and recent life events. For example, a depressed mood is appropriate in the context of a recent **death** or other sad event in the patient's family but inappropriate in the context of a recent pay raise. Speech patterns are often influenced by racial or ethnic background as well as by occupation or schooling. In general, however, the absence of obvious delusions, hallucinations, or thought disorders together with the presence of insight, good judgment, and socially appropriate appearance and behavior are considered normal results. A normal numerical score for the MMSE is between 28 and 30.

Abnormal results

Abnormal results for a mental status examination include:

- Any evidence of organic brain damage.
- Evidence of thought disorders.
- A mood or affect that is clearly inappropriate to its context.
- Thoughts of suicide.

KEY TERMS

Aphasia—The loss of the ability to speak, or to understand written or spoken language. A person who cannot speak or understand language is said to be aphasic.

Cognition—The act or process of knowing or perceiving.

Coma—A state of prolonged unconsciousness in which a person cannot respond to spoken commands or mildly painful physical stimuli.

Delusion—A belief that is resistant to reason or contrary to actual fact. Common delusions include delusions of persecution, delusions about one's importance (sometimes called delusions of grandeur), or delusions of being controlled by others.

Dementia—A decline in a person's level of intellectual functioning. Dementia includes memory loss as well as difficulties with language, simple calculations, planning or decision-making, and motor (muscular movement) skills.

Dissociation—The splitting off of certain mental processes from conscious awareness. Specific symptoms of dissociation include feelings of unreality, depersonalization, and confusion about one's identity.

Hallucination—A sensory experience, usually involving either sight or hearing, of something that does not exist outside the mind.

Illusion—A false visual perception of an object that others perceive correctly. A common example is the number of sightings of "UFOs" that turn out to be airplanes or weather balloons.

Obsession—Domination of thoughts or feelings by a persistent idea, desire, or image.

Organic brain disorder—An organic brain disorder refers to impaired brain function due to damage or deterioration of brain tissue.

- Disturbed speech patterns.
- Dissociative symptoms.
- Delusions or hallucinations.

A score below 27 on the MMSE usually indicates an organic brain disorder.

Resources

BOOKS

Beers, Mark H., MD, and Robert Berkow, MD, editors. "Neurologic Disorders: Neurologic Examination." In *The Merck Manual of Diagnosis and Therapy.*

Whitehouse Station, NJ: Merck Research Laboratories, 2004.

Eisendrath, Stuart J., MD, and Jonathan E. Lichtmacher, MD. "Psychiatric Disorders: Psychiatric Assessment." In *Current Medical Diagnosis & Treatment 2001*, edited by L. M. Tierney, Jr., MD, et al., 40th ed. New York: Lange Medical Books/McGraw-Hill, 2001.

Rebecca J. Frey, PhD

Mesothelioma

Definition

Mesothelioma is an uncommon disease that causes malignant **cancer** cells to form within the lining of the chest, abdomen, or around the heart. Its primary cause is believed to be exposure to asbestos.

Description

Malignant mesothelioma is also known as asbestos cancer or simply "meso." Mesothelioma causes cancerous cells to develop in the body's mesothelium, where they can spread to and damage vital organs and tissue. These malignant cells can also metastasize to other regions of the body. Mesothelioma is very difficult to diagnose and responds poorly to most treatment modalities, accounting for a poor prognosis.

The disease derives its name from the mesothelium, a sac-like membrane that protects most of the body's internal organs. It is divided into two distinct protective layers of cells: the visceral (the layer directly surrounding the organ) and the parietal (a sac around the body cavity). By releasing a lubricating fluid, the mesothelium allows the organs to move more freely within the body cavity; for example, the contraction and expansion of the lungs. The mesothelium is also referred to according to where it is located in the body: pleura (chest), peritoneum (abdomen), and pericardium (heart).

Over two-thirds of all mesothelioma cases begin in the pleura region. Pleural mesothelioma spreads through the chest cavity, occasionally developing in the lungs as well. The disease most commonly causes **pleural effusion**, an excess build-up of fluid inside the chest cavity. This excess fluid increases pressure on the lungs and restricts breathing. In addition, malignant cells can cause the pleural lining to thicken and restrict the breathing space even further.

Peritoneal mesothelioma is the second most common form of the disease, accounting for less than 30% of all cases. Malignant cells form in the peritoneum, affecting the abdomen, bowel, liver, and spleen. Similar to pleural mesothelioma, the disease also causes a build up of excess fluid in the abdominal cavity. Normal bodily functions, such as digestion, can be hindered by the obstruction of organ movement.

Very rare forms of mesothelioma occur in the pericardium, as well as the mesothelium of the male and female reproductive organs. Cystic mesothelioma of the peritoneum, another rare form of the disease, occurs predominantly in women and is more benign in nature.

Malignant mesothelioma takes the form of one of three cell-types: epithelioid (50% to 70% of cases), sarcomatous (7% to 20% of cases), and biphasic/mixed (20% to 35% of cases). Of these cell-types, epithelioid mesothelioma carries the most favorable prognosis, followed by biphasic, and finally sarcomatous (very aggressive).

Mesothelioma remains relatively uncommon in the United States, with approximately 2,500 new cases reported annually. The incidence rates are much higher in Western Europe (over 5,000 cases reported annually). These numbers are expended to climb dramatically over the next 20 years. Older males (median age 60 at diagnosis) are three to five times more likely to develop mesothelioma than women. This is most like do to male predominance in those professions with an increased risk of asbestos exposure.

Causes & symptoms

Approximately 80% of all mesothelioma patients have a history of asbestos exposure. The majority of these patients were employed in an industry that involved the use of asbestos in some fashion. In addition to occupational exposure, household exposure of family members is not uncommon. An exposed individual can carry the asbestos particles on their clothing, skin, and in their hair when they return home, resulting in paraoccupational exposure. Even brief exposure to asbestos, as little as one to two months, can result in long-term consequences. Although the dangers of asbestos have been known for decades, the long latency period of mesothelioma (30 to 40 years) means that majority of patients were already exposed as far back as the 1950s. It is estimated that up to eight million Americans have already been exposed. Several industries, in particular, show a higher incidence of asbestos exposure:

- Insulators (Asbestos workers)
- Boilermakers
- Ship-fitters
- Steel workers
- Maintenance workers
- Plumbers
- Brake mechanics

Symptoms

Mesothelioma is very aggressive once it truly takes hold. However, its initial symptoms are generally non-specific in nature and/or mimic other conditions, such as persistent **pneumonia** or gastronomical disorders. Some patients will exhibit no symptoms at all. As such, proper evaluation and diagnosis are commonly delayed and must be confirmed by a doctor.

Patients suffering from pleural mesothelioma most commonly exhibit signs of dyspnea, pleural effusions, and/or chest **pain**. The majority of pleural effusion symptoms will exhibit in the right lung (60% of the time). Patients may also exhibit persistent **cough**, weight loss, weakness, **fever**, and difficulty swallowing.

Patients suffering from peritoneal mesothelioma most commonly exhibit signs of pain and/or swelling in the abdomen from fluid retention or tumor growth. Weight loss, **nausea**, bowel obstruction, anemia, fever, and swelling in the legs and/or feet are also known symptoms.

Diagnosis

Only a physician can properly diagnose mesothelioma. A review of the patient's medical history, including any past exposure to asbestos, should be conducted for any patient displaying dyspnea, chest pain, fluid build-up, or pain and/or swelling in the abdomen. This review is followed up with a complete **physical examination**, which should involve the use of imaging techniques. X rays, computed tomography (CT) scans, and magnetic resonance (MRI) scans of the chest and/or abdomen, as well as lung function, can provide the doctor with critical diagnostic information. Although **positron emission tomography** scans are expensive and not covered under most insurance, this diagnostic tool has proven very useful in determining tumor sites and staging of the disease.

If indicated, the doctor may wish to internally examine the patient's chest and/or abdominal cavity. These diagnostic procedures, known as **thoracoscopy** (chest) and peritoneoscopy (abdomen), are usually conducted in a hospital setting. Both procedures involve a fiber-optic imaging tool being inserted into the patient through an incision. These endoscopic tools will provide the doctor with a closer look at the body cavity, and any abnormal tissue or fluid build-up found therein. Excess fluid can be suctioned out through a needle or tube, in a process known as **thoracentesis** (for the chest) or **paracentesis** (for the abdomen). Additionally, the doctor may perform a biopsy of any abnormal tissue they discover during this time. Pathological examination of abnormal tissue, as well as fluid, remains the only effective method of confirming the diagnosis of mesothelioma. Biopsy will also assist the doctor in properly staging the disease's progression.

Once a confirmation of malignant mesothelioma has been established, the doctor will conduct further tests to determine the extent to which the primary disease has spread. This diagnostic process is known as "staging." Malignant pleural mesothelioma of can be broken into four stages:

- Localized Malignant Mesothelioma (Stage 1)—Cancer is present in the right or left pleura. May involve the lung, the pericardium, or diaphragm on that side.
- Advanced Malignant Mesothelioma (Stage 2)—Cancer has spread beyond the right or left pleura to lymph nodes on that side. May involve the lung, the pericardium, or diaphragm on that side.
- Advanced Malignant Mesothelioma (Stage 3)—Cancer has spread into the chest wall, diaphragm, ribs, heart, esophagus, or through the abdominal lining. Nearby lymph nodes may or may not be involved.
- Advanced Malignant Mesothelioma (Stage 4)—Cancer shows evidence of metastasis or spread through the bloodstream to distant organs and/or tissues.

Recurrent malignant mesothelioma may also occur, where the cancer returns in its original location or elsewhere in the body even after treatment.

Treatment

There are three traditional treatment modalities for mesothelioma: surgery, **radiation therapy**, and **chemotherapy**. The location and the stage of the disease, as well as the patient's age and general health, will determine which treatment should be utilized. Additionally, these modalities can be combined if indicated. Indeed, the multimodality approach appears to provide the most positive results for treating mesothelioma.

Surgery, the most common treatment, involves the removal of the tumor. In the early stages of mesothelioma, this only involves removal of a section of the mesothelium and surrounding tissue, but may require removing part of the diaphragm as well. For more advanced stages of the disease, removing the entire lung may be the only option, which is known as pneumonectomy.

Radiation therapy, also known as radiotherapy, destroys and shrinks the cancer cells through various types of radiation. Both external (such as a machine) and internal (such as radioisotopes) radiation therapies can be utilized effectively to treat malignant mesothelioma.

Finally, chemotherapy, a systemic treatment modality, uses **anticancer drugs** to destroy the cancerous cells throughout the body. The majority of drugs used to treat mesothelioma are delivered intravenously. The effectiveness of intracavitary chemotherapy, the process of directly injecting the drugs into the chest or abdominal cavity, is being studied.

Pain and other symptoms caused by fluid build-up around the chest and/or abdomen can be treated by drain excess fluid through a needle or tube. These procedures are known as thoracentesis (chest) and paracentesis (abdomen). Drugs, radiotherapy, and surgery can also relieve or prevent further fluid accumulation.

Physicians are currently studying other treatment modalities, such as immunotherapy, **gene therapy**, and intraoperative photodynamic therapy.

Alternative treatment

Due to the poor prognosis associated with mesothelioma, regardless of proper treatment, in many cases palliative care is the preferred, and only, option available to patients. This is particularly true for the advanced stages of the disease. By treating the symptoms rather than the disease itself, the goal of this approach is to obtain "quality" of life instead of "quantity" of life. Palliative care aims to relieve the patient s discomfort caused by dyspnea and pain. Chemotherapy, radiation, and/or surgical pleurodeis, in combination with effective management of pain and respiratory function should form the basis of proper palliative care of mesothelioma. Techniques to reduce **stress**, such as **acupuncture**, **aromatherapy**, massage, and **reflexology**, can provide addition benefit to the patient's sense of well-being.

Prognosis

The stage and location, what cell-type is involved, as well as the patient's age and histology factor greatly

KEY TERMS

Asbestos—A naturally occurring mineral, utilized worldwide for its durability and heat resistant qualities. Extremely fibrous in nature, asbestos particles can easily enter the respiratory system and damage sensitive tissue. This damage can result in asbestosis, mesothelioma, and lung cancer.

Dyspnea—A difficulty in breathing or shortness of breath, typically associated with some form of heart or lung disease. Also known as air hunger.

Mesothelium—A membrane/sac that that protects the body's major internal organs and allows them freedom of movement (for example, lung contractions). The mesothelium is comprised of several regions, including the abdominal cavity (peritoneum), the chest cavity (pleura), and pericardium (heart).

Pleural effusion—An abnormal accumulation of fluid in the pleura, a fibrous membrane that lines the inside of the chest cavity and protects the lungs. This accumulation can cause shortness of breath, cough, and chest pain.

on life expectancy. Unfortunately, even with aggressive treatment, the prognosis for mesothelioma patients is poor. Pleural mesothelioma offers a median survival time of approximately 16 to 17 months after initial symptoms. Prognosis for peritoneal mesothelioma is poorer and has a median survival time of only ten months after initial symptoms. Unfortunately, the more advanced stages of mesothelioma may offer as little as four or five month's survival time.

The survival time for patients with localized mesothelioma can be extended several months with aggressive therapy, with roughly 20% of patients surviving past the five-year mark. Therapy programs recently developed at leading cancer centers have extended this survival time even further. Dr. Sugarbaker, of the Brigham and Women's Center in Boston, has achieved a median of 40% survival rate at five years with his treatment regimen for pleural mesothelioma, as reported in the *Journal of Thoracic and Cardiovascular Surgery*. Other programs are also exhibiting favorable results. However, despite such successes, no cure for mesothelioma currently exists.

Prevention

Avoiding or limiting exposure to asbestos is the best way to prevent mesothelioma. Unfortunately, because of the significant delay between exposure and onset (30 to 40 years), it is probably too late to prevent the development of mesothelioma for most patients. Not **smoking** may slow the disease's progression and/or prevent other further complications associated with asbestos exposure.

Resources

BOOKS

Jaurand, Marie-Claude, and Jean Bignon (eds). *The Mesothelial Cell and Mesothelioma.* New York: Marcel Dekker, 1994.

Robinson, Bruce, and A. Philippe Chahinian (eds). *Mesothelioma.* London: Martin Dunitz, 2002.

PERIODICALS

Pistolesi, Massimo, and James Rusthoven. "Malignant Pleural Mesothelioma."*Chest* 126 (October, 2004): 1318-1329

Sugarbaker, David, et al. "Resection Margins, Extrapleural Nodal Status, and Cell Type Determine Postoperative Long-Term Survival in Trimodality Therapy of Malignant Pleural Mesothelioma."*Journal of Thoracic and Cardiovascular Surgery* 117 (January, 1999): 54-65

van Ruth, Serge, Paul Baas, and Frans Zoetmulder. "Surgical Treatment of Malignant Pleural Mesothelioma." *Chest* 123 (February, 2003): 551-561

ORGANIZATIONS

Mesothelioma Research Foundation of America. 5716 Corsa Ave., Suite 203, Westlake Village, CA 91362. (800) 281-9804. < http://www.mesothelioma-rfa.org >.

The Mesothelioma Center. 1030 Fifth Ave., Pittsburgh, PA 15219. (412) 471-3980. < http://mesotheliomacenter.org >.

OTHER

"Malignant Mesothelioma." *National Cancer Institute* < http://www.nci.nih.gov/cancertopics/types/malignantmesothelioma/ >.

"Mesothelioma."*Mesothelioma Information* < http://www.mesoinfo.com >.

"Mesothelioma."*Mesothelioma Web* < http://www.mesotheliomaweb.org >.

Jason Fryer

Metabolic acidosis

Definition

Metabolic acidosis is a pH imbalance in which the body has accumulated too much acid and does not have enough bicarbonate to effectively neutralize the effects of the acid.

Description

Metabolic acidosis, as a disruption of the body's acid/base balance, can be a mild symptom brought on by a lack of insulin, a **starvation** diet, or a gastrointestinal disorder like **vomiting** and **diarrhea**. Metabolic acidosis can indicate a more serious problem with a major organ like the liver, heart, or kidneys. It can also be one of the first signs of **drug overdose** or **poisoning**.

Causes and symptoms

Metabolic acidosis occurs when the body has more acid than base in it. Chemists use the term "pH" to describe how acidic or basic a substance is. Based on a scale of 14, a pH of 7.0 is neutral. A pH below 7.0 is an acid; the lower the number, the stronger the acid. A pH above 7.0 is a base; the higher the number, the stronger the base. Blood pH is slightly basic (alkaline), with a normal range of 7.36-7.44.

Acid is a natural by-product of the breakdown of fats and other processes in the body; however, in some conditions, the body does not have enough bicarbonate, an acid neutralizer, to balance the acids produced. This can occur when the body uses fats for energy instead of carbohydrates. Conditions where metabolic acidosis can occur include chronic **alcoholism**, **malnutrition**, and **diabetic ketoacidosis**. Consuming a diet low in carbohydrates and high in fats can also produce metabolic acidosis. The disorder may also be a symptom of another condition like kidney failure, liver failure, or severe diarrhea. The build up of lactic acid in the blood due to such conditions as **heart failure**, **shock**, or **cancer**, induces metabolic acidosis. Some poisonings and overdoses (**aspirin**, methanol, or ethylene glycol) also produce symptoms of metabolic acidosis.

In mild cases of metabolic acidosis, symptoms include **headache**, lack of energy, and sleepiness. Breathing may become fast and shallow. **Nausea**, vomiting, diarrhea, **dehydration**, and loss of appetite are also associated with metabolic acidosis. Diabetic patients with symptoms of metabolic acidosis may also have breath that smells fruity. The patient may lose consciousness or become disoriented. Severe cases can produce **coma** and **death**.

Diagnosis

Metabolic acidosis is suspected based on symptoms, but is usually confirmed by laboratory tests on blood and urine samples. Blood pH below 7.35 confirms the condition. Levels of other blood components, including potassium, glucose, ketones, or lactic acid, may also be above normal ranges. The level of bicarbonate in the blood will be low, usually less than 22 mEq/L. Urine pH may fall below 4.5 in metabolic acidosis.

Treatment

Treatment focuses first on correcting the acid imbalance. Usually, sodium bicarbonate and fluids will be injected into the blood through a vein. An intravenous line may be started to administer fluids and allow for the quick injection of other drugs that may be needed. If the patient is diabetic, insulin may be administered. Drugs to regulate blood pressure or heart rate, to prevent seizures, or to control **nausea and vomiting** might be given. Vital signs like pulse, respiration, blood pressure, and body temperature will be monitored. The underlying cause of the metabolic acidosis must also be diagnosed and corrected.

Prognosis

If the metabolic acidosis is recognized and treated promptly, the patient may have no long-term complications, however, the underlying condition that caused the acidosis needs to be corrected or managed. Severe metabolic acidosis that is left untreated will lead to coma and death.

Prevention

Diabetic patients need to routinely test their urine for sugar and acetone, strictly follow their appropriate diet, and take any medications or insulin to prevent metabolic acidosis. Patients receiving **tube feedings** or intravenous feedings must be monitored to prevent

dehydration or the accumulation of ketones or lactic acid.

Resources

BOOKS

"Fluid, Electrolyte, and Acid-Base Disorders." In *Family Medicine Principles and Practices*. 5th ed. New York: Springer-Verlag, 1998.

Altha Roberts Edgren

Metabolic alkalosis

Definition

Metabolic alkalosis is a pH imbalance in which the body has accumulated too much of an alkaline substance, such as bicarbonate, and does not have enough acid to effectively neutralize the effects of the alkali.

Description

Metabolic alkalosis, as a disturbance of the body's acid/base balance, can be a mild condition, brought on by **vomiting**, the use of steroids or diuretic drugs, or the overuse of **antacids** or **laxatives**. Metabolic alkalosis can also indicate a more serious problem with a major organ such as the kidneys.

Causes and symptoms

Metabolic alkalosis occurs when the body has more base than acid in the system. Chemists use the term "pH" to decribe how acidic or alkaline (also called basic) a substance is. Based on a scale of 14, a pH of 7.0 is neutral. A pH below 7.0 is an acid; the lower the number, the stronger the acid. A pH above 7.0 is alkaline; the higher the number, the stronger the alkali. Blood pH is slightly alkaline, with a normal range of 7.36-7.44. Conditions that lead to a reduced amount of fluid in the body, like vomiting or excessive urination due to use of diuretic drugs, change the balance of fluids and salts. The blood levels of potassium and sodium can decrease dramatically, causing symptoms of metabolic alkalosis.

In cases of metabolic alkalosis, slowed breathing may be an initial symptom. The patient may have episodes of apnea (not breathing) that may go on 15 seconds or longer. **Cyanosis**, a bluish or purplish discoloration of the skin, may also develop as a sign of inadequate oxygen intake. **Nausea**, vomiting, and **diarrhea** may also occur. Other symptoms can include irritability, twitching, confusion, and picking at bedclothes. Rapid heart rate, irregular heart beats, and a drop in blood pressure are also symptoms. Severe cases can lead to convulsions and **coma**.

Diagnosis

Metabolic alkalosis may be suspected based on symptoms, but often may not be noticeable. The condition is usually confirmed by laboratory tests on blood and urine samples. Blood pH above 7.45 confirms the condition. Levels of other blood components, including salts like potassium, sodium, and chloride, fall below normal ranges. The level of bicarbonate in the blood will be high, usually greater than 29 mEq/L. Urine pH may rise to about 7.0 in metabolic alkalosis.

Treatment

Treatment focuses first on correcting the imbalance. An intravenous line may be started to administer fluids (generally normal saline, a salt water solution) and allow for the quick injection of other drugs that may be needed. Potassium chloride will be administered. Drugs to regulate blood pressure or heart rate, or to control **nausea and vomiting** might be given. Vital signs like pulse, respiration, blood pressure, and body temperature will be monitored. The underlying cause of the metabolic alkalosis must also be diagnosed and corrected.

Prognosis

If metabolic alkalosis is recognized and treated promptly, the patient may have no long-term complications; however, the underlying condition that caused the alkalosis needs to be corrected or managed.

Severe metabolic alkalosis that is left untreated will lead to convulsions, **heart failure**, and coma.

Prevention

Patients receiving **tube feedings** or intravenous feedings must be monitored to prevent an imbalance of fluids and salts, particularly potassium, sodium, and chloride. Overuse of some drugs, including **diuretics**, laxatives, and antacids, should be avoided.

Resources

BOOKS

Bennett, J. Claude, and Fred Plum, eds. "Acid-Base Disturbances." In *Cecil Textbook of Medicine.* Philadelphia: W. B. Saunders Co., 1996.

DuBose, Thomas D., Jr. "Acidosis and Alkalosis" In *Harrison's Principles of Internal Medicine,* ed. Anthony S. Fauci, et al. New York: McGraw-Hill, 1997.

"Fluid, Electrolyte, and Acid-Base Disorders." In *Family Medicine Principles and Practices.* 5th ed. New York: Springer-Verlag, 1998.

"Fluid & Electrolyte Disorders." In *Current Medical Diagnosis and Treatment, 1998*. 37th ed. Ed. Stephen McPhee, et al. Stamford: Appleton & Lange, 1997.

Altha Roberts Edgren

Metabolic encephalopahty *see* **Delirium**

Meth *see* **Muscle relaxants**

Methadone

Definition

Methadone is a powerful narcotic drug in the same class as heroin. This class is known as the opioids.

Purpose

Methadone, formerly known as dolophine, is a psycho-active drug, meaning that it affects the mind or behavior. It belongs to the class of opioids, drugs that share some of the analgesic properties, and mimic the action of some of the body's naturally occurring chemicals called peptides, such as endorphins and enkephalines.

Methadone is used to relieve chronic **pain** in **cancer** patients and as a maintenance drug to control withdrawal symptoms in people undergoing treatment for opiate **addiction**.

In opiate addiction treatment, methadone blocks the opioid receptors of the brain that bind opiates such as heroin. The blocking of these receptors leads to two major effects:

- because these chemical receptors remain blocked by methadone for up to 24 hours, even if a person addicted to heroin takes heroin after the administration of methadone, this person is not likely to feel the same effects of the heroin as he or she previously felt;

- because the action of methadone is associated with slower and less intense withdrawal symptoms than those of heroin, the patient can experience milder opiate effects while the addiction is being treated and avoid the unpleasant withdrawal symptoms associated with heroin.

Methadone has also been shown to reduce cravings for heroin while not altering a person's mood.

Precautions

Methadone magnifies the effects of alcohol and other **central nervous system depressants**, such as **antihistamines**, cold medicines, sedatives, tranquilizers, other prescription and over-the-counter (OTC) pain medications, **barbiturates**, seizure medications, **muscle relaxants**, and certain anesthetics including some dental anesthetics. Alcohol and other central nervous system depressants should not be taken or consumed while methadone is being taken.

Methadone is a powerful narcotic. It can cause some people to feel drowsy, dizzy, or light-headed. People taking methadone should not drive a car or operate machinery.

Intentional or accidental overdose of methadone can lead to unconsciousness, **coma**, or **death**. The signs of methadone overdose include confusion, difficulty speaking, seizures, severe nervousness or restlessness, severe **dizziness**, severe drowsiness, and/or slow or troubled breathing. These symptoms are increased by alcohol or other central nervous system (CNS) depressants. Anyone who feels that he or she, or someone else, may have overdosed on methadone, or a combination of methadone and other central nervous system depressants, should seek emergency medical attention for that person at once.

Description

A typical adult dosage for methadone is 5–20 mg as an oral solution, 2.5–10 mg as an oral tablet or injection, every four to eight hours as necessary for pain. When used for **detoxification**, methadone is initially given in a dose of 15–100 mg per day as an oral solution. This dose is then decreased until the patient no longer requires the medication. The injection form of methadone is only used for detoxification in patients who are unable to take the medication by mouth.

Preparation

No preparation is generally necessary prior to the intake of methadone as a pain reliever. In cases of maintenance treatments, it is important to be sure that the patient is not currently intoxicated by alcohol, heroin, other opioids, or taking other central nervous system depressants.

Aftercare

Patients receiving methadone should be monitored for adverse reactions to this drug, and/or possible accidental overdose.

Risks

Methadone can interfere with or exacerbate certain medical conditions. For these reasons, it is important that the prescribing physician be informed of any current case, or history of:

- alcohol abuse
- brain disease or head injury
- colitis
- drug dependency, particularly of **narcotics**
- emotional problems
- emphysema, **asthma**, or other chronic lung disease
- enlarged prostate
- gallstones or gallbladder disease
- heart disease
- kidney disease
- liver disease
- problems with urination
- seizures
- underactive thyroid

Side effects

The most common side effects of methadone include:

- constipation
- dizziness

- drowsiness

- itching

- nausea

- urine retention

- vomiting

    Less common side effects of methadone include:

- abnormally fast or slow heartbeat

- blurred or double vision

- cold, clammy skin

- depression or other mood changes

- dry mouth

- fainting

- hallucinations

- hives

- loss of appetite

- nightmares or unusual dreams

- pinpoint pupils of the eyes

- redness or flushing of the face

- restlessness

- rigid muscles

- ringing or buzzing in the ears

- seizure

- severe drowsiness

- skin reaction at the site of injection

- stomach cramps or pain

- sweating

- trouble sleeping (insomnia)

- yellowing of the skin or whites of the eyes

Normal results

Normal results after the administration of methadone to treat chronic pain is the alleviation of that patient's pain, at least to the point where the pain is bearable.

Normal results of methadone treatment to control heroin addiction, is that the patient reduces heroin intake almost immediately upon starting methadone treatments, followed by complete abstinence, usually within two weeks after starting treatment.

Resources

PERIODICALS

Sadovsky, Richard. "Methadone Maintenance Therapy." *American Family Physician* July 15, 2000.

ORGANIZATIONS

National Alliance of Methadone Advocates (NAMA). 435 Second Avenue, New York, NY, 10010. (212) 595-6262. < http://www.methadone.org/ >.

National Clearinghouse for Alcohol and Drug Information. 11426-28 Rockville Pike, Suite 200, Rockville, MD 20852. (800) 729-6686. < http://www.health.org/ >.

Paul A. Johnson, Ed.M.

Methemoglobinemia

Definition

When excessive hemoglobin in the blood is converted to another chemical that cannot deliver oxygen to tissues, called methemoglobin.

Description

The molecule hemoglobin in the blood is responsible for binding oxygen to give to the body. When hemoglobin is oxidized to methemoglobin its structure changes and it is no longer able to bind oxygen. Hemoglobin is constantly under oxidizing stresses; however, normally less than 1% of a person's hemoglobin is in the methemoglobin state. This is due to the body's systems that reduce methemoglobin back to hemoglobin. Infants have a higher risk of acquiring methemoglobinemia because infant hemoglobin is more prone to be oxidized to methemoglobin.

Causes and symptoms

Methemoglobinemia can either be congenital or acquired.

There are two causes of the congenital form. One cause is a defect in the body's systems to reduce methemoglobin to hemoglobin. The other cause is a mutant form of hemoglobin called hemoglobin M that cannot bind to oxygen. Both of these forms are typically benign.

Acquired methemoglobinemia is caused by an external source, usually a drug or medication. Some of these medications include benzocaine, lidocaine and prilocaine. These medications can inhibit the body's systems of reducing methemoglobin to hemoglobin resulting in methemoglobinemia.

With a methemoglobin level of 3-15% skin can turn to a pale gray or blue (**cyanosis**). With levels above 25% the following symptoms may be present:

- Cyanosis unaffected by oxygen administration
- Blood that is dark or chocolate in color that will not change to red in the presence of oxygen
- Headache
- Weakness
- Confusion
- Chest pain

When methemoglobin levels are above 70% **death** may result if not treated immediately.

Diagnosis

Diagnosis is based on the symptoms and history. If these are indicative of methemoglobinemia blood tests are performed to confirm the presence and level of methemoglobin.

Treatment

For acquired methemoglobinemia the typical treatment is with methylene blue. This is administered with an IV over a five-minute period and results are typically seen within 20 minutes. Methylene blue reduces methemoglobin back to hemoglobin.

Though congenital methemoglobinemia is usually benign, the form due to a defective reducing system can be treated with ascorbic acid (vitamin C) taken daily. The other congenital form due to hemoglobin M has no treatment as of late.

Alternative treatment

There are not any known alternative treatments for methemoglobinemia. Methylene blue, or a similar treatment, is needed to reduce methemoglobin to hemoglobin.

Prognosis

If found early, acquired methemoglobinemia can be easily treated with no side effects. After treatment with methylene blue the patient can expect a full recovery.

Congenital methemoglobinemia is typically benign and should be observed. If methemoglobinemia symptoms occur the person should be taken to the hospital for treatment.

Prevention

If a person gets methemoglobinemia from a certain medication that medication should be avoided at

2432

all costs in the future. For people with congenital methemoglobinemia medications or other things that are known to oxidize hemoglobin should be avoided.

Resources

BOOKS

Beutler, Ernest. "Methemoglobinemia and Other Causes of Cyanois." In *Williams Hematology*. 6th ed. New York: McGraw-Hill, 2001, pp. 611-17.

PERIODICALS

Wilburn-Goo, Dawn, and Lloyd. "When Patients Become Cyanotic: Acquired Methemoglobinemia." *Journal of the American Dental Association* June 1999: 826-31.

Wright, Lewander, and Woolf. "Methemoglobinemia: Etiology, Pharmacology, and Clinical Management." *Annals of Emergency Medicine* November 1999: 646-56.

OTHER

eMedicine. Website. 2001. < http://www.emedicine.com >.

Thomas Scott Eagan
Ronald Watson, PhD

Methylphenidate *see* **Central nervous system stimulants**

Metoprolol *see* **Beta blockers**

Metronidazole *see* **Antiprotozoal drugs**

Micronaz *see* **Antifungal drugs, topical**

Microphthalmia and anophthalmia

Definition

Anophthalmia is the complete absence of an eye. Microphthalmia is an eye that has an abnormal smallness.

Description

Anophthalmia is caused by a defect in embryonic development. The total absence of an eye is extremely rare and often a clinical sign associated with a broad range of genetic disorders or, more commonly, a sporadic mutation. Sporadic transmission occurs in the affected individual due to a genetic abnormality. It is not passed on from the parents, but usually due to a combination of environmental and genetic influences. More commonly anophthalmia clinically presents as a small cyst. The defect, which causes anophthalmia, is an absence of the optic vesicle, a structure important for eye development. The genetic abnormality usually occurs during weeks one to three after conception. It is estimated that the incidence of microphthalmia occurs 0.22 times per 1,000 live births. Anophthalmia can occur during adult life but not associated with a genetic cause.

Microphthalmia refers to an abnormally small eye. This clinical sign is often associated with autosomal dominant or recessively transmitted genetic disorders. Most disorders dominantly inherited with microphthalmia are associated with some visual capabilities in infancy and early childhood. Microphthalmia may be isolated (the only presenting sign) or associated with a range of ocular or systemic abnormalities. Isolated cases of microphthalmia may be sporadic or inherited. There is a variable degree of **visual impairment**. Microphthalmia occurs due to autosomal recessive transmission and is part of a syndrome associated with abnormalities in the retina or systemic lesions. Microphthalmia results from a developmental defect after formation of the optic vesicle. The developmental abnormality causes the optic vesicle to fold inwards, resulting in the formation of a cyst. The cyst will progressively swell from birth, and it may be situated along the optic nerve. The cyst may also be situated along other important eye structures.

Causes and symptoms

Microphthalmia and anophthalmia can be caused by sporadic or genetic mutations. Anophthalmia is characterized by a total absence of an eye. Anophthalmia in an adult is usually caused by trauma, infection, tumor, or advanced eye disease.

Diagnosis

Microscope examination confirms the diagnosis of true anophthalmia. The clinician examines a piece of tissue taken from the eye and notes eviscerated tissue. For microphthalmia the confirmation can be established by eye measurements. Eyes, which have an axial length <21 mm in an adult, or <19 mm in a one-year-old child are described as having microphthalmia.

Treatment

Large cysts causing microphthalmia should be aspirated or removed surgically. There is no known cure for anophthalmia or microphthalmia. For anophthalmia a prosthetic eye can be fitted which may involve surgery. Treatment for microphthalmia depends on the complexity of eye involvement.

Prognosis

For anophthalmia, prosthetic eyes should be seen by a specialist two to three times per year to assess fit, mobility, and smoothness. They are usually well tolerated and have good appearance and mobility. The clinical course for microphthalmia depends on the extent of smallness, but usually patients progress favorably without major treatment. Since the smallness is distinctly noticeable, there may be individual cosmetic considerations.

Prevention

There is no known prevention for either, since these clinical signs are commonly associated with genetic inheritance.

Resources

BOOKS

Yanoff, Myron, et al, editors. *Ophthalmology*. 1st ed. Mosby International Ltd., 1999.

PERIODICALS

Mills, M. "The Eye in Childhood." *American Family Physician* 60 (September 1999).

ORGANIZATIONS

American Society of Human Genetics. Administrative Office. 9650 Rockville Pike Bethesda, Maryland 20814-3998. (301) 571-1825. 2001. < http://www.faseb.org/genetics/ashg/moreinfo.htm >.

Laith Farid Gulli, M.D.

Middle ear infection *see* **Otitis media**

Mifeprex *see* **Mifepristone**

Mifepristone

Definition

Mifepristone is a pill that can be taken as an alternative to a surgical abortion.

Purpose

This medication most often is used for ending early pregnancies. In 2003, studies were surfacing reporting other possible uses for mifepristone, at least at low doses. These studies included its possible use in treating psychotic depression. Low-dose mifepristone also showed success as a treatment for **uterine fibroids**, or benign growths in the muscular tissue of a woman's uterus. However, many uses of the drug other than for abortions were still experimental, even if promising.

Mifespristone's primary use for medical abortions is preferred by many over surgical approaches to abortions. It has emerged as a form of **emergency contraception** when taken at low does within a short time period following possible conception.

Precautions

Women who are more than seven weeks pregnant (or 49 days since their last menstrual period) should not take mifepristone. Other reasons to avoid mifepristone include: use of an intrauterine device (**IUD**), **ectopic pregnancy**, use of blood thinners, bleeding disorders, use of steroid medications, **allergies** to mifepristone or similar drugs and lack of access to medical help within two weeks after the treatment. When the drug is used at low doses as emergency **contraception**, it poses few side effects.

Description

Mifepristone, sold commercially under the name Mifeprex, also is known as RU-486, the abortion pill, the early option pill for medical abortion. While it has been used for many years in Europe, mifepristone has only been available for use in the United States since the U.S. Food and Drug Administration (FDA) approved it in 2000 for use in abortion. More than 37,000 abortions were performed using the pill in the first six months of 2001.

This drug causes **pregnancy** to end by blocking the female hormone progesterone. The lack of progesterone makes the uterus shed its lining, which causes bleeding similar to a menstrual period. Three days after taking mifepristone, women are given a second drug, misprostol, to cause uterine contractions that expel the contents of the uterus. Most women are able remain in their own home while they pass the fetus.

Preparation

Before taking mifepristone, health care providers likely will give the woman a urine or blood test to be sure that she is, in fact, pregnant. They also may give her some counseling and support. Once she has made the decision to use mifepristone, they will ask her to sign a written statement that she has decided to end her pregnancy.

Aftercare

Using mifepristone and misoprostol causes heavy bleeding and cramping. Doctors can offer **pain** medicine, such as Motrin, to ease the cramps. For two weeks after treatment with mifepristone, health care providers likely will ask patients to abstain from sexual intercourse, heavy lifting and strenuous **exercise**. They also may advise against breast-feeding, since scientists are not sure if the drug is present in breast milk.

Physicians require patients to come in for a follow-up visit 14 days after their first dose of mifepristone to verify that they are no longer pregnant and that they are properly healing.

Risks

Other common side effects include: **fatigue**, headaches, **dizziness**, **nausea**, **vomiting**, **diarrhea** and low-back pain.

Since pregnancy hormones are in flux after a medical abortion, many women have emotional

KEY TERMS

Dilation and curettage (D and C)—During this surgical procedure, a physician dilates the cervix, then uses an instrument to scrape tissue away from the walls of the uterus.

Misprostol—A drug used in combination with mifepristone to cause uterine contractions that expel the contents of the uterus.

side-effects, such as mood swings, depression or a mild case of the blues. These feelings usually subside when hormones stabilize a few weeks later. For those who feel stuck in their grief or anger about the situation, counseling or support groups may offer relief.

Normal results

Most women feel better after about two weeks. Bleeding and spotting usually occurs for 9-16 days, but may last for a month.

Abnormal results

In some cases, mifepristone does not completely end the pregnancy. If the fetus is still left inside the uterus, a doctor may recommend a surgical abortion, or a procedure called dilation and curettage (D and C). About five to eight of every 100 women who take mifepristone go on to have a surgical abortion, according to the FDA. During a D and C, which usually is done at a hospital or clinic under a local anesthetic, a physician dilates the cervix, then uses an instrument to scrape any residual tissue away from the walls of the uterus. This allows the heavy bleeding to eventually stop so a woman can return to her normal cycle sooner.

Resources

PERIODICALS

"Abortion Pills Account For 5% of U.S. Abortions." *Medical Letter on the CDC and FDA* February 9, 2003: 7.

"The Abortion Pill's Grim Progress." *Mother Jones* 24 (January 1, 1999).

Grimes, David A, Mitchell D. Creinin. "Induced Abortion: an Overview for Internists." *Annals of Internal Medicine* April 20, 2004: 620–627.

"Low-dose Mifepristone Blocks Pregnancy by Altering Ovarian Function." *Drug Week* March 5, 2004: 107.

"Treatments for Depression with Psychosis." *Harvard Mental Health Letter* August 2003.

Walling, Anne D. "Low-dose Mifepristone Shrinks Uterine Fibroids." *American Family Physician* September 1, 2003: 956.

Melissa Knopper
Teresa G. Odle

Migraine headache

Definition

Migraine is a type of **headache** marked by severe head **pain** lasting several hours or more.

Description

Migraine is an intense and often debilitating type of headache. Migraines affect as many as 24 million people in the United States, and are responsible for billions of dollars in lost work, poor job performance, and direct medical costs. Approximately 18% of women and 6% of men experience at least one migraine attack per year. More than three million women and one million men have one or more severe headaches every month. Migraines often begin in adolescence, and are rare after age 60.

Two types of migraine are recognized. Eighty percent of migraine sufferers experience "migraine without aura" (common migraine). In "migraine with aura," or classic migraine, the pain is preceded or accompanied by visual or other sensory disturbances, including **hallucinations**, partial obstruction of the visual field, **numbness** or **tingling**, or a feeling of heaviness. Symptoms are often most prominent on one side of the head or body, and may begin as early as 72 hours before the onset of pain.

Causes and symptoms

Causes

The physiological basis of migraine has proved difficult to uncover. Genetics appear to play a part for many, but not all, people with migraine. There are a multitude of potential triggers for a migraine attack, and recognizing one's own set of triggers is the key to prevention.

PHYSIOLOGY. The most widely accepted hypothesis of migraine suggests that a migraine attack is precipitated when pain-sensing nerve cells in the brain (called nociceptors) release chemicals called neuropeptides. At least one of the neurotransmitters, substance P, increases the pain sensitivity of other nearby nociceptors.

Other neuropeptides act on the smooth muscle surrounding cranial blood vessels. This smooth muscle regulates blood flow in the brain by relaxing or contracting, thus constricting the enclosed blood vessels and stimulating adjacent pain receptors. At the onset of a migraine headache, neuropeptides are thought to cause muscle relaxation, allowing vessel dilation and increased blood flow. Other neuropeptides increase the leakiness of cranial vessels, allowing fluid leak, and promote inflammation and tissue swelling. The pain of migraine is though to result from this combination of increased pain sensitivity, tissue and vessel swelling, and inflammation. The aura seen during a migraine may be related to constriction in the blood vessels that dilate in the headache phase.

GENETICS. Susceptibility to some types of migraine is inherited. A child of a migraine sufferer has as much as a 50% chance of developing migraines. If both parents are affected, the chance rises to 70%. In 2002, a team of Australian researchers identified a region on human chromosome 1 that influences susceptibility to migraine. It is likely that more than one gene is involved in the inherited forms of the disorder. Many cases of migraine, however, have no obvious familial basis. It is likely that the genes that are involved set the stage for migraine, and that full development requires environmental influences, as well.

Two groups of Italian researchers have recently identified two loci on human chromosomes 1 and 14 respectively that are linked to migraine headaches. The locus on chromosome 1q23 has been linked to familial hemiplegic migraine type 2, while the locus on chromosome 14q21 is associated with migraine without aura.

TRIGGERS. A wide variety of foods, drugs, environmental cues, and personal events are known to trigger migraines. It is not known how most triggers set off the events of migraine, nor why individual migraine sufferers are affected by particular triggers but not others.

Common food triggers include:

- cheese
- alcohol
- **caffeine** products, and caffeine withdrawal
- chocolate
- intensely sweet foods

- dairy products
- fermented or pickled foods
- citrus fruits
- nuts
- processed foods, especially those containing nitrites, sulfites, or monosodium glutamate (msg)

Environmental and event-related triggers include:

- **stress** or time pressure
- menstrual periods, **menopause**
- sleep changes or disturbances, oversleeping
- prolonged overexertion or uncomfortable posture
- hunger or **fasting**
- odors, smoke, or perfume
- strong glare or flashing lights

Drugs which may trigger migraine include:

- oral contraceptives
- estrogen replacement therapy
- nitrates
- theophylline
- reserpine
- nifedipine
- indomethicin
- cimetidine
- decongestant overuse
- analgesic overuse
- benzodiazepine withdrawal

Symptoms

Migraine without aura may be preceded by elevations in mood or energy level for up to 24 hours before the attack. Other pre-migraine symptoms may include **fatigue**, depression, and excessive yawning.

Aura most often begins with shimmering, jagged arcs of white or colored light progressing over the visual field in the course of 10-20 minutes. This may be preceded or replaced by dark areas or other visual disturbances. **Numbness and tingling** is common, especially of the face and hands. These sensations may spread, and may be accompanied by a sensation of weakness or heaviness in the affected limb.

The pain of migraine is often present only on one side of the head, although it may involve both, or switch sides during attacks. The pain is usually throbbing, and may range from mild to incapacitating. It is often accompanied by **nausea** or **vomiting**, painful

sensitivity to light and sound, and intolerance of food or odors. Blurred vision is common.

Migraine pain tends to intensify over the first 30 minutes to several hours, and may last from several hours to a day or longer. Afterward, the affected person is usually weary, and sensitive to sudden head movements.

Diagnosis

Ideally, migraine is diagnosed by a careful medical history. Unfortunately, migraine is underdiagnosed because many doctors tend to minimize its symptoms as "just a headache." According to a 2003 study, 64% of migraine patients in the United Kingdom and 77% of those in the United States never receive a correct medical diagnosis for their headaches.

So far, laboratory tests and such imaging studies as computed tomography (CT scan) or **magnetic resonance imaging** (MRI) scans have not been useful for identifying migraine. However, these tests may be necessary to rule out a **brain tumor** or other structural causes of migraine headache in some patients.

Treatment

Once a migraine begins, the person will usually seek out a dark, quiet room to lessen painful stimuli. Several drugs may be used to reduce the pain and severity of the attack.

Nonsteroidal anti-inflammatory drugs (NSAIDs) are helpful for early and mild headache. NSAIDs include **acetaminophen**, ibuprofen, naproxen, and others. A recent study concluded that a combination of acetaminophen, **aspirin**, and caffeine could effectively relieve symptoms for many migraine patients. One such over-the-counter preparation is available as Exedrin Migraine.

More severe or unresponsive attacks may be treated with drugs that act on serotonin receptors in the smooth muscle surrounding cranial blood vessels. Serotonin, also known as 5-hydroxytryptamine, constricts these vessels, relieving migraine pain. Drugs that mimic serotonin and bind to these receptors have the same effect. The oldest of them is ergotamine, a derivative of a common grain fungus. Ergotamine and dihydroergotamine are used for both acute and preventive treatment. Derivatives with fewer side effects have come onto the market in the past decade, including sumatriptan (Imitrex). Some of these drugs are available as nasal sprays, intramuscular injections, or rectal suppositories for patients in whom vomiting precludes oral administration. Other drugs used for acute attacks include meperidine and metoclopramide.

Studies are showing that rizatriptan is a promising drug for the treatment of migraines. One study showed that 10mg of rizatriptan provided relief to 90% of the patients in the study group and kept 50% of them pain-free 2 hours after taking the medication. Sumatriptan has been on the market since 1993, while rizatriptan became available in 1998.

Sumatriptan and other triptan drugs (zolmitriptan, rizatriptan, naratriptan, almotriptan, and frovatriptan) should not be taken by people with any kind of vascular disease because they cause coronary artery narrowing. Otherwise these drugs have been shown to be very safe.

Continued use of some **antimigraine drugs** can lead to "rebound headache," marked by frequent or chronic headaches, especially in the early morning hours. Rebound headache can be avoided by using antimigraine drugs under a doctor's supervision, with the minimum dose necessary to treat symptoms. Tizanidine (Zanaflex) has been reported to be effective in treating rebound headaches when taken together with an NSAID.

Alternative treatments

Alternative treatments are aimed at prevention of migraine. Migraine headaches are often linked with **food allergies** or intolerances. Identification and elimination of the offending food or foods can decrease the frequency of migraines and/or alleviate these headaches altogether. Herbal therapy with feverfew (*Chrysanthemum parthenium*) may lessen the frequency of attacks. Learning to increase the flow of blood to the extremities through **biofeedback** training may allow a patient to prevent some of the vascular changes once a migraine begins. During a migraine, keep the lights low; put the feet in a tub of hot water and place a cold cloth on the occipital region (the back of the head). This treatment draws the blood to the feet and decreases the pressure in the head.

Prognosis

Most people with migraines can bring their attacks under control through recognizing and avoiding triggers, and by use of appropriate drugs when migraine occurs. Some people with severe migraines do not respond to preventive or drug therapy. Migraines usually wane in intensity by age 60 and beyond.

KEY TERMS

Aura—A group of visual or other sensations that precedes the onset of a migraine attack.

Coenzyme Q$_{10}$—A substance used by cells in the human body to produce energy for cell maintenance and growth. It is being studied as a possible preventive for migraine headaches.

Nociceptor—A specialized type of nerve cell that senses pain.

Prevention

The frequency of migraine may be lessened by avoiding triggers. It is useful to keep a headache journal, recording the particulars and noting possible triggers for each attack. Specific measures which may help include:

- Eating at regular times, and not skipping meals.
- Reducing the use of caffeine and pain-relievers.
- Restricting physical exertion, especially on hot days.
- Keeping regular sleep hours, but not oversleeping.
- Managing one's time efficiently in order to avoid stress at work and home.

Some drugs can be used for migraine prevention, including specific members of these drug classes:

- beta blockers
- tricyclic antidepressants
- calcium channel blockers
- selective serotinin reuptake inhibitors (SSRIs)
- monoamine oxidase inhibitors (MAOIs)
- serotonin antagonists

One substance that is being studied as a possible migraine preventive is coenzyme Q$_{10}$, a compound used by cells to produce energy needed for cell growth and maintenance. Coenzyme Q$_{10}$ has been studied as a possible complementary treatment for **cancer**. Its use in preventing migraines is encouraging and merits further study.

A study published in early 2003 reported that three drugs currently used to treat disorders of muscle tone are being explored as possible preventive treatments for migraine. They are botulinum toxin type A (Botox), baclofen (Lioresal), and tizanidine (Zanaflex). Early results of open trials of these medications are positive.

Anti-epileptic drugs, which are also known as anticonvulsants, are also being studied as possible migraine preventives. As of 2003, sodium valproate (Epilim) is the only drug approved by the Food and Drug Administration (FDA) for prevention of migraine. Such newer anticonvulsants as gabapentin (Neurontin) and topiramate (Topamax) are presently being evaluated as migraine preventives.

A natural preparation made from butterbur root (*Petasites hybridus*) has been sold in Germany since the 1970s as a migraine preventive under the trade name Petadolex. Petadolex has been available in the United States since December 1998 and has passed several clinical safety and postmarketing surveillance trials.

Resources

BOOKS

Beers, Mark H., MD, and Robert Berkow, MD, editors. "Migraine." Section 14, Chapter 168. In *The Merck Manual of Diagnosis and Therapy*. Whitehouse Station, NJ: Merck Research Laboratories, 2004.

Pelletier, Kenneth R., MD. *The Best Alternative Medicine*, Part II, "CAM Therapies for Specific Conditions: Headaches." New York: Simon & Schuster, 2002.

Rakel, Robert. *Conn's Current Therapy: Latest Approved Methods of Treatment for the Practicing Physician*. Philadelphia: W.B. Saunders Company, 2001.

Tierney, Lawrence, et al. *Current Medical Diagnosis and Treatment*. Los Altos, CA: Lange Medical Publications, 2001.

PERIODICALS

Bendtsen, L. "Sensitization: Its Role in Primary Headache." *Current Opinion in Investigational Drugs* 3 (March 2002): 449–453.

Corbo, J. "The Role of Anticonvulsants in Preventive Migraine Therapy." *Current Pain and Headache Reports* 7 (February 2003): 63–66.

Danesch, U., and R. Rittinghausen. "Safety of a Patented Special Butterbur Root Extract for Migraine Prevention." *Headache* 43 (January 2003): 76–78.

Diamond, S., and R. Wenzel. "Practical Approaches to Migraine Management." *CNS Drugs* 16 (2002): 385–403.

Freitag, F. G. "Preventative Treatment for Migraine and Tension-Type Headaches: Do Drugs Having Effects on Muscle Spasm and Tone Have a Role?" *CNS Drugs* 17 (2003): 373–381.

Lea, R. A., A. G. Shepherd, R. P. Curtain, et al. "A Typical Migraine Susceptibility Region Localizes to Chromosome 1q31." *Neurogenetics* 4 (March 2002): 17–22.

Lipton, R. B., A. I. Scher, T. J. Steiner, et al. "Patterns of Health Care Utilization for Migraine in England and in the United States." *Neurology* 60 (February 11, 2003): 441–448.

Marconi, R., M. De Fusco, P. Aridon, et al. "Familial Hemiplegic Migraine Type 2 is Linked to 0.9Mb Region on Chromosome 1q23." *Annals of Neurology* 53 (March 2003): 376–381.

Rozen, T. D., M. L. Oshinsky, C. A. Gebeline, et al. "Open Label Trial of Coenzyme Q$_{10}$ as a Migraine Preventive." *Cephalalgia* 22 (March 2002): 137–141.

Sheftell, F. D., and S. J. Tepper. "New Paradigms in the Recognition and Acute Treatment of Migraine." *Headache* 42 (January 2002): 58–69.

Sinclair, Steven. "Migraine Headaches: Nutritional, Botanical and Other Alternative Approaches." *Alternative Medicine Review* 4 (1999): 86–95.

Soragna, D., A. Vettori, G. Carraro, et al. "A Locus for Migraine Without Aura Maps on Chromosome 14q21.2-q22.3." *American Journal of Human Genetics* 72 (January 2003): 161–167.

Tepper, S. J., and D. Millson. "Safety Profile of the Triptans." *Expert Opinion on Drug Safety* 2 (March 2003): 123–132.

ORGANIZATIONS

American Council for Headache Education. 19 Mantua Road, Mt. Royal, NJ 08061. (609) 423-0043 or (800) 255-2243. < http://www.achenet.org >.

National Headache Foundation. 428 West St. James Place, Chicago, IL 60614. (773) 388-6399 or (800) 843-2256. < http://www.headaches.org >.

U. S. Food and Drug Administration (FDA). 5600 Fishers Lane, Rockville, MD 20857. (888) 463-6332. < http://www.fda.gov >.

OTHER

American Medical Association. "Migraine." < http://www.ama-assn.org/special/migraine/ >.

Kim A. Sharp, M.Ln.
Rebecca J. Frey, PhD

Miliaria *see* **Prickly heat**

Mineral deficiency

Definition

The term mineral deficiency means a condition where the concentration of any one of the **minerals** essential to human health is abnormally low in the body. In some cases, an abnormally low mineral concentration is defined as that which leads to an impairment in a function dependent on the mineral. In other cases, the convention may be to define an abnormally low mineral concentration as a level lower than that found in a specific healthy population.

The mineral nutrients are defined as all the inorganic elements or inorganic molecules that are required for life. As far as human **nutrition** is concerned, the inorganic nutrients include water, sodium, potassium, chloride, calcium, phosphate, sulfate, magnesium, iron, copper, zinc, manganese, iodine, selenium, and molybdenum. Some of the inorganic nutrients, such as water, do not occur as single atoms, but occur as molecules. Other inorganic nutrients that are molecules include phosphate, sulfate, and selenite. Phosphate contains an atom of phosphorus. Sulfate contains an atom of sulfur. We do not need to eat sulfate, since the body can acquire all the sulfate it needs from protein. Selenium occurs in foods as selenite and selenate.

There is some evidence that other inorganic nutrients, such as chromium and boron, play a part in human health, but their role is not well established. Fluoride has been proven to increase the strength of bones and teeth, but there is little or no reason to believe that is needed for human life.

The mineral content of the body may be measured by testing samples of blood plasma, red blood cells, or urine. In the case of calcium and phosphate deficiency, the diagnosis may also involve taking x rays of the skeleton. In the case of iodine deficiency, the diagnosis may include examining the patient's neck with the eyes and hands. In the case of iron deficiency, the diagnosis may include the performance of a stair-stepping test by the patient. Since all the minerals serve strikingly different functions in the body, the tests for the corresponding deficiency are markedly different from each other.

Description

Laboratory studies with animals have revealed that severe deficiencies in any one of the inorganic nutrients can result in very specific symptoms, and finally in **death**, due to the failure of functions associated with that nutrient. In humans, deficiency in one nutrient may occur less often than deficiency in several nutrients. A patient suffering from **malnutrition** is deficient in a variety of nutrients. In the United States, malnutrition is most often found among severe alcoholics. In part, this is because the alcohol consumption may supply half of the energy requirement, resulting in a mineral and vitamin intake of half the expected level. Deficiencies in one nutrient do occur, for example, in human populations living in iodine-poor regions of the world, and in iron deficient persons who lose excess iron by abnormal bleeding.

Inorganic nutrients have a great variety of functions in the body. Water, sodium, and potassium deficiencies are most closely associated with abnormal nerve action and cardiac **arrhythmias**. Deficiencies in these nutrients tend to result not from a lack of content in the diet, but from excessive losses due to severe **diarrhea** and other causes. Iodine deficiency is a global public health problem. It occurs in parts of the world with iodine-deficient soils, and results in **goiter**, which involves a relatively harmless swelling of the neck, and cretinism, a severe birth defect. The only use of iodine in the body is for making thyroid hormone. However, since thyroid hormone has a variety of roles in development of the embryo, iodine deficiency during **pregnancy** results in a number of **birth defects**.

Calcium deficiency due to lack of dietary calcium occurs only rarely. However, calcium deficiency due to **vitamin D deficiency** can be found among certain populations. Vitamin D is required for the efficient absorption of calcium from the diet, and hence vitamin D deficiency in growing infants and children can result in calcium deficiency.

Dietary phosphate deficiency is rare because phosphate is plentiful in plant and animal foods, but also because phosphate is efficiently absorbed from the diet into the body. Iron deficiency causes anemia (lack of red blood cells), which results in tiredness and **shortness of breath**.

Dietary deficiencies in the remaining inorganic nutrients tend to be rare. Magnesium deficiency is uncommon, but when it occurs it tends to occur in chronic alcoholics, in persons taking diuretic drugs, and in those suffering from severe and prolonged diarrhea. Magnesium deficiency tends to occur with the same conditions that provoke deficiencies in sodium and potassium. Zinc deficiency is rare, but it has been found in impoverished populations in the Middle East, who rely on unleavened whole wheat bread as a major food source. Copper deficiency is also rare, but dramatic and health-threatening changes in copper metabolism occur in two genetic diseases, Wilson's disease and Menkes' disease.

Selenium deficiency may occur in regions of the world where the soils are poor in selenium. Low-selenium soils can produce foods that are also low in selenium. Premature infants may also be at risk for selenium deficiency. Manganese deficiency is very rare. Experimental studies with humans fed a manganese deficient diet have revealed that the deficiency produces a scaly, red rash on the skin of the upper torso. Molybdenum deficiency has probably never occurred, but indirect evidence suggests that if molybdenum deficiency could occur, it would result in **mental retardation** and death.

Causes and symptoms

Sodium deficiency (**hyponatremia**) and water deficiency are the most serious and widespread deficiencies in the world. These deficiencies tend to arise from excessive losses from the body, as during prolonged and severe diarrhea or **vomiting**. Diarrheal diseases are a major world health problem, and are responsible for about a quarter of the 10 million infant deaths that occur each year. Nearly all of these deaths occur in impoverished parts of Africa and Asia, where they result from contamination of the water supply by animal and human feces.

The main concern in treating diarrheal diseases is **dehydration**, that is, the losses of sodium and water which deplete the fluids of the circulatory system (the heart, veins, arteries, and capillaries). Severe losses of the fluids of the circulatory system result in **shock**. Shock nearly always occurs when dehydration is severe enough to produce a 10% reduction in body weight. Shock, which is defined as inadequate supply of blood to the various tissues of the body, results in a lack of oxygen to all the cells of the body. Although diarrheal fluids contain a number of electrolytes, the main concern in avoiding shock is the replacement of sodium and water.

Sodium deficiency and potassium deficiency also frequently result during treatment with drugs called **diuretics**. Diuretics work because they cause loss of sodium from the body. These drugs are used to treat high blood pressure (**hypertension**), where the resulting decline in blood pressure reduces the risk for cardiovascular disease. However, diuretics can lead to sodium deficiency, resulting in low plasma sodium levels. A side effect of some diuretics is excessive loss of potassium, and low plasma potassium (**hypokalemia**) may result.

Iodine deficiency tends to occur in regions of the world where the soil is poor in iodine. Where soil used in agriculture is poor in iodine, the foods grown in the soil will also be low in iodine. An iodine intake of 0.10-0.15 mg/day is considered to be nutritionally adequate, while iodine deficiency occurs at below 0.05 mg/day. Goiter, an enlargement of the thyroid gland (located in the neck), results from iodine deficiency. Goiter continues to be a problem in eastern Europe, parts of India and South America, and in Southeast Asia. Goiter has been eradicated in the United States because of the fortification of foods with iodine. Iodine deficiency during pregnancy results in cretinism in the newborn. Cretinism involves mental retardation, a large tongue, and sometimes deafness, muteness, and lameness.

Iron deficiency occurs due to periods of dietary deficiency, rapid growth, and excessive loss of the body's iron. Human milk and cow milk both contains low levels of iron. Infants are at risk for acquiring iron deficiency because their rapid rate of growth needs a corresponding increased supply of dietary iron, for use in making blood and muscles. Human milk is a better source of iron than cow milk, since about half of the iron in human breast milk is absorbed by the infant's digestive tract. In contrast, only 10% of the iron in cow milk is absorbed by the infant. Surveys of lower-income families in the United States have revealed that about 6% of the infants are anemic indicating a deficiency of iron in their **diets**. Blood loss that occurs with menstruation in women, as well as with a variety of causes of intestinal bleeding is a major cause of iron deficiency. The symptoms of iron deficiency are generally limited to anemia, and the resulting tiredness, weakness, and a reduced ability to perform physical work.

Calcium and phosphate are closely related nutrients. About 99% of the calcium and 85% of the phosphate in the body occur in the skeleton, where they exist as crystals of solid calcium phosphate. Both of these nutrients occur in a great variety of foods. Milk, eggs, and green, leafy vegetables are rich in calcium and phosphate. Whole cow milk, for example, contains about 1.2 g calcium and 0.95 g phosphorus per kg of food. Broccoli contains 1.0 g calcium and 0.67 g phosphorus per kg food. Eggs supply about one third of the calcium and phosphate of the overall population of the United States. Dietary deficiencies in calcium (**hypocalcemia**) or phosphate are extremely rare throughout the world. Vitamin D deficiency can be found among young infants, the elderly, and others who may be shielded from sunshine for prolonged periods of time. Vitamin D deficiency impairs the absorption of calcium from the diet, and in this way can provoke calcium deficiency even when the diet contains adequate calcium.

Zinc deficiency has been found among peasant populations in rural areas of the Middle East. Unleavened whole wheat bread can account for 75% of the energy intake in these areas. This diet, which does not contain meat, does contain zinc, but it also contains phytic acid at a level of about 3 g/day. The phytic acid, which naturally occurs in wheat, inhibits zinc absorption. The yeast used to leaven bread produces enzymes that inactivate the phytic acid. Unleavened bread does not contain yeast, and therefore, contains intact phytic acid. The symptoms of zinc deficiency include lack of sexual maturation, lack of pubic hair, and small stature. The amount of phytic acid in a typical American diet cannot provoke zinc deficiency.

Zinc deficiency is relatively uncommon in the United States, but it may occur in adults with **alcoholism** or intestinal malabsorption problems. Low plasma zinc has been found in patients with alcoholic **cirrhosis**, **Crohn's disease**, and **celiac disease**. Experimental studies with humans have shown that the signs of zinc deficiency are detectable after two to five weeks of consumption of the zinc-free diet. The signs include a rash and diarrhea. The rash occurs on the face, groin, hands, and feet. These symptoms can easily be reversed by administering zinc. An emerging concern is that increased calcium intake can interfere with zinc absorption or retention. Hence, there is some interest in the question of whether persons taking calcium to prevent **osteoporosis** should also take zinc supplements.

Severe alterations in copper metabolism occur in two genetic diseases, Wilson's disease and Menkes' disease. Both of these diseases are rare and occur in about one in 100,000 births. Both diseases involve mutations in copper transport proteins, that is, in special channels that allow the passage of copper ions through cell membranes. Menkes' disease is a genetic disease involving mental retardation and death before the age of three years. The disease also results in steely or kinky hair. The hair is tangled, grayish, and easily broken. Menkes' disease involves a decrease in copper levels in the serum, liver, and brain, and increases in copper in the cells of the intestines and kidney.

Selenium deficiency may occur in premature infants, since this population naturally tends to have low levels of plasma selenium. Full term infants have plasma selenium levels of about 0.001-0.002 mM, while premature infants may have levels about one third this amount. Whether these lower levels result in adverse consequences is not clear. Selenium deficiency occurs in regions of the world containing low-selenium soils. These regions include Keshan Province in China, New Zealand, and Finland. In Keshan Province, a disease (Keshan disease) occurs which results in deterioration of regions of the heart and the development of fibers in these regions. Keshan disease, which may be fatal, is thought to result from a combination of selenium deficiency and a virus.

Diagnosis

The diagnosis of deficiencies in water, sodium, potassium, iron, calcium, and phosphate involve chemical testing of the blood plasma, urine, and red blood cells.

Iodine deficiency can be diagnosed by measuring the concentration of iodine in the urine. A urinary level greater than 0.05 mg iodine per gram creatinine means adequate iodine status. Levels under 0.025 mg iodine/g creatinine indicate a serious risk.

Normal blood serum magnesium levels are 1.2-2.0 mM. Magnesium deficiency results in hypomagnesemia, which is defined as serum magnesium levels below 0.8 mM. Magnesium levels below 0.5 mM provoke a decline in serum calcium levels. Hypomagnesemia can also result in low serum potassium. Some of the symptoms of hypomagnesemia, which include twitching and convulsions, actually result from the hypocalcemia. Other symptoms of hypomagnesemia, such as cardiac arrhythmias, result from the low potassium levels.

There is no reliable test for zinc deficiency. When humans eat diets containing normal levels of zinc (16 mg/day), the level of urinary zinc is about 0.45 mg/day, while humans consuming low-zinc diets (0.3 mg/day) may have urinary levels of about 0.150 mg/day. Plasma zinc levels tend to be maintained during a dietary deficiency in zinc. Plasma and urinary zinc levels can be influenced by a variety of factors, and for this reason cannot provide a clear picture of zinc status.

Selenium deficiency may be diagnosed by measuring the selenium in plasma (70 ng/mL) or red blood cells (90 ng/mL), where the normal values are indicated. There is also some interest in measuring the activity of an enzyme in blood platelets, in order to assess selenium status. This enzyme is glutathione peroxidase. Platelets are small cells of the bloodstream which are used mainly to allow the clotting of blood after an injury.

Treatment

The treatment of deficiencies in sodium, potassium, calcium, phosphate, and iron usually involves intravenous injections of the deficient mineral.

Iodine deficiency can be easily prevented and treated by fortifying foods with iodine. Table salt is fortified with 100 mg potassium iodide per kg sodium chloride. Goiter was once common in the United States in areas from Washington State to the Great Lakes region, but this problem has been eliminated by iodized salt. Public health programs in impoverished countries have involved injections of synthetic oils containing iodine. Goiter is reversible but, cretinism is not.

Magnesium deficiency can be treated with a magnesium rich diet. If magnesium deficiency is due to a

KEY TERMS

Recommended Dietary Allowance—The Recommended Dietary Allowances (RDAs) are quantities of nutrients that are required each day to maintain human health. RDAs are established by the Food and Nutrition Board of the National Academy of Sciences and may be revised every few years. A separate RDA value exists for each nutrient.

prolonged period of depletion, treatment may include injections of magnesium sulfate (2.0 mL of 50% MgSO₄). Where magnesium deficiency is severe enough to provoke convulsions, magnesium needs to be administered by injections or infusions. For infusion, 500 mL of a 1% solution (1 gram/100 mL) of magnesium sulfate is gradually introduced into a vein over the course of about five hours.

Zinc deficiency and copper deficiency are quite rare, but when they are detected or suspected, they can be treated by consuming zinc or copper, on a daily basis, at levels defined by the RDA.

Selenium deficiency in adults can be treated by eating 100 mg selenium per day for a week, where the selenium is supplied as selenomethionine. The incidence of Keshan disease in China has been reduced by supplementing children with 1.0 mg sodium selenite per week.

Prognosis

In iodine deficiency, the prognosis for treating goiter is excellent, however cretinism cannot be reversed. The effects of iron deficiency are not life-threatening and can be easily treated. The prognosis for treating magnesium deficiency is excellent. The symptoms may be relieved promptly or, at most, within two days of starting treatment. In cases of zinc deficiency in Iran and other parts of the Middle East, supplementation of affected young adults with zinc has been found to provoke the growth of pubic hair and enlargement of genitalia to a normal size within a few months.

Prevention

In the healthy population, all mineral deficiencies can be prevented by the consumption of inorganic nutrients at levels defined by the Recommended Dietary Allowances (RDA). Where a balanced diet is not available, government programs for treating individuals, or for fortifying the food supply, may be used. Government sponsored programs for the prevention of iron deficiency and iodine deficiency are widespread throughout the world. Selenium treatment programs have been used in parts of the world where selenium deficiency exists. Attention to potassium status, and to the prevention of potassium deficiency, is an issue mainly in patients taking diuretic drugs. In many cases of mineral deficiency, the deficiency occurs because of disease, and individual medical attention, rather than preventative measures, is used. The prevention of calcium deficiency is generally not an issue or concern, however calcium supplements are widely used with the hope of preventing osteoporosis. The prevention of deficiencies in magnesium, zinc, copper, manganese, or molybdenum are not major health issues in the United States. Ensuring an adequate intake of these minerals, by eating a balanced diet or by taking mineral supplements, is the best way to prevent deficiencies.

Resources

BOOKS

Brody, Tom. *Nutritional Biochemistry.* San Diego: Academic Press, 1998.

Tom Brody, PhD

Mineral excess *see* **Mineral toxicity**

Mineral toxicity

Definition

The term mineral toxicity means a condition where the concentration in the body of any one of the **minerals** is abnormally high, and where there is an adverse effect on health.

Description

In general, mineral toxicity results when there is an accidental consumption of too much of any mineral, as with drinking ocean water (sodium toxicity) or with overexposure to industrial pollutants, household chemicals, or certain drugs. Mineral toxicity may also apply to toxicity that can be the result of certain diseases or injuries. For example, **hemochromatosis** leads to iron toxicity; Wilson's disease results in copper toxicity; severe trauma can lead to **hyperkalemia** (potassium toxicity).

The mineral nutrients are defined as all the inorganic elements or inorganic molecules that are required for life. As far as human **nutrition** is concerned, the inorganic nutrients include water, sodium, potassium, chloride, calcium, phosphate, sulfate, magnesium, iron, copper, zinc, manganese, iodine, selenium, and molybdenum.

The mineral content of the body may be measured by testing samples of blood plasma, red blood cells, and urine.

Causes and symptoms

An increase in the concentrations of sodium in the bloodstream can be toxic. The normal concentration of sodium in the blood plasma is 136-145 mM, while levels over 152 mM can result in seizures and **death**. Increased plasma sodium, which is called **hypernatremia**, causes various cells of the body, including those of the brain, to shrink. Shrinkage of the brain cells results in confusion, **coma**, **paralysis** of the lung muscles, and death. Death has occurred where table salt (sodium chloride) was accidently used, instead of sugar, for feeding infants. Death due to sodium toxicity has also resulted when baking soda (sodium bicarbonate) was used during attempted therapy of excessive **diarrhea** or **vomiting**. Although a variety of processed foods contain high levels of sodium chloride, the levels used are not enough to result in sodium toxicity.

The normal level of potassium in the bloodstream is in the range of 3.5-5.0 mM, while levels of 6.3-8.0 mM (severe hyperkalemia) result in cardiac **arrhythmias** or even death due to cardiac arrest. Potassium is potentially quite toxic, however toxicity or death due to potassium **poisoning** is usually prevented because of the vomiting reflex. The consumption of food results in mild increases in the concentration of potassium in the bloodstream, but levels of potassium do not become toxic because of the uptake of potassium by various cells of the body, as well as by the action of the kidneys transferring the potassium ions from the blood to the urine. The body's regulatory mechanisms can easily be overwhelmed, however, when potassium chloride is injected intravenously, as high doses of injected potassium can easily result in death.

Iodine toxicity can result from an intake of 2.0 mg of iodide per day. The toxicity results in impairment of the creation of thyroid hormone, resulting in lower levels of thyroid hormone in the bloodstream. The thyroid gland enlarges, as a consequence, and **goiter** is produced. This enlargement is also called **hyperthyroidism**. Goiter is usually caused by iodine deficiency. In addition to goiter, iodine toxicity produces ulcers on the skin. This condition has been called "kelp acne," because of its association with eating kelp, an ocean plant, which contains high levels of iodine. Iodine toxicity occurs in Japan, where large amounts of seaweed are consumed.

Iron toxicity is not uncommon, due to the wide distribution of iron pills. A lethal dose of iron is in the range of 200-250 mg iron/kg body weight. Hence, a child who accidently eats 20 or more iron tablets may die as a result of iron toxicity. Within six hours of ingestion, iron toxicity can result in vomiting, diarrhea, abdominal **pain**, seizures, and possibly coma. A latent period, where the symptoms appear to improve, may occur but it is followed by **shock**, low blood glucose, liver damage, convulsions, and death, occuring 12-48 hours after toxic levels of iron are ingested.

Nitrite poisoning should be considered along with iron toxicity, since nitrite produces its toxic effect by reacting with the iron atom of hemoglobin. Hemoglobin is an iron-containing protein that resides within the red blood cells. This protein is responsible for the transport of nearly all of the oxygen, acquired from the lungs, to various tissues and organs of the body. Hemoglobin accounts for the red color of our red blood cells. A very small fraction of our hemoglobin spontaneously oxidizes per day, producing a protein of a slightly different structure, called methemoglobin. Normally, the amount of methemoglobin constitutes less than 1% of the total hemoglobin. Methemoglobin can accumulate in the blood as a result of nitrite poisoning. Infants are especially susceptible to poisoning by nitrite.

Nitrate, which is naturally present in green leafy vegetables and in the water supply is rapidly converted to nitrite by the naturally occurring bacteria residing on our tongue, as well as in the intestines, and then absorbed into the bloodstream. The amount of nitrate that is supplied by leafy vegetables and in drinking water is generally about 100-170 mg/day. The amount of nitrite supplied by a typical diet is much less, that is, than 0.1 mg nitrite/day. Poisoning by nitrite, or nitrate after its conversion to nitrite, results in the inability of hemoglobin to carry oxygen throughout the body. This condition can be seen by the blue color of the skin. Adverse symptoms occur when over 30% of the hemoglobin has been converted to methemoglobin, and these symptoms include cardiac arrhythmias, **headache**, **nausea and vomiting**, and in severe cases, seizures.

Calcium and phosphate are closely related nutrients. Calcium toxicity is rare, but overconsumption of calcium supplements may lead to deposits of calcium phosphate in the soft tissues of the body. Phosphate toxicity can occur with overuse of **laxatives** or **enemas** that contain phosphate. Severe phosphate toxicity can result in **hypocalcemia**, and in various symptoms resulting from low plasma calcium levels. Moderate phosphate toxicity, occurring over a period of months, can result in the deposit of calcium phosphate crystals in various tissues of the body.

Zinc toxicity is rare, but it can occur in metal workers who are exposed to fumes containing zinc. Excessive dietary supplements of zinc can result in **nausea**, vomiting, and diarrhea. The chronic intake of excessive zinc supplements can result in copper deficiency, as zinc inhibits the absorption of copper.

Severe alterations in copper metabolism occur in two genetic diseases, Wilson's disease and Menkes' disease. Both of these diseases are rare and occur in about one in 100,000 births. Both diseases involve mutations in the proteins that transport copper, that is, in special channels that allow the passage of copper ions through cell membranes. Wilson's disease tends to occur in teenagers and in young adults, and then remain for the lifetime. Copper accumulates in the liver, kidney, and brain, resulting in damage to the liver and nervous system. Wilson's disease can be successfully controlled by lifelong treatment with d-penicillamine. Treatment also involves avoiding foods that are high in copper, such as liver, nuts, chocolate, and mollusks. After an initial period of treatment with penicillamine, Wilson's disease may be treated with zinc (150 mg oral Zn/day). The zinc inhibits the absorption of dietary copper.

Selenium toxicity occurs in regions of the world, including some parts of China, where soils contain high levels of selenium. A daily intake of 0.75-5.0 mg selenium may occur in these regions, due to the presence of selenium in foods and water. Early signs of selenium toxicity include nausea, weakness, and diarrhea. With continued intake of selenium, changes in fingernails and hair loss results, and damage to the nervous system occurs. The breath may acquire a garlic odor, as a result of the increased production of dimethylselenide in the body, and its release via the lungs.

Manganese toxicity occurs in miners in manganese mines, where men breath air containing dust bearing manganese at a concentration of 5-250 mg/cubic meter. Manganese toxicity in miners has been documented in Chile, India, Japan, Mexico, and elsewhere. Symptoms of manganese poisoning typically occur within several months or years of exposure. These symptoms include a mental disorder resembling **schizophrenia**, as well as hyperirritability, violent acts, **hallucinations**, and difficulty in walking.

Diagnosis

The initial diagnosis of mineral toxicity involves questioning the patient in order to determine any unusual aspects of the diet, unusual intake of drugs and chemicals, and possible occupational exposure. Diagnosis of mineral toxicities also involves measuring the metal concentration in the plasma or urine. Concentrations that are above the normal range can confirm the initial, suspected diagnosis.

Treatment

Iron toxicity is treated by efforts to remove remaining iron from the stomach, by use of a solution of 5% sodium bicarbonate. Where plasma iron levels are above 0.35 mg/dL, the patient is treated with deferoxamine. Treatment of manganese toxicity involves removal of the patient from the high manganese environment, as well as lifelong doses of the drug L-dopa. The treatment is only partially successful. Treatment of nitrite or nitrate toxicity involves inhalation of 100% oxygen for several hours. If oxygen treatment is not effective, then methylene blue may be injected, as a 1.0% solution, in a dose of 1.0 mg methylene blue/kg body weight.

Prognosis

The prognosis for treating toxicity due to sodium, potassium, calcium, and phosphate is usually excellent. Toxicity due to the deposit of calcium phosphate crystals is not usually reversible. The prognosis for treating iodine toxicity is excellent. For any mineral overdose that causes coma or seizures, the prognosis for recovery is often poor, and death results in a small fraction of patients. For any mineral toxicity that causes nerve damage, the prognosis is often fair to poor.

Prevention

When mineral toxicity results from the excessive consumption of mineral supplements, toxicity can be prevented by not using supplements. In the case of manganese, toxicity can be prevented by avoiding work in manganese mines. In the case of iodine, toxicity can be prevented by avoiding overconsumption of seaweed or kelp. In the case of selenium toxicity that arises due to high-selenium soils, toxicity can be prevented by relying on food and water acquired from a low-selenium region.

Resources

BOOKS

Brody, Tom. *Nutritional Biochemistry*. San Diego: Academic Press, 1998.

Tom Brody, PhD

Minerals

Definition

The minerals (inorganic nutrients) that are relevant to human **nutrition** include water, sodium, potassium, chloride, calcium, phosphate, sulfate, magnesium, iron, copper, zinc, manganese, iodine, selenium, and molybdenum. Cobalt is a required mineral for human health, but it is supplied by vitamin B_{12}. Cobalt appears to have no other function, aside from being part of this vitamin. There is some evidence that chromium, boron, and other inorganic elements play some part in human nutrition, but the evidence is indirect and not yet convincing. Fluoride seems not to be required for human life, but its presence in the diet contributes to long term dental health. Some of the minerals do not occur as single atoms, but occur as molecules. These include water, phosphate, sulfate, and selenite (a form of selenium). Sulfate contains an atom of sulfur. We do not need to eat sulfate, since the body can acquire all the sulfate it needs from protein.

The statement that various minerals, or inorganic nutrients, are required for life means that their continued supply in the diet is needed for growth, maintenance of body weight in adulthood, and for reproduction. The amount of each mineral that is needed to support growth during infancy and childhood, to maintain body weight and health, and to facilitate **pregnancy** and **lactation**, are listed in a table called the Recommended Dietary Allowances (RDA). This table was compiled by the Food and Nutrition Board, a committee that serves the United States government. All of the values listed in the RDA indicate the daily amounts that are expected to maintain health throughout most of the general population. The actual levels of each inorganic nutrient required by any given individual is likely to be less than that stated by the RDA. The RDAs are all based on studies that provided the exact, minimal requirement of each mineral needed to maintain health. However, the RDA values are actually greater than the minimal requirement, as determined by studies on small groups of healthy human subjects, in order to accomodate the variability expected among the general population.

The RDAs for adult males are 800 mg of calcium, 800 mg of phosphorus, 350 mg of magnesium, 10 mg of iron, 15 mg of zinc, 0.15 mg of iodine, and 0.07 mg of selenium. The RDA for sodium is expressed as a range (0.5-2.4 g/day). The minimal requirement for chloride is about 0.75 g/day, and the minimal requirement for potassium is 1.6-2.0 g/day, though RDA values have not been set for these nutrients. The RDAs for several other minerals has not been determined, and here the estimated safe and adequate daily dietary intake has been listed by the Food and Nutrition Board. These values are listed for copper (1.5-3.0 mg), manganese (2-5 mg), fluoride (1.5-4.0 mg), molybdenum (0.075-0.25 mg), and chromium (0.05-0.2 mg). In noting the appearance of chromium in this list, one should note that the function of chromium is essentially unknown, and evidence for its necessity exists only for animals, and not for human beings. In considering the amount of any mineral used for treating **mineral deficiency**, one should compare the recommended level with the RDA for that mineral. Treatment at a level that is one tenth of the RDA might not be expected to be adequate, while treatment at levels ranging from 10-1,000 times the RDA might be expected to exert a toxic effect, depending on the mineral. In this way, one can judge whether any claim of action, for a specific mineral treatment, is likely to be adequate or appropriate.

Purpose

People are treated with minerals for several reasons. The primary reason is to relieve a mineral deficiency, when a deficiency has been detected. Chemical tests suitable for the detection of all mineral deficiencies are available. The diagnosis of the deficiency is often aided by tests that do not involve chemical reactions, such as the **hematocrit** test for the red blood cell content in blood for iron deficiency, the visual examination of the neck for iodine deficiency, or the examination of bones by densitometry for calcium deficiency. Mineral treatment is conducted after a test and diagnosis for iron-deficiency anemia, in the case of iron, and after a test and diagnosis for hypomagnesemia, in the case of magnesium, to give two examples.

A second general reason for mineral treatment is to prevent the development of a possible or expected deficiency. Here, minerals are administered when tests for possible mineral deficiency are not given. Examples include the practice of giving young infants iron supplements, and of the food industry's practice of supplementing infant formulas with iron. The purpose here is to reduce the risk for **iron deficiency anemia**. Another example is the practice of many women of taking calcium supplements, with the hope of reducing the risk of **osteoporosis**.

Most minerals are commercially available at supermarkets, drug stores, and specialty stores. There is reason to believe that the purchase and consumption of most of these minerals is beneficial to health for some, but not all, of the minerals. Potassium supplements are useful for reducing blood pressure, in cases of persons with high blood pressure. The effect of potassium varies from person to person. The consumption of calcium supplements is likely to have some effect on reducing the risk for osteoporosis. The consumption of selenium supplements is expected to be of value only for residents of Keshan Province, China, because of the established association of selenium deficiency in this region with "Keshan disease."

Precautions

During emergency treatment of sodium deficiency (**hyponatremia**), potassium deficiency (**hypokalemia**), and calcium deficiency (**hypocalcemia**) with intravenous injections, extreme caution must be taken to avoid producing toxic levels of each of these minerals (**hypernatremia, hyperkalemia,** and **hypercalcemia**), as **mineral toxicity** can be life-threatening in some instances. The latter three conditions can be life threatening. Selenium is distinguished among most of the nutrients in that dietary intakes at levels only ten times that of the RDA can be toxic. Hence, one must guard against any overdose of selenium. Calcium and zinc supplements, when taken orally, are distinguished among most of the other minerals in that their toxicity is relatively uncommon.

Description

Minerals are used in treatments by three methods, namely, by replacing a poor diet with a diet that supplies the RDA, by consuming oral supplements, or by injections or infusions. Injections are especially useful for infants, for mentally disabled persons, or where the physician wants to be totally sure of compliance. Infusions, as well as injections, are essential for medical emergencies, as during mineral deficiency

situations like hyponatremia, hypokalemia, hypocalcemia, and hypomagnesemia. Oral mineral supplements are especially useful for mentally alert persons who otherwise cannot or will not consume food that is a good mineral source, such as meat. For example, a vegetarian who will not consume meat may be encouraged to consume oral supplements of iron, as well as supplements of vitamin B_{12}.

Iron treatment is used for young infants, given as supplements of 7 mg of iron per day to prevent anemia. Iron is also supplied to infants via the food industry's practice of including iron at 12 mg/L in cow milk-based infant formulas, as well as adding powdered iron at levels of 50 mg iron per 100 g dry infant cereal.

Calcium supplements, along with estrogen and calcitonin therapy, are commonly used in the prevention and treatment of osteoporosis. Estrogen and calcitonin are naturally occurring hormones. Bone loss occurs with **diets** supplying under 400 mg Ca/day. Bone loss can be minimized with the consumption of the RDA for calcium. There is some thought that all postmenopausal women should consume 1,000–1,500 mg of calcium per day. These levels are higher than the RDA. There is some evidence that such supplementation can reduce bone losses in some bones, such as the elbow (ulna), but not in other bones. Calcium absorption by the intestines decreases with **aging**, especially after the age of 70. The regulatory mechanisms of the intestines that allow absorption of adequate calcium (500 mg Ca/day or less) may be impaired in the elderly. Because of these changes, there is much interest in increasing the RDA for calcium for older women.

Fluoride has been proven to reduce the rate of **tooth decay**. When fluoride occurs in the diet, it is incorporated into the structure of the teeth, and other bones. The optimal range of fluoride in drinking water is 0.7-1.2 mg/L. This level results in a reduction in the rate of tooth decay by about 50%. The American Dental Association recommends that persons living in areas lacking fluoridated water take fluoride supplements. The recommendation is 0.25 mg F/day from the ages of 0-2 years, 0.5 mg F/day for 2-3 years, and 1.0 mg F/day for ages 3-13 years.

Magnesium is often used to treat a dangerous condition, called **eclampsia**, that occasionally occurs during pregnancy. In this case, magnesium is used as a drug, and not to relieve a deficiency. High blood pressure is a fairly common disorder during pregnancy, affecting 1-5% of pregnant mothers. **Hypertension** during pregnancy can result in increased release of protein in the urine. In pregnancy, the combination of hypertension with increased urinary protein is called **preeclampsia**. Preeclampsia is a concern during pregnancies as it may lead to eclampsia. Eclampsia involves convulsions and possibly **death** to the mother. Magnesium sulfate is the drug of choice for preventing the convulsions of eclampsia.

Treatment with cobalt, in the form of vitamin B_{12}, is used for relieving the symptoms of **pernicious anemia**. Pernicious anemia is a relatively common disease which tends to occur in persons older than 40 years. Free cobalt is never used for the treatment of any disease.

Preparation

Evaluation of a patient's mineral levels requires a blood sample, and the preparation of plasma or serum from the blood sample. An overnight fast is usually recommended as preparation prior to drawing the blood and chemical analysis. The reason for this is that any mineral present in the food consumed at breakfast may artificially boost the plasma mineral content beyond the normal **fasting** level, and thereby mask a mineral deficiency. In some cases, red blood cells are used for the mineral status assay.

Aftercare

The healthcare provider assesses the patient's response to mineral treatment. A positive response confirms that the diagnosis was correct. Lack of response indicates that the diagnosis was incorrect, that the patient had failed to take the mineral supplement, or that a higher dose of mineral was needed. The response to mineral treatment can be monitored by chemical tests, by an examination of red blood cells or white blood cells, or by physiological tests, depending on the exact mineral deficiency.

Risks

There are few risks associated with mineral treatment. In treating emergency cases of hyponatremia, hypokalemia, or hypocalcemia by intravenous injections, there exists a very real risk that giving too much sodium, potassium, or calcium, can result in hypernatremia, hyperkalemia, or hypercalcemia, respectively. Risk for toxicity is rare where treatment is by dietary means. This is because the intestines act as a barrier, and absorption of any mineral supplement is gradual. The gradual passage of any mineral through the intestines, especially when the mineral supplement is taken with food, allows the various organs of the body to acquire the mineral. Gradual passage of the mineral

into the bloodstream also allows the kidneys to excrete the mineral in the urine, should levels of the mineral rise to toxic levels in the blood.

Resources

BOOKS

Brody, Tom. *Nutritional Biochemistry*. San Diego: Academic Press, 1998.

Tom Brody, PhD

Minnesota multiphasic personality inventory (MMPI-2)

Definition

The Minnesota Multiphasic Personality Inventory (MMPI-2; MMPI-A) is a written psychological assessment, or test, used to diagnose mental disorders.

Purpose

The MMPI is used to screen for personality and **psychosocial disorders** in adults and adolescents. It is also frequently administered as part of a neuropsychological test battery to evaluate cognitive functioning.

Precautions

The MMPI should be administered, scored, and interpreted by a clinical professional trained in its use, preferably a psychologist or psychiatrist. The MMPI is only one element of psychological assessment, and should never be used alone as the sole basis for a diagnosis. A detailed history of the test subject and a review of psychological, medical, educational, or other relevant records are required to lay the groundwork for interpreting the results of any psychological measurement.

Cultural and language differences in the test subject may affect test performance and may result in inaccurate MMPI results. The test administrator should be informed before psychological testing begins if the test taker is not fluent in English and/or has a unique cultural background.

Description

The original MMPI was developed at the University of Minnesota and introduced in 1942. The current standardized version for adults 18 and over, the MMPI-2, was released in 1989, with a subsequent revision of certain test elements in early 2001. The MMPI-2 has 567 items, or questions, and takes approximately 60 to 90 minutes to complete. There is a short form of the test that is comprised of the first 370 items on the long-form MMPI-2. There is also a version of the inventory for adolescents age 14 to 18, the MMPI-A.

The questions asked on the MMPI are designed to evaluate the thoughts, emotions, attitudes, and behavioral traits that comprise personality. The results of the test reflect an individual's personality strengths and weaknesses, and may identify certain disturbances of personality (psychopathologies) or mental deficits caused by neurological problems.

There are six validity scales and ten basic clinical or personality scales scored in the MMPI-2, and a number of supplementary scales and subscales that may be used with the test. The validity scales are used to determine whether the test results are actually valid (i.e., if the test-taker was truthful, answered cooperatively and not randomly) and to assess the test-taker's response style (i.e., cooperative, defensive). Each clinical scale uses a set or subset of MMPI-2 questions to evaluate a specific personality trait. The MMPI should always be administered in a controlled environment by a psychologist or other qualified mental health professional trained in its use.

Preparation

The administrator should provide the test subject with information on the nature of the test and its intended use, complete standardized instructions to taking the MMPI (including any time limits, and information on the confidentiality of the results).

Normal results

The MMPI should be scored and interpreted by a trained professional. When interpreting test results for test subjects, the test administrator will review what the test evaluates, its precision in evaluation and any margins of error involved in scoring, and what the individual scores mean in the context of overall norms for the test and the background of the test subject.

Resources

BOOKS

Graham, John R. *MMPI-2: Assessing Personality and Psychopathology*. 3rd ed. New York: Oxford University Press, 1999.

ORGANIZATIONS

ERIC Clearinghouse on Assessment and Evaluation. 1131 Shriver Laboratory Bldg 075, University of Maryland, College Park, MD 20742. (800) 464-3742. <http://www.ericae.net>.

Paula Anne Ford-Martin

Minor tranquilizers *see* **Antianxiety drugs**

Minority health

Definition

Minority health addresses the special medical and/or health needs associated with specific ethnic groups.

Description

The United States, as well as many other countries, experiences cultural diversity. This poses specific health issues that are specific to ethnic groups. Additionally, the propensity for certain diseases or illnesses is of concern in certain minority groups. These specific health issues include infant mortality rates, **cancer**, cardiovascular disease, diabetes, HIV infection, and immunizations.

DR. ANTONIA NOVELLO (1944–)

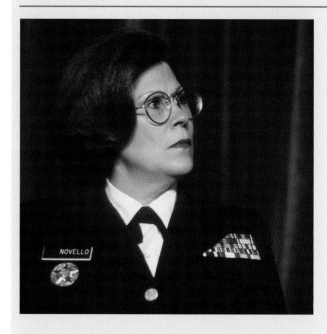

(Gamma Liaison. Reproduced by permission.)

Born Antonia Coello was born in Fajardo, Puerto Rico, on August 23, 1944, the oldest of three children. At eight years old, she suffered two blows that she would carry all of her life. Her father, Antonio Coello, died, leaving her mother, Ana Delia Flores Coello, to raise her children alone until she later remarried Ramon Flores, an electrician. Novello was also diagnosed with a chronic condition called congenital megacolon, an illness in which her colon was overly large and not functioning properly, which required regular hospitalization. Although an operation would have helped Novello, it was not performed until she was 18 years old, and even after the surgery, complications followed her for years. Because of her childhood illness, Novello grew up wanting to be a doctor.

On October 17, 1989, President George Bush officially nominated Novello for Surgeon General. The fourteenth United States Surgeon General, Novello, sworn in on March 9, 1990, remarked that "the American dream is well and alive...today the West Side Story comes to the West Wing." Novello was the first woman and the first Hispanic to be appointed Surgeon General of the United States. Noted for her philosophy of "good science, good sense" and for her approachability, Novello was dedicated to the prevention of AIDS, substance abuse, and smoking, as well as to the education of the American public. Her special concerns were for women, children, and hispanics— populations often overlooked by public health services.

Infant mortality rates

Infant mortality rates (IMRs) in the United States and in all countries worldwide are an accurate indicator of health status. They provide information concerning programs about **pregnancy** education and counseling, technological advances, and procedures and aftercare. IMRs vary among racial groups. African Americans had an IMRs of 14.2 per 1,000 live births in 1996, approximately 2.5 times higher than Caucasians. The IMRs among American Native Indian groups varies greatly, with some communities possessing IMRs about two times more than national rates. Additionally Hispanic IMRs (7.6 per 1,000 live births) are also diverse for separate groups, since the IMRs for example among Puerto Ricans is higher (8.9 per 1,000 live births).

Cancer

Cancer is a serious national, worldwide, and minority health concern. It is the second cause of **death** in the United States, claiming over half a million lives each year. Approximately 50% of persons who develop cancer will die. There is great disparity among the cancer rates in minority groups. Across genders, cancer death rates for African Americans are 35% higher when compared to statistics for Caucasians. The death rates for **prostate cancer** (two times more) and lung cancer (27 times more) are disproportionately higher when compared to Caucasians. There are also gender differences among ethnic groups and specific cancers. Lung cancers in African American and Hawaiian men are evaluated compared with Caucasian males. Vietnamese females who live in the United States have five times more new cases of **cervical cancer** when compared to Caucasian women. Hispanic females also have a greater incidence of cervical cancer than Caucasian females. Additionally, Alaskan native men and women have a greater propensity for cancers in the rectum and colon than do Caucasians.

Cardiovascular disease

Cardiovascular disease is responsible for the leading cause of disability and death rates about equal to death from all other diseases combined. Cardiovascular disease can affect the patient's lifestyle and function in addition to having an impact on family members. The financial costs are very high. Among ethnic and racial groups cardiovascular disease is the leading cause of death. **Stroke** is the leading cause of cardiovascular related death, which occurs in higher numbers for Asian-American males when compared to Caucasian men. Mexican-American men and women and African-American males have a higher incidence of **hypertension**. African-American women have higher rates of being overweight, which is a major risk factor of cardiovascular disease.

Diabetes

Diabetes—a serious health problem in Americans and ethnic groups—is the seventh leading cause of death in the United States. The prevalence of diabetes in African Americans is about 70% higher than Caucasians.

HIV

HIV infection/AIDS is the most common cause of death for all persons age 25 to 44 years old. Ethnic groups account for 25% of the United States population and 54% of all **AIDS** cases. In addition to sexual transmission there is an increase in HIV among ethnic groups related to intravenous drug usage.

Immunizations

Immunization, the reduction of preventable disease by **vaccination**, was lower in 1996, but the there has been a rapid increase in African Americans taking vaccinations. The coverage for immunization among African Americans and Hispanics for persons age 65 and over is currently below the general population. This may increase the death rates due to respiratory infections.

Causes and symptoms

IMRs are correlated with prenatal care. Women who receive adequate prenatal care tend to have better pregnancy outcomes when compared to little or no care. Women who receive inadequate prenatal care also have increased chances of delivering a very low birth weight (VLBW) infant, which is linked to risk of early death.

Cancer is related to several preventable lifestyle choices. Tobacco use, diet, and exposure to sun (skin cancer) can be prevented by lifestyle modifications. Additionally many cancers can occur due to lack of interest and/or lack of availability for screening and educational programs.

Cardiovascular diseases are higher among persons with high blood cholesterol and high blood pressure. Certain lifestyle choices may increase the chance for heart disease includes lack of **exercise**, overweight, and cigarette **smoking**. Cardiovascular disease is responsible for over 50% of the deaths in persons with diabetes.

HIV occurs at a higher frequency among homosexuals (the number of African-American males who have AIDS through sex with men has increased). Additionally unprotected sexual intercourse and sharing used needles for IV drug injection are strongly correlated with infection.

Vaccinations are an effective method of preventing certain disease such as **polio**, **tetanus**, pertussis, **diphtheria**, **influenza**, **hepatitis b**, and pneumococcal infections. Approximately 90% of influenza related mortality is associated with persons aged 65 and older. This is mostly due to neglect of vaccinations. About 45,000 adults each year die of diseases related to hepatitis B, pneumococcal, and influenza infections.

Diagnosis

The diagnosis of VLBW is by weight. Infants who weigh 1,500 g are at high risk for death. For cancer, the diagnosis can be made through screening procedures such as **mammography** (for **breast cancer**), PAP smear (for cervical cancer), and lifestyle modifications such as avoidance of sun, cigarette smoking, balanced **diets**, and adequate **nutrition**. Other specific screening tests (PSA, prostate surface antigen) are helpful for diagnosing prostate cancer. Cardiovascular diseases can be detected by medical check-up. Blood pressure and cholesterol levels can be measured. **Obesity** can be diagnosed by assessing a persons weight relative to height. Diabetes and its complications can be detected by blood tests, in-depth eye examinations and studies that assess the flow of blood through blood vessels in legs. HIV can be detected through a careful history/ physical examination and analysis of blood using a special test called a western blot. Infections caused by lack of immunizations can either be detected by careful **physical examination** and culturing the specific microorganism in the laboratory.

Treatment

Treatment is directed at the primary causes(s) that minorities have increased chances of developing disease(s). Cancer may require treatment utilizing surgery, radiotherapy, or **chemotherapy**. Cardiovascular diseases may require surgical procedures for establishing a diagnosis and initiating treatment. Depending on the extent of disease cardiovascular management can become complicated requiring medications and daily lifestyle modifications. Treatment usually includes medications, dietary modifications, and—if complications arise—specific interventions tailored to alleviating the problem. HIV can be treated with specific medications and more often than not with symptomatic treatment as reported complications arise. Diseases caused by lack of immunizations are treated based on the primary disease. The best method of treatment is through prevention and generating public awareness through educational awareness.

Alternative treatment

Alternative therapies do exist, but more research is needed to substantiate present data. The diseases that relate to minority health are best treated with nationally accepted standards of care.

Prognosis

Generally the prognosis is related to the diagnosis, patients state of health, age, and if there is another disease or complication in addition to the presenting problem. The course for IMRs is related to educational programs and prenatal care, which includes medical and psychological treatments. The prognosis for chronic diseases such as cardiovascular problems, high blood pressure, cancer, and diabetes is variable. These diseases are not cured and control is achieved by standardized treatment options. Eventually complications, even with treatment can potentially occur. For HIV the clinical course at present is death even though this process may take years. Educational programs with an emphasis on disease prevention can potentially improve outcomes concerning pediatric and geriatric diseases.

Prevention

Prevention is accomplished best through educational programs specific to target populations. IMRs can be prevented by increasing awareness, interest, and accessibility for prenatal care that address a comprehensive approach for the needs of each patient. Regular physicals and special screening tests ca potentially prevent certain cancers in high-risk groups. Educational programs concerning lifestyle modifications, diet, exercise, and testing may prevent the development of cardiovascular disease and diabetes. Educational programs assemble to illicit IV drug abusers and persons who engage in unprotected sexual intercourse may decrease the incidence of HIV infection.

Resources

ORGANIZATIONS

Office of Minority Health. 2001. < http://www.omhrc.gov/rah/3rdpgBlue/Cardio/3pgGoalsCardio.htm >.

Laith Farid Gulli, M.D.
Nicole Mallory, M.S.

Minoxidil

Definition

Minoxidil is a drug available in two forms to treat different conditions. Oral minoxidil is used to treat high blood pressure and the topical solution form is used to treat hair loss and baldness.

Purpose

Minoxidil was the first drug approved by the FDA for the treatment of androgenetic **alopecia** (hair loss). Before that, minoxidil had been used as vasodilator drug prescribed as oral tablet to treat high blood pressure, with side effects that included hair growth and reversal of male baldness. In the 1980s, UpJohn Corporation came out with a topical solution of 2% minoxidil, called Rogaine, for the specific treatment of androgenetic alopecia. Since the 1990s, numerous generic forms of minoxidil have become available to treat hair loss while the oral form is still used to treat high blood pressure.

The popularity hair loss treatment is due to the general preference in the overall population for the cosmetic appearance of a full head of hair. Minoxidil is used to stimulate hair growth in areas of the scalp that have stopped growing hair. As of early 2001, the exact mechanism of action of minoxidil is not known.

Precautions

People who have had a prior unusual or allergic reaction to either minoxidil or propylene glycol, a non-active chemical in the Rogaine solution, should not use topical minoxidil. People who have had a previous allergic reaction to preservatives or dyes may also be at risk for having an allergic reaction to minoxidil.

People who are using cortisone, or cortisone-like drugs (**corticosteroids**), petroleum jelly (Vaseline), or tretinoin (Retin-A) on their scalps should consult their doctors prior to using minoxidil. The use of any of these products in conjunction with minoxidil may cause excessive minoxidil absorption into the body and increase the risk of side effects.

Also, people who have skin problems or irritations of the scalp, including **sunburn**, may absorb too much minoxidil and increase their risk of side effects.

As for oral minoxidil, the form prescribed for high blood pressure, patients should use minoxidil only under medical supervision to ensure that excessive amounts of the drug are not absorbed into their bodies. Large amounts of minoxidil may increase the severity of the symptoms and side effects of **hypertension**.

Minoxidil may pass from mother to child through breast milk. Therefore, women who are breastfeeding should not use minoxidil.

Description

For the treatment of hair loss, minoxidil is available as a topical solution that is generally either 2% or 5% minoxidil in propylene glycol. The propylene glycol ensures that the applied minoxidil is evenly spread across the affected area and easily absorbed through the skin. As of early 2001, the 5% solution is only approved by the FDA for use on men. Approximately 1 milliliter of minoxidil solution is applied to the scalp once a day using the fingertips or a pump spray. It should be applied from the center of the area being treated outward.

In the treatment of high blood pressure, oral minoxidil is usually prescribed when other medications have failed to treat the condition. Dosage is usually 2.5-100 mg per day as a single dose for adults and 200 micrograms to 1 mg per kg of body weight for children.

Preparation

Before using topical minoxidil, the hair and scalp should be clean and dry before the minoxidil solution is applied.

Aftercare

Hands, and any other areas of the body where hair growth is not desired that may have come into contact with topical minoxidil, should be washed immediately after applying the minoxidil solution on the scalp. Once applied, topical minoxidil should be allowed to air-dry for at least two to four hours before clothing are pulled on or off over the head, a hat is worn, or the patient goes to bed. Prior to this, the minoxidil solution may stain clothing, hats, or bed linens; or, it may be accidentally transferred from the patient's head to one of these objects, then back to other parts of the patient's body where hair growth is not desired. A blow dryer, or other drying methods, should not be used to speed the drying of the minoxidil as this may interfere with the absorption of the medicine. People using minoxidil should also not shampoo, wash, or rinse their hair for at least 4 hours after minoxidil is applied.

Risks

The most common side effects of topical minoxidil use are **itching** and skin irritation of the treated area of the scalp. Unwanted hair growth may also occur adjacent to treated areas or in areas where the medicine has been inadvertently transferred several times. This unwanted hair growth adjacent to the treatment area may be particularly distressing to women when the face is involved. The itching and irritation usually subside after the drug has been used for approximately two weeks. If symptoms persist after this time, minoxidil use should be halted until a physician has been consulted.

Extremely rare side effects that may occur if too much topically or orally administered minoxidil is being absorbed in the body include:

- changes in vision, most commonly blurred vision
- chest pain
- very low blood pressure
- decreased sexual desire
- fast or irregular heartbeat
- flushing of the skin
- headache
- lightheadedness
- numbness or **tingling** in the hands, feet, or face
- partial, or complete, impotence
- rapid weight gain
- swelling of the hands, feet, lower legs, or face

KEY TERMS

Androgenetic alopecia—Hair loss that develops into baldness and affects both men and women.

Hypertension—Persistently high arterial blood pressure.

Scalp—That part of the head that is usually covered with hair.

Topical drug—Drug or medication applied to a specific area of the skin and affecting only the area to which it is applied.

Vasodilation—The increase in the diameter of a blood vessel resulting from relaxation of smooth muscle within the wall of the vessel. Vasodilation activates the blood flow.

Vasodilators—Drugs or substances that cause vasodilation.

Normal results

Topical minoxidil is much more effective at treating baldness that occurs on the top, or crown, of the head than it is at causing hair growth on other parts of the head. Minoxidil does not work for everyone and there is no predictor, in early 2001, of whether or not it will be effective in any particular person. Clinical tests on the effectiveness of topical minoxidil in men with baldness on the top of the head showed that 48% of men who had used minoxidil for one year reported moderate to dense re-growth of hair within the treated area. Thirty-six percent reported minimal re-growth. While 16% reported no re-growth. Similar percentages have been reported in women.

In both men and women, hair re-growth generally does not begin until the medicine has been used for at least four months. The first signs that minoxidil may be effective in a particular person usually occur after approximately 90 days of treatment, when the patient notices that he or she is losing (shedding) much less hair than prior to beginning treatment.

When new growth begins, the first hairs may be soft and barely visible. For some patients, this is the extent to the effectiveness of this medication. For others, this down-like hair develops into hair of the same color and thickness as the other hairs on their heads.

Minoxidil is a treatment for hair loss, it is not a cure. Once a patient stops taking minoxidil, he or she will most likely lose all of the re-grown hair within

90 days of stopping the medication and no further hair growth will occur.

Resources

PERIODICALS

Bowser, Andrew. "Treatments Abound for Female Hair Loss." *Dermatology Times* June 1999.

Scow, Dean Thomas. "Medical Treatments for Balding in Men." *American Family Physician* April 15, 1999.

ORGANIZATIONS

American Academy of Dermatology. 930 N. Meacham Road, PO Box 4014, Schaumburg, IL 60168-4014. (847) 330-0230. Fax: 847-330-0050. < http://www.aad.org/ >.

American Hair Loss Council. 30 Grassy Plain Road, Bethel, CT 06801. (888) 873-9719. < http://www.ahlc.org/ >.

Paul A. Johnson, Ed.M.

Miscarriage

Definition

Miscarriage means loss of an embryo or fetus before the 20th week of **pregnancy**. Most miscarriages occur during the first 14 weeks of pregnancy. The medical term for miscarriage is spontaneous abortion.

Description

Miscarriages are very common. Approximately 20% of pregnancies (one in five) end in miscarriage. The most common cause is a genetic abnormality of the fetus. Not all women realize that they are miscarrying and others may not seek medical care when it occurs.

A miscarriage is often a traumatic event for both partners, and can cause feelings similar to the loss of a child or other member of the family. Fortunately, 90% of women who have had one miscarriage subsequently have a normal pregnancy and healthy baby; 60% are able to have a healthy baby after two miscarriages. Even a woman who has had three miscarriages in a row still has more than a 50% chance of having a successful pregnancy the fourth time.

Causes and symptoms

There are many reasons why a woman's pregnancy ends in miscarriage. Often the cause is not clear. However, more than half the miscarriages that occur in the first eight weeks of pregnancy involve serious chromosomal abnormalities or **birth defects** that would make it impossible for the baby to survive. These are different from inherited genetic diseases. They probably occur during development of the specific egg or sperm, and therefore are not likely to occur again.

In about 17% of cases, miscarriage is caused by an abnormal hormonal imbalance that interferes with the ability of the uterus to support the growing embryo. This is known as luteal phase defect. In another 10% of cases, there is a problem with the structure of the uterus or cervix. This can especially occur in women whose mothers used diethylstilbestrol (DES) when pregnant with them.

The risk of miscarriage is increased by:

• **Smoking** (up to a 50% increased risk)

• Infection

• Exposure to toxins (such as arsenic, lead, formaldehyde, benzene, and ethylene oxide)

• Multiple pregnancy

• Poorly-controlled diabetes.

The most common symptom of miscarriage is bleeding from the vagina, which may be light or heavy. However, bleeding during early pregnancy is common and is not always serious. Many women have slight vaginal bleeding after the egg implants in the uterus (about 7-10 days after conception), which can be mistaken for a threatened miscarriage. A few women bleed at the time of their monthly periods through the pregnancy. However, any bleeding in the first three months of pregnancy (first trimester) is considered a threat of miscarriage.

Women should not ignore vaginal bleeding during early pregnancy. In addition to signaling a threatened miscarriage, it could also indicate a potentially life-threatening condition known as **ectopic pregnancy**. In an ectopic pregnancy, the fetus implants at a site other than the inside of the uterus. Most often this occurs in the fallopian tube.

Cramping is another common sign of a possible miscarriage. The cramping occurs because the uterus attempts to push out the pregnancy tissue. If a pregnant woman experiences both bleeding and cramping the possibility of miscarriage is more likely than if only one of these symptoms is present.

If a woman experiences any sign of impending miscarriage, she should be examined by a practitioner. The doctor or nurse will perform a **pelvic exam** to check if the cervix is closed as it should be. If the cervix is open, miscarriage is inevitable and nothing can

preserve the pregnancy. Symptoms of an inevitable miscarriage may include dull relentless or sharp intermittent **pain** in the lower abdomen or back. Bleeding may be heavy. Clotted material and tissue (the placenta and embryo) may pass from the vagina.

A situation in which only some of the products in the uterus have been expelled is called an incomplete miscarriage. Pain and bleeding may continue and become severe. An incomplete miscarriage requires medical attention.

A "missed abortion" occurs when the fetus has died but neither the fetus nor placenta is expelled. There may not be any bleeding or pain, but the symptoms of pregnancy will disappear. The physician may suspect a missed abortion if the uterus does not continue to grow. The physician will diagnose a missed abortion with an ultrasound examination.

A woman should contact her doctor if she experiences any of the following:

• Any bleeding during pregnancy.

• Pain or cramps during pregnancy.

• Passing of tissue.

• Fever and chills during or after miscarriage.

Diagnosis

If a woman experiences any sign of impending miscarriage she should see a doctor or nurse for a pelvic examination to check if the cervix is closed, as it should be. If the cervix is open, miscarriage is inevitable.

An ultrasound examination can confirm a missed abortion if the uterus has shrunk and the patient has had continual spotting with no other symptoms.

Treatment

Threatened miscarriage

For women who experience bleeding and cramping, bed rest is often ordered until symptoms disappear. Women should not have sex until the outcome of the threatened miscarriage is determined. If bleeding and cramping are severe, women should drink fluids only.

Miscarriage

Although it may be psychologically difficult, if a woman has a miscarriage at home she should try to collect any material she passes in a clean container for analysis in a laboratory. This may help determine why the miscarriage occurred.

An incomplete miscarriage or missed abortion may require the removal of the fetus and placenta by a D&C (**dilatation and curettage**). In this procedure the contents of the uterus are scraped out. It is performed in the doctor's office or hospital.

After miscarriage, a doctor may prescribe rest or **antibiotics** for infection. There will be some bleeding from the vagina for several days to two weeks after miscarriage. To give the cervix time to close and avoid possible infection, women should not use tampons or have sex for at least two weeks. Couples should wait for one to three normal menstrual cycles before trying to get pregnant again.

Prognosis

A miscarriage that is properly treated is not life-threatening, and usually does not affect a woman's ability to deliver a healthy baby in the future.

Feelings of grief and loss after a miscarriage are common. In fact, some women who experience a miscarriage suffer from major depression during the six months after the loss. This is especially true for women who don't have any children or who have had depression in the past. The emotional crisis can be similar to that of a woman whose baby has died after birth.

Prevention

The majority of miscarriages cannot be prevented because they are caused by severe genetic problems determined at conception. Some doctors advise women who have a threatened miscarriage to rest in bed for a day and avoid sex for a few weeks after the bleeding stops. Other experts believe that a healthy woman (especially early in the pregnancy) should continue normal activities instead of protecting a pregnancy that may end in miscarriage later on, causing even more profound distress.

If miscarriage was caused by a hormonal imbalance (luteal phase defect), this can be treated with a hormone called progesterone to help prevent subsequent miscarriages. If structural problems have led to repeated miscarriage, there are some possible procedures to treat these problems. Other possible ways to prevent miscarriage are to treat genital infections, eat a well-balanced diet, and refrain from smoking and using recreational drugs.

Resources

ORGANIZATIONS

American College of Obstetricians and Gynecologists. 409 12th Street, S.W., P.O. Box 96920.

Hygeia Foundation, Inc. P.O. Box 3943 New Haven, CT 06525. (203) 387-3589. < http://www.hygeia.org >.

Carol A. Turkington

Mitral incompetence *see* **Mitral valve insufficiency**

Mitral regurgitation *see* **Mitral valve insufficiency**

Mitral stenosis *see* **Mitral valve stenosis**

Mitral valve insufficiency

Definition

Mitral valve insufficiency is a term used when the valve between the upper left chamber of the heart (atrium) and the lower left chamber (ventricle) does not close well enough to prevent back flow of blood when the ventricle contracts. Mitral valve insufficiency is also known as mitral valve regurgitation or mitral valve incompetence.

Description

Normally, blood enters the left atrium of the heart from the lungs and is pumped through the mitral valve into the left ventricle. The left ventricle contracts to pump the blood forward into the aorta. The aorta is a large artery that sends oxygenated blood through the circulatory system to all of the tissues in the body. If the mitral valve is leaky due to mitral valve insufficiency, it allows some blood to get pushed back into the atrium. This extra blood creates an increase in pressure in the atrium, which then increases blood pressure in the vessels that bring the blood from the lungs to the heart. Increased pressure in these vessels can result in increased fluid buildup in the lungs.

Causes and symptoms

In the past, **rheumatic fever** was the most common cause of mitral valve insufficiency. However, the increased use of **antibiotics** for **strep throat** has made rheumatic **fever** rare in developed countries. In these countries, mitral valve insufficiency caused by rheumatic fever is seen mostly in the elderly. In countries with less developed health care, rheumatic fever is still common and is often a cause of mitral valve insufficiency.

Heart attacks that damage the structures that support the mitral valve are a common cause of mitral valve insufficiency. Myxomatous degeneration can cause a "floppy" mitral valve that leaks. In other cases, the valve simply deteriorates with age and becomes less efficient.

People with mitral valve insufficiency may not have any symptoms at all. It is often discovered during a doctor's visit when the doctor listens to the heart sounds.

Both the left atrium and left ventricle tend to get a little bigger when the mitral valve does not work properly. The ventricle has to pump more blood so it gets bigger to increase the force of each beat. The atrium gets bigger to hold the extra blood. An enlarged ventricle can cause **palpitations**. An enlarged atrium can develop an erratic rhythm (atrial fibrillation), which reduces its efficiency and can lead to **blood clots** forming in the atrium.

Diagnosis

When the doctor listens to the heart sounds, mitral valve insufficiency is generally recognized by the sound the blood makes as it leaks backward. It sounds like a regurgitant murmur. The next step is generally a **chest x ray** and an electrocardiogram (ECG) to see if the heart is enlarged. The most definitive noninvasive test is **echocardiography**, a test that uses sound waves to make an image of the heart. This

test gives a picture of the valve in action and shows the severity of the problem.

Treatment

A severely impaired valve needs to be repaired or replaced. Either option will require surgery. Repairing the valve can fix the problem completely or reduce it enough to make it bearable and prevent damage to the heart. Valves can be replaced with either a mechanical valve or one that is partly mechanical and partly from a pig's heart.

Mechanical valves are effective but can increase the incidence of blood clots. To prevent blood clots from forming, the patient will need to take drugs that prevent abnormal blood clotting (anticoagulants). The valves made partly from a pigs heart do not have as great a risk of blood clots but don't last as long as fully mechanical valves. If a valve wears out, it must be replaced again.

Damaged heart valves are easily infected. Anytime a procedure is contemplated that might allow infectious organisms to enter the blood, the person with mitral valve insufficiency should take antibiotics to prevent possible infection.

Prognosis

The diagnostic, medical and surgical procedures available to the person with mitral valve insufficiency are all likely to produce good results.

Prevention

The only possible way to prevent mitral valve insufficiency is to prevent rheumatic fever. This can be done by evaluating sore throats for the presence of the bacteria that causes strep throat. Strep throat is easily treated with antibiotics.

Resources

ORGANIZATIONS

American Heart Association. 7320 Greenville Ave. Dallas, TX 75231. (214) 373-6300. <http://www.americanheart.org>.

OTHER

The Meck Page. <http://www.merck.com>.

Dorothy Elinor Stonely

Mitral valve prolapse

Definition

Mitral valve prolapse (MVP) is a ballooning of the support structures of the mitral heart valve into the left upper collection chamber of the heart.

Description

Other names for MVP include floppy valve and Barlow's syndrome. The mitral valve is located on the left side of the heart between the top chamber (left atrium) and the bottom chamber (left ventricle). The valve opens and closes according to the heartbeat and the pressure that is exerted upon it from the blood in both chambers.

The valve has supporting structures that attach to the heart muscle to help it open and close properly. When these structures weaken or lengthen abnormally, the valve may balloon into the left atrium. Sometimes this can cause the mitral valve to leak blood backward.

This condition may be inherited and occurs in approximately 10% of the population. It affects more women than men and often peaks after the age of 40.

Causes and symptoms

MVP may occur due to rheumatic heart disease but is usually found in healthy people. Changes that occur in the valve are caused by rapid multiplication of cells in the middle layer that presses on the outer layer. The outer layer weakens, causing a prolapse of the valve toward the left atrium.

Most persons do not have symptoms. Those that do may experience sharp, left-sided chest **pain**. Some complain of **fatigue**, or a pounding feeling in the chest. Others can have an irregular heart beat and even pass out. Some persons may experience difficulty breathing, ankle swelling and fluid in the lungs. Other symptoms may include **anxiety**, headaches, morning tiredness and constantly cold hands and feet. **Death** from this condition is rare.

Diagnosis

The diagnosis of MVP is based on symptoms and physical exam. During the exam, the physician may hear a click and/or heart murmur with a stethoscope.

The best diagnostic test for MVP is the echocardiogram. The test reflects sound waves through the chest wall to give two-dimensional color flow pictures of the heart, its size, position, motion, chambers, and valves. Unfortunately, during the early 1980s, this diagnosis was often made excessively from faulty echocardiographic criteria prevalent at that time.

Any person with symptoms or family history of MVP should consider having an echocardiogram. The test takes 15-20 minutes and is done in doctor's offices and hospitals. It is performed by trained technicians and is read by cardiologists. Family physicians, internists, cardiologists, and nurse practitioners can treat MVP. Echocardiograms are recommended periodically depending on the extent of valve leakage.

Treatment

Persons who experience certain types of an irregular heartbeat with MVP should be treated. Propranolol (Inderal) or other **beta blockers** or digoxin (Lanoxin) are often helpful. Persons who develop moderate to severe symptoms with a leaky mitral valve may require repair or replacement of the mitral valve with an artificial heart valve. Persons with MVP and a leaky valve need to protect themselves from heart or heart valve infections. **Antibiotics** should be taken before any surgical, dental or oral procedures according to the American Heart Association recommendations.

Other treatments include drinking lots of fluids during strenuous activity and hot weather. Water pills, **caffeine** and donating blood may aggravate the symptoms of MVP.

Prognosis

MVP is usually not a serious condition. However, dangerous, untreated irregular heartbeats may rarely cause sudden death. These persons should be carefully monitored.

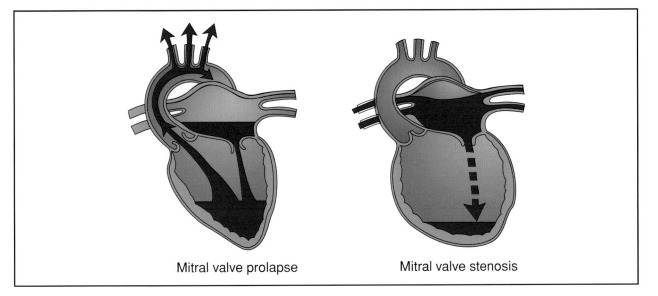

Mitral valve prolapse   Mitral valve stenosis

Mitral valve prolapse occurs when the mitral valve does not open and close properly. When this happens, the valve may balloon into the left atrium of the heart, causing the mitral valve to leak blood backward. Mitral valve stenosis refers to the narrowing of the mitral valve, in which the flow of blood from the atrium to the ventricle becomes restricted. *(Illustration by Electronic Illustrators Group.)*

Resources

PERIODICALS

McGrath, Dicey. "Mitral Valve Prolapse." *American Journal of Nursing* May 1997: 40-41.

Lisa Papp, RN

Mitral valve stenosis

Definition

The term stenosis means an abnormal narrowing of an opening. Mitral valve stenosis refers to a condition in the heart in which one of the valve openings has become narrow and restricts the flow of blood from the upper left chamber (left atrium) to the lower left chamber (left ventricle).

Description

In the heart, the valve that regulates the flow of blood between the left atrium and the left ventricle is called the mitral valve. If the mitral valve is abnormally narrow, due to disease or birth defect, blood flow from the atrium to the ventricle is restricted. This restricted flow leads to an increase in the pressure of blood in the left atrium. Over a period of time, this back pressure causes fluid to leak into the lungs. It can also lead to an abnormal heart rhythm (atrial fibrillation), which further decreases the efficiency of the pumping action of the heart.

Causes and symptoms

Mitral valve stenosis is almost always caused by **rheumatic fever**. As a result of rheumatic **fever**, the leaflets that form the opening of the valve are partially fused together. Mitral valve stenosis can also be present at birth. Babies born with this problem usually require surgery if they are to survive. Sometimes, growths or tumors can block the mitral valve, mimicking mitral valve stenosis.

If the restriction is severe, the increased blood pressure can lead to **heart failure**. The first symptoms of heart failure, which are **fatigue** and **shortness of breath**, usually appear only during physical activity. As the condition gets worse, symptoms may also be felt even during rest. A person may also develop a deep red coloring in the cheeks.

Diagnosis

Mitral valve stenosis is usually detected by a physician listening to heart sounds. Normal heart valves open silently to permit the flow of blood. A stenotic valve makes a snapping sound followed by a "rumbling" murmur. The condition can be confirmed with a **chest x ray** and an electrocardiogram, both of which will show an enlarged atrium. **Echocardiography**, which produces images of the heart's structure, is also helpful in making the diagnosis. If surgery is necessary, **cardiac catheterization** may be done to fully evaluate the heart before the operation.

Treatment

Drug therapy may help to slow the heart rate, strengthen the heart beat, and control abnormal heart rhythm. Drugs such as **beta blockers**, **calcium channel blockers**, and digoxin may be prescribed. A drug that prevents abnormal blood clotting (anticoagulant) called warfarin (Coumadin) may be recommended. If drug therapy does not produce satisfactory results, valve repair or replacement may be necessary.

Repair can be accomplished in two ways. In the first method, **balloon valvuloplasty**, the doctor will try to stretch the valve opening by threading a thin tube (catheter) with a balloon tip through a vein and into the heart. Once the catheter is positioned in the valve, the balloon is inflated, separating the fused areas. The second method involves opening the heart and surgically separating the fused areas.

If the valve is damaged beyond repair, it can be replaced with a mechanical valve or one that is partly mechanical and partly made from a pig's heart.

Prognosis

Procedures available to treat mitral valve stenosis, whether medical or surgical, all produce effective results.

Prevention

The only possible way to prevent mitral valve stenosis is to prevent rheumatic fever. This can be done by evaluating sore throats for the presence of

---

KEY TERMS

Atrium—One of the two upper chambers of the heart.

Beta blocker—A drug that can be used to reduce blood pressure.

Rheumatic fever—An illness which sometimes follows a streptococcal infection of the throat.

Ventricle—One of the two lower chambers of the heart.

---

the bacteria that causes **strep throat**. Strep throat is easily treated with **antibiotics**.

Resources

ORGANIZATIONS

American Heart Association. 7320 Greenville Ave. Dallas, TX 75231. (214) 373-6300. < http:// www.americanheart.org >.

OTHER

The Meck Page. < http://www.merck.com >.

Dorothy Elinor Stonely

Molar pregnancy *see* **Hydatidiform mole**

Moles

Definition

A mole (nevus) is a pigmented (colored) spot on the outer layer of the skin (epidermis).

Description

Moles can be round, oval, flat, or raised. They can occur singly or in clusters on any part of the body. Most moles are brown, but colors can range from pinkish flesh tones to yellow, dark blue, or black.

Everyone has at least a few moles. They generally appear by the time a person is 20 and resemble freckles at first. A mole's color and shape don't usually change. Changes in hormone levels that occur during **puberty** and **pregnancy** can make moles larger and darker. New moles may also appear during this period.

A mole usually lasts about 50 years before beginning to fade. Some moles disappear completely, and

---

some never lighten at all. Some moles develop stalks that raise them above the skin's surface; these moles eventually drop off.

Types of moles

About 1–3% of all babies have one or more moles when they are born. Moles that are present at birth are called congenital nevi.

Other types of moles include:

- Junctional moles, which are usually brown and may be flat or slightly raised.

- Compound moles, which are slightly raised, range in color from tan to dark brown, and involve pigment-producing cells (melanocytes) in both the upper and lower layers of the skin (epidermis and dermis).

- Dermal moles, which range from flesh-color to brown, are elevated, most common on the upper body, and may contain hairs.

- Sebaceous moles, which are produced by over-active oil glands and are yellow and rough-textured.

- Blue moles, which are slightly raised, colored by pigment deep within the skin, and most common on the head, neck, and arms of women.

Most moles are benign, but atypical moles (dysplastic nevi) may develop into **malignant melanoma**, a potentially fatal form of skin **cancer**. Atypical moles are usually hereditary. Most are bigger than a pencil eraser, and the shape and pigmentation are irregular.

Congenital nevi are more apt to become cancerous than moles that develop after birth, especially if they are more than eight inches in diameter. Lentigo maligna (melanotic freckle of Hutchinson), most common on the face and after the age of 50, first appears as a flat spot containing two or more shades of tan. It gradually becomes larger and darker. One in three of these moles develop into a form of skin cancer known as lentigo maligna melanoma.

Causes and symptoms

The cause of moles is unknown, although atypical moles seem to run in families and result from exposure to sunlight.

In the past several years, researchers have identified two genes known as CDKN2A and CDK4 that govern susceptibility to melanoma in humans. Other susceptibility genes are being sought as of early 2003. Most experts, however, think that these susceptibility genes are not sufficient by themselves to account for moles becoming cancerous but are influenced by a combination of other inherited traits and environmental factors.

Diagnosis

Only a small percentage of moles require medical attention. A mole that has the following symptoms should be evaluated by a dermatologist (a physician spealizing in skin diseases).

- Appears after the age of 20

- Bleeds

- Itches

- Looks unusual or changes in any way.

A doctor who suspects skin cancer will remove all or part of the mole for microscopic examination. This procedure, which is usually performed in a doctor's office, is simple, relatively painless, and does not take more than a few minutes. It does leave a scar.

The doctor may also use a dermatoscope to examine the mole prior to removal. The dermatoscope, which can be used to distinguish between benign moles and melanomas, is an instrument that resembles an ophthalmoscope. An immersion oil is first applied to the mole to make the outer layers of skin transparent.

A combination of high-frequency ultrasound and color Doppler studies has also been shown to have a high degree of accuracy in distinguishing between melanomas and benign moles.

Treatment

If laboratory analysis confirms that a mole is cancerous, the dermatologist will remove the rest of the mole. Patients should realize that slicing off a section of a malignant mole will not cause the cancer to spread.

Removing a mole for cosmetic reasons involves numbing the area and using scissors or a scalpel to remove the elevated portion. The patient is left with a flat mole the same color as the original growth. Cutting out parts of the mole above and beneath the surface of the skin can leave a scar more noticeable than the mole.

Scissors or a razor can be used to temporarily remove hair from a mole. Permanent hair removal, however, requires electrolysis or surgical removal of the mole.

Prognosis

Moles are rarely cancerous and, once removed, unlikely to recur. A dermatologist should be consulted if a mole reappears after being removed.

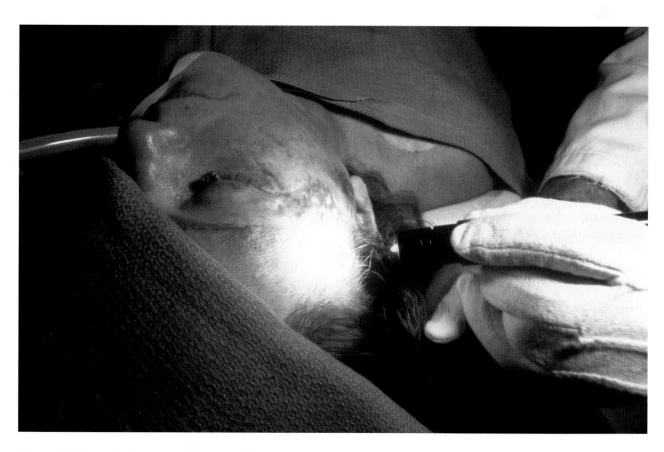

Woman's birthmark being removed by laser. *(Photograph by Alexander Tsiaras, Photo Researchers, Inc. Reproduced by permission.)*

Prevention

Wearing a sunscreen and limiting sun exposure may prevent some moles. Anyone who has moles should examine them every month and see a dermatologist if changes in size, shape, color, or texture occur or if new moles appear.

A team of researchers at Duke University reported in 2003 that topical application of a combination of 15% vitamin C and 1% vitamin E over a four-day period offered significant protection against **sunburn**. The researchers suggest that this combination may protect skin against **aging** caused by sunlight as well.

Anyone with a family history of melanoma should see a dermatologist for an annual skin examination. Everyone should know the ABCDEs of melanoma:

- A: Asymmetry, which occurs when the two halves of the mole are not identical

- B: Borders that are irregular or indistinct

- C: Color that varies in a single mole

- D: Diameter, which should be no larger than a pencil eraser (about 6 mm)

- E: Elevated above the surrounding tissue.

A mole with any of these characteristics should be evaluated by a dermatologist.

KEY TERMS

Dermatology—The branch of medicine that studies and treats disorders of the skin.

Malignant melanoma—A potentially fatal form of skin cancer that develops from melanocytes, which are skin cells containing melanin.

Melanin—A dark insoluble pigment found in humans in the skin, hair, choroid layer of the eye, and a part of the brain called the substantia nigra.

Nevus (plural, nevi)—The medical term for any anomaly of the skin that is present at birth, including moles and birthmarks.

Advances in photographic technique have now made it easier to track the development of moles with the help of whole-body photographs. A growing number of hospitals are offering these photographs as part of outpatient mole-monitoring services.

Resources

BOOKS

Beers, Mark H., MD, and Robert Berkow, MD, editors. "Dermatologic Disorders: Malignant Tumors." Section 10, Chapter 126. In *The Merck Manual of Diagnosis and Therapy*. Whitehouse Station, NJ: Merck Research Laboratories, 2004.

Beers, Mark H., MD, and Robert Berkow, MD, editors. "Dermatologic Disorders: Moles." Section 10, Chapter 125. In *The Merck Manual of Diagnosis and Therapy*. Whitehouse Station, NJ: Merck Research Laboratories, 2004.

Beers, Mark H., MD, and Robert Berkow, MD, editors. "Dermatologic Disorders: Reactions to Sunlight." Section 10, Chapter 119. In *The Merck Manual of Diagnosis and Therapy*. Whitehouse Station, NJ: Merck Research Laboratories, 2004.

PERIODICALS

Bennett, D. C. "Human Melanocyte Senescence and Melanoma Susceptibility Genes." *Oncogene* 22 (May 19, 2003): 3063–3069.

Bessoud, B., N. Lassau, S. Koscielny, et al. "High-Frequency Sonography and Color Doppler in the Management of Pigmented Skin Lesions." *Ultra sound in Medicine & Biology* 6 (June 2003): 875-879.

Bray, C. "The Development of an Improved Method of Photography for Mole-Monitoring at the University Hospital of North Durham." *Journal of Audiovisual Media in Medicine* 26 (June 2003): 60–66.

Hall, Daniel J., MD, and Michael Holtel, MD. "Malignant Melanoma of the Face and Neck." *eMedicine* July 3, 2003. < http://www.emedecine.com.ent/topic27.htm >.

Lin, J. Y., M. A. Selim, C. R. Shea, et al. "UV Photoprotection by Combination Topical Antioxidants Vitamin C and Vitamin E." *Journal of the American Academy of Dermatology* 48 (June 2003): 866-874.

Tucker, M. A., and A. M. Goldstein. "Melanoma Etiology: Where Are We?" *Oncogene* 22 (May 19, 2003): 3042–3052.

ORGANIZATIONS

American Academy of Dermatology. 930 N. Meacham Road, P.O. Box 4014, Schaumburg, IL 60168-4014. (847) 330-0230. Fax: (847) 330-0050. < http://www.aad.org >.

American Cancer Society. 1599 Clifton Road NE, Atlanta, GA 30329. (800) ACS-2345.

National Cancer Institute (NCI). NCI Public Inquiries Office, Suite 3036A, 6116 Executive Boulevard, MSC8332, Bethesda, MD 20892-8322. (800) 4-CANCER or (800) 332-8615 (TTY). < http://www.nci.nih.gov >.

Nevus Outreach, Inc. 1601 Madison Blvd., Bartesville, OK 74006. (877) 426-3887. < http://www.nevus.org >.

Maureen Haggerty
Rebecca J. Frey, PhD

Molybdenum excess *see* **Mineral toxicity**

Mometasone *see* **Corticosteroids**

Moncytic ehrlichiosis *see* **Ehrlichiosis**

Mongolism *see* **Down syndrome**

Moniliasis *see* **Candidiasis**

Monkeypox

Definition

Monkeypox is an infectious disease caused by an orthopoxvirus. Orthopoxviruses are a genus of viruses that include the disease agents that cause human **smallpox**, cowpox, and camelpox as well as monkeypox. Monkeypox, which was first identified in humans in an outbreak in Africa in 1970, usually produces a less severe illness with fewer fatalities than smallpox. However, its symptoms are similar: **fever**, pus-filled blisters all over the body, and respiratory problems.

Monkeypox is classified as a **zoonosis**, which means that it is a disease of animals that can be transmitted to humans under natural conditions. The first cases of monkeypox reported in humans involved contact between humans and animals in the African rain forest. The outbreak that made headlines in the United States in June 2003, however, involved animals purchased as pets from pet stores. In nature, monkeypox has been found in monkeys, chimpanzees, rabbits, prairie dogs, Gambian rats, ground squirrels, and mice. It is not known as of late 2003 whether other wild or domestic animals can contract monkeypox.

Description

Prior to 2003, most monkeypox cases were diagnosed in remote areas of central and west Africa. Between February 1996 and October 1997, however, there were 511 suspected cases of monkeypox in the Democratic Republic of the Congo (DRC, formerly Zaire). This outbreak, the largest ever, raised fears that the virus had mutated and become more infectious.

In late 1997, the U.S. Centers for Disease Control and Prevention (CDC) and the World Health Organization (WHO) announced that this relatively large outbreak was likely due to human behavior, rather than virus mutation. During the outbreak, the DRC was embroiled in civil war. Food shortages increased reliance on hunting and raised chances that people would come into contact with infected animals.

The 2003 outbreak in the United States, which was the first confirmed instance of community-acquired monkeypox in North America, came to the attention of the CDC in early June, when a laboratory in Wisconsin identified the monkeypox virus in samples taken from the skin of an infected patient and lymph node tissue from the patient's pet prairie dog. By the end of June, cases of monkeypox in humans had been identified in six Midwestern states (Illinois, Indiana, Kansas, Missouri, Ohio, and Wisconsin). The patients acquired the virus from infected prairie dogs purchased as pets, which in turn were infected through contact with animals imported from Africa that were sold in the same pet stores.

Monkeypox is less severe than smallpox and can sometimes be confused with **chickenpox**. It seems partly preventable with smallpox **vaccination**, but vaccination programs were discontinued in the late 1970s. (Barring samples stored in laboratories, smallpox has been eradicated.) People under the age of 16—those born after smallpox vaccination ended—seem the most susceptible to monkeypox. During the 1996-97 outbreak, approximately 85% of the cases were in this age group.

Although the monkeypox virus is related to the smallpox virus, experts do not think (as of late 2003) that it is likely to be cultivated as an agent of bioterrorism. Monkeypox is much less easily transmitted person-to-person than smallpox and has a much lower fatality rate.

Causes and symptoms

The monkeypox virus is transmitted to humans through an infected animal's blood, body sores, or bite; or through handling an infected animal's bedding or cage. Initial symptoms of monkeypox in humans include fever, a bodywide rash (exanthem) of pus-filled blisters, and flu-like muscle aches and **fatigue**. These symptoms can be accompanied by **diarrhea**, swollen lymph nodes, a **sore throat**, and mouth sores. In some cases, a victim may experience trouble breathing. Symptoms are at their worst for 3–7 days, after which the fever lessens and blisters begin to form crusts.

The symptoms of monkeypox in pet rabbits, rats, or mice include inflammation of the eyes, a nasal discharge, fever, loss of appetite, a skin rash, and tiredness. Pet monkeys typically develop a rash with pus-filled lesions on the palms of the hands, trunk, and tail. They may also have mouth ulcers.

Diagnosis

Since the symptoms of monkeypox resemble other diseases caused by orthopox viruses, definitive diagnosis may require laboratory testing to uncover the virus or evidence (from antibodies in the blood) that it is present. As of 2003, laboratory techniques that can be used to identify the monkeypox virus include electron microscopy, polymerase chain reaction (PCR), immunohistochemistry, and ELISA testing.

Treatment

Like most viruses, monkeypox cannot be resolved with medication. The only treatment option is symptomatic—that is, patients are made as comfortable as possible. In March 1998, the U.S. Army Medical Research Institute for Infectious Diseases reported that an antiviral drug called cidofovir may combat monkeypox infection. As of 2003, additional studies report that cidofovir appears to be safe and effective as a treatment for monkeypox in humans. The drug has worked successfully in primates, but further research is needed to determine its effectiveness in humans.

Prognosis

Children are more likely to contract the disease and have the highest **death** rate. Monkeypox is not as lethal as smallpox, but the death rate among young children may reach 2–10%. In some cases, hospitalization is required. Recovery is good among survivors, although some scarring may result from the blisters.

Prevention

Monkeypox is one of the diseases that physicians, veterinarians, and public health officials are required by law to report to the CDC.

Although smallpox vaccination offers some protection against monkeypox, experts do not generally recommend getting a smallpox vaccination simply to guard against monkeypox if one has not been exposed to it. However, the CDC recommends as of June 2003 that anyone who has had close contact with humans or animals infected with monkeypox, or has helped to care for them, should be vaccinated against smallpox. The vaccination can be administered as late as 14 days after exposure to the virus. In addition, veterinarians

KEY TERMS

Antiviral—Refers to a drug that can destroy viruses and help treat illnesses caused by them.

Bioterrorism—The intentional use of disease-causing microbes or other biologic agents to intimidate or terrorize a civilian population for political or military reasons.

Mutation—A change in an organism's genetic code that causes it to develop new characteristics.

Orthopoxvirus—The genus of viruses that includes monkeypox, smallpox, cowpox, and camelpox.

Symptomatic—Refers to treatment that addresses the symptoms of an illness, but not its underlying cause.

Zoonosis (plural, zoonoses)—Any disease of animals that can be transmitted to humans under natural conditions. Monkeypox is a zoonosis.

or public health personnel conducting field investigations should be vaccinated before any exposure to monkeypox.

As of late 2003, no cases of monkeypox were identified in cats or dogs belonging to people infected by the June outbreak. The American Veterinary Medicine Association (AVMA) recommends, however, that cats, dogs, or other mammals that have been in contact with an animal known to have monkeypox should be kept in quarantine for 30 days from the date of exposure.

People who have a pet with symptoms of monkeypox should *not* take it to an animal shelter or release it into the wild. They should isolate it from humans and other animals, and take it to a veterinarian in a closed, chew-proof container with air holes.

On June 11, 2003, the CDC and the Food and Drug Administration (FDA) issued a joint order prohibiting the importation of rats and other rodents from Africa. In addition, the agencies banned the sale and distribution of prairie dogs and six species of African rodents in the United States.

Resources

PERIODICALS

Altman, Larry K., MD, and Jodi Wilgoren. "20 Cases of Disease Related to Smallpox Detected in the U.S." *New York Times* June 9, 2003.

Centers for Disease Control and Prevention. "Multistate Outbreak of Monkeypox—Illinois, Indiana, and Wisconsin, 2003." *Morbidity and Mortality Weekly Report* 52 (June 13, 2003): 537–540.

Centers for Disease Control and Prevention. "Update: Multistate Outbreak of Monkeypox—Illinois, Indiana, Kansas, Missouri, Ohio, and Wisconsin, 2003." *Morbidity and Mortality Weekly Report* 52 (June 20, 2003): 561–564.

Centers for Disease Control and Prevention. "Update: Multistate Outbreak of Monkeypox—Illinois, Indiana, Kansas, Missouri, Ohio, and Wisconsin, 2003." *Morbidity and Mortality Weekly Report* 52 (June 27, 2003): 589–590.

Rosen, T., and J. Jablon. "Infectious Threats from Exotic Pets: Dermatological Implications." *Dermatologic Clinics* 21 (April 2003): 229–236.

Smee, D. F., K. W. Bailey, and R. W. Sidwell. "Comparative Effects of Cidofovir and Cyclic HPMPC on Lethal Cowpox and Vaccinia Virus Respiratory Infections in Mice." *Chemotherapy* 49 (June 2003): 126–131.

ORGANIZATIONS

American Veterinary Medical Association (AVMA). 1931 North Meacham Road, Suite 100, Schaumburg, IL 60173-4360. <http://www.avma.org>.

Centers for Disease Control and Prevention. 1600 Clifton Rd., NE, Atlanta, GA 30333. (800) 311-3435, (404) 639-3311. <http://www.cdc.gov>.

OTHER

American Veterinary Medical Association (AVMA). "Foreign Animal Disease Alert: Investigation Uncovers First Outbreak of Monkeypox Infection in the Western Hemisphere," June 23, 2003. <http://www.avma.org/pubhlth/monkeypox/default.asp>.

American Veterinary Medical Association (AVMA). *Monkeypox Backgrounder.* Schaumburg, IL: AVMA, June 2003.

Centers for Disease Control and Prevention (CDC). *Fact Sheet: Basic Information About Monkeypox.* Atlanta, GA: CDC, June 2003.

Centers for Disease Control and Prevention (CDC). *Fact Sheet: Embargoed Animals and Monkeypox Virus.* Atlanta, GA: CDC, June 2003.

Julia Barrett
Rebecca J. Frey, PhD

Monoamine oxidase inhibitors

Definition

Monoamine oxidase inhibitors (MAO inhibitors) are medicines that relieve certain types of mental depression.

Purpose

MAO inhibitors are a type of antidepressant and are used to treat mental depression. Like other **antidepressant drugs**, MAO inhibitors help reduce the extreme sadness, hopelessness, and lack of interest in life that are typical in people with depression. MAO inhibitors are especially useful in treating people whose depression is combined with other problems such as **anxiety**, panic attacks, **phobias**, or the desire to sleep too much.

Description

Discovered in the 1950s, MAO inhibitors work by correcting chemical imbalances in the brain. Normally, natural chemicals called neurotransmitters carry signals from one brain cell to another. Some neurotransmitters, such as serotonin and norepinephrine, play important roles in controlling mood. But other substances in the brain may interfere with mood control by breaking down these neurotransmitters. Researchers believe that MAO inhibitors work by blocking the chemicals that break down serotonin and norepinephrine. This gives the neurotransmitters more time to do their important work.

Because MAO inhibitors also affect other chemicals throughout the body, these drugs may produce many unwanted side effects. They can be especially dangerous when taken with certain foods, beverages and medicines. Anyone taking these drugs should ask his or her physician or pharmacist for a list of products to avoid.

MAO inhibitors are available only with a physician's prescription. They are sold in tablet form. Some commonly used MAO inhibitors are isocarboxazid (Marplan), phenelzine (Nardil), and tranylcypromine (Parnate).

Recommended dosage

The recommended dosage depends on the type of MAO inhibitor and the type of depression for which it is being taken. Dosages may be different for different patients. Check with the physician who prescribed the drug or the pharmacist who filled the prescription for the correct dosage.

Always take MAO inhibitors exactly as directed by your physician. Never take larger or more frequent doses, and do not take the drug for longer than directed. See the physician regularly while taking this medicine, especially in the first few months of treatment. The physician will check to make sure the medicine is working as it should and will note unwanted side effects. The physician may also need to adjust the dosage during this period.

Several weeks may be needed for the effects of this medicine to be felt. Be sure to keep taking it as directed, even if it does not seem to be helping.

Do not stop taking this medicine suddenly. Tapering the dose may be necessary to reduce the chance of withdrawal symptoms. If it is necessary to stop taking the drug, check with the physician who prescribed it for instructions on how to stop.

MAO inhibitors may be taken with or without food, on a full or empty stomach. Check package directions or ask the physician or pharmacist for instructions on how to take the medicine. Remember that some foods and beverages must be avoided during treatment with MAO inhibitors.

Precautions

The effects of this medicine may continue for 2 weeks or more after patients stop taking it. All precautions should be observed during this period, as well as throughout treatment with MAO inhibitors.

MAO inhibitors may cause serious and possibly life-threatening reactions, such as sudden high blood pressure, when taken with certain foods, beverages, or medicines. The dangerous reactions may not begin until several hours after consuming these things. Aged cheeses, red wines, smoked or pickled meats, chocolate, caffeinated beverages, and foods containing monosodium glutamate (MSG) are among the foods and drinks to be avoided. Be sure to get a complete list from the physician who prescribed the medicine or the pharmacist who filled the prescription.

Do not drink any alcoholic beverages or reduced-alcohol or alcohol-free beer or wine while taking this medicine.

Anyone who is taking MAO inhibitors should not use any other medicine unless it has been approved or prescribed by a physician who knows that they are taking MAO inhibitors. This includes nonprescription (over-the-counter) medicines such as sleep aids; medicines for colds, **cough**, hay **fever**, or **asthma** (including nose drops or sprays); medicines to increase alertness or keep from falling asleep; and appetite control products.

Because MAO inhibitors work on the central nervous system, they may add to the effects of alcohol and other drugs that slow down the central nervous system, such as **antihistamines**, cold medicine, allergy medicine, sleep aids, medicine for seizures, tranquilizers, some **pain** relievers, and **muscle relaxants**. Anyone taking MAO inhibitors should check with his or her physician before taking any of the above.

MAO inhibitors may interact with medicines used during surgery, dental procedures, or emergency treatment. These interactions could increase the chance of side effects. Anyone who is taking MAO inhibitors should be sure to tell the health care professional in charge before having any surgical or dental procedures or receiving emergency treatment.

Some people feel drowsy, dizzy, lightheaded, or less alert when using MAO inhibitors. The drugs may also cause blurred vision. For these reasons, anyone who takes these drugs should not drive, use machines or do anything else that might be dangerous until they have found out how the drugs affect them.

These medicines also make some people feel lightheaded, dizzy, or faint when they get up after sitting or lying down. To lessen the problem, get up gradually and hold onto something for support if possible.

Older people may be especially sensitive to the effects of MAO inhibitors. This may increase the chance of side effects, such as **dizziness** or lightheadedness.

Special conditions

People with certain medical conditions or who are taking certain other medicines can have problems if they take MAO inhibitors. Before taking these drugs, be sure to let the physician know about any of these conditions:

ALLERGIES. Anyone who has had unusual reactions to MAO inhibitors in the past should let his or her physician know before taking the drugs again. The physician should also be told about any **allergies** to foods, dyes, preservatives, or other substances.

PREGNANCY. Studies suggest that taking MAO inhibitors during **pregnancy** may increase the risk of **birth defects** or problems in the newborn after birth. Women who are pregnant or who may become pregnant should check with their physicians before using MAO inhibitors.

BREASTFEEDING. MAO inhibitors may pass into breast milk, but no problems have been reported in nursing babies whose mothers took the medicine. Women who are breastfeeding their babies should check with their physicians before using this medicine.

DIABETES. MAO inhibitors may affect blood sugar levels. Persons with diabetes who are taking this medicine and notice changes in their blood or urine tests should check with their physicians.

ANGINA. MAO inhibitors may make people feel unusually energetic and healthy. People with **angina** (chest pain) should be careful not to overexert themselves and should check with their physicians before increasing their levels of activity or **exercise**.

OTHER MEDICAL CONDITIONS. Before using MAO inhibitors, people with any of these medical problems should make sure their physicians are aware of their conditions:

• Alcohol **abuse**

• High blood pressure

• Recent **heart attack** or **stroke**

• Heart or blood vessel disease

• Liver disease

• Kidney disease

• Frequent or severe headaches

• Epilepsy

• Parkinson's disease

• Current or past mental illness

• Asthma or **bronchitis**

• Overactive thyroid

• Pheochromocytoma (a tumor of the adrenal gland).

USE OF CERTAIN MEDICINES. Taking MAO inhibitors with certain other drugs may affect the way the drugs work or may increase the chance of side effects.

Side effects

The most common side effects are dizziness, lightheadedness, drowsiness, tiredness, weakness, blurred vision, shakiness or trembling, restlessness, sleep problems or twitching during sleep, increased appetite (especially for sweets), weight gain, decreased sexual ability, decreased amount of urine, and mild **headache**. These problems usually go away as the body adjusts to the drug and do not require medical treatment unless they interfere with normal activities.

More serious side effects may occur. If any of the following side effects occur, stop taking the medicine and get emergency medical attention immediately:

• Severe chest pain

• Severe headache

• Stiff, sore neck

• Enlarged pupils

• Increased sensitivity of eyes to light

• Fast or slow heartbeat

- Sweating, with or without fever or cold, clammy skin
- Nausea and vomiting.

Other side effects may occur. Anyone who has unusual or troublesome symptoms after taking MAO inhibitors should get in touch with his or her physician.

Interactions

MAO inhibitors may interact with many other medicines. When this happens, the effects of one or both of the drugs may change or the risk of side effects may be greater. *Anyone who takes MAO inhibitors must check with his or her physician before taking any other prescription or nonprescription (over-the-counter) medicine.* Among the drugs that may interact with MAO inhibitors are:

- Central nervous system (CNS) depressants such as medicine for allergies, colds, hay fever, and asthma; sedatives; tranquilizers; prescription pain medicine; muscle relaxants; medicine for seizures; sleep aids; **barbiturates**; and anesthetics

- Medicine for high blood pressure

- Other antidepressants, including **tricyclic antidepressants** (such as Tofranil and Norpramin), antidepressants that raise serotonin levels (such as Prozac and Zoloft), and bupropion (Wellbutrin)

- Diabetes medicines taken by mouth
- Insulin
- Water pills (diuretics).

The list above does not include every drug that may interact with MAO inhibitors. Check with a physician or pharmacist before combining MAO inhibitors with any other prescription or nonprescription (over-the-counter) medicine.

Nancy Ross-Flanigan

Mononucleosis *see* **Infectious mononucleosis**

Montezuma's revenge *see* **Traveler's diarrhea**

Mood disorders

Definition

Mood disorders are mental disorders characterized by periods of depression, sometimes alternating with periods of elevated mood.

Description

While many people go through sad or elated moods from time to time, people with mood disorders suffer from severe or prolonged mood states that disrupt their daily functioning. Among the general mood disorders classified in the fourth edition (1994) of the *Diagnostic and Statistical Manual of Mental Disorders* (*DSM-IV*) are major depressive disorder, **bipolar disorder**, and dysthymia.

In classifying and diagnosing mood disorders, doctors determine if the mood disorder is unipolar or bipolar. When only one extreme in mood (the depressed state) is experienced, this type of depression is called unipolar. Major depression refers to a single severe period of depression, marked by negative or hopeless thoughts and physical symptoms like **fatigue**. In major depressive disorder, some patients have isolated episodes of depression. In between these episodes, the patient does not feel depressed or have other symptoms associated with depression. Other patients have more frequent episodes.

Bipolar depression or bipolar disorder (sometimes called manic depression) refers to a condition in which people experience two extremes in mood. They alternate between depression (the "low" mood) and **mania** or hypomania (the "high" mood). These patients go from depression to a frenzied, abnormal elevation in mood. Mania and hypomania are similar, but mania is usually more severe and debilitating to the patient.

Dysthymia is a recurrent or lengthy depression that may last a lifetime. It is similar to major depressive disorder, but dysthymia is chronic, long-lasting, persistent, and mild. Patients may have symptoms that are not as severe as major depression, but the symptoms last for many years. It seems that a mild form of the depression is always present. In some cases, people also may experience a major depressive episode on top of their dysthymia, a condition sometimes referred to as a "double depression."

Causes and symptoms

Mood disorders tend to run in families. These disorders are associated with imbalances in certain chemicals that carry signals between brain cells (neurotransmitters). These chemicals include serotonin, norepinephrine, and dopamine. Women are more vulnerable to unipolar depression than are men. Major life stressors (like divorce, serious financial problems, **death** of a family member, etc.) will often provoke the symptoms of depression in susceptible people.

Major depression is more serious than just feeling "sad" or "blue." The symptoms of major depression may include:

- Loss of appetite
- A change in sleep patterns, like not sleeping (**insomnia**) or sleeping too much
- Feelings of worthlessness, hopelessness, or inappropriate guilt
- Fatigue
- Difficulty in concentrating or making decisions
- Overwhelming and intense feelings of sadness or grief
- Disturbed thinking. The person may also have physical symptoms like stomachaches or headaches.

Bipolar disorder includes mania or hypomania. Mania is an abnormal elevation in mood. The person may be excessively cheerful, have grandiose ideas, and may sleep less. He or she may talk nonstop for hours, have unending enthusiasm, and demonstrate poor judgement. Sometimes the elevation in mood is marked by irritability and hostility rather than cheerfulness. While the person may at first seem normal with an increase in energy, others who know the person well see a marked difference in behavior. The patient may seem to be in a frenzy and often will make poor, bizarre, or dangerous choices in his/her personal and professional lives. Hypomania is not as severe as mania and does not cause the level of impairment in work and social activities that mania can.

Diagnosis

Doctors diagnose mood disorders based on the patient's description of the symptoms as well as the patient's family history. The length of time the patient has had symptoms also is important. Generally patients are diagnosed with dysthymia if they feel depressed more days than not for at least two years. The depression is mild but long lasting. In major depressive disorder, the patient is depressed almost all day nearly every day of the week for at least two weeks. The depression is severe. Sometimes laboratory tests are performed to rule out other causes for the symptoms (like thyroid disease). The diagnosis may be confirmed when a patient responds well to medication.

Treatment

The most effective treatment for mood disorders is a combination of medication and psychotherapy. In fact, a 2003 report revealed that people on medication for bipolar disorder had better results if they also participated in family-focused therapy. The four different classes of drugs used in mood disorders are:

- Heterocyclic antidepressants (HCAs), like amitriptyline (Elavil)
- Selective serotonin reuptake inhibitors (**SSRI** inhibitors), like fluoxetine (Prozac), paroxetine (Paxil), and sertraline (Zoloft)
- Monoamine oxidase inhibitors (MAOI inhibitors), like phenelzine sulfate (Nardil) and tranylcypromine sulfate (Parnate)
- Mood stabilizers, like lithium carbonate (Eskalith) and valproate, often used in people with bipolar mood disorders.

A number of psychotherapy approaches are useful as well. Interpersonal psychotherapy helps the patient recognize the interaction between the mood disorder and interpersonal relationships. **Cognitive-behavioral therapy** explores how the patient's view of the world may be affecting his or her mood and outlook.

When depression fails to respond to treatment or when there is a high risk of **suicide**, **electroconvulsive** therapy (ECT) sometimes is used. ECT is believed to affect neurotransmitters like the medications do. Patients are anesthetized and given **muscle relaxants** to minimize discomfort. Then low-level electric current is passed through the brain to cause a brief convulsion. The most common side effect of ECT is mild, short-term memory loss.

Alternative treatment

There are many alternative therapies that may help in the treatment of mood disorders, including **acupuncture**, botanical medicine, homeopathy, **aromatherapy**, constitutional **hydrotherapy**, and light therapy. The therapy used is an individual choice. Short-term clinical studies have shown that the herb **St. John's wort** (*Hypericum perforatum*) can effectively treat some types of depression. Though it appears very safe, the herb may have some side effects and its long-term effectiveness has not been proven. It has not been tested in patients with bipolar disorder. Despite uncertainty concerning its effectiveness, a 2003 report said acceptance of the treatment continues to increase. A poll showed that about 41% of 15,000 science professionals in 62 countries said they would use St. John's wort for mild to moderate depression. Although St. John's wort appears to be a safe alternative to conventional antidepressants, care should be taken, as the herb can interfere with the actions of some pharmaceuticals. The usual dose is 300 mg three times daily. St. John's wort and **antidepressant drugs** should not be taken simultaneously, so patients should tell their doctor if they are taking St. John's wort.

Prognosis

Most cases of mood disorders can be successfully managed if properly diagnosed and treated.

Prevention

People can take steps to improve mild depression and keep it from becoming worse. They can learn **stress** management (like relaxation training or breathing exercises), **exercise** regularly, and avoid drugs or alcohol.

Resources

PERIODICALS

"Family-focused Therapy May Reduce Relapse Rate." *Health & Medicine Week* September 29, 2003: 70.

"St. John's Wort Healing Reputation Upheld." *Nutraceuticals International.* September 2003.

ORGANIZATIONS

American Psychiatric Association. 1400 K Street NW, Washington DC 20005. (888) 357-7924. <http://www.psych.org>.

National Depressive and Manic Depressive Association (NDMDA). 730 N. Franklin St., Ste. 501, Chicago, IL 60610. (800) 826-3632. <http://www.ndmda.org>.

National Institute of Mental Health. Mental Health Public Inquiries, 5600 Fishers Lane, Room 15C-05, Rockville, MD 20857. (888) 826-9438. <http://www.nimh.nih.gov>.

Robert Scott Dinsmoor
Teresa G. Odle

Morning after pill *see* **Mifepristone**

Motion sickness

Definition

Motion sickness is the uncomfortable **dizziness**, **nausea**, and **vomiting** that people experience when their sense of balance and equilibrium is disturbed by constant motion. Riding in a car, aboard a ship or boat, or riding on a swing all cause stimulation of the vestibular system and visual stimulation that often leads to discomfort. While motion sickness can be bothersome, it is not a serious illness, and can be prevented.

PATRICIA SUZANNE COWINGS
(1948–)

Patricia Suzanne Cowings was born on December 15, 1948, in New York City. She was one of four children born to Sadie and Albert Cowings, a grocery store owner. Cowings showed interest in science by the time she was eleven years old. She enrolled in the State University of New York at Stony Brook, earning her bachelor's degree with honors in 1970. She began her graduate work at the University of California at Davis where she was awarded both her master's and her doctoral degrees in 1973. Cowings also received an associateship from the National Research Council that same year, which allowed her to complete two years of research at NASA's Ames Research Center. She has held a position as a researcher with Ames since 1977.

Cowings's work at Ames' Psychophysiological Research Laboratory led to major breakthroughs for astronauts. Her pioneering experiments with bio-feedback as a method to control bodily functions has proven very effective for astronaut crews who experience "zero-gravity sickness syndrome." Her program was finally used during the 1992 *Endeavour* space flight. Presently, Cowings is researching exercises that will allow astronauts to maintain muscle strength while in zero gravity. She has published numerous papers with her colleague and husband, William B. Toscano. In addition, she has written articles including *The Relationship of Motion Sickness Susceptibility to Learned Autonomic Control for Symptom Suppression* (1982), *Autogenic-Feedback Training as a Preventive Method for Space Adaptation Syndrome* (1985), and *Autogenic-Feedback Training: A Preventive Method for Motion and Space Sickness* (1990).

Description

Motion sickness is a common problem, with nearly 80% of the general population suffering from it at one time in their lives. People with migraine headaches or Ménière's syndrome, however, are more likely than others to have recurrent episodes of motion sickness. Researchers at the Naval Medical Center in San Diego, California, reported in 2003 that 70% of research subjects with severe motion sickness had abnormalities of the vestibular system; these abnormalities are often found in patients diagnosed with migraines or **Ménière's disease**.

While motion sickness may occur at any age, it is more common in children over the age of two, with the majority outgrowing this susceptibility.

When looking at why motion sickness occurs, it is helpful to understand the role of the sensory organs. The sensory organs control a body's sense of balance by telling the brain what direction the body is pointing, the direction it is moving, and if it is standing still or turning. These messages are relayed by the inner ears (or labyrinth); the eyes; the skin pressure receptors, such as in those in the feet; the muscle and joint sensory receptors, which track what body parts are moving; and the central nervous system (the brain and spinal cord), which is responsible for processing all incoming sensory information.

Motion sickness and its symptoms surface when conflicting messages are sent to the central nervous system. An example of this is reading a book in the back seat of a moving car. The inner ears and skin receptors sense the motion, but the eyes register only the stationary pages of the book. This conflicting information may cause the usual motion sickness symptoms of dizziness, **nausea and vomiting**.

Causes and symptoms

While all five of the body's sensory organs contribute to motion sickness, excess stimulation to the vestibular system within the inner ear (the body's "balance center") has been shown to be one of the primary reasons for this condition. Balance problems, or vertigo, are caused by a conflict between what is seen and how the inner ear perceives it, leading to confusion in the brain. This confusion may result in higher heart rates, rapid breathing, nausea and sweating, along with dizziness and vomiting.

Pure optokinetic motion sickness is caused solely by visual stimuli, or what is seen. The optokinetic system is the reflex that allow the eyes to move when an object moves. Many people suffer when what they view is rotating or swaying, even if they are standing still.

Additional factors that may contribute to the occurrence of motion sickness include:

- Poor ventilation.

- Anxiety or fear. Both have been found to lower a person's threshold for experiencing motion sickness symptoms.

- Food. It is recommended that a heavy meal of spicy and greasy foods be avoided before and during a trip.

- Alcohol. A drink is often thought to help calm the nerves, but in this case it could upset the stomach further. A hangover for the next morning's trip may also lead to motion sickness.

- Genetic factors. Research suggests that some people inherit a predisposition to motion sickness. This predisposition is more marked in some ethnic groups than in others; one study published in 2002 found that persons of Chinese or Japanese ancestry are significantly more vulnerable to motion sickness than persons of British ancestry.

- **Pregnancy**. Susceptibility in women to vomiting during pregnancy appears to be related to motion sickness, although the precise connections are not well understood as of 2004.

Often viewed as a minor annoyance, some travelers are temporarily immobilized by motion sickness, and a few continue to feel its effects for hours and even days after a trip (the "mal d'embarquement" syndrome).

Diagnosis

Most cases of motion sickness are mild and self-treatable disorders. If symptoms such as dizziness become chronic, a doctor may be able to help alleviate the discomfort by looking further into a patient's general health. Questions regarding medications, head injuries, recent infections, and other questions about the ear and neurological system will be asked. An examination of the ears, nose, and throat, as well as tests of nerve and balance function, may also be completed.

Severe cases of motion sickness symptoms, and those that become progressively worse, may require additional, specific tests. Diagnosis in these situations deserves the attention and care of a doctor with specialized skills in diseases of the ear, nose, throat, equilibrium, and neurological system.

Treatment

There are a variety of medications to help ease the symptoms of motion sickness, and most of these are available without a prescription. Known as over-the-counter (OTC) medications, it is recommended that these be taken 30-60 minutes before traveling to prevent motion sickness symptoms, as well as during an extended trip.

Drugs

The following OTC drugs consist of ingredients that have been considered safe and effective for the treatment of motion sickness by the Food and Drug Administration:

- Marezine (and others). Includes the active ingredient cyclizine and is not for use in children under age 6.

- Benadryl (and others). Includes the active ingredient diphenhydramine and is not for use in children under age 6.

- Dramamine (and others). Includes the active ingredient dimenhydrinate and is not for use in children under age 2.

- Bonine (and others). Includes the active ingredient meclizine and is not for use in children under age 12.

Each of the active ingredients listed above are **antihistamines** whose main side effect is drowsiness. Caution should be used when driving a vehicle or operating machinery, and alcohol should be avoided when taking any drug for motion sickness. Large doses of OTC drugs for motion sickness may also cause **dry mouth** and occasional blurred vision.

The side effects of cinnarizine and the other antihistamine antiemetics indicate that they should not be used by members of flight crews responsible for the control of aircraft or for other tasks that require sustained attention and alertness.

The Food and Drug Administration (FDA) recommends that people with **emphysema**, chronic **bronchitis**, **glaucoma**, or difficulty urinating due to an **enlarged prostate** do not use OTC drugs for motion sickness unless directed by their doctor.

Longer trips may require a prescription medication called scopolamine (Transderm Scop). Formerly used in the transdermal skin patch (now discontinued), travelers must now ask their doctor to prescribe it in the form of a gel. In gel form, scopolamine is most effective when smeared on the arm or neck and covered with a bandage.

Another prescription drug that is sometimes given for motion sickness is ondansetron (Zofran), which was originally developed to treat nausea associated with **cancer chemotherapy**. Unlike cyclizine, ondansetron appears to be safe for use in children under the age of six.

Several newer antiemetic medications are under development as of early 2004. The most promising of these newer drugs is a class of compounds known as neurokinin-1 (substance P) antagonists. The neurokinins are being tested for the control of nausea following cancer chemotherapy as well as nausea related to motion sickness. In March 2003 the FDA approved the first of this new class of antiemetic drugs. Known as aprepitant, it is sold under the trade name Emend.

Alternative treatment

Alternative treatments for motion sickness have become widely accepted as a standard means of care. Ginger (*Zingiber officinale*) in its various forms is often used to calm the stomach, and it is now known that the oils it contains (gingerols and shogaols) appear to relax the intestinal tract in addition to mildly depressing the central nervous system. Some of the most effective forms of ginger include the powdered, encapsulated form; ginger tea prepared from sliced ginger root; or candied pieces. All forms of ginger should be taken on an empty stomach.

Placing manual pressure on the Neiguan or Pericardium-6 **acupuncture** point (located about three finger-widths above the wrist on the inner arm), either by acupuncture, **acupressure**, or a mild, electrical pulse, has shown to be effective against the symptoms of motion sickness. Elastic wristbands sold at most drugstores are also used as a source of relief due to the pressure it places in this area. Pressing the small intestine 17 (just below the earlobes in the indentations behind the jawbone) may also help in the functioning of the ear's balancing mechanism.

There are several homeopathic remedies that work specifically for motion sickness. They include *Cocculus*, *Petroleum*, and *Tabacum*.

Prognosis

While there is no cure for motion sickness, its symptoms can be controlled or even prevented. Most people respond successfully to the variety of treatments, or avoid the unpleasant symptoms through prevention methods.

Prevention

Because motion sickness is easier to prevent than treat once it has begun, the best treatment is prevention. The following steps may help deter the unpleasant symptoms of motion sickness before they occur:

- Avoid reading while traveling, and do not sit in a backward facing seat.

- Always ride where the eyes may see the same motion that the body and inner ears feel. Safe positions include the front seat of the car while looking at distant scenery; the deck of a ship where the horizon can be seen; and sitting by the window of an airplane. The least motion on an airplane is in a seat over the wings.

- Maintain a fairly straight-ahead view.

> ## KEY TERMS
>
> **Acupressure**—Often described as acupuncture without needles, acupressure is a traditional Chinese medical technique based on theory of *qi* (life energy) flowing in energy meridians or channels in the body. Applying pressure with the thumb and fingers to acupressure points can relieve specific conditions and promote overall balance and health.
>
> **Acupuncture**—Based on the same traditional Chinese medical foundation as acupressure, acupuncture uses sterile needles inserted at specific points to treat certain conditions or relieve pain.
>
> **Neurological system**—The tissue that initiates and transmits nerve impulses including the brain, spinal cord, and nerves.
>
> **Optokinetic**—A reflex that causes a person's eyes to move when their field of vision moves.
>
> **Vertigo**—The sensation of moving around in space, or objects moving around a person. It is a disturbance of equilibrium.
>
> **Vestibular system**—The brain and parts of the inner ear that work together to detect movement and position.

- Eat a light meal before traveling, or if already nauseated, avoid food altogether.

- Avoid watching or talking to another traveler who is having motion sickness.

- Take motion sickness medicine at least 30-60 minutes before travel begins, or as recommended by a physician.

- Learn to live with the condition. Even those who frequently endure motion sickness can learn to travel by anticipating the conditions of their next trip. Research also suggests that increased exposure to the stimulation that causes motion sickness may help decrease its symptoms on future trips.

Resources

BOOKS

Pelletier, Dr. Kenneth R. *The Best Alternative Medicine.* New York: Simon and Schuster, 2002.

PERIODICALS

Black, F. O. "Maternal Susceptibility to Nausea and Vomiting of Pregnancy: Is the Vestibular System

Involved?" *American Journal of Obstetrics and Gynecology* 185, Supplement 5 (May 2002): S204-S209.

Bos, J. E., W. Bles, and B. de Graaf. "Eye Movements to Yaw, Pitch, and Roll About Vertical and Horizontal Axes: Adaptation and Motion Sickness." *Aviation, Space, and Environmental Medicine* 73 (May 2002): 434-444.

Hamid, Mohamed, MD, PhD, and Nicholas Lorenzo, MD. "Dizziness, Vertigo, and Imbalance." *eMedicine* September 17, 2002. < http://emedicine.com/neuro/topic693.htm >.

Harm, D. L., and T. T. Schlegel. "Predicting Motion Sickness During Parabolic Flight." *Autonomic Neuroscience* 31 (May 2002): 116-121.

Hoffer, M. E., K. Gottshall, R. D. Kopke, et al. "Vestibular Testing Abnormalities in Individuals with Motion Sickness." *Otology and Neurotology* 24 (July 2003): 633–636.

Keim, Samuel, MD, and Michael Kent, MD. "Vomiting and Nausea." *eMedicine* April 29, 2002. < http://emedicine.com/aaem/topic476.htm >.

Liu, L., L. Yuan, H. B. Wang, et al. "The Human Alpha(2A)-AR Gene and the Genotype of Site -1296 and the Susceptibility to Motion Sickness." [in Chinese] *Sheng Wu Hua Xue Yu Sheng Wu Wu Li Xue Bao (Shanghai)* 34 (May 2002): 291-297.

Loewen, P. S. "Anti-Emetics in Development." *Expert Opinion on Investigational Drugs* 11 (June 2002): 801-805.

Nicholson, A. N., et al. "Central Effects of Cinnarizine: Restricted Use in Aircrew" *Aviation, Space, and Environmental Medicine* 73 (June 2002): 570-574.

O'Brien, C. M., G. Titley, and P. Whitehurst. "A Comparison of Cyclizine, Ondansetron and Placebo as Prophylaxis Against Postoperative Nausea and Vomiting in Children." *Anaesthesia* 58 (July 2003): 707–711.

Patel, L., and C. Lindley. "Aprepitant—A Novel NK1-Receptor Antagonist." *Expert Opinion in Pharmacotherapy* 4 (December 2003): 2279–2296.

ORGANIZATIONS

Civil Aerospace Medical Institute. P. O. Box 20582, Oklahoma City, OK 73125. (202) 366-4000. < http://www.cami.jccbi.gov >.

National Aeronautics and Space Administration. Office of Biological and Physical Research. < http://www.spaceresearch.nasa.gov >.

Vestibular Disorders Association. P.O. Box 4467, Portland, OR 97208-4467. (800) 837-8428. < http://www.teleport.com/~veda >.

Beth A. Kapes
Rebecca J. Frey, PhD

Mountain sickness *see* **Altitude sickness**

Mouth cancer *see* **Head and neck cancer**

Movement disorders

Definition

Movement disorders are a group of diseases and syndromes affecting the ability to produce and control movement.

Description

Though it seems simple and effortless, normal movement in fact requires an astonishingly complex system of control. Disruption of any portion of this system can cause a person to produce movements that are too weak, too forceful, too uncoordinated, or too poorly controlled for the task at hand. Unwanted movements may occur at rest. Intentional movement may become impossible. Such conditions are called movement disorders.

Abnormal movements themselves are symptoms of underlying disorders. In some cases, the abnormal movements are the only symptoms. Disorders causing abnormal movements include:

- Parkinson's disease
- Parkinsonism caused by drugs or poisons
- Parkinson-plus syndromes (**progressive supranuclear palsy**, multiple system atrophy, and cortical-basal ganglionic degeneration)
- Huntington's disease
- Wilson's disease
- Inherited ataxias (**Friedreich's ataxia**, Machado-Joseph disease, and spinocerebellar ataxias)
- **Tourette syndrome** and other tic disorders
- Essential tremor
- Restless leg syndrome
- Dystonia
- Stroke
- **Cerebral palsy**
- Encephalopathies
- Intoxication
- Poisoning by carbon monoxide, cyanide, methanol, or manganese.

Causes and symptoms

Causes

Movement is produced and coordinated by several interacting brain centers, including the motor cortex, the cerebellum, and a group of structures in the inner portions of the brain called the basal ganglia. Sensory information provides critical input on the current position and velocity of body parts, and spinal nerve cells (neurons) help prevent opposing muscle groups from contracting at the same time.

To understand how movement disorders occur, it is helpful to consider a normal voluntary movement, such as reaching to touch a nearby object with the right index finger. To accomplish the desired movement, the arm must be lifted and extended. The hand must be held out to align with the forearm, and the forefinger must be extended while the other fingers remain flexed.

THE MOTOR CORTEX. Voluntary motor commands begin in the motor cortex located on the outer, wrinkled surface of the brain. Movement of the right arm is begun by the left motor cortex, which generates a large volley of signals to the involved muscles. These electrical signals pass along upper motor neurons through the midbrain to the spinal cord. Within the spinal cord, they connect to lower motor neurons, which convey the signals out of the spinal cord to the surface of the muscles involved. Electrical stimulation of the muscles causes contraction, and the force of contraction pulling on the skeleton causes movement of the arm, hand, and fingers.

Damage to or death of any of the neurons along this path causes weakness or **paralysis** of the affected muscles.

ANTAGONISTIC MUSCLE PAIRS. This picture of movement is too simple, however. One important refinement to it comes from considering the role of opposing, or antagonistic, muscle pairs. Contraction of the biceps muscle, located on the top of the upper arm, pulls on the forearm to flex the elbow and bend the arm. Contraction of the triceps, located on the opposite side, extends the elbow and straightens the arm. Within the spine, these muscles are normally wired so that willed (voluntary) contraction of one is automatically accompanied by blocking of the other. In other words, the command to contract the biceps provokes another command within the spine to prevent contraction of the triceps. In this way, these antagonist muscles are kept from resisting one another. Spinal cord or brain injury can damage this control system and cause involuntary simultaneous contraction and spasticity, an increase in resistance to movement during motion.

THE CEREBELLUM. Once the movement of the arm is initiated, sensory information is needed to guide the finger to its precise destination. In addition to sight,

the most important source of information comes from the "position sense" provided by the many sensory neurons located within the limbs (proprioception). Proprioception is what allows you to touch your nose with your finger even with your eyes closed. The balance organs in the ears provide important information about posture. Both postural and proprioceptive information are processed by a structure at the rear of the brain called the cerebellum. The cerebellum sends out electrical signals to modify movements as they progress, "sculpting" the barrage of voluntary commands into a tightly controlled, constantly evolving pattern. Cerebellar disorders cause inability to control the force, fine positioning, and speed of movements (ataxia). Disorders of the cerebellum may also impair the ability to judge distance so that a person under- or over-reaches the target (dysmetria). Tremor during voluntary movements can also result from cerebellar damage.

THE BASAL GANGLIA. Both the cerebellum and the motor cortex send information to a set of structures deep within the brain that help control involuntary components of movement (basal ganglia). The basal ganglia send output messages to the motor cortex, helping to initiate movements, regulate repetitive or patterned movements, and control muscle tone.

Circuits within the basal ganglia are complex. Within this structure, some groups of cells begin the action of other basal ganglia components and some groups of cells block the action. These complicated feedback circuits are not entirely understood. Disruptions of these circuits are known to cause several distinct movement disorders. A portion of the basal ganglia called the substantia nigra sends electrical signals that block output from another structure called the subthalamic nucleus. The subthalamic nucleus sends signals to the globus pallidus, which in turn blocks the thalamic nuclei. Finally, the thalamic nuclei send signals to the motor cortex. The substantia nigra, then, begins movement and the globus pallidus blocks it.

This complicated circuit can be disrupted at several points. For instance, loss of substantia nigra cells, as in Parkinson's disease, increases blocking of the thalamic nuclei, preventing them from sending signals to the motor cortex. The result is a loss of movement (motor activity), a characteristic of Parkinson's.

In contrast, cell loss in early Huntington's disease decreases blocking of signals from the thalamic nuclei, causing more cortex stimulation and stronger but uncontrolled movements.

Disruptions in other portions of the basal ganglia are thought to cause tics, **tremors**, dystonia, and a variety of other movement disorders, although the exact mechanisms are not well understood.

Some movement disorders, including Huntington's disease and inherited ataxias, are caused by inherited genetic defects. Some disease that cause sustained muscle contraction limited to a particular muscle group (focal dystonia) are inherited, but others are caused by trauma. The cause of most cases of Parkinson's disease is unknown, although genes have been found for some familial forms.

Symptoms

Abnormal movements are broadly classified as either hyperkinetic–too much movement–and hypokinetic–too little movement. Hyperkinetic movements include:

- Dystonia. Sustained muscle contractions, often causing twisting or repetitive movements and abnormal postures. Dystonia may be limited to one area (focal) or may affect the whole body (general). Focal dystonias may affect the neck (cervical dystonia or **torticollis**), the face (one-sided or hemifacial spasm, contraction of the eyelid or blepharospasm, contraction of the mouth and jaw or oromandibular dystonia, simultaneous spasm of the chin and eyelid or Meige syndrome), the vocal cords (laryngeal dystonia), or the arms and legs (writer's cramp, occupational cramps). Dystonia may be painful as well as incapacitating.

- Tremor. Uncontrollable (involuntary) shaking of a body part. Tremor may occur only when muscles are relaxed or it may occur only during an action or holding an active posture.

- Tics. Involuntary, rapid, nonrhythmic movement or sound. Tics can be controlled briefly.

- Myoclonus. A sudden, shock-like muscle contraction. Myoclonic jerks may occur singly or repetitively. Unlike tics, myoclonus cannot be controlled even briefly.

- Chorea. Rapid, nonrhythmic, usually jerky movements, most often in the arms and legs.

- Ballism. Like chorea, but the movements are much larger, more explosive and involve more of the arm or leg. This condition, also called ballismus, can occur on both sides of the body or on one side only (hemiballismus).

- Akathisia. Restlessness and a desire to move to relieve uncomfortable sensations. Sensations may include a feeling of crawling, **itching**, stretching, or creeping, usually in the legs.

- Athetosis. Slow, writhing, continuous, uncontrollable movement of the arms and legs.

Hypokinetic movements include:

- Bradykinesia. Slowness of movement.

- Freezing. Inability to begin a movement or involuntary stopping of a movement before it is completed.

- Rigidity. An increase in muscle tension when an arm or leg is moved by an outside force.

- Postural instability. Loss of ability to maintain upright posture caused by slow or absent righting reflexes.

Diagnosis

Diagnosis of movement disorders requires a careful medical history and a thorough physical and neurological examination. Brain imaging studies are usually performed. Imaging techniques include computed tomography scan (CT scan), **positron emission tomography (PET)**, or **magnetic resonance imaging** (MRI) scans. Routine blood and urine analyses are performed. A lumbar puncture (spinal tap) may be necessary. Video recording of the abnormal movement is often used to analyze movement patterns and to track progress of the disorder and its treatment. **Genetic testing** is available for some forms of movement disorders.

Treatment

Treatment of a movement disorder begins with determining its cause. Physical and occupational therapy may help make up for lost control and strength. Drug therapy can help compensate for some imbalances of the basal ganglionic circuit. For instance, levodopa (L-dopa) or related compounds can substitute for lost dopamine-producing cells in Parkinson's disease. Conversely, blocking normal dopamine action is a possible treatment in some hyperkinetic disorders, including tics. Oral medications can also help reduce overall muscle tone. Local injections of botulinum toxin can selectively weaken overactive muscles in dystonia and spasticity. Destruction of peripheral nerves through injection of phenol can reduce spasticity. All of these treatments may have some side effects.

Surgical destruction or inactivation of basal ganglionic circuits has proven effective for Parkinson's disease and is being tested for other movement disorders. Transplantation of fetal cells into the basal ganglia has produced mixed results in Parkinson's disease.

KEY TERMS

Botulinum toxin—Any of a group of potent bacterial toxins or poisons produced by different strains of the bacterium *Clostridium botulinum*. The toxins cause muscle paralysis, and thus force the relaxation of a muscle in spasm.

Cerebral palsy—A movement disorder caused by a permanent brain defect or injury present at birth or shortly after. It is frequently associated with premature birth. Cerebral palsy is not progressive.

Computed tomography (CT)—An imaging technique in which cross-sectional x rays of the body are compiled to create a three-dimensional image of the body's internal structures.

Encephalopathy—An abnormality in the structure or function of tissues of the brain.

Essential tremor—An uncontrollable (involuntary) shaking of the hands, head, and face. Also called familial tremor because it is sometimes inherited, it can begin in the teens or in middle age. The exact cause is not known.

Fetal tissue transplantation—A method of treating Parkinson's and other neurological diseases by grafting brain cells from human fetuses onto the basal ganglia. Human adults cannot grow new brain cells but developing fetuses can. Grafting fetal tissue stimulates the growth of new brain cells in affected adult brains.

Hereditary ataxia—One of a group of hereditary degenerative diseases of the spinal cord or cerebellum. These diseases cause tremor, spasm, and wasting of muscle.

Huntington's disease—A rare hereditary condition that causes progressive chorea (jerky muscle movements) and mental deterioration that ends in dementia. Huntington's symptoms usually appear in patients in their 40s. There is no effective treatment.

Levodopa (L-dopa)—A substance used in the treatment of Parkinson's disease. Levodopa can cross the blood-brain barrier that protects the brain. Once in the brain, it is converted to dopamine and thus can replace the dopamine lost in Parkinson's disease.

Magnetic resonance imaging (MRI)—An imaging technique that uses a large circular magnet and radio waves to generate signals from atoms in the body. These signals are used to construct images of internal structures.

Parkinson's disease—A slowly progressive disease that destroys nerve cells in the basal ganglia and thus causes loss of dopamine, a chemical that aids in transmission of nerve signals (neurotransmitter). Parkinson's is characterized by shaking in resting muscles, a stooping posture, slurred speech, muscular stiffness, and weakness.

Positron emission tomography (PET)—A diagnostic technique in which computer-assisted x rays are used to track a radioactive substance inside a patient's body. PET can be used to study the biochemical activity of the brain.

Progressive supranuclear palsy—A rare disease that gradually destroys nerve cells in the parts of the brain that control eye movements, breathing, and muscle coordination. The loss of nerve cells causes palsy, or paralysis, that slowly gets worse as the disease progresses. The palsy affects ability to move the eyes, relax the muscles, and control balance.

Restless legs syndrome—A condition that causes an annoying feeling of tiredness, uneasiness, and itching deep within the muscle of the leg. It is accompanied by twitching and sometimes pain. The only relief is in walking or moving the legs.

Tourette syndrome—An abnormal condition that causes uncontrollable facial grimaces and tics and arm and shoulder movements. Tourette syndrome is perhaps best known for uncontrollable vocal tics that include grunts, shouts, and use of obscene language (coprolalia).

Wilson's disease—An inborn defect of copper metabolism in which free copper may be deposited in a variety of areas of the body. Deposits in the brain can cause tremor and other symptoms of Parkinson's disease.

Alternative treatment

There are several alternative therapies that can be useful when treating movement disorders. The progress made will depend on the individual and his/her condition. Among the therapies that may be helpful are **acupuncture**, homeopathy, touch therapies, postural alignment therapies, and **biofeedback**.

Prognosis

The prognosis for a patient with a movement disorder depends on the specific disorder.

Prevention

Prevention depends on the specific disorder.

Resources

ORGANIZATIONS

Worldwide Education and Awareness for Movement Disorders. One Gustave L. Levy Place, Box 1052, New York, NY 10029. (800) 437-6683. < http:// www.wemove.org >.

Richard Robinson

Movement therapy

Definition

Movement therapy refers to a broad range of Eastern and Western movement approaches used to promote physical, mental, emotional, and spiritual well-being.

Purpose

The physical benefits of movement therapy include greater ease and range of movement, increased balance, strength and flexibility, improved muscle tone and coordination, joint resiliency, cardiovascular conditioning, enhanced athletic performance, stimulation of circulation, prevention of injuries, greater longevity, **pain** relief, and relief of rheumatic, neurological, spinal, **stress**, and respiratory disorders. Movement therapy can also be used as a **meditation** practice to quiet the mind, foster self-knowledge, and increase awareness. In addition, movement therapy is beneficial in alleviating emotional distress that is expressed through the body. These conditions include eating disorders, excessive clinging, and **anxiety** attacks. Since movements are related to thoughts and feelings, movement therapy can also bring about changes in attitude and emotions. People report an increase in self-esteem and self-image. Communication skills can be enhanced and tolerance of others increased. The physical openness facilitated by movement therapy leads to greater emotional openness and creativity.

Description

Origins

Movement is fundamental to human life. In fact movement is life. Contemporary physics tells us that the universe and everything in it is in constant motion. We can move our body and at the most basic level our body is movement. According to the somatic educator Thomas Hanna, "The living body is a moving body—indeed, it is a constantly moving body." The poet and philosopher Alan Watts eloquently states a similar view, "A living body is not a fixed thing but a flowing event, like a flame or a whirlpool." Centuries earlier, the great Western philosopher Socrates understood what modern physics has proven, "The universe is motion and nothing else."

Since the beginning of time, indigenous societies around the world have used movement and dance for individual and community healing. Movement and song were used for personal healing, to create community, to ensure successful crops, and to promote fertility. Movement is still an essential part of many healing traditions and practices throughout the world.

Western movement therapies generally developed out of the realm of dance. Many of these movement approaches were created by former dancers or choreographers who were searching for a way to prevent injury, attempting to recover from an injury, or who were curious about the effects of new ways of moving. Some movement therapies arose out of the fields of physical therapy, psychology, and bodywork. Other movement therapies were developed as way to treat an incurable disease or condition.

Eastern movement therapies, such as **yoga**, **qigong**, and t'ai chi began as a spiritual or self-defense practices and evolved into healing therapies. In China, for example, Taoist monks learned to use specific breathing and movement patterns in order to promote mental clarity, physical strength, and support their practice of meditation. These practices, later known as qigong and t'ai chi eventually became recognized as ways to increase health and prolong life.

There are countless approaches to movement therapy. Some approaches emphasize awareness and attention to inner sensations. Other approaches use movement as a form of psychotherapy, expressing and working through deep emotional issues. Some approaches emphasize alignment with gravity and specific movement sequences, while other approaches encourage spontaneous movement. Some approaches are primarily concerned with increasing the ease and efficiency of bodily movement. Other approaches address the reality of the body "as movement" instead of the body as only something that runs or walks through space.

The term movement therapy is often associated with dance therapy. Some dance therapists work privately with people who are interested in personal growth. Others work in mental health settings with autistic, brain injured and learning disabled children, the elderly, and disabled adults.

Laban movement analysis (LMA), formerly known as Effort-Shape is a comprehensive system for discriminating, describing, analyzing, and categorizing movements. LMA can be applied to dance, athletic coaching, fitness, acting, psychotherapy, and a variety of other professions. Certified movement analysts can "observe recurring patterns, note movement preferences, asses physical blocks and dysfunctional movement patterns, and the suggest new movement patterns." As a student of Rudolf Laban, Irmgard Bartenieff developed his form of movement analysis into a system of body training or reeducation called Bartenieff fundamentals (BF). The basic premise of this work is that once the student experiences a physical foundation, emotional, and intellectual expression become richer. BF uses specific exercises that are practiced on the floor, sitting, or standing to engage the deeper muscles of the body and enable a greater range of movement.

Authentic movement (AM) is based upon Mary Starks Whitehouse's understanding of dance, movement, and depth psychology. There is no movement instruction in AM, simply a mover and a witness. The mover waits and listens for an impulse to move and then follows or "moves with" the spontaneous movements that arise. These movements may or may not be visible to the witness. The movements may be in response to an emotion, a dream, a thought, pain, joy, or whatever is being experienced in the moment. The witness serves as a compassionate, non judgmental mirror and brings a "special quality of attention or presence." At the end of the session the mover and witness speak about their experiences together. AM is a powerful approach for self development and awareness and provides access to preverbal memories, creative ideas, and unconscious movement patterns that limit growth.

Gabrielle Roth (5 Rhythms movement) and Anna Halprin have both developed dynamic movement practices that emphasize personal growth, awareness, expression, and community. Although fundamentally different forms, each of these movement/dance approaches recognize and encourage our inherent desire for movement.

Several forms of movement therapy grew out of specific bodywork modalities. **Rolfing** movement integration (RMI) and Rolfing rhythms are movement forms which reinforce and help to integrate the structural body changes brought about by the hands-on work of Rolfing (structural integration). RMI uses a combination of touch and verbal directions to help develop greater awareness of one's vertical alignment and habitual movement patterns. RMI teacher Mary Bond says, "The premise of Rolfing Movement Integration... is that you can restore your structure to balance by changing the movement habits that perpetuate imbalance." Rolfing rhythms is a series of lively exercises designed to encourage awareness of the Rolfing principles of ease, length, balance, and harmony with gravity.

The movement education component of **Aston-Patterning** bodywork is called neurokinetics. This movement therapy teaches ways of moving with greater ease throughout every day activities. These movement patterns can also be used to release tension in the body. Aston fitness is an **exercise** program which includes warm-up techniques, exercises to increase muscle tone and stability, stretching, and cardiovascular fitness.

Rosen method movement (an adjunct to Rosen method bodywork) consists of simple fun movement exercises done to music in a group setting. Through gentle swinging, bouncing, and stretching every joint in the body experiences a full range of movement. The movements help to increase balance and rhythm and create more space for effortless breathing.

The movement form of **Trager psychophysical integration** bodywork, Mentastics, consists of fun, easy swinging, shaking, and stretching movements. These movements, developed by Dr. **Milton Trager**, create an experience of lightness and freedom in the body, allowing for greater ease in movement. Trager also worked successfully with **polio** patients.

Awareness through movement, the movement therapy form of the **Feldenkrais method**, consists of specific structured movement experiences taught as a group lesson. These lessons reeducate the brain without tiring the muscles. Most lessons are done lying down on the floor or sitting. **Moshe Feldenkrais** designed the lessons to "improve ability ... turn the impossible into the possible, the difficult into the easy, and the easy into the pleasant."

Ideokinesis is another movement approach emphasizing neuromuscular reeducation. Lulu Sweigart based her work on the pioneering approach of her teacher Mabel Elsworth Todd. Ideokinesis uses imagery to train the nervous system to stimulate the right muscles for the intended movement. If one continues to give the nervous system a clear mental picture of the movement intended, it will automatically select the best way to perform the movement. For example, to enhance balance in standing, Sweigart taught people to visualize "lines of movement" traveling through their bodies. Sweigart did not train teachers in ideokinesis but some individuals use ideokinetic imagery in the process of teaching movement.

The Mensendieck system of functional movement techniques is both corrective and preventative. Bess Mensendieck, a medical doctor, developed a series of exercises to reshape, rebuild and revitalize the body. A student of this approach learns to use the conscious will to relax muscles and releases tension. There are more than 200 exercises that emphasize correct and graceful body movement through everyday activities. Unlike other movement therapy approaches this work is done undressed or in a bikini bottom, in front of mirrors. This allows the student to observe and feel where a movement originates. Success has been reported with many conditions including Parkinson's disease, muscle and joint injuries, and repetitive strain injuries.

The **Alexander technique** is another functional approach to movement therapy. In this approach a teacher gently uses hands and verbal directions to subtly guide the student through movements such as sitting, standing up, bending and walking. The Alexander technique emphasizes balance in the neck-head relationship. A teacher lightly steers the students head into the proper balance on the tip of the spine while the student is moving in ordinary ways. The student learns to respond to movement demands with the whole body, in a light integrated way. This approach to movement is particularly popular with actors and other performers.

Pilates or physical mind method is also popular with actors, dancers, athletes, and a broad range of other people. Pilates consists of over 500 exercises done on the floor or primarily with customized exercise equipment. The exercises combine sensory awareness and physical training. Students learn to move from a stable, central core. The exercises promote strength, flexibility, and balance. Pilates training is increasingly available in sports medicine clinics, fitness centers, dance schools, spas, and physical therapy offices.

Many approaches to movement therapy emphasize awareness of internal sensations. Charlotte Selver, a student of somatic pioneer Elsa Gindler, calls her style of teaching sensory awareness (SA). This approach has influenced the thinking of many innovators, including Fritz Perls, who developed **gestalt therapy**. Rather than suggesting a series of structured movements, visualizations, or body positions, in SA the teacher outlines experiments in which one can become aware of the sensations involved in any movement. A teacher might ask the student to feel the movement of her breathing while running, sitting, picking up a book, etc. This close attunement to inner sensory experience encourages an experience of body-mind unity in which breathing becomes less restricted and posture, coordination, flexibility, and balance are improved. There may also be the experience of increased energy and aliveness.

Gerda Alexander Eutony (GAE) is another movement therapy approach that is based upon internal awareness. Through GAE one becomes a master of self-sensing and knowing which includes becoming sensitive to the external environment, as well. For example, while lying on the floor sensing the breath, skin or form of the body, one also senses the connection with the ground. GAE is taught in group classes or private lessons which also include hands-on therapy. In 1987, after two years of observation in clinics throughout the world, GAE became the first mind-body discipline accepted by the World Health Organization (WHO) as an alternative health-care technique.

Kinetic awareness developed by dancer-choreographer Elaine Summers, emphasizes emotional and physical inquiry. Privately or in a group, a teacher sets up situations for the student to explore the possible causes of pain and movement restrictions within the body. Rubber balls of various sizes are used as props to focus attention inward, support the body in a stretched position and massage a specific area of the body. The work helps one to deal with chronic pain, move easily again after injuries and increase energy, flexibility, coordination, and comfort.

Body-mind centering (BMC) was developed by Bonnie Bainbridge Cohen and is a comprehensive educational and therapeutic approach to movement. BMC practitioners use movement, touch, **guided imagery**, developmental repatterning, dialogue, music, large balls, and other props in an individual session to meet the needs of each person. BMC encourages people to develop a sensate awareness and experience of the ligaments, nerves, muscles, skin, fluids, organs, glands, fat, and fascia that make up one's body. It has been effective in preventing and rehabilitating from chronic injuries and in improving neuromuscular response in children with **cerebral palsy** and other neurological disorders.

Continuum movement has also been shown to be effective in treating neurological disorders including spinal chord injury. Developed by Emilie Conrad and Susan Harper, continuum movement is an inquiry into the creative flux of our body and all of life. Sound, breath, subtle and dynamic movements are explored that stimulate the brain and increase resonance with the fluid world of movement. The emphasis is upon unpredictable, spontaneous or spiral movements rather than a linear movement pattern. According to Conrad, "Awareness changes how we physically move. As we become more fluid and resilient so do the mental, emotional, and spiritual movements of our lives."

Eastern movement therapies such as yoga, t'ai chi, and qigong are also effective in healing and preventing a wide range of physical disorders, encouraging emotional stability, and enhancing spiritual awareness. There are a number of different approaches to yoga. Some emphasize the development of physical strength, flexibility, and alignment. Other forms of yoga emphasize inner awareness, opening, and meditation.

Precautions

People with acute injuries and chronic physical and mental conditions need to be careful when choosing a form of movement therapy. It is best to consult with a knowledgeable physician, physical therapist, or mental health therapist.

A special form of movement therapy known as constraint-induced movement therapy, or CIMT, is being used as of the early 2000s to rehabilitate the upper limbs of patients who have suffered a **stroke**, traumatic brain injury, or damage to the spinal cord. In CIMT, the arm that has been less affected by the injury is constrained by a sling for 90% of the patient's waking hours for a period of two weeks. The sling forces the patient to use the weaker arm more often; in addition, a physical therapist works with the patient to practice repetitive motions with the weaker arm. CIMT also appears to be useful in treating children with muscular weakness on one side of the body caused by cerebral palsy.

Research and general acceptance

Although research has documented the beneficial effects of dance therapy, qigong, t'ai chi, yoga, Alexander technique, awareness through movement (Feldenkrais), and Rolfing, other forms of movement therapy have not been as thoroughly researched.

CIMT has become widely accepted in **rehabilitation** medicine since its introduction in the mid-1990s, although some doctors still consider it experimental. Further research in CIMT is being carried out by the National Institute of Neurological Disorders and Stroke (NINDS), one of the National Institutes of Health.

Resources

BOOKS

Halprin, Anna. *Dance as a Healing Art: Returning to Health Through Movement and Imagery*. Life Rhythm, 1999.

PERIODICALS

Bunch, W. "Dancing through the Pain. Physician Executive Launches New Business to Treat Patients with Chronic Pain." *Physician Executive* 30 (January-February 2004): 30–33.

Cottingham, John T., and Jeffrey Maitland. "Integrating Manual and Movement Therapy With Philosophical Counseling for Treatment of a Patient With Amyotrophic Lateral Sclerosis: A Case Study That Explores the Principles of Holistic Intervention." *Alternative Therapies Journal* March 2000: 120-128.

Mark, V. W., and E. Taub. "Constraint-Induced Movement Therapy for Chronic Stroke Hemiparesis and Other Disabilities." *Restorative Neurology and Neuroscience* 22 (March 2004): 317–336.

Page, S. J., S. Sisto, P. Levine, and R. E. McGrath. "Efficacy of Modified Constraint-Induced Movement Therapy in Chronic Stroke: A Single-Blinded Randomized Controlled Trial." *Archives of Physical Medicine and Rehabilitation* 85 (January 2004): 14–18.

Taub, E., S. L. Ramey, S. DeLuca, and K. Echols. "Efficacy of Constraint-Induced Movement Therapy for Children with Cerebral Palsy with Asymmetric Motor Impairment." *Pediatrics* 113 (February 2004): 305–312.

ORGANIZATIONS

National Institute of Neurological Disorders and Stroke (NINDS). NIH Neurological Institute, P. O. Box 5801, Bethesda, MD 20824. (800) 352-9424 or (301) 496-5751. < http://www.ninds.nih.gov >.

Linda Chrisman
Rebecca J. Frey, PhD

Mpell disease *see* **Ankylosing spondylitis**

MR *see* **Magnetic resonance imaging**

MRI *see* **Magnetic resonance imaging**

MS *see* **Multiple sclerosis**

M's disease *see* **Waldenström's macroglobulinemia**

Mucopolysaccharidoses

Definition

Mucopolysaccharidosis (MPS) is a general term for a number of inherited diseases that are caused by the accumulation of mucopolysaccharides, resulting in problems with an individual's development. With each condition, mucopolysaccharides accumulate in the cells and tissues of the body because of a deficiency of a specific enzyme. The specific enzyme that is deficient or absent is what distinguishes one type of MPS from another. However, before these enzymes were identified, the MPS disorders were diagnosed by the signs and symptoms that an individual expressed. The discovery of these enzymes resulted in a reclassification of some of the MPS disorders. These conditions are often referred to as MPS I, MPS II, MPS III, MPS IV, MPS VI, MPS VII, and MPS IX. However, these conditions are also referred to by their original names, which are Hurler, Hurler-Scheie, Scheie (all MPS I), Hunter (MPS II), Sanfilippo (MPS III), Morquio (MPS IV), Maroteaux-Lamy (MPS VI), Sly (MPS VII), and Hyaluronidase deficiency (MPS IX).

Description

Mucopolysaccharides are long chains of sugar molecules that are essential for building the bones, cartilage, skin, tendons, and other tissues in the body. Normally, the human body continuously breaks down and builds mucopolysaccharides. Another name for mucopolysaccharides is glycosaminoglycans (GAGs). There are many different types of GAGs and specific GAGs are unable to be broken down in each of the MPS conditions. There are several enzymes involved in breaking down each GAG and a deficiency or absence of any of the essential enzymes can cause the GAG to not be broken down completely and result in its accumulation in the tissues and organs in the body. In some MPS conditions, in addition to the GAG being stored in the body, some of the incompletely broken down GAGs can leave the body via the urine. When too much GAG is stored, organs and tissues can be damaged or not function properly.

Genetic profile

Except for MPS II, the MPS conditions are inherited in an autosomal recessive manner. MPS conditions occur when both of an individual's genes that produce the specific enzyme contain a mutation, causing them to not work properly. When both genes do not work properly, either none or a reduced amount of

the enzyme is produced. An individual with an autosomal recessive condition inherits one of those nonworking genes from each parent. These parents are called "carriers" of the condition. When two people are known carriers for an autosomal recessive condition, they have a 25% chance with each **pregnancy** to have a child affected with the disease. Some individuals with MPS do have children of their own. Children of parents who have an autosomal recessive condition are all carriers of that condition. These children are not at risk to develop the condition unless the other parent is a carrier or affected with the same autosomal recessive condition.

Unlike the other MPS conditions, MPS II is inherited in an X-linked recessive manner. This means that the gene causing the condition is located on the X chromosome, one of the two sex chromosomes. Since a male has only one X chromosome, he will have the disease if the X chromosome inherited from his mother carries the defective gene. Females, because they have two X chromosomes, are called "carriers" of the condition if only one of their X chromosomes has the gene that causes the condition, while the other X chromosome does not.

Causes and symptoms

Each type of MPS is caused by a deficiency of one of the enzymes involved in breaking down GAGs. It is the accumulation of the GAGs in the tissues and organs in the body that cause the wide array of symptoms characteristic of the MPS conditions. The accumulating material is stored in cellular structures called lysosomes, and these disorders are also known as lysosomal storage diseases.

MPS I

MPS I is caused by a deficiency of the enzyme alpha-L-iduronidase. Three conditions, Hurler, Hurler-Scheie, and Scheie syndromes, all are caused by a deficiency of this enzyme. Initially, these three conditions were felt to be separate because each were associated with different physical symptoms and prognoses. However, once the underlying cause of these conditions was identified, it was realized that these three conditions were all variants of the same disorder. The gene involved with MPS I is located on chromosome 4p16.3.

MPS I H (HURLER SYNDROME). It has been estimated that approximately one baby in 100,000 will be born with Hurler syndrome. Individuals with Hurler syndrome tend to have the most severe form of MPS I. Symptoms of Hurler syndrome are often evident within the first year or two after birth. Often these infants begin to develop as expected, but then reach a point where they begin to loose the skills that they have learned. Many of these infants may initially grow faster than expected, but their growth slows and typically stops by age three. Facial features also begin to appear "coarse." They develop a short nose, flatter face, thicker skin, and a protruding tongue. Additionally, their heads become larger and they develop more hair on their bodies with the hair becoming coarser. Their bones are also affected, with these children usually developing joint **contractures** (stiff joints), **kyphosis** (a specific type of curve to the spine), and broad hands with short fingers. Many of these children experience breathing difficulties, and respiratory infections are common. Other common problems include heart valve dysfunction, thickening of the heart muscle (**cardiomyopathy**), enlarged spleen and liver, clouding of the cornea, **hearing loss**, and **carpal tunnel syndrome**. These children typically do not live past age 12.

MPS I H/S (HURLER-SCHEIE SYNDROME). Hurler-Scheie syndrome is felt to be the intermediate form of MPS I, meaning that the symptoms are not as severe as those in individuals who have MPS I H but not as mild as those in MPS I S. Approximately one baby in 115,000 will be born with Hurler-Scheie syndrome. These individuals tend to be shorter than expected, and they can have normal intelligence, however, some individuals with MPS I H/S will experience learning difficulties. These individuals may develop some of the same physical features as those with Hurler syndrome, but usually they are not as severe. The prognosis for children with MPS I H/S is variable with some individuals dying during childhood, while others living to adulthood.

MPS I S (SCHEIE SYNDROME). Scheie syndrome is considered the mild form of MPS I. It is estimated that approximately one baby in 500,000 will be born with Scheie syndrome. Individuals with MPS I S usually have normal intelligence, but there have been some reports of individuals with MPS I S developing psychiatric problems. Common physical problems include corneal clouding, heart abnormalities, and orthopedic difficulties involving their hands and back. Individuals with MPS I S do not develop the facial features seen with MPS I H and usually these individuals have a normal life span.

MPS II (Hunter syndrome)

Hunter syndrome is caused by a deficiency of the enzyme iduronate-2-sulphatase. All individuals with Hunter syndrome are male, because the gene that causes the condition is located on the X chromosome, specifically Xq28. Like many MPS conditions, Hunter syndrome is divided into two groups, mild and severe. It has been estimated that approximately 1 in 110,000 males are born with Hunter syndrome, with the severe form being three times more common than the mild form. The severe form is felt to be associated with progressive **mental retardation** and physical disability, with most individuals dying before age 15. In the milder form, most of these individuals live to adulthood and have normal intelligence or only mild mental impairments. Males with the mild form of Hunter syndrome develop physical differences similar to the males with the severe form, but not as quickly. Men with mild Hunter syndrome can have a normal life span and some have had children. Most males with Hunter syndrome develop joint stiffness, chronic **diarrhea**, enlarged liver and spleen, heart valve problems, hearing loss, kyphosis, and tend to be shorter than expected. These symptoms tend to progress at a different rate depending on if an individual has the mild or severe form of MPS II.

MPS III (Sanfilippo syndrome)

MPS III, like the other MPS conditions, was initially diagnosed by the individual having certain physical characteristics. It was later discovered that the physical symptoms associated with Sanfilippo syndrome could be caused by a deficiency in one of four enzymes. Each type of MPS III is now subdivided into four groups, labeled A-D, based on the specific enzyme that is deficient. All four of these enzymes are involved in breaking down the same GAG, heparan sulfate. Heparan sulfate is mainly found in the central nervous system and accumulates in the brain when it cannot be broken down because one of those four enzymes are deficient or missing.

MPS III is a variable condition with symptoms beginning to appear between ages two and six years of age. Because of the accumulation of heparan sulfate in the central nervous system, the central nervous system is severely affected. In MPS III, signs that the central nervous system is degenerating usually are evident in most individuals between ages six and 10. Many children with MPS III will develop seizures, sleeplessness, thicker skin, joint contractures, enlarged tongues, cardiomyopathy, behavior problems, and mental retardation. The life expectancy in MPS III is also variable. On average, individuals with MPS III live until they are teenagers, with some living longer and others not that long.

MPS IIIA (SANFILIPPO SYNDROME TYPE A). MPS IIIA is caused by a deficiency of the enzyme heparan

N-sulfatase. Type IIIA is felt to be the most severe of the four types, in which symptoms appear and **death** occurs at an earlier age. A study in British Columbia estimated that one in 324,617 live births are born with MPS IIIA. MPS IIIA is the most common of the four types in Northwestern Europe. The gene that causes MPS IIIA is located on the long arm of chromosome 17 (location 17q25).

MPS IIIB (SANFILIPPO SYNDROME TYPE B). MPS IIIB is due to a deficiency in N-acetyl-alpha-D-glucosaminidase (NAG). This type of MPS III is not felt to be as severe as Type IIIA and the characteristics vary. Type IIIB is the most common of the four in southeastern Europe. The gene associated with MPS IIIB is also located on the long arm of chromosome 17 (location 17q21).

MPS IIIC (SANFILIPPO SYNDROME TYPE C). A deficiency in the enzyme acetyl-CoA-alpha-glucosaminide acetyltransferase causes MPS IIIC. This is considered a rare form of MPS III. The gene involved in MPS IIIC is believed to be located on chromosome 14.

MPS IIID (SANFILIPPO SYNDROME TYPE D). MPS IIID is caused by a deficiency in the enzyme N-acetylglucosamine-6-sulfatase. This form of MPS III is also rare. The gene involved in MPS IIID is located on the long arm of chromosome 12 (location 12q14).

MPS IV (Morquio syndrome)

As with several of the MPS disorders, Morquio syndrome was diagnosed by the presence of particular signs and symptoms. However, it is now known that the deficiency of two different enzymes can cause the characteristics of MPS IV. These two types of MPS IV are called MPS IV A and MPS IV B. MPS IV is also variable in its severity. The intelligence of individuals with MPS IV is often completely normal. In individuals with a severe form, skeletal abnormalities can be extreme and include dwarfism, kyphosis (backward-curved spine), prominent breastbone, flat feet, and knock-knees. One of the earliest symptoms seen in this condition usually is a difference in the way the child walks. In individuals with a mild form of MPS IV, limb stiffness, and joint **pain** are the primary symptoms. MPS IV is one of the rarest MPS disorders, with approximately one baby in 300,000 born with this condition.

MPS IV A (MORQUIO SYNDROME TYPE A). MPS IV A is the "classic" or the severe form of the condition and is caused by a deficiency in the enzyme galactosamine-6-sulphatase. The gene involved with MPS IV A is located on the long arm of chromosome 16 (location 16q24.3).

MPS IV B (MORQUIO SYNDROME TYPE B). MPS IV B is considered the milder form of the condition. The enzyme, beta-galactosidase, is deficient in MPS IV B. The location of the gene that produces beta-galactosidase is located on the short arm of chromosome 3 (location 3p21).

MPS VI (Maroteaux-Lamy syndrome)

MPS VI, which is another rare form of MPS, is caused by a deficiency of the enzyme N-acetylglucosamine-4-sulphatase. This condition is also variable; individuals may have a mild or severe form of the condition. Typically, the nervous system or intelligence of an individual with MPS VI is not affected. Individuals with a more severe form of MPS VI can have airway obstruction, develop **hydrocephalus** (extra fluid accumulating in the brain) and have bone changes. Additionally, individuals with a severe form of MPS VI are more likely to die while in their teens. With a milder form of the condition, individuals tend to be shorter than expected for their age, develop corneal clouding, and live longer. The gene involved in MPS VI is believed to be located on the long arm of chromosome 5 (approximate location 5q11-13).

MPS VII (Sly syndrome)

MPS VII is an extremely rare form of MPS and is caused by a deficiency of the enzyme beta-glucuronidase. It is also highly variable, but symptoms are generally similar to those seen in individuals with Hurler syndrome. The gene that causes MPS VII is located on the long arm of chromosome 7 (location 7q21).

MPS IX (Hyaluronidase deficiency)

MPS IX is a condition that was first described in 1996 and has been grouped with the other MPS conditions by some researchers. MPS IX is caused by the deficiency of the enzyme hyaluronidase. In the few individuals described with this condition, the symptoms are variable, but some develop soft-tissue masses (growths under the skin). Also, these individuals are shorter than expected for their age. The gene involved in MPS IX is believed to be located on the short arm of chromosome 3 (possibly 3p21.3-21.2)

Many individuals with an MPS condition have problems with airway constriction. This constriction may be so serious as to create significant difficulties in administering **general anesthesia**. Therefore, it is recommended that surgical procedures be performed under **local anesthesia** whenever possible.

KEY TERMS

Cardiomyopathy—A thickening of the heart muscle.

Enzyme—A protein that catalyzes a biochemical reaction or change without changing its own structure or function.

Joint contractures—Stiffness of the joints that prevents full extension.

Kyphosis—An abnormal outward curvature of the spine, with a hump at the upper back.

Lysosome—Membrane-enclosed compartment in cells, containing many hydrolytic enzymes; where large molecules and cellular components are broken down.

Mucopolysaccharide—A complex molecule made of smaller sugar molecules strung together to form a chain. Found in mucous secretions and intercellular spaces.

Recessive gene—A type of gene that is not expressed as a trait unless inherited by both parents.

X-linked gene—A gene carried on the X chromosome, one of the two sex chromosomes.

Diagnosis

While a diagnosis for each type of MPS can be made on the basis of the physical signs described above, several of the conditions have similar features. Therefore, enzyme analysis is used to determine the specific MPS disorder. Enzyme analysis usually cannot accurately determine if an individual is a carrier for a MPS condition. This is because the enzyme levels in individuals who are not carriers overlaps the enzyme levels seen in those individuals who are carrier for a MPS. With many of the MPS conditions, several mutations have been found in each gene involved that can cause symptoms of each condition. If the specific mutation is known in a family, DNA analysis may be possible.

Once a couple has had a child with an MPS condition, prenatal diagnosis is available to them to help determine if a fetus is affected with the same MPS as their other child. This can be accomplished through testing samples using procedures such as an **amniocentesis** or **chorionic villus sampling** (CVS). Each of these procedures has its own risks, benefits, and limitations.

Treatment

There is no cure for mucopolysaccharidosis. There are several types of experimental therapies that are being investigated. Typically, treatment involves trying to relieve some of the symptoms. For MPS I and VI, **bone marrow transplantation** has been attempted as a treatment option. In those conditions, bone marrow transplantation has sometimes been found to help slow down the progression or reverse some of symptoms of the disorder in some children. The benefits of a bone marrow transplantation are more likely to be noticed when performed on children under two years of age. However it is not certain that a bone marrow transplant can prevent further damage to certain organs and tissues, including the brain. Furthermore, bone marrow transplantation is not felt to be helpful in some MPS disorders and there are risks, benefits, and limitations with this procedure. In 2000, ten individuals with MPS I received recombinant human alpha-L-iduronidase every week for one year. Those individuals showed an improvement with some of their symptoms. Additionally, there is ongoing research involving gene replacement therapy (the insertion of normal copies of a gene into the cells of patients whose gene copies are defective).

Prevention

No specific preventive measures are available for genetic diseases of this type. For some of the MPS diseases, biochemical tests are available that will identify healthy individuals who are carriers of the defective gene, allowing them to make informed reproductive decisions. There is also the availability of prenatal diagnosis for all MPS disease to detect affected fetuses.

Resources

PERIODICALS

Caillud, C., and L. Poenaru. "Gene Therapy in Lysosomal Diseases." *Biomed & Pharmacother* 54 (2000): 505–512.

Kakkis, E. D., et al. "Enzyme-Replacement Therapy in Mucopolysaccharidosis I." *The New England Journal of Medicine* 344 (2001): 182–188.

ORGANIZATIONS

Canadian Society for Mucopolysaccharide and Related Diseases. PO Box 64714, Unionville, ONT L3R-OM9. Canada (905) 479-8701 or (800) 667-1846. <http://www.mpssociety.ca>.

Children Living with Inherited Metabolic Diseases. The Quadrangle, Crewe Hall, Weston Rd., Crewe, Cheshire, CW1-6UR. UK 127 025 0221. Fax: 0870-7700-327. <http://www.climb.org.uk>.

Metabolic Information Network. PO Box 670847, Dallas, TX 75367-0847. (214) 696-2188 or (800) 945-2188.

National MPS Society. 102 Aspen Dr., Downingtown, PA 19335. (610) 942-0100. Fax: (610) 942-7188. info@mpssociety.org. < http://www.mpssociety.org >.

National Organization for Rare Disorders (NORD). PO Box 8923, New Fairfield, CT 06812-8923. (203) 746-6518 or (800) 999-6673. Fax: (203) 746-6481. < http:// www.rarediseases.org >.

Society for Mucopolysaccharide Diseases. 46 Woodside Rd., Amersham, Buckinghamshire, HP6 6AJ. UK +44 (01494) 434156. < http://www.mpssociety.co.uk >.

Zain Hansen MPS Foundation. 23400 Henderson Rd., Covelo, CA 95420. (800) 767-3121.

OTHER

National Library of Medicine. National Institutes of Health. < http://www.nlm.nih.gov/ >.

"NINDS Mucopolysaccharidoses Information Page." The National Institute of Neurological Disorders and Stroke. National Institutes of Health. < http:// www.ninds.nih.gov/health_and_medical/disorders/ mucopolysaccharidoses.htm >.

Online Mendelian Inheritance in Man (OMIM). National Center for Biotechnology Information. < http:// www.ncbi.nlm.nih.gov/Omim/ >.

Sharon A. Aufox, MS, CGC

Mucormycosis

Definition

Mucormycosis is a rare but often fatal disease caused by certain fungi. It is sometimes called zygomycosis or phycomycosis. Mucormycosis is an opportunistic infection that typically develops in patients with weakened immune systems, diabetes, kidney failure, organ transplants, or **chemotherapy** for **cancer**. It may also develop in patients receiving an iron chelating drug called desferrioxamine (Desferal) as treatment for acute iron **poisoning**.

Description

In the United States, mucormycosis is most likely to develop in the patient's nasal area or in the lungs; however, it may also develop on the skin or in the digestive tract. Gastrointestinal disease usually develops only in severely malnourished patients. Cutaneous mucormycosis is most likely to develop under occlusive surgical dressings. Occlusive dressings are intended to keep air out of incisions or other **wounds**, but they also trap body heat and moisture.

The incidence of the disease is difficult to evaluate because it is very rare; however, the rate seems to be increasing. One American cancer center reported in 2000 that mucormycosis was found in 0.7% of patients at **autopsy** and in 20 patients per 100,000 admissions to the center. The most recent mortality statistics from the Centers for Disease Control and Prevention (CDC) indicate that a total of 22 Americans died from mucormycosis in 2001—1 from pulmonary mucormycosis, 5 from rhinocerebral mucormycosis, 2 from disseminated mucormycosis, and 14 from unspecified forms of the disease.

As far as is known, mucormycosis affects members of either sex and all races equally, although the pulmonary form of the disease is somewhat more common in men than in women. Mucormycosis may develop in patients in any age group, including newborns.

Rhinocerebral mucormycosis

Rhinocerebral mucormycosis is an infection of the nose, eyes, and brain. The fungus destroys the tissue of the nasal passages, sinuses, or hard palate, producing a black or pus-filled discharge and visible patches of dying tissue. The patient will typically have **fever**, **pain**, and forward bulging of the eyes (proptosis). The fungus then invades the tissues around the eye socket and eventually the brain. At that point the patient may have convulsions or **paralysis** on one side of the body.

Pulmonary mucormycosis

Most patients with the pulmonary form of the disease are being treated for leukemia. The fungus enters the patient's lungs, where it eventually invades a major blood vessel, causing the patient to **cough** up blood or hemorrhage into the lungs.

Gastrointestinal mucormycosis

Gastrointestinal mucormycosis has been reported in premature or low-birth-weight infants as well as malnourished adults. It may lead to intestinal perforation and other complications requiring immediate surgery. A Spanish hospital reported in 2004 on an outbreak of gastrointestinal mucormycosis that affected five patients in an ICU over a 14-week period. Two of the patients died. The outbreak was eventually traced to a supply of wooden tongue depressors that had been contaminated by two species of *Rhizopus* fungi.

Causes and symptoms

Mucormycosis is caused by fungi of several different species, including *Mucor*, *Rhizopus*, *Absidia*, and *Rhizomucor*. When these organisms gain access to the mucous membranes of the patient's nose or lungs, they multiply rapidly and invade the nearby blood vessels. The fungi destroy soft tissue and bone, as well as the walls of blood vessels.

The early symptoms of rhinocerebral mucormycosis include fever, sinus pain, **headache**, and **cellulitis**. As the fungus reaches the eye tissues, the patient develops dilated pupils, drooping eyelids, a bulging eye, and eventually hemorrhage of the blood vessels in the brain– causing convulsions, partial paralysis, and **death**.

The symptoms of pulmonary mucormycosis include fever and difficulty breathing, with eventual bleeding from the lungs.

The symptoms of gastrointestinal mucormycosis are not unique to the disease, which may complicate diagnosis. Patients typically complain of pressure or pain in the abdomen, **nausea**, and **vomiting**.

Diagnosis

Diagnosis is usually based on a combination of the patient's medical history and a visual examination of the nose, throat, and eyes. The doctor will take a tissue sample for biopsy, or a PAS, potassium hydroxide (KOH), or Calcofluor stain in order to make a tentative diagnosis. Confirmation requires a laboratory culture.

Imaging studies are not needed to make the diagnosis. If the patient has mucormycosis, however, **magnetic resonance imaging** (MRI) and **computed tomography scans** (CT scans) will usually show the destruction of soft tissue or bone in patients with advanced disease. Chest x rays will sometimes show a cavity in the lung or an area filled with tissue fluid if the patient has pulmonary mucormycosis.

Treatment

Treatment is usually begun without waiting for laboratory reports because of the rapid spread and high mortality rate of the disease. Therapy includes intravenous amphotericin B (Fungizone); surgical removal of infected tissue; and careful monitoring of the disorder or condition that is responsible for the patient's vulnerability. Most patients who survive require a 4–6-week course of treatment.

Follow-up care includes educating patients about the signs of recurrent mucormycosis—particularly

facial swelling and a black discharge from the nose—and telling them to see a doctor at once if they notice these symptoms.

Patients who survive rhinocerebral mucormycosis are often left with severe facial disfigurement and usually require **plastic surgery** to restore their appearance.

Prognosis

The prognosis for recovery from mucormycosis is poor. The mortality rate is 30%–50% of patients with the rhinocerebral form, and even higher for patients with pulmonary mucormycosis. The disease is almost 100% fatal for patients with **AIDS**.

Prevention

Prevention depends on protecting high-risk patients from contact with sugary foods, decaying plants, moldy bread, manure, and other breeding grounds for fungi. In addition, health care professionals treating hospital inpatients should be careful to change occlusive dressings frequently and check the underlying skin for any signs of possible fungal infection.

Resources

BOOKS

Beers, Mark H., MD, and Robert Berkow, MD, editors. "Mucormycosis." Section 13, Chapter 158. In *The Merck Manual of Diagnosis and Therapy*. Whitehouse Station, NJ: Merck Research Laboratories, 2004.

PERIODICALS

Eisen, Damon, MD. "Mucormycosis." *eMedicine* December10, 2001. < http://www.emedicine.com/med/topic1513.htm >.

Maravi-Poma, E., J. L. Rodriguez-Tudela, J. G. de Jalon, et al. "Outbreak of Gastric Mucormycosis Associated with the Use of Wooden Tongue Depressors in Critically Ill Patients." *Intensive Care Medicine* 30 (April 2004): 724–728.

Numa, W. A., Jr, P. K. Foster, J. Wachholz, et al. "Cutaneous Mucormycosis of the Head and Neck with Parotid Gland Involvement: First Report of a Case." *Ear, Nose, and Throat Journal* 83 (April 2004): 282–286.

Siu, K. L., and W. H. Lee. "A Rare Cause of Intestinal Perforation in an Extreme Low Birth Weight Infant—Gastrointestinal Mucormycosis: A Case Report." *Journal of Perinatology* 24 (May 2004): 319–321.

Wolf, O., Z. Gil, L. Leider-Trejo, et al. "Tracheal Mucormycosis Presented as an Intraluminal Soft Tissue Mass." *Head and Neck* 26 (June 2004): 541–543.

ORGANIZATIONS

Centers for Disease Control. 1600 Clifton Rd., NE, Atlanta, GA 30333. (800) 311-3435, (404) 639-3311. < http://www.cdc.gov >.

Rebecca J. Frey, PhD

Mucoviscidosis *see* **Cystic fibrosis**

MUGA scan *see* **Multiple-gated acquisition (MUGA) scan**

Multiple-gated acquisition (MUGA) scan

Definition

The multiple-gated acquisition (MUGA) scan is a non-invasive nuclear test that uses a radioactive isotope called technetium to evaluate the functioning of the heart's ventricles.

Purpose

The MUGA scan is performed to determine if the heart's left and right ventricles are functioning properly and to diagnose abnormalities in the heart wall. It can be ordered in the following patients:

- With known or suspected **coronary artery disease**, to diagnose the disease and predict outcomes
- With lesions in their heart valves
- Who have recently had a **heart attack**, to assess damage to heart tissue and predict the likelihood of future cardiac events
- With congestive **heart failure**

- Who have undergone percutaneous transluminal coronary **angioplasty**, **coronary artery bypass graft surgery**, or medical therapy, to assess the efficacy of the treatment
- With low cardiac output after open-heart surgery
- Who are undergoing **chemotherapy**.

Precautions

Pregnant women and those who are breastfeeding should not be exposed to technetium.

Description

The MUGA scan measures the heart's function and the flow of blood through it. The strongest chamber in the heart is the left ventricle, which serves as the main pump of blood through the body. The left ventricular is assessed by measuring the amount of blood pumped with each heartbeat (the ejection fraction), ventricle filling, and the blood flow into the pumping chamber. A normal ejection fraction is 50% or more. The heart's ejection fraction is one of the most important measures of its performance. The right ventricle's ability to pump blood to the lungs is also assessed, and any abnormalities in the heart wall are identified. The MUGA scan is the most accurate, non-invasive test available to assess the heart's ventricles.

MUGA is a nuclear heart scan, which means that it involves the use of a radioactive isotope that targets the heart and a radionuclide detector that traces the absorption of the radioactive isotope. The isotope is injected into a vein and absorbed by healthy tissue at a known rate during a certain time period. The radionuclide detector, in this case a gamma scintillation camera, picks up the gamma rays emitted by the isotope.

During the MUGA scan, electrodes are placed on the patient's body so that an electrocardiogram (ECG) can be conducted. The imaging equipment and computer are synchronized with the ECG so that images of the heart can be recorded without motion or blur. Then a small amount of a mildly radioactive isotope called technetium Tc99m stannous pyrophosphate, usually called technetium, is injected, usually into an arm vein. While the patient lies motionless on the test table, a gamma scintillation camera follows the movement of the technetium through the blood circulating in the heart. The camera, which looks like an x-ray machine and is suspended above the table, moves back and forth over the patient. It displays multiple images of the heart in motion and records them on a computer for later analysis.

The MUGA scan is usually performed in a hospital's nuclear medicine department, but it can also be performed in an outpatient facility or at the patient's bedside if equipment is available. The scan is done immediately after injection of the technetium and usually takes about 30 minutes to one hour. It is also called multigated graft acquisition, multigated acquisition scan, cardiac blood-pool imaging, and equilibrium radionuclide **angiography**. Test results can be affected by patient movement during the test, electrocardiogram abnormalities, an irregular heartbeat, or long-acting nitrates.

The MUGA scan can be done with the patient at rest or exercising (called a **stress** MUGA). The stress MUGA is often performed in patients who have or are suspected of having coronary artery disease. The resting MUGA is compared to the stress MUGA and changes in the heart's pumping performance are analyzed. In some cases, the rest MUGA is compared to a nitroglycerin MUGA, in which a strong heart drug called nitroglycerin is administered to the patient before the scan. For the nitroglycerin MUGA, a cardiologist should be present.

The MUGA scan is not dangerous. The technetium is completely gone from the body within a few days of the test. The scan itself exposes the patient to about the same amount of radiation as a **chest x ray**. The patient can resume normal activities immediately after the test.

Normal results

If the patient's heart is normal, the technetium will appear to be evenly distributed in the scans. In a stress MUGA, patients with normal hearts will exhibit an increase in ejection fraction or no change.

Abnormal results

An uneven distribution of technetium in the heart indicates that the patient has coronary artery disease, a **cardiomyopathy**, or blood shunting within the heart. Abnormalities in a resting MUGA usually indicate a heart attack, while those that occur during **exercise** usually indicate **ischemia**. In a stress MUGA, patients with coronary artery disease may exhibit a decrease in ejection fraction.

Resources

ORGANIZATIONS

American Heart Association. 7320 Greenville Ave. Dallas, TX 75231. (214) 373-6300. < http:// www.americanheart.org >.

KEY TERMS

Ejection fraction—The fraction of all blood in the ventricle that is ejected at each heartbeat. One of the main advantages of the MUGA scan is its ability to measure ejection fraction, one of the most important measures of the heart's performance.

Electrocardiogram—A test in which electronic sensors called electrodes are placed on the body to record the heart's electrical activities.

Heart attack—A cardiac emergency that occurs when a clot blocks blood flow in one or more of the heart's arteries. Oxygen supply to the heart muscle is cut off, resulting in the death of heart tissue in the affected area.

Ischemia—A decreased supply of oxygenated blood to a body part or organ, often marked by pain and organ dysfunction, as in ischemic heart disease.

Non-invasive—A procedure that does not penetrate the body.

Radioactive isotope—One of two or more atoms with the same number of protons but a different number of neutrons with a nuclear composition. In nuclear scanning, radioactive isotopes are used as a diagnostic agent.

Technetium—A radioactive isotope frequently used in radionuclide scanning of the heart and other organs. It is produced during nuclear fission reactions.

Ventricles—The heart's lower chambers are called the left and right ventricles. They send blood to the lungs and throughout the body. The MUGA scan is performed to evaluate the ventricles.

Texas Heart Institute. Heart Information Service. P.O. Box 20345, Houston, TX 77225-0345. < http:// www.tmc.edu/thi >.

Lori De Milto

Multiple chemical sensitivity

Definition

Multiple chemical sensitivity—also known as MCS syndrome, environmental illness, idiopathic environmental intolerance, chemical **AIDS**, total allergy syndrome, or simply MCS—is a disorder in which a person develops symptoms from exposure to chemicals in the environment. With each incidence of exposure, lower levels of the chemical will trigger a reaction and the person becomes increasingly vulnerable to reactions triggered by other chemicals.

Medical experts disagree on the cause of the syndrome, and as to whether MCS is a clinically recognized illness. In a 1992 position statement that remained unchanged as of early 2000, the American Medical Association's Council on Scientific Affairs did not recognize MCS as a clinical condition due to a lack of accepted diagnostic criteria and controlled studies on the disorder. A more recent discussion of methodological problems in published studies of MCS, as well as recommendations for patient care, may be found in the 1999 position paper on MCS drafted by the American College of Occupational and Environmental Medicine (ACOEM). As of 2003, however, many researchers in Europe as well as the United States regard MCS as a contemporary version of neurasthenia, a concept first introduced by a physician named George Miller Beard in 1869.

Description

Multiple chemical sensitivity typically begins with one high-dose exposure to a chemical, but it may also develop with long-term exposure to a low level of a chemical. Chemicals most often connected with MCS include: formaldehyde; pesticides; solvents; petrochemical fuels such as diesel, gasoline, and kerosene; waxes, detergents, and cleaning products; latex; tobacco smoke; perfumes and fragrances; and artificial colors, flavors, and preservatives. People who develop MCS are commonly exposed in one of the following situations: on the job as an industrial worker; residing or working in a poorly ventilated building; or living in conditions of high air or water pollution. Others may be exposed in unique incidents.

Because MCS is difficult to diagnose, estimates vary as to what percentage of the population develops MCS. However, most MCS patients are female. The median age of MCS patients is 40 years old, and most experienced symptoms before they were 30 years old. There is also a large percentage of Persian Gulf War veterans who have reported symptoms of chemical sensitivity since their return from the Gulf in the early 1990s.

Causes and symptoms

Chemical exposure is often a result of indoor air pollution. Buildings that are tightly sealed for energy conservation may cause a related illness called sick building syndrome, in which people develop symptoms from chronic exposure to airborne environmental chemicals such as formaldehyde from the furniture, carpet glues, and latex caulking. A person moving into a newly constructed building, which has not had time to degas, may experience the initial high-dose exposure that leads to MCS.

As of late 2002, the specific biochemical and physiological mechanisms in humans that lead to MCS are not well understood. A recent hypothesis, however, suggests that MCS is the end result of four different mechanisms of sensitization acting to reinforce one another. Further research is required to test this hypothesis.

The symptoms of MCS vary from person to person and are not chemical-specific. Symptoms are not limited to one physiological system, but primarily affect the respiratory and nervous systems. Symptoms commonly reported are **headache**, **fatigue**, weakness, difficulty concentrating, short-term memory loss, **dizziness**, irritability and depression, **itching**, **numbness**, burning sensation, congestion, **sore throat**, hoarseness, **shortness of breath**, **cough**, and stomach pains.

One commonly reported symptom of MCS is a heightened sensitivity to odors, including a stronger emotional reaction to them. A Japanese study published in late 2002 reported that patients diagnosed with MCS can identify common odors as accurately as most people, but regard a greater number of them as unpleasant.

One test that has been devised to evaluate patients with MCS is the capsaicin inhalation test. Capsaicin is an alkaloid found in hot peppers that is sometimes used in topical creams and rubs for the treatment of arthritis. When inhaled, capsaicin causes coughing in healthy persons as well as those with **allergies** that affect the airway; however, persons with MCS cough more deeply and frequently than control subjects when given a dose of capsaicin. Although the test is not diagnostic in the strict sense, it has been shown to be an effective way of identifying patients with MCS.

Diagnosis

Multiple chemical sensitivity is a twentieth-century disorder, becoming more prevalent as more human-made chemicals are introduced into the environment in greater quantities. It is especially difficult to diagnose because it presents no consistent or measurable set of symptoms and has no single diagnostic test or marker. For example, a 2002 study of **PET** scans of

MCS patients found no significant functional changes in the patients' brain tissues. Physicians are often either unaware of MCS as a condition, or refuse to accept that MCS exists. They may be unable to diagnose it, or may misdiagnose it as another degenerative disease, or may label it as a psychosomatic illness (a physical illness that is caused by emotional problems). Their lack of understanding generates frustration, **anxiety**, and distrust in patients already struggling with MCS. However, a new specialty of medicine is evolving to address MCS and related illnesses: occupational and environmental medicine. A physician looking for MCS will take a complete patient history and try to identify chemical exposures.

Some MCS patients may be helped by a psychologic evaluation, particularly if they show signs of panic attacks or other **anxiety disorders**. It is known that many patients with MCS suffer from comorbid depression and anxiety. In addition, MCS patients appear to have high rates of **mood disorders** compared to **asthma** patients as well as normal test subjects.

Treatment

While doctors may recommend **antihistamines**, **analgesics**, and other medications to combat the symptoms, the most effective treatment is to avoid those chemicals which trigger the symptoms. This becomes increasingly difficult as the number of offending chemicals increases, and people with MCS often remain at home where they are able to control the chemicals in their environment. This isolation often limits their abilities to work and socialize, so supportive counseling may also be appropriate.

Alternative treatment

Some MCS patients find relief with **detoxification** programs of **exercise** and sweating, and chelation of heavy metals. Others support their health with nutritional regimens and immunotherapy vaccines. Some undergo food-allergy testing and testing for accumulated pesticides in the body to learn more about their condition and what chemicals to avoid. Homeopathy and **acupuncture** can give added support to any treatment program for MCS patients. Botanical medicine can help to support the liver and other involved organs.

Prognosis

Once MCS sets in, sensitivity continues to increase and a person's health continues to deteriorate. Strictly avoiding exposure to triggering chemicals for a year or more may improve health.

KEY TERMS

Capsaicin—An alkaloid found in hot peppers that is used in an inhalation test to identify patients with MCS.

Degas—To release and vent gases. New building materials often give off gases and odors and the air should be well circulated to remove them.

Neurasthenia—A term coined in the late nineteenth century to refer to a condition of chronic mental and physical weakness and fatigue. Some researchers regard MCS as a twentieth-century version of neurasthenia.

Sick building syndrome—An illness related to MCS in which a person develops symptoms in response to chronic exposure to airborne environmental chemicals found in a tightly sealed building.

Prevention

Multiple chemical sensitivity is difficult to prevent because even at high-dose exposures, different people react differently. Ensuring adequate ventilation in situations with potential for acute high-dose or chronic low-dose chemical exposure, as well as wearing the proper protective equipment in industrial situations, will minimize the risk.

Resources

BOOKS

American Psychiatric Association.*Diagnostic and Statistical Manual of Mental Disorders*. 4th ed., revised. Washington, DC: American Psychiatric Association, 2000.

Beers, Mark H., MD, and Robert Berkow, MD, editors. "Multiple Chemical Sensitivity Syndrome." Section 21, Chapter 287. In *The Merck Manual of Diagnosis and Therapy*. Whitehouse Station, NJ: Merck Research Laboratories, 2004.

Gibson, Pamela. *Multiple Chemical Sensitivity: A Survival Guide*. Oakland, CA: New Harbinger Publications, 2000.

PERIODICALS

Bornschein, S., C. Hausteiner, A. Drzezga, et al. "PET in Patients With Clear-Cut Multiple Chemical Sensitivity (MCS)." *Nuklearmedizin* 41 (December 2002): 233–239.

Bornschein, S., C. Hausteiner, T. Zilker, and H. Forstl. "Psychiatric and Somatic Disorders and Multiple Chemical Sensitivity (MCS) in 264 'Environmental Patients'." *Psychological Medicine* 32 (November 2002): 1387–1394.

Caccappollo-vanVliet, E., K. Kelly-McNeil, B. Natelson, et al. "Anxiety Sensitivity and Depression in Multiple Chemical Sensitivities and Asthma." *Journal of*

Occupational and Environmental Medicine 44 (October 2002): 890–901.

Johansson, A., O. Lowhagen, E. Millqvist, and M. Bende. "Capsaicin Inhalation Test for Identification of Sensory Hyperreactivity." *Respiratory Medicine* 96 (September 2002): 731–735.

Ojima, M., H. Tonori, T. Sato, et al. "Odor Perception in Patients with Multiple Chemical Sensitivity." *Tohoku Journal of Experimental Medicine* 198 (November 2002): 163–173.

Pall, M. L. "NMDA Sensitization and Stimulation by Peroxynitrite, Nitric Oxide, and Organic Solvents as the Mechanism of Chemical Sensitivity in Multiple Chemical Sensitivity." *FASEB Journal* 16 (September 2002): 1407–1417.

Schafer, M. L. "On the History of the Concept Neurasthenia and Its Modern Variants Chronic-Fatigue-Syndrome, Fibromyalgia and Multiple Chemical Sensitivities" [in German] *Fortschritte der Neurologie-Psychiatrie* 70 (November 2002): 570–582.

Ternesten-Hasseus, E., M. Bende, and E. Millqvist. "Increased Capsaicin Cough Sensitivity in Patients with Multiple Chemical Sensitivity." *Journal of Occupational and Environmental Medicine* 44 (November 2002): 1012–1017.

ORGANIZATIONS

American Academy of Environmental Medicine. P.O. Box CN 1001-8001, New Hope, PA 18938. (215) 862-4544.

American College of Occupational and Environmental Medicine (ACOEM). 1114 North Arlington Heights Road, Arlington Heights, IL 60004. (847) 818-1800. < www.acoem.org >.

OTHER

"Multiple Chemical Sensitivities: Idiopathic Environmental Intolerance." Position Statement by the American College of Occupational and Environmental Medicine (ACOEM), April 26, 1999. < www.acoem.org/position/statements.asp?CATA_ID = 46 >.

Bethany Thivierge
Rebecca J. Frey, PhD

Multiple endocrine adenomatosis *see* **Multiple endocrine neoplasia syndromes**

Multiple endocrine neoplasia syndromes

Definition

The multiple endocrine neoplasia (MEN) syndromes are three related disorders affecting the thyroid and other hormonal (endocrine) glands of the body. MEN has previously been known as familial endocrine adenomatosis.

Description

The three forms of MEN are MEN1 (Wermer's syndrome), MEN2A (Sipple syndrome), and MEN2B (previously known as MEN3). Each is an autosomal dominant genetic condition which predisposes to hyperplasia (excessive growth of cells) and tumor formation in a number of endocrine glands.

Causes and symptoms

MEN1 patients experience hyperplasia or tumors of several endocrine glands, including the parathyroids, the pancreas, and the pituitary. The most frequent symptom of MEN1 is **hyperparathyroidism**. Overgrowth of the parathyroid glands leads to over secretion of parathyroid hormone, which leads to elevated blood calcium levels, **kidney stones**, weakened bones, and nervous system depression. Almost all MEN1 patients show parathyroid symptoms by age 40.

Tumors of the pancreas known as gastrinomas are also common in MEN1. Excessive secretion of gastrin (a hormone secreted into the stomach to aid in digestion) by these tumors can cause upper gastrointestinal ulcers. The anterior pituitary and the adrenal glands can also be affected. Unlike MEN2, the thyroid gland is rarely involved in MEN1 symptoms.

Patients with MEN2A and MEN2B experience two main symptoms, medullary **thyroid cancer** (MTC) and a tumor of the adrenal gland medulla known as **pheochromocytoma**. MTC is a slow-growing **cancer**, but one that can be cured in less than 50% of cases. Pheochromocytoma is usually a benign tumor that causes excessive secretion of adrenal hormones, which, in turn, can cause life-threatening **hypertension** and cardiac arrhythmia.

The two forms of MEN2 are distinguished by additional symptoms. MEN2A patients have a predisposition to increase in size (hypertrophy) and to develop tumors of the parathyroid gland. Although similar to MEN1, less than 20% of MEN2A patients will show parathyroid involvement.

MEN2B patients show a variety of additional conditions: a characteristic facial appearance with swollen lips; tumors of the mucous membranes of the eye, mouth, tongue, and nasal cavity; enlarged colon; and skeletal abnormalities. Symptoms develop early in life (often under five years of age) in cases of MEN2B and the tumors are more aggressive. MEN2B is about ten-fold less common than MEN2A.

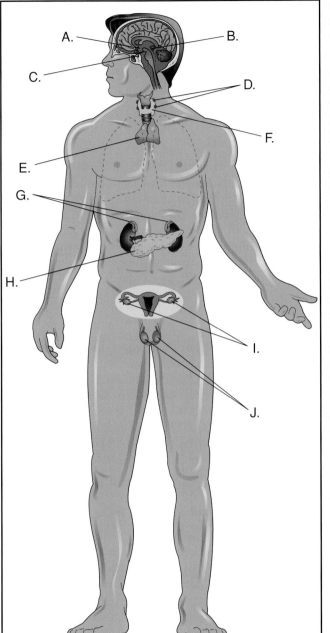

The human endocrine system: A. Hypothalamus. B. Pineal. C. Pituitary. D. Parathyroid. E. Thymus. F. Thyroid. G. Adrenals. H. Pancreas. I. Ovaries (female). J. Testes (male). *(Illustration by Electronic Illustrators Group.)*

MEN1 is caused by mutation at the PYGM gene. PYGM is one of a group of genes known as tumor suppressor genes. A patient who inherits one defective copy of a tumor suppressor gene from either parent has a strong predisposition to the disease because of the high probability of incurring a second mutation in at least one dividing cell. That cell no longer possesses even one normal copy of the gene. When both copies are defective, tumor suppression fails and tumors develop.

Both types of MEN2 are caused by mutations in another gene, known as RET. A mutation in only one copy of the RET gene is sufficient to cause disease. A number of different mutations can lead to MEN2A, but only one specific genetic alteration leads to MEN2B.

For all types of MEN, the children of an affected individual have a 50% chance of inheriting the defective gene.

Diagnosis

Classical diagnosis of MEN is based on clinical features and on testing for elevated hormone levels. For MEN1, the relevant hormone is parathyroid hormone. For both types of MEN2, the greatest concern is development of medullary thyroid cancer. MTC can be detected by measuring levels of the thyroid hormone, calcitonin. Numerous other hormone levels can be measured to assess the involvement of the various other endocrine glands.

Diagnosis of MEN2B can be made by **physical examination** alone. However, MEN2A shows no distinct physical features and must be identified by measuring hormone levels or by finding endocrine tumors.

Since 1994, genetic screening using DNA technology has been available for both MEN1 and MEN2. This new methodology allows diagnosis prior to the onset of symptoms.

In the past, there was no way of definitively identifying which children had inherited the defective gene. As a result, all children had to be considered at risk. In the case of MEN2A and MEN2B, children would undergo frequent calcitonin testing. Molecular techniques now allow a positive distinction to be made between children who are and are not actually at risk.

Children who are identified as carriers of the RET gene can be offered total **thyroidectomy** on a preventative (prophylactic) basis to prevent the development of MTC.

Treatment

No comprehensive treatment is available for genetic conditions such as MEN. However, some of the consequences of MEN can be symptomatically treated.

Pheochromocytoma in both types of MEN 2 can be cured by surgical removal of this slow growing tumor.

KEY TERMS

Endocrine—A term used to describe the glands that produce hormones in the body.

Hyperplasia—An overgrowth of normal cells within an organ or tissue.

Medullary thyroid cancer (MTC)—A slow-growing tumor associated with MEN.

Neoplasm—An abnormal formation of tissue; for example, a tumor.

Pheochromocytoma—A tumor of the medullary of the adrenal gland.

Treatment of MTC is by surgical removal of the thyroid, although doctors may disagree at what stage to remove the thyroid. After thyroidectomy, the patient will receive normal levels of thyroid hormone orally or by injection.

Even when surgery is performed early, metastatic spread of the cancer may have already occurred. Since this cancer is slow growing, metastasis may not be obvious. Metastasis is very serious in MTC because **chemotherapy** and **radiation therapy** are not effective in controlling its spread.

Prognosis

Diagnosed early, the prognosis for the MEN diseases is reasonably good, even for MEN2B, the most dangerous of the three forms. Even in the absence of treatment, a few individuals with MEN2A mutations will never show any symptoms at all. Analysis of at-risk family members using molecular genetic techniques will lead to earlier treatment and improved outcomes.

Prevention

One of the most serious consequences of MEN is MTC, which can be prevented by thyroidectomy. There is no preventive measure to block the occurrence of genetic mutations such as those that cause MEN.

Resources

ORGANIZATIONS

Canadian MEN Society. P.O. Box 100, Meola, Saskatchewan SOM 1XO. (306) 892-2080.

Victor Leipzig, PhD

Multiple myeloma

Definition

Multiple myeloma is a **cancer** in which antibody-producing plasma cells grow in an uncontrolled and invasive (malignant) manner.

Description

Multiple myeloma, also known as plasma cell myeloma, is the second-most common cancer of the blood. It is the most common type of plasma cell neoplasm. Multiple myeloma accounts for approximately 1% of all cancers and 2% of all deaths from cancer. Multiple myeloma is a disease in which malignant plasma cells spread through the bone marrow and hard outer portions of the large bones of the body. These myeloma cells may form tumors called plasmacytomas. Eventually, multiple soft spots or holes, called osteolytic lesions, form in the bones.

Bone marrow is the spongy tissue within the bones. The breastbone, spine, ribs, skull, pelvic bones, and the long bone of the thigh all are particularly rich in marrow. Bone marrow is a very active tissue that is responsible for producing the cells that circulate in the blood. These include the red blood cells that carry oxygen, the white blood cells that develop into immune system cells, and platelets, which cause blood to clot.

Plasma cells and immunoglobulins

Plasma cells develop from B-lymphocytes or B-cells, a type of white blood cell. B-cells, like all blood cells, develop from unspecialized stem cells in the bone marrow. Each B-cell carries a specific antibody that recognizes a specific foreign substance called an antigen. Antibodies are large proteins called immunoglobulins (Igs), which recognize and destroy foreign substances and organisms such as bacteria. When a B-cell encounters its antigen, it begins to divide rapidly to form mature plasma cells. These plasma cells are all identical (monoclonal). They produce large amounts of identical antibody that are specific for the antigen.

Malignant plasma cells

Multiple myeloma begins when the genetic material (DNA) is damaged during the development of a stem cell into a B-cell in the bone marrow. This causes the cell to develop into an abnormal or malignant plasmablast, a developmentally early form of plasma cell. Plasmablasts produce adhesive molecules that allow them to bond to the inside of the bone marrow. A growth factor, called interleukin-6, promotes uncontrolled growth of these myeloma cells in the bone marrow and prevents their natural death. Whereas normal bone marrow contains less than 5% plasma cells, bone marrow of an individual with multiple myeloma contains over 10% plasma cells.

In most cases of multiple myeloma, the malignant plasma cells all make an identical Ig. Igs are made up of four protein chains that are bonded together. Two of the chains are light and two are heavy. There are five classes of heavy chains, corresponding to five types of Igs with different immune system functions. The Igs from myeloma cells are nonfunctional and are called paraproteins. All of the paraproteins from any one individual are monoclonal (identical) because the myeloma cells are identical clones of a single plasma cell. Thus, the paraprotein is a monoclonal protein or M-protein. The M-proteins crowd out the functional Igs and other components of the immune system. They also cause functional antibodies, which are produced by normal plasma cells, to rapidly break down. Thus, multiple myeloma depresses the immune system.

In about 75% of multiple myeloma cases, the malignant plasma cells also produce monoclonal light chains, or incomplete Igs. These are called Bence-Jones proteins and are secreted in the urine. Approximately 1% of multiple myelomas are called nonsecretors because they do not produce any abnormal Ig.

Osteolytic lesions

About 70% of individuals with multiple myeloma have soft spots or lesions in their bones. These lesions can vary from quite small to grapefruit-size. In part, these lesions occur because the malignant plasma cells rapidly outgrow the normal bone-forming cells. In addition, malignant myeloma cells produce factors that affect cells called osteoclasts. These are the cells that normally destroy old bone, so that new bone can be produced by cells called osteoblasts. The myeloma cell factors increase both the activation and the growth of osteoclasts. As the osteoclasts multiply and migrate, they destroy healthy bone and create lesions. **Osteoporosis**, or widespread bone weakness, may develop.

There are more than 40,000 multiple myeloma patients in the United States. The American Cancer Society predicts an additional 14,400 new cases in 2001. About 11,200 Americans will die of the disease in 2001. Multiple myeloma is one of the leading causes of cancer deaths among African Americans.

In Western industrialized countries, approximately four people in 100,000 develop multiple myeloma. The incidence of multiple myeloma among African Americans is 9.5 per 100,000, about twice that of Caucasians. Asians have a much lower incidence of the disease. In China, for example, the incidence of multiple myeloma is only one in 100,000. The offspring and siblings of individuals with multiple myeloma are at a slightly increased risk for the disease.

At diagnosis, the average age of a multiple myeloma patient is 68 to 70. Although the average age at onset is decreasing, most multiple myelomas still occur in people over 40. This cancer is somewhat more prevalent in men than in women.

Causes and symptoms

Associations

The cause of multiple myeloma has not been determined. However, a number of possible associations have been identified:

- decreased immune system function; the immune systems of older individuals may be less efficient at detecting and destroying cancer cells

- genetic (hereditary) factors, suggested by the increased incidence in some ethnic groups and among family members

- occupational factors, suggested by the increased incidence among agricultural, petroleum, wood, and leather workers, and cosmetologists

- long-term exposure to herbicides, pesticides, petroleum products, heavy metals, plastics, and dusts such as asbestos

- radiation exposure, as among Japanese atomic bomb survivors, nuclear weapons workers, and medical personnel such as radiologists

- Kaposi's sarcoma-associated herpes virus (also called human herpes virus-8 or HHV-8), found in the blood and bone marrow cells of many multiple myeloma patients

Early symptoms

The accumulation of malignant plasma cells can result in tiny cracks or **fractures** in bones. Malignant plasma cells in the bone marrow can suppress the formation of red and white blood cells and platelets. About 80% of individuals with multiple myeloma are anemic due to low red blood cell formation. Low white blood cell formation results in increased susceptibility to infection, since new, functional antibodies are not produced. In addition, normal circulating antibodies are rapidly destroyed. Low platelet formation can result in poor blood clotting. It is rare, however, that insufficient white blood cell and platelet formations are presenting signs of multiple myeloma.

These factors cause the early symptoms of multiple myeloma:

- **pain** in the lower back or ribs
- fatigue and paleness due to anemia (low red blood cell count)
- frequent and recurring infections, including bacterial **pneumonia**, urinary-tract and kidney infections, and shingles
- bleeding

Bone destruction

Bone pain, particularly in the backbone, hips, and skull, is often the first symptom of multiple myeloma. As malignant plasma cells increase in the bone marrow, replacing normal marrow, they exert pressure on the bone. As overly-active osteoclasts (large cells responsible for the breakdown of bone) remove bone tissue, the bone becomes soft. Fracture and spinal cord compression may occur.

Plasmacytomas (malignant tumors of plasma cells) may weaken bones, causing fractures. Fractured bones or weak or collapsed spinal bones, in turn, may place unusual pressure on nearby nerves, resulting in nerve pain, burning, or **numbness** and muscle weakness. Proteins produced by myeloma cells also may damage nerves.

Calcium from the destroyed bone enters the blood and urine, causing **hypercalcemia**, a medical condition in which abnormally high concentrations of calcium compounds exist in the bloodstream. High calcium affects nerve cell and kidney function. The symptoms of hypercalcemia include:

- weakness and fatigue
- depression
- mental confusion
- constipation
- increased thirst
- icreased urination
- nausea and vomiting
- kidney pain
- kidney failure

Hypercalcemia affects about one-third of multiple myeloma patients.

Serum proteins

The accumulation of M-proteins in the serum (the liquid portion of the blood) may cause additional complications, such as hyperviscosity syndrome, or thickening of the blood (though rare in multiple myeloma patients). Symptoms of hyperviscosity include:

- fatigue
- headaches
- shortness of breath
- mental confusion
- chest pain
- kidney damage and failure
- vision problems
- Raynaud's phenomenon

Poor blood circulation, or Raynaud's phenomenon, can affect any part of the body, but particularly the fingers, toes, nose, and ears.

Cryoglobulinemia occurs when the protein in the blood forms particles under cold conditions. These particles can block small blood vessels and cause pain and numbness in the toes, fingers, and other extremities during cold weather.

Amyloidosis is a rare complication of multiple myeloma. It usually occurs in individuals whose plasma cells produce only Ig light chains. These Bence-Jones proteins combine with other serum proteins to form amyloid protein. This starchy substance can invade tissues, organs, and blood vessels. In particular, amyloid proteins can accumulate in the kidneys, where they block the tiny tubules that are the kidney's filtering system. Indicators of amyloidosis include:

- carpal tunnel syndrome
- kidney failure
- liver failure
- heart failure

Diagnosis

Blood and urine tests

Often, the original diagnosis of multiple myeloma is made from routine blood tests that are performed for other reasons. Blood tests may indicate:

- anemia
- abnormal red blood cells
- high serum protein levels
- how levels of normal antibody

- high calcium levels

- high blood urea nitrogen (BUN) levels

- high creatinine levels

Urea and creatinine normally are excreted in the urine. High levels of urea and creatinine in the blood indicate that the kidneys are not functioning properly to eliminate these substances.

Protein electrophoresis is a laboratory technique that uses an electrical current to separate the different proteins in the blood and urine on the basis of size and charge. Since all of the multiple myeloma M-proteins in the blood and urine are identical, electrophoresis of blood and urine from a patient with multiple myeloma shows a large M-protein spike, corresponding to the high concentration of monoclonal Ig. Electrophoresis of the urine also can detect Bence-Jones proteins.

Bones

A **bone marrow aspiration** utilizes a very thin, long needle to remove a sample of marrow from the hip bone. Alternatively, a **bone marrow biopsy** with a larger needle removes solid marrow tissue. The marrow is examined under the microscope for plasma cells and tumors. If 10% to 30% of the cells are plasma cells, multiple myeloma is the usual diagnosis.

X rays are used to detect osteoporosis, osteolytic lesions, and fractures. Computer-assisted tomography (CAT or CT) scans can detect lesions in both bone and soft tissue. **Magnetic resonance imaging** (MRI) may give a more detailed image of a certain bone or a region of the body.

Treatment

Related disorders

Monoclonal gammopathy of undetermined significance (MGUS) is a common condition in which a monoclonal Ig is detectable. However, there are no tumors or other symptoms of multiple myeloma. MGUS occurs in about 1% of the general population and in about 3% of those over age 70. Over a period of years, about 16% to 20% of those with MGUS will develop multiple myeloma or a related cancer called malignant lymphoma.

Occasionally, only a single plasmacytoma develops, either in the bone marrow (isolated plasmacytoma of the bone) or other tissues or organs (extramedullary plasmacytoma). Some individuals with solitary plasmacytoma may develop multiple myeloma.

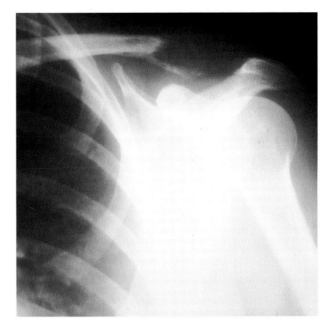

This x ray of the patient's left clavicle indicates an occurrence of myelomas in the bone. *(Custom Medical Stock Photo. Reproduced by permission.)*

Clinical stages

The Durie-Salmon system is used to stage multiple myeloma. Stage I multiple myeloma requires all of the following (1 gram = approx. 0.02 pints, 1 deciliter = approx. 0.33 ounces):

- hemoglobin (the oxygen-transporting molecule of red blood cells) above 10 grams/deciliter (g/dl)

- serum calcium below 12 mg/dl

- normal bone structure or only isolated plasmacytoma

- low M-protein, based on established guideline levels of Ig protein chains

Approximately 5% of multiple myeloma cases are not progressing at diagnosis, and may not progress for months or years. This is called smoldering myeloma. These patients have stage I blood chemistry but no symptoms.

Stage II multiple myeloma fits neither stage I nor stage III. Stage III multiple myeloma meets one or more the following criteria:

- hemoglobin below 8.5 g/dl

- serum calcium above 12 mg/dl

- advanced bone lesions

- high M-protein

Each stage is subclassified as A or B, based on serum creatinine indicators of normal or abnormal kidney function. Most patients have stage III multiple myeloma at diagnosis.

Prognostic indicators

Prognostic indicators for multiple myeloma may be used instead of, or in addition to, the staging system described above. Prognostic indicators are laboratory tests that help to define the stage of the disease at diagnosis, and its progression during treatment. These indicators are:

- plasmablastic multiple myeloma (presence of plasmablasts, the precursor malignant plasma cells)
- plasma cell labeling index (the percentage of plasma cells that are actively dividing)
- beta 2-microglobulin, a protein secreted by B-cells that correlates with the myeloma cell mass (also indicates kidney damage)

Since multiple myeloma often progresses slowly, and since the treatments can be toxic, the disease may not be treated until M-protein levels in the blood are quite high. In particular, MGUS and smoldering myeloma may be followed closely but not treated. Solitary plasmacytomas are treated with radiation and/or surgery and followed closely with examinations and laboratory tests.

Chemotherapy

Chemotherapy, or treatment with anti-cancer drugs, is used for multiple myeloma. MP, a combination of the drugs melphalan and prednisone, is the standard treatment. Usually, the drugs are taken by mouth every 3 to 4 weeks for 6 to 9 months or longer, until the M-protein levels in the blood stop decreasing. MP usually results in a 50% reduction in M-protein.

Dexamethasone, a corticosteroid, sometimes is used to treat the elderly or those in poor health. It can drop the M-protein levels by 40% in untreated individuals and by 20% to 40% in patients who have not responded to previous treatment. Other chemotherapy drugs, including cyclophosphamide, carmustine, doxorubicin, vincristine, and chlorambucil, may be used as well.

Multiple myeloma usually recurs within a year after the end of chemotherapy. Although the chemotherapy can be repeated after each recurrence, it is progressively less responsive to treatment.

Side effects of chemotherapy may include:

- anemia
- hair loss
- nausea
- vomiting
- diarrhea
- mood swings
- swelling
- acne

These side effects disappear after treatment is discontinued.

Other drug treatments

Bisphosphonates are drugs that inhibit the activity of osteoclasts. These drugs can slow the progression of bone disease, reduce pain, and help prevent bone fractures. Different types of bisphosphonates inhibit osteoclasts in different ways. They also reduce the production of interleukin-6 by bone marrow cells. Laboratory studies suggest that bisphosphonates may kill or inhibit the growth of multiple myeloma cells. Pamidronate is the most common bisphosphonate for treating multiple myeloma.

The drug thalidomide appears to have several anti-myeloma activities. Thalidomide affects the immune system in various ways and it appears to inhibit myeloma cells, both directly and indirectly. It also inhibits the growth of new blood vessels that are needed by tumors. However, if thalidomide is taken during **pregnancy**, it an cause severe **birth defects** or death of the fetus.

The drug allopurinol may be used to reduce high blood levels of uric acid that result from kidney dysfunction. **Diuretics** can improve kidney function. Infections require prompt treatment with **antibiotics**.

BONE AND PERIPHERAL BLOOD STEM CELL TRANSPLANTATION. Bone marrow or peripheral blood stem cell transplantations (PBSCT) are used to replace the stem cells of the bone marrow following high-dosage chemotherapy. Chemotherapy destroys the bone marrow stem cells that are necessary to produce new blood cells. In an autologous transplant, the patient's bone marrow stem cells or peripheral blood stem cells (immature bone marrow cells found in the blood) are collected, treated with drugs to kill any myeloma cells, and frozen prior to chemotherapy. Growth factors are used to increase the number of peripheral stem cells prior to collection. A procedure called apheresis is used to collect the peripheral stem cells. Following high-dosage chemotherapy, the stem cells are reinjected into the individual. In an allogeneic

KEY TERMS

Amyloidosis—A complication of multiple myeloma in which amyloid protein accumulates in the kidneys and other organs, tissues, and blood vessels.

Anemia—Any condition in which the red blood cell count is below normal.

Antibody—Immunoglobulin produced by immune system cells that recognizes and binds to a specific foreign substance (antigen).

Antigen—Foreign substance that is recognized by a specific antibody.

B-cell (B-lymphocyte)—Type of white blood cell that produces antibodies.

Bence-Jones protein—Light chain of an immunoglobulin that is overproduced in multiple myeloma and is excreted in the urine.

Beta 2-microglobulin—Protein produced by B-cells; high concentrations in the blood are indicative of multiple myeloma.

Cryoglobulinemia—Condition in which protein in the blood forms particles in the cold, blocking blood vessels, leading to pain and numbness of the extremities.

Electrophoresis—Use of an electrical field to separate proteins in a mixture (such as blood or urine), on the basis of the size and electrical charge of the proteins.

Hemoglobin—Protein in red blood cells that carries oxygen.

Hypercalcemia—Abnormally high levels of calcium in the blood.

Hyperviscosity—Thick, viscous blood, caused by the accumulation of large proteins, such as immunoglobulins, in the serum.

Immunoglobulin (Ig)—Antibody; large protein produced by B-cells that recognizes and binds to a specific antigen.

M-protein—Monoclonal or myeloma protein; paraprotein; abnormal antibody found in large amounts in the blood and urine of individuals with multiple myeloma.

Malignant—A characteristic of cancer cells that grow uncontrollably and invade other tissues.

Monoclonal—Identical cells or proteins; cells (clones) derived from a single, genetically-distinct cell, or proteins produced by these cells.

Monoclonal gammopathy of undetermined significance (MGUS)—Common condition in which M-protein is present, but there are no tumors or other symptoms of disease.

Neoplasm—Tumor made up of cancer cells.

Osteoblast—Bone-forming cell.

Osteoclast—Cell that absorbs bone.

Osteolytic lesion—Soft spot or hole in bone caused by cancer cells.

Osteoporosis—Condition in which the bones become weak and porous, due to loss of calcium and destruction of cells.

Paraprotein—M-protein; abnormal immunoglobulin produced in multiple myeloma.

Plasma cell—Type of white blood cell that produces antibodies; derived from an antigen-specific B-cell.

Platelet—Cell that is involved in blood clotting.

Stem cell—Undifferentiated cell that retains the ability to develop into any one of numerous cell types.

transplant, the donor stem cells come from a genetically-related individual such as a sibling.

Other treatments

Blood transfusions may be required to treat severe anemia.

Plasmapheresis, or plasma exchange **transfusion**, may be used to thin the blood to treat hyperviscosity syndrome. In this treatment, blood is removed and passed through a machine that separates the plasma, containing the M-protein, from the red and white blood cells and platelets. The blood cells are transfused back into the patient, along with a plasma substitute or donated plasma.

Multiple myeloma may be treated with high-energy x rays directed at a specific region of the body. **Radiation therapy** is used for treating bone pain.

Alternative treatment

Interferon alpha, an immune-defense protein that is produced by some white blood cells and bone marrow cells, can slow the growth of myeloma cells. It usually is given to patients following chemotherapy, to prolong their remission. However, interferon may have toxic effects in older individuals with multiple myeloma.

Once multiple myeloma is in remission, calcium and vitamin D supplements can improve bone density. It is important not to take these supplements when the myeloma is active. Individuals with multiple myeloma must drink large amounts of fluid to counter the effects of hyperviscous blood.

Prognosis

The prognosis for individuals with MGUS or solitary plasmacytoma is very good. Most do not develop multiple myeloma. However, approximately 15% of all patients with multiple myeloma die within three months of diagnosis. About 60% respond to treatment and live for an average of two and a half to three years following diagnosis. Approximately 23% of patients die of other illnesses associated with advanced age.

The prognosis for a given individual may be based on the prognostic indicators described above. The median survival for those without plasmablasts, and with a low plasma cell labeling index (PCLI) and low beta 2-microglobulin, is 5.5 years. The median survival for patients with plasmablastic multiple myeloma, or with a high PCLI (1% or greater) and high beta 2-microglobulin (4 or higher), is 1.9 and 2.4 years, respectively. Many multiple myeloma patients are missing part or all of chromosome 13. The deletion of this chromosome, along with high beta 2-microglobulin, leads to a poor prognosis.

With treatment, multiple myeloma may go into complete remission. This is defined as:

- M-protein absent from the blood and urine
- myeloma cells not detectable in the bone marrow
- no clinical symptoms
- negative laboratory tests

However, with very sensitive testing, a few myeloma cells are usually detectable and eventually lead to a recurrence of the disease, in the bone or elsewhere in the body.

Prevention

There are no clearly-established risk factors for multiple myeloma and it is possible that a combination of factors interact to cause the disease. Thus, there is no method for preventing multiple myeloma.

Resources

BOOKS

Holland, Jimmie C., and Sheldon Lewis. *The Human Side of Cancer: Living with Hope, Coping with Uncertainty.* New York: HarperCollins, 2000.

ORGANIZATIONS

Multiple Myeloma Research Foundation. 11 Forest Street, New Canaan, CT 06840. (203) 972-1250. < http:// www.multiplemyeloma.org >. Information and research funding.

OTHER

"About Myeloma." *Multiple Myeloma Research Foundation.* April 16, 2001. [cited June 15,2001]. < http://www.multiplemyeloma.org/ aboutmyeloma.html >.

Complementary and Alternative Therapies for Leukemia, Lymphoma, Hodgkin's Disease and Myeloma. The Leukemia and Lymphoma Society. March 27, 2001. [cited June 15, 2001]. < http://www.leukemia-lymphoma.org >.

Facts and Statistics About Leukemia, Lymphoma, Hodgkin's Disease and Myeloma. The Leukemia and Lymphoma Society. March 15, 2001. [cited Mar27, 2001]. < http:// www.leukemia-lymphoma.org >.

"Multiple Myeloma and Other Plasma Cell Neoplasms." *CancerNet* National Cancer Institute. March 2001. [cited April 16, 2001]. < http://cancernet.nci.nih.gov >.

"Multiple Myeloma." *Cancer Resource Center.* American Cancer Society. April 16, 2001. [cited June 15, 2001]. < http://www3.cancer.org/cancerinfo >.

Margaret Alic, Ph.D.

Multiple personality disorder

Definition

Multiple personality disorder, or MPD, is a mental disturbance classified as one of the **dissociative disorders** in the fourth edition of the *Diagnostic and Statistical Manual of Mental Disorders* (*DSM-IV*). It has been renamed dissociative identity disorder (DID). MPD or DID is defined as a condition in which "two or more distinct identities or personality states" alternate in controlling the patient's consciousness and behavior. Note: "Split personality" is not an accurate term for DID and should not be used as a synonym for **schizophrenia**.

Description

The precise nature of DID (MPD) as well as its relationship to other mental disorders is still a subject of debate. Some researchers think that DID may be a relatively recent development in western society. It may be a culture-specific syndrome found in western society, caused primarily by both childhood **abuse** and unspecified long-term societal changes. Unlike depression or **anxiety disorders**, which have been recognized, in some form, for centuries, the earliest cases of persons reporting DID symptoms were not recorded until the 1790s. Most were considered medical oddities or curiosities until the late 1970s, when increasing numbers of cases were reported in the United States. Psychiatrists are still debating whether DID was previously misdiagnosed and underreported, or whether it is currently over-diagnosed. Because childhood trauma is a factor in the development of DID, some doctors think it may be a variation of **post-traumatic stress disorder** (PTSD). DID and PTSD are conditions where dissociation is a prominent mechanism. The female to male ratio for DID is about 9:1, but the reasons for the gender imbalance are unclear. Some have attributed the imbalance in reported cases to higher rates of abuse of female children; and some to the possibility that males with DID are underreported because they might be in prison for violent crimes.

The most distinctive feature of DID is the formation and emergence of alternate personality states, or "alters." Patients with DID experience their alters as distinctive individuals possessing different names, histories, and personality traits. It is not unusual for DID patients to have alters of different genders, sexual orientations, ages, or nationalities. Some patients have been reported with alters that are not even human; alters have been animals, or even aliens from outer space. The average DID patient has between two and 10 alters, but some have been reported with over one hundred.

Causes and symptoms

The severe dissociation that characterizes patients with DID is currently understood to result from a set of causes:

- An innate ability to dissociate easily

- Repeated episodes of severe physical or sexual abuse in childhood

- The lack of a supportive or comforting person to counteract abusive relative(s)

- The influence of other relatives with dissociative symptoms or disorders

The relationship of dissociative disorders to childhood abuse has led to intense controversy and lawsuits concerning the accuracy of childhood memories. The brain's storage, retrieval, and interpretation of childhood memories are still not fully understood.

The major dissociative symptoms experienced by DID patients are **amnesia**, depersonalization, derealization, and identity disturbances.

Amnesia

Amnesia in DID is marked by gaps in the patient's memory for long periods of their past, in some cases, their entire childhood. Most DID patients have amnesia, or "lose time," for periods when another personality is "out." They may report finding items in their house that they can't remember having purchased, finding notes written in different handwriting, or other evidence of unexplained activity.

Depersonalization

Depersonalization is a dissociative symptom in which the patient feels that his or her body is unreal, is changing, or is dissolving. Some DID patients experience depersonalization as feeling to be outside of their body, or as watching a movie of themselves.

Derealization

Derealization is a dissociative symptom in which the patient perceives the external environment as unreal. Patients may see walls, buildings, or other objects as changing in shape, size, or color. DID patients may fail to recognize relatives or close friends.

Identity disturbances

Identity disturbances in DID result from the patient's having split off entire personality traits or characteristics as well as memories. When a stressful or traumatic experience triggers the reemergence of these dissociated parts, the patient switches—usually within seconds—into an alternate personality. Some patients have histories of erratic performance in school or in their jobs caused by the emergence of alternate personalities during examinations or other stressful situations. Patients vary with regard to their alters' awareness of one another.

Diagnosis

The diagnosis of DID is complex and some physicians believe it is often missed, while others feel it is over-diagnosed. Patients have been known to have been treated under a variety of other psychiatric diagnoses for a long time before being re-diagnosed with DID. The average DID patient is in the mental health care system for six to seven years before being diagnosed as a person with DID. Many DID patients are misdiagnosed as depressed because the primary or "core" personality is subdued and withdrawn, particularly in female patients. However, some core personalities, or alters, may genuinely be depressed, and may benefit from antidepressant medications. One reason misdiagnoses are common is because DID patients may truly meet the criteria for **panic disorder** or somatization disorder.

Misdiagnoses include schizophrenia, borderline personality disorder, and, as noted, somatization disorder and panic disorder. DID patients are often frightened by their dissociative experiences, which can include losing awareness of hours or even days of time, meeting people who claim to know them by another name, or feeling "out of body." Persons with the disorder may go to emergency rooms or clinics because they fear they are going insane.

When a doctor is evaluating a patient for DID, he or she will first rule out physical conditions that sometimes produce amnesia, depersonalization, or derealization. These conditions include head injuries; brain disease, especially seizure disorders; side effects from medications; **substance abuse** or intoxication; **AIDS dementia** complex; or recent periods of extreme physical **stress** and sleeplessness. In some cases, the doctor may give the patient an electroencephalograph (EEG) to exclude epilepsy or other seizure disorders. The physician also must consider whether the patient is **malingering** and/or offering fictitious complaints.

If the patient appears to be physically normal, the doctor will next rule out psychotic disturbances, including schizophrenia. Many patients with DID are misdiagnosed as schizophrenic because they may "hear" their alters "talking" inside their heads. If the doctor suspects DID, he or she can use a screening test called the Dissociative Experiences Scale (DES). If the patient has a high score on this test, he or she can be evaluated further with the Dissociative Disorders Interview Schedule (DDIS) or the Structured Clinical Interview for *DSM-IV* Dissociative Disorders (SCID-D). The doctor may also use the Hypnotic Induction Profile (HIP) or a similar test of the patient's hypnotizability.

Treatment

Treatment of DID may last for five to seven years in adults and usually requires several different treatment methods.

Psychotherapy

Ideally, patients with DID should be treated by a therapist with specialized training in dissociation. This specialized training is important because the patient's personality switches can be confusing or startling. In

addition, many patients with DID have hostile or suicidal alter personalities. Most therapists who treat DID patients have rules or contracts for treatment that include such issues as the patient's responsibility for his or her safety. Psychotherapy for DID patients typically has several stages: an initial phase for uncovering and "mapping" the patient's alters; a phase of treating the traumatic memories and "fusing" the alters; and a phase of consolidating the patient's newly integrated personality.

Most therapists who treat multiples, or DID patients, recommend further treatment after personality integration, on the grounds that the patient has not learned the social skills that most people acquire in adolescence and early adult life. In addition, **family therapy** is often recommended to help the patient's family understand DID and the changes that occur during personality reintegration.

Many DID patients are helped by group as well as individual treatment, provided that the group is limited to people with dissociative disorders. DID patients sometimes have setbacks in mixed therapy groups because other patients are bothered or frightened by their personality switches.

Medications

Some doctors will prescribe tranquilizers or antidepressants for DID patients because their alter personalities may have **anxiety** or **mood disorders**. However, other therapists who treat DID patients prefer to keep medications to a minimum because these patients can easily become psychologically dependent on drugs. In addition, many DID patients have at least one alter who abuses drugs or alcohol, substances which are dangerous in combination with most tranquilizers.

Hypnosis

While not always necessary, hypnosis is a standard method of treatment for DID patients. Hypnosis may help patients recover repressed ideas and memories. Further, hypnosis can also be used to control problematic behaviors that many DID patients exhibit, such as **self-mutilation**, or eating disorders like **bulimia nervosa**. In the later stages of treatment, the therapist may use hypnosis to "fuse" the alters as part of the patient's personality integration process.

Alternative treatment

Alternative treatments that help to relax the body are often recommended for DID patients as an adjunct to psychotherapy and/or medication. These

KEY TERMS

Alter—An alternate or secondary personality in a patient with DID.

Amnesia—A general medical term for loss of memory that is not due to ordinary forgetfulness. Amnesia can be caused by head injuries, brain disease, or epilepsy as well as by dissociation.

Depersonalization—A dissociative symptom in which the patient feels that his or her body is unreal, is changing, or is dissolving.

Derealization—A dissociative symptom in which the external environment is perceived as unreal.

Dissociation—A psychological mechanism that allows the mind to split off traumatic memories or disturbing ideas from conscious awareness.

Dissociative identity disorder (DID)—Term that replaced Multiple Personality Disorder (MPD). A condition in which two or more distinctive identities or personality states alternate in controlling a person's consciousness and behavior.

Hypnosis—An induced trance state used to treat the amnesia and identity disturbances that occur in dissociative identity disorder (DID).

Multiple personality disorder (MPD)—The former, though often still used, term for dissociative identity disorder (DID).

Primary personality—The core personality of an DID patient. In women, the primary personality is often timid and passive, and may be diagnosed as depressed.

Trauma—A disastrous or life-threatening event that can cause severe emotional distress. DID is associated with trauma in a person's early life or adult experience.

treatments include **hydrotherapy**, botanical medicine (primarily herbs that help the nervous system), therapeutic massage, and **yoga**. Homeopathic treatment can also be effective for some people. **Art therapy** and the keeping of journals are often recommended as ways that patients can integrate their past into their present life. **Meditation** is usually discouraged until the patient's personality has been reintegrated.

Prognosis

Some therapists believe that the prognosis for recovery is excellent for children and good for most adults. Although treatment takes several years, it is often ultimately effective. As a general rule, the earlier the patient is diagnosed and properly treated, the better the prognosis.

Prevention

Prevention of DID requires intervention in abusive families and treating children with dissociative symptoms as early as possible.

Resources

BOOKS

Eisendrath, Stuart J. "Psychiatric Disorders." In *Current Medical Diagnosis and Treatment, 1998*, edited by Stephen McPhee, et al., 37th ed. Stamford: Appleton & Lange, 1997.

Rebecca J. Frey, PhD

Multiple pregnancy

Definition

Multiple **pregnancy** is a pregnancy where more than one fetus develops simultaneously in the womb.

Description

Twins happen naturally about one in every 100 births. There are two types of twinning—identical and fraternal. Identical twins represent the splitting of a single fertilized zygote (union of two gametes or male/female sex cells that produce a developing fetus) into two separate individuals. They usually, but not always, have identical genes. When they do not separate completely, the result is Siamese (or conjoined) twins. Fraternal twins are three times as common as identical twins. They occur when two eggs are fertilized by separate sperm. Each has a different selection of its parents' genes. The natural incidence of multiple pregnancy has been upset by advances in fertility treatments, resulting in higher rates of multiple births in the United States. All these children are fraternal; they each arose from a separate egg and a separate sperm. Cloning produces identical twins.

The human female is designed to release one egg every menstrual cycle. A hormone called progesterone, released by the first egg to be produced, prevents any other egg from maturing during that cycle. When this control fails, fertilization of more than one egg is

LOUIS GERALD KEITH (1935–)

Louis Gerald Keith and his twin brother, Donald, were born on April 24, 1935, to Russian immigrants. Although the boys received much attention due to their status as twins, their parents encouraged them to pursue their own goals, and at age twelve, Louis decided he wanted to become a doctor. After completing his bachelor of science degree at the University of Illinois, Keith entered the Chicago Medical school, graduating with his degree in 1960. He joined the U.S. Public Health Service and was stationed in Puerto Rico after completing his residency and internship at Cook County Hospital. Keith returned to Chicago after receiving his certification in obstetrics and gynecology in 1967 and worked as a professor and a physician.

Keith began his research on twins when a friend's twin brother died of lymphoma. The fact that Keith was a twin made his research more personally fulfilling and worthwhile to him. Keith and Donald founded the Center for the Study of Multiple Birth in 1977 located in Chicago. The center, a non-profit facility, was the first multiple birth research organization in the United States. Keith has delivered many speeches and has published various study results. In addition to books and scientific articles written individually and cooperatively, he was co-author of *Multiple Pregnancy: Epidemiology, Gestation and Prenatal Outcome* (1996) with his brother Donald, and others. He is currently the chief obstetrician at the Prentice Women's Hospital and Maternity Center in Chicago.

possible. Fertility drugs inhibit these controls, allowing multiple pregnancy to occur. Multiple pregnancy is more difficult and poses more health risks than single pregnancy. Premature birth is greater with each additional fetus.

The problem with multiple births is that there is only so much room in even the most accommodating womb (uterus). Babies need to reach a certain size and gestational age before they can survive outside the uterus. **Prematurity** is the constant threat of multiple pregnancies. Twins have five times the **death** rate of single births. Triplets and higher die even more often. The principle threat of prematurity is that the lungs are not fully developed. A disease called hyaline membrane disease afflicts premature infants. Their lungs do not stay open after their first breath because they lack a chemical called **surfactant**. Survival of premature infants was greatly improved when surfactant was finally synthesized in a form that could be of benefit to premature babies. Tiny babies also have trouble regulating their body temperature.

KEY TERMS

Amniotic membranes—A thin membrane surrounding the fetus and containing serous fluid.

Genes—Hereditary determinants of identifying characteristics.

Gestational—Refers to pregnancy.

Ovulate—To release a mature egg for fertilization.

Zygote—The earliest stage of a fertilized egg.

Causes and symptoms

Fertility drugs prevent the normal process of single ovulation by permitting more than one egg at a time to mature and ovulate (move from the ovary to the uterus in anticipation of fertilization). This happens naturally to produce fraternal twins. The first drug to accomplish this was clomiphene. Subsequently, two natural hormones—follicle stimulating hormone and chorionic gonadotrophin—were developed and used.

Diagnosis

Multiple pregnancies cause the uterus to grow faster than usual. Obstetricians can detect this unusually rapid growth as the pregnancy progresses. Before birth, an ultrasound will also detect multiple babies in the uterus. After birth, physical appearance or a careful examination of the placenta and amniotic membranes will usually reveal whether the babies were in the same water bag or separate ones. One bag means identical twins.

A multiple pregnancy almost always means increased monitoring and surveillance for complications. This often means more frequent visits to the healthcare provider, serial ultrasounds to make sure that the babies are growing adequately, **amniocentesis** to check for lung development, and close monitoring for preterm labor.

Treatment

Mothers may be put on bedrest during a multiple pregnancy, in order to try to try to prevent pre-term labor and delivery. If preterm labor is impossible to control at home, the mother may be hospitalized, and medication may be used to attempt to control contractions and dilatation of the cervix. Multiple pregnancies more often end in cesarean deliveries than singleton pregnancies.

Babies from multiple pregnancies are often born early, and may require longer-than-normal hospitalization. The babies may need assistance with breathing, careful control of body temperature within an

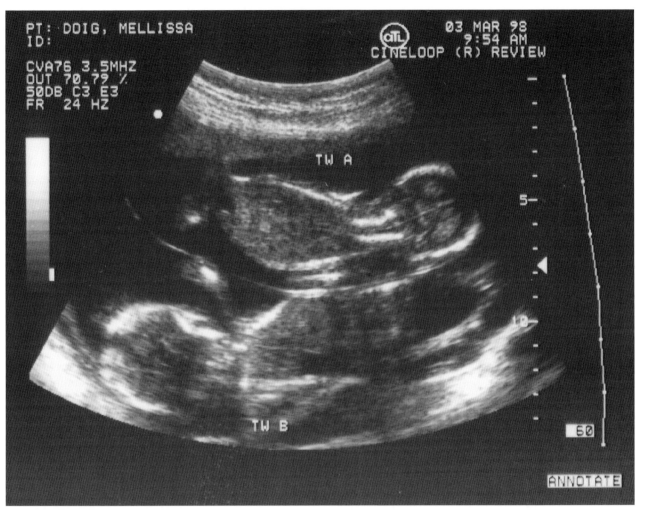

An ultrasound image of identical twin male fetuses. The distortion is due to "twin B" being closer to the monitor. *(Courtesy of Melissa Walsh Doig.)*

incubator, and surveillance for other complications that frequently beset pre-term babies. While premature babies are fragile in many other ways, modern methods of intensive care have successfully stabilized babies as small as one pound.

Alternative treatment

There are no specific treatments to alleviate medical difficulties caused by multiple pregnancies, however there are supportive measures that may help both mother and children recover from the birthing process. There are treatments to encourage breast milk production and to combat postpartum difficulties. Various homeopathic remedies and massage can be helpful to both mother and children during the early adjustment period after birth.

Prognosis

With modern medical advances and excellent prenatal care, many multiple pregnancies reach fruition without difficulties. If the babies are born prematurely, immediate medical care increases the chance of survival without any complications.

Resources

PERIODICALS

Evans, M.I., et al. "What Are the Ethical and Technical Problems Associated with Multifetal Pregnancy Reduction." *Clinical Obstetrics and Gynecology* 41 (March 1998): 46-54.

Rosalyn Carson-DeWitt, MD

Multiple sclerosis

Definition

Multiple sclerosis (MS) is a chronic autoimmune disorder affecting movement, ensation, and bodily functions. It is caused by destruction of the myelin insulation covering nerve fibers (neurons) in the central nervous system (brain and spinal cord).

Description

MS is a nerve disorder caused by destruction of the insulating layer surrounding neurons in the brain and spinal cord. This insulation, called myelin, helps electrical signals pass quickly and smoothly between the brain and the rest of the body. When the myelin is destroyed, nerve messages are sent more slowly and less efficiently. Patches of scar tissue, called plaques, form over the affected areas, further disrupting nerve communication. The symptoms of MS occur when the brain and spinal cord nerves no longer communicate properly with other parts of the body. MS causes a wide variety of symptoms and can affect vision, balance, strength, sensation, coordination, and bodily functions.

Multiple sclerosis affects more than a quarter of a million people in the United States. Most people have their first symptoms between the ages of 20 and 40; symptoms rarely begin before 15 or after 60. Women are almost twice as likely to get MS as men, especially in their early years. People of northern European heritage are more likely to be affected than people of other racial backgrounds, and MS rates are higher in the United States, Canada, and Northern Europe than in other parts of the world. MS is very rare among Asians, North and South American Indians, and Eskimos.

Causes and symptoms

Causes

Multiple sclerosis is an autoimmune disease, meaning its cause is an attack by the body's own immune system. For unknown reasons, immune cells attack and destroy the myelin sheath that insulates neurons in the brain and spinal cord. This myelin sheath, created by other brain cells called glia, speeds transmission and prevents electrical activity in one cell from short-circuiting to another cell. Disruption of communication between the brain and other parts of the body prevent normal passage of sensations and control messages, leading to the symptoms of MS.

The demyelinated areas appear as plaques, small round areas of gray neuron without the white myelin covering. The progression of symptoms in MS is correlated with development of new plaques in the portion of the brain or spinal cord controlling the affected areas. Because there appears to be no pattern in the appearance of new plaques, the progression of MS can be unpredictable.

Despite considerable research, the trigger for this autoimmune destruction is still unknown. At various times, evidence has pointed to genes, environmental factors, viruses, or a combination of these.

The risk of developing MS is higher if another family member is affected, suggesting the influence of genetic factors. In addition, the higher prevalence of MS among people of northern European background suggests some genetic susceptibility.

The role of an environmental factor is suggested by studies of the effect of migration on the risk of developing MS. Age plays an important role in determining this change in risk—young people in low-risk groups who move into countries with higher MS rates display the risk rates of their new surroundings, while older migrants retain the risk of their original home country. One interpretation of these studies is that an environmental factor, either protective or harmful, is acquired in early life; the risk of disease later in life reflects the effects of the early environment.

These same data can be used to support the involvement of a slow-acting virus, one that is acquired early on but begins its destructive effects much later. Slow viruses are known to cause other diseases, including **AIDS**. In addition, viruses have been implicated in other autoimmune diseases. Many claims have been made for the role of viruses, slow or otherwise, as the trigger for MS, but as of 2001 no strong candidate has emerged.

How a virus could trigger the autoimmune reaction is also unclear. There are two main models of virally induced autoimmunity. The first suggests the immune system is actually attacking a virus (one too well-hidden for detection in the laboratory), and the myelin damage is an unintentional consequence of fighting the infection. The second model suggests the immune system mistakes myelin for a viral protein, one it encountered during a prior infection. Primed for the attack, it destroys myelin because it resembles the previously-recognized viral invader.

Either of these models allows a role for genetic factors, since certain genes can increase the likelihood of autoimmunity. Environmental factors as well might change the sensitivity of the immune system or interact with myelin to provide the trigger for the secondary immune response. Possible environmental triggers that have been invoked in MS include viral infection, trauma, electrical injury, and chemical exposure, although controlled studies do not support a causative role.

Symptoms

The symptoms of multiple sclerosis may occur in one of three patterns:

- The most common pattern is the "relapsing-remitting" pattern, in which there are clearly defined symptomatic attacks lasting 24 hours or more, followed by complete or almost complete improvement. The period between attacks may be a year or more at the beginning of the disease, but may shrink to several months later on. This pattern is especially common in younger people who develop MS.

- In the "primary progressive" pattern, the disease progresses without remission or with occasional plateaus or slight improvements. This pattern is more common in older people.

- In the "secondary progressive" pattern, the person with MS begins with relapses and remissions, followed by more steady progression of symptoms.

Between 10–20% of people have a benign type of MS, meaning their symptoms progress very little over the course of their lives.

Because plaques may form in any part of the central nervous system, the symptoms of MS vary widely from person-to-person and from stage-to-stage of the disease. Initial symptoms often include:

- Muscle weakness, causing difficulty walking
- Loss of coordination or balance
- **Numbness**, "pins and needles," or other abnormal sensations
- Visual disturbances, including blurred or double vision.

Later symptoms may include:

- **Fatigue**
- Muscle spasticity and stiffness
- Tremors
- Paralysis
- **Pain**
- Vertigo
- Speech or swallowing difficulty
- Loss of bowel and bladder control
- Incontinence, **constipation**
- Sexual dysfunction
- Cognitive changes.

Weakness in one or both legs is common, and may be the first symptom noticed by a person with MS. Muscle spasticity, or excessive tightness, is also common and may be more disabling than weakness.

Double vision or eye tremor (**nystagmus**) may result from involvement of the nerve pathways controlling movement of the eye muscles. Visual disturbances result from involvement of the optic nerves (optic neutritis) and may include development of blind spots in one or both eyes, changes in color vision, or blindness. **Optic neuritis** usually involves only one eye at a time and is often associated with movement of the effected eye.

More than half of all people affected by MS have pain during the course of their disease, and many experience chronic pain, including pain from spasticity. Acute pain occurs in about 10% of cases. This pain may be a sharp, stabbing pain especially in the face, neck, or down the back. Facial numbness and weakness are also common.

Cognitive changes, including memory disturbances, depression, and personality changes, are found in people affected by MS, though it is not entirely clear whether these changes are due primarily to the disease or to the psychological reaction to it. Depression may be severe enough to require treatment in up to 25% of those with MS. A smaller number of people experience disease-related euphoria, or abnormally elevated mood, usually after a long disease duration and in combination with other psychological changes.

Symptoms of MS may be worsened by heat or increased body temperature, including **fever**, intense physical activity, or exposure to sun, hot baths, or showers.

Diagnosis

There is no single test that confirms the diagnosis of multiple sclerosis, and there are a number of other diseases with similar symptoms. While one person's diagnosis may be immediately suggested by her symptoms and history, another's may not be confirmed without multiple tests and prolonged observation. The distribution of symptoms is important: MS affects multiple areas of the body over time. The pattern of symptoms is also critical, especially evidence of the relapsing-remitting pattern, so a detailed medical history is one of the most important parts of the diagnostic process. A thorough search to exclude other causes of a patient's symptoms is especially important if the following features are present: 1) family history of neurologic disease, 2) symptoms and findings attributable to a single anatomic location, 3) persistent back pain, 4) age of onset over 60 or under 15 years of age, or 5) progressively worsening disease.

In addition to the medical history and a standard neurological exam, several lab tests are used to help confirm or rule out a diagnosis of MS:

- Magnetic resonance imaging (MRI) can reveal plaques on the brain and spinal cord. Gadolinium enhancement can distinguish between old and new plaques, allowing a correlation of new plaques with new symptoms. Plaques may be seen in several other diseases as well, including encephalomyelitis, neurosarcoidosis, and cerebral lupus. Plaques on MRI may be difficult to distinguish from small strokes, areas of decreased blood flow, or changes seen with trauma or normal **aging**.

- A lumbar puncture, or spinal tap, is done to measure levels of immune proteins, which are usually elevated in the cerebrospinal fluid of a person with MS. This test may not be necessary if other tests are diagnostic.

- Evoked potential tests, electrical tests of conduction speed in the nerves, can reveal reduced speeds consistent with the damage caused by plaques. These tests may be done with small electrical charges applied to the skin (somatosensory evoked potential), with light patterns flashed on the eyes (visual evoked potential), or with sounds presented to the ears (auditory evoked potential).

The clinician making the diagnosis, usually a neurologist, may classify the disease as "definite MS," meaning the symptoms and test results all point toward MS as the cause. "Probable MS" and "possible MS" reflect less certainty and may require more time to pass to observe the progression of the disease and the distribution of symptoms.

Treatment

The three major drugs previously approved for the treatment of MS affect the course of the disease. None of these drugs is a cure, but they can slow disease progression in many patients.

Known as the ABC drugs, Avonex and Betaseron are forms of the immune system protein beta interferon, while Copaxone is glatiramer acetate (formerly called copolymer-1). All three have been shown to reduce the rate of relapses in the relapsing-remitting form of MS. Different measurements from tests of each have demonstrated other benefits as well: Avonex may slow the progress of physical impairment, Betaseron may reduce the severity of symptoms,

and Copaxone may decrease disability. All three drugs are administered by injection

Two major clinical studies were recently completed that focused on the question of whether disease-modifying therapy known to slow the disease, can postpone the development of clinically definitive MS in high risk patients. Data presented at the annual meeting of the American Academy of Neurology in May, 2000, highlighted the different effects of interferon therapy when it was initiated at the earliest recognizable stages of MS versus later. Previous studies with interferon beta-1b (Betaseron) and interferon beta-1a (Avonex, Rebif) clearly demonstrated benefits in patients with relapsing forms of MS. Moreover, previous treatment with High-dose **corticosteroids** also delays, but does not prevent the ultimate development of MS. The encouraging message from the CHAMPS study in the United states and the ETOMS study in Europe is that early intervention can reduce the probability of developing clinically definitive MS.

Although the ABC drugs stop relapses and may keep patients in relatively good health for the short-term, their long-term success has not been proven and they don't work well for patients who have reached a steadily progressive stage of MS. In the meantime, new approaches to using current therapies are being researched especially using combinations of different types of agents when one agent alone is not effective. Clinical trials are now evaluating the safety and efficacy of combining cyclophosphamide (Cytoxan) and methylprednisolone (Medrol) in patients who do not respond to the ABC drus, and of adding mitoxantrone (Novantrone), prednisone (Prelone), azathioprine (Imuran), or methotrexate (Rheumatrex) to beta-interferon for further benefit.

In addition, Miloxzantrone HCI (novantrone), a drug approved for **cancer** treatment, has been approved for treating patients with advanced or chronic multiple sclereosis.In clinical trials, mitoxantrone reduced the number of relapse episodes and slowed down the disease. Reserved for progressive forms of MS, it is given intravenously by a doctor to help maintain mobility and reduce the number of flare-ups. However, there are serious side effects with the drug including heart problems, **nausea**, and hair thinning.

As reported in the Spring, 2001, Volume 19, No 2 issue of InsideMS, the FDA recently approved the Copaxone Autoject and the Mixject vial adapters to help people using Copaxone self administer the drug. The autoject keeps the syringe steady and hides the needle. The same syringe may be used for both mixing

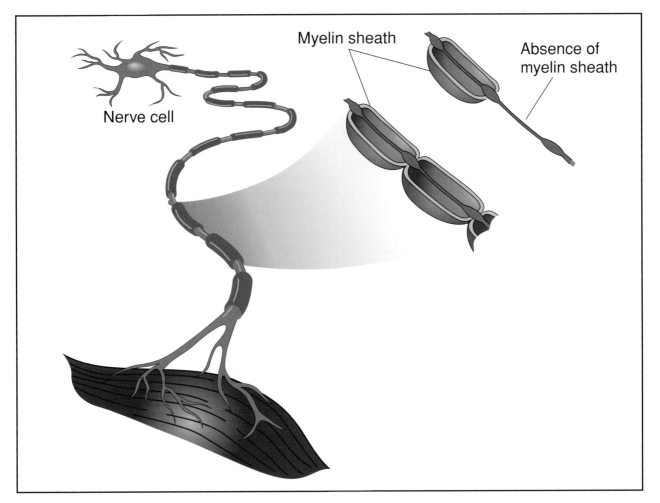

Nerve cell

Myelin sheath

Absence of myelin sheath

Multiple sclerosis (MS) is an autoimmune disease in which immune cells attack and destroy the myelin sheath which stimulates neurons in the brain and spinal cord. When the myelin is destroyed, nerve messages are sent more slowly and less efficiently. Scar tissue then forms over the affected areas, disrupting nerve communication. MS symptoms occur when the brain and spinal cord nerves cease to communicate properly with other parts of the body. *(Illustration by Electronic Illustrators Group.)*

and injecting with the Mixject vial adapters. A similar device is available for patients using Betassseron. Some patients are using the needlefree Biojector 2000 which uses a CO_2 cartridge to deliver doses of medication through the skin. The FDA has not approved its use and patients should discuss this with their physician for its use with either Copaxone or Betaseron. Avonex must be injected in the muscle.

Immunosuppressant drugs have been used for many years to treat acute exacerbations (relapses). Drugs used include corticosteroids such as prednisone and methylprednisone; the hormone adrenocorticotropic hormone (ACTH); and azathioprine. Recent studies indicate that several days of intravenous methylprednisone may be more effective than other immunosuppressant treatments for acute symptoms. This treatment may require hospitalization.

MS causes a large variety of symptoms, and the treatments for these are equally diverse. Most symptoms can be treated and complications avoided with good care and attention from medical professionals. Good health and **nutrition** remain important preventive measures. **Vaccination** against **influenza** can prevent respiratory complications, and contrary to earlier concerns, is not associated with worsening of symptoms. Preventing complications such as **pneumonia**, bed sores, injuries from falls, or urinary infection requires attention to the primary problems which may cause them. Shortened life spans with MS are almost always due to complications rather than primary symptoms themselves.

Physical therapy helps the person with MS to strengthen and retrain affected muscles; to maintain range of motion to prevent muscle stiffening; to learn to use assistive devices such as canes and walkers; and to learn safer and more energy-efficient ways of moving, sitting, and transferring. **Exercise** and stretching programs are usually designed by the physical therapist and taught to the patient and caregivers for use at home. Exercise is an important part of maintaining function for the person with MS. Swimming is often recommended, not only for its low-impact workout, but also because it allows strenuous activity without overheating.

Occupational therapy helps the person with MS adapt to her environment and adapt the environment to her. The occupational therapist suggests alternate strategies and assistive devices for activities of daily living, such as dressing, feeding, and washing, and evaluates the home and work environment for safety and efficiency improvements that may be made.

Training in bowel and bladder care may be needed to prevent or compensate for incontinence. If the urge to urinate becomes great before the bladder is full, some drugs may be helpful, including propantheline bromide (Probanthine), oxybutynin chloride (Ditropan), or imipramine (Tofranil). Baclofen (Lioresal) may relax the sphincter muscle, allowing full emptying. Intermittent catheterization is effective in controlling bladder dysfunction. In this technique, a catheter is used to periodically empty the bladder.

Spasticity can be treated with oral medications, including baclofen and diazepam (Valium), or by injection with botulinum toxin (Botox). Spasticity relief may also bring relief from chronic pain. Other more acute types of pain may respond to carbamazepine (Tegretol) or diphenylhydantoin (Dilantin). **Low back pain** is common from increased use of the back muscles to compensate for weakened legs. Physical therapy and over-the-counter pain relievers may help.

Fatigue may be partially avoidable with changes in the daily routine to allow more frequent rests. Amantadine (Symmetrel) and pemoline (Cylert) may improve alertness and lessen fatigue. Visual disturbances often respond to corticosteroids. Other symptoms that may be treated with drugs include seizures, vertigo, and tremor.

Myloral, an oral preparation of bovine myelin, has recently been tested in clinical trials for its effectiveness in reducing the frequency and severity of relapses. Preliminary data indicate no difference between it and placebo.

Alternative treatment

Bee venom has been suggested as a treatment for MS, but no studies or objective reports support this claim.

In British studies, **marijuana** has been shown to have variable effects on the symptoms of MS. Improvements have been documented for tremor, pain, and spasticity, and worsening for posture and balance. Side effects have included weakness, dizziness, relaxation, and incoordination, as well as euphoria. As a result, marijuana is not recommended as an alternative treatment.

Some studies support the value of high doses of **vitamins**, **minerals**, and other dietary supplements for controlling disease progression or improving symptoms. Alpha-linoleic and linoleic acids, as well as selenium and vitamin E, have shown effectiveness in the treatment of MS. The selenium and vitamin E act as antioxidants. In addition, the Swank diet (low in saturated fats), maintained over a long period of time, may retard the disease process.

Removal of mercury fillings has been touted as a possible cure, but is of no proven benefit.

Studies have also shown that t'ai chi can be an effective therapy for MS because it works to improve balance and increase strength.

There are conflicting views about **Echinacea** and its benefit to MS. Some medicine books recommend Echinacea for people with MS. However, Echinacea appears to stimulate different parts of the immune system, particularly immune cells known as macrophages. In MS these cells are very active already and further stimulation could worsen the disease.

Prognosis

It is difficult to predict how multiple sclerosis will progress in any one person. Most people with MS will be able to continue to walk and function at their work for many years after their diagnosis. The factors associated with the mildest course of MS are being female, having the relapsing-remitting form, having the first symptoms at a younger age, having longer periods of remission between relapses, and initial symptoms of decreased sensation or vision rather than of weakness or incoordination.

Less than 5% of people with MS have a severe progressive form, leading to **death** from complications within five years. At the other extreme, 10–20% have a benign form, with a very slow or no progression of their symptoms. The most recent studies show that

KEY TERMS

Clinical trial—All new drugs undergo clinical trials before approval. Clinical trials are carefully conducted tests in which effectiveness and side effects are studied, with the placebo effect eliminated.

Evoked potentials—Tests that measure the brain's electrical response to stimulation of sensory organs (eyes or ears) or peripheral nerves (skin). These tests may help confirm the diagnosis of multiple sclerosis.

Myelin—A layer of insulation that surrounds the nerve fibers in the brain and spinal cord.

Plaque—Patches of scar tissue that form where the layer of yelin covering the nerve fibers is destroyed by the multiple sclerosis disease process.

Primary progressive—A pattern of symptoms of multiple sclerosis in which the disease progresses without remission, or with occasional plateaus or slight improvements.

Relapsing-remitting—A pattern of symptoms of multiple sclerosis in which symptomatic attacks occur that last 24 hours or more, followed by complete or almost complete improvement.

Secondary progressive—A pattern of symptoms of multiple sclerosis in which there are relapses and remissions, followed by more steady progression of symptoms.

about seven out of 10 people with MS are still alive 25 years after their diagnosis, compared to about nine out of 10 people of similar age without disease. On average, MS shortens the lives of affected women by about six years, and men by 11 years. **Suicide** is a significant cause of death in MS, especially in younger patients.

The degree of disability a person experiences five years after onset is, on average, about three-quarters of the expected disability at 10–15 years. A benign course for the first five years usually indicates the disease will not cause marked disability.

Prevention

There is no known way to prevent multiple sclerosis. Until the cause of the disease is discovered, this is unlikely to change. Good nutrition; adequate rest; avoidance of **stress**, heat, and extreme physical exertion; and good bladder hygiene may improve quality of life and reduce symptoms.

Resources

BOOKS

Kraft, Georg H., and Marci Catanzaro. *Living with Multiple Sclerosis: A Wellness Approach.* Demos Medical Publishing, 2000.

Ruthan Brodsky

Mumps

Definition

Mumps is a relatively mild short-term viral infection of the salivary glands that usually occurs during childhood. Typically, mumps is characterized by a painful swelling of both cheek areas, although the person could have swelling on one side or no perceivable swelling at all. The salivary glands are also called the parotid glands, therefore, mumps is sometimes referred to as an inflammation of the parotid glands (epidemic parotitis). The word mumps comes from an old English dialect, meaning lumps or bumps within the cheeks.

Description

Mumps is a very contagious infection that spreads easily in such highly populated areas as day care centers and schools. Although not as contagious as **measles** or **chickenpox**, mumps was once quite common. Prior to the release of a mumps vaccine in the United States in 1967, approximately 92% of all children had been exposed to mumps by the age of 15. In these pre-vaccine years, most children contracted mumps between the ages of four and seven. Mumps epidemics came in two to five year cycles. The greatest mumps epidemic was in 1941 when approximately 250 cases were reported for every 100,000 people. In 1968, the year after the live mumps vaccine was released, only 76 cases were reported for every 100,000 people. By 1985, less than 3,000 cases of mumps were reported throughout the entire United States, which works out to about 1 case per 100,000 people. The reason for the decline in mumps was the increased usage of the mumps vaccine. However, 1987 noted a five-fold increase in the incidence of the disease because of the reluctance of some states to adopt comprehensive school immunization laws. Since then, state-enforced school entry requirements have achieved student immunization rates of nearly 100% in kindergarten and first grade. In 1996, the Centers for Disease

Control and Prevention (CDC) reported only 751 cases of mumps nationwide, or, in other words, about one case for every five million people.

Causes and symptoms

The paramyxovirus that causes mumps is harbored in the saliva and is spread by sneezing, coughing, and other direct contact with another person's infected saliva. Once the person is exposed to the virus, symptoms generally occur in 14-24 days. Initial symptoms include chills, **headache**, loss of appetite, and a lack of energy. However, an infected person may not experience these initial symptoms. Swelling of the salivary glands in the face (parotitis) generally occurs within 12-24 hours of the above symptoms. Accompanying the swollen glands is **pain** on chewing or swallowing, especially with acidic beverages, such as lemonade. A **fever** as high as 104°F (40°C) is also common. Swelling of the glands reaches a maximum on about the second day and usually disappears by the seventh day. Once a person has contracted mumps, they become immune to the disease, despite how mild or severe their symptoms may have been.

While the majority of cases of mumps are uncomplicated and pass without incident, some complications can occur. Complications are, however, more noticeable in adults who get the infection. In 15% of cases, the covering of the brain and spinal cord becomes inflamed (**meningitis**). Symptoms of meningitis usually develop within four or five days after the first signs of mumps. These symptoms include a stiff neck, headache, **vomiting**, and a lack of energy. Mumps meningitis is usually resolved within seven days, and damage to the brain is exceedingly rare.

The mumps infection can spread into the brain causing inflammation of the brain (**encephalitis**). Symptoms of mumps encephalitis include the inability to feel pain, seizures, and high fever. Encephalitis can occur during the parotitis stage or one to two weeks later. Recovery from mumps encephalitis is usually complete, although complications, such as seizure disorders, have been noted. Only about 1 in 100 with mumps encephalitis dies from the complication.

About one-quarter of all post-pubertal males who contract mumps can develop a swelling of the scrotum (**orchitis**) about seven days after the parotitis stage. Symptoms include marked swelling of one or both testicles, severe pain, fever, **nausea**, and headache. Pain and swelling usually subside after five to seven days, although the testicles can remain tender for weeks.

Girls occasionally suffer an inflammation of the ovaries, or oophoritis, as a complication of mumps, but this condition is far less painful than orchitis in boys.

As of late 2002, some researchers in Europe are studying the possibility that mumps increases a person's risk of developing inflammatory bowel disease (IBD) in later life. This hypothesis will require further research, as present findings are inconclusive.

Diagnosis

When mumps reaches epidemic proportions, diagnosis is relatively easy on the basis of the physical symptoms. The doctor will take the child's temperature, gently palpate (touch) the skin over the parotid glands, and look inside the child's mouth. If the child has mumps, the openings to the ducts inside the mouth will be slightly inflamed and have a "pouty" appearance. With so many people vaccinated today, a case of mumps must be properly diagnosed in the event the salivary glands are swollen for reasons other than viral infection. For example, in persons with poor **oral hygiene**, the salivary glands can be infected with bacteria. In these cases, **antibiotics** are necessary. Also in rare cases, the salivary glands can become blocked, develop tumors, or swell due to the use of certain drugs, such as iodine. A test can be performed to determine whether the person with swelling of the salivary glands actually has the mumps virus.

As of late 2002, researchers in London have reported the development of a bioassay for measuring mumps-specific IgG. This test would allow a doctor to check whether an individual patient is immune to mumps, and allow researchers to measure the susceptibility of a local population to mumps in areas with low rates of **vaccination**.

Treatment

When mumps does occurs, the illness is usually allowed to run its course. The symptoms, however, are treatable. Because of difficulty swallowing, the most important challenge is to keep the patient fed and hydrated. The individual should be provided a soft diet, consisting of cooked cereals, mashed potatoes, broth-based soups, prepared baby foods, or foods put through a home food processor. **Aspirin, acetaminophen**, or ibuprofen can relieve some of the pain due to swelling, headache, and fever. Avoid fruit juices and other acidic foods or beverages that can irritate the salivary glands. Avoid dairy products that can be hard to digest. In the event of complications, a physician

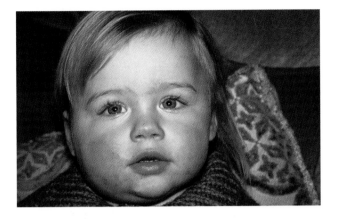

A young child with mumps. *(Photo Researchers. Reproduced by permission.)*

should be contacted at once. For example, if orchitis occurs, a physician should be called. Also, supporting the scrotum in a cotton bed on an adhesive-tape bridge between the thighs can minimize tension. Ice packs are also helpful.

Alternative treatment

Acupressure can be used effectively to relieve pain caused by swollen glands. The patient can, by using the middle fingers, gently press the area between the jawbone and the ear for two minutes while breathing deeply.

A number of homeopathic remedies can be used for the treatment of mumps. For example, belladonna may be useful for flushing, redness, and swelling. Bryonia (wild hops) may be useful for irritability, lack of energy, or thirst. Phytolacca (poke root) may be prescribed for extremely swollen glands. A homeopathic physician should always be consulted for appropriate doses for children, and remedies that do not work within one day should be stopped. A homeopathic preparation of the mumps virus can also be used prophylactically or as a treatment for the disease.

Several herbal remedies may be useful in helping the body recover from the infection or may help alleviate the discomfort associated with the disease. **Echinacea** (*Echinacea* spp.) can be used to boost the immune system and help the body fight the infection. Other herbs taken internally, such as cleavers (*Galium aparine*), calendula (*Calendula officinalis*), and phytolacca (poke root), target the lymphatic system and may help to enhance the activity of the body's internal filtration system. Since phytolacca can be toxic, it should only be used by patients under the care of a skilled practitioner. Topical applications are also useful in relieving the discomfort of mumps. A cloth dipped in a heated mixture of vinegar and cayenne (*Capsicum frutescens*) can be wrapped around the neck several times a day. Cleavers or calendula can also be combined with vinegar, heated, and applied in a similar manner.

Prognosis

When mumps is uncomplicated, prognosis is excellent. However, in rare cases, a relapse occurs after about two weeks. Complications can also delay complete recovery.

Prevention

A vaccine exists to protect against mumps. The vaccine preparation (MMR) is usually given as part of a combination injection that helps protect against measles, mumps, and **rubella**. MMR is a live vaccine administered in one dose between the ages of 12-15 months, 4-6 years, or 11-12 years. Persons who are unsure of their mumps history and/or mumps vaccination history should be vaccinated. Susceptible health care workers, especially those who work in hospitals, should be vaccinated. Because mumps is still prevalent throughout the world, susceptible persons over age one who are traveling abroad would benefit from receiving the mumps vaccine.

The mumps vaccine is extremely effective, and virtually everyone should be vaccinated against this disease. There are, however, a few reasons why people should *not* be vaccinated against mumps:

- Pregnant women who contract mumps during **pregnancy** have an increased rate of **miscarriage**, but not **birth defects**. As a result, pregnant women should not receive the mumps vaccine because of the possibility of damage to the fetus. Women who have had the vaccine should postpone pregnancy for three months after vaccination.

- Unvaccinated persons who have been exposed to mumps should not get the vaccine, as it may not provide protection. The person should, however, be vaccinated if no symptoms result from the exposure to mumps.

- Persons with minor fever-producing illnesses, such as an upper respiratory infection, should not get the vaccine until the illness has subsided.

- Because mumps vaccine is produced using eggs, individuals who develop **hives**, swelling of the mouth or throat, **dizziness**, or breathing difficulties after eating eggs should not receive the mumps vaccine.

KEY TERMS

Asymptomatic—Persons who carry a disease and may be capable of transmitting the disease but who do not exhibit symptoms of the disease are said to be asymptomatic.

Autism—A severe developmental disorder that usually begins before three years of age and affects a child's social as well as intellectual development. Some researchers theorized that immunization with the MMR vaccine was a risk factor for autism.

Encephalitis—Inflammation of the brain.

Epidemic parotitis—The medical name for mumps.

Immunoglobulin G (IgG)—A group of antibodies against certain viral infections that circulate in the bloodstream. One type of IgG is specific against the mumps paramyxovirus.

Meningitis—Inflammation of the membranes covering the brain and spinal cord.

Orchitis—Inflammation or swelling of the scrotal sac containing the testicles.

Paramyxovirus—A genus of viruses that includes the causative agent of mumps.

Parotitis—Inflammation and swelling of the salivary glands.

• Persons with immune deficiency diseases and/or those whose immunity has been suppressed with anti-cancer drugs, **corticosteroids**, or radiation should not receive the vaccine. Family members of immunocompromised people, however, should get vaccinated to reduce the risk of mumps.

• The CDC recommends that all children infected with human **immunodeficiency** disease (HIV) who are asymptomatic should receive an the MMR vaccine at 15 months of age.

The mumps vaccine has been controversial in recent years because of concern that its use was linked to a rise in the rate of childhood **autism**. The negative publicity given to the vaccine in the mass media led some parents to refuse to immunize their children with the MMR vaccine. One result has been an increase in the number of mumps outbreaks in several European countries, including Italy and the United Kingdom.

In the fall of 2002, the *New England Journal of Medicine* published a major Danish study disproving the hypothesis of a connection between the MMR vaccine and autism. A second study in Finland showed that the vaccine is not associated with aseptic meningitis or encephalitis as well as autism. Since these studies were published, American primary care physicians have once again reminded parents of the importance of immunizing their children against mumps and other childhood diseases.

Resources

BOOKS

Beers, Mark H., MD, and Robert Berkow, MD, editors. "Viral Infections: Mumps." Section 19, Chapter 265. In *The Merck Manual of Diagnosis and Therapy.* Whitehouse Station, NJ: Merck Research Laboratories, 2004.

PERIODICALS

Gabutti, G., M. C. Rota, S. Salmaso, et al. "Epidemiology of Measles, Mumps and Rubella in Italy." *Epidemiology and Infection* 129 (December 2002): 543–550.

Kimmel, S. R. "Vaccine Adverse Events: Separating Myth From Reality." *American Family Physician* 66 (December 1, 2002): 2113–2120.

Madsen, K. M., A. Hviid, M. Vestergaard, et al. "A Population-Based Study of Measles, Mumps, and Rubella Vaccination and Autism." *New England Journal of Medicine* 347 (November 7, 2002): 1477–1482.

Makela, A., J. P. Nuorti, and H. Peltola. "Neurologic Disorders After Measles-Mumps-Rubella Vaccination." *Pediatrics* 110 (November 2002): 957–963.

McKie, A., D. Samuel, B. Cohen, and N. A. Saunders. "A Quantitative Immuno-PCR Assay for the Detection of Mumps-Specific IgG." *Journal of Immunological Methods* 270 (December 1, 2002): 135–141.

Nielsen, S. E., O. H. Nielsen, B. Vainer, and M. H. Claesson. "Inflammatory Bowel Disease—Do Microorganisms Play a Role?" [in Danish] *Ugeskrift for laeger* 164 (December 9, 2002): 5947–5950.

Pugh, R. N., B. Akinosi, S. Pooransingh, et al. "An Outbreak of Mumps in the Metropolitan Area of Walsall, UK." *International Journal of Infectious Diseases* 6 (December 2002): 283–287.

ORGANIZATIONS

American Academy of Pediatrics (AAP). 141 Northwest Point Boulevard, Elk Grove Village, IL 60007. (847) 434-4000. <www.aap.org>.

Centers for Disease Control and Prevention. 1600 Clifton Rd., NE, Atlanta, GA 30333. (800) 311-3435, (404) 639-3311. <http://www.cdc.gov>.

Ron Gasbarro, PharmD
Rebecca J. Frey, PhD

Munchausen syndrome

Definition

Munchausen syndrome is a psychiatric disorder that causes an individual to self-inflict injury or illness or to fabricate symptoms of physical or mental illness, in order to receive medical care or hospitalization. In a variation of the disorder, Munchausen by proxy (MSBP), an individual, typically a mother, intentionally causes or fabricates illness in a child or other person under her care.

Description

Munchausen syndrome takes its name from Baron Karl Friederich von Munchausen, an 18th century German military man known for his tall tales. The disorder first appeared in psychiatric literature in the early 1950s when it was used to describe patients who sought hospitalization by inventing symptoms and complicated medical histories, and/or inducing illness and injury in themselves. Categorized as a factitious disorder (a disorder in which the physical or psychological symptoms are under voluntary control), Munchausen's syndrome seems to be motivated by a need to assume the role of a patient. Unlike **malingering**, there does not seem to be any clear secondary gain (e.g., money) in Munchausen syndrome.

Individuals with Munchausen by proxy syndrome use their child (or another dependent person) to fulfill their need to step into the patient role. The disorder most commonly victimizes children from birth to 8 years old. Parents with MSBP may only exaggerate or fabricate their child's symptoms, or they may deliberately induce symptoms through various methods, including **poisoning**, suffocation, **starvation**, or infecting the child's bloodstream.

Causes and symptoms

The exact cause of Munchausen syndrome is unknown. It has been theorized that Munchausen patients are motivated by a desire to be cared for, a need for attention, dependency, an ambivalence toward doctors, or a need to suffer. Factors that may predispose an individual to Munchausen's include a serious illness in childhood or an existing personality disorder.

The Munchausen patient presents a wide array of physical or psychiatric symptoms, usually limited only by their medical knowledge. Many Munchausen patients are very familiar with medical terminology

and symptoms. Some common complaints include fevers, **rashes**, abscesses, bleeding, and **vomiting**. Common Munchausen by proxy symptoms include apnea (cessation of breathing), **fever**, vomiting, and **diarrhea**. In both Munchausen and MSBP syndromes, the suspected illness does not respond to a normal course of treatment. Patients or parents may push for invasive diagnostic procedures and display an extraordinary depth of knowledge of medical procedures.

Diagnosis

Because Munchausen sufferers often go from doctor to doctor, gaining admission into many hospitals along the way, diagnosis can be difficult. They are typically detected rather than diagnosed. During a course of treatment, they may be discovered by a hospital employee who encountered them during a previous hospitalization. Their caregivers may also notice that symptoms such as high fever occur only when the patient is left unattended. Occasionally, unprescribed medication used to induce symptoms is found with the patient's belongings. When the patient is confronted, they often react with outrage and check out of the hospital to seek treatment at another facility with a new caregiver.

Treatment

There is no clearly effective treatment for Munchausen syndrome. Extensive psychotherapy may be helpful with some Munchausen patients. If Munchausen syndrome co-exists with other mental disorders, such as a personality disorder, the underlying disorder is typically treated first.

Prognosis

The infections and injuries Munchausen patients self-inflict can cause serious illness. Patients often undergo countless unnecessary surgeries throughout their lifetimes. In addition, because of their frequent hospitalizations, they have difficulty holding down a job. Further, their chronic health complaints may damage interpersonal relationships with family and friends. Children victimized by sufferers of MSBP are at a real risk for serious injury and possible **death**. Those who survive physically unscathed may suffer developmental problems later in life.

Prevention

Because the cause of Munchausen syndrome is unknown, formulating a prevention strategy is difficult. Some medical facilities and healthcare practitioners have attempted to limit hospital admissions for Munchausen patients by sharing medical records. While these attempts may curb the number of hospital admissions, they do not treat the underlying disorder and may endanger Munchausen sufferers that have made themselves critically ill and require treatment. Children who are found to be victims of persons with Munchausen by proxy syndrome should be immediately removed from the care of the abusing parent or guardian.

Resources

ORGANIZATIONS

American Psychiatric Association. 1400 K Street NW, Washington DC 20005. (888) 357-7924. < http://www.psych.org >.
American Psychological Association (APA). 750 First St. NE, Washington, DC 20002-4242. (202) 336-5700. < ttp://www.apa.org >.
National Alliance for the Mentally Ill (NAMI). Colonial Place Three, 2107 Wilson Blvd., Ste. 300, Arlington, VA 22201-3042. (800) 950-6264. < http://www.nami.org >.
National Institute of Mental Health. Mental Health Public Inquiries, 5600 Fishers Lane, Room 15C-05, Rockville, MD 20857. (888) 826-9438. < http://www.nimh.nih.gov >.

Paula Anne Ford-Martin

Mupirocin *see* **Antibiotics, topical**

Murine (endemic) typhus *see* **Typhus**

Muscle cramps *see* **Muscle spasms and cramps**

Muscle relaxants

Definition

Skeletal muscle relaxants are drugs that relax striated muscles (those that control the skeleton).

They are a separate class of drugs from the muscle relaxant drugs used during intubations and surgery to reduce the need for anesthesia and facilitate intubation.

Purpose

Skeletal muscle relaxants may be used for relief of spasticity in neuromuscular diseases, such as **multiple sclerosis**, as well as for **spinal cord injury** and **stroke**. They may also be used for **pain** relief in minor strain injuries and control of the muscle symptoms of **tetanus**. Dantrolene (Dantrium) has been used to prevent or treat malignant hyperthermia in surgery.

Description

Although the muscle relaxants may be divided into only two groups, centrally acting and peripherally acting, the centrally acting group, which appears to act on the central nervous system, contains 10 drugs which are chemically different, while only dantrolene has a direct action at the level of the nerve-muscle connection.

Baclofen (Lioresal) may be administered orally or intrathecally for control of spasticity due to neuromuscular disease.

Carisoprodol (Soma), chlorphenesin (Maolate), chlorzoxazone (Paraflex), cyclobenzaprine (Flexeril), diazepam (Valium), metaxalone (Skelaxin), methocarbamol (Robaxin), and orphenadrine (Norflex) are used primarily as an adjunct for rest in management of acute **muscle spasms** associated with **sprains**. Muscle relaxation may also be an adjunct to physical therapy in **rehabilitation** following stroke, spinal cord injury, or other musculoskeletal conditions.

Diazepam and methocarbamol are also used by injection for relief of tetanus.

Recommended dosage

Dose varies with the drug, route of administration, and purpose. There may be individual variations in absorption that require doses higher than those usually recommended, particularly with methocarbamol. Consult specific references for further information.

Precautions

All drugs in this class may cause **sedation**. Baclofen, when administered intrathecally, may cause severe central nervous system (CNS) depression with cardiovascular collapse and **respiratory failure**.

Diazepam may be addictive. It is a controlled substance under federal law.

Dantrolene has a potential for hepatotoxicity. The incidence of symptomatic hepatitis is dose related, but may occur even with a short period of doses at or above. Even short periods of doses at or above 800 mg per day greatly increases the risk of serious liver injury. Overt hepatitis has been most frequently observed between the third and twelfth months of therapy. Risk of hepatic injury appears to be greater in women, in patients over 35 years of age and in patients taking other medications in addition to dantrolene.

Tizanidine may cause low blood pressure, but this may be controlled by starting with a low dose and increasing it gradually. The drug may rarely cause liver damage.

Methocarbamol and chlorzoxazone may cause harmless color changes in urine—orange or reddish-purple with chlorzoxazone and purple, brown, or green with methocarbamol. The urine will return to its normal color when the patient stops taking the medicine.

Most drugs in this class are well tolerated.

Not all drugs in this group have been evaluated for safety in **pregnancy** and breast feeding.

Baclofen is pregnancy category C. It has caused fetal abnormalities in rats at doses 13 times above the human dose. Baclofen passes into breast milk, and breast feeding while taking baclofen is not recommended.

Diazepam is category D. All **benzodiazepines** cross the placenta. Although the drugs appear to be safe for use during the first trimester of pregnancy, use later in pregnancy may be associated with **cleft lip and palate**. Diazepam should not be taken while breast feeding. Infants who were breast fed while their mothers took diazepam were excessively sleepy and lethargic.

Dantrolene is category C. In animal studies it has reduced the rate of survival of the newborn when given in doses seven times the normal human dose. Mothers should not breast feed while receiving dantrolene.

Interactions

Skeletal muscle relaxants have many potential **drug interactions**. Individual references should be consulted.

Because these drugs cause sedation, they should be used with caution with other drugs that may also cause drowsiness.

KEY TERMS

Central nervous system—The brain and spinal cord.

Intrathecal—Introduced into or occurring in the space under the arachnoid membrane which covers the brain and spinal cord.

Pregnancy category—A system of classifying drugs according to their established risks for use during pregnancy. Category A: Controlled human studies have demonstrated no fetal risk. Category B: Animal studies indicate no fetal risk, but no human studies, or adverse effects in animals, but not in well-controlled human studies. Category C: No adequate human or animal studies, or adverse fetal effects in animal studies, but no available human data. Category D: Evidence of fetal risk, but benefits outweigh risks. Category X: Evidence of fetal risk. Risks outweigh any benefits.

Sedative—Medicine used to treat nervousness or restlessness.

Spasm—Sudden, involuntary tensing of a muscle or a group of muscles.

Tranquilizer (minor)—A drug that has a calming effect and is used to treat anxiety and emotional tension.

The activity of diazepam may be increased by drugs that inhibit its metabolism in the liver. These include: Cimetidine, oral contraceptives, Disulfiram, Fluoxetine, Isoniazid, Ketoconazole, Metoprolol, Propoxyphene, Propranolol, and Valproic acid.

Dantrolene may have an interaction with estrogens. Although no interaction has been demonstrated, the rate of liver damage in women over the age of 35 who were taking estrogens is higher than in other groups.

Samuel D. Uretsky, PharmD

Muscle spasms and cramps

Definition

Muscle spasms and cramps are spontaneous, often painful muscle contractions.

Description

Most people are familiar with the sudden **pain** of a muscle cramp. The rapid, uncontrolled contraction, or spasm, happens unexpectedly, with either no stimulation or some trivially small one. The muscle contraction and pain last for several minutes, and then slowly ease. Cramps may affect any muscle, but are most common in the calves, feet, and hands. While painful, they are harmless, and in most cases, not related to any underlying disorder. Nonetheless, cramps and spasms can be manifestations of many neurological or muscular diseases.

The terms cramp and spasm can be somewhat vague, and they are sometimes used to include types of abnormal muscle activity other than sudden painful contraction. These include stiffness at rest, slow muscle relaxation, and spontaneous contractions of a muscle at rest (fasciculation). Fasciculation is a type of painless muscle spasm, marked by rapid, uncoordinated contraction of many small muscle fibers. A critical part of diagnosis is to distinguish these different meanings and to allow the patient to describe the problem as precisely as possible.

Causes and symptoms

Causes

Normal voluntary muscle contraction begins when electrical signals are sent from the brain through the spinal cord along nerve cells called motor neurons. These include both the upper motor neurons within the brain and the lower motor neurons within the spinal cord and leading out to the muscle. At the muscle, chemicals released by the motor neuron stimulate the internal release of calcium ions from stores within the muscle cell. These calcium ions then interact with muscle proteins within the cell, causing the proteins (actin and myosin) to slide past one another. This motion pulls their fixed ends closer, thereby shortening the cell and, ultimately, the muscle itself. Recapture of calcium and unlinking of actin and myosin allows the muscle fiber to relax.

Abnormal contraction may be caused by abnormal activity at any stage in this process. Certain mechanisms within the brain and the rest of the central nervous system help regulate contraction. Interruption of these mechanisms can cause spasm. Motor neurons that are overly sensitive may fire below their normal thresholds. The muscle membrane itself may be over sensitive, causing contraction without stimulation. Calcium ions may not be recaptured quickly enough, causing prolonged contraction.

Interuption of brain mechanisms and overly sensitive motor neurons may result from damage to the nerve pathways. Possible causes include **stroke**, **multiple sclerosis**, **cerebral palsy**, neurodegenerative diseases, trauma, **spinal cord injury**, and nervous system poisons such as strychnine, **tetanus**, and certain insecticides. Nerve damage may lead to a prolonged or permanent muscle shortening called contracture.

Changes in muscle responsiveness may be due to or associated with:

- Prolonged **exercise**. Curiously, relaxation of a muscle actually requires energy to be expended. The energy is used to recapture calcium and to unlink actin and myosin. Normally, sensations of pain and **fatigue** signal that it is time to rest. Ignoring or overriding those warning signals can lead to such severe energy depletion that the muscle cannot be relaxed, causing a cramp. The familiar advice about not swimming after a heavy meal, when blood flow is directed away from the muscles, is intended to avoid this type of cramp. Rigor mortis, the stiffness of a corpse within the first 24 hours after **death**, is also due to this phenomenon.

- **Dehydration** and salt depletion. This may be brought on by protracted **vomiting** or **diarrhea**, or by copious sweating during prolonged exercise, especially in high temperatures. Loss of fluids and salts—especially sodium, potassium, magnesium, and calcium—can disrupt ion balances in both muscle and nerves. This can prevent them from responding and recovering normally, and can lead to cramp.

- Metabolic disorders that affect the energy supply in muscle. These are inherited diseases in which particular muscle enzymes are deficient. They include deficiencies of myophosphorylase (McArdle's disease), phosphorylase b kinase, phosphofructokinase, phosphoglycerate kinase, and lactate dehydrogenase.

- Myotonia. This causes stiffness due to delayed relaxation of the muscle, but does not cause the spontaneous contraction usually associated with cramps. However, many patients with myotonia do experience cramping from exercise. Symptoms of myotonia are often worse in the cold. Myotonias include **myotonic dystrophy**, myotonia congenita, paramyotonia congenita, and neuromyotonia.

Fasciculations may be due to fatigue, cold, medications, metabolic disorders, nerve damage, or neurodegenerative disease, including **amyotrophic lateral sclerosis**. Most people experience brief, mild fasciculations from time to time, usually in the calves.

Symptoms

The pain of a muscle cramp is intense, localized, and often debilitating Coming on quickly, it may last for minutes and fade gradually. **Contractures** develop more slowly, over days or weeks, and may be permanent if untreated. Fasciculations may occur at rest or after muscle contraction, and may last several minutes.

Diagnosis

Abnormal contractions are diagnosed through a careful medical history, physical and neurological examination, and **electromyography** of the affected muscles. Electromyography records electrical activity in the muscle during rest and movement.

Treatment

Most cases of simple cramps require no treatment other than patience and stretching. Gently and gradually stretching and massaging the affected muscle may ease the pain and hasten recovery.

More prolonged or regular cramps may be treated with drugs such as carbamazepine, phenytoin, or quinine. Fluid and salt replacement, either orally or intravenously, is used to treat dehydration. Treatment of underlying metabolic or neurologic disease, where possible, may help relieve symptoms.

Alternative treatment

Cramps may be treated or prevented with Gingko (*Ginkgo biloba*) or Japanese quince (*Chaenomeles speciosa*). Supplements of vitamin E, niacin, calcium, and magnesium may also help. Taken at bedtime, they may help to reduce the likelihood of night cramps.

Prognosis

Occasional cramps are common, and have no special medical significance.

Prevention

The likelihood of developing cramps may be reduced by eating a healthy diet with appropriate levels of **minerals**, and getting regular exercise to build up energy reserves in muscle. Avoiding exercising in extreme heat helps prevent heat cramps. Heat cramps can also be avoided by taking salt tablets and water before prolonged exercise in extreme heat. Taking a warm bath before bedtime may increase circulation to the legs and reduce the incidence of nighttime leg cramps.

Resources

BOOKS

Bradley, Walter G., et al. *Neurology in Clinical Practice.* 2nd ed. Woburn, MA: Butterworth-Heinemann, 1995.

Richard Robinson

Muscular dystrophy

Definition

Muscular dystrophy is the name for a group of inherited disorders in which strength and muscle bulk gradually decline. Nine types of muscular dystrophies are generally recognized.

Description

The muscular dystrophies include:

- Duchenne muscular dystrophy (DMD): DMD affects young boys, causing progressive muscle weakness, usually beginning in the legs. It is the most severe form of muscular dystrophy. DMD occurs in about 1 in 3,500 male births, and affects approximately 8,000 boys and young men in the United States. A milder form occurs in very few female carriers.

- Becker muscular dystrophy (BMD): BMD affects older boys and young men, following a milder course than DMD. BMD occurs in about 1 in 30,000 male births.

- Emery-Dreifuss muscular dystrophy (EDMD): EDMD affects young boys, causing **contractures** and weakness in the calves, weakness in the shoulders and upper arms, and problems in the way electrical impulses travel through the heart to make it beat (heart conduction defects). Fewer than 300 cases of EDMD have been identified.

- Limb-girdle muscular dystrophy (LGMD): LGMD begins in late childhood to early adulthood and affects both men and women, causing weakness in the muscles around the hips and shoulders. It is the most variable of the muscular dystrophies, and there are several different forms of the disease now recognized. Many people with suspected LGMD have probably been misdiagnosed in the past, and therefore the prevalence of the disease is difficult to estimate. The number of people affected in the United States may be in the low thousands.

- Facioscapulohumeral muscular dystrophy (FSH): FSH, also known as Landouzy-Dejerine disease, begins in late childhood to early adulthood and affects both men and women, causing weakness in the muscles of the face, shoulders, and upper arms. The hips and legs may also be affected. FSH occurs in about 1 out of every 20,000 people, and affects approximately 13,000 people in the United States.

- **Myotonic dystrophy**: also known as Steinert's disease, affects both men and women, causing generalized weakness first seen in the face, feet, and hands. It is accompanied by the inability to relax the affected muscles (myotonia). Symptoms may begin from birth through adulthood. It is the most common form of muscular dystrophy, affecting more than 30,000 people in the United States.

- Oculopharyngeal muscular dystrophy (OPMD): OPMD affects adults of both sexes, causing weakness in the eye muscles and throat. It is most common among French Canadian families in Quebec, and in Spanish-American families in the southwestern United States.

- Distal muscular dystrophy (DD): DD begins in middle age or later, causing weakness in the muscles of the feet and hands. It is most common in Sweden, and rare in other parts of the world.

- Congenital muscular dystrophy (CMD): CMD is present from birth, results in generalized weakness, and usually progresses slowly. A subtype, called Fukuyama CMD, also involves **mental retardation**. Both are rare; Fukuyama CMD is more common in Japan.

Causes and symptoms

Causes

Several of the muscular dystrophies, including DMD, BMD, CMD, and most forms of LGMD, are due to defects in the genes for a complex of muscle proteins. This complex spans the muscle cell membrane to unite a fibrous network on the interior of the cell with a fibrous network on the outside. Current theory holds that by linking these two networks, the complex acts as a "shock absorber," redistributing and evening out the forces generated by contraction of the muscle, thereby preventing rupture of the muscle membrane. Defects in the proteins of the complex lead to deterioration of the muscle. Symptoms of these diseases set in as the muscle gradually exhausts its ability to repair itself. Both DMD and BMD are caused by flaws in the gene for the protein called dystrophin. The flaw leading to DMD prevents the formation of any dystrophin, while that of BMD allows some protein to be made, accounting for the differences in severity and onset between the two diseases. Differences among the other diseases in the muscles involved and the ages of onset are less easily explained.

The causes of the other muscular dystrophies are not as well understood:

- One form of LGMD is caused by defects in the gene for a muscle enzyme, calpain. The relationship between this defect and the symptoms of the disease is unclear.

- EDMD is due to a defect in the gene for a protein called emerin, which is found in the membrane of a cell's nucleus, but whose exact function is unknown.

- Myotonic dystrophy is linked to gene defects for a protein that may control the flow of charged particles within muscle cells. This gene defect is called a triple repeat, meaning it contains extra triplets of DNA code. It is possible that this mutation affects nearby genes as well, and that the widespread symptoms of myotonic dystrophy are due to a range of genetic disruptions.

- The gene for OPMD appears to also be mutated with a triple repeat. The function of the affected protein may involve translation of genetic messages in a cell's nucleus.

- The cause of FSH is unknown. Although the genetic region responsible for it has been localized on its chromosome, the identity and function of the gene or genes involved had not been determined as of 1997.

- The gene responsible for DD has not yet been found.

Genetics and patterns of inheritance

The muscular dystrophies are genetic diseases, meaning they are caused by defects in genes. Genes, which are linked together on chromosomes, have two functions: They code for the production of proteins, and they are the material of inheritance. Parents pass along genes to their children, providing them with a complete set of instructions for making their own proteins.

Because both parents contribute genetic material to their offspring, each child carries two copies of almost every gene, one from each parent. For some diseases to occur, both copies must be flawed. Such diseases are called autosomal recessive diseases. Some forms of LGMD and DD exhibit this pattern of inheritance, as does CMD. A person with only one flawed copy, called a carrier, will not have the disease, but may pass the flawed gene on to his children. When two carriers have children, the chances of having a child with the disease is one in four for each **pregnancy**.

Other diseases occur when only one flawed gene copy is present. Such diseases are called autosomal dominant diseases. Other forms of LGMD exhibit this pattern of inheritance, as do DM, FSH, OPMD, and some forms of DD. When a person affected by the disease has a child with someone not affected, the chances of having an affected child is one in two.

Because of chromosomal differences between the sexes, some genes are not present in two copies. The chromosomes that determine whether a person is male or female are called the X and Y chromosomes. A person with two X chromosomes is female, while a person with one X and one Y is male. While the X chromosome carries many genes, the Y chromosome carries almost none. Therefore, a male has only one copy of each gene on the X chromosome, and if it is flawed, he will have the disease that defect causes. Such diseases are said to be X-linked. X-linked diseases include DMD, BMD, and EDMD. Women aren't usually affected by X-linked diseases, since they will likely have one unaffected copy between the two chromosomes. Some female carriers of DMD suffer a mild form of the disease, probably because their one unaffected gene copy is shut down in some of their cells.

Women carriers of X-linked diseases have a one in two chance of passing the flawed gene on to each child born. Daughters who inherit the disease gene will be carriers. A son born without the disease gene will be free of the disease and cannot pass it on to his children. A son born with the defect will have the disease. He will pass the flawed gene on to each of his daughters, who will then be carriers, but to none of his sons (because they inherit his Y chromosome).

Not all genetic flaws are inherited. As many as one third of the cases of DMD are due to new mutations that arise during egg formation in the mother. New mutations are less common in other forms of muscular dystrophy.

Symptoms

All of the muscular dystrophies are marked by muscle weakness as the major symptom. The distribution of symptoms, age of onset, and progression differ significantly. **Pain** is sometimes a symptom of each, usually due to the effects of weakness on joint position.

DMD. A boy with Duchenne muscular dystrophy usually begins to show symptoms as a pre-schooler. The legs are affected first, making walking difficult and causing balance problems. Most patients walk three to six months later than expected and have difficulty running. Later on, the boy with DMD will push his hands against his knees to rise to a standing position, to compensate for leg weakness. About the same time, his calves will begin to swell, though with fibrous tissue rather than with muscle, and feel firm and rubbery; this condition gives DMD one of its alternate names, pseudohypertrophic muscular dystrophy. He will widen his stance to maintain balance, and walk with a waddling gait to advance his weakened legs. Contractures (permanent muscle tightening) usually begin by age five or six, most severely in the calf muscles. This pulls the foot down and back, forcing the boy to walk on tip-toes, called equinus, and further decreases balance. Frequent falls and broken bones are common beginning at this age. Climbing stairs and rising unaided may become impossible by age nine or ten, and most boys use a wheelchair for mobility by the age of 12. Weakening of the trunk muscles around this age often leads to **scoliosis** (a side-to-side spine curvature) and **kyphosis** (a front-to-back curvature).

The most serious weakness of DMD is weakness of the diaphragm, the sheet of muscles at the top of the abdomen that perform the main work of breathing and coughing. Diaphragm weakness leads to reduced energy and stamina, and increased lung infection because of the inability to **cough** effectively. Young men with DMD often live into their twenties and beyond, provided they have mechanical ventilation assistance and good respiratory hygiene.

About one third of boys with DMD experience specific learning disabilities, including trouble learning by ear rather than by sight and trouble paying attention to long lists of instructions. Individualized educational programs usually compensate well for these disabilities.

BMD. The symptoms of BMD usually appear in late childhood to early adulthood. Though the progression of symptoms may parallel that of DMD, the symptoms are usually milder and the course more variable. The same pattern of leg weakness, unsteadiness, and contractures occur later for the young man with BMD, often allowing independent walking into the twenties or early thirties. Scoliosis may occur, but is usually milder and progresses more slowly. Heart muscle disease (**cardiomyopathy**), occurs more commonly in BMD. Problems may include irregular heartbeats (**arrhythmias**) and congestive **heart failure**. Symptoms may include **fatigue**, **shortness of breath**, chest pain, and **dizziness**. Respiratory weakness also occurs, and may lead to the need for mechanical ventilation.

EDMD. This type of muscular dystrophy usually begins in early childhood, often with contractures preceding muscle weakness. Weakness affects the shoulder and upper arm originally, along with the calf muscles, leading to foot-drop. Most men with EDMD survive into middle age, although a defect in the heart's rhythm (**heart block**) may be fatal if not treated with a pacemaker.

LGMD. While there are at least a half-dozen genes that cause the various types of LGMD, two major clinical forms of LGMD are usually recognized. A severe childhood form is similar in appearance to DMD, but is inherited as an autosomal recessive trait. Symptoms of adult-onset LGMD usually appear in a person's teens or twenties, and are marked by progressive weakness and wasting of the muscles closest to the trunk. Contractures may occur, and the ability to walk is usually lost about 20 years after onset. Some people with LGMD develop respiratory weakness that requires use of a ventilator. Lifespan may be somewhat shortened. (Autosomal dominant forms usually occur later in life and progress relatively slowly.)

FSH. FSH varies in its severity and age of onset, even among members of the same family. Symptoms most commonly begin in the teens or early twenties, though infant or childhood onset is possible. Symptoms tend to be more severe in those with earlier onset. The disease is named for the regions of the body most severely affected by the disease: muscles of the face (facio-), shoulders (scapulo-), and upper arms (humeral). Hips and legs may be affected as well. Children with FSH often develop partial or complete deafness.

The first symptom noticed is often difficulty lifting objects above the shoulders. The weakness may be greater on one side than the other. Shoulder weakness also causes the shoulder blades to jut backward, called scapular winging. Muscles in the upper arm often lose bulk sooner than those of the forearm, giving a "Popeye" appearance to the arms. Facial weakness may lead to loss of facial expression, difficulty closing the eyes completely, and inability to drink through a straw, blow up a balloon, or whistle. A person with FSH may not develop strong facial wrinkles. Contracture of the calf muscles may cause foot-drop, leading to frequent tripping over curbs or rough spots. People with earlier onset often require a wheelchair for mobility, while those with later onset rarely do.

MYOTONIC DYSTROPHY. Symptoms of Myotonic dystrophy include facial weakness and a slack jaw, drooping eyelids (**ptosis**), and muscle wasting in the forearms and calves. A person with this dystrophy has difficulty relaxing his grasp, especially if the object is cold. Myotonic dystrophy affects heart muscle, causing arrhythmias and heart block, and the muscles of the digestive system, leading to motility disorders and **constipation**. Other body systems are affected as well: Myotonic dystrophy may cause **cataracts**, retinal degeneration, low IQ, frontal balding, skin disorders, testicular atrophy, **sleep apnea**, and **insulin resistance**. An increased need or desire for sleep is common, as is diminished motivation. Severe disability affects most people with this type of dystrophy within 20 years of onset, although most do not require a wheelchair even late in life.

OPMD. OPMD usually begins in a person's thirties or forties, with weakness in the muscles controlling the eyes and throat. Symptoms include drooping eyelids, difficulty swallowing (dysphagia), and weakness progresses to other muscles of the face, neck, and occasionally the upper limbs. Swallowing difficulty may cause aspiration, or the introduction of food or saliva into the airways. **Pneumonia** may follow.

DD. DD usually begins in the twenties or thirties, with weakness in the hands, forearms, and lower legs. Difficulty with fine movements such as typing or fastening buttons may be the first symptoms. Symptoms progress slowly, and the disease usually does not affect life span.

CMD. CMD is marked by severe muscle weakness from birth, with infants displaying "floppiness" and very little voluntary movement. Nonetheless, a child with CMD may learn to walk, either with or without some assistive device, and live into young adulthood or beyond. In contrast, children with Fukuyama CMD are rarely able to walk, and have severe mental retardation. Most children with this type of CMD die in childhood.

Diagnosis

Diagnosis of muscular dystrophy involves a careful medical history and a thorough physical exam to determine the distribution of symptoms and to rule out other causes. Family history may give important clues, since all the muscular dystrophies are genetic conditions (though no family history will be evident in the event of new mutations).

Lab tests may include:

- Blood level of the muscle enzyme creatine kinase (CK). CK levels rise in the blood due to muscle damage, and may be seen in some conditions even before symptoms appear.

- Muscle biopsy, in which a small piece of muscle tissue is removed for microscopic examination. Changes in the structure of muscle cells and presence of fibrous tissue or other aberrant structures are characteristic of different forms of muscular dystrophy. The muscle tissue can also be stained to detect the presence or absence of particular proteins, including dystrophin.

- Electromyogram (EMG). This electrical test is used to examine the response of the muscles to stimulation. Decreased response is seen in muscular dystrophy. Other characteristic changes are seen in DM.

- Genetic tests. Several of the muscular dystrophies can be positively identified by testing for the presence of the mutated gene involved. Accurate genetic tests are available for DMD, BMD, DM, several forms of LGMD, and EDMD.

- Other specific tests as necessary. For EDMD and BMD, for example, an electrocardiogram may be needed to test heart function, and hearing tests are performed for children with FSH.

For most forms of muscular dystrophy, accurate diagnosis is not difficult when done by someone familiar with the range of diseases. There are exceptions, however. Even with a muscle biopsy, it may be difficult to distinguish between FSH and another muscle disease, **polymyositis**. Childhood-onset LGMD is often mistaken for the much more common DMD, especially when it occurs in boys. BMD with an early onset appears very similar to DMD, and a genetic test may be needed to accurately distinguish them. The muscular dystrophies may be confused with diseases involving the motor neurons, such as spinal muscular atrophy; diseases of the neuromuscular junction, such as **myasthenia gravis**; and other muscle diseases, as all involve generalized weakening of varying distribution.

Treatment

Drugs

There are no cures for any of the muscular dystrophies. Prednisone, a corticosteroid, has been shown to delay the progression of DMD somewhat, for reasons that are still unclear. Prednisone is also prescribed for BMD, though no controlled studies have tested its benefit. A related drug, deflazacort, appears to have similar benefits with fewer side effects. It is available and is prescribed in Canada and Mexico, but is unavailable in the United States. Albuterol, an adrenergic agonist, has shown some promise for FSH in small trials; larger trials are scheduled for 1998. No other drugs are currently known to have an effect on the course of any other muscular dystrophy.

Treatment of muscular dystrophy is mainly directed at preventing the complications of weakness, including decreased mobility and dexterity, contractures, scoliosis, heart defects, and respiratory insufficiency.

Physical therapy

Physical therapy, in particular regular stretching, is used to maintain the range of motion of affected muscles and to prevent or delay contractures. Braces are used as well, especially on the ankles and feet to prevent equinus. Full-leg braces may be used in DMD to prolong the period of independent walking. Strengthening other muscle groups to compensate for weakness may be possible if the affected muscles are few and isolated, as in the earlier stages of the milder muscular dystrophies. Regular, nonstrenuous **exercise** helps maintain general good health. Strenuous exercise is usually not recommended, since it may damage muscles further.

Surgery

When contractures become more pronounced, tenotomy surgery may be performed. In this operation, the tendon of the contractured muscle is cut, and the limb is braced in its normal resting position while the tendon regrows. In FSH, surgical fixation of the scapula can help compensate for shoulder weakness. For a person with OPMD, surgical lifting of the eyelids may help compensate for weakened muscular control. For a person with DM, sleep apnea may be treated surgically to maintain an open airway. Scoliosis surgery is often needed in DMD, but much less often in other muscular dystrophies. Surgery is recommended at a much lower degree of curvature for DMD than for scoliosis due to other conditions, since the decline in respiratory function in DMD makes surgery at a later time dangerous.

In this surgery, the vertebrae are fused together to maintain the spine in the upright position. Steel rods are inserted at the time of operation to keep the spine rigid while the bones grow together.

When any type of surgery is performed in patients with muscular dystrophy, anesthesia must be carefully selected. People with MD are susceptible to a severe reaction, known as malignant hyperthermia, when given halothane anesthetic.

Occupational therapy

The occupational therapist suggests techniques and tools to compensate for the loss of strength and dexterity. Strategies may include modifications in the home, adaptive utensils and dressing aids, compensatory movements and positioning, wheelchair accessories, or communication aids.

Nutrition

Good **nutrition** helps to promote general health in all the muscular dystrophies. No special diet or supplement has been shown to be of use in any of the conditions. The weakness in the throat muscles seen especially in OPMD and later DMD may necessitate the use of a **gastrostomy** tube, inserted in the stomach to provide nutrition directly.

Cardiac care

The arrhythmias of EDMD and BMD may be treatable with antiarrhythmia drugs such as mexiletine or nifedipine. A pacemaker may be implanted if these do not provide adequate control. Heart transplants are increasingly common for men with BMD.

Respiratory care

People who develop weakness of the diaphragm or other ventilatory muscles may require a mechanical ventilator to continue breathing deeply enough. Air may be administered through a nasal mask or mouthpiece, or through a tracheostomy tube, which is inserted through a surgical incision through the neck and into the windpipe. Most people with muscular dystrophy do not need a tracheostomy, although some may prefer it to continual use of a mask or mouthpiece. Supplemental oxygen is not needed. Good hygiene of the lungs is critical for health and longterm survival of a person with weakened ventilatory muscles. Assisted cough techniques provide the strength needed to clear the airways of secretions; an assisted cough machine is also available and provides excellent results.

Experimental treatments

Two experimental procedures aiming to cure DMD have attracted a great deal of attention in the past decade. In myoblast transfer, millions of immature muscle cells are injected into an affected muscle. The goal of the treatment is to promote the growth of the injected cells, replacing the defective host cells with healthy new ones. Despite continued claims to the contrary by a very few researchers, this procedure is widely judged a failure. Modifications in the technique may change that in the future.

Gene therapy introduces good copies of the dystrophin gene into muscle cells. The goal is to allow the existing muscle cells to use the new gene to produce the dystrophin it cannot make with its flawed gene. Problems have included immune rejection of the virus used to introduce the gene, loss of gene function after several weeks, and an inability to get the gene to enough cells to make a functional difference in the affected muscle. Nonetheless, after a number of years of refining the techniques in mice, researchers are beginning human trials in 1998.

Prognosis

The expected lifespan for a male with DMD has increased significantly in the past two decades. Most young men will live into their early or mid-twenties. Respiratory infections become an increasing problem as their breathing becomes weaker, and these infections are usually the cause of **death**.

The course of the other muscular dystrophies is more variable; expected life spans and degrees of disability are hard to predict, but may be related to age of onset and initial symptoms. Prediction is made more difficult because, as new genes are discovered, it is becoming clear that several of the dystrophies are not uniform disorders, but rather symptom groups caused by different genes.

People with dystrophies with significant heart involvement (BMD, EDMD, Myotonic dystrophy) may nonetheless have almost normal life spans, provided that cardiac complications are monitored and treated aggressively. The respiratory involvement of BMD and LGMD similarly require careful and prompt treatment.

Prevention

There is no way to prevent any of the muscular dystrophies in a person who has the genes responsible for these disorders. Accurate genetic tests, including

KEY TERMS

Autosomal dominant—Diseases that occur when a person inherits only one flawed copy of the gene.

Autosomal recessive —Diseases that occur when a person inherits two flawed copies of a gene—one from each parent.

Becker muscular dystrophy (BMD)—A type of muscular dystrophy that affects older boys and men, and usually follows a milder course than DMD.

Contractures—A permanent shortening (as of muscle, tendon, or scar tissue) producing deformity or distortion.

Distal muscular dystrophy (DD)—A form of muscular dystrophy that usually begins in middle age or later, causing weakness in the muscles of the feet and hands.

Duchenne muscular dystrophy (DMD)—The most severe form of muscular dystrophy, DMD usually affects young boys and causes progressive muscle weakness, usually beginning in the legs.

Dystrophin—A protein that helps muscle tissue repair itself. Both DMD and BMD are caused by flaws in the gene that instructs the body how to make this protein.

Facioscapulohumeral muscular dystrophy (FSH)—This form of muscular dystrophy, also known as Landouzy-Dejerine disease, begins in late childhood to early adulthood and affects both men and women, causing weakness in the muscles of the face, shoulders, and upper arms.

Limb-girdle muscular dystrophy (LGMD)—This form of muscular dystrophy begins in late childhood to early adulthood and affects both men and women, causing weakness in the muscles around the hips and shoulders.

Myotonic dystrophy—This type of muscular dystrophy, also known as Steinert's disease, affects both men and women, causing generalized weakness first seen in the face, feet, and hands. It is accompanied by the inability to relax the affected muscles (myotonia).

Oculopharyngeal muscular dystrophy (OPMD)—This type of muscular dystrophy affects adults of both sexes, causing weakness in the eye muscles and throat.

prenatal tests, are available for some of the muscular dystrophies. Results of these tests may be useful for purposes of family planning.

Resources

ORGANIZATIONS

Muscular Dystrophy Association. 3300 East Sunrise Drive, Tucson, AZ 85718. (800) 572-1717. <http://www.mdausa.org>.

Richard Robinson

Mushroom poisoning

Definition

Mushroom **poisoning** refers to the severe and often deadly effects of various toxins that are found in certain types of mushrooms. One type known as *Amanita phalloides*, appropriately called "death cap," accounts for the majority of cases. The toxins initially cause severe abdominal cramping, **vomiting**, and watery **diarrhea**, and then lead to liver and kidney failure.

Description

The highest reported incidences of mushroom poisoning occur in western Europe, where a popular pastime is amateur mushroom hunting. Since the 1970s, the United States has seen a marked increase in mushroom poisoning due to an increase in the popularity of "natural" foods, the use of mushrooms as recreational hallucinogens, and the gourmet qualities of wild mushrooms. About 90% of the deaths due to mushroom poisoning in the United States and western Europe result from eating *Amanita phalloides*. This mushroom is recognized by its metallic green cap (the color may vary from light yellow to greenish brown), white gills (located under the cap), white stem, and bulb-shaped structure at the base of the stem. A pure white variety of this species also occurs. Poisoning results from ingestion of as few as one to three mushrooms. Higher **death** (mortality) rates of more than 50% occur in children less than 10 years of age.

Causes and symptoms

Poisonous mushrooms contain at least two different types of toxins, each of which can cause death if taken in large enough quantities. Some of the toxins found in poisonous mushrooms are among the most potent ever discovered. One group of poisons, known as amatoxins, blocks the production of DNA, the basis of cell reproduction. This leads to the death of many cells, especially those that reproduce frequently such as in the liver, intestines, and kidney. Other mushroom poisons affect the proteins needed for muscle contraction, and therefore reduce the ability of certain muscle groups to perform.

Symptoms of *Amanita* poisoning occur in different stages or phases. These include:

- First phase. Abdominal cramping, **nausea**, vomiting, and severe watery diarrhea occur anywhere from 6-24 hours after eating the mushroom and last for about 24 hours. These intestinal symptoms can lead to **dehydration** and low blood pressure (hypotension).

- Second phase. A period of remission of symptoms that lasts 1-2 days. During this time, the patient feels better, but blood tests begin to show evidence of liver and kidney damage.

- Third phase. Liver and kidney failure develop at this point and either lead to death within about a week or recovery within 2-3 weeks.

Other symptoms are due to either a decrease in blood clotting factors that leads to internal bleeding or reduced muscle function, with the development of weakness and **paralysis**.

Diagnosis

In most cases, the fact that the patient has recently eaten wild mushrooms is the clue to the cause of symptoms. Moreover, the identification of any remaining mushrooms by a qualified mushroom specialist (mycologist) can be a key to diagnosis. When in doubt, the toxin known as alpha-amantin can be found in the blood, urine, or stomach contents of an individual who has ingested poisonous *Amanita* mushrooms.

Treatment

It is important to remember that there is no specific antidote for mushroom poisoning. However, several advances in therapy have decreased the death rate over the last several years. Early replacement of lost body fluids has been a major factor in improving survival rates.

Therapy is aimed at decreasing the amount of toxin in the body. Initially, attempts are made to remove toxins from the upper gastrointestinal tract by inducing vomiting or by gastric lavage (stomach

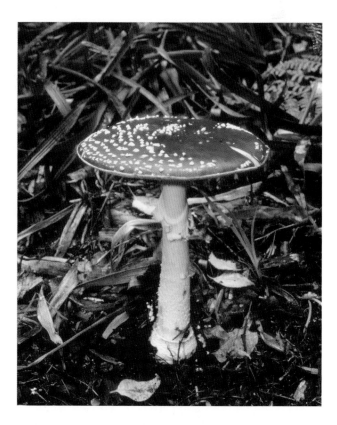

A poisonous mushroom, *Amanita muscaria* *(Photo Researchers. Reproduced by permission.)*

pumping). After that continuous aspiration of the upper portion of the small intestine through a nasogastric tube is done and oral charcoal (every four hours for 48 hours) is given to prevent absorption of toxin. These measures work best if started within six hours of ingestion.

In the United States, early removal of mushroom poison by way of an artificial kidney machine (dialysis) has become part of the treatment program. This is combined with the correction of any imbalances of salts (electrolytes) dissolved in the blood, such as sodium or potassium. An enzyme called thioctic acid and **corticosteroids** also appear to be beneficial, as well as high doses of penicillin. In Europe, a chemical taken from the milk thistle plant, *Silybum marianum* , is also part of treatment. When liver failure develops, **liver transplantation** may be the only treatment option.

Prognosis

The mortality rate has decreased with improved and rapid treatment. However, according to some medical reports death still occurs in 20-30% of cases, with a higher mortality rate of 50% in children less than 10 years old.

Prevention

The most important factor in preventing mushroom poisoning is to avoid eating wild or noncultivated mushrooms. For anyone not expert in mushroom identification, there are generally no easily recognizable differences between nonpoisonous and poisonous mushrooms. It is also important to remember that most mushroom poisons are not destroyed or deactivated by cooking, canning, freezing, drying, or other means of food preparation.

Resources

OTHER

"Alerts from the CDC." *Experience Lab Page.* < http://www.medsitenavigator.com >.

"Cyclopeptide-Containing Mushroom Toxicity." *The Toxikon Multimedia Project Page.* < http://www.uic.edu/com/er/toxikon/mushroo.htm >.

"Mushroom Poisoning in Children." *American Association of Family Physicians.* < http://www.aafp.org/patient-info/mushroom.html >.

Mushroom Toxins from the FDA. < http://vm.cfsan.fda.gov/~mow/chap40.html >.

David Kaminstein, MD

Music therapy

Definition

Music therapy is a technique of complementary medicine that uses music prescribed in a skilled manner by trained therapists. Programs are designed to help patients overcome physical, emotional, intellectual, and social challenges. Applications range from improving the well being of geriatric patients in nursing homes to lowering the **stress** level and **pain** of women in labor. Music therapy is used in many settings, including schools, **rehabilitation** centers, hospitals, hospice, nursing homes, community centers, and sometimes even in the home.

Purpose

Music can be beneficial for anyone. Although it can be used therapeutically for people who have physical, emotional, social, or cognitive deficits, even those who are healthy can use music to relax, reduce stress, improve mood, or to accompany **exercise**.

There are no potentially harmful or toxic effects. Music therapists help their patients achieve a number of goals through music, including improvement of communication, academic strengths, attention span, and motor skills. They may also assist with behavioral therapy and **pain management**.

Physical effects

Brain function physically changes in response to music. The rhythm can guide the body into breathing in slower, deeper patterns that have a calming effect. Heart rate and blood pressure are also responsive to the types of music that are listened to. The speed of the heartbeat tends to speed or slow depending on the volume and speed of the auditory stimulus. Louder and faster noises tend to raise both heart rate and blood pressure; slower, softer, and more regular tones produce the opposite result. Music can also relieve muscle tension and improve motor skills. It is often used to help rebuild physical patterning skills in rehabilitation clinics. Levels of endorphins, natural pain relievers, are increased while listening to music, and levels of stress hormones are decreased. This latter effect may partially explain the ability of music to improve immune function. A 1993 study at Michigan State University showed that even 15 minutes of exposure to music could increase interleukin-1 levels, a consequence which also heightens immunity.

Mental effects

Depending on the type and style of sound, music can either sharpen mental acuity or assist in relaxation. Memory and learning can be enhanced, and this used with good results in children with learning disabilities. This effect may also be partially due to increased concentration that many people have while listening to music. Better productivity is another outcome of an improved ability to concentrate. The term "Mozart effect" was coined after a study showed that college students performed better on math problems when listening to classical music.

Emotional effects

The ability of music to influence human emotion is well known, and is used extensively by moviemakers. A variety of musical moods may be used to create feelings of calmness, tension, excitement, or romance. Lullabies have long been popular for soothing babies to sleep. Music can also be used to express emotion nonverbally, which can be a very valuable therapeutic tool in some settings.

Description

Origins

Music has been used throughout human history to express and affect human emotion. In biblical accounts, King Saul was reportedly soothed by David's harp music, and the ancient Greeks expressed thoughts about music having healing effects as well. Many cultures are steeped in musical traditions. It can change mood, have stimulant or sedative effects, and alter physiologic processes such as heart rate and breathing. The apparent health benefits of music to patients in Veterans Administration hospitals following World War II lead to it being studied and formalized as a complementary healing practice. Musicians were hired to continue working in the hospitals. Degrees in music therapy became available in the late 1940s, and in 1950, the first professional association of music therapists was formed in the United States. The National Association of Music Therapy merged with the American Association of Music Therapy in 1998 to become the American Music Therapy Association.

Goals

Music is used to form a relationship with the patient. The music therapist sets goals on an individual basis, depending on the reasons for treatment, and selects specific activities and exercises to help the patient progress. Objectives may include development of communication, cognitive, motor, emotional, and social skills. Some of the techniques used to achieve this are singing, listening, instrumental music, composition, creative movement, **guided imagery**, and other methods as appropriate. Other disciplines may be integrated as well, such as dance, art, and psychology. Patients may develop musical abilities as a result of therapy, but this is not a major concern. The primary aim is to improve the patient's ability to function.

Techniques

Learning to play an instrument is an excellent musical activity to develop motor skills in individuals with developmental delays, brain injuries, or other motor impairment. It is also an exercise in impulse control and group cooperation. Creative movement is another activity that can help to improve coordination, as well as strength, balance, and gait. Improvisation facilitates the nonverbal expression of emotion. It encourages socialization and communication about feelings as well. Singing develops articulation, rhythm, and breath control. Remembering lyrics and melody is an exercise in sequencing for **stroke** victims and others who may be intellectually impaired.

Composition of words and music is one avenue available to assist the patient in working through fears and negative feelings. Listening is an excellent way to practice attending and remembering. It may also make the patient aware of memories and emotions that need to be acknowledged and perhaps talked about. Singing and discussion is a similar method, which is used with some patient populations to encourage dialogue. Guided Imagery and Music (GIM) is a very popular technique developed by music therapist Helen Bonny. Listening to music is used as a path to invoke emotions, picture, and symbols from the patient. This is a bridge to the exploration and expression of feelings.

Music and children

The sensory stimulation and playful nature of music can help to develop a child's ability to express emotion, communicate, and develop rhythmic movement. There is also some evidence to show that speech and language skills can be improved through the stimulation of both hemispheres of the brain. Just as with adults, appropriately selected music can decrease stress, **anxiety**, and pain. Music therapy in a hospital environment with those who are sick, preparing for surgery, or recovering postoperatively is appropriate and beneficial. Children can also experience improved self-esteem through musical activities that allow them to succeed.

Newborns may enjoy an even greater benefit of music. Those who are premature experience more rapid weight gain and hospital discharge than their peers who are not exposed to music. There is also anecdotal evidence of improved cognitive function.

Music and rehabilitation

Patients with brain damage from stroke, traumatic brain injury, or other neurologic conditions have been shown to exhibit significant improvement as a result of music therapy. This is theorized to be partially the result of entrainment, which is the synchronization of movement with the rhythm of the music. Consistent practice leads to gains in motor skill ability and efficiency. Cognitive processes and language skills often benefit from appropriate musical intervention.

Music and the elderly

The geriatric population can be particularly prone to anxiety and depression, particularly in nursing home residents. Chronic diseases causing pain are also not uncommon in this setting. Music is an excellent outlet to provide enjoyment, relaxation, relief from pain, and an opportunity to socialize and reminisce about music that has had special importance to the individual. It can have a striking effect on patients with **Alzheimer's disease**, even sometimes allowing them to focus and become responsive for a time. Music has also been observed to decrease the agitation that is so common with this disease. One study shows that elderly people who play a musical instrument are more physically and emotionally fit as they age than their nonmusical peers are.

Music and the mentally ill

Music can be an effective tool for the mentally or emotionally ill. **Autism** is one disorder that has been particularly researched. Music therapy has enabled some autistic children to relate to others and have improved learning skills. **Substance abuse**, **schizophrenia**, **paranoia**, and disorders of personality, anxiety, and affect are all conditions that may be benefited by music therapy. In these groups, participation and social interaction are promoted through music. Reality orientation is improved. Patients are helped to develop coping skills, reduce stress, and express their feelings.

Music and hospice

Pain, anxiety, and depression are major concerns with patients who are terminally ill, whether they are in hospice or not. Music can provide some relief from pain, through release of endorphins and promotion of relaxation. It can also provide an opportunity for the patient to reminisce and talk about the fears that are associated with **death** and dying. Music may help regulate the rapid breathing of a patient who is anxious, and soothe the mind. The Chalice of Repose project, headquartered at St. Patrick Hospital in Missoula, Montana, is one organization that attends and nurtures dying patients through the use of music, in a practice they called music-thanatology by developer Therese Schroeder-Sheker. Practitioners in this program work to relieve suffering through music prescribed for the individual patient.

Music and labor

Research has proven that mothers require less pharmaceutical pain relief during labor if they make use of music. Using music that is familiar and associated with positive imagery is the most helpful. During early labor, this will promote relaxation. Maternal movement is helpful to get the baby into a proper birthing position and dilate the cervix. Enjoying some "music to move by" can encourage the mother to stay active for as long as possible during labor. The rhythmic auditory stimulation may also prompt the body to release endorphins, which are a

---

KEY TERMS

Entrainment—The patterning of body processes and movements to the rhythm of music

Physiologic—Characteristic of normal, healthy functioning

---

natural form of pain relief. Many women select different styles of music for each stage of labor, with a more intense, or faster piece feeling like a natural accompaniment to the more difficult parts of labor. Instrumental music is often preferred.

Precautions

Patients making use of music therapy should not discontinue medications or therapies prescribed by other health providers without prior consultation.

Research and general acceptance

There is little disagreement among physicians that music can be of some benefit for patients, although the extent to which it can have physical effects is not as well acknowledged in the medical community. Research has shown that listening to music can decrease anxiety, pain, and recovery time. There is also good data for the specific subpopulations discussed. A therapist referral can be made through the AMTA.

Resources

ORGANIZATIONS

American Music Therapy Association, Inc. 8455 Colesville Road, Suite 1000 Silver Spring, ML 20910. (301) 589-3300. < http://www.musictherapy.org >.

Chalice of Repose Project at St. Patrick Hospital. 312 East Pine Street, Missoula, MT 59802. (406) 329-2810. Fax: (406) 329-5614. < http://www.saintpatrick.org/chalice/ >.

Judith Turner

Mutism

Definition

Mutism is a rare childhood condition characterized by a consistent failure to speak in situations where talking is expected. The child has the ability to converse normally, and does so, for example, in the home, but consistently fails to speak in specific situations such as at school or with strangers. It is estimated that one in every 1,000 school-age children are affected.

Description

Experts believe that this problem is associated with **anxiety** and fear in social situations such as in school or in the company of adults. It is therefore often considered a type of social phobia. This is not a communication disorder because the affected children can converse normally in some situations. It is not a developmental disorder because their ability to talk, when they choose to do so, is appropriate for their age level. This problem has been linked to anxiety, and one of the major ways in which both children and adults attempt to cope with anxiety is by avoiding whatever provokes the anxiety.

Affected children are typically shy, and are especially so in the presence of strangers and unfamiliar surroundings or situations. However, the behaviors of children with this condition go beyond **shyness**.

Causes and symptoms

Mutism is believed to arise from anxiety experienced in social situations where the child may be called upon to speak. Refusing to speak, or speaking in a whisper, spares the child from the possible humiliation or embarrassment of "saying the wrong thing." When asked a direct question by teachers, for example, the affected child may act as if they are unable to answer. Some children may communicate via gestures, nodding, or very brief utterances. Additional features may include excessive shyness, oppositional behavior, and impaired learning at school.

Diagnosis

The diagnosis of mutism is fairly easy to make because the signs amd symptoms are clear-cut and easily observable. However, other social disorders effecting social speech, such as **autism** or **schizophrenia**, must be considered in the diagnosis.

Treatment

There are two recommended treatments for mutism: behavior modification therapy and antidepressant medication. Treatment is most effective when individualized to each patient. It has been suggested that speech pathologists may also be able to help these children.

Prognosis

The prognosis for mutism is good. Sometimes it disappears suddenly on its own. The negative impact on learning and school activities may, however, persist into adult life.

Prevention

Mutism cannot be prevented because the cause is not known. However, family conflict or problems at school contribute to the seriousness of the symptoms.

Resources

BOOKS

Diagnostic and Statistical Manual of Mental Disorders. 4th ed. Washington, DC: American Psychiatric Association, 1994.

Donald G. Barstow, RN

MVP *see* **Mitral valve prolapse**

Myasthenia gravis

Definition

Myasthenia gravis is an autoimmune disease that causes muscle weakness.

Description

Myasthenia gravis (MG) affects the neuromuscular junction, interrupting the communication between nerve and muscle, and thereby causing weakness. A person with MG may have difficulty moving their eyes, walking, speaking clearly, swallowing, and even breathing, depending on the severity and distribution of weakness. Increased weakness with exertion, and improvement with rest, is a characteristic feature of MG.

About 30,000 people in the United States are affected by MG. It can occur at any age, but is most common in women who are in their late teens and early twenties, and in men in their sixties and seventies.

Causes and symptoms

Myasthenia gravis is an autoimmune disease, meaning it is caused by the body's own immune system. In MG, the immune system attacks a receptor on the surface of muscle cells. This prevents the muscle from receiving the nerve impulses that normally make it respond. MG affects "voluntary" muscles, which are those muscles under conscious control responsible for movement. It does not affect heart muscle or the "smooth" muscle found in the digestive system and other internal organs.

A muscle is stimulated to contract when the nerve cell controlling it releases acetylcholine molecules onto its surface. The acetylcholine lands on a muscle protein called the acetylcholine receptor. This leads to rapid chemical changes in the muscle which cause it to contract. Acetylcholine is then broken down by acetylcholinesterase enzyme, to prevent further stimulation.

In MG, immune cells create antibodies against the acetylcholine receptor. Antibodies are proteins normally involved in fighting infection. When these antibodies attach to the receptor, they prevent it from receiving acetylcholine, decreasing the ability of the muscle to respond to stimulation.

Why the immune system creates these self-reactive "autoantibodies" is unknown, although there are several hypotheses:

- During fetal development, the immune system generates many B cells that can make autoantibodies, but B cells that could harm the body's own tissues are screened out and destroyed before birth. It is possible that the stage is set for MG when some of these cells escape detection.

- Genes controlling other parts of the immune system, called MHC genes, appear to influence how susceptible a person is to developing autoimmune disease.

- Infection may trigger some cases of MG. When activated, the immune system may mistake portions of the acetylcholine receptor for portions of an invading virus, though no candidate virus has yet been identified conclusively.

- About 10% of those with MG also have thymomas, or benign tumors of the thymus gland. The thymus is a principal organ of the immune system, and

researchers speculate that thymic irregularities are involved in the progression of MG.

Some or all of these factors (developmental, genetic, infectious, and thymic) may interact to create the autoimmune reaction.

The earliest symptoms of MG often result from weakness of the extraocular muscles, which control eye movements. Symptoms involving the eye (ocular symptoms) include double vision (diplopia), especially when not gazing straight ahead, and difficulty raising the eyelids (**ptosis**). A person with ptosis may need to tilt their head back to see. Eye-related symptoms remain the only symptoms for about 15% of MG patients. Another common early symptom is difficulty chewing and swallowing, due to weakness in the bulbar muscles, which are in the mouth and throat. **Choking** becomes more likely, especially with food that requires extensive chewing.

Weakness usually becomes more widespread within several months of the first symptoms, reaching their maximum within a year in two-thirds of patients. Weakness may involve muscles of the arms, legs, neck, trunk, and face, and affect the ability to lift objects, walk, hold the head up, and speak.

Symptoms of MG become worse upon exertion, and better with rest. Heat, including heat from the sun, hot showers, and hot drinks, may increase weakness. Infection and **stress** may worsen symptoms. Symptoms may vary from day to day and month to month, with intervals of no weakness interspersed with a progressive decline in strength.

"Myasthenic crisis" may occur, in which the breathing muscles become too weak to provide adequate respiration. Symptoms include weak and shallow breathing, **shortness of breath**, pale or bluish skin color, and a racing heart. Myasthenic crisis is an emergency condition requiring immediate treatment. In patients treated with anticholinesterase agents, myasthenic crisis must be differentiated from cholinergic crisis related to overmedication.

Pregnancy worsens MG in about one third of women, has no effect in one third, and improves symptoms in another third. About 12% of infants born to women with MG have "neonatal myasthenia," a temporary but potentially life-threatening condition. It is caused by the transfer of maternal antibodies into the fetal circulation just before birth. Symptoms include weakness, floppiness, feeble cry, and difficulty feeding. The infant may have difficulty breathing, requiring the use of a ventilator. Neonatal myasthenia usually clears up within a month.

Diagnosis

Myasthenia gravis is often diagnosed accurately by a careful medical history and a neuromuscular exam, but several tests are used to confirm the diagnosis. Other conditions causing worsening of bulbar and skeletal muscles must be considered, including drug-induced myasthenia, thyroid disease, Lambert-Eaton myasthenic syndrome, **botulism**, and inherited muscular dystrophies.

MG causes characteristic changes in the electrical responses of muscles that may be observed with an electromyogram, which measures muscular response to electrical stimulation. Repetitive nerve stimulation leads to reduction in the height of the measured muscle response, reflecting the muscle's tendency to become fatigued.

Blood tests may confirm the presence of the antibody to the acetylcholine receptor, though up to a quarter of MG patients will not have detectable levels. A **chest x ray** or chest computed tomography scan (CT scan) may be performed to look for **thymoma**.

Treatment

While there is no cure for myasthenia gravis, there are a number of treatments that effectively control symptoms in most people.

Edrophonium (Tensilon) blocks the action of acetylcholinesterase, prolonging the effect of acetylcholine and increasing strength. An injection of edrophonium rapidly leads to a marked improvement in most people with MG. An alternate drug, neostigmine, may also be used.

Pyridostigmine (Mestinon) is usually the first drug tried. Like edrophonium, pyridostigmine blocks acetylcholinesterase. It is longer-acting, taken by mouth, and well-tolerated. Loss of responsiveness and disease progression combine to eventually make pyridostigmine ineffective in tolerable doses in many patients.

Thymectomy, or removal of the thymus gland, has increasingly become standard treatment for MG. Up to 85% of people with MG improve after thymectomy, with complete remission eventually seen in about 30%. The improvement may take months or even several years to fully develop. Thymectomy is not usually recommended for children with MG, since the thymus continues to play an important immune role throughout childhood.

Immune-suppressing drugs are used to treat MG if response to pyridostigmine and thymectomy are not adequate. Drugs include **corticosteroids** such as prednisone, and the non-steroids azathioprine (Imuran) and cyclosporine (Sandimmune).

Plasma exchange may be performed to treat myasthenic crisis or to improve very weak patients before thymectomy. In this procedure, blood plasma is removed and replaced with purified plasma free of autoantibodies. It can produce a temporary improvement in symptoms, but is too expensive for long-term treatment. Another blood treatment, intravenous immunoglobulin therapy, is also used for myasthenic crisis. In this procedure, large quantities of purified immune proteins (immunoglobulins) are injected. For unknown reasons, this leads to symptomatic improvement in up to 85% of patients. It is also too expensive for long-term treatment.

People with weakness of the bulbar muscles may need to eat softer foods that are easier to chew and swallow. In more severe cases, it may be necessary to obtain **nutrition** through a feeding tube placed into the stomach (**gastrostomy** tube).

Prognosis

Most people with MG can be treated successfully enough to prevent their condition from becoming debilitating. In some cases, however, symptoms may worsen even with vigorous treatment, leading to generalized weakness and disability. MG rarely causes early **death** except from myasthenic crisis.

Prevention

There is no known way to prevent myasthenia gravis. Thymectomy improves symptoms significantly in many patients, and relieves them entirely in some. Avoiding heat can help minimize symptoms.

Some drugs should be avoided by people with MG because they interfere with normal neuromuscular function.

Drugs to be avoided or used with caution include:

- Many types of **antibiotics**, including erythromycin, streptomycin, and ampicillin
- Some cardiovascular drugs, including Verapamil, betaxolol, and propranolol
- Some drugs used in psychiatric conditions, including chlorpromazine, clozapine, and lithium

Many other drugs may worsen symptoms as well, so patients should check with the doctor who treats their MG before taking any new drugs.

A Medic-Alert card or bracelet provides an important source of information to emergency

KEY TERMS

Antibody—An immune protein normally used by the body for combating infection and which is made by B cells.

Autoantibody—An antibody that reacts against part of the self.

Autoimmune disease—A disease caused by a reaction of the body's immune system.

Bulbar muscles—Muscles that control chewing, swallowing, and speaking.

Neuromuscular junction—The site at which nerve impulses are transmitted to muscles.

Pyridostigmine bromide (Mestinon)—An anticholinesterase drug used in treating myasthenia gravis.

Tensilon test—A test for diagnosing myasthenia gravis. Tensilon is injected into a vein and, if the person has MG, their muscle strength will improve for about five minutes.

Thymus gland—A small gland located just above the heart, involved in immune system development.

providers about the special situation of a person with MG. They are available from health care providers.

Resources

ORGANIZATIONS

Muscular Dystrophy Association. 3300 East Sunrise Drive, Tucson, AZ 85718. (800) 572-1717. < http://www.mdausa.org >.

Myasthenia Gravis Foundation of America. 222 S. Riverside Plaza, Suite 1540, Chicago, IL 60606. (800) 541-5454. < http://www.med.unc.edu >.

Richard Robinson

Mycetoma

Definition

Mycetoma, or maduromycosis, is a slow-growing bacterial or fungal infection focused in one area of the body, usually the foot. For this reason—and because the first medical reports were from doctors in Madura, India—an alternate name for the disease is Madura

foot. The infection is characterized by an abnormal tissue mass beneath the skin, formation of cavities within the mass, and a fluid discharge. As the infection progresses, it affects the muscles and bones; at this advanced stage, disability may result.

Description

Although the bacteria and fungi that cause mycetoma are found in soil worldwide, the disease occurs mainly in tropical areas in India, Africa, South America, Central America, and southeast Asia. Mycetoma is an uncommon disease, affecting an unknown number of people annually.

There are more than 30 species of bacteria and fungi that can cause mycetoma. Bacteria or fungi can be introduced into the body through a relatively minor skin wound. The disease advances slowly over months or years, typically with minimal **pain**. When pain is experienced, it is usually due to secondary infections or bone involvement. Although it is rarely fatal, mycetoma causes deformities and potential disability at its advanced stage.

Causes and symptoms

Owing to a wound, bacteria or fungi gain entry into the skin. Approximately one month or more after the injury, a nodule forms under the skin surface. The nodule is painless, even as it increases in size over the following months. Eventually, the nodule forms a tumor, or mass of abnormal tissue. The tumor contains cavities—called sinuses—that discharge blood- or pus-tainted fluid. The fluid also contains tiny grains, less than two thousandths of an inch in size. The color of these grains depends on the type of bacteria or fungi causing the infection.

As the infection continues, surrounding tissue becomes involved, with an accumulation of scarring and loss of function. The infection can extend to the bone, causing inflammation, pain, and severe damage. Mycetoma may be complicated by secondary infections, in which new bacteria become established in the area and cause an additional set of problems.

Diagnosis

The primary symptoms of a tumor, sinuses, and grain-flecked discharge often provide enough information to diagnose mycetoma. In the early stages, prior to sinus formation, diagnosis may be more difficult and a biopsy, or microscopic examination of the tissue, may be necessary. If bone involvement is

KEY TERMS

Biopsy—A medical procedure in which a small piece of tissue is surgically removed for microscopic examination.

Grains—Flecks of hardened material such as bacteria or fungi spores.

Nodule—A hardened area or knot sometimes associated with infection.

Secondary infection—Illness caused by new bacteria, viruses, or fungi becoming established in the wake of an initial infection.

Sinuses—Cavities or hollow areas.

Tumor—A mass or clump of abnormal tissue, not necessarily caused by a cancer.

suspected, the area is x rayed to determine the extent of the damage. The species of bacteria or fungi at the root of the infection is identified by staining the discharge grains and inspecting them with a microscope.

Treatment

Combating mycetoma requires both surgery and drug therapy. Surgery usually consists of removing the tumor and a portion of the surrounding tissue. If the infection is extensive, **amputation** is sometimes necessary. Drug therapy is recommended in conjunction with surgery. The specific prescription depends on the type of bacteria or fungi causing the disease. Common medicines include antifungal drugs, such as ketoconazole and **antibiotics** (streptomycin sulfate, amikacin, sulfamethoxazole, penicillin, and rifampin).

Prognosis

Recovery from mycetoma may take months or years, and the infection recurs after surgery in at least 20% of cases. Drug therapy can reduce the chances of a re-established infection. The extent of deformity or disability depends on the severity of infection; the more deeply entrenched the infection, the greater the damage. By itself, mycetoma is rarely fatal, but secondary infections can be fatal.

Prevention

Mycetoma is a rare condition that is not contagious.

Resources

PERIODICALS

McGinnis, Michael R. "Mycetoma." *Dermatologic Clinics* 14, no. 1 (January 1996): 97.

Julia Barrett

Mycobacterial infections, atypical

Definition

Atypical mycobacterial infections are infections caused by several types of mycobacteria similar to the germ that causes **tuberculosis**. These atypical mycobacterial infections are a frequent complication in patients with human **immunodeficiency** virus (HIV) infection or **AIDS**.

Description

Mycobacteria are a group of rod-shaped bacteria that cause several diseases, among them **leprosy** and tuberculosis. For some time, scientists have known of bacteria that are similar to *Mycobacterium tuberculosis*, the cause of tuberculosis, but that grow and act differently. When tuberculosis was a much more widespread problem and microbiology was much less able to tell the difference between similar microbes, these atypical mycobacteria were ignored. Today, they have been classified more precisely as members of the same species and called atypical (or nontuberculosis) mycobacteria.

Although the medical profession has known about these atypical infections for a long time, they were not considered a serious problem until the early 1980s. It was then that many of these atypical infections were noticed among homosexuals and intravenous drug users in New York City. These bacteria rarely cause infection in humans other than those with HIV or AIDS.

Causes and symptoms

Although there are more than a dozen species of atypical mycobacteria, the two most common are *Mycobacterium kansasii* and *M. avium-intracellulare*. These microbes are found in many places in the environment: tap water, fresh and ocean water, milk, bird droppings, soil, and house dust. The manner in which these bacteria are transmitted is not completely understood. There is no evidence that they are transmitted from person to person.

M. avium-intracellulare (MAC or MAI) is a rare cause of lung disease in otherwise healthy humans but a frequent cause of infection among those whose resistance has been lowered by another disorder (opportunistic infection). According to some experts, MAC infection is an almost inevitable complication of HIV. The infection is caused by one of two similar organisms, *M. avium* and *M. intracellulare.*

AIDS patients are almost always attacked by these mycobacteria. Once inside the body, the atypical mycobacterial organisms colonize and grow in the lungs like tuberculosis. Because AIDS patients have a poorly functioning immune system, the microbes multiply because they aren't stopped by the body's normal response to infection. Once they have colonized the lungs, the organisms enter the bloodstream and spread throughout the body, affecting almost every organ. These devastating infections can invade the lymph nodes, liver, spleen, bone marrow, gastrointestinal tract, skin, and brain.

Symptoms include **shortness of breath**, **fever**, night sweats, weight loss, appetite loss, **fatigue**, and progressively severe **diarrhea**, stomach **pain**, **nausea and vomiting**. If the infection spreads to the brain, the patient may experience weakness, headaches, vision problems, and loss of balance.

MAC and *M. kansasii* sometimes cause lung infections in middle-aged and elderly people with chronic lung conditions. MAC, *M. kansasii*, and *M. scrofulaceum* may cause inflammation of the lymph nodes in otherwise healthy young children. *M. fortuitum* and *M. chelonae* cause skin and wound infections and abscesses after trauma or surgical procedures. *M. marinum* causes a nodular inflammation, usually on the arms and legs. This infection is called "swimming pool granuloma" because it is associated with swimming pools, fish tanks, and other bodies of water. *M. ulcerans* infection causes chronic skin ulcerations, usually on an arm or leg. Atypical mycobacteria infections can also occur without causing any symptoms. In such cases, a **tuberculin skin test** may be positive.

Diagnosis

The diagnosis is made from the patient's symptoms and organisms grown in culture from the site of infection. In cases of lung infection, a diagnostic workup will include a **chest x ray** and tests on discharges from the respiratory passages (sputum).

KEY TERMS

Culture—A test in which a sample of body fluid, such as prostatic fluid, is placed on materials specially formulated to grow microorganisms. A culture is used to learn what type of bacterium is causing infection.

Human immunodeficiency virus (HIV)—The virus that causes AIDS.

Treatment

These nontypical mycobacteria are not easy to treat in any patient and the problem is complicated when the person has AIDS. **Antibiotics** are not particularly effective, although rifabutin (a cousin of the anti-tuberculosis drug rifampin) and clofazimine (an anti-leprosy drug) have helped some patients. It is also possible to contain the infection to some degree by combining different drugs, including ethionamide, cycloserine, ethambutol, and streptomycin.

Prognosis

Because drug therapy is not easily effective, the overwhelming infections caused by these mycobacteria in AIDS patients can be fatal.

Prevention

People with HIV infection can prevent or delay the onset of MAC by taking disease-preventing drugs such as rifabutin.

AIDS patients and persons with tissue damage, such as skin **wounds** or pulmonary disease, can make a number of lifestyle changes to help prevent MAC infection. Since these mycobacteria are found in most city water systems, in hospital water supplies, and in bottled water, at-risk persons should boil drinking water. Persons at risk should also avoid raw foods, especially salads, root vegetables, and unpasteurized milk or cheese. Fruits and vegetables should be peeled and rinsed thoroughly. Conventional cooking (baking, boiling or steaming) destroys mycobacteria, which are killed at 176°F (80°C).

Finally, at-risk patients should avoid contact with animals, especially birds and bird droppings. Pigeons in particular can transmit MAC.

Resources

ORGANIZATIONS

National AIDS Treatment Advocacy Project. 580
    Broadway, Ste. 403, New York, NY 10012. (888) 266-
    2827. < http://www.natap.org >.

Carol A. Turkington

Mycobacterium leprae infection *see* **Leprosy**

Mycobacterium tuberculosis see
Tuberculosis

Mycoplasma infections

Definition

Mycoplasma are the smallest of the free-living organisms. (Unlike viruses, mycoplasma can reproduce outside of living cells.) Many species within the genus *Mycoplasma* thrive as parasites in human, bird, and animal hosts. Some species can cause disease in humans.

Description

Mycoplasma are found most often on the surfaces of mucous membranes. They can cause chronic inflammatory diseases of the respiratory system, urogenital tract, and joints. The most common human illnesses caused by mycoplasma are due to infection with *M. pneumoniae,* which is responsible for 10-20% of all pneumonias. This type of **pneumonia** is also called atypical pneumonia, walking pneumonia, or community-acquired pneumonia. Infection moves easily among people in close contact because it is spread primarily when infected droplets circulate in the air (that is, become aerosolized), usually due to coughing, spitting, or sneezing.

Causes and symptoms

Atypical pneumonias can affect otherwise healthy people who have close contact with one another. Pneumonia caused by *M. pneumoniae* may start out with symptoms of an upper respiratory infection, probably a **sore throat** progressing to a dry **cough** within a few days. Gradually, **fever**, **fatigue**, muscle aches, and a cough that produces thin sputum (spit or phlegm) will emerge. Nonrespiratory symptoms may occur too: abdominal **pain**, **headache**, and **diarrhea**; about 20% of patients may have ear pain.

Another mycoplasma species, *M. hominis*, is common in the mucous membranes of the genital area (including the cervix), and can cause infection in both males and females. Its presence does not always result in symptoms.

Diagnosis

Usually, mycoplasma pneumonia will be identified after other common diagnoses are set aside. For example, a type of antibiotic known as a beta-lactam might be prescribed for a respiratory infection producing fever and cough. If symptoms do not improve in 3-5 days, the organism causing the disease is not a typical one and not susceptible to these **antibiotics**. If a Gram's stain (a common test done on sputum) does not indicate a gram-positive pathogen, the doctor will suspect a gram-negative organism, such as mycoplasma. The actual underlying organism may not be identified (it is not in almost 50% of cases of atypical pneumonia). Although it is rare, a rash may appear along with pneumonia symptoms. This should trigger suspicion of mycoplasma pneumonia, even if laboratory tests are inconclusive.

Standard x rays may reveal a patchy material that has entered the tissue; this can be evident for months. Laboratory tests include cold agglutinins, complement fixation, culture, and enzyme immunoassay. The presence of infection with *M. pneumoniae* would be indicated by a fourfold rise in *M. pneumoniae*-specific antibody in serum, during the illness or convalescence. Highly sophisticated and specific polymerase chain reaction methods (PCR) have been developed for many respiratory pathogens, including *M. pneumoniae*. They are not readily available and are very expensive.

Treatment

A 2-3 week course of certain antibiotics (erythromycin, azithromycin, clarithromycin, dirithromycin, or doxycycline) is generally prescribed for atypical pneumonia. This disease is infectious for weeks, even after the patient starts antibiotics. A persistent cough may linger for 6 weeks.

Prognosis

Mycoplasma pneumonia may be involved in the onset of **asthma** in adults; other rare complications include meningoencephalitis, **Guillain-Barré syndrome**, mononeuritis multiplex, **myocarditis**, or **pericarditis**. This may increase the risk of acute **arrhythmias** leading to **sudden cardiac death**. However, with proper treatment and rest, recovery should be complete.

Prevention

At this time, there are no vaccines for mycoplasma infection. It is difficult to control its spread, especially in a group setting. The best measures are still the simplest ones. Avoid exposure to people with respiratory infections whenever possible. A person who has a respiratory infection should cover the face while coughing or sneezing.

Resources

BOOKS

Cassell, Gail H., Gregory G. Gray, and K. B. Waites. "Mycoplasma Infections." In *Harrison's Principles of Internal Medicine*, edited by Anthony S. Fauci, et al. New York: McGraw-Hill, 1997.

Jill S. Lasker

Mycoplasmal pneumonia *see* **Mycoplasma infections**

Myelocytic leukemia, acute *see* **Leukemias, acute**

Myelodysplastic syndrome

Definition

Myelodysplastic syndrome (MDS) is a disease that is associated with decreased production of blood cells. Blood cells are produced in the bone marrow, and the blood cells of people with MDS do not mature normally. There are three major types of blood cells — red blood cells, white blood cells and platelets. Patients with MDS can have decreased production of one, two, or all three types of blood cells.

Description

Blood cells are used in the body for many different and important functions, such as carrying oxygen (red blood cells), fighting infection (white blood cells), and controlling bleeding (platelets). Blood cells are formed and stored in the bone marrow, which is the spongy tissue inside large bones. Stem cells, or immature blood cells, are stored in the bone marrow and have the ability to develop into all three types of mature blood cells. When the body needs a specific type of blood cell, the bone marrow uses its stockpile of stem cells to produce the kind of mature cells needed for that particular situation.

In patients who have MDS, blood cells fail to mature normally. In other words, the bone marrow is unable to develop a normal amount of mature blood cells, and is also not able to increase blood cell production when mature cells are needed. Sometimes, even the cells that are produced do not function normally. The marrow eventually becomes filled with the immature cells and there is not room for the normal cells to grow and develop. MDS therefore causes a shortage of functional blood cells.

Subtypes of MDS

MDS is divided into five different subtypes that are classified according to the number and appearance of blast cells in the bone marrow. It is important for doctors to know the type of MDS a patient has, because each subtype affects patients differently and requires specific treatment. The International Prognostic Scoring System (IPSS) can help the doctor to determine the best treatment for an individual patient. The subtypes are as follows:

- Refractory anemia (RA). Bone marrow with less than 5% blast cells and abnormal red blood cell blasts

- Refractory anemia with ring sideroblasts (RARS). Bone marrow with less than 5% blasts and characteristic abnormalities in red blood cells

- Refractory anemia with excess blasts (RAEB). Bone marrow with 5-20% blast cells, and higher risk of changing into acute leukemia over time

- Refractory anemia with excess blasts in transformation (RAEBT). Bone marrow with 21-30% blast cells. This form is most likely to change into acute leukemia.

- Chronic myelomonocytic leukemia (CMMoL). Marrow with 5-20% blasts and excess monocytes (a specific type of white blood cell).

Approximately 15,000 new cases are diagnosed annually in the United States. The average age at diagnosis is 70. The most common types are RA and

RARS. It is rare to have MDS before age 50. MDS is slightly more common in males than in females.

Causes and symptoms

Causes

There is no clear cause for the majority of MDS cases, which is referred to as primary or *de novo* myelodysplastic syndrome. In some cases, however, MDS results from earlier **cancer** treatments such as radiation and/or **chemotherapy**. This type of MDS is called secondary or treatment related MDS, is often seen 3 to 7 years after the exposure, and usually occurs in younger people.

Other possible causative agents for MDS include exposure to radiation, cigarette smoke or toxic chemicals such as benzene. Children with pre-existing chromosomal abnormalities such as **Down syndrome** have a higher risk of developing MDS. MDS does not appear to run in families, nor can it be spread to other individuals.

Symptoms

MDS symptoms are related to the type of blood cells that the body is lacking. The earliest symptoms are usually due to anemia, which results from a shortage of mature red blood cells. Anemia causes patients to feel tired and out of breath because there is a lack of cells transporting oxygen throughout the body. MDS may also lead to a shortage of white blood cells resulting in an increased likelihood of infections. Another symptom of MDS is increased bleeding (e.g., blood in stool, nose bleeds, increased **bruises** or bleeding gums) which is due to low level of platelets. These symptoms can occur in any combination, depending on a given patient's specific subtype of MDS.

Diagnosis

Blood tests

People who have MDS usually visit their primary care doctor first, with symptoms of **fatigue**, and are then referred to a hematologist (a physician who specializes in diseases of the blood). The diagnosis of MDS requires a complete analysis of the patient's blood and bone marrow, which is done by the hematologist. A complete **blood count** (CBC) is done to determine the number of each blood cell type within the sample. Low numbers of red blood cells, white blood cells, and or platelets are signs that a patient has MDS. Numerous other medical problems such as bleeding, nutritional deficiencies, or adverse reaction to a medication can also cause low blood counts. The hematologist will investigate other causes for low blood counts before assigning a diagnosis of MDS. Blood cells in patients with MDS can also be abnormal when viewed under the microscope.

Bone marrow aspiration and biopsy

A **bone marrow biopsy** is required to confirm the diagnosis of MDS and determine the correct MDS subtype. This procedure involves a needle used to take a sample of marrow from inside the bone. The area of the skin where the needle is inserted is numbed and sometimes the patient is also sedated. Patients may experience some discomfort but the procedure is safe and is over fairly quickly. Marrow samples are usually taken from the back of the hip bone (iliac crest). A sample of the marrow, known as an aspirate, and a small piece of bone are both removed with the needle.

A hematologist or a pathologist (a specialist in diagnosing diseases through cell examination) will carefully examine the bone marrow sample through a microscope. Microscopic examination allows the doctor to determine the number and type of blast cells (immature cells) within the marrow in order to identify the MDS subtype. Cells from the bone marrow are also sent for cytogenetic testing, which analyzes the cells' chromosomes. Forty to seventy percent of MDS patients have abnormal bone marrow chromosomes as a result of the disease. The pattern of these abnormalities can be used to predict how a patient will respond to a particular treatment. Thus, the full set of information provided by a bone marrow biopsy and CBC will ultimately allow the doctor to recommend the most effective treatment plan.

International Prognostic Scoring System (IPSS) for MDS

Once a diagnosis of MDS is established, the doctor will calculate the IPSS score for each individual patient. The bone marrow blast percentage, chromosomal abnormalities and number of different blood types that are reduced determine the score. A score of 0 to 3.5 is assigned to each patient. Patients with lower score have a better prognosis and usually should not undertake treatment upon initial diagnosis. Patients with a higher score have more aggressive disease and should consider more aggressive treatment.

Treatments

Supportive care

Treatment for MDS is tailored to the patient's age, general health, specific MDS subtype, and IPSS score. Treatment varies for each patient, but most treatment strategies are designed to control the symptoms of MDS. This approach is called supportive care and aims to improve the patient's quality of life.

Supportive care for the MDS patients commonly includes red blood cell transfusions to relieve symptoms related to anemia. Red cell transfusions are relatively safe and the physician will review risks and benefits with this approach. Transfusions of any type only last a certain amount of time and therefore need to be repeated at certain intervals. Platelet transfusions can also be a way to control excessive bleeding. The doctor will decide with each individual patient when it is appropriate to give a **transfusion**. **Antibiotics** are used when needed to combat infections that can occur more frequently in patients with low white blood cell counts.

Bone marrow transplantation

Bone marrow transplantation (BMT) is a type of treatment that attempts to provide MDS patients with a cure. This strategy requires the patients to be in fairly good health and are therefore more likely to be used in younger patients. Bone marrow transplantation (BMT) has been found to be a successful treatment for MDS patients under the age of 50 (and some over 50 in good health). Following BMT, many patients are able to achieve long-term, disease-free survival. Unfortunately, most MDS patients cannot receive a traditional bone marrow transplant because of older age or because they do not have a suitable donor. Bone marrow donors are usually siblings or are obtained from the national bone marrow registry. "Mini"-bone marrow transplants use less intense chemotherapy, and are currently being tested in older patients who would otherwise not be candidates for traditional bone marrow transplants.

Chemotherapy

Chemotherapy has been used to treat some MDS patients; however, the disease often recurs after a period of time. This type of therapy uses cell-killing drugs that may also damage healthy cells in the body. Most chemotherapy drugs are associated with some side effects. For these reasons, chemotherapy is generally not used until the MDS becomes more aggressive or the patient has a high IPSS score.

Growth factors

Growth factors are natural proteins that the body normally uses to control blood production. These substances stimulate the patient's bone marrow to produce healthy blood cells. Growth factors that stimulate white cell production are G-CSF (also called neupogen or filgrastim) and GMCSF (Leukine, sargramostim). In order to increase red cell production another growth factor, erythropoietin (Procrit) is used. These growth factors are safe with few side effects and are available only in the injectable form. The physician will decide if this treatment is appropriate for an individual patient.

Alternative treatment

There are no alternative therapies that have been proven to successfully treat MDS. Some of the available alternative drugs can have adverse side effects and therefore a physician should be informed if they are being used.

Prognosis

The prognosis for MDS patients depends on the subtype of their disease and the IPSS score. Patients with RA, RARS or low IPSS score rarely develop leukemia and may live with disease for some years. The higher-risk patients including those with RAEB, RAEBt, CMMoL or high IPSS scores progress more rapidly, and require intensive therapy to control the disease.

Managing MDS requires frequent doctor appointments to monitor disease progression and to evaluate the response to treatment. Fortunately for many patients, recent advances in therapy have significantly enhanced their ability to cope with MDS. Experimental drugs and a better understanding of the disease are likely to improve the overall prognosis in the future.

Prevention

MDS is usually impossible to prevent. Being careful about daily activities and avoiding the use of aspirin-like products that thin the blood may prevent secondary complications of MDS such as bruising and bleeding. Practicing good hygiene and avoiding crowds or people with infections can sometimes prevent infections. A well balanced diet is recommended to increase overall energy.

Resources

BOOKS

Aguayo, Alvaro, Jorge Cortes, and Hagop Kantarjian. "Myelodysplastic Syndromes." In *Cancer Management: A Multidisciplinary Approach*, edited by Richard Pazdur, et al., 4th ed. PRR, Inc, 2000.

ORGANIZATIONS

Aplastic Anemia Foundation of America. P.O. Box 613, Annapolis, MD 21404. (800) 747-2820. < http://www.aplastic.org >.

Leukemia Society of America. 600 Third Avenue, New York, NY 10016. (800) 955-4572. < http://www.leukemia.org >.

Myelodysplastic Syndromes Foundation. 464 Main Street, P.O. Box 477, Crosswicks, NJ 08515. (800) MDS-0839. < http://www.mds-foundation.org >.

Andrea Ruskin, M.D.

Myelofibrosis

Definition

Myelofibrosis is a rare disease of the bone marrow in which collagen builds up fibrous scar tissue inside the marrow cavity. This is caused by the uncontrolled growth of a blood cell precursor, which results in the accumulation of scar tissue in bone marrow. Myelofibrosis goes by many names including idiopathic myelofibrosis, agnogenic myeloid metaplasia, chronic myelosclerosis, aleukemic megakaryocytic myelosis, and leukoerythroblastosis.

Description

Myelofibrosis can be associated with many other conditions including **breast cancer**, **prostate cancer**, **Hodgkin's disease**, non-Hodgkin's lymphoma, acute myeloid leukemia, acute lymphocytic leukemia, **hairy cell leukemia**, **multiple myeloma**, myeloproliferative diseases, **tuberculosis**, Gaucher's disease, and **Paget's disease of bone**. Myelofibrosis typically becomes progressively worse and can cause **death**.

In myelofibrosis, abnormal cells (hematopoietic stem cells) grow out of control and begin to produce both immature blood cells and excess scar (fibrous) tissue. The fibrous tissue builds up (fibrosis) primarily in the bone marrow, the place where blood cells are produced. The fibrous tissue interferes with the production of normal blood cells. The outcome of this is that the blood made by the bone marrow is of poor quality. To compensate for this, blood cell production occurs in other parts of the body (extramedullary hematopoiesis), but most notably in the spleen and liver. This causes enlargement of the spleen (splenomegaly) and the liver (hepatomegaly). Extramedullary hematopoiesis is not effective and, combined with the reduced production of blood cells by the bone marrow, a condition called anemia results.

The abnormal stem cells can spread throughout the body, settle in other organs, and form tumors that produce more abnormal blood cells and fibrous tissue. These tumors are most commonly found in the adrenals, kidneys, lymph nodes, breast, lungs, skin, bowel, thymus, thyroid, prostate, and urinary tract.

Most patients with myelofibrosis are over 50 years old; the average age at diagnosis is 65 years. However, myelofibrosis can occur at any age. Myelofibrosis occurs with equal frequency in women and men, but in children it affects girls twice as often as it does boys.

Causes and symptoms

Myelofibrosis is caused by an abnormality in a single stem cell, which causes it to grow out of control. Myelofibrosis tumors that have originated from a single cell are called monoclonal. The cause of the stem cell abnormality is unknown. Persons who were exposed to benzene or high doses of radiation have developed myelofibrosis. There may be an association between myelofibrosis and autoimmune diseases, such as **systemic lupus erythematosus** and **scleroderma**, in which the immune system treats certain molecules of the body as foreign invaders.

Symptoms usually appear slowly over a long period of time. About one quarter of all patients with myelofibrosis have no symptoms (asymptomatic). An enlarged spleen discovered at an annual medical examination may be the first clue. Symptoms of myelofibrosis include:

- fatigue
- weight loss
- paleness
- fever
- sweating
- weakness
- heart palpitations
- shortness of breath
- itchiness
- feeling full after eating a small amount of food
- stomach **pain** or discomfort
- pain in the left shoulder or upper left portion of the body
- unexpected bleeding
- bone pain, especially in the legs

Diagnosis

Because symptoms are similar to other diseases (mostly leukemias), myelofibrosis is not easy to diagnose. The doctor would use his or her hands to feel (palpate) for enlargement of the spleen and liver. Blood tests and urine tests would be performed. **Bone marrow aspiration and biopsy** can help make a diagnosis, but they often fail because of the fibrosis. X-ray imaging and **magnetic resonance imaging** (MRI) may be performed.

Treatment

Many asymptomatic patients, if stable, do not require treatment. There is no cure for myelofibrosis, although **bone marrow transplantation** is curative in some cases. Treatment is aimed at reducing symptoms and improving quality of life.

Medications

Male hormones (androgens) can be used to treat anemia but, in women, these drugs can cause the development of male characteristics (e.g., hair growth on the face and body). Glucocorticoid therapy is also an effective treatment of anemia and can improve myelofibrosis in children. Nutrients that stimulate blood formation (hematinics), such as iron, **folic acid**, and vitamin B_{12}, may reduce anemia. **Cancer chemotherapy** (usually hydroxyurea) can decrease splenomegaly and hepatomegaly, reduce symptoms of myelofibrosis, lessen anemia, and sometimes reduce bone marrow fibrosis. The bone marrow of myelofibrosis patients is often not strong enough to withstand the harsh chemotherapy drugs, so this treatment is not always an option. Interferon-alpha has been shown to reduce spleen size, reduce bone pain, and, in some cases, increase the number of blood platelets (structures involved in blood clotting).

Other treatments

In certain cases, the enlarged spleen may be removed (**splenectomy**). Conditions that warrant splenectomy include spleen pain, the need for frequent blood **transfusion**, very low levels of platelets (**thrombocytopenia**), and extreme pressure in the blood vessels of the liver (portal **hypertension**).

Radiation therapy is used to treat splenomegaly, spleen pain, bone pain, tumors in certain places such as next to the spinal cord, and fluid accumulation inside the abdomen (**ascites**). Patients who are not strong enough to undergo splenectomy are often treated with radiation therapy.

Bone marrow transplantation may be used to treat some patients with myelofibrosis. This procedure may be performed on patients who are less than 50 years old, have a poor life expectancy, and have a brother or sister with blood-type similarities.

Patients with severe anemia may require blood transfusions.

Prognosis

Similar to leukemias, myelofibrosis is progressive and often requires therapy to control the disease. Myelofibrosis can progress to acute lymphocytic leukemia or lymphoma. Although a number of factors to predict the survival time have been proposed, advanced age or severe anemia are consistently associated with a poor prognosis. The average survival rate of patients diagnosed with myelofibrosis is five years. Death is usually caused by infection, bleeding, complications of splenectomy, **heart failure**, or progression to leukemia. Spontaneous remission is rare.

Prevention

Persons who have been exposed to radiation, benzene, or radioactive thorium dioxide (a chemical used during certain diagnostic radiological procedures) are at risk for myelofibrosis.

KEY TERMS

Anemia—Low numbers of red blood cells in the blood.

Benzene—A colorless volatile flammable toxic liquid hydrocarbon used as a solvent and as a motor fuel.

Biopsy—Surgical removal of tissue for microscopic examination.

Fibrosis—Buildup of scar tissue.

Glucocorticoid therapy—Treatment using corticoids that are anti-inflammatory and immunosuppressive.

Leukemia—Cancer of white blood cells.

Portal hypertension—Extreme pressure on the blood vessels of the liver.

Stem cell—A cell that has the ability to become many different specialized cells.

Resources

BOOKS

Lichtman, Marshall. "Idiopathic Myelofibrosis (Agnogenic Myeloid Metaplasia)." In *Williams Hematology*, edited by Ernest Beutler, et al. New York: McGraw Hill, 2001, pp.1125-36.

Mavroudis, Dimitrios and John Barrett. "Myelofibrosis (Agnogenic Myeloid Metaplasia)." In *Bone Marrow Failure Syndromes*, edited by Neal Young. Philadelphia: W.B. Saunders Company, 2000, pp.122-34.

Peterson, Powers. "Myelofibrosis." In *Practical Diagnosis of Hematologic Disorders*, edited by Carl Kjeldsberg. Chicago: ASCP Press, 2000, pp.477-9.

Belinda Rowland, Ph.D.
J. Ricker Polsdorfer, MD

Myelogram *see* **Myelography**

Myelography

Definition

Myelography is an x-ray examination of the spinal canal. A contrast agent is injected through a needle into the space around the spinal cord to display the spinal cord, spinal canal, and nerve roots on an x ray.

Purpose

The purpose of a myelogram is to evaluate the spinal cord and/or nerve roots for suspected compression. Pressure on these delicate structures causes **pain** or other symptoms. A myelogram is performed when precise detail about the spinal cord is needed to make a definitive diagnosis. In most cases, myelography is used after other studies, such as **magnetic resonance imaging** (MRI) or a computed tomography scan (CT scan), have not yielded enough information to be sure of the disease process. Sometimes myelography followed by CT scan is an alternative for patients who cannot have an MRI scan, because they have a pacemaker or other implanted metallic device.

A herniated or ruptured intervertebral disc, popularly known as a slipped disc, is one of the most common causes for pressure on the spinal cord or nerve roots. Discs are pads of fiber and cartilage that contain rubbery tissue. They lie between the vertebrae, or individual bones, which make up the spine. Discs act as cushions, accommodating **strains**, shocks, and position changes. A disc may rupture suddenly, due to

injury, or a sudden straining with the spine in an unnatural position. In other cases, the problem may come on gradually as a result of progressive deterioration of the discs with **aging**. The lower back is the most common area for this problem, but it sometimes occurs in the neck, and rarely in the upper back. A myelogram can help accurately locate the disc or discs involved.

Myelography may be used when a tumor is suspected. Tumors can originate in the spinal cord, or in tissues surrounding the cord. Cancers that have started in other parts of the body may spread or metastasize in the spine. It is important to precisely locate the mass causing pressure, so effective treatment can be undertaken. Patients with known **cancer** who develop back pain may require a myelogram for evaluation.

Other conditions that may be diagnosed using myelography include arthritic bony growths, known as spurs, narrowing of the spinal canal, called **spinal stenosis**, or malformations of the spine.

Precautions

Patients who are unable to lie still or cooperate with positioning should not have this examination. Severe congenital spinal abnormalities may make the examination technically difficult to carry out. Patients with a history of severe allergic reaction to contrast material (x-ray dye) should report this to their physician. Pretreatment with medications to minimize the risk of severe reaction may be recommended.

Description

Myelograms can be performed in a hospital x-ray department or in an outpatient radiology facility. The patient lies on the x-ray table on his or her stomach. The radiologist first looks at the spine under fluoroscopy, where the images appear on a monitor screen. This is done to find the best location to position the needle. The skin is cleaned, then numbed with local anesthetic. The needle is inserted. Occasionally, a small amount of cerebrospinal fluid, the clear fluid which surrounds the spinal cord and brain, may be withdrawn through the needle and sent for laboratory studies. Then contrast material is injected. The contrast material (dye) is a liquid that shows up on x rays.

The x-ray table is tilted slowly. This allows the contrast material to reach different levels in the spinal canal. The flow is observed under fluoroscopy, then x rays are taken with the table tilted at various angles. A footrest and shoulder straps or supports will keep the patient from sliding.

In many instances, a CT scan of the spine will be performed immediately after a myelogram, while the contrast material is still in the spinal canal. This helps outline internal structures most clearly.

A myelogram takes approximately 30-60 minutes. A CT scan adds about another hour to the examination. If the procedure is done as an outpatient exam, some facilities prefer the patient to stay in a recovery area for up to four hours.

Preparation

Patients should be well hydrated at the time of a myelogram. Increasing fluids the day before the study is usually recommended. All food and fluid intake should be stopped approximately four hours before the myelogram.

Certain medications may need to be stopped for one to two days before myelography is performed. These include some antipsychotics, antidepressants, blood thinners, and diabetic medications. Patients should consult with their physician and/or the facility where the study is to be done.

Patients who smoke may be asked to stop the day before the test. This helps decrease the chance of **nausea** or headaches after the myelogram. Immediately before the examination, patients should empty their bowels and bladder.

Aftercare

After the examination is completed, the patient usually rests for several hours, with the head elevated. Extra fluids are encouraged, to help eliminate the contrast material and prevent headaches. A regular diet and routine medications may be resumed. Strenuous physical activity, especially any which involve bending over, may be discouraged for one or two days. The doctor should be notified if a **fever**, excessive **nausea and vomiting**, severe **headache**, or stiff neck develops.

Risks

Headache is a common complication of myelography. It may begin several hours to several days after the examination. The cause is thought to be changes in cerebrospinal fluid pressure, not a reaction to the dye. The headache may be mild and easily alleviated with rest and increased fluids. Sometimes, nonprescription medicine are recommended. In some instances, the headache may be more severe and require stronger medication or other measures for relief. Many factors influence whether the patient develops this problem.

These include the type of needle used and the age and sex of the patient. Patients with a history of chronic or recurrent headache are more likely to develop a headache after a myelogram.

The chance of reaction to the contrast material is a very small, but potentially significant risk with myelography. It is estimated that only 5-10% of patients experience any effect from contrast exposure. The vast majority of reactions are mild, such as sneezing, nausea, or **anxiety**. These usually resolve by themselves. A moderate reaction, like **wheezing** or **hives**, may be treated with medication, but is not considered life threatening. Severe reactions, such as heart or **respiratory failure**, happen very infrequently. These require emergency medical treatment.

Rare complications of myelography include injury to the nerve roots from the needle, or from bleeding into the spaces around the roots. Inflammation of the delicate covering of the spinal cord, called arachnoiditis, or infections, can also occur. Seizures are another very uncommon complication reported after myelography.

Normal results

A normal myelogram would show a spinal canal of normal width, with no areas of constriction or obstruction.

Abnormal results

A myelogram may reveal a **herniated disk**, tumor, bone spurs, or narrowing of the spinal canal (spinal stenosis).

Resources

ORGANIZATIONS

Spine Center. 1911 Arch St., Philadelphia, PA 19103. (215) 665-8300. < http://www.thespinecenter.com >.

Ellen S. Weber, MSN

Myeloma *see* **Multiple myeloma**

Myers-Briggs type indicator

Definition

The Myers-Briggs Type Indicator (MBTI) is a widely-used personality inventory, or test, employed in vocational, educational, and psychotherapy settings to evaluate personality type in adolescents and adults age 14 and older.

Purpose

In an educational setting, the MBTI may be performed to assess student learning style. Career counselors use the test to help others determine what occupational field they might be best suited for, and it is also used in organizational settings to assess management skills and facilitate teamwork and problem-solving, including communication difficulties. Because the MBTI is also a tool for self-discovery, mental health professionals may administer the test in counseling sessions to provide their patients with insight into their behavior.

As of the early 2000s, the MBTI is also being used in the mental health field to assess vulnerability to **anxiety disorders** and depression. Preliminary results indicate that some of the 16 types are more susceptible to **mood disorders** than others. ISFPs, for example, are overrepresented among patients in treatment for unipolar depression, while the four ST types appear to be more vulnerable to **anxiety** states.

Precautions

The MBTI should be administered, scored, and interpreted only by a professional trained in its use. Cultural and language differences in the test subject may affect performance and may result in inaccurate test results. The test administrator should be informed before testing begins if the test taker is not fluent in English and/or he has a unique cultural background.

Description

In 2000, an estimated two million people took the MBTI, making it the most frequently used personality inventory available. The test was first introduced in 1942, the work of a mother and daughter, Katharine Cook Briggs and Isabel Briggs Myers. There are now several different versions of the test available. Form M, which contains 93 items, is the most commonly used.

The Myers-Briggs inventory is based on Carl Jung's theory of types, outlined in his 1921 work *Psychological Types*. Jung's theory holds that human beings are either *introverts* or *extraverts*, and their behavior follows from these inborn psychological types. He also believed that people take in and process information different ways, based on their personality traits.

The Myers-Briggs evaluates personality type and preference based on the four Jungian psychological types:

- extraversion (E) or introversion (I)
- sensing (S) or intuition (N)
- thinking (T) or feeling (F)
- judging (J) or perceiving (P)

Preparation

Prior to the administration of the MBTI, the test subject should be fully informed about the nature of the test and its intended use. He or she should also receive standardized instructions for taking the test and any information on the confidentiality of the results.

Normal results

Myers-Briggs results are reported as a four-letter personality type (e.g., ESTP, ISFJ). Each letter corresponds to an individual's preference in each of the four pairs of personality indicators (i.e., E or I, S or N, T or F, and J or P). There are a total of sixteen possible combinations of personality types on the MBTI.

Letter One: E or I

Extraverts focus more on people and things in the outside world, introverts on internal thoughts and ideas.

Letter Two: S or N

Sensing dominant personalities prefer to perceive things through sight, sound, taste, touch, and smell, while intuition dominant types look to past experience and are more abstract in their thinking.

Letter Three: T or F

The third subtype is a measure of how people use judgment. Thinking types use logic to judge the world, while feeling types tend to view things on the basis of what emotions they elicit.

Letter Four: J or P

Everyone judges and perceives, but those who are judging dominant are said to be more methodical and results-oriented, while perceiving dominant personalities are good at multitasking and are flexible.

Resources

BOOKS

Quenck, Naomi. *Essentials of Myers-Briggs Type Indicator Assessment.* New York: John Wiley & Sons, 1999.

PERIODICALS

Clack, G. B., J. Allen, D. Cooper, and J. O. Head. "Personality Differences between Doctors and Their Patients: Implications for the Teaching of Communication Skills." *Medical Education* 38 (February 2004): 177–186.

Janowsky, D. S., E. Hong, S. Morter, and L. Howe. "Myers Briggs Type Indicator Personality Profiles in Unipolar Depressed Patients." *World Journal of Biological Psychiatry* 3 (October 2002): 207–215.

Kameda, D. M., and J. L. Nyland. "Relationship between Psychological Type and Sensitivity to Anxiety." *Perceptual and Motor Skills* 97 (December 2003): 789–793.

Paula Anne Ford-Martin
Rebecca J. Frey, PhD

Myocardial biopsy

Definition

Myocardial biopsy is a procedure wherein a small portion of tissue is removed from the heart muscle for testing. This test is also known as endomyocardial biopsy.

Purpose

The main reason for a biopsy is to secure tissue samples that will be useful in the diagnosis, treatment, and care of heart muscle disorders. The test is also used to detect rejection after a **heart transplantation** procedure.

Precautions

This procedure is not used when the patient is taking blood-thinning medication (anticoagulant therapy). It should not be done when the patient has leukemia and **aplastic anemia** or if there is a blood clot on the interior wall of the heart.

Description

A long, flexible tube, called a catheter, is inserted into a vein and threaded up into the heart. The doctor can guide the catheter by watching its movement on a TV monitor showing an x-ray image of the area. The tip of the catheter is fitted with tiny jaws that the doctor can open and close. Once the catheter is in place, the doctor will take several small snips of muscle for microscopic examination.

Preparation

Preparation for myocardial biopsy is quite extensive. The patient will be asked not to eat for several hours before the procedure. A technician will shave the hair from the area of the incision and will also insert an intravenous line in the arm. The patient will be given a sedative to relax but will not be fully anesthetized. The patient will be connected to an electrocardiograph (ECG) to monitor the heart, and a blood-pressure cuff will be placed. Finally, the patient will be covered with sterile drapes, so that the area of the biopsy is kept free of germs. The cardiologist will numb the area where the catheter will be inserted.

Aftercare

At the end of the biopsy, the catheter will be removed and pressure will be applied at the site where it entered the blood vessel in order to encourage healing. The patient will then be taken to the recovery room. It is advisable to remain flat and not to move about for 6-8 hours. After that time, most people begin walking around. Swelling and bruising at the puncture site are common and usually go away without need for further attention.

Risks

The risks involved with myocardial biopsy are small because the patient is monitored closely and attended by well-trained staff. Racing of the heart (**palpitations**) and quivering of the heart muscles (atrial fibrillation) are both possible during the procedure.

Resources

ORGANIZATIONS

American Heart Association. 7320 Greenville Ave. Dallas, TX 75231. (214) 373-6300. <http://www.americanheart.org>.

Dorothy Elinor Stonely

Myocardial infarction *see* **Heart attack**

Myocardial resection

Definition

Myocardial resection is a surgical procedure in which a portion of the heart muscle is removed.

Purpose

Myocardial resection is done to improve the stability of the heart function or rhythm. Also known as endocardial resection, this open-heart surgery is done to destroy or remove damaged areas of the heart that cause life-threatening heart rhythms. This procedure is often performed in people who have had a **heart attack**, in order to prevent future rapid heart rates. It is also used in people who have **Wolff-Parkinson-White syndrome** (a condition resulting in abnormal heart rhythm).

Precautions

This is major surgery and should be the treatment of choice only after medications have failed and the

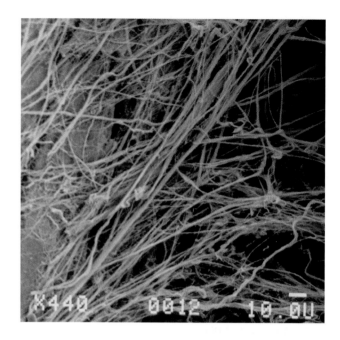

Once the catheter is threaded up into the heart, the surgeon will take several small samples of muscle for laboratory analysis. *(Custom Medical Stock Photo. Reproduced by permission.)*

use of an **implantable cardioverter-defibrillator** (a device that delivers electrical shock to control heart rhythm) has been ruled out.

Description

After receiving a general anesthetic, an incision will be made in the chest to expose the heart. When the exact source of the abnormal rhythm is identified, it is removed. If there are areas around the source that may contribute to the problem, they can be frozen with a special probe to further insure against dangerous heart rates. The amount of tissue removed is so small, usually only 2 or 3 millimeters, that there is no damage to the structure of the heart. On some occasions, aneurysms of the heart wall are removed as well.

Preparation

Prior to surgery, the physician will explain the procedure, routine blood tests will be completed, and consent forms will be signed.

Aftercare

Immediately after surgery, the patient will be moved to a recovery room until the affects of anesthesia have worn off. The patient will then be transferred to the intensive care unit for further recovery. In the

KEY TERMS

Implantable cardioverter-defibrillator—A device placed in the body to deliver an electrical shock to the heart in response to a serious abnormal rhythm.

Wolff-Parkinson-White syndrome—An abnormal, rapid heart rhythm, due to an extra pathway for the electrical impulses to travel from the atria to the ventricles.

intensive care unit, the heart will be monitored for any disturbances in rhythm and the patient will be watched for any signs of post-operative problems.

Risks

The risks of myocardial resection are based in large part on the person's underlying heart condition and, therefore, vary greatly. The procedure involves opening the heart, so the person is at risk for the complications associated with major heart surgery such as **stroke**, shock, infection, and hemorrhage.

Normal results

Anywhere from 5-25% of post-heart attack patients do not survive open-heart surgery. The survivors have a 90% arrhythmia-free one-year survival rate, (arrthymia is an irregular heart beat).

Resources

ORGANIZATIONS

American Heart Association. 7320 Greenville Ave. Dallas, TX 75231. (214) 373-6300. < http://www.americanheart.org >.

Dorothy Elinor Stonely

Myocarditis

Definition

Myocarditis is an inflammatory disease of the heart muscle (myocardium) that can result from a variety of causes. While most cases are produced by a viral infection, an inflammation of the heart muscle may also be instigated by toxins, drugs, and hypersensitive immune reactions. Myocarditis is a rare but serious condition that affects both males and females of any age.

Description

Most cases of myocarditis in the United States originate from a virus, and the disease may remain undiagnosed by doctors due to its general lack of initial symptoms. The disease may also present itself as an acute, catastrophic illness that requires immediate treatment. Although the inflammation or degeneration of the heart muscle that myocarditis causes may be fatal, this disease often goes undetected. It may also disguise itself as ischemic, valvular, or hypertensive heart disease.

An inflammation of the heart muscle may occur as an isolated disorder or be the dominating feature of a systemic disease (one that affects the whole body, like **systemic lupus erythematosus**).

Causes and symptoms

While there are several contributing factors that may lead to myocarditis, the primary cause is viral. Myocarditis usually results from the Coxsackie B virus, and may also result from **measles**, **influenza**, chicken pox, hepatitis virus, or the adenovirus in children. If an acute onset of severe myocarditis occurs, a patient may display the following symptoms:

- Rhythm disturbances of the heart
- Rapid heartbeat (**Ventricular tachycardia**)
- Left or right ventricular enlargement
- **Shortness of breath** (Dyspnea)
- Pulmonary **edema** (the accumulation of fluid in the lungs due to left-sided **heart failure**)
- Swollen legs.

Additional causes of myocarditis include:

- Bacterial infections, such as **tetanus**, **gonorrhea**, or **tuberculosis**
- Parasite infections, such as **Chagas' disease** (which is caused by an insect-borne protozoan most commonly seen in Central and South America)
- Rheumatic **fever**
- Surgery on the heart
- Radiation therapy for **cancer** that is localized in the chest, such as breast or lung cancer
- Certain medications.

As of 1996, research has shown that illegal drugs and toxic substances may also produce acute or

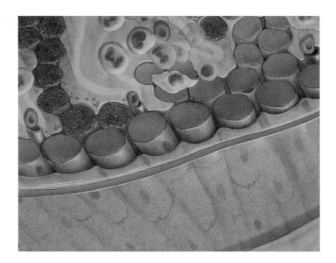

This illustration depicts the inflammation of the myocarditis, the middle muscular layer of the heart wall. *(Custom Medical Stock Photo. Reproduced by permission.)*

chronic injury to the myocardium. These studies also indicate an increase in the incidence of toxic results from the use of **cocaine**. This illegal drug causes coronary artery spasm, myocardial infarction (**heart attack**), and **arrhythmias**, as well as myocarditis.

Further studies conducted in 1996 indicate that **malnutrition** encourages the Coxsackie B virus to flourish, leading to the potential development of myocarditis. Human **immunodeficiency** virus (HIV) is also now recognized as a cause of myocarditis, though its prevalence is not known.

Symptoms of myocarditis may start as **fatigue**, shortness of breath, fever and aching of the joints, all characteristic of a flu-like illness. In contrast to this type of mild appearance, myocarditis may also appear suddenly in the form of heart failure, or **sudden cardiac death** without any prior symptoms. If an inflammation of the heart muscle leads to congestive heart failure, symptoms such as swollen feet and ankles, distended neck veins, a rapid heartbeat, and difficulty breathing while reclining may all appear.

Diagnosis

The best way to diagnose myocarditis may be through a person's observation of his or her own symptoms, followed by a thorough medical history and physical exam conducted by a doctor. Further tests usually include laboratory blood studies and **echocardiography**. An electrocardiogram (ECG) is also routinely used due to its ability to detect a mild case of the disease. **Cardiac catheterization** and **angiography** are additional diagnostic tests used to determine the presence of myocarditis, or to rule out other possible heart diseases that may lead to heart failure.

Another measure used to diagnosis myocarditis is the endomyocardial biopsy procedure. This invasive catheterization procedure examines a biopsied, or "snipped," piece of the endocardium (the lining membrane of the inner surface of the heart). The tissue sample is examined to verify the presence of the disease, as well as to try to determine the infective cause. An approach used only with a patient's consent, this procedure may also confirm acute myocarditis, allowing close monitoring of potential congestive heart failure.

Treatment

While myocarditis is a serious condition, there is no medical treatment necessary if it results from a general viral infection. The only steps to recovery include rest and avoidance of physical exertion. Adequate rest becomes more important to recovery if the case is severe myocarditis with signs of dilated **cardiomyopathy** (disease of the heart muscles). In this case, medical treatment for congestive heart failure may include the following medications: angiotensin converting enzyme (ACE) inhibitors, **diuretics** to reduce fluid retention, digitalis to stimulate a stronger heartbeat, and low-dose beta-blockers.

If myocarditis is caused by a bacterial infection, the disease is treated with **antibiotics** to fight the infection. If severe rhythm disturbances are involved, cardiac assist devices, an "artificial heart," or **heart transplantation** may be the only option for complete recovery.

Prognosis

The outlook for a diagnosed case of myocarditis caused by a viral infection is excellent, with many cases healing themselves spontaneously. Severe or acute myocarditis may be controlled with medication to prevent heart failure. Because this disease may be mild or may be extreme and cause serious arrhythmias, the prognosis varies. Cases of myocarditis may vary from complete healing (with or without significant scarring), to severe congestive heart failure leading to **death** or requiring a heart transplant.

Inflammation of the myocardium may also cause acute **pericarditis** (inflammation of the outer lining of the heart). Due to the potential effects of the disease, including sudden death, it is imperative that proper medical attention is obtained.

KEY TERMS

Adenovirus—One type of virus that can cause upper respiratory tract infections.

Angiography—A procedure which uses x ray after injecting a radiopaque substance to examine the blood vessels and lymphatics.

Arrhythmia—An irregular heartbeat or action.

Cardiac catheterization—A diagnostic procedure that gives a comprehensive examination of how the heart and its blood vessels function; performed by inserting one or more catheters through a peripheral blood vessel in the arm or leg.

Coxsackie B virus—A mild virus belonging to a group of viruses (coxsackievirus) that may produce a variety of illnesses, including myocarditis.

Echocardiography—A noninvasive diagnostic procedure that uses ultrasound to examine internal cardiac structures.

Electrocardiogram—A record of the electrical activity of the heart, with each wave being labeled as P, Q, R, S, and T waves. Often used in the diagnosis of cases of abnormal cardiac rhythm and myocardial damage.

Hypertensive heart disease—High blood pressure resulting in a disease of the heart.

Ischemic heart disease—Insufficient blood supply to the heart muscle (myocardium).

Valvular heart disease—A disease of any one of the four valves that controls blood flow into, through, and out of the heart.

Ventricular tachycardia— An abnormally rapid heartbeat. It includes a series of at least three beats arising from a ventricular area at a rate of more than 100 beats per minute, usually ranging from 150-200 beats per minute.

Prevention

Although myocarditis is an unpredictable disease, the following measures may help prevent its onset. Individuals should:

- Take extra measures to avoid infections, and obtain appropriate treatment for infections.

- Limit alcohol consumption to no more than one or two drinks a day, if any.

- Maintain current immunizations against **diphtheria**, tetanus, measles, **rubella**, and **polio**.

- Avoid anything that may cause the abnormal heart to work too hard, including salt and vigorous exercise.

Resources

ORGANIZATIONS

American Heart Association. 7320 Greenville Ave. Dallas, TX 75231. (214) 373-6300. <http://www.americanheart.org>.

National Heart, Lung and Blood Institute. P.O. Box 30105, Bethesda, MD 20824-0105. (301) 251-1222. <http://www.nhlbi.nih.gov>.

Beth A. Kapes

Myoglobin test

Definition

Myoglobin is a protein found in muscle. Myoglobin tests are done to evaluate a person who has symptoms of a **heart attack** (myocardial infarction) or other muscle damage.

Purpose

Myoglobin holds oxygen inside heart and skeletal muscle (muscles that attach to and move bones). It is continually released into the blood in small amounts due to normal turnover of muscle cells. Kidneys discard the myoglobin into urine.

When muscle is damaged, as in a heart attack, larger amounts of myoglobin are released and blood levels rise rapidly. Myoglobin is one of the first tests done to determine if a person with chest **pain** is having a heart attack, as it may be one of the first blood tests to become abnormal.

Damage or injury to skeletal muscle also causes myoglobin to be released into the blood.

Description

Heart attack must be diagnosed quickly. Medications to prevent heart damage are effective only within a limited number of hours. Yet, because of their risk for excessive bleeding, these medications are given only after a diagnosis of heart attack is made.

Myoglobin is one of several cardiac markers used to make the diagnosis. Cardiac markers are substances in blood whose levels rise in the hours following a heart attack. Increased levels help diagnose a heart attack; persistent normal levels rule it out.

Each cardiac marker rises, peaks, and returns to a normal level according to its own timeline, or diagnostic window. Myoglobin is useful because it has the earliest diagnostic window. It is the first marker to rise after chest pain begins. Myoglobin levels rise within two to three hours, and sometimes as early as 30 minutes. They peak after six to nine hours. The levels return to normal within 24-36 hours.

Although a rise in myoglobin supports a diagnosis of heart attack, it is not conclusive. Simultaneous skeletal muscle damage could also cause the increase. Myoglobin rules out, rather than proves, a diagnosis in the following way. If myoglobin levels have not risen after more than five hours, a heart attack in unlikely. Normal levels in the first two to three hours do not rule out an infarction.

The myoglobin test is sometimes repeated every one to two hours to watch for the rise and peak. Results are available within 30 minutes.

Myoglobin in large amounts is toxic to the kidney. When a person has high amounts of myoglobin in the blood, kidney function must be monitored.

Preparation

This test requires 5 ml of blood. Collection of the sample takes only a few minutes. A urine myoglobin test requires 1 ml of urine collected into a urine collection cup.

Aftercare

Discomfort or bruising may occur at the puncture site or the person may feel dizzy or faint. Pressure to the puncture site until the bleeding stops reduces bruising. Warm packs to the puncture site relieve discomfort.

Normal results

Normal results vary based on the laboratory and method used.

Abnormal results

Myoglobin levels and levels of other cardiac markers are usually considered before finally confirming a diagnosis of heart attack. A level that has doubled after one to two hours, even if the level is still in the normal range, indicates a significant rise that may be due to heart attack.

Increased levels are also found with skeletal muscle damage or disease, such as an injury, **muscular dystrophy**, or **polymyositis**. Myoglobin levels also rise during renal failure because kidneys lose their ability to clear myoglobin from blood.

Resources

BOOKS

Wu, Alan, editor. *Cardiac Markers*. Washington, DC: American Association of Clinical Chemistry (AACC) Press, 1998.

Nancy J. Nordenson

Myomas *see* **Uterine fibroids**

Myomectomy

Definition

Myomectomy is the removal of fibroids (noncancerous tumors) from the wall of the uterus. Myomectomy is the preferred treatment for symptomatic fibroids in women who want to keep their uterus. Larger fibroids must be removed with an abdominal incision, but small fibroids can be taken out using **laparoscopy** or **hysteroscopy**.

Purpose

A myomectomy can remove **uterine fibroids** that are causing symptoms. It is an alternative to surgical removal of the whole uterus (**hysterectomy**). The procedure can relieve fibroid-induced menstrual symptoms that have not responded to medication. Myomectomy also may be an effective treatment for **infertility** caused by the presence of fibroids.

Precautions

There is a risk that removal of the fibroids may lead to such severe bleeding that the uterus itself will have to be removed. Because of the risk of blood loss during a myomectomy, patients may want to consider banking their own blood before surgery.

Description

Usually, fibroids are buried in the outer wall of the uterus and abdominal surgery is required. If they are on the inner wall of the uterus, uterine fibroids can be removed using hysteroscopy. If they are on a stalk (pedunculated) on the outer surface of the uterus, laparoscopy can be performed.

Removing fibroids through abdominal surgery is a more difficult and slightly more risky operation than a hysterectomy. This is because the uterus bleeds from the sites where the fibroids were, and it may be difficult or impossible to stop the bleeding. This surgery is usually performed under **general anesthesia**, although some patients may be given a spinal or epidural anesthesia.

The incision may be horizontal (the "bikini" incision) or a vertical incision from the navel downward. After separating the muscle layers underneath the skin, the surgeon makes an opening in the abdominal wall. Next, the surgeon makes an incision over each fibroid, grasping and pulling out each growth.

Every opening in the uterine wall is then stitched with sutures. The uterus must be meticulously repaired in order to eliminate potential sites of bleeding or infection. Then, the surgeon sutures the abdominal wall and muscle layers above it with absorbable stitches, and closes the skin with clips or nonabsorbable stitches.

When appropriate, a laparoscopic myomectomy may be performed. In this procedure, the surgeon removes fibroids with the help of a viewing tube (laparoscope) inserted into the pelvic cavity through an incision in the navel. The fibroids are removed through a tiny incision under the navel that is much smaller than the 4 or 5 inch opening required for a standard myomectomy.

If the fibroids are small and located on the inner surface of the uterus, they can be removed with a thin telescope-like device called a hysteroscope. The hysteroscope is inserted into the vagina through the cervix and into the uterus. This procedure does not require any abdominal incision, so hospitalization is shorter.

Preparation

Surgeons often recommend hormone treatment with a drug called leuprolide (Lupron) two to six months before surgery in order to shrink the fibroids. This makes the fibroids easier to remove. In addition, Lupron stops menstruation, so women who are anemic have an opportunity to build up their **blood count**. While the drug treatment may reduce the risk of excess blood loss during surgery, there is a small risk that temporarily-smaller fibroids might be missed during myomectomy, only to enlarge later after the surgery is completed.

Aftercare

Patients may need four to six weeks of recovery following a standard myomectomy before they can return to normal activities. Women who have had laparoscopic or hysteroscopic myomectomies, however, can leave the hospital the day after surgery and usually recovery completely within two to three days to one to three weeks.

Risks

The risks of a myomectomy performed by a skilled surgeon are about the same as hysterectomy (one of the most common and safest surgeries). Removing multiple fibroids is more difficult and slightly more risky.

Possible complications include:

- Infection.
- Blood loss.
- The wall of the uterus may be weakened if the removal of a large fibroid leaves a wound that extends the complete thickness of the wall. Special precautions may be needed in future pregnancies. For example, the delivery may need to be performed surgically (Caesarean section).
- Adverse reactions to anesthesia.
- Internal scarring (and possible infertility).

Since fibroids tend to appear and grow as a woman ages (until **menopause**), it is possible that new fibroids will appear after myomectomy.

Resources

OTHER

Toaff, Michael E. "Myomectomy." *Alternatives to Hysterectomy Page.* < http://www.netreach.net/~hysterectomyedu/myomecto.htm >.

Carol A. Turkington

Myopathies

Definition

Myopathies are diseases of skeletal muscle which are not caused by nerve disorders. These diseases cause the skeletal or voluntary muscles to become weak or wasted.

Description

There are many different types of myopathies, some of which are inherited, some inflammatory, and some caused by endocrine problems. Myopathies are rare and not usually fatal. Typically, effects are mild, largely causing muscle weakness and movement problems, and many are transitory. Only rarely will patients become dependent on a wheelchair. However, **muscular dystrophy** (which is technically a form of myopathy) is far more severe. Some types of this disease are fatal in early adulthood.

Causes and symptoms

Myopathies are usually degenerative, but they are sometimes caused by drug side effects, chemical **poisoning**, or a chronic disorder of the immune system.

Genetic myopathies

Among their many functions, genes are responsible for overseeing the production of proteins important in maintaining healthy cells. Muscle cells produce thousands of proteins. With each of the inherited myopathies, a genetic defect is linked to a lack of, or problem with, one of the proteins needed for normal muscle cell function.

There are several different kinds of myopathy caused by defective genes:

- Central core disease
- Centronuclear (myotubular) myopathy
- Myotonia congenita

- Nemaline myopathy
- Paramyotonia congenita
- Periodic **paralysis** (hypokalemic and hyperkalemic forms)
- Mitochondrial myopathies.

Most of these genetic myopathies are dominant, which means that a child needs to inherit only one copy of the defective gene from one parent in order to have the disease. The parent with the defective gene also has the disorder, and each of this parent's children has a 50% chance of also inheriting the disease. Male and female children are equally at risk.

However, one form of myotonia congenita and some forms of nemaline myopathy must be inherited from both parents, each of whom carry a recessive defective gene but who do not have symptoms of the disease. Each child of such parents has a 25% chance of inheriting both genes and showing signs of the disease, and a 50% chance of inheriting one defective gene from only one parent. If the child inherited just one defective gene, he or she would be a carrier but would not show signs of the disease.

A few forms of centronuclear myopathy develop primarily in males. Females who inherit the defective gene are usually carriers without symptoms, like their mothers, but they can pass on the disease to their sons. Mitochondrial myopathies are inherited through the mother, since sperm do not contain mitochondria. (Mitochondria play a key role in energy production in the body's cells.)

The major symptoms associated with the genetic myopathies include:

- Central core disease: mild weakness of voluntary muscles, especially in the hips and legs; hip displacement; delays in reaching developmental motor milestones; problems with running, jumping, and climbing stairs develop in childhood
- Centronuclear myopathy: weakness of voluntary muscles including those on the face, arms, legs, and trunk; drooping upper eyelids; facial weakness; foot drop; affected muscles almost always lack reflexes
- Myotonia congenita: voluntary muscles of the arms, legs, and face are stiff or slow to relax after contracting (myotonia); stiffness triggered by **fatigue**, **stress**, cold, or long rest periods, such as a night's sleep; stiffness can be relieved by repeated movement of the affected muscles
- Nemaline myopathy: moderate weakness of voluntary muscles in the arms, legs, and trunk; mild weakness of facial muscles; delays in reaching developmental

motor milestones; decreased or absent reflexes in affected muscles; long, narrow face; high-arched palate; jaw projects beyond upper part of the face

- Paramyotonia congenita: stiffness (myotonia) of voluntary muscles in the face, hands, and forearms; attacks spontaneous or triggered by cold temperatures; stiffness made worse by repeated movement; episodes of stiffness last longer than those seen in myotonia congenita

- Periodic paralysis: attacks of temporary muscle weakness (muscles work normally between attacks); in the hypokalemic (low calcium) form, attacks triggered by vigorous **exercise**, heavy meals (high in carbohydrates), insulin, stress, alcohol, infection, **pregnancy**; in the hyperkalemic (normal/high calcium) form, attacks triggered by vigorous exercise, stress, pregnancy, missing a meal, steroid drugs, high potassium intake

- Mitochondrial myopathies: symptoms vary quite widely with the form of the disease and may include progressive weakness of the eye muscles (ocular myopathy), weakness of the arms and legs, or multisystem problems primarily involving the brain and muscles.

Endocrine-related myopathies

In some cases, myopathies can be caused by a malfunctioning gland (or glands), which produces either too much or too little of the chemical messengers called hormones. Hormones are carried by the blood and one of their many functions is to regulate muscle activity. Problems in producing hormones can lead to muscle weakness.

Hyperthyroid myopathy and hypothyroid myopathy affect different muscles in different ways. Hyperthyroid myopathy occurs when the thyroid gland produces too much thyroxine, leading to muscle weakness, some muscle wasting in hips and shoulders, and, sometimes, problems with eye muscles. The hypothyroid type occurs when too little hormone is produced, leading to stiffness, cramps, and weakness of arm and leg muscles.

Inflammatory myopathies

Some myopathies are inflammatory, leading to inflamed, weakened muscles. Inflammation is a protective response of injured tissues characterized by redness, increased heat, swelling, and/or **pain** in the affected area. Examples of this type include **polymyositis**, **dermatomyositis**, and **myositis** ossificans.

Dermatomyositis is a disease of the connective tissue that also involves weak, tender, inflamed muscles. In fact, muscle tissue loss may be so severe that the person may be unable to walk. Skin inflammation is also present. The cause is unknown, but viral infection and **antibiotics** are associated with the condition. In some cases, dermatomyositis is associated with rheumatologic disease or **cancer**. Polymyositis involves inflammation of many muscles usually accompanied by deformity, swelling, sleeplessness, pain, sweating, and tension. It, too, may be associated with cancer. Myositis ossificans is a rare inherited disease in which muscle tissue is replaced by bone, beginning in childhood.

Muscular dystrophy

While considered to be a separate group of diseases, the muscular dystrophies also technically involve muscle wasting and can be described as myopathies. These relatively rare diseases appear during childhood and adolescence, and are caused by muscle destruction or degeneration. They are a group of genetic disorders caused by problems in the production of key proteins.

The forms of muscular dystrophy (MD) differ according to the way they are inherited, the age of onset, the muscles they affect, and how fast they progress. The most common type is Duchenne MD, affecting one or two in every 10,000 boys. Other types of MD include Becker's, **myotonic dystrophy**, limb-girdle MD, and facioscapulohumeral MD.

Diagnosis

Early diagnosis of myopathy is important so that the best possible care can be provided as soon as possible. An experienced physician can diagnose a myopathy by evaluating a person's medical history and by performing a thorough physical exam. Diagnostic tests can help differentiate between the different types of myopathy, as well as between myopathy and other neuromuscular disorders. If the doctor suspects a genetic myopathy, a thorough family history will also be taken.

Diagnostic tests the doctor may order include:

- Measurements of potassium in the blood

- Muscle biopsy

- Electromyogram (EMG).

Treatment

Treatment depends on the specific type of myopathy the person has:

- Periodic paralysis: medication and dietary changes

- Hyperthyroid or hypothyroid myopathy: treatment of the underlying thyroid abnormality

- Myositis ossificans: medication may prevent abnormal bone formation, but there is no cure following onset

- Central core disease: no treatment

- Nemaline myopathy: no treatment

- Centronuclear (myotubular) myopathy: no treatment

- Paramyotonia congenita: treatment often unnecessary

- Myotonia congenita: drug treatment (if necessary), but drugs do not affect the underlying disease, and attacks may still occur.

Prognosis

The prognosis for patients with myopathy depends on the type and severity of the individual disease. In most cases, the myopathy can be successfully treated and the patient returned to normal life.

Muscular dystrophy, however, is generally a much more serious condition. Duchenne's MD is usually fatal by the late teens; Becker's MD is less serious and may not be fatal until the 50s.

Resources

ORGANIZATIONS

Muscular Dystrophy Association. 3300 East Sunrise Drive, Tucson, AZ 85718. (800) 572-1717. <http://www.mdausa.org>.

Carol A. Turkington

Myopia

Definition

Myopia is the medical term for nearsightedness. People with myopia see objects more clearly when they are close to the eye, while distant objects appear blurred or fuzzy. Reading and close-up work may be clear, but distance vision is blurry.

Description

To understand myopia it is necessary to have a basic knowledge of the main parts of the eye's focusing system: the cornea, the lens, and the retina. The cornea is a tough, transparent, dome-shaped tissue that covers the front of the eye (not to be confused with the white, opaque sclera). The cornea lies in front of the iris (the colored part of the eye). The lens is a transparent, double-convex structure located behind the iris. The retina is a thin membrane that lines the rear of the eyeball. Light-sensitive retinal cells convert incoming light rays into electrical signals that are sent along the optic nerve to the brain, which then interprets the images.

In people with normal vision, parallel light rays enter the eye and are bent by the cornea and lens (a process called refraction) to focus precisely on the retina, providing a crisp, clear image. In the myopic eye, the focusing power of the cornea (the major refracting structure of the eye) and the lens is too great with respect to the length of the eyeball. Light rays are bent too much, and they converge in front of the retina. This inaccuracy is called a refractive error. In other words, an overfocused fuzzy image is sent to the brain.

There are many types of myopia. Some common types include:

- Physiologic
- Pathologic
- Acquired.

By far the most common form, physiologic myopia develops in children sometime between the ages of 5-10 years and gradually progresses until the eye is fully grown. Physiologic myopia may include refractive myopia (the cornea and lens-bending properties are too strong) and axial myopia (the eyeball is too long). Pathologic myopia is a far less common abnormality. This condition begins as physiologic myopia, but rather than stabilizing, the eye continues to enlarge at an abnormal rate (progressive myopia). This more advanced type of myopia may lead to degenerative changes in the eye (degenerative myopia). Acquired myopia occurs after infancy. This condition may be seen in association with uncontrolled diabetes and certain types of **cataracts**. **Antihypertensive drugs** and other medications can also affect the refractive power of the lens.

Genetic profile

Eyecare professionals have debated the role of genetics in the development of myopia for many years. Some believe that a tendency toward myopia may be inherited, but the actual disorder results from a combination of environmental and genetic factors. Environmental factors include close work; work with computer monitors or other instruments that emit some light (electron microscopes, photographic equipment, lasers, etc.); emotional **stress**; and eye strain.

A variety of genetic patterns for inheriting myopia have been suggested. One explanation for lack of agreement is that the genetic profile of high myopia (defined as a refractive error greater than -6 diopters) may differ from that of low myopia. Some researchers think that high myopia is determined by genetic factors to a greater extent than low myopia.

Another explanation for disagreement regarding the role of heredity in myopia is the sensitivity of the human eye to very small changes in its anatomical structure. Since even small deviations from normal structure cause significant refractive errors, it may be difficult to single out any specific genetic or environmental factor as their cause.

Since 1992, genetic markers that may be associated with genes for myopia have been located on human chromosomes 1, 2, 12, and 18. There is some genetic information on the short arm of chromosome 2 in highly myopic people. Genetic information for low myopia appears to be located on the short arm of chromosome 1, but it is not known whether this information governs the structure of the eye itself or vulnerability to environmental factors.

In 1998 a team of American researchers presented evidence that a gene for familial high myopia with an autosomal dominant transmission pattern could be mapped to human chromosome 18 in eight North American families. The same group also found a second locus for this form of myopia on human chromosome 12 in a large German/Italian family. In 1999 a group of French researchers found no linkage between chromosome 18 and 32 French families with familial high myopia. These findings have been taken to indicate that more than one gene is involved in the transmission of the disorder.

It has been known for some years that a family history of myopia is one of the most important risk factors for developing the condition. Only 6%-15% of children with myopia come from families in which neither parent is myopic. In families with one myopic parent, 23%-40% of the children develop myopia. If both parents are myopic, the rate rises to 33%-60% for their children. One American study found that children with two myopic parents are 6.42 times as likely to develop myopia themselves as children with only one or no myopic parents. The precise interplay of genetic and environmental factors in these family patterns, however, is not yet known.

One multigenerational study of Chinese subjects indicated that subjects in the third generation had a higher risk of developing myopia even if their parents were not myopic. The researchers concluded that, at least in China, the genetic factors in myopia have remained constant over the past three generations while the environmental factors have intensified. The increase in the percentage of people with myopia over the last 50 years in the United States has led American researchers to the same conclusion.

The debate continued with more recent reports. In the summer of 2004, one report said that scientists were close to identifying the myopia gene, located on chromosome 11. Another report reviewed several studies and claimed that lifestyle was to blame for myopia. For instance, a study found that 80% of 14- to 18-year old boys studying in schools in Israel that emphasize reading religious texts have myopia, while the rates for boys in state school was just 30%. It is likely that genes and environment play a role.

Myopia is the most common eye disorder in humans around the world. It affects between 25% and 35% of the adult population in the United States and the developed countries, but is thought to affect as much as 40% of the population in some parts of Asia. Some researchers have found slightly higher rates of myopia in women than in men.

The age distribution of myopia in the United States varies considerably. Five-year-olds have the lowest rate of myopia (less than 5%) of any age group. The prevalence of myopia rises among children and adolescents in school until it reaches the 25%-35% mark in the young adult population. It declines slightly in the over-45 age group; about 20% of 65-year-olds have myopia. The figure drops to 14% for Americans over 70.

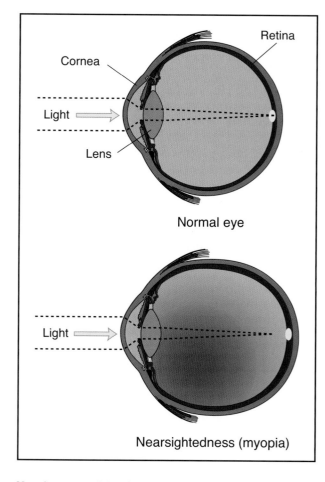

Normal eye

Nearsightedness (myopia)

Myopia, or nearsightedness, is a condition of the eye in which objects are seen more clearly when close to the eye while distant objects appear blurred or fuzzy. *(Illustration by Electronic Illustrators Group.)*

Other factors that affect the demographic distribution of myopia are income level and education. The prevalence of myopia is higher among people with above-average incomes and educational attainments. Myopia is also more prevalent among people whose work requires a great deal of close focusing, including work with computers.

Causes and symptoms

Myopia is said to be caused by an elongation of the eyeball. This means that the oblong (as opposed to normal spherical) shape of the myopic eye causes the cornea and lens to focus at a point in front of the retina. A more precise explanation is that there is an inadequate correlation between the focusing power of the cornea and lens and the length of the eye.

People are generally born with a small amount of **hyperopia** (farsightedness), but as the eye grows this

decreases and myopia does not become evident until later. This change is one reason why some researchers think that myopia is an acquired rather than an inherited trait.

The symptoms of myopia are blurred distance vision, eye discomfort, squinting, and eye strain.

Diagnosis

The diagnosis of myopia is typically made during the first several years of elementary school when a teacher notices a child having difficulty seeing the chalkboard, reading, or concentrating. The teacher or school nurse often recommends an **eye examination** by an ophthalmologist or optometrist. An ophthalmologist—M.D. or D.O. (Doctor of Osteopathy)—is a medical doctor trained in the diagnosis and treatment of eye problems. Ophthalmologists also perform eye surgery. An optometrist (O.D.) diagnoses and manages and/or treats eye and visual disorders. In many states, optometrists are licensed to use diagnostic and therapeutic drugs.

A patient's distance vision is tested by reading letters or numbers on a chart posted a set distance away (usually 20 ft). The doctor asks the patient to view images through a variety of lenses to obtain the best correction. The doctor also examines the inside of the eye and the retina. An instrument called a slit lamp is used to examine the cornea and lens. The eyeglass prescription is written in terms of diopters (D), which measure the degree of refractive error. Mild to moderate myopia usually falls between -1.00D and -6.00D. Normal vision is commonly referred to as 20/20 to describe the eye's focusing ability at a distance of 20 ft from an object. For example, 20/50 means that a myopic person must stand 20 ft away from an eye chart to see what a normal person can see at 50 ft. The larger the bottom number, the greater the myopia.

Treatment

People with myopia have three main options for treatment: eyeglasses, contact lenses, and for those who meet certain criteria, refractive eye surgery.

Eyeglasses

Eyeglasses are the most common method used to correct myopia. Concave glass or plastic lenses are placed in frames in front of the eyes. The lenses are ground to the thickness and curvature specified in the eyeglass prescription. The lenses cause the light rays to diverge so that they focus further back, directly on the retina, producing clear distance vision.

Contact lenses

Contact lenses are a second option for treatment. Contact lenses are extremely thin round discs of plastic that are worn on the eye in front of the cornea. Although there may be some initial discomfort, most people quickly grow accustomed to contact lenses. Hard contact lenses, made from a material called PMMA, are virtually obsolete. Rigid gas permeable lenses (RGP) are made of plastic that holds its shape but allows the passage of some oxygen into the eye. Some believe that RGP lenses may halt or slow the progression of myopia because they maintain a constant, gentle pressure that flattens the cornea. As of 2001, the National Eye Institute is conducting an ongoing study of RGP lenses called the Contact Lens and Myopia Progression (CLAMP) Study, with results to be published in 2003.

A procedure called orthokeratology acts on this principle of "corneal molding." However, when contact lenses are discontinued for a period of time, the cornea will generally go back to its original shape. Rigid gas permeable lenses offer crisp, clear, sight. Soft contact lenses are made of flexible plastic and can be up to 80% water. Soft lenses offer increased comfort and the advantage of extended wear; some can be worn continuously for up to one week. While oxygen passes freely through soft lenses, bacterial contamination and other problems can occur, requiring replacement of lenses on a regular basis. It is very important to follow the cleaning and disinfecting regimens prescribed because protein and lipid buildup can occur on the lenses, causing discomfort or increasing the risk of infection. Contact lenses offer several benefits over glasses, including: better vision, less distortion, clear peripheral vision, and cosmetic appeal. In addition, contacts do not steam up from perspiration or changes in temperature.

Refractive eye surgery

For people who find glasses and contact lenses inconvenient or uncomfortable, and who meet selection criteria regarding age, degree of myopia, general health, etc., refractive eye surgery is a third treatment alternative. There are three types of corrective surgeries available as of 2001: 1) **radial keratotomy** (RK), 2) photorefractive keratectomy (PRK), and 3) laser-assisted in-situ keratomileusis (LASIK). Refractive eye surgery improves myopic vision by permanently changing the shape of the cornea so that light rays focus properly on the retina. These procedures are performed on an outpatient basis and generally take 10-30 minutes. LASIK is approved by the

FDA, though certain lasers are in various stages of approval at a given time. Patients should check with the FDA and ask for patient references when choosing a LASIK provider.

RADIAL KERATOTOMY. Radial keratotomy (RK), the first of these procedures made available, has a high associated risk. It was first developed in Japan and the Soviet Union, and introduced into the United States in 1978. The surgeon uses a delicate diamond-tipped blade, a microscope, and microscopic instruments to make several spoke-like "radial" incisions in the non-viewing (peripheral) portion of the cornea. As the incisions heal, the slits alter the curve of the cornea, making it more flat, which may improve the focus of images onto the retina.

PHOTOREFRACTIVE KERATECTOMY. Photorefractive keratectomy (PRK) involves the use of a computer to measure the shape of the cornea. Using these measurements, the surgeon applies a computer-controlled laser to make modifications to the cornea. The PRK procedure flattens the cornea by vaporizing small amounts of tissue from the cornea's surface. It is important to make sure the laser being used is FDA approved. Photorefractive keratectomy can be used to treat mild to moderate forms of myopia. The cost is approximately $2,000 per eye.

LASER-ASSISTED IN-SITU KERATOMILEUSIS. Laser-assisted in-situ keratomileusis (LASIK) is the newest of these procedures. It is recommended for moderate to severe cases of myopia. A variation on the PRK method, LASIK uses lasers and a cutting tool called a microkeratome to cut a circular flap on the cornea. The flap is flipped back to expose the inner layers of the cornea. The cornea is treated with a laser to change the shape and focusing properties, then the flap is replaced.

Risks

All of these surgical procedures carry risks, the most serious being corneal scarring, corneal rupture, infection, cataracts, and loss of vision. In addition, a study published in March 2001 warned that mountain climbers who have had LASIK surgery should be aware of possible changes in their vision at high altitudes. The lack of oxygen at high altitudes causes temporary changes in the thickness of the cornea.

Since refractive eye surgery does not guarantee 20/20 vision, it is important to have realistic expectations before choosing this treatment. In a 10-year study conducted by the National Eye Institute between 1983 and 1993, more than 50% of people with radial keratotomy gained 20/20 vision, and 85% passed a

KEY TERMS

Accommodation—The ability of the lens to change its focus from distant to near objects. It is achieved through the action of the ciliary muscles that change the shape of the lens.

Cornea—The transparent structure of the eye over the lens that is continous with the sclera in forming the outermost, protective, layer of the eye.

Diopter (D)—A unit of measure for describing refractive power.

Laser-assisted in-situ keratomileusis (LASIK)—A procedure that uses a cutting tool and a laser to modify the cornea and correct moderate to high levels of myopia.

Lens—The transparent, elastic, curved structure behind the iris (colored part of the eye) that helps focus light on the retina.

Ophthalmologist—A physician specializing in the medical and surgical treatment of eye disorders.

Optic nerve—A bundle of nerve fibers that carries visual messages from the retina in the form of electrical signals to the brain.

Optometrist—A medical professional who examines and tests the eyes for disease and treats visual disorders by prescribing corrective lenses and/or vision therapy. In many states, optometrists are licensed to use diagnostic and therapeutic drugs to treat certain ocular diseases.

Orthokeratology—A method of reshaping the cornea using a contact lens. It is not considered a permanent method to reduce myopia.

Peripheral vision—The ability to see objects that are not located directly in front of the eye. Peripheral vision allows people to see objects located on the side or edge of their field of vision.

Photorefractive keratectomy (PRK)—A procedure that uses an excimer laser to make modifications to the cornea and permanently correct myopia.

Radial keratotomy (RK)—A surgical procedure involving the use of a diamond-tipped blade to make several spoke-like slits in the peripheral (nonviewing) portion of the cornea to improve the focus of the eye and correct myopia by flattening the cornea.

Refraction—The bending of light rays as they pass from one medium through another. Used to describe the action of the cornea and lens on light rays as they enter they eye. Also used to describe the determination and measurement of the eye's focusing system by an optometrist or ophthalmologist.

Refractive eye surgery—A general term for surgical procedures that can improve or correct refractive errors by permanently changing the shape of the cornea.

Retina—The light-sensitive layer of tissue in the back of the eye that receives and transmits visual signals to the brain through the optic nerve.

Visual acuity—The ability to distinguish details and shapes of objects.

---

driving test (requiring 20/40 vision) after surgery, without glasses or contact lenses. Even if the patient gains near-perfect vision, however, there are potentially irritating side effects, such as postoperative **pain**, poor night vision, variation in visual acuity, light sensitivity and glare, and optical distortion. Refractive eye surgeries are considered elective procedures and are not always covered by insurance plans.

Myopia treatments under research include corneal implants and permanent surgically placed contact lenses.

Alternative treatments

Some eye care professionals recommend treatments to help improve circulation, reduce eye strain, and relax the eye muscles. It is possible that by combining exercises with changes in behavior, the progression of myopia may be slowed or prevented. Alternative treatments include: visual therapy (also referred to as **vision training** or eye exercises); discontinuing close work; reducing eye strain (taking a rest break during periods of prolonged near vision tasks); and wearing bifocals to decrease the need to accommodate when doing close-up work.

Prognosis

Glasses and contact lenses can (but not always) correct the patient's vision to 20/20. Refractive surgery can make permanent improvements for the right candidates.

While the genetic factors that influence the transmission and severity of myopia cannot be changed, some environmental factors can be modified. They include reducing close work; reading and working in good light; taking frequent breaks when working at a computer or microscope for long periods of time; maintaining good **nutrition**; and practicing visual therapy (when recommended).

Eye strain can be prevented by using sufficient light for reading and close work, and by wearing corrective lenses as prescribed. Everyone should have regular eye examinations to see if their prescription has changed or if any other problems have developed. This is particularly important for people with high (degenerative) myopia who are at a greater risk of developing **retinal detachment**, retinal degeneration, **glaucoma**, or other problems.

Resources

PERIODICALS

"Blame lifestyle for myopia, not genes." *Biotech Week* July 28, 2004: 65.

Naiglin. L., et al. "Familial high myopia: evidence of an autosomal dominant mode of inheritance and genetic heterogeneity." *Annals of Genetics* 42, no. 3 (1999): 140-146.

Pacell, R, et al. "Role of genetic factors in the etiology of juvenile-onset myopia based on a longitudinal study of refractive error." *Optometry and Visual Science* 76 (June 1999): 381-386.

Saw, SM, et al. "Myopia: gene-environment interaction." *Annals of the Academy of Medicine of Singapore* 29 (May 2000): 290-297.

"Scientists close to identifying myopia gene." *Chemistry and Industry* August 16, 2004: 7.

Wu, MM, and MH Edwards. "The effect of having myopic parents: an analysis of myopia in three generations." *Optometry and Visual Science* 76 (June 1999): 341-342.

ORGANIZATIONS

American Academy of Ophthalmology. PO Box 7424, San Francisco, CA 94120-7424. (415) 561-8500. < http://www.eyenet.org >.

American Optometric Association. 243 North Lindbergh Blvd., St. Louis, MO 63141. (314) 991-4100. < http://www.aoanet.org >.

International Myopia Prevention Association. RD No. 5, Box 171, Ligonier, PA 15658. (412) 238-2101.

Myopia International Research Foundation. 1265 Broadway, Room 608, New York, NY 10001. (212) 684-2777.

National Eye Institute. Bldg. 31 Rm 6A32, 31 Center Dr., MSC 2510, Bethesda, MD 20892-2510. (301) 496-5248. 2020@nei.nih.gov. < http://www.nei.nih.gov >.

Rebecca J. Frey, PhD
Risa Palley Flynn
Teresa G. Odle

Myositis

Definition

Myositis is a rare disease in which the muscle fibers and skin are inflamed and damaged, resulting in muscle weakness. There are several types of myositis that affect different parts of the body.

Description

The persistent inflammation that is associated with myositis develops slowly over weeks to months and often years, with progressive weakening of the muscles. Later in the course of the disease development muscle wasting or shortening (contracture) may develop. Myositis can range in severity from mild to debilitating.

The forms of myositis include:

- **Polymyositis** (PM) inflames and weakens muscles in many parts of the body, and especially those parts closest to the trunk. With polymyositis, dysphagia (difficulty, discomfort or **pain** in speaking or swallowing), **fatigue**, and pain in the muscles are common. PM rarely affects people under the age of 20, with the peak onset between the ages of 30 and 60.

- **Dermatomyositis** (DM) affects both the muscle fibers and skin by damaging the tiny blood vessels (capillaries) that supply blood to the muscle and skin, resulting in muscle weakness, pain, and fatigue. In addition the affected person develops a distinctive patchy, reddish rash on the eyelids, cheeks, bridge of the nose, back or upper chest, elbows, knees, and knuckles. There may also be hardened, tender bumps (possibly caused by inflammation of fat) under the skin. DM can occur at any age and is more common in females than males.

- Inclusion Body Myositis (IBM) typically begins after age 50, and is characterized by gradual weakening of muscles throughout the body, including the wrists or fingers, development of dysphagia, and atrophy of forearms and/or thigh muscles. Unlike the other types of myositis, IBM occurs more often in men than women, and also does not respond very well to drug therapy.

- Juvenile myositis (JM) involves muscle weakness, skin rash, and dysphagia in children. A common characteristic of JM is the formation of calcium deposits in the muscle (calcinosis). These deposits are hard and sometimes painful lumps of calcium under the skin that appear on the child's fingers, hands, elbows, and knees. Painful sores may appear if the lumps break through the skin. The child may also suffer from **contractures**, which is muscle shortening that results in joints staying bent. About half of the children with JM will have pain in their muscles.

Myositis is rare, affecting about 10 in one million people each year. DM and PM affect mostly women in the forties and fifties but men and children can also affect be affected, some at a young age (between the ages of 5 and 15). About 40,000 people in the United States may have this disease, with about 3,000 to 5,000 children affected.

Causes and symptoms

Myositis is thought to be an autoimmune disease. The body normally fights infections and disease by producing antibodies and white blood cells called lymphocytes in a process called the immune response. In an autoimmune disease, the immune response is overactive, and the immune system attacks and destroys the body's own normal healthy tissues. There is no known cause to the autoimmune response that results in myositis. However, investigators are studying whether the disease is triggered by such environmental agents as the organism that causes **toxoplasmosis**, *Toxoplasma gondii*, the **Lyme disease** organism, *Borrelia burgdorferi*, the coxsackievirus, or by **food allergies**. Some cases of IBM are thought to be inherited.

The first symptoms of most types of myositis are weakness and pain in the muscles of the hips and shoulders. The affected person may have trouble getting up from a chair, lifting the arms above the head, or climbing stairs, and may be too tired to walk or stand. DM and PM mostly affects muscles that are close to and within the trunk of the body, while IBM involves a wider range of muscles. Myositis may make it difficult for the person to speak or swallow. When the disease affects the lungs or chest muscles, the person may have difficulty breathing. If the person has DM, they may develop characteristic **rashes**. Other symptoms may include **fever** and joint pain and swelling.

The first signs of JM is usually a red and patchy skin rash and/or a red or purplish rash on the eyelids or cheeks that look like **allergies**. Weak muscles may develop at the same time as the rash, or may develop days, weeks, or months after the appearance of the rash. Other symptoms of JM include falling, a weaker voice (dysophonia), or dysphagia. Calcinosis usually develops later during the course of the disease.

Diagnosis

Myositis can a difficult disease to diagnose, because it is rare, because the symptoms develop slowly, and because it can be mistaken for other diseases causing muscle weakness such as limb-girdle **muscular dystrophy**. Many cases of myositis go undiagnosed for years. The health care provider must rule out other conditions such as **hypothyroidism**, toxin exposure, drug reactions, and genetic disorders that can also affect muscles. The **physical examination** will include a complete medical history focusing on symptoms and when they occurred, and blood tests for autoantibodies and muscle enzymes (for example, creatine kinase (CK), which when present in the blood indicates muscle damage). Specialized tests may also be performed, including:

- an electromyogram, which measures the electrical pattern of the muscles

- a muscle biopsy, in which a small piece of muscle is removed, stained, and examined by microscopic techniques to determine if muscle fibers are damaged and whether the muscle fibers are being infiltrated by cells of the immune system

- magnetic resonance imaging (MRI) to identify areas of muscle inflammation.

Treatment

There is no cure for myositis. However, prompt and aggressive treatment may reduce muscle inflammation and prevent muscle weakness from progressing. Because of the many different kinds of symptoms and a wide range of reactions to different drugs, each person's treatment for myositis should be individualized.

Drugs that are used for treatment include **corticosteroids**, such as prednisone, to reduce inflammation and improve the body's reaction to infections. Corticosteroids are usually taken in the form of pills, but may also be injected. The amount of creatine kinase (CK) levels in the blood are monitored to determine how well the medicine is working. Corticosteroids may produce a number of side effects, such as weight gain, difficulties in fighting infections, psychiatric changes, sleeping troubles, water retention, bone thinning, facial swelling, diabetes, and **cataracts**. Corticosteroid therapy usually leads to improvement in myositis symptoms within two to three months, after which the dose can be lowered to avoid the side effects. If the dose of corticosteriods is going to be reduced, it is essential to lower the dose over a period of time.

Immunosuppressant drugs are used to slow down the immune system's attack on healthy tissue and improve skin rashes. Persons may be prescribed these drugs to control myositis if they are unable to tolerate corticosteroids or if the corticosteroids are not accomplishing the desired degree of treatment. Immunosuppressant drugs may also be used in conjunction with corticosteroids so that lower doses of corticosteroids can be used. Immunosuppressant drugs include azathioprine, methotrexate, cyclosporine, tacrolimus, etanercept, and mycophenolate mofetil.

Intravenous immunoglobulin (IVIg) appears to aid in improving muscle strength in many persons with myositis, particularly those with DM. It may be less effective in PM, and its role in treating IBM requires more study, although it has been shown to help some patients with IBM if they are diagnosed early. Immunoglobulins are normal proteins in the blood that attack anything foreign in the body, such as viruses and bacteria. IVIg is made from donated blood plasma from people with normal immune systems. Side effects from the the use of IVIg include **headache** and flu-like symptoms.

Topical cream or ointment forms of some of the medicines, such as prednisone and tacrolimus, can be used to heal and soothe the rash associated with DM. Non-steriodal anti-inflammatory drugs (NSAIDS) such as **aspirin** or ibuprofen can be used for pain relief. Calcinosis can be treated with prednisone, plaquenil (also called hydroxychloroquine), intravenous immunoglobin (IVIG), cyclosporine, and methotrexate.

After drug treatment results in improvement, the affected person begins a program of regular stretching exercises to maintain range of motion in the weakened arms and legs. Physical therapy may be used to prevent permanent muscle shortening. Whirlpool baths, heat, and gentle massages may also provide relief. Adequate rest is necessary, and affected persons should take frequent breaks throughout the day and limit their activity.

Patients with throat problems should be evaluated by a speech therapist who can evaluate the swallowing-related problems and make recommendations regarding diet changes and safe swallowing techniques.

Before a woman with myositis becomes pregnant, she should discuss the medicines that she is taking with her health care provider and evaluate the possible risks that she and the baby face if she does become pregnant. Many of the drugs used in the treatment of myositis may be harmful to the fetus or to a breast-fed baby.

It is recommended that a doctor experienced in the treatment of myositis, assisted by a rheumatologist, dermatologist, or neurologist, be consulted. Oftentimes a patient may have to be treated at a major medical center, where the disease has been seen and treated before.

Alternative treatment

Various supplements may be used in conjunction with traditional treatment to offset side effects of conventional drug treatment. The use of these suppplements should be approved by the primary health care provider.

Immunosuppressant drugs such as methotroxate and cyclophosphamide increase the risk of infection, so a healthy well-balanced diet is required. Methotroxate impairs the body's ability to absorb **folic acid**, so foods high in folic acid, such as leafy green vegetables, fruits, and folate-fortified breads and cereals are recommended. The use of folate supplements may also be recommended by the health care provider. **Vitamins** C and E can be used to help with the pain and infections associated with calcinosis.

Corticosteroids may have multiple side effects when taken for long periods of time at high doses. Calcium and Vitamin D are recommended to lower the risk of **osteoporosis**, a common side effect of prednisone use. **Hypertension** and fluid retention may be controlled by a diet low in salt. Steroid-induced diabetes (hyperglycemia) can be aided by a diet low in sugar and other simple carbohydrates. Proteinuria, in which the body breaks down protein faster than normal, may mean that more protein should be included in the diet.

Weight gain associated with the use of corticosteroids can be managed by the use of the DASH (Dietary Approach to Stop Hypertension) diet, which is high in fruits, vegetables, dietary fiber, and low-fat dairy products. Information concerning this diet, developed by the National Institutes of Health, can be found at [www.nhlbi.nih.gov/health/public/heart/hbp/dash/]. Weight gain can overtax weakened muscles and should be avoided if possible.

Prognosis

The progression of PM and DM varies from person to person, but the lifespan of an affected person is not usually significantly affected. DM responds more favorably to therapy than PM. Overall, many patients do improve and have a functional recovery. About half of the patients recover and can discontinue treatment within 5 years of beginning treatment. In children the chances of a cure are better than in adults, although some children do suffer a relapse. Of the remaining 50%, about 20% will still have the active disease and will require ongoing treatment, while up to 30% may have some remaining muscle weakness. However, IBM is disabling, and most patients will require the use of an assistive device such as a cane, walker, or wheel chair. The older the patient is when contracting IBM, the more rapidly the disease progresses.

Prevention

There is no known way to prevent myositis.

Resources

BOOKS

Kilpatrick, James R. (Compiler). *Coping with a Myositis Disease. Written by Myositis Patients Telling Their Personal Story of Dealing with this Muscle Disease.* Athens, TX: Kilpatrick Publishing Company, 2000.

Icon Health Publications. *Myositis: A Medical Dictionary, Bibliography, and Annotated Research Guide to Internet Resources.* San Diego, CA: Icon Health Publications, 2004.

Icon Health Publications. *The Official Patient's Sourcebook on Dermatomyositis: A Revised and Updated Directory for the Internet Age.* San Diego, CA: Icon Health Publications, 2002.

Icon Health Publications. *The Official Patient's Sourcebook on Inclusion Body Myositis: A Revised and Updated Directory for the Internet Age.* San Diego, CA: Icon Health Publications, 2002.

ORGANIZATIONS

Muscular Dystrophy Association - USA, National Headquarters. 3300 E. Sunrise Drive, Tucson, AZ 85718. Telephone: (800) 572-1717. Web site: www.mdausa.org/

Myositis Support Group. 205 Laurel Road, Athens, TX 75751. Telephone: (903) 675-6825. Fax: (903) 675-6823. Web site: www.myositissupportgroup.org/

The Myositis Association (TMA). 1233 20th St. NW, Suite 402Washington, DC 20036. Telephone: (202) 887-0082; Fax: (202) 466-8940; Web site: www.myositis.org/

OTHER

Progressive Management. *21st Century Complete Medical Guide to Myositis, including Dermatomyositis and Polymyositis, Authoritative Government Documents, Clinical References, and Practical Information for Patients and Physicians.* (CD-ROM). Washington, DC: Progressive Management, 2004.

Judith Sims

Myositis *see* **Myopathies**

Myotonia atrophica *see* **Myotonic dystrophy**

Myotonic dystrophy

Definition

Myotonic dystrophy is a progressive disease in which the muscles are weak and are slow to relax after contraction.

Description

Myotonic dystrophy (DM), also called dystrophia myotonica, myotonia atrophica, or Steinert's disease, is a common form of **muscular dystrophy**. DM is an inherited disease, affecting males and females approximately equally. About 30,000 people in the United States are affected. Symptoms may appear at any time from infancy to adulthood. DM causes general weakness, usually beginning in the muscles of the hands, feet, neck, or face. It slowly progresses to involve other muscle groups, including the heart. DM affects a wide variety of other organ systems as well.

A severe form of DM, congenital myotonic dystrophy or Thomsen's disease, may appear in newborns of mothers who have DM. Congenital means that the condition is present from birth. The incidence of congenital myotonic dystrophy is thought to be about 1:20,000.

DM occurs in about 1 per 7,000–8,000 people and has been described in people from all over the world.

Causes and symptoms

The most common type of DM is called DM1 and is caused by a mutation in a gene called myotonic dystrophy protein kinase (DMPK). The DMPK gene is located on chromosome 19q. When there is a mutation in this gene, a person develops DM1. The specific mutation that causes DM1 is called a trinucleotide repeat expansion.

Some families with symptoms of DM do not have a mutation in the DMPK gene. As of early 2001, scientists have found that the DM in many of these families is caused by a mutation in a gene on chromosome 3. These families are said to have DM2.

Congenital myotonic dystrophy has been linked to a region on chromosome 7 that contains a muscle chloride channel gene.

Trinucleotide repeats

In the DMPK gene, there is a section of the genetic code called a CTG repeat. The letters stand for three nucleotides (complex organic molecules) known as cytosine, thymine, and guanine, and are repeated a certain number of times. In people who have DM1, this sequence of nucleotides is repeated too many times—more than the normal number of 37 times—and thus this section of the gene is too big. This enlarged section of the gene is called a trinucleotide repeat expansion.

People who have repeat numbers in the normal range will not develop DM1 and cannot pass it to their children. Having more than 50 repeats causes DM1. People who have 38–49 repeats have a premutation and will not develop DM1, but can pass DM1 onto their children. Having repeats numbers greater than 1000 causes congenital myotonic dystrophy.

In general, the more repeats in the affected range that someone has, the earlier the age of onset of symptoms and the more severe the symptoms. However, this is a general rule. It is not possible to look at a person's repeat number and predict at what age they will begin to have symptoms or how their condition will progress.

Exactly how the trinucleotide repeat expansion causes myotonia, the inability to relax muscles, is not yet understood. The disease somehow blocks the flow of electrical impulses across the muscle cell membrane. Without proper flow of charged particles, the muscle cannot return to its relaxed state after it has contracted.

Since 2001 it has been discovered that DM2 is caused by a CCTG (cytosine-cytosine-thymine-guanine) expansion on chromosome 3 at locus 3q21, but as of 2004 it is not known how this repeat affects muscle cell function.

Anticipation

Sometimes when a person who has repeat numbers in the affected or premutation range has children, the expansion grows larger. This is called anticipation. A larger expansion can result in an earlier age of onset in children than in their affected parent. Anticipation happens more often when a mother passes DM1 onto her children then when it is passed from the father. Occasionally repeat sizes stay the same or even get smaller when they are passed to a person's children.

Inheritance

DM is inherited through autosomal dominant inheritance. This means that equal numbers of males and females are affected. It also means that only one gene in the pair needs to have the mutation in order for a person to be affected. Since a person only passes one copy of each gene onto their children, there is a 50% or one in two chance that a person who has DM will pass it onto each of their children. This percentage is not changed by results of other pregnancies. A person with a premutation also has a 50%, or one in two, chance of passing the altered gene on to each of their children. However, whether or not their children will develop DM1 depends on whether the trinucleotide repeat becomes further expanded. A person who has repeat numbers in the normal range cannot pass DM1 onto their children.

There is a range in the severity of symptoms in DM and not everyone will have all of the symptoms listed here.

Myotonic dystrophy causes weakness and delayed muscle relaxation called myotonia. Symptoms of DM include facial weakness and a slack jaw, drooping eyelids called **ptosis**, and muscle wasting in the forearms and calves. A person with DM has difficulty relaxing his or her grasp, especially in the cold. DM affects the heart muscle, causing irregularities in the heartbeat. It also affects the muscles of the digestive system, causing **constipation** and other digestive problems. DM may cause **cataracts**, retinal degeneration, low IQ, frontal balding, skin disorders, atrophy of the testicles, and diabetes. It can also cause sleep apnea—a condition in which normal breathing is interrupted during sleep. DM increases the need for sleep and decreases motivation. Severe disabilities do not set in until about 20 years after symptoms begin. Most people with myotonic dystrophy maintain the ability to walk, even late in life.

A severe form of DM, congenital myotonic dystrophy, may appear in newborns of mothers who have DM1. Congenital myotonic dystrophy is marked by severe weakness, poor sucking and swallowing responses, respiratory difficulty, delayed motor development, and **mental retardation**. **Death** in infancy is common in this type.

Some people who have a trinucleotide repeat expansion in their DMPK gene do not have symptoms or have very mild symptoms that go unnoticed. It is not unusual for a woman to be diagnosed with DM after she has an infant with congenital myotonic dystrophy.

Predictive testing

It is possible to test someone who is at risk for developing DM1 before they are showing symptoms to see whether they inherited an expanded trinucleotide repeat. This is called predictive testing. Predictive testing cannot determine the age of onset that someone will begin to have symptoms, or the course of the disease.

Diagnosis

Diagnosis of DM is not difficult once the disease is considered. However, the true problem may be masked because symptoms can begin at any age, can be mild or severe, and can occur with a wide variety of associated complaints. Diagnosis of DM begins with a careful medical history and a thorough physical exam to determine the distribution of symptoms and to rule out other causes. A family history of DM or unexplained weakness helps to establish the diagnosis.

A definitive diagnosis of DM1 is done by **genetic testing**, usually by taking a small amount of blood. The DNA in the blood cells is examined and the number of repeats in the DMPK gene is determined. Various other tests may be done to help establish the diagnosis, but only rarely would other testing be needed. An electromyogram (EMG) is a test is used to examine the response of the muscles to stimulation. Characteristic changes are seen in DM that helps distinguish it from other muscle diseases. Removing a small piece of muscle tissue for microscopic examination is called a muscle biopsy. DM is marked by characteristic changes in the structure of muscle cells that can be seen on a muscle biopsy. An electrocardiogram could be performed to detect characteristic abnormalities in heart rhythm associated with DM. These symptoms often appear later in the course of the disease.

Prenatal testing

Testing a **pregnancy** to determine whether an unborn child is affected is possible if genetic testing in a family has identified a DMPK mutation. This can be done at 10–12 weeks gestation by a procedure called **chorionic villus sampling** (CVS) that involves removing a tiny piece of the placenta and analyzing DNA from its cells. It can also be done by **amniocentesis** after 14 weeks gestation by removing a small amount of the amniotic fluid surrounding the baby and analyzing the cells in the fluid. Each of these procedures has a small risk of **miscarriage** associated with it and those who are interested in learning more should check with their doctor or genetic counselor.

There is also another procedure called preimplantation diagnosis that allows a couple to have a child that is unaffected with the genetic condition in their family. This procedure is experimental and not widely available. Those interested in learning more about this procedure should check with their doctor or genetic counselor.

A group of researchers in Houston, Texas, reported in 2004 that they have successfully developed a technique for detecting the CCTG expansion that causes DM2 and estimating the size of the repeat expansion.

Treatment

Myotonic dystrophy cannot be cured, and no treatment can delay its progression. As of the early 2000s there is no standardized treatment for these disorders because the precise reasons for muscle weakness are not yet fully understood. However, many of the symptoms can be treated. Physical therapy can help preserve or increase strength and flexibility in muscles. Ankle and wrist braces can be used to support weakened limbs. Occupational therapy is used to develop tools and techniques to compensate for loss of strength and dexterity. A speech-language pathologist can provide retraining for weakness in the muscles controlling speech and swallowing.

Irregularities in the heartbeat may be treated with medication or a pacemaker. A yearly electrocardiogram is usually recommended to monitor the heartbeat. **Diabetes mellitus** in DM is treated in the same way that it is in the general population. A high-fiber diet can help prevent constipation. **Sleep apnea** may be treated with surgical procedures to open the airways or with nighttime ventilation. Treatment of sleep apnea may reduce drowsiness. Lens replacement surgery is available when cataracts develop. Pregnant woman should be followed by an obstetrician familiar with the particular problems of DM because complications can occur during pregnancy, labor and delivery.

Wearing a medical bracelet is advisable. Some emergency medications may have dangerous effects on the heart rhythm in a person with DM. Adverse reactions to **general anesthesia** may also occur.

Prognosis

The course of myotonic dystrophy varies. When symptoms appear earlier in life, disability tends to become more severe. Occasionally people with DM may require a wheelchair later in life. Children with congenital DM usually require special educational programs and physical and occupational therapy. For both types of DM, respiratory infections pose a danger when weakness becomes severe.

Resources

BOOKS

Beers, Mark H., MD, and Robert Berkow, MD, editors. "Myotonic Disorders." Section 14, Chapter 184. In *The Merck Manual of Diagnosis and Therapy*. Whitehouse Station, NJ: Merck Research Laboratories, 2004.

PERIODICALS

International Myotonic Dystrophy Consortium (IMDC). "New Nomenclature and DNA Testing Guidelines for Myotonic Dystrophy Type 1 (DM1)." *Neurology* 54 (2000): 1218–1221.

Meola, G., and V. Sansone. "Treatment in Myotonia and Periodic Paralysis." *Revue neurologique (Paris)* 160, no. 5, Part 2 (May 2004): S55–S69.

Meola, Giovanni. "Myotonic Dystrophies." *Current Opinion in Neurology* 13 (2000): 519–525.

Ranum, L. P., and J. W. Day. "Myotonic dystrophy: RNA Pathogenesis Comes into Focus." *American Journal of Human Genetics* 74 (May 2004): 793–804.

Sallinen, R., A. Vihola, L. L. Bachinski, et al. "New Methods for Molecular Diagnosis and Demonstration of the (CCTG)n Mutation in Myotonic Dystrophy Type 2 (DM2)." *Neuromuscular Disorders* 14 (April 2004): 274–283.

ORGANIZATIONS

Muscular Dystrophy Association. 3300 East Sunrise Dr., Tucson, AZ 85718. (520) 529-2000 or (800) 572-1717. < http://www.mdausa.org >.

OTHER

Gene Clinics. < http://www.geneclinics.org >.
Myotonic Dystrophy Website. < http://www.umd.necker.fr/myotonic_dystrophy.html >.
NCBI Genes and Disease Web Page. < http://www.ncbi.nlm.nih.gov/disease/Myotonic.html >.

Karen M. Krajewski, M.S., C.G.C.
Rebecca J. Frey, Ph.D.

Myringotomy and ear tubes

Definition

Myringotomy is a surgical procedure in which a small incision is made in the eardrum (the tympanic membrane), usually in both ears. The word comes from *myringa,* modern Latin for drum membrane, and *tomē,* Greek for cutting. It is also called myringocentesis, tympanotomy, tympanostomy, or **paracentesis** of the tympanic membrane. Fluid in the middle ear can be sucked out through the incision.

Ear tubes, or tympanostomy tubes, are small tubes, open at both ends, that are inserted into the incisions in the eardrums during myringotomy. They come in various shapes and sizes and are made of plastic, metal, or both. They are left in place until they fall out by themselves or until they are removed by a doctor.

Purpose

Myringotomy with the insertion of ear tubes is an optional treatment for inflammation of the middle ear with fluid collection (effusion), also called glue ear, that lasts more than three months (chronic **otitis media** with effusion) and does not respond to drug treatment. It is the recommended treatment if the condition lasts four to six months. Effusion is the collection of fluid that escapes from blood vessels or the lymphatic system. In this case, the fluid collects in the middle ear.

Initially, acute inflammation of the middle ear with effusion is treated with one or two courses of **antibiotics**. **Antihistamines** and **decongestants** have been used, but they have not been proven effective unless there is also hay **fever** or some other allergic inflammation that contributes to the problem. Myringotomy with or without the insertion of ear tubes is NOT recommended for initial treatment of otherwise healthy children with middle ear inflammation with effusion.

In about 10% of children, the effusion lasts for three months or longer, when the disease is considered chronic. In children with chronic disease, systemic steroids may help, but the evidence is not clear, and there are risks.

When medical treatment does not stop the effusion after three months in a child who is one to three years old, is otherwise healthy, and has **hearing loss** in both ears, myringotomy with insertion of ear tubes becomes an option. If the effusion lasts for four to six months, myringotomy with insertion of ear tubes is recommended.

The purpose of myringotomy is to relieve symptoms, to restore hearing, to take a sample of the fluid to examine in the laboratory in order to identify any microorganisms present, or to insert ear tubes.

Ear tubes can be inserted into the incision during myringotomy and left there. The eardrum heals around them, securing them in place. They usually fall out on their own in 6-12 months or are removed by a doctor.

While they are in place, they keep the incision from closing, keeping a channel open between the middle ear and the outer ear. This allows fresh air to reach the middle ear, allowing fluid to drain out, and preventing pressure from building up in the middle ear. The patient's hearing returns to normal immediately and the risk of recurrence diminishes.

Parents often report that children talk better, hear better, are less irritable, sleep better, and behave better after myringotomy with the insertion of ear tubes.

Description

The procedure is usually done in an ambulatory surgical unit under **general anesthesia**, although some physicians do it in the office with **sedation** and **local**

anesthesia, especially in older children. The ear is washed, a small incision made in the eardrum, the fluid sucked out, a tube inserted, and the ear packed with cotton to control bleeding.

There has been an effort to design ear tubes that are easier to insert or to remove, and to design tubes that stay in place longer. Therefore, ear tubes come in various shapes and sizes.

Preparation

The child may not have food or water for four to six hours before anesthesia. Antibiotics are usually not needed.

Aftercare

Use of antimicrobial drops is controversial. Water should be kept out of the ear canal until the eardrum is intact. A doctor should be notified if the tubes fall out.

Risks

The risks include:

- Cutting the outer ear
- Formation at the myringotomy site of granular nodes due to inflammation
- Formation of a mass of skin cells and cholesterol in the middle ear that can grow and damage surrounding bone (cholesteatoma)
- Permanent perforation of the eardrum.

The risk of persistent discharge from the ear (otorrhea) is 13%.

If the procedure is repeated, structural changes in the eardrum can occur, such as loss of tone (flaccidity), shrinkage or retraction, or hardening of a spot on the eardrum (typmanosclerosis). The risk of hardening is 51%; its effects on hearing are not known, but they are probably insignificant.

It is possible that the incision will not heal properly, leaving a permanent hole in the eardrum, which can cause some hearing loss and increases the risk of infection.

It is also possible that the ear tube will move inward and get trapped in the middle ear, rather than move out into the external ear, where it either falls out on its own or can be retrieved by a doctor. The exact incidence of tubes moving inward is not known, but it could increase the risk of further episodes of middle-ear inflammation, inflammation of the eardrum or the part of the skull directly behind the ear, formation of a

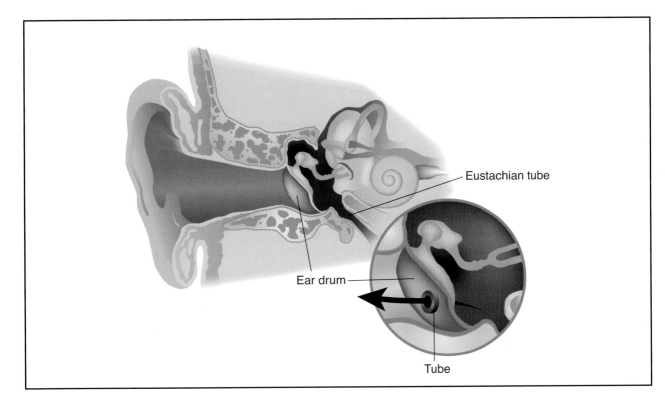

Eustachian tube

Ear drum

Tube

The insertion of ear tubes in the eardrum helps to alleviate chronic middle ear infections. *(Illustration by Argosy, Inc.)*

mass in the middle ear, or infection due to the presence of a foreign body.

The surgery may not be a permanent cure. As many as 30% of children undergoing myringotomy with insertion of ear tubes need to undergo another procedure within five years.

The other risks include those associated with sedatives or general anesthesia.

An additional element of post-operative care is the recommendation by many doctors that the child use ear plugs to keep water out of the ear during bathing or swimming, to reduce the risk of infection and discharge.

Resources

BOOKS

Lim, David J., et al., editors. *Recent Advances in Otitis Media: Proceedings of the Sixth International Symposium, June 4-8, 1995, Marriott Harbot Beach, Ft. Lauderdale, Florida.* Hamilton, Ontario: B. C. Decker Inc., 1996.

Mary Zoll, PhD

Myxedema *see* **Hypothyroidism**

KEY TERMS

Acute otitis media—Inflammation of the middle ear with signs of infection lasting less than three months.

Chronic otitis media—Inflammation of the middle ear with signs of infection lasting three months or longer.

Effusion—The escape of fluid from blood vessels or the lymphatic system and its collection in a cavity, in this case, the middle ear.

Middle ear—The cavity or space between the eardrum and the inner ear. It includes the eardrum, the three little bones (hammer, anvil, and stirrup) that transmit sound to the inner ear, and the eustachian tube, which connects the inner ear to the nasopharynx (the back of the nose).

Tympanic membrane—The eardrum. A thin disc of tissue that separates the outer ear from the middle ear.

Tympanostomy tube—Ear tube. A small tube made of metal or plastic that is inserted during myringotomy to ventilate the middle ear.

GALE ENCYCLOPEDIA OF MEDICINE

Myxoma

Definition

A myxoma is a rare, usually noncancerous, primary tumor (a new growth of tissue) of the heart. It is the most common of all benign heart tumors.

Description

Myxoma is an intracardiac tumor; it is found inside the heart. Seventy five percent of all myxomas are found in the left atrium, and almost all other myxomas are found in the right atrium. It is very rare for a myxoma to be found in either of the ventricles. The tumor takes one of two general shapes: a round, firm mass, or an irregular shaped, soft, gelatinous mass. They are attached to the endocardium, the inside lining of the heart. The cells that make up the tumor are spindle-shaped cells and are embedded in a matrix rich in mucopolysaccharides (a group of carbohydrates). Myxomas may contain calcium, which shows up on x rays. The tumor gets its blood supply from capillaries that bring blood from the heart to the tumor. Thrombi (**blood clots**) may be attached to the outside of the myxoma.

There are three major syndromes linked to myxomas: embolic events, obstruction of blood flow, and constitutional syndromes. Embolic events happen when fragments of the tumor, or the thrombi attached to the outside of the tumor, are released and enter the blood stream. Gelatinous myxomas are more likely to embolize than the more firm form of this tumor.

Myxomas may also obstruct blood flow in the heart, usually at a heart valve. The mitral valve is the heart valve most commonly affected. Blood flow restrictions can lead to pulmonary congestion and heart valve disease. Embolization can lead to severe consequences. In cases of left atrial myxoma, 40-50% of patients experience embolization. Emboli usually end up in the brain, kidneys, and extremities.

The third syndrome linked to myxomas are called constitutional syndromes, nonspecific symptoms caused by the myxoma.

Causes and symptoms

There is no known causative agent for myxoma. The main symptoms, if any, produced by myxoma are

generic and not specific. These include **fever**, weight loss, anemia, elevated white blood cell (WBC) count, decreased **platelet count** and Raynaud's phenomenon. Most patients with myxoma are between 30-60 years of age.

Diagnosis

Diagnosis is made following a suspicion that a myxoma might be present, and can usually be confirmed by echocardiogram

Treatment

Surgery is used to remove the tumor. Myxomas can regrow if they are not completely removed. The survival rate for this operation is excellent.

Prognosis

Successful removal of the tumor rids the patient of this disease. Emboli from a myxoma may survive in other areas of the body. However, there is no evidence that myxoma is truly metastatic (able to transfer disease from one area to another), causing tumors in other areas of the body.

Resources

OTHER

"Myxoma, Intracardiac." *OMIM Home Page, Online Mendelian Inheritance in Man.* <http://www.ncbi.nlm.nih.gov/Omim>.

John T. Lohr, PhD